A Textbook of Children's and Young People's Nursing

Senior Commissioning Editor: *Ninette Premdas*
Development Editor: *Carole McMurray*
Project Manager: *Frances Affleck*
Designer: *Kirsteen Wright*
Illustration buyer: *Merlyn Harvey*
Cover Images: *Tin Wheeler*

A Textbook of Children's and Young People's Nursing

SECOND EDITION

Edited by

E Alan Glasper
Professor, School of Health Sciences,
University of Southampton, Southampton, UK

Jim Richardson
Head of Division (Family Care),
Faculty of Health, Sport and Science,
University of Glamorgan, Pontypridd, Wales, UK

CHURCHILL LIVINGSTONE
ELSEVIER

CHURCHILL
LIVINGSTONE
ELSEVIER

An imprint of Elsevier Limited

First published 2006
Second edition 2010

ISBN 9780 7020 3183 0

British Library Cataloguing in Publication Data
A catalogue record for this book is available from the British Library

Library of Congress Cataloging in Publication Data
A catalog record for this book is available from the Library of Congress

Notice
Medical knowledge is constantly changing. Standard safety precautions must be followed, but as new research and clinical experience broaden our knowledge, changes in treatment and drug therapy may become necessary or appropriate. Readers are advised to check the most current product information provided by the manufacturer of each drug to be administered to verify the recommended dose, the method and duration of administration, and contraindications. It is the responsibility of the practitioner, relying on experience and knowledge of the patient, to determine dosages and the best treatment for each individual patient. Neither the Publisher nor the Editors assumes any liability for any injury and/or damage to persons or property arising from this publication.

The Publisher

Printed in Spain

Contents

Contributors

Penny Aitken
Sister, Paediatric Emergency Assessment Unit, Child Health Directorate, Southampton General Hospital, Southampton, UK

Jennifer Allison AAS RN RSCN MICR
Senior Nurse Manager, Wellcome Trust Clinical Research Facility, Southampton General Hosptial, Southampton, UK

Marion Aylott BSc (Hons) MA RGN RM RSCN
Lecturer Child Health Nursing, School of Nursing and Midwifery, University of Southampton, Southampton, UK

Clare Barrow BSc Neonatology
Advanced Neonatal Nurse Practitioner, NICU Singleton Hopsital, Swansea, Wales, UK

Cathryn Battrick MSc RGN RSCN
Matron for Children's Services, Southampton Children's Hospital, Southampton, UK

Maureen Bradshaw RGN RSCn MSc DipN CertEd (FE)
Formerly Children's Nursing Lecturer, School of Nursing and Midwifery, University of Sheffield, Sheffield, UK

Mary Brophy MSc RSCN RN RNT ENB405 ENB 998
Child Health Lecturer, School of Health Sciences, University of Wales, Cardiff, Wales, UK

Peter Callery MSc PhD BA (Hons) RGN RSCN
Chair in Children's Nursing, University of Manchester School of Nursing, Midwifery and Social Work, Manchester, UK

Anne Campbell BA (Hons) MSc RGN RSCN DN RNT
Senior Lecturer in Children's Nursing, Division Faculty of Health, South Bank University, Whipps Cross University Hospital, London, UK

Anne Casey MSc RSCN FRCN
Advisor, Royal College of Nursing, London, UK

Sonya Clarke PGCert BSc (Hons) RGN RN(Child)
Senior Teaching Fellow (Children's & Orthopaedic/Trauma Nursing), School of Nursing and Midwifery, Queen's University Belfast, Belfast, Northern Ireland, UK

Valerie Coleman MA BSc RSCN RGN Cert Ed (FE)
Formerly Children's Nursing Lecturer, School of Nursing and Midwifery, University of Sheffield, Sheffield, UK

Michael Cooper
Formerly School of Nursing and Midwifery, University of Southampton, Southampton, UK

Sue Courtman
Community Children's Nurse, Diabetes Nurse Specialist, East and North Hertfordshire NHS Trust, UK

Annette K Dearmun PhD BSc (Hons) RSCN RGN DN DNE RNT ITGE
Principal Lecturer/Practitioner, Children's Medical Ward, John Radcliffe Hospital, Oxford, UK

Barbara Elliott MSc BNurs RGN RSCN RHV DNCert PGCHE
Lecturer, Faculty of Health and Social Care, University of Hull, Hull, UK

Sarah Dowle RGN RSCN DipN (Paediatric Intensive Care) BSc (Hons)
Advanced Paediatric Nurse Practitioner, Paediatric Unit, Diana, Princess of Wales Hospital, Grimsby, UK

Sue Fallon RGN MA RSCN PhD
Lecturer in Paediatric Oncology Nursing, University of Leeds, Leeds, UK

Terri Fletcher
Lecturer, Child Health, St. Mary's Hospital, Portsmouth, UK

E Alan Glasper
Professor, Child Health Nursing, University of Southampton School of Nursing and Midwifery, Southampton, UK

Liz Gormley-Fleming,
Senior Lecturer, Children's Nursing, University of Hertfordshire, UK

Rachel E A Haggarty RGN RSCN
Sister, Children's Surgical Unit, Child Health Directorate, Southampton General Hospital, Southampton, UK

Tom C A Hain
Formerly Helpful Health Trust, Winchester, UK

Maureen Harrison MSc BSc CertEd RGN RSCN RNT
Lecturer in Child Health, School of Nursing and Midwifery, University of Southampton, Southampton, UK

Anna L Hemphill MSc BSc (Hons) RSCN RGN CTHE Dip Management
Senior Lecturer, Child Health Nursing, Oxford Brookes University, Oxford, UK

Susan Hooton OBE RSCN RGN BSc (Hons) MA RNT
Assistant Director Governance, Performance and Patient Safety, Five Boroughs NHS Partnership Trust, UK

Lorraine Ireland SRN RSCN MSc BSc (Hons) RCNT RNT PGCEA
Lecturer in Child Health Nursing, School of Health Sciences, University of Southampton, Southampton, UK

Victoria Jones BA (Hons) PGCE RNLD
Senior Lecturer, Unit for Development in Intellectual Disability, Faculty of Health, Sport and Science, University of Glamorgan, Pontypridd, Wales, UK

Agnes B Kanneh MSc BSc (Hons) PGCEA RCNT RSCN RM RGN ENB
Lecturer in Applied Biological Sciences, City University, School of Community Health Sciences, St Bartholomew School of Nursing, London, UK

Janet Kelsey MSc BSc (Hons) Adv Dip Ed PGCE RSCN RGN RNT
Senior Lecturer, Faculty of Health, University of Plymouth, Plymouth, Devon, UK

Kate Khair
Nurse Consultant, Great Ormond Street Hospital, London, UK

Rosemary King RGN RN (Child) PGCert Allergy
Children's Allergy Nurse Specialist, Southampton University Hospital NHS Trust, Southampton, UK

Maggie Kirk PhD BSc (Hons) RGN DipN
Professor of Genetics Education and Lead Professional Specialist (Nursing), NHS National Genetics Education and Development Centre, University of Glamorgan, Pontypridd, Wales, UK

Susan Lowson
Nurse Advisor to the Ombudsman, Office of the Health Service Ombudsman, London, UK

Gill McEwing RGN RSCN MSc RNT
Lecturer in Nursing, Faculty of Health, University of Plymouth, Plymouth, UK

Kevin McFarlane RSCN B ed Masters Child Health RSCN
Lecturer, School of Nursing, Dundee University, Ninewells Hospital, Dundee, UK

Marisa McFarlane RGN RSCN BSc (Hons)
Paediatric Macmillan Nurse, Royal Belfast Hospital for Children, Belfast, Northern Ireland, UK

Catherine Martin
Staff Nurse, Regional Paediatric and Adolescent Oncology unit, St James's Hospital, Leeds, UK

Janet Matthews RGN RM RSCN RNT MSc Nursing
Senior Lecturer, Napier University, School of Community Health, Edinburgh, UK

Donna Mead
Professor and Dean, Child Health Nursing, University of Glamorgan, Pontypridd, Wales, UK

Ruth M Mitchell RSCN RGN SCM RCNT DipCNE RNT Cert Ed MSc
Lecturer, Child Health, Faculty of Health and Life Sciences, Napier University, Edinburgh, UK

Julie Mould RGN RSCN BSc MSc
Lecturer/Practitioner, Faculty of Health and Social Care, University of Hull, UK

Philomena Morrow BSc (Hons) Nursing MSc Nursing Dip Nursing RGN RSCN
Nurse Lecturer, School of Nursing and Midwifery, Queen's University Belfast, Belfast, Northern Ireland, UK

Gary Mountain MA BA (Hons) RGN RSCn RCNT RNT
Senior Child Health Lecturer, School of Healthcare Studies, The University of Huddersfield, Huddersfield, UK

Sarah Neill MSc PGDE BSc (Hons) RGN RSCN
Senior Lecturer in Children's Nursing, Centre Healthcare Education, University College, Northampton General Hospital, Northampton

Colman Noctor
Lecturer, School of Nursing, Midwifery & Health Systems, Health Sciences Centre, Belfield, Dublin, Ireland

Ruth Northway PhD MSc (Econ) RNCD CertEd FRCN
Professor of Learning Disability Nursing, School of Care Sciences, University of Glamorgan, Pontypridd, Wales, UK

Barbara V Novak MSc (Comp Phys) B Ed (Hons) RSCN RN RM RNT
Senior Lecturer in Applied Biological Sciences, Education head for NM Independent and Supplementary Prescribing, City University, School of Community and Health Sciences, London, UK

Arija Nikola Parker BA (Hons) RGN RSCN PGCE
Senior Lecturer, Division of Children's Nursing, University of Central Lancashire, Preston, UK

Emer Parker BSc (Hons) Psych RGN RSCN Cert Ed (FE)
Senior Lecturer, Genomics Policy Unit, University of Glamorgan, Cardiff, Wales, UK

Jackie Parkes PhD BNurs (Hons) RSCN RGN NONCert
Senior Lecturer, School of Nursing and Midwifery, Queen's University Belfast, Belfast, Northern Ireland

Jayne Price MSc BSc (Hons) PGDipEd RGN RN (Child)
Senior Teaching Fellow, School of Nursing and Midwifery, Queen's University Belfast, Belfast, Northern Ireland, UK

Gill Prudhoe
Lecturer in Children's and Young People's Nursing, University of Southampton, Southampton, UK

Catherine Powell PhD BNSc (Hons) RGN RSCN RHV
Lecturer in Child Health Nursing/Honorary Child Protection Nurse Specialist, School of Nursing and Midwifery, University of Southampton, Southampton, UK

Jim Richardson
Head of Division (Family Care), Faculty of Health, Sport and Science, University of Glamorgan, Pontypridd, Wales, UK

Helen Rushforth PhD BA(Hons) RSCn RGN RNT Nurse Teacher (Recorded)
Senior Lecturer, School of Health Sciences, University of Southampton, Southampton, UK

Kathy Scanlon BSc (Hons) DPSN PGDip Health Ethics RGN RM RSCN RNT
Formerly Senior Lecturer in Children's Nursing, Division of Children's Nursing, University of Central Lancashire, Preston, UK

Diane Scott SRN RSCN BSc MSc
Nurse Consultant, Child Health Directorate, East Lancashire Hospitals NHS Trust, Burnley, UK

Beth Sepion
School of Nursing and Midwifery, University of Southampton, Southampton, UK

Linda Shields PhD FRCNA
Professor of Paediatric and Child Health Nursing, Curtin University and Child and Adolescent Health Service, Perth, Australia

Jo Sibert
Professor of Child Health, University of Cardiff, Cardiff, Wales, UK

Sally R Siddall RN RCNT RSCN BA (Hons) MSc
Lecturer in Health Sciences, Department of Health Sciences, University of Hull, Hull, UK

Brian Silverwood MA (Health Care Law) RGN RSCN ENB
Healthcare Assessor, Care Quality Commission, UK

Sandie Skinner RGN RSCN ANNP BN MSc
Consultant Nurse Winchester, Lead Nurse, South Central Newborn Network, BOOST II Regional Nurse Wales SW England

Anna-Lisa Sorrentino BSc (Hons) RGN RSCN ENB998 PGCE
Lecturer/Practitioner, Division of Children's Nursing, University of Central Lancashire, Preston, UK

Joanna Smith MSc BSc (Hons) RNT RSCN RGN
Lecturer, Child Health, School of Child Health, University of Leeds, Leeds, UK

Lynda Smith MA Ed BA (Hons) RGN PhD RSCN
Senior Lecturer, Sheffield Hallam University, Faculty Of Health and Wellbeing, Department of Nursing and Midwifery, Sheffield, UK

Jennifer Stinson RN PhD CPNP
Clinical Scientist, Child Health Evaluative Sciences, The Hospital for Sick Children, Assistant Professor, Lawrence S. Bloomberg Faculty of Nursing, University of Toronto, Toronto, Canada

Ann Tanner MHlth Sc (Hlth Prom)
Registered Nurse, Children's Theatre, Royal Brisbane Children's Hospital, Brisbane, Australia

Louise Terry PhD LLB RIIBMS
Senior Lecturer, Faculty of Health, Southbank University, Essex, UK

Alison Twycross RGn RMN RSCN MSc DMS CertEd(HE)
Course Director for Dip HE Nursing and Principal Lecture in Children's Nursing, Faculty of Health and Social Care Sciences, Kingston University, St George's University of London, London, UK

Janice Watson RGNRSCNBsc (Hons) Msc
Lecturer, Child Health Nursing, School of Nursing and Midwifery, University of Southampton, Southampton, UK

Mark Whiting MSc B Nursing RGN RSCN Dn HV PGDipEd RNT
Senior Lecturer in Community Children's Nursing, Division Faculty of Health, South Bank University, Whipps Cross University Hospital, London, UK

Maureen Wiltshire RSCN RGN Dip HE
Formerly Sister, Paediatric Emergency Assessment Unit, Child Health Directorate, Southampton General Hospital, Southampton, UK

Julia Winter MSc BSc RNT RSCN RGN
Joint Programme Lead/Senior Lecturer Children's Nursing, Oxford Brookes University, Oxford, UK

Barbara Wood EdD RGN RSCN Dip Nursing RNT RCNT
Principal Lecturer, School of Human and Helth Sciences, University of Huddersfield, Huddersfield, UK

Foreword

It is a privilege to be a children's nurse, trusted on a daily basis by children and young people and their families, to provide the best possible care that will help them to live their lives to the full. This privilege does not however come without the professional - and indeed personal - responsibility to ensure every aspect of our professional practice is underpinned by the knowledge and expertise that enables us to care in whatever setting that care is being delivered.

Whether in an acute ward or in a home setting, infants and children require increasingly complex interventional care as technological advancements facilitate the long-term survival of children; but with this remains the vital necessity that children's nurses never forget that the child is an individual, and also that their role is one of a caring professional.

This book commences with an important consideration of the historical perspectives of children's nursing in the UK, since its inception in 1852. This includes consideration of the changing concepts of childhood and how the recognition of the specific needs of children supported the evolution of children's nursing. Through the discursive and reflective approach the authors attempt to instil in practitioners today the need to continue protecting the recognition of children's' nursing as a distinct field of nursing practice. Children's nursing requires from its practitioners a commitment to understanding every influence upon the health and wellbeing of children. Understanding the influences and professional challenges of the past will allow children's professionals to inform and protect the future.

'Children's nurses' is actually a misnomer for this complex role, which is essentially about the care of children as *part of a family*. The psychosocial development and needs of a child or a young person cannot be considered without a systematic approach to considering a child or young person in the context of their family, the culture within which they exist, and indeed in wider society. The gathering and interpretation of such psychosocial information to inform the care of children and young people is what has for years been considered as constituting a family-centred care approach. This actually requires a level of sociological and social policy knowledge, and acumen that goes beyond 'rote' or 'moment in time' learning, to an acceptance of the constant need to keep abreast of health and social policy as it relates to child health. Children's nurses must have insight but, in addition, they should have the conviction that they can change policies of the future.

As well as family-centred care, professionals must remember that above all, excellence in care must be focused upon meeting the needs of each individual child or young person. The psychological and physical needs of children and young people are complex to understand, and indeed to meet, and are forever expanding (see, for example, a consideration of this in the chapter focusing on genetics). However, all professional care should be provided based on the best available evidence. Such evidence-based good practice must commence from the child's first contact with the health service, for example at the point of access or even before, preparing children effectively for contact with the health service. Evidence-based care must then be provided wherever and whenever received, and for whatever condition, and this is discussed in the later (condition- or system-) specific chapters of the book. This should also be without practitioners ever losing the aspiration that children will be helped *and not adversely affected by* the healthcare they receive. To ensure that children and families experience no psychological, social and physical harm, requires continuous reflection on practice, and this is supported throughout the book by case studies. These case studies will, in practice, assist the assessing of cases presenting, and also the careful planning and implementing of care, incorporating lessons learned. Indeed safeguarding children does require not only a professional approach to all care but also an overarching realisation of such things as what may or can harm children, including recognising risk factors and listening to and hearing from the children themselves. Communication goes beyond hearing speech to being receptive about how physical and psychological responses may be portrayed in every age group. This requires not only knowledge but also the professional commitment to empower young people and to be receptive. A challenge for children's nurses generally is to understand the growth and development of children including how this effects children's coping mechanisms and the impact of family.

An appreciation of psychological and personality development theories presented in this book will help with interpretation and with the subsequent delivery of quality care.

Overall the key focus of children's nursing is the provision of quality care. Policy drivers and national bodies suggest that there is accepted quality practice against which to transform and audit current practice. What is most evidently needed, however, is increased research activity to arrive within policy at statements of definitive good practice, although the moral and ethical minefield of undertaking research with children needs to be actively managed.

Research upon which to base evidence-based practice is more available in areas of practice that have a primarily physiological basis, but even these areas of practice fall short in having an underpinning knowledge base when considering the impact of psychological and social stressors upon the child's and family's experiences.

This book capitalises on the expertise of leaders in the field of children's nursing, allowing the reader to benefit from the authors' commitment to excellence in practice. It encourages a contemporary and reflexive style that supports a change in approach of the readership to want to continue to develop their own knowledge and expertise, thus attempting to ensure children and young people will continue to benefit from forward-focused and well-informed professionals.

Professor Judith Ellis MBE
Director of Nursing and Education,
Great Ormond Street Hospital for Children, London
December 2009

Section 1

Essentials of children's nursing

Historical perspectives of children's nursing

1

E Alan Glasper Ruth M Mitchell

ABSTRACT

The primary aim of this chapter and its companion PowerPoint presentation is to consider the historical perspectives of children's nursing, in the UK, since its inception in 1852. To do this, the origins of children's nursing are explored in the context of the changing concepts of childhood. Details of the fight for registration in the latter part of the 19th century, and of the evolution of children's nursing in the 19th and 20th centuries, provide the reader with an account of key developments. The final section includes an overview of the educational provision necessary to equip practitioners with the necessary knowledge and skills to care for children and families and the current issues in children's nursing that inform the curriculum.

LEARNING OUTCOMES

- Consider the origins of children's nursing in the context of the changing concepts of childhood.
- Understand the fight for registration and the subsequent evolution of children's nursing.
- Explore the developments in nurse education designed to ensure that children's nurses are fit for practice and purpose.
- Examine some of the key challenges facing child health nurses in the 21st century.

Introduction

Children in our present society are given 'rights' that were not accorded to children in previous generations. In Victorian times it was often said that children should be 'seen but not heard'. In today's society, children have rights under the United Nations Convention on the Rights of the Child (United Nations General Assembly 1989). This sets out the basic human rights that all children are entitled to without discrimination. The Convention is underpinned by four guiding principles, which are those of non-discrimination (Article 2), the best interests of the child (Article 3), survival and development (Article 6) and participation (Article 12). The British government ratified the document in 1991 and, by so doing, committed itself to protecting and ensuring children's rights and agreed to hold itself accountable before the international community. Although in itself it is not a legal statute, the United Nations Convention on the Rights of the Child can be used to support the rights of children. Legislation, which builds on the Articles contained in the Convention on the Rights of the Child, seeks to offer further protection to one of the most vulnerable groups within our society.

The Children Act (1989), which applies in England and Wales, is based on the principle that the child's welfare is the paramount consideration and that effective interventions should be in place to ensure the safety and well-being of children who are at risk of harm. It states that children should, wherever possible, be brought up and cared for within their own family, with both parents playing a full part in their lives, without resorting to legal proceedings. Only in situations where there is fundamental disagreement between parents, or concerns about the child's welfare, will the Courts make orders about a child's place of residence and contact arrangements. The Act emphasises the rights of children to be kept informed about issues that affect them.

The Children (Scotland) Act (1995), which applies in Scotland, is based on the following key principles:

- Each child has a right to be treated as an individual.
- Each child who can form his or her views on matters affecting him or her has the right to express those views if he or she wishes.
- Parents should normally be responsible for the upbringing of their children and should share that responsibility.
- Each child has the right to the protection from all forms of abuse, neglect or exploitation.
- In decisions relating to the protection of a child, every effort should be made to keep the child in the family home.

DOI: 10.1016/B978-0-7020-3183-0.10001-3

- Any intervention by a public authority in the life of a child should be properly supported by services from all relevant agencies working in collaboration.

WWW

Check out the UN convention on:

- http://www.unicef.org/crc/fulltext.htm

With the introduction of the Human Rights Act (DoH 1998) some of the rights set out in the European Convention for the Protection of Human Rights and Fundamental Freedoms (1950) became part of British law. Many rights are set out in the Act but of particular relevance to children's nurses, and indeed to all health professionals, are:

- the right to life: Article 2
- the right not to be subjected to degrading treatment: Article 3
- the right to a fair hearing: Article 5
- the right to respect for private and family life: Article 6
- the right not to suffer discrimination in relation to any of the other basic rights: Article 14.

The Human Rights Act, which is central to the right to self-determination by children and young people, includes their right to consent to or refuse treatment (Lowden 2002). However, the Children Act (1989) and the Children (Scotland) Act (1995), although providing legislation that relates to the care of children and their upbringing and protection from harm, do not go beyond establishing their right to be involved in decision making about their welfare. The Human Rights Act enables action to be taken if it is proved that children's rights have been infringed (Power 2002).

PowerPoint

Access the companion PowerPoint presentation and look up the following web pages and consider the extent of the material on children's rights:

- http://www.unhchr.ch/html/menu3/b/k2crc.htm
- http://www.hmso.gov.uk/acts/acts1998/19980042.htm

Children in our society are without a political voice and, until recently, played no significant role in the political processes that impact and influence their lives.

The recent appointment of Children's Commissioners in Wales, Northern Ireland and Scotland is a response to the need to address the rights of children. England delayed the appointment of a children's commissioner after lengthy discussions about the proposed role and powers. The role was felt to fall short of the United Nations international guidelines. In the interim, Margaret Hodge, the Minister for Children in England, held responsibility for children's services, childcare and the protection of the under-fives as part of her portfolio. Al Aynsley-Green was appointed Commissioner for Children in England in March 2005. The appointment of Peter Clarke in Wales, Nigel Williams in Northern Ireland and Kathleen Marshall in Scotland ensures that children in these countries have an advocate in all matters that affect them, either directly or indirectly. Part of the role of the Commissioner is to monitor all proposed legislation to ensure that the needs and best interests of children are met. They will also have a remit in relation to child protection (see Chapter 19). Undertaking and commissioning research is another strand of their work. This activity should contribute to the body of knowledge on which sound decisions can be made on matters affecting children.

WWW

Look up the following web pages and read about the role and remit of the recently appointed Children's Commissioners:

- http://www.crights.org.uk/commissioner/commissioner.html
- http://www.niccy.org/
- http://www.childcom.org.uk/english/index.html
- http://www.scottish.parliament.uk/news/news-04/pa04-008.htm

With rights come societal responsibilities and subsequently new challenges for nurses caring for children and their families in hospital and community. In the past, children were considered as individuals with needs, whereas in contemporary society they are considered to be individuals with rights. The two standpoints are not mutually exclusive. However, the task facing children's nurses today is very different from the task faced by those caring for children at the time of the inception of children's nursing in 1852.

The changing concepts of childhood

The material that follows traces the origins of children's nursing in the UK in the context of changing concepts of childhood. Consideration will be given to the fight for registration for sick children's nurses and the evolution of children's nursing in response to greater understanding of the needs of children and their families. Consideration will be given to the educational provision that seeks to ensure that the children's nurses of tomorrow are equipped to provide high standards of care for children and families. Finally, an overview will be given of some of the challenges currently facing children's nurses in the UK.

Children's nursing has undergone a number of fundamental changes since its inception in the mid-18th century. The changes reflect developments within the nursing profession but also changes in societal views towards children themselves and to the needs of children and families. Reference to the sociological analysis of childhood provides substantial evidence of the ambivalent attitude of the British towards children (Scraton 1997). Indeed, this began to change in the time of the European Enlightenment when, rather than looking at children as poor and weak, whose survival was little valued, society increasingly recognised that children were its future and that their healthy survival was essential for the continuation of society (Seidler 1990). However, there is continued evidence of a lack of respect for children and their specific needs within society in general, and this attitude is even more evident in the NHS than in the general population.

It is generally agreed that the perspective from which they are considered influences perceptions about children and childhood. Writers on the subject rarely reach a consensus. Thomas, cited by Avery & Briggs (1989), highlights the difficulties of unravelling the concept of childhood by suggesting that historians and modern writers continue to write the history of adults' attitudes towards children rather than the history of childhood. This can still be seen in society today, when debates about what constitutes the best interests of children often centre on what adults define as 'best interests'.

One of the most influential writers on the subject of childhood is Aries (1962), a French historian. He and de Mause (1995) are referred to in many childcare texts. Aries' (1962) views are often misrepresented, as he did not consider the absence of a concept of childhood as detrimental to children. He noted that children in the Middle Ages mingled with adults and spent considerable time in their presence, working and playing. In his opinion the separation of adults from children occurred in the 17th century, with the start of education dominated by religion-based morality. Not all historians agree with this view and, in his writings, de Mause makes the dramatic statement:

> The historical record points to childhood being a nightmare from which we have only begun to awaken. The further back in history one goes, the lower the levels of childcare, the more likely children are to be killed, abandoned, beaten, terrorised and sexually abused
>
> (de Mause 1982)

During the 18th century the needs of children were increasingly recognised and by the 19th century children were considered valuable and therefore in need of protection (Stone 1977). It was this change in attitude that led to the establishment of foundling hospitals and dispensaries for children. In the 20th century the individuality of the child has become more evident. Family life has become increasingly important. The status of the child has increased significantly with the introduction of the European Convention on the Rights of the Child in 1989 and the Human Rights Act (1998). In our society today children have the right to expect protection from harm and a right to self-determination. This is in stark contrast to the Victorian view of children, whom they considered should be seen and not heard. It has been suggested that changing perceptions of childhood over the years can be analysed by studying the themes of play, art and literature (Watt & Mitchell 1995).

Children throughout history and in all cultures engage in some form of play through which they learn to make sense of the world of which they are part. They use imitation and experimentation to learn and experience essential social roles and values. Before the 17th century, little evidence exists for children's play, although in the 4th century BC Aristotle – a proponent of play as a prerequisite to health – advocated that children under the age of 5 years should not work. He considered that to do so would be detrimental to their health and well-being. Singer (1973) suggests that it is likely that children did play but, as it was not considered an important activity, adults did not comment upon it.

According to Aries (1962) there were few attempts to portray childhood in art before the 12th century. This reflected society at that time and the place of children within it. In some of the early artwork images children were depicted as miniature adults. It was not until the 15th and 16th centuries that it became popular to portray children in a social context. The Dutch artist Rembrandt achieved popular acclaim for his work, which included portraits of individual children.

Activity

Go to the website below and work through the different sections of the exhibition 'The new child'. This exhibition from Berkeley, USA, depicts British Art and Origins of Modern Childhood 1730–1830.

- http://www.bampfa.berkeley.edu/exhibits/newchild/index.html

There is limited evidence of children's literature prior to the 18th century. Orbis Sensualism Pictus by Comenius, which was printed in 1658, is said to be the earliest illustrated book specifically designed for children. Much of the early children's literature was written to appeal to adults and often contained moral messages. Der Stuwwelpeter, is a good example of this. Heinrich Hoffman (1809–1894), a German psychiatrist, wrote and illustrated it in 1845 for his son.

Activity

Look at the following extract from Der Struwwlpeter and compare it with an extract from a contemporary children's storybook. Consider what messages the books convey to young readers.

The story of little suck-a-thumb

One day, Mamma said, 'Conrad dear,
I must go out and leave you here.
But mind now, Conrad, what I say,
Don't suck your thumb while I'm away.
The great tall tailor always comes
To little boys who suck their thumbs:
And ere they dream what he's about,
He takes his great sharp scissors out
And cuts their thumbs off, and then,
You know, they never grow again.'
Mamma had scarcely turn'd her back,
The thumb was in, Alack! Alack!
The door flew open, in he ran,
The great, long, red-legged scissor-man.
Oh! Children, see! The tailor's come
And caught out little Suck-a-Thumb.
Snip! Snap! Snip! the scissors go;
And Conrad cries out - Oh! Oh! Oh!
Snip! Snap! Snip! They go so fast
That both his thumbs are off at last.
Mamma comes home; there Conrad stands
And looks quite sad and shows his hands
'Ah!' said Mamma, 'I knew he'd come
To naughty little Suck-a-Thumb.'

Look up the following website and read more about some of the early children's books:

- http://www.sc.edu/library/spcoll/kidlit/kidlit/kidlit.html

The following website contains details of the original illustrations which Dr Hoffman included in the original version of Der Struwwelpeter.

- http://www.fln.vcu.edu/struwwel/struwwel.html

This brief overview of the changing concept of childhood provides some insight into the nature of children's lives in earlier centuries.

The origins of foundling hospitals and dispensaries

In Britain in the mid-18th century, many parents – faced with extreme poverty – abandoned their infants and children. They did so in the hope that they would be taken by adults who were in a better position to love, nurture and care for them (Schwartzman 1978). Interestingly, the mortality rate among children who remained with their natural families was higher than among those who were abandoned and subsequently taken in by other adults. This was because the original home conditions for many children were squalid, with poor sanitation, overcrowding and high levels of poverty (Kosky & Lunnon 1991). It is estimated that during the 1850s, 50,000 deaths occurred each year, of which over 21,000 were children less than 10 years of age.

Activity

Consider the aims set out by Charles West in 1852 for the Sick Children's Hospital, Great Ormond Street (Miles 1986a, b), and reflect on how they compare with the aims of the Alder Hey Children's Hospital, Liverpool, at the beginning of the 21st century.

The Sick Children's Hospital, Great Ormond Street

- To provide for the reception and maintenance and medical treatment of children of the poor during sickness and to furnish them with advice, that is, the mothers of those who cannot be admitted into the hospital.
- To promote the advancement of medical science generally with reference to the diseases of children and, in particular, to provide for the more efficient instruction of students in this department of medical knowledge.
- To disseminate among all classes of the community, but chiefly among the poor, a better acquaintance with the management of infants and children during illness by employing and training of women in the special duties of children's nursing.

Alder Hey Children's Hospital (2003)

- Aim:
  - To provide a comprehensive, high-quality child health service that promotes the integration of hospital and community care in a family-centred, friendly and safe environment.
- Guiding principles:
  - A range of services will be provided to meet all child health needs with the least possible delay.
  - Parents will be involved with professionals in the planning and provision of care.
  - Parents shall be encouraged to stay with their children in hospital at all times.
  - Recreation, play activities and education will be provided according to individual needs.
  - Opportunities for development and training will be provided to ensure highly motivated, well-trained and educated staff.
  - Equal care and consideration will be given to all our patients so that their privacy, dignity and beliefs are respected at all times.
  - Children and parents will be told the name and status of any person caring for them.
- http://www.alderhey.com/RLCH/home.asp

Thomas Coram (1668–1751) was born in Dorset and spent much of his life at sea. After working in the ship-building business he moved to London, where by 1732 he was a successful merchant. The sight of abandoned infants and children appalled Thomas Coram and in response to what he saw he applied for and was granted a Royal Charter by George II to open the Foundling Hospital, in Hatton Gardens in London in 1741 (Franklin 1964). By taking abandoned infants and children into the Foundling Hospital, Coram wanted to prevent the murder of infants at birth and to stop the practice of parents abandoning their infants and children to die on the streets of London. The primary aim of the Foundling Hospital, which was not a hospital as we know it today, was the provision of care and education. The visionary work of Thomas Coram was widely recognised and many famous artists became patrons and governors of the hospital. Some of their artwork was displayed in the Foundling Hospitals during the 18th century. Today examples of the work of Hogarth, Reynolds and Gainsborough are now on view in the Foundling Museum, established in London in 1998.

There were many such hospitals and, as the name suggests, they were places to which children who were the illegitimate offspring of the poor or who had been abandoned by their parents were taken. Members of the public viewed the foundling hospitals with a high degree of suspicion, considering them to be places of death because of their high mortality rates. In 1756 the governors appealed to the House of Commons for financial assistance. Although granted, the assistance was conditional and required that the governors accepted all children offered to them. The number of sick and seriously debilitated infants and children arriving at the hospital increased dramatically. According to Franklin (1964), the indiscriminate admission of 14,934 babies over a 46-month period in the 1760s resulted in 10,389 deaths. The majority of the infants who died were under 6 months of age. Increasingly it was recognised that children who survived until their second birthday had a significantly improved chance of surviving childhood.

In the UK, the response to the growing problem of sick children involved the setting up of charitable dispensaries. Dr George Armstrong (1719–1789), a Scottish surgeon, is credited with the establishment of the first dispensary or 'ambulatorium' in Red Lion Square, London, in 1769. His work is an early example of ambulatory care and some today consider him to be the 'father of ambulatory care'. The main aim of dispensaries was to lower the toll of mortality among infants and children by providing advice and administering medicines to children of the poor, from birth to 10–12 years of age. This provision was designed to meet the needs of infants and children who, at that time, were often refused admission by most hospitals. Children were acknowledged to be susceptible to infection often as a result of poor nutrition.

As well as keeping children out of hospital, the work of Dr George Armstrong was based on the belief that to separate children from their families was to 'break their heart' (Miles 1985). Accounts about the dispensaries suggest that cost of hospital care was a factor for many parents. Armstrong shared the concern that the economic pressure of looking after a child in hospital would place an intolerable financial burden on many parents. However, the overriding view of Armstrong was that children should 'remain at home, however humble, surrounded and affectionately nursed by their dearest relations, and by those who feel a natural and earnest interest in their welfare' (Miles 1986a, b).

John Bunnell Davis founded the Universal Dispensary for Children in 1816. In 1823 it became the Royal Universal Dispensary, located in Waterloo Road in London (Franklin 1964). It was intended to provide a centre-point of medical attention for the investigation of diseases in children and young people. Although initially teaching and home visits appeared central to the work of the dispensary, these elements gradually ceased. Other cities throughout the UK opened dispensaries based on similar principles, for example in Manchester in 1829 and Liverpool in 1851. The figures from the Universal Dispensary for Children during the first 3.5 years after its introduction demonstrate a significant improvement on the statistics from the foundling hospitals. It is reported that during this time 7820 sick infants were treated and 7030 cured, 300 vaccinated, 130 died and the remainder continued to receive ongoing care (Franklin 1964). Charles West, the founder of the Hospital for Sick Children, Great Ormond Street, worked for almost 10 years as the physician from 1842. John Bunnell Davis died at the young age of 44 but is credited with being one of the most important influences on British paediatrics, having established an early version of a school of medicine linked to the Universal Dispensary for Children that he founded (Franklin 1964).

Although dispensaries met with some success in reducing the mortality rate amongst infants and children, physicians were forming the opinion that specialist inpatient care was becoming increasingly necessary. In their first argument for such a provision they cited examples of the European cities where children's hospitals were already established. The number of children's hospitals in Europe had increased steadily throughout the 17th, 18th and 19th centuries, starting with the La Maison de l'enfant Jesus (which was an orphanage, although reported by some writers to be a foundling hospital; Guthrie 1960), which opened in 1679. This institution was subsequently converted to L'Hôpital des Enfants Malades in 1802 at the Rue de Sevres in Paris. Other European cities that opened hospitals include St Petersburg in 1834, Vienna in 1837, Budapest in 1839 and Moscow in 1842. However, the mortality in such places was a cause for concern. The high mortality rate reported in L'Hôpital des Enfants Malades was attributed to infectious diseases and the scarcity of nurses with the necessary knowledge and skills (Lomax 1996). Around this time, Louis Pasteur's work on microorganisms was gaining momentum and the knowledge and understanding of microorganisms and cross-infection steadily increased (Craig 1977). Pasteur (1822–1895) provided the impetus for microbiology and contributed to the development of the first vaccines.

Seminar discussion topic

In your study group, discuss the following questions:

1. What are the fundamental differences between a foundling hospital and a modern children's hospital?
2. Why did it take so long for the concept of a children's hospital to spread worldwide?

After your discussion go the following website and read the article by Retureta et al (2003) about foundling and children's hospitals in other parts of the world:

- http://www.int-pediatrics.org/Volume%2013/133hist.htm

The establishment of children's hospitals

In London in 1850 it was estimated that children under the age of 10 years occupied approximately 3% of available hospital beds but that the deaths in the same age group accounted for 50% of all deaths in London (Franklin 1964). In 1851, a public meeting approved the idea of establishing a children's hospital and the Hospital for Sick Children, in Great Ormond Street, opened in 1852 with 10 beds (Arton 1982). In 1858 the purchase of a second house adjacent to the original provided much needed additional accommodation and the number of children who could be admitted rose to 75. The novelist Charles Dickens, a close friend of Charles West – the founder of the Hospital for Sick Children, Great Ormond Street – was himself a strong advocate of the idea of a children's hospital and his depiction of the nurse Sairey Gamp in his novel 'Martin Chuzzelwit' (Dickens 1984) has been credited with providing ammunition that undermined the early working-class domiciliary nursing movement in favour of a medically dominated, nurse subservient workforce (Rafferty 1995). Queen Victoria, who subscribed to the project, subsequently became its patron (Arton 1982) and Lord Shaftesbury (1801–1885), the factory reformer and philanthropist, was another supporter of the venture to build a children's hospital. The slogan used at the time of fundraising in the late 19th century was 'children's health, the nation's wealth'. Today, as the Hospital for Sick Children, Great Ormond Street plans new and exciting developments, the centrality of the child continues to be reflected in its mission statement 'the child first and always'.

During his time at the Universal Dispensary for Children, West had had the opportunity to visit the homes of sick children and was aware of the acute problems, such as overcrowding and lack of ventilation, that made the home environment unsuitable for many of the children. Before establishing the Hospital for Sick Children, Great Ormond Street, he also visited the National Children's Hospital in Dublin, the first hospital in Britain entirely dedicated to the care of sick children.

Activity

Access the companion PowerPoint presentation and, using the map available at the website, identify the location of children's services throughout the UK (include children's hospitals and children's wards within District General Hospitals).
Suggested website:

- http://coursework.org.uk/essentials/ukmap.html

The aims outlined by West in 1852 formed the basis for other similar institutions throughout the UK. They reflected a change in emphasis from reducing mortality to a stronger focus on teaching. This shift in emphasis acknowledged that specially trained children's nurses would be vital in the overall efficiency of care of sick children. By 1888 it was estimated that there were 38 hospitals for sick children in the UK (Franklin 1964). Many general hospitals dedicated wards to the care of sick children. The newly founded children's hospitals, in common with adult hospitals, were voluntary hospitals that relied entirely on public money for support.

Activity

Consider what other circumstances, faced by parents in the mid-18th century, might have contributed to their decision to abandon their children. Consider some of the possible consequences for the children by reflecting on what happened to children in Romania prior to the overthrow of the Romanian dictator, Nicolae Ceausescu.

The growth of children's hospitals

Many hospitals were established during the 19th and early 20th centuries. One such was the Royal Manchester Children's Hospital, which was founded in 1829 as a dispensary and became a six-bedded hospital in 1855. Like many other early children's hospital, the demands on the hospital were great and in 1873 it moved to its present site to the north of the city centre. Booth Hall Infirmary, now known as Booth Hall Children's Hospital, opened in 1909 but its designation as a children's hospital came 6 years later in 1915 and Royal Patronage was granted in 1923.

PowerPoint

Access the companion PowerPoint presentation and look at the website for Manchester Children's Hospital for further details of its history and planned developments:

- http://www.cmht.nwest.nhs.uk

Nottingham Children's Hospital, originally referred to as the Free Hospital for Sick Children, was founded in 1869. The aims of the hospital included the reception, maintenance and provision of medical treatment to children less than 10 years of age. The hospital moved to a new site shortly after its opening and, in 1978, moved again to its present site as part of the University Hospital, Queens Medical Centre (Crothall 1978). Like many children's hospitals across the UK, it has an informative website detailing information about its history and current initiatives and future plans.

PowerPoint

Access the companion PowerPoint presentation and look at the website for Nottingham Children's Hospital:

- http://www.mss.library.nottingham.ac.uk/isad/uhc.html

In Oxford, plans are in place to build a new children's hospital as part of the John Radcliffe Hospital. The new children's hospital will be linked to the new John Radcliffe Hospital and will provide centralised services for children.

PowerPoint

Access the companion PowerPoint presentation and look at the website for Oxford Children's Hospital:

- http://www.chox.org.uk/plans/

Dr William Jackson Cleaver established the Sheffield Free Hospital for Sick Children in a rented property, Brightmore House, in 1867. The opening of the hospital met with some degree of opposition, and the hospital accommodation was soon inadequate for the demands placed on it (Harvey 1976). Like so many other children's hospitals it moved to a new site a few years later.

The Southampton Children's Hospital, the only dedicated children's hospital in the Hampshire region, was established in 1884, initially as The Shirley Children's Hospital and Dispensary for Women. In reality, the hospital was little more than a small house in Church Street, Shirley – then an outlying village of Southampton. Although the hospital moved to larger premises in Winchester Road, Southampton, in 1912, it was not until 1920, when a new wing was built, that the name was changed to the Southampton Children's Hospital and Dispensary for Women. Although the General Nursing Council established the Register for Nurses in 1919, the Southampton Children's Hospital did not found its own school to train Registered Sick Children's Nurses (RSCN) until 1936. The nurses undertook a 3-year course leading to part 8 of the professional register. Probationers following the Registered Sick Children's Nursing course at the hospital had to work, attending lectures and studying in their own free time. The classroom was very small and the nurses were educated in the art and science of children's nursing by the resident Sister Tutor.

The RSCN course was suspended during the early years of the Second World War and recommenced in 1944, the same year that the hospital became the Southampton Children's Hospital. Although the hospital flourished after the inauguration of the National Health Service in 1948, the training of Registered Sick Children's Nurses was discontinued in 1960, after the General Nursing Council decreed that the hospital was too small to adequately train RSCNs. For a short time the Children's Hospital continued to offer training for Enrolled Nurses. The hospital was closed in 1974, transferring its children to the newly built east wing of Southampton General Hospital. Since then, children's services at Southampton have grown and, as in Oxford, there are plans for a separate children's hospital.

In Ireland, the Adelaide, Meath and National Children's Hospitals were all voluntary hospitals. The Meath was founded early – in 1753. In 1821 a group of doctors from Dublin founded the first hospital in Ireland (also the first in Britain) entirely devoted to the care of children. It was this hospital that Charles West visited before setting up the Hospital for Sick Children, Great Ormond Street. The Adelaide was founded in 1839 and opened a school of nursing in 1859, the year in which 'Notes on Nursing' was published. The three institutions amalgamated in 1998.

In Wales, the opening of a new children's hospital early in 2005 replaced a multisite service with services for children and their families at a central location. With a strong emphasis on creating a suitable environment for children and appropriate facilities for parents, the new hospital offers a wide range of specialist services to the children of Cardiff, south of Wales and beyond.

From 1860 to 1883, three children's hospitals opened in Scotland. The Hospital for Sick Children in Edinburgh opened in early 1860 and credit for the founding of this hospital is given to two members of the medical profession – Charles Wilson and John Smith (Guthrie 1960). John Smith visited the Paris Children's Hospital and is reported to have stated:

> There is no question whatever that it seemed inconceivable and altogether unaccountable that while almost every municipality on the continent of Europe possesses at least one, if not two, hospitals devoted to children's diseases, no such institution was to be found in the famous medical centre of Edinburgh
>
> (Birrell 1995)

The development of the Hospital for Sick Children was similar to the development of the Great Ormond Street hospital: it started with limited facilities and gradually acquired larger premises. Guthrie (1960), writing about the early days of the hospital, notes that when it was first opened children were, to some extent, still regarded as miniature adults, with little or no consideration given to the unique diseases from which they suffered.

PowerPoint

Access the companion PowerPoint presentation and look up the history of the Royal Hospital for Sick Children in Edinburgh and then view the silent film on childcare in the 1930s, in particular section 2:

- http://www.lhsa.lib.ed.ac.uk/images/hc/healthycity. html

The Aberdeen Children's Hospital opened in 1877 to provide services for children in the city of Aberdeen, the surrounding counties of Aberdeen, Kincardine, Banff, Moray and the islands of Orkney and Shetland. It moved to a site at Foresterhill in Aberdeen in 1929. A new children's hospital, built within the Foresterhill complex, opened early in 2004 and is one of the UK's newest children's hospitals.

The Glasgow Hospital for Sick Children, which later became the Royal Hospital for Sick Children, opened in 1883. It moved to its Yorkhill site in 1914 and is the largest children's hospital in Scotland.

PowerPoint

Access the companion PowerPoint presentation and view the archive material from the Royal Hospital for Sick Children in Glasgow, which provides an interesting account of nurses' training, working and living conditions 1883–1920.

Children's hospitals also opened in other parts of the world in the later part of the 19th century. Examples include the Children's Hospital of Philadelphia, which is the oldest hospital in the USA solely dedicated to the care of children. It was founded in 1895 during the Industrial Revolution. Francis West Lewis visited the Hospital for Sick Children, Great Ormond Street and on his return to the USA decided to open a similar institution devoted to the care of sick children and to finding cures and treating illnesses and injuries specific to children. The innovative research programmes have led to developments such as fetal surgery techniques and the hospital is recognised to be a leader in its field.

PowerPoint

Access the companion PowerPoint presentation and look at the website for further information on the Children's Hospital of Philadelphia, which has detailed information about its contribution to developments in children's health care:

- http://www.chop.edu/consumer/index.jsp

Allan Campbell founded the Adelaide Children's Hospital in 1876. The hospital is now merged with the Queen Victoria Hospital and is the first fully integrated Women's and Children's Hospital in Australia.

In 1904, the Children's Memorial Hospital opened in Montreal, Canada. It was the first hospital in Montreal whose sole mandate was the provision of care for sick children. Five years after it opened a new hospital was built and in 1920 the hospital became part of a teaching hospital affiliated to McGill University; it is now part of the McGill University Health Centre. It is a multicultural, bilingual institution that serves an increasingly diverse community.

PowerPoint

Access the companion PowerPoint presentation and look at the website of the Children's Hospital of Montreal to explore the features of a multicultural/bilingual institution:

- http://www.thechildren.com

The origins of education and registration of children's nurses

Undoubtedly, Charles West, the Founder of Great Ormond Street Children's Hospital, was a formidable individual. Before founding Great Ormond Street Children's Hospital, he worked in The Universal Dispensary for Children in London. He resigned when he failed to persuade the management of the need to expand the facilities to include inpatient beds. It was during his time in the dispensary that he came to the conclusion that dispensaries did not have all the necessary facilities to cope with the problems of children. In his opinion, the dispensaries served only to accentuate the need for specialist hospitals (Miles 1986a, b). Franklin, in his account of children's hospitals in the UK, pays this tribute to West, describing the way he dealt with children: 'the fractious or frightened child could not long resist the magic of his smile or the winning gentleness of his manner' (Franklin 1964). Charles West's book 'How to nurse sick children' contains much of interest and he is very direct in his observation about what he considers to be the qualities of a sick children's nurse (West 1854). This book was published 5 years before 'Notes on nursing' by Florence Nightingale. West's book formed the basis of the theoretical teaching at Great Ormond Street. Although only 52 pages in length, it was considered very comprehensive and for many years remained the mainstay of teaching within the hospital, continuing in print until 1907 (Arton 1982). It was recently reprinted by Great Ormond Street Children's Hospital.

Seminar discussion topic

Read this extract from West's book and discuss what qualities children's nurses need in order to be able to provide effective care for children and families in the 21st century.

> *Indeed, if any of you have entered on your office without a feeling of very earnest love to little children – a feeling which makes you long to be with them, to help them – you have made a great mistake in undertaking such duties as you are now engaged in: and the sooner you seek some other mode of gaining an honest livelihood, the better. I do not mean this unkindly, for you may be very good, very respectable women, and yet be very bad nurses. You may be feeble in health, and then you will be unable to bear the confinement and fatigue upon attending upon the sick; or you may be fretful in temper, and may find your greatest trial to consist in the difficulty of subduing it, and in being as thankful to God for all his daily mercies, and as friendly with those who you live amongst as you ought to be; or you may naturally have low spirits and a child's prattle, instead of refreshing, may weary you. Now if any of these things are really the case with you, I would advise you not to be a children's nurse, and especially not to be a nurse in the Hospital for Sick Children*
>
> (West 1854).

In 1856, 2 years after the publication of his book, Charles West appointed a superintendent to oversee the training of pupil nurses. Catherine Jane Wood wrote the book entitled 'A handbook for nursing', which was considered an important adjunct to the original text written by West. Wood had many innovative ideas about how nursing should be organised and proposed patient allocation and an early version of the nursing process (Arton 1982).

Activity

Consider the following extract from West's book 'How to nurse sick children'. How valid are the comments in the light of current knowledge about the care of sick children?

> *At the Children's Hospital you know it is customary, unless otherwise ordered by the doctor, to place a child on its admission in a warm bath. For this now there are several reasons in addition to the very evident one of ensuring the child's perfect cleanliness. The warmth of the water is grateful and soothing to its feverishness, and that is one advantage; but another is than when stripped for the bath the nurse has the opportunity of carefully examining the whole of the child's body and thus of seeing whether there is any rash, or eruption as it is called, upon it, while the bath moreover helps to throw out any rash if it were about to appear.*

Although part of the initial strategy, it was almost 26 years after the opening of Hospital for Sick Children, Great Ormond Street, before the first purpose-built training school for sick children's nurses opened under the tutelage of Catherine Jane Wood. She stated that 'sick children require special nurses and sick children's nurses need special training' (Wood 1888) and demonstrated great determination in her efforts to ensure that children received appropriate care. Often forgotten in the general discussion about the origins of nurse training is the fact that children's nurse training started almost 10 years before the training of adult nurses (Miles 1986a, b).

Florence Nightingale, on her return from the Crimea, was suffering from what many now believe to be post-traumatic stress syndrome. However, she and colleagues such as Mary Seacole were determined to professionalise nursing. Although Nightingale remained preoccupied with general nursing, she does make mention of the needs of children in her book 'Notes on nursing', in which she states 'children; they are affected by the same things (as adults) but much more quickly and seriously' (Nightingale 1859). However, she saw no need for a children's hospital, although it is known that she corresponded with Charles West, possibly because she was considered the 'official voice of nursing' at that time. There is evidence from the archives of Hospital for Sick Children, Great Ormond Street, that West and Nightingale corresponded on matters such as the optimum way to nurse children. This is surprising in view of the fact that Nightingale's knowledge of children, sick or well, was considered to be scant. This pattern of prominent individuals seeking advice about children from nurses who do not hold the requisite qualification or knowledge continues to the current day.

Nightingale used money given to her by the State, in recognition of her contribution during the Crimean war, to develop a school of nursing. The Nightingale School at St Thomas' Hospital in London contributed to the ascendancy of the generalist nurse with the subsequent denigration of other types of nursing, including children's nursing. The seeds of generic nurse preparation were sown and, like hydra's teeth of Greek mythology, have returned to haunt the profession in the years since.

The battle for training and a professional recordable qualification continued for many years. Florence Nightingale opposed registration and its introduction occurred only after her death in 1910 (Baly 1973). Baly describes how the Midwives Act, passed in 1902 and which mandated all midwives to undergo a period of formal training and to subsequently register with the Central Midwives Board, made the registration of general nurses an inevitability. The First World War slowed the progression towards registration but did not stop it. Mrs Bedford Fenwick, who was responsible for founding the British Nurses' Association, worked for more than two decades to develop a register and continued despite many obstacles, such as the introduction of Private Members bills during the war years. She, together with other colleagues, did not support the inclusion of children's nurses in the Registration Act (1919).

Conflict among the 'branches' of nursing was precipitated when the College of Nursing was founded in 1916. This organisation became the Royal College of Nursing; it was considered to be a rival group to the British Nurses' Association and had the backing of the medical royal colleges. The College of Nursing and the British Nurses' Association decided that nurses who had undergone training only in a children's hospital should not have their names included in the proposed register of nurses. There was also no attempt to include the names of children's nurses in the proposed supplementary register that was set up to include the names of male nurses, mental and fever nurses.

With little support from the nurses' organisations, staff in the sick children's hospitals took action. The matrons of the London children's hospitals produced a petition opposing the idea by the British Nurses' Association for a supplementary register without the names of children's nurses. The petition from the children's hospitals had the support of an eminent paediatrician from Great Ormond Street, Arthur Frances Voelcker. According to Twistington-Higgins (1952), Voelcker wrote in the petition that 'serious injury will be caused not only to children's nurses but to children's hospitals and the Empire'. He considered that to exclude the names of children's nurses from the supplementary register would be disadvantageous in terms of status, prestige and financial remuneration.

In 1919, the unified Nurses Registration Bill was presented to the House of Lords. In addition to the general part of the register, there were a number of supplementary parts, including one containing the names of nurses trained in the nursing of sick children. The supplementary part of the Register for sick children's nurses now remains part of the Register of Nurses in the UK (Barlow & Swanick 1994). The supplementary register was set up to recognise the specialist nursing required by children, although the records of the debate that preceded its establishment suggest that at least one Member of Parliament was keen to ensure that sick children's nurses should not masquerade as registered nurses! The Registration Bill, passed in December 1919, enabled the setting up of the General Nursing Council (GNC) for each of the countries in the UK. Initially, a caretaker GNC was formed until elections were arranged from amongst the registered nurses.

One of the remits of the GNC was to create the register of nurses. Those whose names appeared on the register were required to have completed a course of study of a designated length, to an agreed standard and in different areas of nursing. Arton (1988) reports on the opposition to the supplementary register by Bedford Fenwick, who believed that the supplementary register for children's nurses would be short lived. However, after 85 years of existence the future of the children's nurse appears to be assured.

Closer examination of the progress of registration for children's nurses, however, reveals it to be fraught with difficulties. Although the original idea was to ensure that nurses, practising in different disciplines, would be of equal qualification, the struggle to establish equity between the different parts of the register continues to the present day.

The Register opened on 27 July 1921 but the process of compiling it was slow because Mrs Bedford Fenwick insisted on scrutinising each individual application. The first sick children's nurse (RSCN no. 1) to be listed on the Supplementary Register was Evelyn Margaret Hughes, who registered on 28 October 1921 following a 3-year course at Birmingham Children's Hospital. Agnes Coulton (RSCN no. 96) was a member of the caretaker GNC, having trained at the Infirmary for Children in Liverpool. She became the Lady Superintendent of the East London Hospital for Children and was a member of the Registration Committee.

Table 1.1 General nursing council register in 1923 (from Arton 1987)

Type of nurse	Number
General nurses	10,887
Male nurses	24
Mental nurses	639
Sick children's nurses	191
Fever nurses	356
Total	12,097

According to United Kingdom Central Council (UKCC) archives, of the 119 women who registered as a Sick Children's Nurse on the first published register, no fewer than 27 trained at the Hospital for Sick Children, Great Ormond Street. On 10 January 1923 the electorate for the forthcoming election for the GNC comprised all the registered nurses, as shown in Table 1.1. At that time a small victory for children's nurses occurred when Dr Addison, Minister for Health, was persuaded to include onto the GNC two nurses who had experience of caring for sick children.

Another remit of the GNC was to compile a syllabus of topics for examination. One of the criticisms of the English GNC was its generic focus, which from the perspective of sick children's nurses could be demonstrated in the content of the examination set in 1925.

Activity

The GNC examination (Arton 1992)

Read and consider the following questions:

1. Describe a case of acute nephritis. How would you nurse such a case? (Mention diet and nursing that might be ordered.)
2. Describe the nursing of a case of peritonitis.

Activity

The 1931 hospital for sick children examination paper

Read the following questions in the examination paper and compare and contrast them with examination questions in your current programme of study.

1. A child of five has developed an acute attack of asthma. Give the symptoms and nursing care of the immediate attack. What general steps would you take to prevent occurrences?
2. Give in detail the treatment of a child of four years suffering from:
   (a) scabies
   (b) threadworms.

In addition to completing the GNC examination, students were required to undertake a hospital examination before completing their training. A sample examination paper from the Hospital for Sick Children, Great Ormond Street, in 1931 has a clear child focus that is in stark contrast to the GNC questions above.

Many of the issues that emerged at the time of the introduction of registration persisted in the years that followed. The ratification of the Supplementary Register created difficulties for RSCNs striving to maintain equal status with their colleagues on the General Register. Despite the recognition that sick children require specialist nurses, many hospitals insisted that, to be promoted to a Ward Sister post, the individual required a general nurse qualification in addition to the RSCN. The establishment of the Association of Sick Children's Hospital Nurses was an attempt by a group of matrons from Sick Children's Hospitals to further the interests of sick children's hospital nurses by enabling discussion on matters pertaining to the nursing of sick children. The over-riding principle of the Association of Sick Children's Hospital Nurses was that 'children's trained nurses should nurse sick children' (Duncombe 1979). The renaming of the Association of Sick Children's Hospital Nurses in 1953 to the Association of British Paediatric Nurses (ABPN) occurred in recognition that the initial title was too restrictive, focusing only on hospital-based nurses when in fact an increasing number of children were being cared for in the community.

PowerPoint

Access the companion PowerPoint presentation and look at the website for the Association of British Paediatric Nurses. Consider the contribution the association has made to children's nursing since it was founded in 1937:

- http://www.abpn.org.uk/

Between the mid-19th century and the inception of the NHS in 1948, considerable advances were made in the provision of community nursing. Community children's nursing services were first introduced during the latter part of the 19th century (Whiting 2000). The minutes of a meeting at the Nottingham Children's Hospital in the mid-1800s provides some of the earliest accounts of paediatric home care provision (RCN 1984/85). According to Hunt & Whiting (1999), a similar system operated from Great Ormond Street in the 1880s following an application to the Management Committee of the hospital. Similar accounts are found in the records from Liverpool Children's Hospital in 1910 (RCN 1984/85). According to Lomax (1996), there is limited information on the number of hospitals that employed nurses to visit children. Many hospitals found the expense of such schemes prohibitive and discontinued the service on these grounds. Great Ormond Street continued to provide a paediatric nursing service until the introduction of the NHS in 1948.

Following the introduction of the NHS, Rotherham is credited with the first appointment of a nurse involved exclusively in the care for sick children in the community in 1949 (Gillet 1954). Much of the work involved the care of children with acute infections such as pneumonia and bronchitis. Building on the success of Rotherham, other home care schemes emerged (While 1991). As early as the time of the Court Report (Department of Health and Social Security (DHSS) 1976) it was recognised that sick children required community care by nurses with the appropriate knowledge and skills. With the changing pattern of hospital care, including shorter admission stays and day surgery, growing numbers are currently being supported in the community. In addition, increasing numbers of children with complex and long-term needs are now being cared for at home (ACT/RCPCH 1997). In 1998 the government made the decision to introduce community children's nursing teams to commemorate the memory of Diana, Princess of Wales. A qualified children's nurse with a community qualification leads each team. Known as Diana, Princess of Wales Community Child Nursing Teams, there are approximately 110 within the UK. The key aims of the initiative are to:

- support children with life-limiting illnesses and their families
- provide high-quality, seamless care
- involve other agencies
- bring different services together to meet a multitude of needs.

Activity

Consider the above aims and explore the potential benefits of the service to children and their families.

Education of children's nurses

Inevitably, the educational programmes for children's nurses have evolved over the years in response to changing perceptions about children and childhood and the increased knowledge and understanding about children's needs in health and illness. The work of John Bowlby (1952, 1953a, b, 1960, 1971, 1988) and James Robertson (1955, 1968, 1970, 1989), among others, added considerably to the knowledge base about the needs of infants and children, and subsequently to the impact of hospitalisation on these groups. Bowlby (1907–1990) and Roberston (1911–1988) have had a profound influence on how infants and children are cared for in hospital and other settings. In his work, Bowlby provided a theoretical framework to explain the process of attachment (Bowlby 1953a) and separation (Bowlby 1953b). Although some criticised the theories of attachment and separation, the original work provoked further studies that have shown the accuracy of Bowlby's original work on the effects of separation (Alsop-Shields & Mohay 2001). Robertson, influenced by Bowlby's work, became very interested in the effects of hospitalisation on the behaviour of young children. He firmly believed in the need to change practices within children's hospitals and, to this end, produced a series of compelling films as evidence for his claims. His series of films included 'A 2-year-old goes to hospital' (Robertson 1953) and later – in 1969 – 'John, 17 months, 9 days in a residential nursery'. Although professionals initially refused to accept these films, they stimulated a significant amount of discussion and debate.

As concern mounted about the welfare of children in hospital, the government response was to commission a report on the welfare of children in hospital, universally known as the Platt Report (Ministry of Health 1959). This report increased public awareness of the impact of separation on young children and led to the foundation, in 1961, of the organisation that became the National Association for the Welfare of Children in Hospital (NAWCH). This association became the Action For Sick Children (ASC) in 1990 when its role changed from being a pressure group to being an advisory one.

Activity

Obtain a copy of the following article:

- Alsop-Shields L, Mohay H 2001 John Bowlby and James Robertson: theorists, scientists and crusaders for improvements in the care of children in hospital. Journal of Advanced Nursing 35(1):50–58.

To what degree do you consider the work of Bowlby and Robertson influences today's care of children in hospital?

PowerPoint

Access the companion PowerPoint presentation and read the web pages describing the origins of Action For Sick Children and its ongoing contribution to the work with sick children and their families:

- http://www.actionforsickchildren.org

Seminar discussion topic

Does Action For Sick Children still have a role in contemporary child health?

Throughout the years since its inception, children's nursing has faced many threats to its continuation, with many attempts from within the nursing profession to introduce a generic preparation for nurses in the UK. The publication of the RCN-commissioned report chaired by Lord Horder in 1943 (RCN 1946), just 5 years before the introduction of the NHS, made clear recommendations that sick children's nursing should become a post-registration qualification. Although never implemented, few doubt that this did a significant amount of damage to the continuation of the direct entry RSCN programme. Sir Alan Moncrieff, a paediatrician from the Hospital for Sick Children, Great Ormond Street, did much to mitigate the pernicious effects of the Horder Report when he addressed a meeting of the Association of Sick Children's Hospital Nurses in 1944 with a paper entitled 'The future of the nursing of sick children'. Central to his message was the belief that 'paediatric nursing is not a specialty but general nursing at a special age period'. Price (1993) draws attention to the similarities between past discussions about children's nurses and the ongoing debate about the current child health qualification.

In England, the damaging effects of the recommendations of the Horder Report were profound and sustained. As a result, the direct-entry RSCN programme was phased out during the mid-1960s. Many RSCNs holding single qualifications found it difficult to further their careers without obtaining a second

Table 1.2 Geographical breakdown of the register (NMC 2004)

Country	Number on register	Percentage of register
England	470,536	72.89
Northern Ireland	20,968	3.25
Scotland	54,527	8.45
Wales	29,665	4.60
Overseas	28,974	4.48
Postcode not known	40,838	6.33

qualification, usually in adult nursing. The impact of nurses leaving to gain a second qualification proved detrimental to the recruitment and retention of staff in children's hospitals. To alleviate the situation, some of the larger teaching hospitals introduced a 4-year combined course leading to the qualification of SRN on completion of the first 3 years and RSCN on successful completion of the fourth year. However, an unexpected number of nurses leaving on successful completion of 3 years further exacerbated the issue of recruitment to children's nursing. To counter this difficulty, in 1968 several teaching hospitals introduced a new programme lasting 3 years and 8 months. This required students to complete the entire programme with one final examination from which, if successful, they received the award of SRN/RSCN and inclusion on Parts 1 and 8.

The 3-year programme in Ireland was discontinued in 1978 (Love 1998). In Wales, the first recognised courses for RSCN commenced in 1976 with limited post-registration courses. Accelerated courses were introduced in 1990 but were replaced by flexible pathways leading to registration and inclusion on Part 15 of the Register (Davies et al 2001). The Welsh Assembly acknowledged the need to employ additional children's nurses with the scheduled opening of the first Children's Hospital in Wales in 2005.

Only in Scotland did the 3-year direct entry continue. Combined courses leading to the award of RGN/RSCN were run in Scotland between 1950 and 1958. The programmes were 4 years and 3 months in length. The courses were subsequently discontinued in Scotland because of the high attrition rate. Just as the integrated schemes of training were discontinued in Scotland, in England they were gaining in popularity. In 1972 new comprehensive programmes were introduced in which all students gained experience in adult nursing, psychiatric nursing, obstetrics and community nursing.

The introduction of the United Kingdom Central Council and the four National Boards under the auspices of the Nurses, Midwives and Health Visitors Act (1974) led to significant changes in the education and registration of nurses. The culmination of the reforms resulted in the publication of Project 2000 (UKCC 1986), an examination of how nurse education should be changed to meet the predicted demands of society in the forthcoming century. Eve Bendall, a well-known and respected children's nurse and previous head of the School of Nursing at the Hospital for Sick Children, Great Ormond Street, became the Chief Executive of the UKCC and Sheila

Barlow, Director of Nurse Education at the Hospital for Sick Children, Great Ormond Street, became Vice President of the Project 2000 working group. Her efforts resulted in the shaping of the new registration in which children's nursing (Part 15) was introduced as a discrete entity. The English National Board (ENB) approved the first 14 Project 2000 sites in England in the year between April 1989 and April 1990; 10 of these sites offered the new child branch programme leading to inclusion on Part 15 of the Register. The programmes embraced the new educational curriculum in which all nurses followed an 18-month common foundation programme irrespective of their chosen branch.

It was anticipated that the new programmes would give all nurses equal status irrespective of their chosen branch and children's nurses were initially euphoric to see their direct entry register returned to them. But the initial euphoria was short lived, as once again overt discrimination against children's nurses became apparent. In the new programmes, the adult nurse continues to be perceived as a 'general' nurse and children's nurses continue to experience difficulty undertaking shortened programmes such as the one leading to registration as a midwife. Employment overseas remains somewhat problematic for children's nurses. The changes in educational provision increase the opportunities for children's nurses who wish to work in Europe, but with the proviso that it must be a country where there is a reciprocal qualification (Smallman 1998). The lack of equity between branches, to the disadvantage of all but adult nurses, continues to be demonstrated by the adult bias of many common foundation programmes (UKCC 1999).

The publication of the UKCC (2001) document 'Fitness for practice and purpose' reopened the debate about the education of children's nurses. Central to the debate is the question of genericism versus specialism (Glasper 1995). In the generic approach to nurse education, students would be required to undertake a general programme followed by a period of specialist preparation following initial registration (Barr & Sines 1996). Those in favour of genericism argue that children's nursing is a specialism and that education should therefore take place at the post-registration level. However, to suggest that children's nursing is a specialism is to fail to recognise the generic nature of the children's nursing curriculum (Glasper 1995). Those opposed to genericism share the view expressed by Moncrieff (1944) that children's nursing is not a specialty but general nursing at a special age period.

For many years there has been inequity between the branches and, with relatively few registered nurses on Parts 8 and 15 of the Register, they have become a vulnerable group (Glasper 1995). According to the Nursing and Midwifery Council (NMC) statistical analysis, of the 645,508 individuals on the Register (Table 1.2) only 36,314 are children's nurses (NMC 2004). It should be noted that a percentage of these might hold dual qualification.

Gibson et al (2003) acknowledged that there is evidence in literature to support the continuation of a children's nursing qualification and considered the need to make a distinction between generalist and specialist nursing to distinguish children's nursing from all other branches of nursing. To do so, competencies required by generalist children's nurses are first identified and then additional competencies are identified. The competencies cover areas such as knowledge, abilities, values and qualities. Gibson et al contend that the development of these standards provides clear statements of what is required for a children's nurse to practice effectively. They suggest that this information can form the basis for identifying whether children's nursing is indeed a distinct and separate entity (Gibson et al 2003). The debates relating to the future of children's nursing will undoubtedly continue but it is important to stress that each year the evidence base for children's nursing interventions increases.

Despite support for the continuation of a specific child field of practice qualification The Nursing and Midwifery Council (NMC) for the UK commenced a consultation of the future configuration of pre-registration nursing in November 2007. The Association of Chief Children's Nurses (ACCN) of the UK, in preparation for a joint symposium with higher education institute children's nursing academics, undertook a SWOT analysis of the suggested changes to the existing register, with particular reference to one of the NMC's review criteria: 'marks relating to fields of practice (nature and number of branches versus no branches at all)'. Ellis et al (2008) reported on the views of these senior children's and young people's nurses on the future configuration of the register concluded that the existing configuration of the NMC register should remain. This analysis of the NMC consultation was later extended to some of the other criteria of the review and involved members of the children's nursing academic community across the UK. The UK academic children's nursing departments were invited to participate in this review and Richardson et al (2007) after an analysis of the data confirmed that academics favoured the retention of a direct entry children's nursing field of practice. The response to the NMC consultation by the children's and young peoples nursing community was extremely robust. In late 2008 the results of the consultation were published and, to the delight of children's and young people's nurses, the NMC made a decision to retain the field of practice. The debates over future configurations to the UK nursing register will undoubtedly continue.

Summary

The role of historical investigation gives healthcare researchers not only a window to the past but also a vehicle to make judgements about the future. The work of the RCN in promoting the History of Nursing Society is commendable and provides all nurses with the opportunity of learning from the past. Not to do so, to cite Plato, is folly, as those who do not are doomed to repeat the lessons of history.

References

ACT and RCPCH, 1997. A guide to developments of children's palliative care services. Report of a joint working party. Royal College of Paediatrics and Child Health, London.

Alsop-Shields, L., Mohay, H., 2001. John Bowlby and James Robertson: theorists, scientists and crusaders for improvements in care of children in hospital. Journal of Advanced Nursing 35 (1), 50–58.

Aries, P., 1962. Centuries of childhood. Jonathan Cape, London.
Arton, M., 1982. Children first and always. Nursing Times 78 (40), 1687–1688.
Arton, M., 1987. The caretaker general nursing council and sick children's nursing 1920-1923. RCN History of Nursing Bulletin 2 (1), 1–7.
Arton, M., 1988. The supplementary register for sick children's nurses. Accident or Design 2 (4), 24–28.
Arton, M., 1992. Development of sick children's nursing 1919–1939. MPhil thesis, University of Bath.
Avery, G., Briggs, J. (Eds.), 1989. Children and their books, Clarendon Press, Oxford.
Baly, M.E., 1973. Nursing and social change, 3rd edn. Routledge, London.
Barlow, S., Swanick, M., 1994. Supplementary benefits. Paediatric Nursing 6 (3), 16–17.
Barr, D., Sines, D., 1996. The development of the generalist nurse with the pre-registration education in the UK: some points for consideration. Nurse Education Today 16, 74–77.
Birrell, J., 1995. A most perfect hospital. Edinburgh Sick Children's NHS Trust, Edinburgh.
Bowlby, J., 1952. Maternal child care and mental health. World Health Organization, Geneva.
Bowlby, J., 1953a. Child care and the growth of love. Penguin, Harmondsworth.
Bowlby, J., 1953b. Attachment. Penguin, Harmondsworth.
Bowlby, J., 1960. Separation anxiety. International Journal of Psychoanalysis 41, 89–113.
Bowlby, J., 1971. Attachment, vol. 1. Penguin, Harmondsworth.
Bowlby, J., 1988. A secure base: parent–child attachment and health human development. Basic Books Inc., New York.
Children Act, 1989. HMSO, London.
Children (Scotland) Act 1995. HMSO, London.
Craig, J., 1977. A short history of the Royal Aberdeen Children's Hospital. University Press, Aberdeen.
Crothall, L., 1978. Let's begin with the children. Nottingham Children's Hospital, Nottingham.
Davies, A., Earles, C., Eaton, N., et al., 2001. Educating children's nurses in Wales. Paediatric Nursing 13 (6), 21–24.
Department of Health and Social Security (DHSS), 1976. Fit for the Future (the Court Report). The Report of the Committee on Child Health Services. HMSO, London.
Dickens, C., 1984. Martin Chuzzlewitt. Oxford University Press, London.
Duncombe, M.A., 1979. A brief history of the Association of British Paediatric nurses 1938–1975. Association of British Paediatric Nurses, London.
Ellis, J., Glasper, E.A., Horsley, A., McEwing, G., Richardson, J., 2008. The future of preregistration children's and young peoples nursing; a swot analysis. Journal of Children's and Young People's Nursing 2 (2, 06), 56–60.
Franklin, A.W., 1964. Children's hospitals. In: Poynter, F.N.L. (Ed.), The evolution of hospitals in Britain, Pitman Medical, London.
Gibson, F., Fletcher, M., Casey, A., 2003. Classifying general and specialist children's nursing competencies. Journal of Advanced Nursing 44 (6), 591–602.
Gillet, J.A., 1954. Children's nursing unit. British Medical Journal 4863, 684–685.
Glasper, E.A., 1995. The value of children's nursing in the third millennium. British Journal of Nursing 4 (1), 27–30.
Guthrie, D., 1960. The Royal Edinburgh Hospital for Sick Children. Churchill Livingstone, Edinburgh.
Harvey, P., 1976. Up the hill to Western Bank, history of the Children's Hospital Sheffield, 1876–1976. The Centenary Committee. Sheffield Children's Hospital, Sheffield.
Hoffman, H., 1845. Der Struwwlpeter. Kindlers Literaturlexikon. [English version 1994 The Struwwelpeter. Munich in association with Ragged Bears Ltd, Singapore].
Human Rights Act, 1998. HMSO, London.
Hunt, M., Whiting, M., 1999. A re-examination of the history of children's community nursing. Paediatric Nursing 11 (4), 33–36.
Kosky, J., Lunnon, R.J., 1991. Great Ormond Street Hospital and the story of medicine. The Hospitals For Sick Children in association with Granta Editions, London.
Lomax, E., 1996. The control of contagious disease in nineteenth-century British paediatric hospitals. The Society for the Social History of Medicine 7 (3), 383–400.
Love, H., 1998. The Royal Belfast Hospital for Sick Children: a history 1948-1998. Blackstaff Press, Belfast.
Lowden, J., 2002. Children's rights: a decade of dispute. Journal of Advanced Nursing 37 (1), 100–106.
de Mause, L., 1982. Foundations of psychohistory. Creative Roots, New York.
de Mause, L. (Ed.), 1995. The history of childhood: untold story of child abuse, Jason Aronson, Northvale, NJ.
Miles, I., 1985. A suitable case for treatment. Nursing Times May, 48–50.
Miles, I., 1986a. The emergence of sick children's nursing. Part 1: sick children's nursing before the turn of the century. Nurse Education Today 6:82–87
Miles, I., 1986b. The emergence of sick children's nursing. Part 2: the emergence of sick children's nursing. Nurse Education Today 6:133–138
Ministry of Health, 1959. Committee of the Central Health Services Council. Report of the Committee on the Welfare of Children in Hospital (The Plest Report). Ministry of Health, London.
Moncrieff, A., 1944. The future of the nursing of sick children. The Association of Sick Children's Hospital Nurses. Great Ormond Street Archives, London.
Nightingale, F., 1859. Notes on nursing: what it is and what it is not. Duckworth, London (reprinted 1970).
Nursing and Midwifery Council (NMC) 2004 Statistical analysis of the register. 1 April 2002 to 31 March 2003. NMC, London.
Power, K., 1998. 2002 Implications of the Human Rights Act. Paediatric Nursing 14 (4), 14–19.
Price, S., 1993. Children's nursing, lessons from the past. Nursing Standard 7 (50), 31–35.
Rafferty, A.M., 1995. The anomaly of autonomy: space and status in early nursing reform. International History of Nursing Journal 1 (1), 43–45.
Richardson, J., Glasper, E.A., McEwing, G., Ellis, J., Horsely, A., 2007. All change in children's and young people's nurse education: the views of senior practitioners. Journal of Children's and Young People's Nursing 1 (8), 377–383. http://eprints.soton.ac.uk/52546/
Royal College of Nursing (RCN), 1946. Report of the Nursing Reconstruction Committee (Horder Report). RCN, London.
Royal College of Nursing (RCN), 1984/85. Changing provision for sick children and diseases in childhood in Liverpool since 1850. RCN Bulletin 6. RCN, London.
Robertson, J., 1953. A two-year-old goes to hospital. A scientific film record. Concord Film Council. Suffolk, Ipswich.
Robertson, J., 1955. Young children in long-term hospitals. Nursing Times September 23, 63–65.
Robertson, J., 1968. The long-stay children in hospital. Maternal and Child Care 4, 161–166.
Robertson, J., 1969. John 17 months, 9 days in a residential nursery (film). Tavistock Institute for Human Relations, London.
Robertson, J., 1970. Young children in hospital, 2nd edn. Tavistock, London.
Robertson, J., 1989. Separation and the very young. Free Association Books, London.
Schwartzman, H.B., 1978. Transformations. Plenum Press, New York.
Scraton, P. (Ed.), 1997. Childhood in crisis, UCL Press, London.
Seidler, E., 1990. An historical survey of children's hospitals. In: Granshaw, L., Porter, R. (Eds.), The hospital in history. Routledge, London.
Singer, J.L., 1973. The child's world of make-believe. Academic Press, New York.
Smallman, S., 1998. Children's nursing in Europe. Paediatric Nursing 11 (11), 6.
Stone, L., 1977. The family, sex and marriage in England 1500-1800. Harper and Row, New York.

Twistington-Higgins, T., 1952. Great Ormond Street 1852-1952. Odhams Press, Watford.

United Kingdom Central Council (UKCC) 1986 Project, 2000. a new preparation for practice. UKCC, London.

United Kingdom Central Council (UKCC), 1999. Fitness for practice. UKCC, London.

United Kingdom Central Council (UKCC), 2001. Fitness for practice and purpose. UKCC, London.

United Nations General Assembly, 1989. Convention on the rights of the child. UNICEF, Geneva.

Watt, S., Mitchell, R., 1995. Historical perspectives. In: Carter, B., Dearnum, A. (Eds.), Child health care nursing. Concepts, theory and practice. Blackwell Science, Oxford.

West, C., 1854. How to nurse sick children. Brown, Green and Longman, London.

While, A., 1991. An evaluation of a paediatric home care service. Journal of Advanced Nursing 90 (12), 1413–1421.

Whiting, M., 2000. 1888–1988 100 years of community children's nursing. In: Muir, J., Sidey, A. (Eds.), Textbook of community children's nursing. Bailliére Tindall/Royal College of Nursing, London.

Wood, C.J., 1888. The training of nurses for sick children. The Nursing Record December 6, 507–510.

Working with children and families

2

Anna L Hemphill   Annette K Dearmun

ABSTRACT

The primary aim of this chapter and its companion PowerPoint presentation is to introduce ways of assessing the psychosocial needs of children and families and provide some tools that the health professional can draw on when working collaboratively with families. The assessment strategy is underpinned by a family systems approach and by Erikson's (1963) developmental model.

LEARNING OUTCOMES

- Recognise the value of working with the family as a system.
- Appreciate the theoretical concepts underpinning this approach.
- Develop the knowledge base underpinning a psychosocial assessment of the child and family.

Introduction

Since the 1980s there has been a sea change in the nature of children's nursing, from a focus on giving direct, 'hands on' care to working in a partnership with the family, providing support in the family's management of the care of the child and the impact that this has on their lives. There is a growing awareness that this facilitation can be more effective if the needs and resources of the family as a whole are understood (Whyte 1992).

Consideration of the family as the unit of care has been demonstrated for over a decade, in the work of American and Canadian writers (Friedemann 1989, Friedman 1998, Wright & Leahey 1994). More recently, this concept of family nursing entered the British literature through the work of Whyte (1992, 1996, 1997). Although a family-centred approach to the care of the sick child is not new to children's nursing, the family was traditionally seen in relation to its ability to care for the child. In other words, the family was viewed as the context of the child. A family systems approach is a new orientation in that the focus of care is on the needs of the whole family. This demands an understanding of family dynamics in relation to a given situation, and the whole family becomes 'the client' (Friedemann 1989). Consider the needs of the family in the scenario below.

Scenario

Richard, aged 18 months, sustained a head injury in a road traffic accident at the age of 1 year and has been in hospital and ventilated since then. He is to be discharged home. He has two siblings, a newborn baby brother and a 4-year-old sister who is just about to start school. Richard's father has recently started up his own furniture business and his grandmother, who lives locally, has just had a hip replacement.

- What are the stresses on this family?
- What are the strengths and resources?
- What would a health professional need to understand in order to devise a realistic, workable plan of care?

To work with this family in an effective, supportive and empowering way it would be necessary to understand how the family functions on both a practical and an emotional level. This understanding might be gained by spending time with the family and getting to know the individual family members. However, without a clear psychosocial assessment strategy, the family's needs might not be fully explored and important factors that could influence the family's coping might be missed.

Throughout this chapter, a systematic approach to the psychosocial assessment of child and family is advocated. This approach can be used in any setting and is valid for all children and families, including those requiring relatively short-term acute care, for example a child hospitalised for a tonsillectomy, and those requiring longer-term support, for example a child with cystic fibrosis.

DOI: 10.1016/B978-0-7020-3183-0.10002-5

The first part of this chapter explores the principles and beliefs underpinning the family systems approach. This is followed by a discussion of the value of psychosocial assessment. Finally, the elements of assessment are discussed, including relevant theory and practical application.

What is a family?

Activity

- Think about the different types of family.
- Now do the activity on the Evolve website.

It is generally accepted that the family is the basic unit of society. However, many assumptions are made about what constitutes a family. At face value 'the family' might seem to be a very straightforward concept, readily understood but rarely contemplated. However, although families have internalised values and traditions, they do not exist in isolation but are influenced and determined by society and cultural norms. It is important to remember that, as such, they take many diverse forms and are open to many interpretations. In essence, the family is who it identifies itself to be, and therefore a family assessment should start by asking the family 'who is in this family?'.

Understanding the family as a system

Thinking about the family as a system is a helpful way of understanding how families function. Family systems theory underpins the approach to psychosocial assessment taken in this chapter. First postulated by Von Bertalanffy (1968), it provides the theoretical underpinning to family therapy and this in turn has formed the fundamental basis for understanding the family within family nursing (Wright & Leahey 1994). The family is seen as a system of humans in interaction with one another (Jones 1993). It is open, in that interaction occurs with the environment outside it and influences both the family system and the environment. Change in one part of the system, for example a child becoming ill, will influence interactions throughout the system.

Wright & Leahey (1994) have identified five concepts that provide a theoretical foundation for understanding the family as a system. The following explanation draws heavily on their work. Overall, it can be seen that communication and feedback mechanisms are important in the functioning of the family (Whyte 1997):

- **Concept 1: A family system is part of a larger supra-system and is also composed of many subsystems.** The family is part of larger supra-systems, for example its local community. Within the family there will be important subsystems, for example, the parental subsystem and the sibling subsystem. Family systems have emotional boundaries that help to establish what is inside the system and what is outside it.
- **Concept 2: The family as a whole is greater than a sum of its parts.** The family's wholeness is more than just the addition of another member. You can understand an individual better by understanding the way his or her family works.
- **Concept 3: A change in one family member affects all family members.** For example, the illness of a child impacts on all roles and relationships within the family: the mother's role, the father's role, their relationship, the sibling's roles and their relationship to their parents and to the sick sibling.
- **Concept 4: A family is able to create a balance between change and stability.** There is always change within families as individual members develop and change. Families adjust continually to incorporate these changes and maintain some stability. At times, family life can be dominated by change, for example when a family moves to a different country or when a family member dies. At other times stability seems to dominate.
- **Concept 5: Family members' behaviour is best understood from a view of circular rather than linear causality.** This is illustrated in the following scenario.

Scenario

Mary is a 3-year-old girl who has begun to wet the bed again after the birth of her sibling. When she wets the bed her mother gets angry and slaps her.

From the perspective of linear causality, the child wetting the bed causes the mother to slap her: event A causes event B.

However, from the perspective of circular causality, the mother's anger and slap in turn affects the child's bedwetting – the child becomes more anxious and therefore more likely to wet the bed again. Thus the cycle continues: event A affects event B, which in turn affects event A and so on.

From the perspective of circular causality, each person mutually contributes to interactions. This is an empowering rather than blaming perspective in that no one individual is viewed as causing negative situations/problems.

These concepts are further illustrated on the Evolve website, where the family system is influenced by the introduction of an additional family member.

In summary there are there are three important concepts (Whyte 1997):

- change/stability
- circularity
- boundaries.

Undertaking a psychosocial assessment of the family

Assessment is not just about gathering information it is also about establishing a relationship with a family and conveying concern about them as individuals and as a unit. The two core beliefs underpinning the family nursing approach are that:

- the central nursing function is to empower the family
- the family is capable of identifying its own needs and devising ways of meeting them.

The assessment can be a process of discovery for the family as well as for the practitioner. It prompts the family to think and talk about aspects of the family that they might not have discussed together before. Gaining an understanding of the family system will help the practitioner and family to identify ways of managing the family's problems.

The form of assessment discussed here would be helpful to anyone working with children and families. Experience from teaching and practising this form of assessment as part of a multidisciplinary course suggests that it has value for a range of practitioners working in community and acute settings who aim to take a holistic view of the child and family. The approach is strongly influenced by Wright & Leahey's (1994) work on family nursing but also draws on Erikson's (1963) work on psychosocial development. It includes assessment of:

- family structure: using genograms and ecomaps as assessment tools (Wright & Leahey 1994)
- family development: including using an understanding of the family life cycle (Carter & McGoldrick 1989) and individual psychosocial development (Erikson 1963)
- family functioning: including problem solving, values and beliefs, communication, emotional life and alliances and boundaries (Bentovim & Bingley Miller 2001, Whyte 1997).

Each of these aspects will be addressed later in the chapter. Throughout the process, the practitioner works with the family and helps it to identify its problems and mobilise its own coping resources (Whyte 1997).

Guidelines for effective practice

The practitioner shares his or her understanding that the health problem of the child is likely to have an effect on the whole family and that the practitioner is therefore interested in the health of the whole family. When undertaking an assessment it is important to transmit acceptance of the family as it is and to phrase questions in a way that is not discriminatory or value laden.

Reflect on your practice

How do you ask questions when you are undertaking assessment? Look at the following question:

- 'What does your husband do?' (i.e. 'What is your husband's occupation?')

What expectations, judgements and assumptions are conveyed in this question? How could you rephrase the question to remove these?

This question could be conceived to be judgemental on a number of counts. It implies that matrimony and employment of the husband are the only acceptable states. It does not allow for the fact the mother might be unmarried, widowed, divorced or in a same-sex relationship. Perhaps it is important to reflect on the reason for wanting to know about 'the husband'. If the intention is to gain knowledge about possible social support it might be more helpful to ask an open question that has the potential to elicit important information about the other significant family members. For example, 'Does anyone else help you to look after John?'

Assessment of family structure

Genograms and ecomaps

These give information about the internal structure of the family and of its wider context. When assessing family structure the creation of a genogram (family diagram or family tree) is a valuable place to start an assessment for several reasons because it:

- summarises information about a family in a short period of time and in a simple way
- provides a vehicle for gaining insight into family development and functioning
- offers new insights to the family and can be a catalyst for change
- engages children, parents and adolescents in the assessment process.

A genogram broadly follows the conventions of a genetic chart. Usually at least three generations of a family are recorded, each generation occupying a separate horizontal level on the chart (Fig. 2.1).

Activity

Create a genogram for your family:

- Represent males by a square and females by a circle.
- Represent marriage or common-law relationships by a horizontal line joining the partners.
- Denote children by a vertical line dropping down from this horizontal; they should be represented in birth order, eldest to the left.
- Record the name and age of the individual within his or square/circle.

A variety of symbols are used to convey information. Those in common use are shown in Fig. 2.2.

Tips for creating a genogram

The following helpful hints for constructing genograms have been informed by Levac & Leahey (1997):

- Define the extent and nature of the information required because this will determine the number of generations to be included in the genogram. If the concern is to identify support available within the family and/or if the child's health problem is influenced in any way by the grandparents then a three-generational genogram will be useful. When the child/family has minor health needs then a two-generational genogram might suffice. The practitioner should be guided by the family and include those whom the family feels are significant.

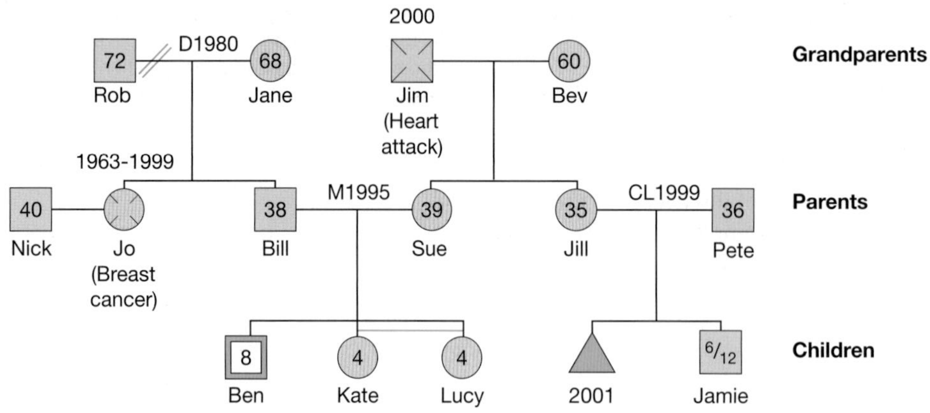

Fig. 2.1 • A genogram of the Taylor family.

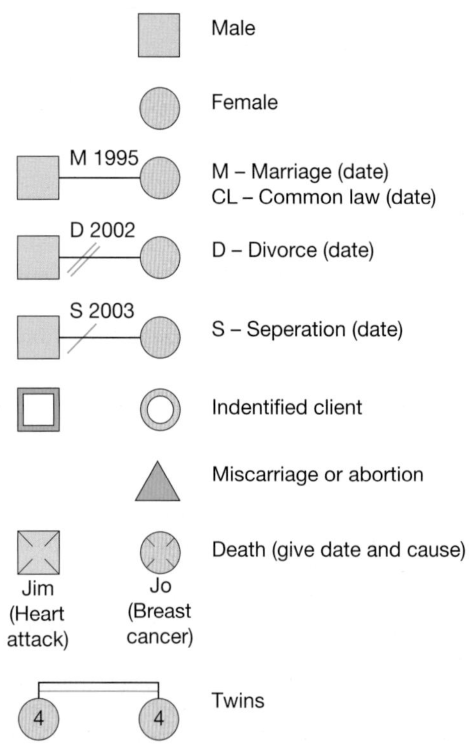

Fig. 2.2 • Common symbols used in genograms.

- Consider ways in which the child and family can be involved in the process. To maximise the value of the genogram as a vehicle to initiate conversation and establish rapport it is important to engage the family in the exercise. This can be achieved via a number of strategies:
  - begin by asking simple and concrete questions, e.g. age, occupation, hobbies, health, school, favourite games
  - when the family appears comfortable, move the discussion to more complex issues, e.g. sibling relationships or parental concerns. If there is a step family it will be relevant to ask questions about custody and contact with the non-custodial parent
  - if appropriate, ask family members how an absent family member might answer the questions
  - overtly value each family member
  - encourage the child's active participation by taking into account his or her developmental age, asking the questions at an appropriate level and interpreting non-verbal as well as verbal responses
  - evaluate the contribution of young people – their inhibitions might prevent them from participating directly and it might be necessary to ask other family members about them.
- Observe the family's non-verbal communication throughout the process and take note of how family members express themselves as well as of the actual content (what is said).

Activity

Consider the ecomap for the Taylor family (Fig. 2.3) together with the information about the family below:

Bill, Sue, Ben, Lucy and Kate are placed in the central circle. Sue gains support from her mother, from her friend and neighbour Nicola, and from her health visitor. She finds her relationship with her sister stressful and demanding. Both Sue and Bill go to church regularly and place a strong value on their life within the church. Bill has strong connections with work. He coaches a boys' football team on Saturday morning. Ben enjoys going along with him to play. Lucy and Kate are twins. They go to nursery where Lucy has settled in well but Kate still finds it stressful and is reluctant to leave Sue.

Ecomaps

Further insight into the family support network can be gained by creating an ecomap. An ecomap depicts the family members' interactions with the wider community. The family genogram is placed in the centre of a circle. Individuals, groups and institutions to whom the family relate are shown around the outside of the circle. Lines are drawn between family members and these outside contacts to show the nature of the relationship. Several lines represent strong connections, single lines represent weaker connections and slashed lines represent stressful relationships. Arrows can be used to illustrate the direction of flow of energy and resources. An ecomap for the Taylor family is shown in Fig. 2.3.

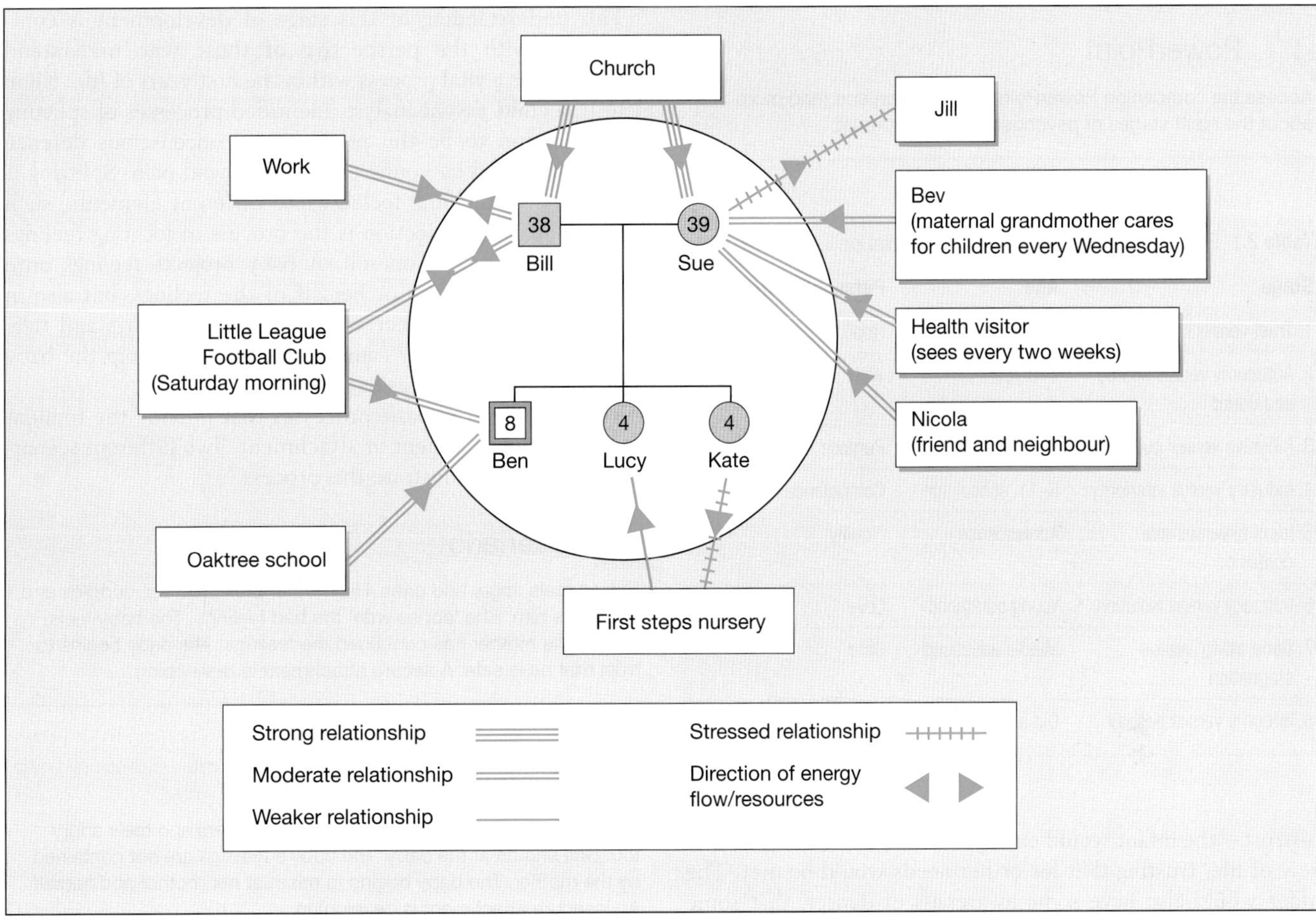

Fig. 2.3 • An ecomap of the Taylor family.

In summary, genograms and ecomaps enable the practitioner to gain awareness of the internal structure of the family and of its wider context. It also provides the opportunity to begin to assess demands on the family, sources of stress and support available to the family.

Assessing child and the family development

Consideration of the psychosocial development of the child and family will give insight into the stresses and challenges faced by individual family members and by the family as a whole. It is important to consider the usual developmental changes that all individuals and families experience over time because these influence and will be influenced by any health problem. In addition, the way in which a child copes with a situation will be influenced by past developmental experiences. Two theories can help with this:

- Erikson's (1963) theory of the psychosocial development of the individual
- family life cycle theory.

Psychosocial development of the individual

Erikson's (1963) theory is still widely accepted and used to aid understanding of children's behaviours and emotions. He presents eight stages of psychosocial development covering the whole life cycle (Table 2.1). The individual is faced with particular developmental tasks at each age-related stage. These tasks are a response to:

- the individual's physical and cognitive maturation
- societal demands
- cultural expectations.

Erikson refers to the individual's experience of working through the task as a crisis. Crisis in this context refers to normal stresses rather than extraordinary life events. The crisis requires the individual to make a fundamental shift in perspective. This experience is characterised both by the individual's increased vulnerability and by his or her heightened potential. The tasks are expressed as a pair of alternative orientations or 'attitudes' towards life, the self and other people. Ideally, the individual achieves a healthy balance between these. For example, in relation to the first stage (0–1 year) – trust versus

PowerPoint

Access the companion PowerPoint presentation and read more about the adult stages of psychosocial development.

Table 2.1 Erikson's eight stages of psychosocial development

Stage	Age	Personality strength
1. Trust versus mistrust	0–1 years	Hope
2. Autonomy versus shame and doubt	1–3 years	Will
3. Initiative versus guilt	3–5: play age	Purpose
4. Industry versus inferiority	6–11: school age	Competence
5. Identity versus role confusion	Adolescence	Fidelity
6. Intimacy versus isolation	Young adulthood	Love
7. Generativity versus stagnation	Middle adulthood	Care
8. Integrity versus despair	Old age	Wisdom

mistrust – the infant would emerge with a generally optimistic view of life, trusting that his or her needs would be met. The infant would also have some awareness of danger, that some people/situations were not to be trusted.

The ages at which individuals experience each developmental stage are likely to vary. Furthermore, the stages are not discrete – they tend to overlap. So, for example, the infant will still be developing a sense of trust at the time when he or she learns to stand up and begins to develop a sense of autonomy. It is also important to acknowledge that each stage is grounded in those that precede it and that issues from previous stages of development can be revisited at any time. The developmental stages of children are discussed in detail below. The stages relating to adulthood are described within the accompanying PowerPoint presentation.

Stages 1 to 5 of Erikson's theory of psychosocial development

1. Trust versus mistrust: age 0–1 year

The foundation of the development of a healthy personality is the establishment of basic trust. Erikson defines this as: 'An essential trustfulness in others as well as a fundamental sense of one's own trustworthiness' (1968 p 96).

The baby's relationship with a mothering figure is central to his or her development of trust. Consistency and dependability are important qualities in the parent. If the baby's physical and psychological needs are sensitively met, i.e. the baby is fed when hungry, reassured when frightened and comforted when in pain, then he or she will learn to trust that needs will be met. This leads to the development of a generally optimistic outlook. Erikson termed this the ego quality of 'hope'.

This understanding of this stage of development is commensurate with the perspective of those who understand attachment as a vital process within the first years of life. Klein (1940), a child psychoanalyst, identified processes of splitting and projection to be the predominant unconscious defence mechanisms used by young children to avoid pain. Splitting is the process of dividing feelings into different elements, such as good and bad. Projection is the process of locating feelings in others rather than oneself. A baby projects feelings onto the mother to rid him- or herself of the feelings, but also in the hope that the mother will contain the feelings and take on board what the baby cannot, and therefore help the baby experience the feelings as bearable.

This is one of the basic processes that provide the foundation for the development of attachment. Two different scenarios can be used to illustrate this process.

Scenario

Robert feels angry and cries. His mother picks him up, cuddles and reassures him. She 'copes with' the bad feelings. The baby feels better. The mother has contained the feelings. The baby begins to trust that he is safe. A secure attachment is developing.

Scenario

Roberta feels angry and cries. The mother hears and feels angry too. She shouts at the baby. The baby's feelings are not contained by the mother. The baby begins to mistrust her mother and herself. An insecure attachment is developing.

It is important, then, that the parent is able to enter the internal world of the baby, to imagine the world from the baby's point of view and use this empathy to respond to the baby's feelings. The baby can then view the world as a safe place. Erikson writes of a favourable ratio between trust and mistrust. It is important that babies have some sense of mistrust if they are to be alert to danger and recognise those who are not trustworthy. If, however, the baby develops an overriding sense of mistrust, of both self and others, the child – and later the adult – might be withdrawn, suspicious and lacking in self-confidence. Related to this, those who have insecure attachments to their primary carers can find it difficult to empathise with the feelings of others and might lack self-esteem.

2. Autonomy versus shame and doubt: age 1–3 years

The neurological and muscular development of the young child facilitates the development of autonomy. Toddlers can walk, explore and 'get into everything'; they are also able to talk, and particularly to say 'no'. At this age they are also able to become continent. A central theme at this stage is 'holding on and letting go'. This does not apply only to bowel control but more globally to the child's struggle for autonomy and self-control. This is reflected in the child's behaviour in many ways. The toddler might cuddle into their mother then aggressively push away from her, they might hoard treasured toys one day then throw them out of the window the next (Erikson 1963). They are primarily trying to exercise a choice (Crain 1988) and to exert their will.

The task is to develop a healthy balance between a sense of autonomy, or self-control, and a sense of shame and doubt, that is, of being 'not good enough'. The child's sense of autonomy comes from within; the sense of shame and doubt comes from the child's social world, through his or her experience of social expectations and regulation. Children need to be able to exert their will while being aware of their capacity for evoking a negative response and of the need to comply with social rules.

Parenting a toddler can be challenging and experienced as a battle of wills (Miller 1993). The aim in relation to Erikson's tasks is to help children learn social behaviour without crushing their will – their desire for free choice (Stevens 1983). Giving children manageable responsibilities, for example, clearing their plate from the table or putting rubbish in the bin, then thanking them respectfully for doing it, will build their confidence in their abilities. Conversely, overcontrolling or critical responses to children's efforts to do things for themselves, or shaming them when they lack self-control (e.g. wet their pants), can lead to feelings that they are not good enough and doubts about their self-control and independence.

3. Initiative versus guilt: age 3–5 years

At this age, children explore what kind of a person they are going to be. They are interested in sex roles, differences and relationships. They consider 'Will I grow up to be a mummy or a daddy?'. They rival the same-sex parent for the love of the other. Girls might transfer affections from their mother to their father, whereas boys compete with their father for their mother's affections. They imitate their parents and want to be like them and do what they do. They are also interested in adult roles and might declare ambitions to be a fireman, nurse or spaceman.

Through play, children learn about taking the initiative, forming and carrying out goals and competing. Their play is imaginative and used to explore roles and act out fantasies. For children to become socialised their drive to take the initiative needs to be tempered by inhibition, so that they learn not to impinge on the rights of others. They develop a conscience (a super ego), so that if they transgress social rules they feel guilty. Again the aim is to achieve a balance. An over-riding sense of guilt can result in over-obedience, conformity and an inability to act out what is desired, so that the individual's emotional self might become hidden. In later years this can result in an inhibited and self-restricted personality (Stevens 1983).

To support children through this stage, Erikson (1963) suggests that parents ease their authority and foster children's desire to 'help' by involving them as equals in interesting projects. Their ambition is then channelled into socially useful activities.

4. Industry versus inferiority: age 6–11 years

The process of learning dominates this stage. This occurs in many settings: school, home, on the street, in clubs and from peers. The child's developing cognitive skills, including operational thinking, memory, problem solving and ability to separate fact from fiction, all facilitate learning and development of social skills.

Children of this age want to engage in tasks and activities and to carry them through to completion. They strive for the sense of competence that their industry can bring them, whether it is by scoring a goal or completing a painting. Their role models are those who know things and how to do things (Erikson 1968), for example, teachers and sports stars. They learn to cooperate with others, to compete and to follow the rules. Children often play within same-sex groups.

Feelings of limitless ability need to be checked by an awareness of one's genuine limitations if optimal development is to occur (Kroger 1996). Children become aware of being judged by their performance. The hurt of failure in class or at play is a common experience and the danger of this stage is that feelings of inadequacy can come to dominate the way children see themselves. These feelings can prevent a child from trying for fear of failure. Unresolved conflicts from previous stages can influence experience so, for example, children who developed more doubt than autonomy in the second stage might be unsure of themselves as they try to master new tasks (Crain 1988).

Erikson (1968) emphasises that parents and teachers play a crucial role in fostering either industry or inferiority. Praise and reward for a job well done will build the child's sense of competence; criticism will undermine it.

5. Identity versus role confusion: adolescence

The central psychosocial task for adolescents is to achieve a unique identity. This involves gaining a clear sense of who they are, what they believe in and the social and occupational roles they wish to pursue (Erikson 1968). Trust, autonomy, initiative and industry all contribute to the young person's identity, which has been forming throughout childhood. Identity formation reaches a crisis in adolescence when young people have to separate from their parents and commit themselves to a set of values, a sexual identity and a vocation (Kroger 1996).

The rapid physical growth and changes of puberty, and the accompanying sexual and aggressive drives, make this a turbulent time when 'trust in the body is shaken' (Wong 1995) and it is hard to know who you are. The following behaviours are typical and normal for young people going through the process of discovering who they are:

- risk-taking behaviour, e.g. smoking, drinking, using drugs, dangerous sports
- healthy assertion and rebellion, e.g. pushing parental boundaries, staying out late
- transferring dependency onto peers and/or a best friend
- trying out new roles, e.g. within religious or political movements
- some rejection of society's norms
- changeable mood, i.e. risking expressing what they feel
- peers alongside parents setting standards
- 'hanging out' with peers
- mobilising energy into action
- deviant self-image they can respect
- privacy and secrecy.

James Marcia (1966) elaborated on Erikson's description of this stage of development through his research on the identity formation process. He identified four identity statuses as described by Miller (1993):

1. **Identity diffusion**. The individual has not yet experienced an identity crisis, nor has he or she made any commitment to a vocation or set of beliefs. There is no indication that he or she is actively trying to make a commitment.
2. **Identity foreclosure**. The individual has not experienced a crisis but nevertheless is committed in his or her goals and beliefs, largely as a result of choices made by others (often parents).
3. **Moratorium**. The individual is in a state of crisis and is actively searching in an attempt to arrive at a choice of identity.
4. **Identity achievement**. The individual has experienced a crisis, has resolved it on his or her own terms and is now firmly committed to an occupation, ideology and social roles.

Those experiencing one of the first three statuses have not formed an independent identity. They are therefore likely to exhibit some of the following features of role confusion:

- intense attachments: typically, difficulty in detaching themselves from parents, particularly the parent of the opposite sex (Marcia 1979)
- dependency on and imitation of parents: common in those with identity foreclosure
- solitary activity: particularly those with identity diffusion
- over-obedience to parents
- unexpressed emotion
- anxiety over puberty
- no idealised future roles
- frustration.

Problems associated with role confusion include anxiety, depression and problems with independence.

As with all the stages of development, individuals will progress through the stages over different periods of time. Some individuals will achieve an identity by late adolescence, others in their early twenties and others might live with role confusion for many years and come to address identity issues later in their adult life.

The value of psychosocial developmental assessment

When trying to understand a child's feelings and psychosocial needs it is helpful to look at both the way the child is now and at his or her developmental history. The following case study illustrates how this aspect of assessment can be useful.

Scenario

Ben is coming into hospital to have a tonsillectomy. Ben is 8 years old and lives with his parents, Sue and Bill, and his younger twin sisters, Lucy and Kate, who are 4 years old (see the genogram of Ben's family in Fig. 2.1). Ben attends primary school, where he enjoys art and playing football, both of which his parents say he is very good at.

Ben's current behaviour

At his preadmission assessment visit, Ben's parents report difficult behaviour that they are struggling to manage, particularly aggression. Ben has anger outbursts during which he might kick furniture or throw things. He doesn't listen, especially when disciplining is involved. He is very active and always on the go or fiddling. At home he rarely sits still for long, except when he's playing his computer games, which he can do for an hour or more. Homework is a difficult time and it is hard to get Ben to do it. His parents have found that sitting next to him and encouraging him from start to finish works. Ben finds it difficult to wait for anything and wants it immediately. He does have friends but finds it difficult to share and compromise.

Developmental history

Ben was born of a planned pregnancy. Sue describes him as being a wriggly, noisy baby who cried a lot. She found him hard to soothe. She breastfed him for 3 months before bottle feeding him. She thinks she had postnatal depression (PND) that was not identified. She found the first 2 years very difficult and felt anxious at times about going out with Ben on her own and embarrassed at not being able to control Ben in front of others. Ben achieved his developmental milestones satisfactorily and attended nursery when he was two and a half.

Review of Ben's development in relation to Erikson's psychosocial stages of development

This assessment can be used to consider Ben's development in relation to the psychosocial tasks.

- *Trust versus mistrust*: from this initial assessment we know that Sue had PND and found her relationship with Ben difficult when he was a baby. Research suggests that mothers with PND find it more difficult to contain their baby's feelings (Goldberg 2000). It is therefore possible that Ben's development of a sense of trust might have been negatively affected. This could have contributed to his anxiety regarding getting his needs met immediately and might have left him lacking self-confidence/esteem.
- *Autonomy versus shame and doubt*: at this stage Sue reports feeling anxious about managing Ben's behaviour, particularly in public. Her doubts in relation to parenting Ben at this stage might have led to rather unclear boundaries. This could explain why Ben does not seem to have achieved a strong sense of self-control. His difficulty in complying with social rules suggests he has doubts about his ability to control himself and the world around him.
- *Initiative versus guilt*: Ben would have been at this stage when his twin sisters were born. His parents have not specifically mentioned Ben's experience of this stage but a nurse might be curious about how he reacted to the changes the birth of his sisters had on the family.
- *Industry versus inferiority*: strengths relating to this current stage include Ben's enjoyment of art and football and the related positive feedback he gets from parents and peers. He seems to have some difficulty starting and sticking at tasks he perceives as challenging, e.g. homework. This might be because his doubts about his ability (stemming from the earlier stage, autonomy versus shame and doubt) have made it difficult for him to risk trying for fear of failure.

Psychosocial development of the family

When undertaking an assessment and supporting a family, consideration of the family's experience of changes as it has developed over time will enhance understanding of its strengths and current sources of stress.

Activity

Implications for Ben's care when in hospital

Think about the psychosocial needs revealed within the above scenario. When Ben comes into hospital for his tonsillectomy, what particular interventions might you use to support Ben and his family?

- Can you think of other interventions that might support Ben?

From this assessment, several interventions can be drawn out which may be supportive to Ben, when caring for him.

Provide boundaries by being clear regarding what you expect Ben to do and by being consistent in your approach.

Aim: to build trust

Give Ben praise and positive attention, particularly when he is faced with new situations or tasks, for example, when having anaesthetic cream applied or when needing to eat and drink postoperatively.

Aim: to build self-esteem

Keep Ben amused with activities he enjoys, such as art.

Aim: to encourage socially acceptable self-expression and build self-esteem

Use behaviour management techniques that encourage Ben to take control such as choices and consequences. For example, 'If you have your bath quickly now there will be time for me to play a game with you before bedtime; if you choose not to have your bath yet there won't be time for a game. Which would you rather do?'

Aim: to build Ben's sense of self-control and autonomy

Encourage Ben to show his sisters around the ward when they visit.

Aim: to strengthen his relationship with his sisters and to build his self-esteem

Encourage Ben to phone, e-mail or write to his friends.

Aim: to strengthen peer relationships

It would be helpful to discuss the potential of these interventions with Ben's parents, to check whether they feel they are appropriate given their knowledge of Ben.

Every family will follow its own unique developmental path, although all families experience changes over time as people enter and leave the family system. Typically, these include events such as birth, raising children, children leaving home, retirement and death.

Family life cycle theory

Family life cycle theory is grounded in the work of Erikson (see above). The family life cycle is a dynamic process of change that includes all the events, and periods of time between events, experienced by a family. Duvall (1977) described this family life cycle using an eight-stage model. Carter & McGoldrick (1989) built on this work to consider three generations of a family system as it moved through time. They recognised that family stress is often greatest at the times of change that mark the transition from one stage to the next within the family, because these are the times when the greatest emotional demands are made on the family.

PowerPoint

Access the companion PowerPoint presentation and look at Table 1, the stages of the family life cycle.

This life cycle model describes an intact American middle-class family. Carter & McGoldrick (1989) recognise that many trends within contemporary Western society affect change in family life cycle patterns. There is a decreasing birth rate, many couples are choosing to have their children when they are older, and life expectancy is increasing. Women's roles have changed, particularly in relation to work, and dual-income households are becoming the norm in many countries. Cohabitation outside marriage, single-parent households, divorce and remarriage are all increasing. Carter & McGoldrick have considered the particular emotional challenges presented by divorce and remarriage. These are discussed within the PowerPoint presentation. Other factors that affect the life cycle include the culture of the family and the economic, political and social context in which they live.

PowerPoint

Access the companion PowerPoint presentation and read about the emotional challenges presented by divorce and remarriage.

Carter & McGoldrick's six-stage model can be criticised for being normative or over-generalised. Nevertheless, it is helpful to have a model to identify the emotional tasks that need to be undertaken. The practitioner can then consider how the unique developmental path of the individual family might have influenced the emotional tasks it faces. When considering the challenges facing a particular family it is helpful to bear in mind that the family's experience might be considerably more complex than the model suggests. For example, the family could include adolescent children from a previous marriage and a young child from the current cohabiting partnership. The practitioner would then have to consider tasks from the two life cycle stages (families with young children and families with adolescents) and the developmental issues for the reconstituted family.

PowerPoint

Access the companion PowerPoint presentation and look at Table 3.

Carter & McGoldrick's six stages in a family life cycle

Stage 1: Leaving home, single young adults

The task for young adults is to separate from their family of origin and establish an independent identity 'without cutting off or attaching reactively to an emotional surrogate' (Friedman 1998). Friedman explains that men and women typically face different challenges at this stage due to the way they are socialised. Both need to achieve a balance between autonomy and attachment in relationships and at work. Men have generally been encouraged to seek their identity through self-expression and therefore are more likely to struggle with attachment and commitment. Women have generally been encouraged to define themselves in terms of their relationships with others, their struggle is therefore more likely to relate to issues of autonomy.

Stage 2: Joining of families, the new couple

The new couple marks the beginning of a new family; it also represents the joining of two families. The partners bring beliefs from their experience of growing up in their own family. The task of the new couple is therefore to decide which beliefs, traditions and rules it is going to adopt from their families of origin, and which it is going to develop for itself. The members of the couple need to develop a new relationship with each set of parents, which is supportive yet protects the autonomy of their partnership. They will also need to make decisions regarding if and when to have children.

Stage 3: Families with young children

This is generally recognised to be the most stressful life transition (Friedman 1998). The parents have to adjust their relationship to make space for the child(ren). There are the extra demands of meeting the child's needs while continuing to meet one another's personal needs. Childrearing, financial and household tasks can all be sources of stress. This stage often coincides with parent's heavy involvement in career development and with financial resources being stretched. Juggling work and childcare is likely to present financial and emotional challenges.

Stage 4: Families with adolescents

The central developmental task of this stage is to balance freedom with responsibility as teenagers mature and become increasingly autonomous. This requires renegotiation of boundaries and demands that parents begin to 'let go' of the adolescent while still providing for his or her dependency needs. For the parents, reduction in the dependency of their child(ren) and the adolescent's questioning of values and life style can refocus their attention on their marriage and career issues, and this phase is usually a time of exploration and refocusing. The ageing of grandparents can bring a change from receiving support from them to needing to support them.

Stage 5: Launching children and moving on

This phase can be a lengthy one, with many exits from and entries into the family. Increasingly, young adults are choosing to live at home with their parents, often for economic reasons. Consequently, the anticipated empty nest can be delayed by several years. There is a need to review and restructure the marital relationship once day-to-day parenting responsibilities cease. Parents and children need to renegotiate their roles so that they relate to one another as adults rather than parent and child. Parents might also need to adjust to include their child's partner and possibly grandchildren within the family. The responsibility for caring for the older generation can make considerable demands on the couple, both practically and emotionally, and might include coping with the death of parents.

Stage 6: Families in later life

This stage begins with the retirement and lasts until both spouses have died. It can span 20 to 30 years and the central process during this time is to accept the shift of generational roles. Tasks during this stage include adapting to new social roles, such as being grandparents, supporting the older generation and coping with loss. Stressors or losses commonly experienced by ageing people and families include economic, housing, social, work and health losses (Friedman 1998).

In summary, a sound knowledge of family development can help a practitioner to think about and assess the stresses experienced by the family. In many cases it helps to look beyond the immediately obvious stresses associated with the family's current circumstances, for example anxiety over the child illness, and to consider other issues that are concerning the family and which need to be acknowledged when helping the family find realistic ways of managing its situation.

Assessing family functioning

The seminal work of Epstein et al (1978) – the McMaster model of family functioning – underpins the assessment of family functioning as described by family nursing writers such as Friedman (1998), Whyte (1997) and Wright & Leahey (1994). The following suggestions for assessing family functioning draw on the work of these writers, and also on Bentovim & Bingley Miller's (2001) work on family assessment. This later work is particularly useful because the writers take the family's ability to meet the needs of children as a central focus within their approach.

The aim of functional assessment is to observe how family members interact and influence each other. In this way, individual family members' behaviour can be understood within the context of the family. It is important to assess the family's strengths as well as its difficulties. Recognition of strengths by the practitioner and, most importantly, by the family members themselves, is helpful because these strengths can be a major resource when working to resolve problems.

Aspects to assess

Problem solving

One of the practitioner's goals is to support the family in solving its problems. It is therefore beneficial to have some insight into the family's problem-solving style and its ability to solve its own problems. A discussion of the way in which the family has managed past problems can give the practitioner and family insight into this. It is helpful to consider both practical and emotional problems:

- **Practical problem solving**: relating to how practical tasks are achieved within the family. For example, if parents both work then ascertaining what they did when their child had chickenpox and had to be off school would give the nurse insight into who takes responsibility for solving problems and also whether the family relies on those within the family (extended family) at times of need or seeks help outside the family.
- **Emotional problem solving**: sometimes problem solving is on an emotional level, an example of this is coping with jealousy between siblings.

Activity

Alice is Jim's younger sister, she is 1 year old and, since her birth, Jim had displayed outward signs of aggression and jealousy.

- Think about questions you could ask to find out how the parents coped with this

The parents' explanation will give insight into how the problem is understood and whether they agree about solutions to emotional problems within the family. It might also give insight into how the parents control their children's behaviour.

Beliefs and values

A family belief system is the family's way of knowing and understanding the world. It is made up of all the shared assumptions, values, myths and traditions that guide the family's behaviour.

Reflect on your practice

Think about your own family:

- Note down any family myths, values and traditions. You might like to think particularly about beliefs in relation to health, education or children.
- How were these beliefs expressed?

For example, in relation to health one family might believe that the best way to manage illnesses is to allow the body to heal itself supported by homeopathic remedies, and thus family members will rarely go to their GP. Another family might believe that it is always safest to get professional advice and will visit the GP regularly, often with minor illnesses.

Beliefs are handed down through families from one generation to the next, and can be a very powerful influence on the way a family copes with stresses. Carter & McGoldrick (1989) conceptualise the flow anxiety in a family as being vertical and horizontal. Vertical, or transgenerational, stresses are the beliefs and patterns of functioning that flow through the generations. These interact with the horizontal stresses experienced by the family in the 'here and now' as a result of both predictable life cycle stresses, such as the birth of a baby, and unpredictable events, such as the baby having a congenital facial disfigurement. In this situation, if, for example, physical beauty is highly prized and a source of power within the family through the generations, then the baby's appearance will create more intensive stress than would have been the case if less importance was attached to physical attractiveness.

Family communication

Communication affects all aspects of family life. The way a family communicates influences the self-esteem of family members and the children's development, particularly in relation to verbal and reading skills. Special care must be taken when working with families with a different first language to your own. It is important to appreciate the cultural expectations regarding communication within the family.

Effective communication requires messages to be clearly expressed and to be received and responded to. In families with communication strengths as identified by Bentovim & Bingley Miller (2001):

- People can express themselves clearly, directly and openly.
- Verbal messages will be matched by non-verbal communication (facial expression, body language) and by tone of voice.
- Family members listen and respond to what others say.
- All family members participate in conversations.
- The family can talk something over and move it on.

Families in which there are communication difficulties might exhibit some of the following problems as identified by Bentovim & Bingley Miller (2001):

- Communications are unclear or inhibited, e.g. whispered or poorly articulated.
- There is a mismatch between what is said and the tone of voice and/or non-verbal messages that accompany it. For example, 'I'm fine' might be said in an angry tone and accompanied by a glare and the slamming of a door as the person exits the room. This type of communication is ambiguous and confusing.
- People do not listen to or acknowledge what others communicate, or respond in inappropriate ways.
- In conversations, one or more family members dominate and others find it difficult to participate or are excluded.
- When the family tries to talk something over it tends to get stuck or it might return to the same topic repeatedly.

Most families will exhibit some strengths and some occasional difficulties. In families in which difficulties dominate it will be difficult for the family members to resolve problems together.

The emotional life of the family

This is not easy to assess but it is important because it colours the whole way that life is experienced within the family. It is useful to consider how feelings are expressed within the family and also, less tangibly, how it might feel to be in the family.

In families in which emotional expression is a strength, a wide range of feelings will be expressed, the intensity of feelings will be appropriate to the situation referred to, and family members recognise each others' feelings and respond to them appropriately. In families in which emotional expression presents difficulties, expression of feelings might be generally discouraged, or certain feelings might not be expressed, for example, anger. The intensity of feelings expressed might not seem to match the situation, being either heightened and possibly overwhelming, or diminished and flat. Feelings expressed by others will not always be responded to helpfully. Physical or psychological symptoms can be a way of expressing feelings in families who have difficulties communicating.

When considering how it might feel to be in the family it is helpful to think about the overall feel of the family and the way family members treat one another. The family atmosphere might be generally warm, safe and reasonably relaxed, allowing family members to express themselves freely. Families with some difficulties are more likely to have a tense atmosphere.

Where painful or negative emotions dominate, the family atmosphere might feel chaotic, dangerous or panicky. The way that family members treat one another might be mostly supportive and understanding of one another. In families with difficulties in the way they treat one another, family members will not feel valued or expect support from one another and attacking, undermining or rejecting relationships might be observed.

Alliances and boundaries

Within the family system are subsystems that consist of a relationship or alliance between two or more people. These can be thought of as teams with particular functions (Bentovim & Bingley Miller 2001). It is useful to identify the important subsystems within the family and to consider how well they work, their strengths and difficulties, to identify any relationships that might require particular support:

- The couple subsystem: in a family with two adults, the quality of their relationship and the way in which the couple meet one another's emotional and sexual needs will influence all other relationships in the family. In families with difficulties there might be lack of support or warmth within the couple relationship and dissatisfaction with it might be expressed as hostility or open conflict.
- The parental subsystem: the task of the parents is to nurture and socialise their children. How well they do this will depend on how well they work as a team. Parents with reasonable strengths will cooperate and support one another, sharing parenting tasks. Difficulties occur when parents disagree about how to deal with the children, undermine one another or are unable to negotiate and compromise.
- The sibling subsystem: children's psychosocial development is influenced by their relationship with their siblings. If relationships are affectionate and supportive they can be a source of strength. It is normal for siblings to quarrel and compete for parental attention but difficulties arise if there is continual fighting and rivalry or if children ignore one another.

The boundaries between the different subsystems can be useful to consider. Clear yet permeable boundaries allow flexibility while maintaining the distinct functions of the subsystems (Minuchin 1974). So, for example, in a family with clear intergenerational boundaries, the parents act as parents and the children act as children most of the time. In a family where this boundary is diffuse the child might be given adult responsibilities and power in decision making (Wright & Leahey 1994), or might even take on a parental role in relation to a child-like parent.

The balance between being able to be an independent individual and having a secure sense of belonging is also important. Family members might become overdependent on one another. This enmeshment can make it difficult for young people to act independently or to separate from some members of the family. Alternatively, when boundaries are rigid, individuals might become isolated and disengaged from the family.

In summary, the interaction of family members and the influence they have on each other and the family as a whole are key components of assessment. Family functioning is not something that can be assessed in one sitting. Assessment involves judgement and it is important that this is based on what has been learned from the family. Furthermore, it needs to be specifically described using evidence gained from talking with and observing the family.

Summary

Drawing on the evidence base, this chapter has argued the value of working with the family as a system and has offered some suggestions of how this could be implemented in practice. When conducting a psychosocial assessment of a child and his or her family, a systematic approach that considers the child's development within the context of the family, and the family structure, development and functioning will give a broad understanding of family strengths and problems. Some practitioners might have the confidence and competence to undertake a more detailed assessment of specific areas of family functioning. The framework presented within this chapter is designed to provide a tool to think with rather than to be prescriptive. Assessment should be a continuous process, rather than a single event and, although the initial gathering of information about the family is important, reflection and analysis of that information is essential to understand family strengths and difficulties. This, in turn, will determine the level of support required to maintain or restore equilibrium within the family.

References

Bentovim, A., Bingley Miller, L., 2001. The family assessment: assessment of family competence, strengths and difficulties. Pavilion Publishing, Brighton.

Carter, B., McGoldrick, M., 1989. The changing family lifecycle, 2nd edn. Allyn & Bacon, London.

Crain, W.C., 1988. Erikson and the eight stages of life. In: Crain, W.C. (Ed.), Theories of development: concepts and applications. Prentice Hall, London.

Duvall, E., 1977. Marriage and family development. Lippincott, Philadelphia.

Epstein, N.B., Bishop, D.S., Levin, S., 1978. The McMaster model of family functioning. Journal of Marriage and Family Counselling 4, 19–31.

Erikson, E.H., 1963. Childhood and society, 2nd edn. Norton, New York.

Erikson, E.H., 1968. Identity: youth and crisis. Norton, New York.

Friedemann, M.L., 1989. The concept of family nursing. Journal of Advanced Nursing 14, 211–216.

Friedman, M.M., 1998. Family nursing: theory and practice, 4th edn. Appleton & Lange, Norwalk, CT.

Goldberg, S., 2000. Attachment and development. Arnold, London.

Jones, E., 1993. Family systems therapy. John Wiley, Chichester.

Klein, M., 1940/1975. Mourning and its relation to manic-depressive states. In: Klein, M. (Ed.), The writings of Melanie Klein, Vol. 1. Hogarth, London.

Kroger, J., 1996. Adolescence as identity synthesis: Erikson's psychosocial approach. In: Kroger, J. (Ed.), Identity in adolescence: overview of major theorists, 2nd revised edn. Routledge, London.

Levac, A.M., Leahey, M., 1997. Children and families: models for assessment and intervention. In: Fox, J. (Ed.), Primary healthcare of children, Mosby, Baltimore, MD.

Marcia, J.E., 1966. Development and validation of ego identity status. Journal of Personality and Social Psychology 3, 551–558.

Marcia, J.E., 1979. Identity status in late adolescence: description and some clinical implications. Identity Development Symposium, Gronigen, the Netherlands, .

Miller, P.H., 1993. Theories of developmental psychology, 3rd edn. WH Freeman, New York.

Minuchin, S., 1974. Families and family therapy. Tavistock, London.

Stevens, R., 1983. The life cycle. In: Stevens, R. (Ed.), Erik Erikson: an introduction. Open University Press, Buckingham.

Von Bertalanffy, L., 1968. General system theory: foundations, development, applications. Brazillier, New York.

Whyte, D., 1992. A family nursing approach to the care of a child with a chronic illness. Journal of Advanced Nursing 17, 317–327.

Whyte, D., 1996. Expanding the boundaries of care. Paediatric Nursing 8 (4), 10–23.

Whyte, D., 1997. Explorations in family nursing. Routledge, London.

Wong, D.L., 1995. Growth and development of children. In: Campbell, S., Glasper, E.A. (Eds.), Whaley and Wong's nursing care of infants and children, 5th edn. CV Mosby, St Louis.

Wright, L.M., Leahey, M., 1994. Nurses and families: a guide to family assessment and intervention, 2nd edn. FA Davis, Philadelphia.

Further Reading

Allmond, B.W., Buckman, W., Gofman, H.F., 1979. The family is the patient. CV Mosby, St Louis.

Cramp, C., Tripp, S., Hughes, N., Dale, J., 2003. Children's home nursing: results of a national survey. Paediatric Nursing 15 (8), 39–43.

Department of Health (DoH), 1991. Welfare of children and young people in hospital. HMSO, London.

Department of Health (DoH), 2003. Getting the right start: National Service Framework for Children and Young People and Maternity Services, Part 1: Standard for Hospital Services. HMSO, London.

Thornes, R., 1993. Bridging the gaps. Action for Sick Children, London.

Contemporary child health policy: the implications for children's nurses

3

E Alan Glasper Susan Lowson

ABSTRACT

The primary aim of this chapter and its companion PowerPoint presentation is to investigate the relationship between child health policy and changes in the pattern of care delivery by children's nurses in the UK since 1959. Although it is not possible to cover all reports or indeed contemporary policy from other countries, a comprehensive range of published reports that demonstrate the complexities of child health policies is reviewed and the success or otherwise of government reforms is discussed. The role of the Health Service Ombudsman is outlined.

LEARNING OUTCOMES

- Recognise the impact of child health policy on changes in care delivery for children and their families.
- Appreciate the role of children's nurses in the translation of policy into practice.
- Recognise the barriers to policy recommendations in contemporary healthcare settings.
- Understand that policies can be a powerful weapon for family advocacy.
- Appreciate the role of the complaint process in the clinical governance agenda.
- Recognise the learning opportunities that arise from complaints.
- Understand the role of the nurse in complaint investigations.
- Recognise the effect of the bereavement process in complaint management.

Introduction

The publication of the now famous government white paper 'Welfare of children in hospital' (Committee of the Central Health Services Council 1959) was a wake-up call for those healthcare workers involved in the care of sick children in hospital. The knowledge and confirmation that children could be harmed by early psychological traumas provided the necessary stimulus for a growing interest in the adverse events of childhood. The work of John Bowlby and James Robertson (Bowlby 1951, Robertson 1962) had been highly influential in bringing to the public domain the negative effects on development that could occur following a child's stay in hospital. Many of the subsequent policy recommendations reiterated the central tenet of the 1959 welfare document now universally known as the Platt report after its chairman Sir Harry Platt. It would be naïve to suggest that all policy documents published since then have taken a proactive stance, as many have been reactive to events or practices that actually harmed children and their families during the process of care. Current practice is therefore the prime beneficiary of the cumulative successes or otherwise of the implementation of the various policies and reports published since 1959. To suggest that health care for sick children is at an optimum level would be imprudent, and this is exemplified through the necessity for periodic public enquiries when and where poor practice flourishes. Child health policy reviews will therefore continue to play an important part in the evolution of optimum child health care.

The role of health policy

The role of health policy is primarily concerned with maintaining or improving the health of individuals or groups within society. Increasingly, such policies are generated at local, national and international forums for the benefit of all. Despite this, it must be acknowledged that there are gross inequalities in health status among childhood populations both within and outside the UK.

Scenario

Louise is a second-year child branch student who, at a meeting of her weekly learning group, reveals that a number of children have been admitted to her ward suffering from chest infections. These sick children are predominately from lower socioeconomic groups.

DOI: 10.1016/B978-0-7020-3183-0.10003-7

Health inequalities

A report published in 1955 by a joint committee of The Institute of Child Health, The Society of Medical Officers of Health and The Population Investigation Committee (University of London 1955) acknowledged that children from disadvantaged, lower socioeconomic, manual labouring families had a higher admission rate to hospital with infections. Overcrowding was cited as a causative agent and was additionally linked to the high level of readmissions in the same group of children. Of historical interest is the reporting of 10% of all admissions being cared for in adult wards and 33% being admitted to wards that allowed no visitors. The final summary point in this report states: 'It is too soon to attempt an assessment of the effects of hospitalisation' (University of London 1955 p 3).

Nearly half a century later, Utting (1997) revealed that approximately 15,300 children spent periods of more than a month per year as hospital inpatients. He particularly highlighted the vulnerability of certain categories of children, such as those with disabilities and emotional or behavioural difficulties. Carter (2002), in stating that children's nurses cannot be complacent about the negative effects of healthcare inequality on children, perhaps reinforces the reality that children's nurses can never be mere bystanders in the determination of health and social policy. To this end, children's nurses are helping in the process of setting and implementing policy, and are not simply following it. Utting's report was commissioned after continuing revelations of wide spread abuse of children living away from home, but especially those living in children's homes. The thrust of Utting's report for the NHS was to establish methods of monitoring and safeguarding the welfare of children in hospitals and other NHS settings.

How do governments respond to policy reviews?

The way in which, for example, the NHS responds to such reports is illuminating and the Utting report (Utting 1997) can serve here as a case in point of how the process works in practice (NHS Executive 1998). The report, under the chairmanship of Sir William Utting, made over 150 recommendations. In response to the report, the government created a ministerial taskforce to advise it on how to respond appropriately to these recommendations. The ministerial taskforce duly reported to the government, which in turn translated some of the key findings into an action plan. This in turn was developed into a Health Service Circular, which was sent for action to, among others all the chief executives of the NHS Trusts in England. (It is important to stress here that Scotland and Wales commission their own policy documents, whereas the Northern Ireland Assembly has thus far primarily followed the English precedent. As a general rule of thumb, UK child health policies are transferable across the four countries of the UK.) The changes, which primarily related to who might or might not work with children, had to be implemented by 1 April 1999. As with other similar reports, the wording used by the NHS Executive was 'Ministers expect' and in this example Regional Offices of the NHS required written confirmation by 31 March 1999 that action had been taken to comply with this circular.

Other reports do not carry the weight of a Health Service Circular and it is for this reason that the reports outlined in this chapter have had mixed success in changing policies towards children requiring health care. For example, the famous Black Report (Department of Health and Social Security (DHSS) 1980) – commissioned by Labour Secretary of State, David Ennals – was predicated on the inability of the NHS to alleviate ill health among the poorest and disadvantaged sectors of society: the reality is that the greatest improvements in health since the foundation of the NHS have been among the upper socioeconomic groups. The working party, under the chairmanship of Sir Douglas Black, an eminent and respected physician, uncovered significant weaknesses in the way that health services were delivered. Black's account recommended sweeping changes, particularly in the child health domain. Among other measures, he advocated increases in child benefit, infant care allowances and free school meals. However, the incoming Conservative government, led by Margaret Thatcher, was not persuaded by the findings and it was to be a further 20 years before the report was taken seriously (Ham 1999).

Black remained a strong supporter of the NHS until his death in 2002 (Tucker 2002) and, eventually, the gauntlet he threw down was picked up by Sir Donald Acheson, the former Chief Medical Officer, whose report – published in 1998 (Department of Health (DoH) 1998) – confirmed that health inequalities still existed. For example in the case of breast feeding, widely acknowledged to be the healthiest option for infants, Acheson revealed a striking difference between those mothers in the upper socioeconomic groups and those in the lower.

UK policy variations

The individual countries within the UK can commission a report after specific problems arise within the child health arena. The Carlile review (National Assembly for Wales 2002) is cited here as an example of how an individual country responds to a crisis within its own children's services.

WWW

The full transcript of the Carlile review can be accessed on the National Assembly for Wales internet site:

- http://www.wales.gov.uk

Seminar discussion topic

Analyse a local, national or international child health policy. In your learning group, discuss if the recommendations are met in your workplace. Are there variations in the way policy recommendations have been implemented?

WWW

Read the Acheson report online:

- http://www.official.documents.co.uk/documents/doh/ ih/ih/htm

The Carlile review (2002)

Welsh Assembly Minister for Health, Jane Hutt, commissioned the Carlile review after allegations of child sexual abuse within NHS child and adolescent inpatient facilities in Wales. Hutt's mandate to appointed chairman Lord Alex Carlile of Berriew was to make recommendations so that proper safeguards could be put in place whenever and wherever a child had contact with the NHS in Wales. Lord Carlile made 150 recommendations based on his enquiry. His emphasis on child health nurses is interesting. For example, recommendation 93:

> We recommend that urgent measures be pursued to increase college places for registered children's nurses including the encouragement of mature nurses to develop their skills and opportunities through training
>
> (National Assembly for Wales 2002 p 141)

Carlile places much emphasis on education and training, believing that all staff who come into contact with children should be taught to recognise the signs of sexual, physical and emotional abuse.

Activity

Access the Carlile review from the PowerPoint presentation.

- How does it apply to you? If you live in Wales, have the recommendations been implemented? What messages does this report have for other countries?

The welfare of children in hospital (1959)

'The welfare of children in hospital', published in 1959 (Committee of the Central Health Services Council 1959), was the first of many reports specifically aimed at alleviating the psychological traumas perpetrated on children during a hospital stay. The main background to the commissioning of the report, chaired by Sir Harry Platt (a famous orthopaedic surgeon), was the growing public concern over the way children were cared for in hospital. The numbers of academic papers suggesting that a stay in hospital could be detrimental to a child's psychological development forced the pace of change and formed a platform upon which the subsequent report would be based. The report was commissioned on 12 June 1956 and the final report was sent to Lord Cohen of Birkenhead, Chair of the Central Health Services Council, on 28 October 1958. The reason given for the delay in reporting was the sheer enormity of the task facing Platt's committee, which included one children's nurse, Miss MW Janes SRN, SCM, RSCN. The primary term of reference given to the committee by the Central Health Services Council was:

> To make a special study of the arrangements made in hospitals for the welfare of ill children – as distinct from their medical and nursing treatment – and to make suggestions which could be passed on to hospital authorities.

Over the two and a half years of the study, the Committee met 20 times to collate the written and verbal evidence. The antecedents of the report have already been covered but suffice to say that the work of Bowlby and Robertson was crucial. Of considerable interest is the revelation within the report that the Central Health Services Council had issued no fewer than three memoranda to hospital authorities to allow daily visiting for children. The failure of some hospitals to implement this recommendation is as pertinent today as it was then and reflects the status and perceived importance of 'topdown' government reports.

PowerPoint

Access the companion PowerPoint presentation and read the full text of the Platt report.

The Platt report had profound and lasting effects on the welfare of children in hospital not only in the UK but also much further afield in countries such as Australia, New Zealand, Canada and The USA. The report made 55 recommendations, the majority of which can be summed up by one (recommendation 52):

> Nurses (and all members of the child health care team) need training not only in the special aspects of disease in children but in the factors that influence the development of the normal child. Part of this training should take the form of practical experience in the care of well children both in nursery schools, etc. and in their homes. The emotional needs of children in hospital should be stressed in refresher courses for ward sisters.

The last point was perhaps an acknowledgement that ward sisters were the gatekeepers who could facilitate or inhibit change. It is therefore ironic that in recommendation 10 Platt sows the seed of the demise of the RSCN direct-entry qualification when he states 'The Sister in charge of the ward should be RSCN as well as SRN'. Platt was not to know that the direct-entry single RSCN qualification was to disappear from England by the early 1960s, leading to shortages in the number of nurses holding a sick children's nursing qualification. If one could travel back in time to have a 1-to-1 with Sir Harry Platt, one could point out to him that the care a sick child receives is only as good as the nurse who delivers it.

Activity

Conduct a SWOT analysis of the Platt report and debate the strengths, weaknesses, opportunities and threats that it posed to healthcare practitioners in the 1960s.

Scenario

Louise is gaining experience in a children's medical unit where some of the nurses do not possess a children's nursing qualification.

PROFESSIONAL CONVERSATION 1

Harriet is a registered children's nurse on Part 15 of the Nursing and Midwifery Council's Professional Register.

Issues affecting skill mix on the children's medical unit

I have been qualified for 4 years and I am really pleased that I decided to undertake a direct-entry children's nursing course. Some of my colleagues who trained some years ago have told me that this option was never open to them and that they had to undertake general nursing first. A few of these colleagues were actually seconded from the children's medical unit to undertake a post-registration children's nursing course. They said that more post-registration child branch places were made available by the workforce confederations in response to policy documents that stated that children should be cared for by people with specific training in the care of sick children. During coffee recently, one of the adult-branch-registered nurses who works on my unit confided to me that she felt uncomfortable working with some of the sicker children because she did not feel that she had the right skills to do so.

- What do child health policy document recommendations have to say about skill mix?

Fit for the future (1976)

'Fit for the future' (Committee on Child Health Services 1976) became known as the Court report, after the chairman of the committee, Professor Donald Court. Among the committee members was Miss Barchard, the Chief Nursing Officer of The Hospital for Sick Children, London. A health visitor was also part of the committee: Miss Bickerton, who subsequently became Professor of Public Health Nursing at The University of Western Sydney in Australia. By the time this report was commissioned (in 1973) more attention than before was being focused on children. Donald Court introduces 'Fit for the future' with a quotation from the novelist Katherine Mansfield:

> By health I mean the power to live a full, adult, living breathing life in close contact with what I love – I want to be all that I am capable of becoming.

This emphasis on letting children grow to their full potential reflected the growing recognition of the harmful effects that a period of ill health could have on a child's development. Although Court reiterates much of the earlier Platt report, as indeed do subsequent policy documents, the emphasis here is on preventing illness among children. Highlighted again is the stark reality that children born into lower socioeconomic groups were dying unnecessarily from preventable 19th century reasons. In the section of the report on nurses, Court gives the number of RSCNs registered with the General Nursing Council as of March 1975 as 20,514. He uses this as evidence of the continuing shortage of children's nurses, adapting a line first used by Catherine Jane Wood, an early matron of London's Hospital For Sick Children: 'sick children should be nursed by nurses who have been trained to do so'.

Activity

Compare the numbers of children's nurses on the register of the Nursing and Midwifery Council (NMC) today. What inferences can you make?

Despite its size, the Court report gives a simple and clear set of recommendations, which can be summarised as:

> We want to see a child- and family-centred service, in which skilled help is readily available and accessible, which is integrated in as much as it sees the child as a whole, and as a continuous developing person. We want to see a service that ensures that this paediatric skill and knowledge are applied in the care of every child whatever his age or disability, and wherever he lives, and we want a service that is increasingly orientated to prevention.

According to Court (Committee on Child Health Services 1976 p 368), all of this could be achieved through an integrated child health service.

Where are the children?

'Where are the children?' (Caring for Children in the Health Services (CCHS) 1987) was the first of a number of important reports published by the organisation CCHS. Founded in 1985, CCHS is a consortium of UK agencies made up of:

- the Royal College of Nursing of the United Kingdom (RCN)
- the British Paediatric Association (BPA), now the College of Paediatrics and Child Health (CPCH)
- Action for Sick Children, formerly the National Association for the Welfare of Children in Hospital (NAWCH)
- the National Association of Health Authorities and Trusts (NAHAT).

The CCHS has proved to be an influential body in improving the quality of child health services across the UK. 'Where are the children?' was predicated on four standards that were first proposed by NAWCH (now called Action for Sick Children) as part of its 10-point Charter for Children in Hospital.

Powerpoint

Access the companion PowerPoint presentation and compare the NAWCH 10-point Charter for Children in Hospital with the ASC Millennium Charter. In what ways do they differ?

www

Visit the Action for Sick Children website:

- http://www.actionforsickchildren.org/index2.html

The four standards selected by CCHS

1. Children shall be admitted to hospital only if the care they require cannot be equally well provided at home or on a day basis.
2. Children shall be cared for with other children of the same age group.
3. Children in hospital shall have the right to have their parents with them at all times provided this is in the best interests of the child. Accommodation should therefore be offered to all parents and they should be encouraged to stay.
4. Children shall enjoy the care of appropriately trained staff, fully aware of the physical and emotional needs of each age group.

This first report from CCHS was motivated by concerns that various government recommendations related to children were being only slowly implemented. The NAWCH Charter had coalesced the recommendations of the Platt Report into 10 key standards and CCHS selected four of these to investigate. These related to where children were cared for and whether children were cared for with other children of a similar age by appropriately trained staff in the presence of parents or relatives.

Summary, findings and recommendations of 'where are the children?'

An analysis of the data collected from the Regional Health Authorities showed that the proportion of children staying in hospital overnight was not decreasing and that paediatric community services had, like with day-case surgery, progressed only sluggishly. The pioneering work of Southampton paediatric surgeon John Atwell and paediatric community nurse Peggy Gow (Atwell & Gow 1985) demonstrated that, in fact, a large proportion of operations could be carried out safely and effectively as day surgery. Importantly, the report reinforced the essential ingredient in day-case surgery for children, that of a team of paediatric community nurses.

Activity

1. Investigate the role of the paediatric community nursing team in your area. Is it linked to day-case surgery?
2. The main finding of 'Where are the children?' was that basic information about children and where they were cared for was lacking. Investigate how information about children is documented in your own clinical area. Has this improved since the publication of this report? Read below the four standards selected by CCHS below and answer the posed questions.

- Standard 1: Children shall be admitted to hospital only if the care they require cannot be equally well provided at home or on a day case basis.

What evidence is available to show that this has improved since this report was published in 1987?

- Standard 2: Children shall be cared for with other children of the same age group.

At the time of this report the data kept by hospitals was inadequate to ascertain if this standard was always met. Is this standard met in your hospital?

- Standard 3: Children in hospital shall have the right to have their parents with them at all times.

Is every parent asked if they wish to stay on your ward? What refreshment, sleeping and bathroom facilities do you have for your parents who stay overnight with their children?

- Standard 4: Children shall enjoy the care of appropriately trained staff.

Are children cared for on your ward by nurses who hold a children's nursing qualification or who have had training in the special needs of children? When children go home do they have the services of a paediatric community nursing team?

Seminar discussion topic

Of interest in this 1987 report is the recommendation that sisters of children's wards hold a children's nursing qualification. It should be noted that this report was published nearly 2 years prior to the full implementation of Project 2000 which led to the reintroduction of the direct entry children's nursing qualification for Part 15 of the Nursing and Midwifery Council register. The authors of this report were undoubtedly conscious of the advocacy role of qualified children's nurses, hence the emphasis on ward sisters holding the appropriate qualification. Additionally, however, is the reality that the post-registration route to prepare children's nurses prior to the advent of Project 2000 was inadequate to provide the numbers necessary.

Other reports from CCHS

Parents staying overnight in hospital with their children (CCHS 1988)

In this report, CCHS studied the success or otherwise of numerous recommendations that children in hospital have the right to the care and comfort of their parents during the process of the admission. A central tenet of these recommendations is the provision of unrestricted visiting and overnight accommodation for parents. This report concentrates on how parents/guardians fare during the process of staying with their children in hospital. In fact, there were wide variations of parental provision in hospital wards across the country, ranging from 20% to 87%. The 'accommodation' available for parents ranged from proper beds or reclining chairs, to mattresses on the floor and, at the extreme, upright wooden chairs.

The main objective of the report was to stimulate enhanced provision for the families of sick children. The report working party recognised that parents were crucial to the care of their children during periods of ill health. Furthermore, it was acknowledged that parents undertake many nursing duties during a child's admission, and that the role of the paediatric nurse changes from direct deliverer of care to facilitator and teacher. To best maximise the parental contribution to care it was accepted that the welfare of parents was important.

Scenario

Louise is admitting a 9-month-old infant who requires an overnight stay. The mother is worried that her 5-year-old son will miss her if she stays in hospital with the baby.

Activity

Consider your own ward or unit and the success or otherwise of parents staying overnight in hospital with their children in changing attitudes towards parents who wish to stay with their sick children in hospital:

- What type of bed is allocated to a parent?
- Where is the bed in relation to the child?
- What toilet and catering facilities are available for resident parents?

- Can all parents or guardians stay if they wish (including fathers)?
- Are parents informed of facilities for overnight accommodation before admission?
- Visit the websites of children's hospitals in North America and investigate parental provision. How do they compare with your own ward or unit?
- What are Ronald Macdonald Houses? (see http://www.ronaldhousecle.org/guest/)

Just for the day (CCHS 1991)

This far-reaching report was undertaken to accelerate the introduction of day care for children. The underlying philosophy was that admitting children as day patients was an excellent way of maintaining the integrity of the family while at the same time avoiding an overnight stay for the child in hospital. However, it is important to note that, in recommending day care services for sick children, CCHS was cognisant of the need to ensure that such services were fully planned in such a way as to avoid exacerbating family stress. Day care for children had been growing since the publication of 'Fit for the future' (Committee on Child Health Services 1976) 15 years earlier, which strongly supported day-case surgery in particular. In 'Just for the day', CCHS was endeavouring to establish national protocols for the delivery of day-care services through the development of quality standards. These standards covered the whole of the family experience, from the preadmission period through to the postdischarge care at home. The project working party, chaired by Lady Lovell-Davies of NAWCH, had two members who were experienced children's nurses. The data collected as part of this work was exhaustive and, in addition to receiving evidence from the Royal Colleges, the professional and voluntary sectors, no less than 230 submissions were received and discussed at the monthly meetings of CCHS.

The mission statement formulated by the project team

Most children, when they are sick, are cared for by their families within their own homes, with the help of GPs and community nurses. Children are more emotionally vulnerable than adults and should be admitted to hospital only if the care they require cannot be provided equally well at home, because hospitalisation can be a distressing and difficult experience. An admission should always be child centred, based on a partnership between the family and healthcare team. Children should not be nursed alongside adults. When hospital care is necessary, children should not be admitted overnight if an equivalent level of care can be provided on a day basis. Such admissions involve parents in additional responsibilities and entail careful preparation and support of the family, and efficient communication between the hospital and primary and/or community services. The planning and delivery of care should recognise the multicultural nature and diverse needs of the population and make provision accordingly (CCHS 1991 p 5).

Activity

- Is this mission statement formulated by the CCHS team still pertinent today?
- How does your clinical area perform in relation to this statement?

Main recommendations

The conclusion of the project working party was that whenever and wherever a child is admitted for day-case treatment a planned package of care should be adopted based on 12 discrete standards relating to:

- overall planning
- preadmission preparation
- the provision of a designated day-case area
- the provision of specific written information
- not mixing children with adults
- designated staff
- staff skilled in day-case work
- organisation of patient care to ensure discharge within the same day
- buildings and equipment that comply with safety standards for children
- a child-friendly environment
- specific documentation
- paediatric community nursing provision after discharge.

Activity

- Does your unit meet these standards set in 1991?
- Does your unit or hospital offer preadmission preparation for families? (See Chapter 5 and companion PowerPoint presentation.)

Bridging the gaps (CCHS 1993)

In this report, which was to spotlight ambulatory care for children as a growing discipline, Rosemary Thornes, on behalf of CCHS, conducted an exploratory study of the interface between primary and specialist care for children within the health services. In particular, the study concentrated on the quality of care provided to children as they moved through the different sectors of the health service. The data that generated the evidence was collected from one Regional Health Authority (Wessex) that agreed to act as a case study for CCHS. The background to this report lay in the frequent accounts of dissatisfaction expressed by the families of sick children, and by professionals, about the inadequacies of the interfaces between hospital and home and the different health agencies within the community at large. During the 9 months of the study the primary aims of the project team were to analyse the failures in care delivery that occur at the point of transfer, to develop principles of care that could be expressed as standards by the differing agencies and to collect examples of good practice to aid in the suggestions for improvement. The report detailed nine key principles, each with detailed suggestions on how best they could be implemented (CCHS & Thornes 1993 pp 19–27):

1. Knowledge and information should be shared between professionals and families, so that the parents and children, when they are able, are in a strong position to take part in planning and decision making.
2. There should be equity in access to, and quality of, services. Particular care should be taken to ensure that vulnerable families receive appropriate services.
3. Consultation, tests and treatment should be provided as close as possible to each child's home. If a child has to travel to a distant hospital, attention should be paid to practical help for the family.
4. Referrals to specialist services, especially those provided by community health agencies, can be made by a range of health professionals who should work to agreed criteria to ensure that care is integrated.
5. The boundary between primary and specialist care, and thus the point of referral, varies from place to place according to the facilities available in the primary setting. The important criterion is for all concerned to accept an agreed standard of care and to ensure that the child is in the right place to receive it.
6. The boundary between care in hospital and at home, and thus the point of referral back to primary carers, should vary from place to place according to the facilities and expertise available in the primary care team and the home. The important criterion is for all to work to a recognised standard of care and to ensure that the child's family has appropriate support to provide it.
7. The steps taken to ensure continuation of the pattern of care should be made explicit to families, so that the parents know who is managing their child's clinical care at every stage and where to go for clinical help.
8. Parents should be quite clear about the care they are expected to provide and at what point to seek clinical help.
9. Communication should be organised in such a way that the professional managing a child's care has sufficient, timely information to continue the care.

Activity

- Bridging the gaps was published in 1993. For each of the nine principles above, consider how well your health service performs now.
- Read Charles-Edwards & Glasper 2002.

Evidence-based practice

The strength of a modern child health policy report is determined to a greater or lesser extent on the evidence offered by the reports authors in seeking to implement or effect change. In 'Bridging the gaps', the report author, Rosemary Thornes, cites evidence taken from a series of interviews with children and their parents. Additionally, data were collected from NHS managers and staff throughout the study area. In this way the researchers attempted to develop a multidisciplinary view, including a patient (family) perspective. In gathering qualitative and quantitative data from different disciplines the report was able to analyse failures as well as successes in care.

The Children Act 1989

'The Children Act. An introductory guide for the NHS Health Publication Unit' (DoH 1989) was written as a guide to staff working with children in the NHS. Although the topic of child abuse and neglect will be covered in detail in Chapter 19, it is worth noting this policy document as one of the most important published by a health service. The language used in this report is much more precise and the word 'duty' figures prominently in the text. The main principle of the Act is that, wherever possible, children should be brought up and cared for within their own families but – and importantly – children should be safe and protected by effective intervention if they are in danger.

The welfare of children and young people in hospital (1991)

Still an industry standard for the care of children in hospital, this report, which was written as a guide (DoH 1991), coalesced many of the previous reports, including those by Platt and Court. Perhaps it was hoped that the status of 'guide' rather than 'report' would enhance compliance with government recommendations. Sadly, a number of tragedies, but principally that of the Allitt case (Glasper & Campbell 1994), would show the extremes of failing to comply with the good practice recommendations of this document. Of interest in this guide are the terms 'advised' and 'should', the former obviously carrying more weight than the latter. To illustrate this, one of the key recommendations of this 'welfare document' is the statement that 'at least two registered sick children's nurses (RSCNs or Project 2000 child branch) should be on duty 24 hours a day in all hospital children's departments or wards' (DoH 1991 p 33). However, this was only advised and has been a contentious issue ever since. This guidance document was an attempt by the DoH to make health districts improve the quality of children's health care. Not all were successful in doing so.

Activity

Read 'The welfare of children and young people in hospital' (DoH 1991) and examine the number of recommendations that are 'advised' or 'should' – compare your own unit's compliance with these recommendations.

Child health in the community (1996)

Published some 5 years after 'The welfare of children and young people in hospital' (DoH 1991), 'Child health in the community' (NHS Executive 1996) was intended to be a companion document reflecting major changes in the way children were managed during illness. Additionally, it highlighted the reality that, for most of the time, most children are cared for in their own homes. This was a reflection of a greater emphasis on preventive measures to avoid illness and therefore hospital admission. This report takes a broader perspective than earlier reports and begins to acknowledge that parenting skills are of paramount importance to the overall health of children. Concerns about falling levels of parenting within families is reflected and cited as one reason for the increase in emotional and behavioural disorders among children. Failure to break the cycle of deprivation when young people start families of their own before they have the skills to do so is highlighted and addressed in this far-reaching report. As in the CCHS report 'Bridging the gaps' (CCHS & Thornes 1993), Child health in the community gives details of how services for children should be targeted and emphasises the importance of good working relationships between hospital and community staff and the value of closer collaboration with other agencies responsible for the welfare of children, including the voluntary sector. In this respect, 'Child health in the community' begins to move the emphasis of care away from simply those children in hospital. As with its companion 'welfare' document 'The welfare of children and young people in hospital' (DoH 1991), 'Child health in the community' uses the terms 'advise' and 'should'.

Activity

During your community placements, investigate through discussion with the paediatric community team whether practice is based on the recommendations of this report?

Children first. A study of hospital services (1993)

As part of its remit to examine the economy, efficiency and effectiveness with which the NHS uses public resources, the Audit Commission conducted 'Children first. A study of hospital services' (Audit Commission 1993). For the first time the effectiveness of treatment regimens and the need for children to be treated in hospital were questioned in the light of the Platt report of 1959 and other subsequent publications. There was a tacit acknowledgement that reports pertaining to the welfare of children had too often not been fully implemented. Crucially, the Audit Commission report did not seek to reiterate the findings of other studies and reports but rather to investigate why these were not being met in some institutions. Children first states six main principles of caring for children in hospital:

1. child- and family-centred care
2. specially skilled staff
3. separate facilities
4. effective treatments
5. appropriate hospitalisation
6. strategic commissioning.

It also identifies the barriers preventing the achievement of good practice. Importantly, the report gives suggestions of how these might be overcome.

In summary, the Audit Commission report advises health agencies to adhere to the guidelines contained within The welfare of children and young people in hospital (DoH 1991).

Activity

- How does your unit measure compliance with national child health policy standards?
- What audit tools are used to gather data for this activity?

The care of sick children. A review of the guidelines in the wake of the Allitt inquiry

This document (RCN 1994) was published in the wake of the Allitt inquiry (Clothier et al 1994), which reported the deaths and injuries among hospitalised children caused by enrolled nurse Beverly Allitt. Recommendation 10 of the 13 made in the Allitt inquiry report recommends that the DoH should take steps to ensure that the policy document 'The welfare of children and young people in hospital' (DoH 1991) be more closely observed. This is similar language to that used by the Audit Commission in its 'Children first' report, published the year before in 1993. The purpose of the RCN guidelines in the wake of Allitt was to bring pressure to bear on purchasers and providers to improve the services offered to sick children by complying with DoH recommendations. The RCN publication reiterates and presents in a digestible format the recommendations of earlier reports, and in particular the need for sick children to be cared for by appropriately qualified staff, pointing out that over half the children in hospital were being cared for by nurses not holding a paediatric nursing qualification. Additionally, Grantham and Kesteven General Hospital, which employed Allitt, was criticised for having a poor appointments procedure (Dyer 1994). Beverly Allitt was reported to be suffering from a disease known as Munchausen syndrome by proxy, although this has subsequently been hotly debated.

Seminar discussion topic

Read and discuss in your learning group the paper:

- Morley CJ 1995 Practical concerns about the diagnosis of Munchausen syndrome by proxy. Archives of Disease in Childhood 72:528–530

Child health rights: implementing the UN Convention on the Rights of the Child within the NHS. A practitioner's guide (1995)

'Child health rights: implementing the UN Convention on the Rights of the Child within the NHS. A practitioners' guide' (British Association for Community Child Health (BACCH) 1995) was published to bring to the attention of all who work with children the mechanisms for the implementation of the UN Convention. This convention on the rights of the child was adopted by the General Assembly of The United Nations in November 1989. It came into force in the UK in January 1992 and its primary aim is to provide a comprehensive set of principles and standards to guide and inform planning and practice for children and young people up to 18 years of age. The BACCH publication attempts to show how it is possible to implement the Convention at local level. A number of other reports on children's rights have been published since and the second report to the UN (DoH 1999) gives details on progress made.

WWW

Read a digestible précis of the UN Convention:

- http://www.unicef.org/crc/

Listening to children. Children, ethics, and social research (1995)

'Listening to children. Children, ethics, and social research' (Alderson 1995) was published as concerns about the ethical aspects of research using children were being increasingly articulated, although the events at Alder Hey and Bristol were yet to hit the newspaper headlines. The whole topic of ethics and children's rights will be covered in a subsequent chapter but Alderson's contribution to the debate must be recognised. In this report, commissioned by Barnardos, Alderson identifies 10 key topics relating to research ethics:

1. the purpose of the research
2. researching with children – the costs and hoped for benefits
3. privacy and confidentiality
4. selection, inclusion and exclusion
5. funding
6. review and revision of the research aims and methods
7. information for children, parents and other carers
8. consent
9. dissemination (of the research findings)
10. impact on children.

Activity

- Identify a research project in your own unit. Are all these 10 principles being adhered to?

Reflect on your practice

As a nurse working in a children's unit where research is carried out, are you accountable even if you are not directly involved?

Government response to the House of Commons Health Committee reports on children and young people (1997)

The official 'Government response to the House of Commons Health Committee reports' (DoH 1997a) is in many respects an endorsement of the original reports and of many of the other reports covered thus far.

Key points

The government welcomed the reports as making a substantial contribution to the debate about child health:

- The response acknowledges that children are different.
- Care should encompass the needs of the whole child, with mental health especially highlighted.
- Fragmentation (between agencies) should be reduced, echoing 'Bridging the gaps' (CCHS & Thornes 1993)
- Endorses 'The welfare of children and young people in hospital' (DoH 1991).
- Endorses 'Child health in the community: a guide to good practice' (NHS Executive 1996).

Although it is beyond the scope of this chapter to consider all aspects, one of the responses to the House of Commons reports highlights the slow development of paediatric community nursing services (House of Commons Health Committee 1997). This point is picked up by Whiting in a subsequent chapter, who discuss the development of a children's community nursing service, highlighting the benefits in terms of a reduction in the length of stay, a reduction in admissions and enhanced family satisfaction.

Activity

Read Chapter 8 by Whiting and review the level of community nursing services in your local area. How does the service operate?

The patient's charter - services for children and young people (the children's charter) (1996)

The patient's charter - services for children and young people (the children's charter) (DoH 1996) was launched as part of the UK government's commitment to accountability in public services. It made a number of innovative pledges to children and their families. These pledges were based on good practice generated through years of published child health policy.

Activity

- Obtain a copy of 'The children's charter' and determine how many of the pledges are honoured in your own area of practice.
- Are copies of the charter freely available to children and their relatives in your clinical area?

A bridge to the future (1997)

The tragic death of a child named Nicholas Geldhart in December 1995 was the precursor to the posing of fundamental questions about the national provision of paediatric intensive care facilities for children across the country. In the aftermath of the negative publicity surrounding this unfortunate child's death, the Chief Nursing Officer's taskforce recognised that demand for paediatric intensive care services for children was growing year on year. Crucial to the debate was the stark reality that there were insufficient paediatric intensive care nurses. The gold-standard qualification to equip paediatric nurses with the skills and knowledge to care for critically ill children was the English (Scottish or Welsh) National Board for Nursing and Midwifery course (ENB) 415 (these validating agency boards no longer exist). Additional intensive care courses and – importantly – student salaries were fully funded in the wake of 'A bridge to the future' (DoH 1997b). To complement this initiative, new paediatric intensive care units were built and equipped. Unlike previous reports, huge amounts of money were invested in achieving improvements to a service that was found to be deficient and politically highly sensitive.

Youth matters: evidence-based best practice for the care of young people in hospital (1998)

'Youth matters' (Viner & Keane 1998), coordinated through the consortium CCHS, aimed to raise awareness of the plight of young people in hospital. The report revealed that only 8% of health authorities contained adolescent provider units in their hospitals. Glasper & Cooper (1999) contrast the prominent position of young people in society with their invisibility in a hospital setting, where they have such a low profile despite the fact that in morbidity terms they continue to be one of the most vulnerable groups in society. This report asked all Health Authorities to conduct a detailed survey to determine what provision should be made for young people in hospital.

Despite a lack of progress following the publication of 'Youth matters', Viner participated in a subsequent policy initiative on behalf of the Royal College of Paediatrics and Child Health, the Royal College of Psychiatrists and others in producing 'Bridging the gaps: health care for adolescents' (2003).

Activity

- Was this survey undertaken in your health area?
- Conduct your own survey in your own hospital or unit. Are you satisfied with the level of adolescent provision?

The facilities for young people in hospital remain poor.

Activity

Access this policy at

- http://www.rcpsych.ac.uk/ publications/cr/council/cr114.pdf.

In your learning group debate the ramifications of this latest adolescent policy.

The Royal Liverpool Children's Inquiry (2001)

'The Royal Liverpool Children's Inquiry' (DoH 2001a) (available online at: http://www.rlcinquiry.org.uk/), chaired by Michael Redfern QC, was initiated after a storm of public protest broke out after revelations that deceased children's body parts had been removed at the Alder Hey Children's Hospital without parental consent. Prior to the publication of this report, Glasper & Powell (2000, 2001) had highlighted the vagueness of the law pertaining to post-mortems, in which some doctors exceeded their mandate. The whole issue of the scandal of Alder Hey revolved around informed consent and the lack of it. Redfern's report has made it clear that consent procedures must be tightened to ensure that a person must have all the information necessary to make an informed decision.

www

Read the report online and consider your own field of practice:

- http://www.rlcinquiry.org.uk/

The Bristol inquiry (2001)

The report of the public inquiry into children's heart surgery (DoH 2001b) (available online at: http://www.bristol-inquiry.org.uk) revealed that the UK health service was badly in need of reform. The inquiry, chaired by Professor Ian Kennedy, was commissioned after it was revealed that success rates for children's heart surgery at the Bristol Royal Infirmary were less than in comparative centres elsewhere in the UK. The inquiry found that much of the criticism levelled at health professionals by parents was the result of a lack of information. Additionally, the report demanded that children in hospital must be cared for in an appropriate, safe environment by competent staff trained in caring for children. Glasper (2001) points out that a plethora of similar reports have made recommendations for prospective change in the health service and yet have achieved less than anticipated.

WWW

Read the report online. How is information given to children and parents in your clinical area?

- http://www.bristol-inquiry.org.uk

The Victoria Climbié inquiry

The death of 8-year-old Victoria Climbié precipitated a national inquiry chaired by Lord Laming, which was eventually published in 2003 (Laming 2003). Although this will be fully covered in Chapter 19, it is important to recognise that in the aftermath of this inquiry it became widely accepted that child maltreatment had become one of the major causes of morbidity in children. Profound changes in policy within all health and social care environments relating to child protection were subsequently introduced in an attempt to prevent such a tragedy from happening again. Powell (2003) highlights the need to ensure that child protection services are commensurate with the scale of the problem in the UK. Children's nurses play a crucial front-line role in the recognition of child maltreatment and this report and its policy recommendations are therefore essential reading.

WWW

Read the report online:

- http//www.victoria-climbie-inquiry.org.uk/finreport/finreport.htm

The National Service Framework for children

The final instalment of the National Service Framework (NSF) for children, young people and maternity services was published in September 2004 (DoH 2004) as part of the government's commitment to children exemplified in its Green Paper, 'Every child matters' (DfES 2003). This sets out proposals for reforming the delivery of services for children, young people and families, augmenting existing measures to ensure that children at risk of harm and neglect are protected and enabled to develop their full potential.

The NSF sets new standards for children and young people across health and social care boundaries in England. Although many elements of health and social care services for children and young people were the subject of much criticism in the Bristol (DoH 2001b) and Victoria Climbié inquiries (Laming 2003) – the primary antecedents to the NSF – this policy document breathes new life into the old adage that the wealth of a nation is invested in the health and welfare of all its children. This will be achieved through the introduction of 11 auditable standards, which are predicated on best evidence-based practice in the care of pregnant women, children and young people. The NSF is presented in three parts:

- Part 1 is concerned with setting standards for well children and young people, and is aimed at keeping them safe and healthy through the provision of optimum life chances.
- Part 2 sets standards for sick children and young people in the community and hospital and for those with mental health problems, disabilities and complex health needs.
- Part 3 addresses maternity services.

In a way that is perhaps reminiscent of the main finding of the Black report (DHSS 1980), which was commissioned by the previous Labour government in 1979, and of 'Tackling health inequalities' (DoH 2003), the introduction to the NSF by John Reid, the Labour Secretary of State for Health, reinforces the reality that inequalities in health and social care still impact on children and young people. His emphasis on child poverty, and on the effect this has on children and young people, forms the backdrop to the whole NSF, commencing perhaps with standard 11 of the report 'maternity services'.

It is known that much ill health and disease in adulthood has its origins before, during and after pregnancy. It is therefore fitting that this NSF standard should highlight the importance of improved preconception care and the role of health promotion in the future well-being of children and young people. The standards of the NSF cover many of the parameters of childhood, such as tackling the growing burden on health of obesity through recommendations to improve school meals and encouraging children to take 60 minutes of exercise daily. This must be tempered with the reality that many school playing fields have been sold for land development. School playing fields are now protected under Section 77 of the School Standards and Framework Act 1998, which empowers the Secretary of State to protect such fields in England from disposal or change of use, and this is an example of how the NSF has the potential to bridge all components of society in the promotion of optimum health for all children and young people. Although the government envisages that the full implementation of the NSF will take up to 10 years, it has stressed that the NHS and local authorities charged with its implementation will be frequently assessed by the Health Care Commission, the Commission for Social Care Inspection and OFSTED to ensure that they are compliant and making progress. Additionally, and of interest to nurses, is the work of the Association of Chief Children's Nurses (ACCN), which regularly posts exemplars of good practice related to the NSF on its website (http://www.accnuk.org)

'The right start: the national service framework for children, young people and maternity services' (DoH 2004, available online at: http://www.doh.gov/childrenstaskforce), the first part of the NSF to be published, was launched as part of the government's commitment to raising standards across the NHS and Social Services departments. In particular, this component of the whole NSF sets rigorous standards for children in hospital, grouped around three main themes:

- child-centred hospital services
- quality and safety of care provided
- quality of setting and environment.

To give robustness to these standards, the Healthcare Commission intends to ensure compliance through inspections. Those hospitals failing to meet these and the other NSF standards will be given appropriate advice on what they need to do to raise standards of care.

Activity

Visit the NSF website (or access it from the PowerPoint presentation) and consider how the compliance to the standards will be audited by the Health Commission, one of whose statutory functions is to monitor and review the implementation of standards set out in the National Service Frameworks.

In summary

This part of the chapter has not been able to consider every report concerning sick children. In the Carlile review (National Assembly for Wales 2002), for example, it was acknowledged that 65 guidance documents with respect to child protection alone were issued to the NHS between 1971 and 2001. The volume of reports commissioned about children in society indicates that much still needs to be achieved.

Getting it right – dealing with complaints

> From one of our most recently constructed hospitals complaints have been made that there were not sufficient nursing conveniences, that nothing was at hand, that everything had to be sought. Where this is the case the hospital administration must be both inefficient and costly
>
> (Florence Nightingale 1863)

Complaints are a fact of life. No organisation or profession can avoid them and it is not desirable to ignore or belittle them. Most complaints, if well handled, can have a very positive outcome. Complaints in the health service often indicate ways in which practice or procedures can be improved or highlight matters that really concern children, families or carers.

If a family makes a complaint about any aspect of their child's care, nurses not only need to be involved in the investigation of that complaint but must also reflect back on the accuracy of their record-keeping, particularly records of any communication that they have had with the child or carers and multidisciplinary colleagues. The Nursing and Midwifery Council (2008) states 'You must keep clear and accurate records of the discussions you have, the assessments you make, the treatment and medicines you give and how effective these have been'. If an aspect of care is not documented, how can there be any evidence that that care has taken place? Often a complaint is made several months after an issue has occurred and it would be difficult for any nurse to recall details of a particular case. Consequently, the nurse is reliant on what is documented.

An effective clinical governance agenda will ensure that complaints are seen and dealt with as part of everyday business and that complaints are used to indicate improvements to services across the whole organisation. If procedures have changed, complainants appreciate being informed of the changes. Consideration needs to be given by Trusts as to the most effective way to encourage staff to change unacceptable practice.

Criteria for investigating complaints

For an investigation under the NHS complaints procedure, a complaint must be about NHS services. Anyone making a complaint under the procedure is entitled to:

- a full and complete explanation of what happened and why, given in a language the complainant can understand
- an apology if there was an error or omission on behalf of the staff
- information about the action that the organisation has taken or is proposing to take, if an error or omission has occurred, to try and prevent it happening again.

Complaints should be dealt with quickly and accurately. Ideally they should be made as soon as possible after the incident has occurred but normally within 6 months of the event or within 6 months from the time that it came to the complainant's notice, providing that not more than 12 months have elapsed since the original event. Occasionally, as a result of bereavement or prolonged illness, a Trust may decide to investigate a complaint if it is outside these time limits.

Stages of the complaints procedure

Prior to April 2009 the stages in the complaints system were:

- local resolution
- the Healthcare Commission
- the Parliamentary and Health Service Ombudsman.

From April 2009, the new NHS Complaints Process will consist of only two stages: Local Resolution and the Parliamentary and Health Service Ombudsman.

Local resolution is an essential stage of the complaint process. This is the stage at which nurses must become involved and take note of when families are becoming anxious or distressed or clearly need to sit down and talk through concerns. How local resolution is handled is for the individual organisation to decide. Staff need to be empowered and trained to act on concerns the moment they receive them. The sooner a complaint is responded to the more likely it is to be resolved. Families often just want to be heard and to express their anxieties and it is at this stage that the Patient Advice and Liaison Service (PALS) can be of great benefit.

Family advocates (PALS) are available to help families. The service is free to all patients, families, carers and friends and they can speak in confidence to trained staff; information will not be disclosed unless permission is given. If it is thought necessary to protect a child from serious harm or injury then a decision needs to be made as to the way forward. PALS can:

- provide a listening ear
- help sort out any problems by liaising with staff
- support families in making their concerns heard
- guide families through the hospital complaints process if they wish to make a formal complaint
- link families to information and support services.

WWW

The PALS team at Great Ormond Street Hospital has implemented this service successfully. Visit their website:

- http://www.goshkids@nhs.uk

Written complaints must receive a written response. A range of individuals can provide this response, often it is a Complaints Manager but sometimes the healthcare professionals themselves will prepare a response for the Complaints Manager, and this will then be collated into a full response for the Chief Executive to sign. This is an important stage for nurses to be involved; they have often been working closely with the families and are able to provide their version of events. It is important to understand the full picture from beginning to end and to hear that story from all the individuals involved. People's perceptions can be very different and it is important to receive a balanced view.

A recommended way to look at the complaint is to actually highlight the questions that the complainant has raised in a letter and then to look at the response and consider whether those particular issues have been answered. The initial letter may well be followed up by a local resolution meeting. It is important that this meeting involves all of the healthcare professionals involved, particularly the nursing staff who can often provide necessary information in an understandable language for the family. Junior nurses will often be represented by a more senior nursing colleague at this local resolution meetings. PALS can often be involved at this stage by supporting a complainant or ensuring that an advocate is available. Talking the issues through and taking time to explain procedures or issues that have been raised can be extremely helpful to complainants.

The final letter at the end of local resolution must advise the complainant of his or her rights. A complainant has the right to request an independent review and needs to indicate by letter which issues he or she considers have not been addressed at local resolution. The request is then passed to the Healthcare Commission.

Finally, if something has gone wrong, the Healthcare Commission (or the Parliamentary and Health Service Ombudsman if the complaint has reached the final stage) must decide whether a Trust has been clear about the steps that have been taken to reduce the chances of a repetition of the event. At this stage it is essential for the investigations teams at the Healthcare Commission or the Ombudsman to take independent clinical advice if the complaint involves clinical issues. The type of advice obtained will depend upon the clinical issues in question, therefore independent advice may be sought from a range of healthcare professionals, for example, nurses, doctors, midwives, dieticians or pharmacists. There are then three options:

- To refer the complaint back to local resolution for further investigation and explanations from the Trust
- The Healthcare Commission undertakes a full independent review
- To fast-track the complaint to the Ombudsman.

If the Healthcare Commission (pre April 2009) agrees that an independent review panel should be held, then the specific issues to be investigated are agreed with the complainant. Issues investigated must be those which have already been raised with the Trust.

Complainants have a right to approach the Parliamentary and Health Service Ombudsman if their request for an independent review panel is refused or if they remain dissatisfied at the end of the current second stage of the NHS Complaints process. The Ombudsman considers the request and decides whether to investigate. As a result, the Ombudsman has become the last resort for a complainant who remains dissatisfied after exhausting the initial two stages of the NHS complaints procedure. The Health Service Ombudsman's powers and duties are set out in the Health Service Commissioner's Act 1993. Jurisdiction was initially confined to the classic Ombudsman territory of maladministration (in the NHS) but was extended in 1996 to include clinical complaints and complaints about family health service practitioners.

WWW

Visit these websites to view these Acts:

- http://www.hmso.gov.uk/acts/acts1993/ Ukpga_19930046_en_2.htm
- http://www.hmso.gov.uk/acts/acts1996/96005--b.htm

The positions of Parliamentary Commissioner, or Ombudsman, came into being in 1967; that of Health Service Ombudsman in 1973. The two offices are always held by the same person, who is appointed by the Queen and answerable to Parliament. The Ombudsman is independent of government and the NHS and is not a member of the medical profession.

If it appears that an investigation may be warranted then the Ombudsman may request that the organisation supplies information about how the complaint was handled and any further information that may help to make a final decision. The Ombudsman is interested to see that the correct procedure has been followed. If the Ombudsman decides to investigate, all the complaints correspondence and clinical records are examined and independent clinical advice will be sought from the Ombudsman's team of clinical advisers prior to producing and full written report, which is then shared with the complainant and those complained about.

An example of a letter copied to the Ombudsman following an investigation is given below. The letter was sent to the Acute Trust involved in the complaint:

> It was also important to us that we receive an apology for what had happened, but it was your policy to refuse point blank to apologise, and adopt the stance that our complaint was not justified. With the publication of the Ombudsman's report, this can now be seen to be an error of judgement on your part, and it has been clearly shown that our complaint was justified. The matter has now entered the public domain through the media, which will do nothing to enhance the reputation of the Health Authority or the hospital in question.

www

General information about the Ombudsman and copies of reports can be found on the following website:

- http://www.ombudsman.org.uk

You are thoroughly recommended to look at these published reports. They provide a valuable learning tool for any healthcare professional.

Key factors leading to complaints involving nursing practice

Communication

Communication – or lack of it – is often a major issue in any complaint. The Nursing and Midwifery Council says very clearly that nurses must listen to the people in their care and respond to concerns. This includes the expectation that nurses will: 'share with people, in a way they can understand, the information they want or need to know about their health' (NMC 2008). Nearly all complaints that the Ombudsman sees involve poor communication. It is widely recognised that what a doctor or nurse believes he or she said might be very different from a child or carer's perception of the same discussion. The importance of documenting such a discussion cannot be over emphasised.

Families who are distressed or vulnerable often fail to hear what is being said to them. It is therefore important to repeat information. Poor communication occurs between nurses and families, nurses and doctors or other healthcare professionals, and nurses and other wards/departments, particularly when patients are transferred from one ward to another. Handover is often extremely poor. This is a stage where often reassessment of the patient is needed to establish a relationship with the patients/carers and ensure all information is clarified.

The simple act of showing family members around a ward, introducing them to staff and being friendly and approachable seems simple but too often staff get this very wrong.

Disappointment

Families do very often have an unrealistic expectation of what can be achieved for their child. This is only natural; it is often their only coping mechanism. However, staff must manage this situation and clear explanations of what is available and what is achievable need to occur. An honest approach to families, particularly in obtaining their consent, is absolutely essential; telling families that there is a 90% chance of success is totally unacceptable. Parents will cling to the 90%, not thinking that there is a possibility that they may be in the 10%.

The disappointment caused by an unpleasant environment or rude staff might seem a minor issue. But it can easily develop into something much more serious that could have been avoided if staff had noticed that the problems were arising:

> At the outset of this complaint when my family and I attended a meeting, my husband was asked in a very aggressive manner what it was we wanted to achieve by this complaint. It was our hope then, and continues to be, that we would achieve something positive, that would bring to your attention a problem within the hospital, and that with the new procedures your service would improve. We are unable to change what happened to our daughter, but we can achieve something positive in her memory.

Fundamental care

It is the fundamental aspects of care which matter to patients: caring, communication, attention to comfort, cleanliness, etc. When these are missing patients and their carers form an enduring and negative impression of the healthcare staff. There are many different examples of when healthcare professionals got the fundamentals of care wrong. Consider the following scenarios:

Scenario

A robust assessment of a patient's skin is not available in any documentation and when the patient develops a sore on their ear on being intubated the family is not only extremely distressed but takes it as evidence of poor risk analysis of the patient.

Involving a dietician or a tissue viability nurse to give expert advice to a child and family often does not occur, even when these professionals are available within an organisation. These experts often have time to talk through the problems that may occur with the family.

Cot sides being left down on beds for a child to fall out are another example of lack of risk analysis.

The quality of nursing documentation, in particular with regard to the recording of communications with the family, were particularly poor. Concerns were raised about care planning and management of K's pressure areas and blisters, the lack of leadership of her care process and poor integration between the palliative care specialist nurses and the ward staff.

The care afforded to K fell well below standard, there was sparsity of record keeping with little evidence of nutritional assessment and fluid intake and output. There was no formal risk assessment or any record of subsequent treatment.

If only

Many families punish themselves with the 'if only' syndrome:

- If only my child hadn't ridden his bike to school …
- If only my child had been seen more quickly in the emergency department …
- If only my child had gone to the intensive care unit sooner …
- If only I had noticed the rash sooner …

Many families need to be helped through this stage of distress but many repeat it constantly in the complaint process and expert attention is needed to move the family on.

Bereavement

Many complaints involve families who are also coping with their bereavement process. If the complaint has involved the death of a child, families sometimes feel that continuing the complaint process almost keeps the child alive for them; that while they are talking about the child they still feel able to cope. However, if the complaint process is closed, how do these families cope?

Bereavement is defined as the normal human reaction to loss and, as a result, medical situations other than death can result in a feeling of loss and bereavement:

- Loss of a body part
- Loss of body image
- Loss of senses
- Loss of function
- Child admitted to care.

People react differently to loss. Some of the more common reactions that are associated with complaints handling are (Gunn 2001):

- anger
- guilt
- shock, numbness and disbelief
- denial
- bargaining
- acceptance
- depression.

An obvious note of anger runs through many of the complaints that have been published and families sometimes seem to need to try to blame a particular individual for what has happened. A particularly moving account of a family working through its bereavement is given below in this anonymised quote from a family's letter:

> Many people have asked me what was the point as at the end of the day it won't bring our daughter back. The investigation has meant justice for her and has allowed us to start grieving for her instead of being so fixated by what happened. The work you have done has given a semblance of sense to what happened as it led to changes, and it has also given our daughter the dignity taken from her during her stay in hospital. The consultant cardiologist works at the private hospital I work at and took time out to talk to me, and give me his true feelings about what happened. He reassured me that the changes were realistic. He said the nature of the complaints procedure was 'confrontational' and he had been unable to speak freely before then. It is a shame that we couldn't all work together to sort things out.

Complaints in the NHS often stem from stressful events at a time when people feel vulnerable and scared. They may at times be unreasonable but must still be assessed objectively. Complaints can also be stressful for NHS staff, who might well feel that they did their best in difficult circumstances and that the only outcome is for them to be criticised. It is essential that Trusts are able to provide support for both the complainant and staff.

Managing complaints on the front line

> The only sustainable option for those in public services is to create a climate of openness. Openness is the only means of establishing public confidence in the Health Service and in the competence of its professionals.
>
> Sir Michael Buckley, Health Service Ombudsman, 1997–2002

It is essential that all staff within a health organisation are trained to handle complainants and complaints. It should be an essential part of induction for all staff.

Handling complaints well

NHS organisations get it right when:

- handling complaints is part of daily clinical practice
- the approach to investigation is sound
- the response is open and complete and action follows.

What should NHS staff do?

Remember that people want:

- to be acknowledged
- to be taken seriously
- an understandable explanation
- an apology where necessary
- to be reassured that it will not happen to anyone else.

The complaint pathway

Ensuring lessons are learnt from complaints in clinical practice (Figs 3.1, 3.2 and 3.3) is important:

> It may seem a strange principle to enunciate as a first requirement in a hospital, that it should do the sick no harm
>
> Florence Nightingale 1863

Complaints are a superb learning tool for all healthcare professionals and should be used in that way to enhance practice and the delivery of care to patients within an organisation. It is also essential that performance is linked to learning and that organisations such as the Nursing and Midwifery Council (NMC), the Healthcare Commission and the National Institute for Clinical Excellence (NICE) all regularly collaborate on issues which may be of concern in health care in order that clinical practice can be reviewed where necessary.

The Ombudsman has clear principles regarding good complaint handling which are identified clearly in a summary of cases – 'Remedy in the NHS' (2008):

- Getting it right will be about getting the right leadership, governance and culture – ownership at the top of the organisation; about equipping and empowering decision makers on complaints; about focusing on outcomes not processes; and about signposting to the Ombudsman in the right way at the right time.
- Being customer focused will be about providing an accessible complaints service, with help to make complaints for those who need it: a service that is simple, speedy, joined-up with other providers, flexible, sensitive and tailored to people's needs – not 'one size fits all'.
- Being open and accountable will be about publicising complaints procedures clearly and well; about keeping proper records of complaints; and about giving reasons for decisions.

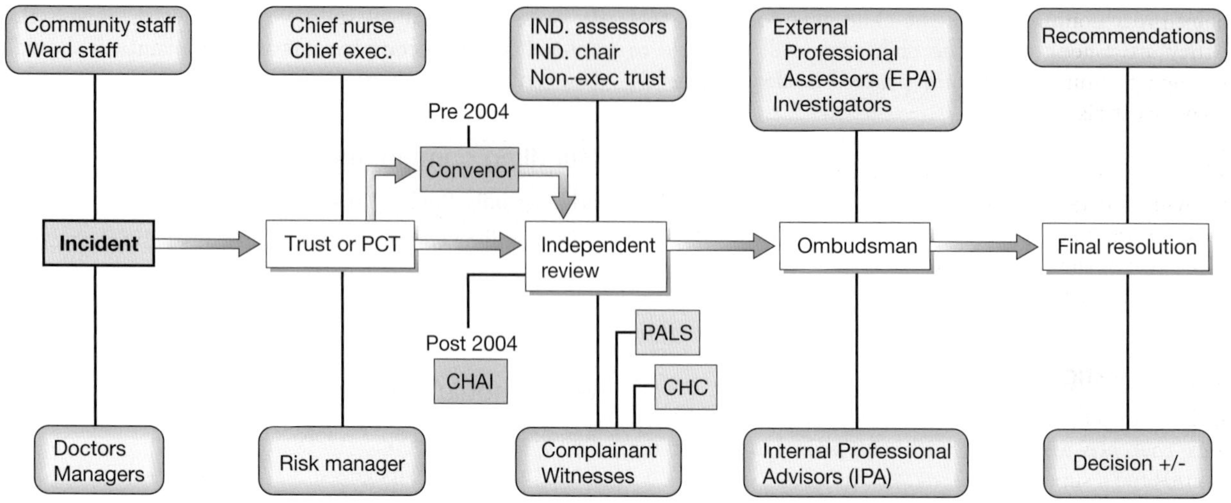

Fig. 3.1 • Complaint pathway.

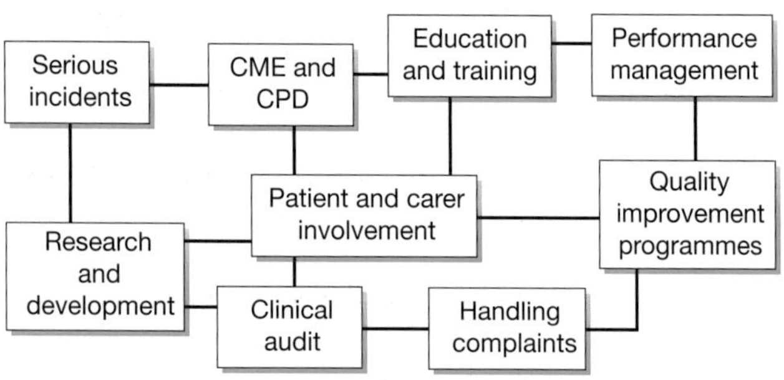

Fig. 3.2 • Linking performance and learning.

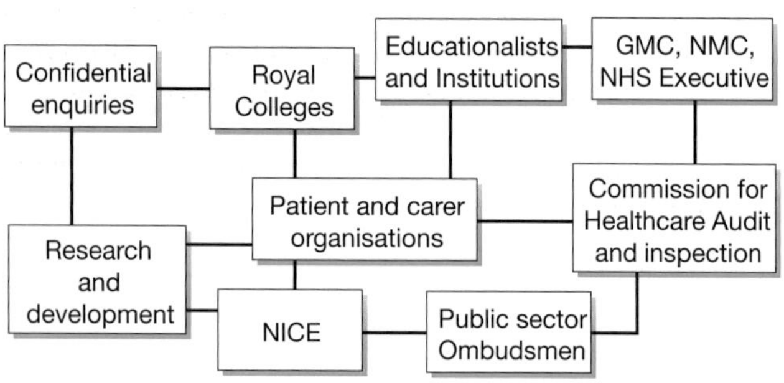

Fig. 3.3 • Linking performance and learning.

- Acting fairly and proportionately will be about decisions being reviewed by someone other than the original decision maker; about natural justice to all the parties; and about not using sledgehammers to crack nuts.
- Putting things right will be about remedy. Not only apologies and explanations (important as they are) and not only changes to prevent a recurrence (important as they are, as well) but, as we have seen, financial remedies where they are justified and appropriate.
- Seeking continuous improvement will be about learning. But it will also be about attitude and culture. Is this an organisation which understands and practises learning from complaints?

Published cases

It is essential for nurses to read complaints and really consider different families' perceptions of healthcare professionals and the image that they portray.

Seminar discussion topic

Read the published cases and discuss them amongst colleagues. The following case is an example: Complaint about the care and treatment of a critically ill child admitted with breathing problems, and complaint about the Commission's subsequent review.

Background to the complaint

Miss A, aged 17, suffered from multiple and severe health problems from birth and her parents were her full-time carers. As she required frequent hospital contact, she had direct access to the paediatric unit. In August 2003 she was admitted to the paediatric unit with shortness of breath and coughing, on the advice of the Paediatric Triage Team, which her parents had contacted. Some hours later, when her condition failed to improve, she was transferred to the Intensive Care Unit; however, sadly, she died an hour later.

The complaint to the Trust and the commission

In January 2004 Mr and Mrs A complained to the Trust about Miss A's care and treatment and in particular her delayed admittance to the Intensive Care Unit, the failure to call the duty consultant when Miss A was admitted and the fact that the consultant was not on the hospital site. They believed that there had been a failure in care and that Miss A had not been adequately reviewed by a senior doctor. They also believed that, had she been transferred to the Intensive Care Unit more quickly, she would have survived.

The Trust's response to the complaint encompassed three letters and two meetings with Mr and Mrs A between February and August 2004. The Trust acknowledged some shortcomings, apologised and highlighted actions arising from the case including the introduction of individualised illness management plans for children with complex conditions; a system of flagging children with special needs on the patient administration system; and developing summary history sheets at the front of patient's notes. The Trust also subsequently reported improved staffing levels.

In November 2004 Mr and Mrs A complained to the Commission, which reviewed the case having taken clinical advice. In February 2006 it concluded that the Trust had taken steps to reduce the risk of similar problems occurring in the future and that there was no scope to take the complaint further.

What we investigated

Mr and Mrs A complained to the Ombudsman in April 2006 and we investigated the complaint as put to the Trust as well as the Commission's subsequent handling.

We had access to Miss A's medical records for the last 5 years of her life and copies of all complaints correspondence. We also took clinical advice from a Senior Nurse with paediatric experience and obtained a full report from a Consultant Paediatrician.

What our investigation found

Our investigation found the following significant failings during Miss A's admission:

- Inadequate monitoring.
- Poor record keeping in terms of both nursing and medical notes.
- Failure to recognise the seriousness of Miss A's condition.
- Delays in seeking and obtaining reviews by senior doctors.
- Delays in contacting the on-call consultant.
- Delay in transferring Miss A to a High Dependency or Intensive Care Unit despite clear indications that she needed more intensive care than was available on the paediatric ward.

We found that the standard of care provided to Miss A during her last illness fell below a reasonable standard. This amounted to service failure on the part of the Trust. We concluded that, while it would never have been possible to say for certain whether Miss A would have survived her illness had she been transferred to the Intensive Care Unit at an earlier stage, there seemed little doubt that her chances would have been improved.

We also found that the Trust had not acknowledged or apologised in relation to several key issues from Mr and Mrs A's original complaint.

We also concluded that the Commission's review was seriously flawed because it was not clear that sufficient clinical advice had been taken from a properly qualified adviser and the clinical advice had not been recorded properly on file (the Commission's files contained only a brief note of a discussion with an adviser which gave no indication of the adviser's qualification and did not make clear if the adviser had seen the relevant clinical records).

The investigation, which concluded in September 2006, upheld the complaints against the Trust and the Commission.

WWW

Visit the website and obtain a copy:

- http://www.doh.gov.uk/essenceofcare

Outcome

As a result of our recommendations the Trust wrote to Mr and Mrs A to apologise for the shortcomings identified in our report.

The Trust also drew up a comprehensive action plan in response to our recommendations which included:

- the commissioning of a designated paediatric high dependency facility;
- the implementation of a paediatric early warning system, which has been integrated with an updated monitoring chart for critically ill children;
- staff induction and training programmes, which include the recognition and resuscitation of critically ill children;
- the regular auditing of new joint medical and nursing notes;
- the appointment of a paediatric clinical practice facilitator; and
- the establishment of professional liaison with the regional paediatric intensive care consortium as a resource for advice, training and service strategy.

The Commission wrote to Mr and Mrs A to apologise for the shortcomings in its review and for any distress or frustration that this had caused. The Commission also explained that its policy now required that clinical advice be recorded in appropriate detail (either the adviser's report or a signed record of a detailed discussion).

References

Alderson, P., 1995. Listening to children. Children, ethics, and social research. Barnardos, London.

Atwell, J., Gow, M.A., 1985. Paediatric trained district nurses in the community: expensive luxury or economic necessity? British Medical Journal 291, 227–229.

Audit Commission, 1993. Children first. A study of hospital services. HMSO, London.

Bowlby, J., 1951. Maternal care and mental health. World Health Organization monograph. Series No. 2. WHO, Geneva.

British Association for Community Child Health (BAACH), 1995. Child health rights, implementing the UN convention on the rights of the child within the National Health Service. A practitioner's guide. BAACH, London.

Caring for Children in the Health Service (CCHS), 1987. Where are the children? NAWCH, London.

Caring for Children in the Health Service (CCHS), 1988. Parents staying overnight in hospital with their children. NAWCH, London.

Caring for Children in the Health Service (CCHS), 1991. Just for the day. NAWCH, London.

Caring for Children in the Health Service (CCHS), Thornes R, 1993. Bridging the gaps. Action for Sick Children, London.

Carter, B., 2002. Health inequalities: a blight on children's lives and futures. Journal of Child Health Care 6 (1), 4–6.

Charles-Edwards, I., Glasper, E.A., 2002. Ethics and children's rights: learning from past mistakes. British Journal of Nursing 11 (17), 1132–1140.

Clothier, C., MacDonald, C.A., Shaw, D.A., 1994. The Allitt inquiry: independent inquiry relating to the deaths and injuries on the children's ward at Grantham and Kesteven General Hospital during the period February to April 1991. HMSO, London.

Committee of the Central Health Services Council, 1959. The welfare of children in hospital (Platt Report). HMSO, London.

Committee on Child Health Services, 1976. Fit for the future. HMSO, London.

Department for Education and Skills (DfES), 2003. Every child matters. The Stationery Office, London.

Department of Health (DoH), 1989. The Children Act. An introductory guide for the NHS Health Publications Unit. HMSO, London.

Department of Health (DoH), 1991. The welfare of children and young people in hospital. HMSO, London.

Department of Health (DoH), 1996. The patient's charter – services for children and young people. HMSO, London.

Department of Health (DoH) 1997a Government response to the reports of the House of Commons Health Committee on health services for children and young people, session 1996-97: The specific health needs of children and young people (307-1); Health services for children and young people in the community, home and school (314-1); Hospital services for children and young people (128-1); Child and adolescent mental health services (26-1). DoH, London

Department of Health (DoH), 1997b. A bridge to the future, nursing standards, education and workforce planning in paediatric intensive care. Report of the Chief Nursing Officer's task force. DoH, London

Department of Health (DoH), 1998. Independent inquiry into inequalities in health report (chairman Sir Donald Acheson). The Stationery Office, London.

Department of Health (DoH), 1999. Convention on the rights of the child. Second report to the UN on the rights of the child by the United Kingdom 1999. Executive Summary. DoH, London.

Department of Health (DoH), 2000. The NHS plan: a plan for investment, a plan for reform. The Stationery Office, London.

Department of Health (DoH), 2001a. The Royal Liverpool children's inquiry: summary and recommendations. The Stationery Office, London

Department of Health (DoH), 2001b. The report of the public inquiry into children's heart surgery at the Bristol Royal Infirmary 1984-1995. Learning from Bristol. DoH, London

Department of Health (DoH), 2001c. Essence of care. DoH, London

Department of Health (DoH), 2003. Tackling health inequalities. A programme for action. Online. Available at: http://www.doh.gov.uk/healthinequalities/programmeforaction [accessed 20 September 2004].

Department of Health (DoH), 2004. The right start: the National Service Framework for children, young people and maternity services. Online. Available at: http://www.doh.gov/childrenstaskforce

Department of Health and Social Security (DHSS), 1980. The Black report: inequalities in health. HMSO, London.

Dyer, C., 1994. Inquiry into serial killer criticises hospital's response. British Medical Journal 308 (6927), 491.

Glasper, E.A., 2001. Nurses must enhance care in the wake of Bristol. British Journal of Nursing 10 (15), 966.

Glasper, E.A., Campbell, S., 1994. Beyond the Clothier inquiry. Nursing Standard 8 (23), 18–19.

Glasper, E.A., Cooper, M., 1999. Hospitals need specialist inpatient adolescent units. British Journal of Nursing 8 (9), 549.

Glasper, E.A., Powell, C., 2000. Children deserve better. British Journal of Health Care Management 6 (1), 3.

Glasper, E.A., Powell, C., 2001. Lessons of Alder Hey: consent must be informed. British Journal of Nursing 10 (4), 213.

Gunn, C., 2001. A practical guide to complaints handling. In the context of clinical governance. Churchill Livingstone, Edinburgh.

Ham, C., 1999. Health policy in Britain, 4th edn. Macmillan, Basingstoke.

House of Commons Health Committee, 1997. Third report: health services for children and young people in the community, home and school. The Stationery Office, London.

Lord Laming 2003 The Victoria Climbie inquiry: report of an inquiry by Lord Laming. The Victoria Climbie Inquiry. Online. Available at: http://www.victoria-climbie-inquiry.org.uk/finreport/finreport.htm

National Assembly for Wales, 2002. A review of safeguards for children and young people treated and cared for by the NHS in Wales. Too serious a thing. The Carlile review. The National Assembly of Wales, Cardiff.

NHS Executive, 1996. Child health in the community: a guide to good practice. DoH, London.

NHS Executive 1998 Health service circular, children's safeguards review: choosing with care. HSC 1998/212. DoH, London. Online. Available at: http://www.open.gov.uk/doh/coinh.htm

Nightingale, F., 1863. Notes on hospitals, 3rd edn. Longmans Green and Co., London.

Powell, C., 2003. Lessons to be learnt from the Victoria Climbie inquiry. British Journal of Nursing 12 (3), 137.

Robertson, J., 1962. Hospitals and children, a parent's eye view. Victor Gollanz, London.

Royal College of Nursing (RCN), 1994. The care of sick children. A review of the guidelines in the wake of the Allitt Inquiry. RCN, London.

Royal College of Paediatrics and Child Health (RCPCH), 2003. Bridging the Gaps: Health Care for Adolescents. RCPCH, London.

Tucker, A., 2002. Sir Douglas Black. The Guardian (Public health) Saturday 14 September 2002

University of London, 1955. An account of hospital admissions in the pre-school period. Joint Committee of The Institute of Child Health, Society of Medical Officers of Health and Population Investigation Committee. University of London, London.

Utting, W., 1997. People like us: the report of the review of safeguards for children living away from home. The Stationery Office, London.

Viner, R., Keane, M., 1998. Youth matters: evidence-based best practice for the care of young people in hospital. Action For Sick Children, London.

Cultural aspects of children's nursing

4

Jim Richardson

ABSTRACT

The primary aim of this chapter and its companion PowerPoint presentation is to explore the ideas of culture, its importance and how these ideas can be applied in everyday practice. By paying due regard to cultural factors when nursing children and families, we can help to ensure that nursing care is personalised and sensitive. Practical strategies for integrating ideas of culture into children's nursing will be introduced. An important element of the chapter is to encourage readers to consider how their own cultural expectations and assumptions might affect their professional decision making and actions.

LEARNING OUTCOMES

- Explore aspects of your own personal culture and the impact these might have on your professional interactions.
- Express what culture means as a term and appreciate the importance of taking culture into account in children's nursing work.
- Recognise what aspects of children's, and their families', responses are determined by their cultural background.
- Identify strategies for using ideas of culture in everyday children's nursing activity.
- Explore the dimensions of cultural safety.

What is culture?

It seems difficult to pin down precisely what we mean by 'culture', although the term is in frequent use. The word contains shades of meaning that include 'race' or 'nationality'; we now talk of multicultural Britain and transcultural nursing. Equally, culture can be taken to mean the creative product of a society such as literature, music, etc.

An examination of what idea of culture this chapter is offering should help to clarify terms from the outset. The Nursing Council of New Zealand (2002 p 3) defines culture quite simply: 'culture refers to the beliefs and practices common to any particular group.'

Helman (2000 p 2) expands on this:

> Culture is … a set of guidelines … which an individual inherits as a member of a particular society and which tells him/her how to view the world and learn how to behave in relation to other people. It also provides him/her with a way of transmitting these guidelines to the next generation.

Helman (2000) goes on to explain that culture can be seen as an acquired lens through which we see the world. This is a useful analogy because culture can be seen in this way as a sort of filter through which our experience of the world passes and which helps us to interpret it. From these definitions some characteristics of culture can be teased out:

- Culture is learned – therefore, it is acquired. Children primarily learn their culture within the family and immediate community. Later, school life and peers contribute to the growing cultural sense of the child. In fact, it might be said that it is beliefs deriving from culture that dictate how we respond to children and our child-rearing practices.
- It is logical, then, that culture is passed from generation to generation. Some aspects of culture seem to change readily between generations (we don't tend to think or behave exactly as our parents or grandparents do!). On the other hand, once we have learned and internalised our cultural norms we might well be quite resistant to any change in these.
- Culture is dynamic – it changes while being passed between the generations (the generation gap). It might also change in response to the time, place and conditions within which a cultural group live.
- Culture helps us to identify the group to which we belong. By extension, it can help us to identify groups to which we do not belong. This can provide a potential source of a sense of solidarity within our group but can also be the origin of friction between groups.

DOI: 10.1016/B978-0-7020-3183-0.10004-9

- Culture helps to identify core beliefs. This can include religious belief and spiritual responses. This aspect can be fundamentally important to people during periods of change, stress or crisis, for example, when a child is sick. This aspect of culture can also determine how people interpret health and ill-health, the causes of ill-health and which treatments should be used.
- Culture helps to define our core values. Culture influences us in how we judge what is 'right' and what is 'wrong' for example.
- Culture has a role to play in the development of our life habits and customs – the way we behave and dress, as well as the food that we eat, are determined by culture. How many of us, in times of stress or tiredness, prefer to eat familiar comforting food from our childhood?
- Culture gives us a pattern for living, it can give us a template for how to respond to crises and difficulties in everyday life.
- Culture is important to us because it dictates how we interpret and respond to the world around us. Without particularly reflecting on this, it can dictate our judgements on the views and actions of others. We tend to regard our own way as correct and might view others as being wrong on the basis of this. For professional people like children's nurses this tendency might seriously affect the quality of our relationships with those we work with.
- Culture is thoroughly internalised. Having learned our culture in childhood, it is an integral part of ourselves and largely subconscious. When we encounter new situations we tend to see them through our cultural 'lens' and make rapid judgements, sometimes without much further thought.

These definitions can be seen to be broad. They indicate that culture is a feature of a wide variety of different groups (Wilkins 1993). One of the bugbears of using cultural ideas in nursing in the past has been the tendency to see culture as being confined to ethnicity. Of course, ethnic groups can be seen as cultural groups but so too can a range of other groups who share beliefs, values and customs. By extension, it is easy then to say that cultural issues concern us all. If we confine our inquiry about cultural aspects to other ethnic groups then we run the risk of not considering our own cultural responses.

If we continue in the vein of considering culture broadly we create the opportunity of seeing a range of cultural groups that we might not otherwise see. It might even be argued that some of the perceived differences in beliefs and behaviours between men and women are based on cultural norms.

Activity

Suggest a range of cultural groups that might not necessarily be based on ethnicity.

If we look at groups based on shared beliefs, values and customs on the list you compiled during the above activity we might find:

- Groups based on age, e.g. the elderly and youth might be seen as cultural or subcultural groups because, although they largely share a world-view with society as a whole, they also have distinctive, slightly different perspectives from the majority.
- Groups based on regional origin, e.g. those originating from the north or the south of England, those from the Midlands and those from the south west all carry with them distinct characteristics of groups from their home region. This is clearly illustrated when someone moves from their home region and is struck by the strange habits of the natives of their new home area.

Activity

- Stretch your imagination a little further and try to think of other areas that could be defined as cultural. An interesting perspective from the point of view of the children's nurse might be a suggestion that subcultures might be formed within the healthcare field.
- Consider, with a view to the definitions of culture given earlier, to what extent children's nurses might form a (sub) cultural group.

If we accept that nurses form a cultural group with a body of shared beliefs, values and customs then, by extension, children and their families do not belong to that group. It will often be observed that 'experienced' mothers – that is mothers whose child's health concerns have brought them into frequent contact with healthcare professionals – often seem to have learned the 'rules' of the culture of the healthcare world, including its language. One parent of a child in hospital observed to me that you could always tell 'experienced' mothers on a hospital ward; they are the ones who always have a packet of biscuits in their handbag!

It makes sense that parents unfamiliar with the healthcare context might find themselves bemused by the unspoken expectations and rules of the healthcare encounter. It is well documented that implementation of child and family care has been complicated by parents feeling uncertain about quite what is expected of them and not being clear about the unwritten 'rules' (Coyne 1995, Darbyshire 1994, Valentine 1998).

Activity

- Think of a family you have cared for who is deemed by healthcare professionals to be 'difficult'.
- To what extent do you think that cultural factors, e.g. beliefs, values and customs common to a group, might have been implicated in this situation?

Examples like this illustrate how cultural misunderstandings or lack of insight can hamper collaborative work or even, in extreme cases, form the basis of conflict situations. From this it can be seen how important culture can be as a factor in the everyday work of children's nurses (Andrews 1995).

Much of what you will read about cultural aspects of health care will appear to contradict this broad reading of what culture is. Many authorities will interpret culture as almost being synonymous with ethnicity. So when commentators describe Britain as being a multicultural society they often mean a multiethnic society. It must be emphasised that the broad reading of what culture is does not negate in any sense the importance of ethnicity in health and social care. Ethnicity is a significant aspect of cultural care issues and caring for children from different ethnic groups often raises very clear cultural questions (Whiting 1999).

www

Find more material about ethnicity and health on the Department of Health website:

- http://www.dh.gov.uk

One of the problems of considering cultural aspects of culture in children's nursing is that it can often seem very abstract, and this is often not helped by the complex, sometimes even obscure, language used to describe cultural concepts (Ahmann 1994). Considering some of these ideas in more detail can be useful in illustrating how facets of cultural thinking can be useful in the everyday, practical world.

Ethnocentrism

Although this word appears fearsome it simply describes the situation where we consider our own personal cultural world-view to be correct in all its detail. As we learn our culture from an early age – an important fact for children's nurses to bear in mind – it tends to be a deeply ingrained part of us. We do not usually consciously consider it when we are making judgements about our experiences. In this way our culture can be compared with Helman's lens, through which we filter everything that happens to us and colours our reaction to these experiences. Anyone who wears glasses will be aware of how quickly you become unaware of the glasses themselves when viewing the world around you.

Activity

Think of a situation in which you have disapproved of something that someone else has said or done. Can you think of why you reacted in this way?

Because the cultural lens, or yardstick, against which you measure your experiences is often virtually subliminal it can form the basis of the 'gut reaction'. Think of how you would feel if you went to eat at a friend's and were offered an unfamiliar or exotic food, such as snake, to eat. Your reaction would be based on your cultural concept of appropriate food to eat, which you learned in childhood. Of course, some of us are more daring and adventurous than others so you might enjoy the opportunity to sample snake! This same kind of 'it's not my way' reaction can occur to any aspect of other people's behaviour. A few years ago I was involved in caring for the child in the scenario below. You can see that it is difficult sometimes to be clear as to quite why we react to situations in the way that we do – this is culture in action.

Scenario

Five-year-old Rachel is being cared for following a traumatic fracture of her left femur. She is confined to bed on balanced traction. She is disorientated by what is happening and is often quite tearful. Her mother breastfeeds her in the morning and when she is settling to sleep in the evening. Many of the nurses on the ward are quite shocked by this.

Activity

- Consider why the nurses might be feeling shocked in this situation?
- What might be the effect of their reacting in this way?

Ethnocentrism could be argued to be a part of all of us and will lead to us responding positively to those with whom we share a culture (Sprott 1994). The other side of the coin is that we can respond negatively to people whose culture orientation leads them to behave or to value things that we do not. Clearly, we do not always demonstrate our reactions to others (nurses traditionally strive not to be judgemental) but it is all too easy for our reactions – positive or negative – to be communicated through channels such as body language. If we disapprove of someone's behaviour, which is based on their cultural orientation, and they become aware of our disapproval then that could have a seriously negative effect on our working together if this occurs in a professional setting. Equally, we might be led to condone behaviours that are culturally acceptable to us but that are not entirely constructive. Alcohol use among young people is widely acceptable within that age group within this community and is often talked of in a 'jokey' fashion.

Ethnocentrism is a natural part of us but it is particularly important for children's nurses to reflect on how it leads us to respond and behave in our work with children and families. Children are especially vulnerable to cultural disapproval because they are learning their family's and community's culture (Chevannes 1997). During this learning process their cultural self might be fragile and vulnerable to the disapproval or scorn of others. Cultural disrespect is potentially damaging. In this way, it can be seen how ethnocentrism can form the basis for prejudice, be it positive or negative. The process of reflecting on our cultural reactions based on ethnocentrism can help to improve our personal self-awareness and help avoid many harmful effects.

www

A range of materials relating to cultural factors in children's nursing along with some exercises can be found on the Royal College of Nursing's website at:

- http://www.rcn.org/resources/transcultural

Scenario

Three-month-old Matty, who was born at 34 weeks' gestation and had a very stormy start to his life, was recently discharged home into the care of his parents and big sister. He has come to outpatients with his mother and 6-year-old sister, Adele. Adele is bored and frustrated with the wait and has just been involved in a noisy disagreement with another child. Her mother reacts strongly and smacks her several times on the legs.

Activity

- How do you feel about children being smacked by their parents?
- To what extent would you think that your views are culturally based?
- What kinds of messages do you give to those you disagree with on this question?

Any discussion about such matters is likely to generate a deal of heat. It could be suggested that this is because such views are often determined by cultural values. The perspective we adopt in relation to such issues is ethnocentric; anyone agreeing with us is right and anyone disagreeing is wrong. Such automatically and unthinkingly assumed polar positions are unhelpful. It could be said that self-awareness is largely cultural self-awareness.

Stereotyping

Stereotyping is a close cousin of ethnocentrism. It can be defined as assuming cultural characteristics of a person (without asking them!) based on our perception of the group that they belong to. An example of this might be when a nurse first meets the father of a child in his or her care. The father is wearing a turban. What does the nurse think? If the reaction is stereotypical it might run something like this:

> Oh, Mr S is a Sikh. I have nursed Sikh people before, they like to do A, B and C and they don't like D, E and F.

Although these assumptions might be correct, they could equally well be quite wrong. People within cultural groups will naturally have individual and subgroup variations. Even within cohesive groups we do not share identical beliefs, values and customs. You need only listen to the sorts of debates that go on around the time of national elections to appreciate this. It is unhelpful to 'pigeonhole' people on the basis of assumed characteristics. The only way to know about people's culturally determined beliefs and habits is to ask them!

Culture shock

Another feature of our cultural understandings being learnt early in life, deeply ingrained and often subconsciously acted on is that we can rely on shared understandings and assumptions when we are within our cultural group. This is a comfortable, secure position to be in. However, if we move outside our group then we can no longer rely on these mutual interpretations. This can feel very disorientating. You might have noticed this when on holiday abroad; it is irritating when people do not do as you expect them to, for example, queue in an orderly fashion in a post office! A South-East Asian refugee to the United States expressed his feeling of culture shock as feeling like a goat in a herd of cows! This is a vivid illustration of how culture shock can make you feel almost visibly different from those around you. Our shared understandings within our own cultural group include many unwritten rules. Everyone in that environment understands and feels comfortable with these conventions; anyone new to the context is likely to feel discomfited.

Activity

Consider your feelings when you first arrived in a clinical area that was quite different from anything you had experienced before, e.g. intensive care unit or operating theatre:

- What were your predominant feelings at that time?
- To what extent do you feel that these reactions were based on culture shock?

Return again to your reflection on the family you thought about in the earlier activity who were considered by healthcare professionals as difficult:

- Do you recognise any features of culture shock in that situation?

It could be argued that the parents of a sick child experience a degree of culture shock when they come into contact with the hospital environment and healthcare professionals. Parents, and patients, often find it difficult to know what is expected of them and the rules that healthcare professionals expect them to abide by. This situation is not helped when children's nurses assume that parents have this knowledge and understanding. More open communication and clarity would go some way towards alleviating the discomfort and stress of culture shock.

Cultural assessment

To be able to use all of these ideas in relation to culture it will be useful to examine a framework of cultural assessment. There are several of these (e.g. Giger & Davidhizar 1995, Purnell & Paulanka 1998, Tripp Reimer et al 1984) and they generally do not vary greatly in terms of content. However, some are more practical than others in terms of clarity and ease of use in practice. Giger & Davidhizar (1995) offer a framework with six dimensions:

1. communication
2. space
3. social organisation
4. time
5. environmental control
6. biological variation.

Giger & Davidhizar believe that each of these dimensions describes an area of human life that is universal, i.e. shared by all cultures, although there might be significant variation between cultural groups. Taken together, these universal dimensions illustrate the major culturally determined differences between people. Therefore, if we use them as a system of assessment for cultural differences then we should identify and capture those issues in the care encounter that require culture sensitivity and understanding.

Communication

Communication is generally agreed to be a central part of the children's nurse's function. Communication is starkly illustrated as an issue when the nurse and patient/family speak different languages. However, it can be just as important when factors such as professional jargon or language that is too complex for the child to understand are used. Often, non-verbal communication is particularly challenging between people from different cultural backgrounds. Gestures carry different meanings in different groups and cultural norms, such as the use of eye contact, can vary a good deal. For some, avoiding eye contact, particularly with authority figures, is seen as simply polite; others would interpret this as shifty behaviour.

Social organisations

How we relate to each other as individuals and groups is strongly culture related. As they grow, children learn how to relate to their elders and parents. This can take the form of small children learning 'good manners', although what constitutes good manners changes over time and between cultural groups. That children should be 'seen and not heard' is not a value promoted in Western cultures today, but it is still a guiding principle for some groups. Similarly, some adults look askance on children behaving exuberantly in a public place, whereas for some groups it is to be positively encouraged. The respective roles adopted by men and women within communities and family groups are also determined largely by cultural norms.

Time

This dimension is important in children's nursing because it takes children a good deal of effort to understand this abstract notion. Small children can struggle with the idea of 'tomorrow' or 'at 2 o'clock'. Some groups value punctuality whereas some are very much less concerned with this. Some cultures have a future orientation (study hard for your exams and you'll get to university then you'll get a good job) and others are more past oriented (what do you want to go to university for? No one in our family ever has done so before). Others again might be present oriented and see the future as impossible to predict, whereas the past is gone and irrelevant. Each of those positions can influence how children and families react to misfortune or ill health.

Environmental control

The variation between groups in terms of how they perceive their ability to affect events in their environment and lives is contained in this dimension. This will affect how they interpret the reason for events, e.g. why a child becomes unwell, what causes this and what should be done about it. Therefore, it will dictate what should be done if a child has, for example, a fever; perhaps nothing will be done – just wait and see – perhaps a drug (e.g. paracetamol) will be given, perhaps the child will be taken to a doctor or to consult a folk healer.

Biological control

This is a very important dimension for nurses because it links to the variations seen under the environmental control category. Factors related to our place and group of origin are aspects of our cultural beliefs and customs in relation to life events. Rituals and required behaviours in the face of difficult challenges are affected by differences between cultures and these are often reflected in religious belief and practice. Dietary aspects also appear in this category – the foods we prefer and the effects we believe foods have on our bodies and health.

Activity

Running through these categories, make a list of factors you and your family/community consider to be important in each dimension, e.g. for the time dimension, do you consider punctuality to be important? Why?

Taking all of these factors together we can begin to get a picture of how complex, subtle and difficult to reveal and analyse cultural factors can be. However, it is not a hopeless picture! There are several approaches to working with cultural aspects in child health care. One is the promotion of cultural safety through self-awareness. This is an attractive idea because, as children's nurses, we seek to ensure the safety and well-being of the children and families in our care. In the past, culture was often not emphasised as a factor in nursing care and the potential for care to be culturally unsafe was considerable. This would occur when the beliefs, values and customs of children were ignored, or even worse scorned. Cultural safety is an orientation with an element of reaction to some previous attempts at developing transcultural nursing models. Some of these, although well meaning, tended to emphasise differences between groups by examining what were sometimes exotically different groups (e.g. the weaning habits of Tibetan yak herders). These also ran the risk of stereotyping people (e.g. all Tibetan yak herders wean their babies at the same age and in the same way). Cultural safety does not concentrate on learning a shopping list of factors that identify a cultural group. Rather, within this framework the children's nurse works to achieve an understanding of her/his own cultural values. This reflection would also consider the nature of power within the nurse–child/family relationship. Obviously, if the nurse is basing professional and personal judgements on personal values, and also holds power in relation to the child and family, then the results could at best be non-constructive and at worst destructive.

Cultural safety consists of a set of ideas that have been evolving for some time in the social sciences and nursing. It is perhaps at its most developed in New Zealand. The context in New Zealand is particular; it is a postcolonial nation where the majority is descended from white European immigrants and the significant minority from the original inhabitants – the Maori. The last three decades of the 20th century saw a wide-ranging debate in New Zealand as to why outcomes for the Maori are worse on almost every dimension – and particularly in health – than for New Zealanders of European origin. The conclusion reached was that cultural oppression was a significant factor in this situation and solutions sought. The key features of cultural safety are (Nursing Council of New Zealand 2002 p 7):

> The effective nursing or midwifery practice of a person or family from another culture, is determined by that person or family. Culture includes, but is not restricted to age or generation; gender; sexual orientation; occupation and socioeconomic status; ethnic origin or migrant experience; religious or spiritual belief; and disability.
>
> The nurse or midwife delivering the nursing or midwifery service will have undertaken a process of reflection on his or her own cultural identity and will recognise the impact that his or her personal culture has on his or her professional practice. Unsafe cultural practice comprises any action which diminishes, demeans or disempowers the cultural identity and wellbeing of an individual.

Cultural safety in this system is based on each nurse gaining a knowledge and understanding of his or her own cultural values rather than trying to learn aspects of the culture of other groups (which runs the risk in any case of being stereotypical). Cultural safety can be said to be achieved when each child/family receives care that is based on all that makes them individual and unique. This can only be defined by those who are receiving that care.

It is not a major leap to appreciating that if this is achieved then the respect, trust and effective communication will be in place on which to base a constructive helping relationship. The Nursing Council New Zealand (2002) proposes a series of stages in learning to integrate culture into care:

- Cultural awareness: simply understanding that people differ on the basis of learnt beliefs and values.
- Cultural sensitivity: acknowledging that these differences are legitimate and gaining awareness of one's own cultural norms and how these might affect others.
- Cultural safety: the care delivered is culturally safe as defined by those receiving care.

Clearly, this represents a theoretical framework that could be further legitimated by testing through research. However, it does offer a number of very thought-provoking insights. It emphasises that culture will be an issue in most caring encounters and that skill in working with cultural aspects will be fundamental for all nurses.

WWW

Read more about the idea of cultural safety on the website of the Nursing Council of NewZealand:

- http://www.nursingcouncil.nz

Consideration of cultural safety practices in care delivery offers the opportunity to develop care skills which are culturally safe and satisfying within a context of child centred care. The following skills will be required to achieve this:

- *Reflection* – this allows the children's nurse to consider themselves as players in care interactions, to learn from positive experiences and to use negative experience to improve future performance.
- *Communication* – this is the key to achieving cultural safety. People who feel undervalued on the basis of their culture may well find it impossible to communicate with some they feel has more power and authority than they do. All elements of communication used within interactions need to be taken into account particularly the non-verbal. It will be important to create an environment and atmosphere conducive to open communication.
- *Use of fundamental values* – care interactions must be based on respect, dignity and kindness.
- *Empathy* – attempting to appreciate the nature another person's viewpoint and experience of a situation or interaction.
- *Motivation* – the desire and commitment to ensuring that care is culturally sensitive and safe.
- *Quality-driven* – the wish to ensure that, in every dimension, care is of the highest quality possible.
- *Leadership* – to define the significance and importance of culturally safe care and to identify a process to lead others through a process of implementing such practices (De & Richardson 2008).

Summary

Culture can be argued to be a significant factor in nursing work and there have been several approaches for nurses to develop their knowledge and skills in this arena. Culture is defined widely as being a characteristic of the beliefs and practices of a wide range of groups, which might include:

- age or generation
- gender
- sexual orientation
- occupation and socioeconomic status
- ethnic origin or immigrant experience
- religious or spiritual belief
- disability.

Taking cultural aspects into account is especially important for children's nurses because of the special and particular nature of children. Because culture is a learnt phenomenon that occurs during childhood, then children will be active learners of their own culture at the time of the care encounter. As a person's individual culture is incompletely learnt until later in childhood, then the child might be at risk of confusion and distress if disrespect is shown towards his or her culturally determined beliefs, values and customs. As active learners of culture, children might also be confused by encountering cultural norms that are at variance with those they are in the process of learning at home and within their community. Failure to take culture into account might result in a discriminatory, insensitive and inappropriate attempt at care, which is bound to fail.

References

Ahmann, E., 1994. 'Chunky stew': appreciating cultural diversity while providing health care for children. Pediatric Nursing 29 (3), 320–324.

Andrews, M.M., 1995. Transcultural perspectives in the nursing care of children and adolescents. In: Andrews, M.M., Boyle, J.S. (Eds.), Transcultural concepts in nursing care, Lippincott, Philadelphia JB.

Chevannes, M., 1997. Nursing care for families – issues in a multicultural society. British Journal of Nursing 6, 161–167.

Coyne, I., 1995. Parental participation in care: a critical review of the literature. Journal of Advanced Nursing 21, 716–722.

Darbyshire, P., 1994. Living with a sick child in hospital: the experiences of parents and nurses. Chapman & Hall, London.

De, D., Richardson, J., 2008. Cultural safety: an introduction. Paediatric Nursing 20 (2), 39–43.

Giger, J.N., Davidhazar, R.E., 1995. Transcultural nursing, 3rd edn. Mosby Year Book, St Louis.

Helman, C.G., 2000. Culture, health and illness, 4th edn. Butterworth Heinemann, Oxford.

Nursing Council of New Zealand, 2002. Guidelines for cultural safety, the treaty of Waitangi and Maori health in nursing and midwifery education and practice. Nursing Council of New Zealand, Wellington.

Purnell, L.D., Paulanka, B.J., 1998. Transcultural healthcare. FA Davis, Philadelphia.

Sprott, J.E., 1994. One person's 'spoiling' is another's freedom to become: overcoming ethnocentric views about parental control. Social Sciences and Medicine 38 (8), 1111–1124.

Tripp-Reimer, T., Brink, P.J., Saunders, J.M., 1984. Cultural assessment: convert and process. Nursing Outlook 32 (2), 78–82.

Valentine, F., 1998. Empowerment: family centred care. Paediatric Nursing 10 (1), 24–27.

Whiting, L., 1999. Caring for children of differing cultures. Journal of Child Health Care 3 (4), 33–37.

Wilkins, H., 1993. Transcultural nursing: a selective review of the literature 1985–1991. Journal of Advanced Nursing 18 (4), 606–612.

The psychological preparation of children for hospitalisation

5

E Alan Glasper   Rachel E A Haggarty

ABSTRACT

Historical and contemporary work identifies that children have fears and anxieties when they are admitted to hospital. After examining the rationale for such anxieties and potential consequences, this chapter concentrates on the various ways in which professionals can help children prepare for and cope with their hospital experience. The role of parents/carers is also identified and questions raised as to the specific needs of children with learning difficulties, communication impairment and chronic illness. Finally, the importance of ongoing staff education is noted.

LEARNING OUTCOMES

- Appreciate why hospitals/healthcare institutions may be a source of anxiety for sick children.
- Explore a typical preadmission programme and discuss the pros and cons of such preparation.
- Describe the full range of interventions and distraction techniques used by children's nurses to allay anxiety preadmission and preprocedurally.
- Understand the ways in which parents/carers can contribute to the preparation of children for hospital procedures, and consider the educational support that parents/carers require.
- Describe how emergency admissions/non-attendees to programmes can be prepared for hospital interventions.
- Consider the specific preparation needs of children with learning difficulties, communication impairment and chronic illness.
- Recognise the importance of ongoing education for healthcare professionals involved in preparing children and families for hospitalisation.

Introduction

This chapter considers issues surrounding the emotional well-being of the sick child, and the psychological preparation of children for hospitalisation. Saile et al (1988 p 109) define psychological preparation as:

> ... any planned strategy used by a professional or trained helper on a child or his family with the purpose of reducing anxiety related to medical procedures, decreasing pain, accelerating the healing process and making it possible for the child to cope adequately with the procedure.

The latter half of the 20th century, and indeed the first few years of the 21st, saw growing recognition within paediatric nursing of the potentially harmful effects that may result from children's hospitalisation. A range of initiatives have been implemented to minimise such harmful effects, including parental participation in care, play specialists, shorter inpatient stays, preadmission preparation programmes and the development of more 'child friendly' hospital environments. It is therefore important that the child health practitioner has a sound understanding of these issues, and of the historical background to these initiatives.

Historical perspectives

The original founders of the UK children's hospitals, which were built during the reign of Queen Victoria, were primarily motivated by the alleviation of the physical elements of illness during childhood. Children's nurses of the past might not always have embraced the concept of family-centred care in the same way as contemporary nurses; this was perhaps a reflection of the poor understanding of the psychological aspects of health and illness prevalent at that time. Despite this, the maxim of the first of these Victorian edifices, the Hospital for Sick Children in London, is 'the child first and always' (Glasper & Charles-Edwards 2002). Indeed, during the 18th century, Dr George Armstrong is credited as being highly influential in delaying the opening of tertiary inpatient facilities for children in London, suggesting that children and their parents should not be separated as doing so would break

DOI: 10.1016/B978-0-7020-3183-0.10005-0

the child's heart (Miles 1986). He believed that parents would not be able to look after their children in hospital because of economic pressures (Glasper & Lowson 1998). However, in reality the appalling sanitary conditions, the overcrowding and the general poverty prevalent at that time ensured that the little care available in the home was also often of a poor quality (Kosky & Lunnon 1991).

It should be remembered that the early children's hospitals were built in the pre-Nightingale era and before the professionalisation of nursing. The Nightingale tradition subtly changed the dynamics of the children's hospitals, and military principles developed by Nightingale in the Crimea began to be applied. The move away from essentially lay care and the development of professional paediatric nursing had some disadvantages, namely the gradual exclusion of parents from the direct participation in care. So although there is evidence from historical drawings of the first ward at Great Ormond Street that parents were able to be with their children in hospital and participate in their care, the military changes eventually resulted in the establishment of strict visiting hours, with parents prohibited from visiting at a time convenient to them. Some hospitals allowed parents to visit only once a week or less often.

Bed rest for children until the advent of antibiotics was long and continuous and the screams and incessant crying bouts that accompanied each weekly visit convinced the nursing staff that parents were generally a hindrance rather than a help. Eventually, parents were perceived to be such an infection risk that some hospitals abandoned visiting altogether. Relatives were therefore often excluded because they were likely harbingers of disease and, perhaps more importantly, potential disturbers of the smoothness of long-established ward routines. The visiting times in many children's hospitals were severely restricted. In the Southampton Children's Hospital, for example, at least up until the outbreak of the First World War, visiting was allowed from 2 to 4 p.m. daily, except Sundays. As the century progressed, it became confined to 1 hour on Wednesday and Sunday afternoons, and then in 1947 was banned completely. Visiting was recommenced in 1950 on a limited basis and parents had to wear face masks. Indeed, looking at the UK as a whole, of the 1300 hospitals in Britain in 1951 that admitted children, only 300 allowed daily visiting (usually limited to 30 minutes) and 150 prohibited visiting altogether (Robertson 1989). The white-coated doctors and the starchly uniformed nurses who were so confident about the rightness of traditional practice often intimidated parents and were inaccessible for discussion. There was little in the curricula of either profession on the emotional aspects of childhood and it was not until after the Second World War that the real detrimental effects of early hospital admission became widely recognised.

There were, however, some enlightened paediatricians who had begun to make observations on the detrimental effects on personality development of institutional care. Sir James Spence, Professor of Child Health at the University of Newcastle's Royal Victoria Hospital, began to allow mothers to stay in hospital with infants and young children, although he did not extend this service to older children (RCPCH 2000).

The recognition that psychological trauma might be perpetrated on children during their hospital stay came about slowly, and in the UK owes much to the work of John Bowlby and James Robertson. Their work was instrumental in providing the precursors necessary for the creation of a much more family-focused approach to the care of hospitalised children.

Theory of attachment

John Bowlby was a London-based psychiatrist who developed a particular interest in developmental psychology. He described the concept of attachment as a tendency of the young to stay in close proximity to the primary care giver, usually the mother in the first instance, and to be comforted by her sight, sound and touch (Gleitman 1986). Bowlby commenced volunteer work with maladjusted children in a residential setting and his lifetime interest in attachment was stimulated through his experience of working with an affectionless teenager who had no familiarity with a permanent mother figure (Bretherton 2002). The century of childhood nursing practice in which parental roles had virtually disappeared was about to change in the light of his work.

Bowlby was heavily influenced by the science of ethology (the study of animal behaviour) and in particular the work of Konrad Lorenz, who first postulated the theory of imprinting in young greylag geese chicks (Gleitman 1986, PSI Café 2002). The process of imprinting is believed to occur in many animals but is graphically evident in animals such as geese or ducks when, shortly after hatching, the chicks form a strong attachment to whatever moving object they see in their line of vision. In the wild this is normally the mother but Lorenz and others substituted natural mothers with moving inanimate objects, such as rubber boots worn by the researchers. Once imprinted, the chicks follow the object wherever it goes throughout their early life.

Bowlby believed that a similar process occurred in human babies and he referred to this as attachment (Rutherford 1998). The crux of Bowlby's theory is that all human infants need to attach to their mothers (or primary caregiver) if they are to develop into healthy, well-adjusted adults. Furthermore he described the concept of 'bonding' as the mother's emotional attachment to the child (Rutherford 1998, Taylor et al 1999). This important process is put at risk by any form of separation between mother and infant. In 1951 Bowlby published a World Health Organization monograph entitled 'Maternal care and mental health', in which he began to articulate the adverse effects on personality development of inadequate maternal care. From this date the tide began to turn, albeit slowly.

Two famous quotations from the WHO monograph still have a resounding impact on contemporary health care, despite the fact that they were published over half a century ago:

> It is essential for mental health that the infant and young child should experience a warm, intimate and continuous relationship with his mother (or mother substitute) in which to find satisfaction and enjoyment.
>
> Motherlove in infancy and childhood is as important for mental health as are vitamins and proteins for physical health.

At the same time that Bowlby was developing his ideas about human attachment, a number of other researchers began a series of primate experiments to investigate attachment under controlled laboratory conditions, studies that continue to this day. Harry Harlow and fellow researchers at the primate laboratory at the University of Wisconsin carried out perhaps the best known of these experiments (Harlow 1958). Harlow demonstrated that nurturing was more important than sustenance when motherless infant monkeys raised in cages with surrogate mothers made of wire or soft cloth chose to spend the majority of their time with the cloth version despite the wire version having embedded within it a feeding bottle. It is important to stress that these monkeys grew into totally dysfunctional adults who were unable to function in primate society. There is no doubt that these studies reinforced Bowlby's assertion that bonding was a testable hypothesis.

If Harlow's work complemented that of Bowlby, it also revealed the inadequacies of the experimental monkeys when they in turn became mothers. These maternally deprived monkeys proved to be either indifferent to their offspring or outright abusive. It is salutary to note that continued research within the field of maternal deprivation using infant monkeys is coming under greater scrutiny and criticism (In Defense of Animals 2002). However, although many now condemn the use of monkeys for the study of maternal deprivation it is sad to reflect that there are children today in many parts of the world who are cared for in suboptimum conditions, often without the benefit of a primary care giver. The situation of the orphanage and hospitalised children in Romania, which became apparent to the outside world only after the overthrow of Nicolae Ceausescu in 1989, is a timely reminder of how appallingly treated children are in some parts of the world, particularly in the aftermath of war (Glasper 1999).

Importantly, Bowlby's theories have been much criticised by other academic researchers, such as Rutter (1981), who believe that Bowlby's emphasis on the constant presence of the mother is overexaggerated, and also that other primary caregivers (most notably the father) also had vital roles. Wolkind & Rutter (1985) argued that infants are capable of 'multiple attachments', and furthermore that these relationships are not necessarily dependent on the amount of time spent with child, but rather on the quality of the interaction. Nevertheless, the concept of attachment and bonding remains the basis for good practice in the care of infants.

Maternal deprivation

As part of Bowlby's work to underpin his theory of attachment, he recruited James Robertson as a research associate to record filmed observations of young hospitalised and institutionalised children who had been separated from their mothers. Among these famous films was 'A two-year-old goes to hospital', which followed 'Laura' through her admission and vividly displayed the adverse effects of maternal separation (Thurtle 1998). Subsequent analysis of these data allowed Bowlby and Robertson to further refine and articulate the stages of separation anxiety that occur during maternal deprivation (Robertson 1970):

- **Protest**: This stage can last from a few hours to a few days. The child has a strong conscious need of the mother and the loud crying exhibited is based on the expectation built on previous experience that the mother will respond to his cries. During this stage of the maternal deprivation sequence the child will cry noisily and look eagerly towards any sound that might be the mother.
- **Despair**: This stage succeeds protest and can best be compared to clinical depression. It is a sign of increasing hopelessness and despondency. The child becomes less active and vocal; in the past this was interpreted by the nursing staff as a sign that the child was settling into the ward.
- **Denial/detachment**: In this the final stage of maternal deprivation the child represses his or her longing for the mother and begins to lose his or her attachment. The child appears, at least superficially, to have settled into the hospital routine and will respond positively, if shallowly, to kind adults who take an interest in him or her. Importantly, the child will react badly to brief reappearances of the mother, as for example during the weekly visiting periods, giving rise to the fallacy that parents actually made matters worse. There is no wonder that generations of children's nurses dreaded 'Sunday afternoon visiting'.

Activity

Obtain and view one of the Robertson videos, e.g. 'A two-year-old goes to hospital'

- How does this scenario compare with your experience today? Clearly there are improvements, but are there any areas of similarity?

Robertson's films were to play a crucial role in improving the conditions under which children were cared for in hospital. His work fuelled concern among the public, which was instrumental in compelling the government of the day to launch a White Paper, chaired by Sir Harry Platt, to investigate the plight of children in hospital. The seminal report 'The welfare of children in hospital' was published in 1959 (Committee of the Central Health Services Council 1959) and it was to fundamentally change practice. Although the Platt report showed the way, subsequent reports began to tackle specific areas of childcare in hospital (Thurtle 1998 p 231 and see Chapter 3).

PowerPoint

Access the companion Chapter 1 PowerPoint presentation and look at the Platt report in full. Does this report still have messages for 21st century children's nurses?

Much of the credit for innovatory change must be attributed to the National Association for the Welfare of Children in Hospital (NAWCH), which is now called Action for Sick Children (ASC). NAWCH was originally founded in 1961 as Mother Care for Children in Hospital. With the support of James Robertson, this parental pressure group thrived and began to campaign for the full implementation of the Platt report. Soon, regional groups were convened all over the UK, which eventually amalgamated in 1963 and became the NAWCH in 1965 (ASC 2002). It is important to stress that, although the Platt report was adopted as an official Ministry of Health policy, in the same way that subsequent Department of Health publications are, hospitals were not legally obliged to implement the recommendations. The gauntlet fell to NAWCH, which has since campaigned with considerable success as an advocate for sick children and their families.

Many generations of parents have expressed feelings of helplessness and inadequacy during their child's admission to hospital, when nurses took over care completely. It would be naïve to believe that this situation changed in the immediate aftermath of the publication of the Platt report, as this unhappy state of affairs continued for many years afterwards in some children's units. However, some children's hospitals began to respond to the White Paper in a positive way. The essential message of the document was that hospitals should take steps to reduce separation of parent and sick child (initially only mothers). This was to be achieved by introducing open and unrestricted visiting, providing parental accommodation and avoiding unnecessary hospital admissions. This would ultimately result in a move towards day surgery, but this did not happen immediately.

Daycare services

Politicians of all political parties have described the health services for children as a potent investment in the country's future. Ambulatory care, of which daycare is a central component, provides the minimum of disruption to the family unit, as a result of shorter hospital stays, and is a potentially powerful weapon in the prevention of psychological trauma caused by an inpatient admission. Many hospitals now have purpose-built day units for children. Such units cater for children undergoing minor surgery, medical therapy, investigative procedures or observation (Ireland & Rushforth 1998). Day units function in a variety of ways; some keep patients for a full day before discharge and others only half a day. For day units to run optimally, a paediatric community nursing service is vital to provide an essential link between hospital and home (Atwell & Gow 1985). Without the provision of such services, the management of children undergoing daycare is fraught with difficulties.

Importance of psychological care

Smith (1986) believes that emotional factors might be an even greater source of concern than the child's physical condition during a hospital admission. Although improvements have occurred since the publication of the Platt report, it is important not to be complacent. The many practical tasks and physical needs required by the child and family can, due to time constraints, all too easily dominate the day. It can therefore be easy to lose sight of the child's psychological needs. In a seminal quote, Jolly (1976 p 1532) recorded the words of a 6-year-old child:

> They looked at my throat and they looked at my ears. They looked at my heart but they didn't look at me.

Fear of the unknown, fear of physical harm and pain, loss of control and identity, uncertainty about what is expected of them and separation from security and family routine are identified by Visintainer & Wolfer (1975) as five key potential threats to a child on admission to hospital. Anecdotal evidence suggests that, 30 years later, these fears are no less real. Anxiety may be displayed in some by, for example, regressive behaviour, tearful/fearful mood, sleep disturbance or changes to eating pattern. Everyone, to a greater or lesser degree, will have concerns, questions and apprehensions when they are admitted to hospital; a child is no exception. In addition to this, the way in which children interact with the world and attempt to understand and interpret what they see and hear is influenced enormously by their age and stage of development (Piaget & Inhelder 1969, and see Chapter 11).

PROFESSIONAL CONVERSATION

James, a 15-year-old boy with a learning disability, is being prepared for surgery.

James clearly understood the concept of the faces pain scale, but then added:

That's all well and good, my physical pain right now is zero but what about a scale on which I can rate my emotions that right now are in a complete scramble?

In contrast to the well-established practice within paediatric nursing of measuring pain, it is interesting to note, as highlighted by James' comments, how rarely nurses explicitly seek to 'measure' children's emotional states. A notable exception is seen in the work of Ellerton & Merriman (1994), who used an 'anxiety faces scale', similar to the well-established 'faces' pain tools, to measure children's emotional anxiety. However, both scales are vulnerable with regard to their accuracy and it is – arguably – important to consider more objective means of measuring anxiety as well.

The link between physiological change and a person's psychological status has been recognised and researched (Hyland & Donaldson 1989). One such early study detected changes in urinary excretion in connection with anxiety responses (Wilson 1981). Additionally, seminal work by Brain & Maclay (1968) showed a higher incidence of complications, such as infection and haemorrhage, in a control group whose mothers were not resident during a child's stay compared with an experimental group whose parents were present. These studies support the fact that disease and illness are not purely a biological phenomenon. However, contemporary research tends to measure anxiety more by behavioural change and attitudinal scales; unfortunately there is a paucity of recent work exploring the physiological manifestations of anxiety.

Activity

Find out about the detailed literature available to complement that provided by hospitals on the website of the National Association of Hospital Play Staff:

- http://www.nahps.org.uk

Scenario

Ollie is 7 years old and his mother is concerned that he is having lots of time off school with frequent sore throats. She arranges for Ollie to be seen by her local family practitioner, who refers him to the local outpatient department.

Preparing children for a hospital admission

On the premise that emotional needs might be as great, if not greater, than a child's physical needs during a hospital admission, a number of different strategies have been developed to help children and their families cope with hospital admission.

Family preparation for day and inpatient surgery is thought to be important in reducing the psychological effects of hospitalisation. Modern child healthcare services require integration between hospital and community. The service should provide for the child as a whole and should meet the social, emotional, spiritual needs of children and their families as well as their physical needs. The growth of paediatric preadmission programmes throughout the UK represents one facet only of this integrated service. Since the publication of the Platt report, paediatric nurses have developed a reputation for endeavouring to improve the care of their patients and families. Attempting to protect children from the stresses of hospital admission may be partially facilitated through the provision of preadmission programmes. Although the evidence base for the efficacy of these programmes has yet to be firmly established, the Commission for Health Audit and Inspection (CHAI, formerly CHI) has developed an audit tool for NHS Trusts to use to measure compliance to the standards of hospital services developed under the auspices of the National Service Framework for Children. One of the paediatric benchmarks that CHAI will audit is related to preparation, and preadmission clubs are specifically cited as examples of best practice.

Activity

Access the companion PowerPoint presentation to see slides of these dolls.

- Use the pattern to make a calico doll yourself.

Preparation programmes

Preadmission preparation programmes offer the child and family the opportunity to visit the hospital to be familiarised with the environment and personnel. At the same time, practical issues can be discussed and the child and family informed about anticipated specific events (Gaughan & Sweeney 1997). Such programmes are conducted either in outpatient departments, when children come in with the family for initial consultation, or in the main hospital at a set time, usually a week before admission. The changes found historically in children's behaviour after hospitalisation underpins the growth of such formal preadmission programmes. A study by Fassler (1980) indicates that a combination of emotional support and information appertaining to the admission appears to be an effective method of reducing preoperative anxiety. Keeton (1999) noted that children who had attended a preparation day settled more quickly in their surroundings and were more relaxed and happy than those who had not. Current work by Keeton is exploring whether preadmission programmes reduce stress and anxiety of family responses at anaesthetic induction in children undergoing day surgery.

PowerPoint

Access the companion PowerPoint presentation and follow the preadmission programme slides.

Scenario

Following Ollie's outpatient appointment, the ENT surgeon has indicated that he requires a tonsillectomy. He is scheduled for surgery within the next 3 months. Before his admission, he and his family receive an invitation to attend the preadmission programme.

The most common type of programme in the UK is conducted in hospital, often at weekends. One of the first preadmission programmes in the UK was developed at the Queen's Medical Centre in Nottingham in 1982. The format established at Nottingham has been emulated in a number of other children's units. Invitations to the programmes are posted to patients with all the other information prior to admission. The programmes often consist of a PowerPoint or video/DVD presentation followed by a visit to the ward/unit to which the child will be admitted. Additionally, children and their carers may have the opportunity of visiting the anaesthetic room, where they can see first hand where they will receive their anaesthetic and – importantly – be reassured that their parent/carer will be allowed to go with them on the day. Therapeutic play programmes and biscuits and juice for the children usually complete the morning's programme. While the children are playing, the parents have coffee and time for 'question and answer', and conversation with other parents, which can yield invaluable peer support. Many children's units give the children a play-pack at the end of the programme consisting of a paper theatre hat, paints, name band, mask and badge, plus a cotton theatre gown which parents are asked to return on admission. Many members of theatre staff participate enthusiastically in preadmission programmes with positive effect (Bonner 1986). The role of the skilled play specialist is another essential element of preadmission preparation, but not to the exclusion of the skilled paediatric nurse. A major benefit of the programmes is that they facilitate interaction between hospital staff and parents/carers, who are encouraged to ask programme workers about their child's admission.

Scenario

Ollie's family is in a position to attend the preadmission programme and join other children one Saturday, 2 weeks before admission

The contents of such programmes are developed primarily from professional values and beliefs together with parental opinions, obtained by means of interviews and questionnaires (Gaughan & Sweeney 1997, Glasper & Stradling 1989). There is invaluable information to be learned by asking and involving the children about their feelings, beliefs and needs, a perspective endorsed by the recently published National Service Framework for Children (DoH 2003). The Commission of Patient and Public Involvement in Health (CPPIH), created in January 2003, will undoubtedly also encourage this.

Fradd (1986) argues that preadmission programmes are an 'undoubted success'. However, not all claims of success can be supported by documentary evidence. Although the principles of such programmes may be seen as positive, one needs to look closely at their content, structure and mode of delivery (Murphy-Taylor 1999). Communication is crucial for effective psychological care and may be considered as the key to its achievement. For example:

- What to say?
- What not to say?
- How to say it?
- When to say it?
- Who should say it?
- Where it should be said?

One significant issue in this respect is that preadmission preparation programmes appear to attempt to teach children of various ages and cultures via a common group programme, thus not allowing or acknowledging individuality, cognitive ability, existing knowledge or previous experience. Such limitations have been recognised by Eiser (1988) and Saile et al (1988). Many misconceptions and fantasies may occur if not handled appropriately by a skilled practitioner. Other limitations include the length of time between preparation programme and actual admission. It could be argued that during the gap between the preparation programme and admission, the child will forget the information or have too much time to worry and panic.

Ward visits offer the opportunity for each child and family to meet, on a one-to-one basis, the staff who will nurse them, and presert an excellent chance to offer personalised, individual preparation; a situation many ward staff make good use of. If, however, a tour of the clinical area is not an appropriately prearranged part of the preadmission programme, families might arrive on the ward unexpectedly. They may be exposed to a busy, noisy atmosphere with people rushing back and forth, seeing other children with beeping monitors attached and 'tubes sticking out of them'. They may be kept waiting while an appropriate member of staff is found to welcome them. The parents in particular may feel uncomfortable in this situation 'taking the nurse away from urgent duties' (Taylor 1991). Although this may be a reality to which they will be exposed in the future, it is not an ideal first impression.

It is noted, though not always clearly highlighted, that – relatively speaking – a minority of children admitted to hospital attend preparation programmes (Gaughan & Sweeney 1997). This could be for a number of reasons. Parents might not be able to spare an extra day from work or family commitment and finances for transport may be limited. Their own beliefs that such preparation is either unnecessary (particularly if their child has been admitted before), or that it could increase their or their child's fear may also prevent them from attending. Interestingly, more under-5s are admitted to hospital than any other age group (Atwell 1997), yet they are not always included in preparation visits (Ellerton & Merriman 1994). Consideration too is needed for those children admitted as an emergency. Thus it is necessary that health professionals look at alternative methods of preparation both prior to and during the admission.

Can the positive impact of preparation be measured in children?

Measuring levels of distress in children can be achieved by using special rating scales. Rice et al (2008) have discussed the use of the Yale Preoperative Anxiety Scale in measuring differences in groups of children attending for day case surgery, some of which had previously attended a preadmission 'Saturday morning club'. They were able to show that attendance at the preadmission programme had a favourable effect on patient anxiety levels, the day ward, the theatre waiting room and the anaesthetic room.

Further key issues in preparation

Play

Children learn through play; it is a natural part of life. Time set aside to play gives the child an ideal opportunity to find out about their hospital experience. In doing so their fears may be allayed and their abilities to cope enhanced. Webster (2000) refers to key policy documents, namely ASC (2000) and the Children Act (DoH 1989), and identifies the recognition in these documents that play preparation allows the child an age-appropriate opportunity to be involved in decisions that are to affect their lives. A knowledge of how children may perceive their internal anatomy, coupled with an understanding of children's cognitive development is clearly essential before embarking on any preparation programme (see Chapter 11). Each child's needs will be unique.

Activity

List a selection of distraction methods and the age groups and situations where they might be appropriate.

There may be different classifications of different types of play. In a helpful paper, Mathison & Butterworth (2001) suggest that play be divided into three types – educative, normative and therapeutic:

- The essence of **educative play** is to give information. This may be in the form of personal letters to the child, indicating in a child-centred way what to bring to hospital. It also includes use of books, pictures and diagram for parents and children to read together to learn more about their hospital admission.
- **Normative play** is 'everyday' play that is offered within the hospital environment to bridge the gap between home and hospital. It offers comfort and security, a sense of familiarity and normality. Frustrations and fears may also be expressed, thus helping the child to gain a feeling of control and confidence in his/her new and potentially threatening environment. It is important to consider that due to their illness and potentially alien environment, the child may need permission, encouragement and assistance to play.
- **Therapeutic play** centres on what the child is about to actually experience or has previously experienced, and uses play to convey information both from the child to the carer, and from the carer to the child (see also Chapter 13). In respect of preparation, when discussing certain procedures involving parts of the anatomy with younger children (especially if they cannot see, hear or touch the relevant part) it is necessary to use things the children can see, hear, touch and relate to concretely, for example anatomical dolls.

Scenario

Ollie's father watches with interest as the nurse uses a doll to explain to Ollie what is going to happen when he attends for surgery and finds this helpful as a tool to ask further questions for himself.

Dolls

The use of dolls is a popular tool in preparing children for specific events. For example Zaadi dolls (Glasper & Thompson 1993), both male and female, are anatomical models developed specifically for children in hospital. These cloth-covered rag dolls have three layers, which peel apart using 'velcro' fastenings to expose the vital organs (note: the dolls have several faces and it is important that the sleeping face is in place before the doll is opened). The body parts are detachable. They can be catheterised and injected, and generally allow the child a visual and tactile experience to support their thoughts and understanding.

Calico dolls (Matthews & Silk 1992) also allow the child an opportunity to explore and learn by vision and touch. The simply made cloth dolls can have a variety of procedures simulated upon them, e.g. skin testing and 'drawing blood' (via plastic tubing attached to a cannula and bag of coloured water). These dolls can also be drawn upon, which can help children to demonstrate where their pain is (Ballentine & Gow 1998). These dolls also have the potential to allow parents/practitioners a visual way of supporting their verbal explanation about a procedure.

Activity

List the various methods of measuring anxiety in children. What evidence is there to suggest that the measurements are valid?

As part of her research to investigate children's knowledge of their internal anatomy, Gaudian (2000) created her own life-sized anatomical rag doll. The internal parts, each made in different-coloured fabric for easy identification, were large enough for the children to compare with their own bodies. She demonstrated that their knowledge of anatomy and physiology was more readily recalled by these three-dimensional prompts than by giving a child a two-dimensional picture to draw on. This suggests the value of such dolls in maximising children's questioning and understanding, and also helping to assess children's existing knowledge accurately before giving explanations.

'Play people' hospital toys are excellent, as are 'doctors and nurses' sets, which contain stethoscopes, auroscopes and fake syringes. It is interesting that dressing up in traditional hospital clothing continues to be popular with children despite the fact that nursing and medical staff no longer wear such uniforms in many children's units. With such toys, as well as standard teddy bears, dolls, paints and plasticine, the child has the opportunity to act out any fears, anxieties or aggressions. Children will often mirror their own experiences through a favourite toy. An observer, be it parent or professional, can gain valuable insight into the child's understanding, potential misconceptions and current feelings, and thus tailor care even more uniquely.

Distraction

Distraction is associated with helping the child cope during a specific event. The purpose of distraction is not purely to divert the child's attention or simply to provide entertainment during a medical or nursing procedure but, more importantly, to use personal, focused and developmentally appropriate play to maximise their coping strategies (Webster 2000). The professional should offer relevant information, assess the child's understanding, guide manageable goals, allow the child some choice and control and ensure emotional support with praise and reward throughout and after the event. The key to distraction is to understand it not as the removal of pain or distress directly, but rather to make the treatment more bearable by taking the focus away from the unpleasant event onto something more interesting or enjoyable (Salantera et al 1999). It may therefore be seen as a powerful intervention to help children cope with stress points/stressful procedures such as venesection/cannulation. Indeed, Willock et al (2004) give consideration to the experience of venepuncture and note the work of Doellman (2003), who describes a wide range of distraction and other supportive interventions that nurses can undertake to help children cope with this stressful procedure. Willcock et al also cite the work of Hodgins & Lander (1997), which categorises the different coping strategies displayed by different children. These range from looking away and wanting to focus on other events, to seeking support (e.g. a hand to hold), to wanting to watch the whole procedure. However, such interventions must be individualised: consider two 3-year-olds, one clinging to her parents and the other actively exploring and interacting inquisitively with the professional.

Individualised care is undoubtedly vital in planning how best to support children through hospital events. Ill-prepared and ill-supported experiences can clearly produce negative effects and distress, as well as a poor ability to cope in the future with similar or associated events.

Activity

Search the literature for different anxiety assessment scales:

- How well do you think these measure anxiety, and how appropriate are they for use with children?
- Create your own emotional rating scale.

To prepare children effectively for hospital events, it is clearly important to have a concept/knowledge of the fears a child may have when hospitalised. The seminal work of Visintainer & Wolfer (1975 p 65) describes this in terms of five key potential threats. In their study they used four variables when preparing children for specific events:

- A control group
- A group that received supportive care
- A group that was given a single session of preparation on Admission
- A group that was prepared immediately before each stressful procedure (stress-point preparation).

Within each group, the children's anxiety response was measured using behaviour upset scales, ease of postoperative fluid intake, medication on recovery, pulse rate and time of first voiding. The group with the optimal outcome was the one that had received stress-point preparation at six key points:

1. Admission
2. Shortly before a blood test
3. Late in the afternoon the day before surgery
4. Shortly before pre-medication
5. Before transfer to theatre
6. Upon return from recovery room.

The children and parents were given 'information, instruction, rehearsal and support from a single nurse who was present at these critical times'. Even for younger children (2–6 years), single preparation was significantly more highly rated than consistent support, suggesting that giving information to such young children can do much to mitigate preoperative stress. However, it must be noted that replications of Visintainer & Wolfer's work have been unable to demonstrate findings of the same quality.

It is positive to note that, although limited, studies are still investigating preparation for specific events. Unlike Visintainer & Wolfer, one such study (Holden et al 1997) showed that there were no differences statistically in the distress experienced by toddlers and young children (and their parents) when a nasogastric tube was passed, whether they received detailed or routine preparation. All were equally unhappy during the procedure. However, Holden et al found a significant difference for older children and adolescents, who showed a more positive response and outcome when prepared for the event as mentioned above.

Using clown humour to help children in hospital

Does humour delivered through clowning benefit children in hospital? The use of humour as a therapy is receiving increasing attention from healthcare professionals who are interested in both the psychological and physical effects on patients well being. Furthermore, some hospitals now routinely use clowns to entertain sick children and the evidence to underpin the efficacy of such interventions is growing. Vagnoli et al (2005) have shown that the use of clowns in alleviating children's anxiety during hospital procedures such as the induction of anaesthesia was significant. Glasper et al (2007), Battrick et al (2007) and Weaver et al (2007) have likewise added to the evidence base supporting clown humour for children in hospital. Weaver et al (2007) in a qualitative study of children's perceptions of hospital clown humour using the 'draw and write' and 'draw and tell' techniques has shown that children appreciate the beneficial effects of a clown visit to them during their hospital stay. The data suggest that clown humour can mitigate some of the negative effects of hospitalisation for sick children – the children interviewed in this study made requests for more frequent clown visits or more clown doctors for children in hospital.

Giving information

It is apparent that the stress of hospital can be alleviated by giving children and their families information before, during and after anxiety-provoking experiences. For many ages of children, verbal explanation alone will be insufficient because of their immature verbal and comprehension skills. The methods discussed (therapeutic play, story books, games, role play and puppet shows) will need to be utilised. When giving information verbally the choice of words and supportive explanation become important. For example, how appropriate is it to refer to an X-ray machine as a camera (Ballentine & Gow 1998)? Or, when taking blood and cannulating, to say that it is like 'a small scratch' or 'a butterfly on your hand'? Such things might be said with the good intention to soothe and reassure, but could cause children confusion, anxiety and even fear of butterflies when they are discharged home. Nurses are often required to translate medical jargon but they also need to consider whether their words and descriptions require greater thought as well (Jolly 1976; see also Chapters 11 and 37).

A further point in respect of giving information is that it is imperative to be sure that it has been understood if it is to be of positive benefit. The best way to assess this, after assessing prior knowledge and having given the relevant information, is by asking questions of the child and parent, encouraging them to ask questions, and observing their interactions in play and conversation. It is also important to go back at a later point to reinforce and re-evaluate. The child and family may feel they should know what to expect so they may not ask for information. If they don't ask it is important not to assume they know. An interesting study by Kiely (1989) found that 80% of parents interviewed about preparation thought they had been given enough information. However, this was not reflected in further interviews when their knowledge was assessed.

We must also be aware that too much information can increase rather than decrease stress (Acharya 1992). As a means of coping, information may be blocked out. When stressed, e.g. learning about the need for an operation, information may be misinterpreted and can be easily forgotten (Taylor et al 1999).

Such considerations might have influenced the work of Sutherland (2003), who sought to explore the value of preparation for cardiac surgery for adolescents in the home environment as opposed to the hospital. This intervention was positively evaluated by those who received it, although the failure to use a matched control makes it impossible to say for certain that this approach is always preferable. Crucially, the opportunity to talk to a knowledgeable practitioner who had the skill to listen well and give information with sensitivity was viewed as the greatest benefit of this approach.

Caress (2003) discusses in depth the many facets of successful communication of information. She considers the benefits of giving information, and raises questions and offers suggestions as to where the information may be given, how it may be given and who is giving and receiving it.

Using written and visual material to prepare children for admission

Hain, Battrick & Glasper (see Chapter 37) show that written and illustrated material can be effective in relieving the stresses of hospitalisation. The use of highly specific information is important to produce accurate expectations in families attending hospital. To this end, a number of books have been written for children about hospital. They can be read as part of a general educational strategy or can be used by parents and others prior to a child's admission. Some are better than others and should be read discerningly by nurses and play specialists before being recommended/made available. At best, they can be perceived as an aid only, but they do fulfil a role as part of an overall preparatory package. Children's books and the use of story telling has been exemplified by Robinson et al (2002), who highlight the health benefits of story telling to address complex issues.

WWW

Go to the following website. Could this North American website be used for children in the UK?

- http://kidshealth.org/index.html

Nicklin (2002) has demonstrated that information needs to be accurate, have provenance and be appropriate for the readership if ambiguity is not to compromise the intentions of the material. The growth in the use of the worldwide web via home computers now gives an increasing number of people the advantage of instant access to material. Although it is often stressed that information is the key to empowerment, not all the information available on the internet is of the highest quality. This is also true of written material produced by health professionals, who are as likely to use 'gobbledegook' as anyone else; there is little point in writing for families if, in turn, they cannot read or understand the information presented.

Other issues to consider include the availability of information in different languages and Braille or on audiotape and the need for professionals to be aware that using family members as translators can raise a confidentiality dilemma. In recent years, it has become customary for many children's units to send out written material in the mail, usually with the letter of admission. Like the books discussed above, this written material can be of varying quality. Some of it attempts to communicate with the parent and some with the child, some do both.

WWW

Go to the following website and click on the information pages. Is the description of glue ear helpful for children and parents/carers?

- http://www.ich.ucl.ac.uk/

Parents interviewed in studies frequently request leaflets giving details of hospital facilities, personnel and routine, and facts about specific medical or surgical conditions (Kiely 1989). It appears that few leaflets actually offer suggestions to parents regarding how to prepare their child psychologically for hospital. Parents in Southampton received such information very positively when a leaflet containing recommendations for preparation was produced (Stone & Glasper 1997) (see also Chapter 37). Murphy-Taylor (1999) also found a desire among parents for more information, and suggested that specific information sheets about individual operations could be included in the mail-out to parents. In this way children could be prepared for surgery through the parents, who are best placed to achieve this.

WWW

Read the new booklet from Queens Medical Centre in Nottingham. Compare this with what is available in your area of work:

- http://www.qmc.nhs.uk/WhatsHappening/ChildrensBooklet.htm

The development of a centre for health information and promotion (CHIP) in Southampton, linked to the outpatient department, offered a valuable resource for families. Such initiatives recognise the importance of empowering families through giving them information (Glasper et al 1995). Perhaps greater links between such services and ward areas are also required to maximise their potential.

Some hospitals have produced video, DVD films or PowerPoint presentations, which can be given to parents and children. Such programmes have been found to be so effective that they are increasingly being developed and used throughout the UK. The complexity of educational material for children is such that healthcare professionals are increasingly using multimedia as a vehicle of delivering material. Children are now very computer literate and McPherson et al (2002) have described how a multimedia package has helped in the delivery of asthma education for children.

The cost of producing professionally edited videotapes is prohibitive for most units, and these products date very quickly. PowerPoint presentations are easier and cheaper to produce and have the added advantage that they can be updated periodically with little difficulty. The flexibility of a PowerPoint presentation is the most effective method of addressing parental concerns about a child's forthcoming hospital admission. PowerPoint slides are easy to produce and can be scanned or imported directly from digital cameras. They are very simple to update and a consistent format can be adopted, perhaps of sequential digital photographs covering the hospital stay from admission to discharge. Ideally, everyone involved in writing the presentation should follow a set script, although the preparation of such is always difficult. In lieu of an agreed script, some units follow an informal approach that takes cues from the PowerPoint slides.

Some hospitals, for example the Hospital for Sick Children in Toronto, have developed very sophisticated virtual tours of clinical areas, which are available for parents and children to view through the hospital website. Hospital-based television programmes may also have a general effect in raising the awareness of preparing children for hospital.

WWW

Go to the following website and take a virtual tour. Discuss this in your learning group:

- http://www.sickkids.on.ca/

Other considerations in parental preparation

Parents are seen as prime informants and interpreters, the people with the most in-depth knowledge about the child. They therefore have a vital need themselves for information and support (Whiting 1993). As discussed earlier, the work of Visintainer & Wolfer (1975) shows favourable parental response to preparation. Parents were more able to cope themselves and thus more effective at supporting their child. Siblings and the wider family also have needs and can also contribute to a child's care, provided education and support from health professionals is available.

The trend to shorter inpatient stays and more day surgery has increased the need for parents to be responsible for both the child's emotional and physical care. Darbyshire (2003) looked at mothers' experiences of their child's recovery both in hospital and at home, and makes important observations regarding the considerable challenges that parents face in caring for their sick child on discharge. One hopes that such work will allow professionals the opportunity to develop preparation programmes and information to suit the client's true needs. Such observations about parental responsibility are also echoed in much of the literature on day surgery (Ireland & Rushforth 1998). It is therefore important that preparation focuses on all stages of the illnesses trajectory, from admission right through to discharge and beyond.

Battrick & Glasper (2004) highlighted the importance of seeking the opinion of the consumers. Such consumer surveys invariably demonstrate that parents are in favour of information. However, whereas some hunger for that information others may avoid it (Miller 1979). In the absence of information, but with their own fears and anxieties, a parent may say nothing to the child and the first the child knows of an admission is walking through the portals of the hospital. Given that parents' informed consent should ideally be sought before any preparation/explanation is given to a younger child, parental refusal to allow the child to be informed about aspects of his or her care places the healthcare professional in a challenging ethical situation to ensure that the child's rights are upheld.

Seminar discussion topic

A parent doesn't want to tell their child they are coming to hospital/ about to undergo surgery. Why might the parent feel like this? As the paediatric nurse and professional advocate for that child and family, how would you approach this situation? (See also Chapter 20)

Just because a certain fact or experience worries an adult it doesn't mean it will worry a child. Both parents and professionals should take care not to impose their fears upon a child. Adults, like children, have different coping strategies. The benefits of parents may be immeasurable in helping a child cope with a stressful event but, paradoxically, an anxious parent is likely to increase the anxiety in their child. This is clarified further by Glasper & Thompson (1993) in their elaboration of 'emotional contagion'.

Emotional contagion, i.e. the transmission of anxiety from an adult to a child, is a major source of concern to those individuals planning any form of supportive programme. Most children depend on emotional support from their parents for help in coping with anxieties. The simplest anxiety is that produced by contagion. This is exemplified by a child who becomes frightened when in close contact with frightened adults. If those whose role is one of protection become frightened themselves, this fear can be transmitted to the child. It may be hypothesised that parents who are frightened are less able to contribute to the psychological welfare of a child who is undergoing a stressful procedure.

In some early work, Campbell (1957) discussed how emotional states in mothers can be communicated to their children. Her investigation, conducted in a well baby clinic, showed that significantly more infants of mothers who received anxiety-arousing instructions cried before immunisation injections than infants of mothers who received neutral instruction. It is thus important to prepare parents as well as children for stressful events to avoid parental anxiety being mirrored in children. Some parents can become frightened about the welfare of their child and sometimes their reaction appears out of proportion to the event at hand. The quality of interaction between an authoritative person, such as a nurse, and a hospitalised child's parent can lower the parent's level of stress and produce changes in the parent's definition of the situation. This in turn can have a demonstrable effect on the child's level of stress, producing a change in his or her social, psychological and physiological behaviour. Children's nurses must learn to recognise the natural resource they have at their disposal in the form of parents and guardians. They must be perceived as partners in the traditional nurse–doctor–patient relationship.

It must be recognised that parents/carers are trying to understand and absorb, in a matter of hours and days, information that professionals have spent years learning. They are expected to trust relative strangers with the life of their child. Professionals need to listen to them, acknowledge their fears and offer factual and practical information with sensitivity and understanding. Parents often fail to ask for advice or help with the daily care needs of their child because they believe the nurse to be too busy in dealing with more important tasks. It is crucial that nurses offer their time to listen to the child and family.

Gibson's (1991) definition of empowerment is one all professionals should emulate:

> Recognising, promoting and enhancing people's ability to meet their own needs, solve their own problems and mobilise their own resources in order to feel in control of their own lives.

Scenario

After surgery, Ollie returns home the following day and, although he makes an uneventful physical recovery, he sleeps less well and remains 'clingy' for several days (see Chapter 8).

Preparation in the community: emergency admissions and non-attendees

By the age of 5 years, 25% of children will have had a stay in hospital, and one-third of these admissions will be caused by accidents (see Chapter 23). Indeed, half of infants aged under 12 months, and a quarter of older children, will attend an A&E over a 1-year period (DoH 2003). Hospitalisation is, therefore, not an uncommon childhood experience. Brett (1983) has indicated that preparation should begin in the classroom and feature as a component of general education.

The needs of children vary with age. It has been suggested that children's fears change with age and cognitive development. Miller (1979) has stated that preschool children are especially frightened of noises, strange persons or events. Schoolchildren's particular fears may be of bodily injury, disease and separation. Vernon et al (1966), in a classic study, collected data that support the hypothesis that children between the ages of 6 months and 4 years of age are the most likely to be upset following hospitalisation. This would suggest that preparation might begin in nursery school or play group. Many nurseries and primary schools have 'hospital play corners' that allow children the opportunity to explore and learn through 'role play'.

Families, like individuals, are unique, each with their own needs, but all appear to profit from a modicum of preparation. Any preparation will be intimately concerned with stress inoculation. Meng & Zastowny (1981) have likened stress inoculation to medical inoculation and indicate that preparatory programmes should achieve this goal. Stress inoculation can be carried out successfully in school classroom situations and the benefit of this approach is that all children can be prepared for the eventuality of being admitted to hospital. School-age children are more likely than preschool children to cope positively with hospitalisation. This is because they are more able to reason, describe and verbalise their feelings than younger children. The school classroom may, therefore, be an excellent environment in which to teach children the skills necessary to cope with hospitalisation. Hospitals in many areas offer schools fairly in-depth and interactive education sessions, both in the hospital setting and with hospital personnel visiting the schools themselves.

Seminar discussion topic

James Robertson, a staunch NAWCH member, stopped the school-wide preparatory programmes because he believed they may cause unnecessary fear and anxiety in children concerning separation, bodily mutilation and the pain of operations. Debate this stance in your action learning group.

Dedicated paediatric areas in emergency departments, with appropriately qualified staff, can clearly provide a more conducive environment for a child. Teddy bears feature highly as a tool for learning. A 'well teddy clinic' in the Emergency Department at the Royal Belfast Hospital for Sick Children proved a great success in helping to allay the fears of children and parents requiring emergency care (Burton 1994). Similarly, a three-day teddy bear community project in Kentucky offered valuable learning for all involved (Santen & Feldman 1994).

Universal preparation for all children facilitated through preschool or school-based programmes may not be the whole answer. Young children are susceptible to fantasy and misunderstanding, and anxiety may even be provoked if ideas of separation from home and family are introduced unnecessarily, leading some critics to question the appropriateness of such blanket preparation. Any preparation for hospital must be carried out accurately and sensitively, with due importance being given to the age and level of cognitive development of the child. The role of the primary healthcare team should also be considered when planning preparatory programmes for children and families. In a typical year, a preschool child will see the GP around six times, and a school-age child two or three times (DoH 2003). It is obvious, therefore, that GPs, health visitors and school nurses are in a good position to supply information about hospitals, especially for elective admissions.

Preparation in the outpatient department has also received attention (Achayra 1992). It is the belief of the authors and their play specialist colleagues that, if handled and organised well, education here – as with formal preparation programmes – can form a firm basis of support and knowledge for the child and family before their ultimate admission to a hospital ward.

First impressions are powerful and lasting. In any year, one in eleven children will be referred to an outpatient department (DoH 2003).

Children with specific preparation needs

Much of the literature with regard to preparation refers to the well and acutely ill child. Particular consideration needs to be given to the children with chronic illnesses, learning difficulties and communication impairment. It might be assumed that a child who regularly attends hospital is better informed than he or she actually is. The practitioner also needs to assess carefully the child's previous experiences, as these will undoubtedly influence his or her behaviour and emotional needs each time they are subsequently admitted to hospital. It is easy to think that everyone else has explained a routine or aspect of care, or indeed that the child and family know what to do, say or feel.

Although much is written about the benefits of preparing the well child for a future period of hospitalisation, it should be stressed that children with chronic conditions and their families may have different and potentially more lasting and serious psychological reactions (Ogden Burke et al 2001). Preparation for such children may be difficult, particularly if the family has experienced prior negative events. The focus of Ogden Burke's study is on using family-centred strategies for coping with stress-point interventions by nurses (SPIN). For children with chronic illness, recognition that others have similar problems, and perhaps the setting-up of peer health groups at ward level and in the community, can offer valuable support. As part of preparation, families in Nottingham are often introduced to another family whose child has had the same surgery (Crawford & Raven 2002).

It is still important for nurses to explain their intended actions, even to children with limited verbal responses who might still be experiencing anxiety and fear. The professional and parents/carers must be aware of children's non-verbal communication and endeavour to interpret and address their needs. The focus may then be on helping them to cope with a potentially frightening experience.

Burgess (2001) offers an interesting perspective on the complementary therapies guided imagery and infant massage as distraction therapy. There was particular emphasis upon such techniques being used to support the child through episodes of pain. Savins (2002) explored the value of art therapy with children in pain and it has also been recognised that music has therapeutic benefits. Music therapy can build a bridge between two worlds – perhaps between those with sight and hearing and those without, and between those with command of speech and those yet to master such skills – in essence, it is a means of non-verbal communication and expression of emotion. Complementary and alternative therapies can help relationships be built and pathways of trust and communication opened. This is clearly a sound basis for preparing and supporting children through new experiences.

The psychological preparation of children whose special needs, e.g. cerebral palsy, result in global developmental delay is beginning to receive attention. Crawford & Raven (2002) offer a multifaceted approach to preparing such children for gastrostomy insertion, which uses many of the interventions previously discussed. They use Minnie and Mickey Mouse dolls, similar to the Zaadi and calico dolls, to allow the child and parent to insert, remove and play with appropriate related pieces of equipment. It was felt important that the characters chosen should not be associated with a particular class, culture or race, or create the image/stereotype of a 'normal' child. Preparation began in the home and continued for some several weeks before hospitalisation and surgery. Another technique used for one particular child in their study was music and massage, which were found to aid relaxation. Also worth highlighting was the introduction of various textures and pressures to the child's abdomen, with the idea that the child could begin to get used to a sensation that later would be associated with their new gastrostomy. This, the mother reported, became a significant and valuable part of her child's care.

Essentially, children with complex needs require no less and no more support and information than any other child in respect of what is offered in preparation for hospital or events within it. The difference will be that professionals need to find out about the specific illness/disability and then tailor and adapt the tools and resources they use to communicate effectively. Interaction with the multidisciplinary team and specialist services will undoubtedly offer valuable information and support. Whoever they are and whatever their circumstances, the children should all be given appropriate opportunities and stimulation, time to respond, to endeavour to share their perspective and develop their strengths and abilities; above all to be respected as unique individuals.

Activity

- Do clown doctors visit your hospital? If yes, endeavour to ascertain from conversation with them their perception of their role.
- Do you think humour has a place in children's units?

Practitioner perspectives

When children are in hospital, the nurse must adopt the role of facilitator and coordinator to all their needs. Continuity and documentation of preparation and information given is imperative if confusion by duplication is to be avoided (Rushforth 1999). Communication is vital, particularly between the nurse and the play specialist, whose skill and knowledge of child development and the therapy of play is of paramount importance. Active participation by the children and families should be encouraged with regard to planning and evaluating their preparation and emotional needs. Praise and rewards by health carers and family members will increase self-esteem and reinforce positive behaviour. Even children who cry or shout should receive acknowledgement that they have done well and tried their best.

Taylor (1991) identified a situation when a child had interactions with 25 people in a 3-hour period. This may be difficult for anyone to assimilate when well, let alone when 4 years old, unwell and most likely feeling somewhat vulnerable. Nurse-led ventures/clinics could be said not only to allow increased professional development and skill for the nurse but, perhaps more importantly, give greater opportunity for trust, security and coping by the child because of an environment in which there is continuity of action, care and management by one or a small number of people (Lawton & Rose 2003). There is a close link here with the concept of primary and named nursing.

It could be argued that clinical psychologists are underutilised in respect of preparing children for hospitalisation. Their role could perhaps be expanded further within the muti-disciplinary team. For example, they could contribute to the formation of protocols of care and advise literature for professionals/carers in respect of the child and families preparation for hospitalisation and emotional needs.

A small-scale study by Rushforth (1996) looked at nurses' beliefs, knowledge and practice regarding children's ability to understand concepts of health and illness. It concluded that nurses' knowledge about a child's conceptual ability, and beliefs in cognitive immaturity, may be adversely influencing practice. Staff education is obviously indicated in this respect, and so too is the need for all those involved in the health care of children to be reminded of how the hospital might be seen through the child's eye (Haggarty & Rushforth 1999).

One tool to achieve this is the video 'A child's eye view' (Haggarty & Rushforth 1996, 1999). The video, recorded at the eye level of a young child, offers an audiovisual encounter of the sights, sounds and experiences of a hospital, offering examples of good and bad practice. The video acts as a catalyst for the viewer to consider what the child might be seeing, hearing and feeling, and how he might react; the video is accompanied by a teaching booklet.

Evaluation data demonstrated a very positive picture with regard to the video as a learning tool. Practitioners felt that their 'habituation' of seeing the hospital world through professional eyes had been challenged and that viewing the video had allowed them to revisit the care situation with 'new eyes', those of the children themselves (Haggarty & Rushforth 1999).

Activity

What are the specific preparation needs of the following groups of children?

- Those with global developmental delay
- Those with communication difficulty, e.g. blindness, deafness
- Those with a chronic illness
- Adolescents.

What specific information is available in the children's nursing literature to guide practitioners in preparing these specific groups of children? Is there any evidence regarding its efficacy? Give examples of your own ideas of other interventions that may address such children's needs (see also Chapters 43, 44 and 47).

Activity

Obtain and view the video 'A child's eye view'. While watching the video, keep note of:

- what you see
- what you hear
- what you are thinking
- how you will act when next with a child.

Summary

It is important that children's and young peoples nurses are constantly aware of the psychological well-being of the children in their care, and that they take every opportunity to maximise the child-centredness of their approach and of the environment in which children are nursed. Such care should be part of the professional's daily routine, not an after-thought or added extra. In particular, the carer (parents and professionals) needs to remember to give children permission to express their emotions and also to negotiate care, with informed consent, to give choices, praise and reward. All details regarding assessment of need, preparation given and outcome for the child should be clearly documented, available for all involved with the family, and appropriately evaluated and modified as the child indicates.

Further development is required to consider the role of a specific person for a child's psychological preparation from assessment of health need through treatment to settling back to normal routine at home. It is important to stress that further work is also needed to look at the specific needs when preparing children with learning difficulties, communication impairment and chronic illness. Information for families about why and how to prepare their child for hospital and how such literature may be disseminated also needs to be expanded.

To conclude this chapter, it would be difficult to find better words than those of Mellish (1969), who pointed out that successful preparation for surgery depends on the attitude of many people, including the surgeon, anaesthetist, and nurses and that:

> ... the criteria for surgical success should not only be measured by intact wounds but also by intact emotions.

Dedication

Rachel Haggarty wishes to dedicate this chapter to the memory of Ben Voller:

> When you reached out, I was privileged to be there for you and to be able to hold your hand.

References

Achayra, S., 1992. Assessing the need for pre-admission visits. Paediatric Nursing 4 (9), 20–23.

ASC 2002 Online. Available at: http://www.actionforsickchildren.org/about_history.html

Atwell, J., 1997. Paediatric surgery. Arnold, London.

Atwell, J., Gow, M., 1985. Paediatric trained district nurses in the community: expensive luxury or economic necessity? British Nursing Journal 291, 227–229.

Ballentine, M., Gow, D., 1998. The value of play in ambulatory settings. In: Glasper, E.A., Lowson, S. (Eds.), Innovations in paediatric ambulatory care. Macmillan, London.

Battrick, C., Glasper, E.A., 2004. The views of children and their families on being in hospital. British Journal of Nursing 12 (6), 36–44.

Battrick, C., Glapser, E.A., Prudhoe, G., Weaver, K., 2007 Clown humour; the perceptions of doctors, nurses, parents and children. JCYPN 1 (4), 174–179.

Bonner, M.L., 1986. Can my friend go with me? Nursing Times October, pp. 75–76.

Bowlby, J., 1951. Maternal care and mental health. WHO monograph, series 2. WHO, Geneva.

Brain, D., Maclay, I., 1968. Cited in Bielby E 1984 A childish concept. Nursing Mirror 159 (18), 26–28.

Bretherton, I., 2002. Online. Available at: http://attachment.edu.ar/bio.html

Brett, A., 1983. Preparing children for hospitalisation – a classroom teaching approach. Journal of School Nursing 53 (9), 561–563.

Burgess, C., 2001. Complementary therapies: guided imagery and infant massage. Paediatric Nursing 13 (6), 37–41.

Burton, R., 1994. How to bear the pain. Child Health April/May, pp. 251–254.

Campbell, E.H., 1957. The effects of mothers' anxiety on infants' behaviour – a dissertation presented to the Faculty of the Graduate School of Yale University. Unpublished doctoral thesis.

Caress, A.L., 2003. Giving information to patients. Nursing Standard 17 (43), 47–54.

Committee of the Central Health Services Council (the Platt report), 1959. The welfare of children in hospital. HMSO, London.

Crawford, C., Raven, K., 2002. Play preparation for children with special needs. Paediatric Nursing 14 (8), 27–29.

Darbyshire, P., 2003. Mothers' experience of their child's recovery in hospital and at home: a qualitative investigation. Journal of Child Health Care 17 (4), 291–309.

Department of Health (DoH), 1989. The Children Act. An introductory guide for the NHS Health Publications Unit. HMSO, London.

Department of Health (DoH), 2003. Getting the right start: national service framework for children, young people and maternity services. DoH, London.

Doellman, D., 2003. Pharmacological vs non pharmacological techniques in reducing venepuncture psychological trauma in pediatric patients. Journal of Infusion Nursing 26 (2), 103–109.

Eiser, C., 1988. Do children benefit from psychological preparation for hospitalisation? Psychology and Health 2, 133–138.

Ellerton, M., Merriam, C., 1994. Preparing children and families psychologically for day surgery: an evaluation. Journal of Advanced Nursing 19, 1057–1062.

Fassler, D., 1980. Reducing preoperative anxiety in children – information versus emotional support. Patient Counselling & Health Education 2 (3), 130–134.

Fradd, E., 1986. Learning about hospital. Nursing Times 82 (3), 28–30.

Gaudian, C., 2000. Children's knowledge of their internal anatomy. In: Glasper, E.A., Ireland, L.M. (Eds.), Evidence-based child health care. Macmillan, Basingstoke.

Gaughan, M., Sweeney, E., 1997. Take heart: setting up a pre-admission day. Paediatric Nursing 9 (1), 22–23.

Gibson, C., 1991. A concept analysis of empowerment. Journal of Advanced Nursing 16 (3), 354–361.

Glasper, E.A., 1999. An evaluation of five years' work in Romania. Paediatric Nursing 11 (8), 32–35.

Glasper, E.A., Charles-Edwards, I., 2002. The child first and always: the registered children's nurse over 150 years. Part one. Paediatric Nursing 14 (4), 38–42.

Glasper, E.A., Lowson, S., 1998. Ambulatory care – the scope of practice. In: Glasper, E.A., Lowson, S. (Eds.), Innovations in paediatric ambulatory care: a nursing perspective. Macmillan, London.

Glasper, E.A., Lowson, S., Manger, R., Phillips, L., 1995. Developing a centre for health information and promotion. British Journal of Nursing 4 (12), 693–697.

Glasper, E.A., Prudhoe, G., Weaver, K., 2007. Does clowning benefit children in hospital? Views of theodora children's trust clown doctors. JCYPN 1 (1), 24–28.

Glasper, E.A., Stradling, P., 1989. Preparing children for admission. Paediatric Nursing July, 18–20.

Glasper, E.A., Thompson, M., 1993. Preparing children for hospital. In: Glasper, E.A., Tucker, A. (Eds.), Advances in child health nursing. Scutari, London.

Gleitman, H., 1986. Psychology, 2nd edn. WW Norton, Ontario.

Haggarty, R., Rushforth, H., 1996. A child's eye view. Video and teaching package. Department of Teaching Media. University of Southampton.

Haggarty, R., Rushforth, H., 1999. A child's eye view. Paediatric Nursing 11 (10), 27–30.

Harlow, H.F., 1958. The nature of love. Address of the President at the sixty-sixth annual Convention of the American Psychological Association, Washington DC, 31 August. Online. Available at: http://psychclassics.yorku.ca/Harlow/love.htm

Hodgins, M., Lander, J., 1997. Children's coping with venepuncture. Journal of Pain and Symptom Management 13 (5), 274–285.

Holden, C.E., Macdonald, A., Ward, M., et al., 1997. Psychological preparation for nasogastric feeding in children. British Journal of Nursing 6 (7), 376–385.

Hyland, M., Donaldson, M., 1989. Psychological care in nursing practice. Scutari Press, London.

In Defense of Animals 2002 Maternal deprivation experiments. Online. Available at: http://www.vivisectioninfo.org/deprivation/

Ireland, L., Rushforth, H., 1998. Paediatric day care and it contribution to ambulatory care nursing. In: Glasper, E.A., Lowson, S. (Eds.), Innovations in paediatric ambulatory care. Macmillan, London.

Jolly, J., 1976. Preparing children for hospital. Nursing Times 72, 1532–1533.

Keeton, D., 1999. Pain, nausea and vomiting: a day surgery audit. Paediatric Nursing 11 (5), 28–32.

Kiely, T., 1989. Preparing children for admission to hospital. Nursing 3 (33), 42–44.

Kosky, J., Lunnon, R.J., 1991. Great Ormond Street and the story of medicine. Granta Editions, London.

Lawton, L.C., Rose, P., 2003. Changing practice in invasive procedures: the experience of the Krishnan Chandran Children's Centre. Journal of Child Health Care 7 (4), 248–257.

Mathison, L., Butterworth, D., 2001. The role of play in the hospitalisation of young children. Neonatal, Paediatric and Child Health Nursing 4 (3), 23–26.

Matthews, M., Silk, G., 1992. Young children, priority one. Cited in: Ballentine, M., Gow, D., 1998. The value of play in ambulatory settings. In: Glasper, E.A., Lowson, S. (Eds.), Innovations in paediatric ambulatory care. Macmillan, London.

McPherson, A., Foster, D., Glazebrook, C., Symth, A., 2002. The asthma files; evaluation of a multimedia package for children's asthma education. Paediatric Nursing 14 (2), 32–35.

Mellish, P.W.R., 1969. Preparation of a child for hospitalisation and surgery. Pediatric Clinics of North America 16 (3), 543–554.

Meng, A., Zastowny, T., 1982. Preparation for hospitalisation: a stress inoculation training program for parents and children. Maternal-Child Nursing Journal 11 (2), 87–94.

Miles, I., 1986. The emergence of sick children's nursing. Part 1. Sick children's nursing before the turn of the century. Nurse Education Today 6, 82–87.

Miller, S., 1979. Children's fears – a review of the literature with implications for nursing research and practice. Nursing Research 28 (4), 217–223.

Murphy-Taylor, C., 1999. The benefits of preparing children and parents for day surgery. British Journal of Nursing 8 (12), 801–804.

Nicklin, J., 2002. Improving the quality of written information for patients. Nursing Standard 16 (49), 39–44.

Ogden Burke, S., Harrison, M.B., Kaufman, E., Wong, C., 2001. effects of stress-point intervention with families of repeatedly hospitalized children. Journal of Family Nursing 7 (2), 128–158.

Piaget, J., Inhelder, B., 1969. The psychology of the child. Routledge and Kegan Paul, London.

PSI Café 2002 A psychology resource site. Online. Available at: http://www.psy.pdx.edu/PsiCafe/KeyTheorists/Lorenz.htm

RCPCH 2000 Online. Available at: http://www.rcpch.ac.uk/publications/recent_publications/Advocacy/advocting.pdf

Rice, M., Glasper, A., Keeton, D., Spargo, P., 2008. The effect of a preoperative education programme on perioperative anxiety in children; an observational study. Pediatric anaesthesia 18, 426–430.

Robertson, J., 1970. Young children in hospital. Tavistock, London.

Robertson, J., 1989. Separation and the very young. Free Association Books, London.

Robinson, S., Hughes, K., Manning, K., 2002. Children's books: a resource for children's nursing. Paediatric Nursing 14 (5), 26–31.

Rushforth, H., 1996. Nurses' knowledge of how children view health and illness. Paediatric Nursing 8 (5), 23–27.

Rushforth, H., 1999. Practitioner review. Communicating with hospitalised children: review and application of research pertaining to children's understanding of health and illness. Journal of Child Psychology and Psychiatry 40 (5), 683–691.

Rutherford, D., 1998. Children's relationships. In: Taylor, J., Woods, M. (Eds.), Early childhood studies, Arnold, London.

Rutter, M., 1981. Maternal deprivation reassessed, 2nd edn. Penguin, Harmondsworth.

Saile, H., Burgemeier, R., Schmidt, L., 1988. A meta-analysis of studies on psychological preparation of children facing medical procedures. Psychology and Health 2, 107–132.

Salantera, S., Lauri, S., Salmi, S., Helenius, T., 1999. Nurses' knowledge about pharmacological and non pharmacological pain management. Journal of Pain and Symptom Management 18 (4), 289–299.

Santen, L., Feldman, T., 1994. A huge community project. American Journal of Maternal-Child Nursing 19, 102–106.

Savins, C., 2002. Therapeutic work with children in pain. Paediatric Nursing 14 (5), 14–16.

Smith, R.M., 1986. Anesthesia for infants and children, 3rd edn. CV Mosby, St Louis.

Stone, K., Glasper, E.A., 1997. Can leaflets assist parents in preparing children for hospital? British Journal of Nursing 6 (18), 1054–1058.

Sutherland, T., 2003. Comparison of hospital and home based preparation for cardiac surgery. Paediatric Nursing 15 (5), 13–16.

Taylor, D., 1991. Prepare for the best. Nursing Times 87 (31), 64–65.

Taylor, J., Muller, D., Wattley, L., Harris, P., 1999. Nursing children: psychology, research and practice, 3rd edn. Stanley Thornes, Cheltenham.

Thurtle, V., 1998. Multi-disciplinary care of the sick child in the community. In: Taylor, J., Woods, M. (Eds.), Early childhood studies. Arnold, London.

Vernon, D.T., Schulman, J.L., Foley, J.M., 1966. Changes in children's behaviour after hospitalisation. American Journal of Diseases of Children 111 (6), 81–93.

Vagnoli, L., Caprilli, S., Robiglio, A., Messeri, A., 2005. Clown doctors as a treatment for preoperative anxiety in children: a randomized, prospective study. Pediatrics 116 (4), e563–e567.

Visintainer, M., Wolfer, J., 1975. Psychological preparation for surgical pediatric patients: the effect on children's and parents' stress responses and adjustments. Pediatrics 56 (2), 187–201.

Weaver, K., Prudhoe, G., Batrrick, C., Glasper, E.A., 2007. Sick children's perceptions of clown humour. JCYPN 1 (8), 359–365.

Webster, A., 2000. The facilitating role of the play specialist. Paediatric Nursing 12 (7), 24–27.

Whiting, M., 1993. Play and surgical patients. Paediatric Nursing 5 (6), 11–13.

Willock, J., Richardson, J., Brazier, A., et al., 2004. Peripheral venepuncture in infants and children. Nursing Standard 18 (27), 43–50.

Wilson, H., 1981. Behavioural preparation for surgery: benefit or harm? Journal of Behavioural Medicine 4, 79–102.

Wolkind, S., Rutter, M., 1985. Separation, loss and family relationships. In: Rutter, M., Hersov, L. (Eds.), Child and adolescent psychiatry. Blackwell Scientific, Oxford.

Family-centred care

6

Lynda Smith Valerie Coleman Maureen Bradshaw

ABSTRACT

The primary aim of this chapter and its companion PowerPoint presentation is to translate the concept of family-centred care into everyday practice for nurses working with children and their families.

LEARNING OUTCOMES

- Understand family-centred care as a concept in children's nursing.
- Understand and appreciate the use of the practice continuum tool in children's nursing practice.
- Use negotiation, empowerment and reflective skills in the delivery of family-centred care.
- Appreciate the challenges of delivering family-centred care in practice.
- Locate family-centred care within the wider context of inter-professional practice
- Understand the value of involving children and young people in decision making in the context of family-centred care
- Understand the professional and legal implications of using a family-centred approach to care.

Glossary

Concept: The way a particular subject is viewed and how it is classified. These views can vary from person to person, which is why family-centred care is difficult to define, because different individuals consider different aspects of family-centred care to be important.

Continuum: A continuum is a continuous whole rather than something that has a defined beginning and end. In this instance, continuum means that there is no start or finish point, that families can be on the continuum at any point and move along it in any direction.

Framework: Identifies and outlines the elements that explicitly belong to a subject, in this instance family-centred care. A number of frameworks describe the different elements or attributes of family-centred care.

Philosophy: An explicit statement of one's beliefs and values. Family-centred care is an explicit statement about the values and beliefs of children's nursing practice, in relation to the children and families in our care.

Self-efficacy: Individuals believe that 'they are capable of performing a given activity' (Tones & Tilford 2001 p 104). In terms of family-centred care, nurses can help families to develop self-efficacy beliefs by negotiating short-term goals related to the care of their children and by providing the appropriate support to enable the families to achieve. Achievement is likely to result in families believing that they are capable of performing this negotiated care and other aspects of their children's care.

Introduction

Family-centred care is a multifaceted concept that has evolved over the past 60 years and remains a significant concept for children's nursing in the 21st century. The concept embraces caring for the child in the context of the family and therefore nurses recognise the central role of the family in the child's life.

Today's healthcare culture, however, continues to present many challenges in translating family-centred care theory into practice, including inter-professional working and involving children and young people in making decisions in the context of family-centred care. The focus of this chapter is to clarify and enhance understanding of family-centred care as a theoretical construct and to discuss how this can be applied in everyday clinical practice using the practice continuum tool, which was developed for this purpose. This is supported by a toolkit of skills that will enable nurses to practice family-centred care effectively.

DOI: 10.1016/B978-0-7020-3183-0.10006-2

Understanding family-centred care as a concept

Different definitions and theoretical frameworks have been used to explain the evolving concept of family-centred care. These definitions and frameworks are all still reflected to some extent in the family-centred care approaches that are currently used by children's nurses in practice. This is because some children's nurses, using their professional judgement, will select the most appropriate family-centred care framework to meet the needs of individual children and their families. Conversely, other children's nurses have not adopted contemporary theoretical family-centred care frameworks for implementation in practice and their approach to care is based on earlier theories. This may be due to choice or because of a lack of knowledge, skills or willingness to adopt new ways of working in practice. Bruce & Ritchie (1997) identify a need for skill development in areas of communication that involve negotiation and the sharing of information with children and their families. These areas of communication are defining characteristics of contemporary family-centred care theoretical frameworks. Bruce et al (2002) advocate the need for continuing education for healthcare professions working with families to further develop these communication skills.

This situation, concerning the use of different family-centred care frameworks in practice, can be confusing, making family-centred care potentially one of 'nursing's most amorphous concepts' (Darbyshire 1994) and 'rather ad hoc and unpredictable' (Callery 1997). Dunst & Trivette (1996) argue that to improve family-centred care practice nurses need to understand the characteristics of using different approaches in their nursing care. Contemporary research/literature reviews have studied different aspects of the concept in an attempt to bring about this improvement, for example parental involvement (Ygge et al 2006); partnership (Lee 2007); negotiation (Corlett & Twycross 2006, McCann et al 2008) and empowerment (Dampier 2002). Several of the examples in recent family-centred care studies use inter-professional examples (Law et al 2003) and others explore children's involvement in decision-making (Coyne 2006) demonstrating the evolving nature of family-centred care.

Whilst the results of the MacKean et al (2005) study challenged the contemporary conceptualisation of family-centred care as 'shifting care, care management and advocacy responsibilities to families' (p 74) instead of collaborative working. It is therefore essential to have an awareness and understanding of functional, holistic, hierarchical and continuum family-centred care theoretical frameworks. Also Bruce et al (2002) and Franck & Callery (2004) recommend rethinking to develop a family-centred care research programme to study the application of family-centred care theory in practice as well as studying understanding of the philosophy (see evidence of recent attempts to evaluate family-centred care in practice, Lewis et al 2007, Murphy & Fealy 2007).

Due to the evolving nature of the concept of family-centred care, different definitions have underpinned the development of these different theoretical frameworks.

Reflect on your practice

- How are families involved in their children's care on your clinical placement?
- Define family-centred care based on this reflection.

Your definition is likely to reflect one of the definitions provided by others to underpin the different family-centred care theoretical frameworks that exist. An early definition was:

> Family-centred care provides an opportunity for the family to care for the hospitalised child under nursing supervision ... The goal of family-centred care is to maintain or strengthen the roles and ties of the family with the hospitalised child in order to promote normality of the family unit
>
> (Brunner & Suddarth 1986 p 66)

This definition suggests that the nurse supervises care and plays a rather passive role with the family and no active role with children. It identifies the opportunity for families to be involved in the care of the hospitalised child and seems to recognise the importance of addressing the psychological needs of the child with regard to promoting normality of the family unit. This definition was largely congruent with societal values and beliefs – and the care of sick children (which predominantly took place in the hospital setting) – up to the early 1980s. However, children are now cared for at home whenever possible and hence family-centred care is likely to have a different meaning, because the context of care has changed. An overarching contemporary definition of family-centred care is:

> The professional support of the child and family through a process of involvement, participation and partnership underpinned by empowerment and negotiation
>
> (Smith et al 2002 p 22)

This definition recognises that family-centred care is not an ad hoc approach to care but that it requires the nurse to make use of professional knowledge and skills to support the child and family, participating in care in both hospital and community settings. It offers different dimensions to family-centred care (involvement, participation and partnership), which are 'each in their own way relevant and provide an opportunity for families to be involved in the care of their child, preferably to an extent of their own choosing through negotiation with nurses' (Smith et al 2002 p 22). In other words, family-centred care does not have to be the same for every family and it may change for individual families at different times during a child's healthcare journey. The implications of this are that it is acceptable for family-centred care to be either nurse-led or family-led, making it significantly different from the earlier definition offered by Brunner & Suddarth (1986), which relied on nursing supervision. The contemporary definition also suggests that an outcome of family-centred care is the empowerment of children and their families, demonstrating its congruence with contemporary health policy in the 21st century, which advocates for child and family empowerment (Department of Health (DoH) 1999, 2000, 2003, 2004).

Other contemporary definitions include Shields et al (2006) which emphasises the need to plan care around the whole family and to recognise them as care recipients as well as carers. The Institute of Family Centered Care (2008) views family-centred care as an approach that is governed by mutually beneficial partnerships between healthcare providers, patients of all ages and families. Whilst this chapter refers to family-centred care there has been a change in policy (DfES 2004, DoH 2004) and literature to child-centred care to conceptualise/define children as central to and as active participants in their own care.

www

Read 'Getting the right start: national service framework for children standard for hospital services' (DoH 2003) online:

- http://www.doh.gov.uk/nsf/children/standardhospservicein dex.htm

This emphasises the need to work in partnership with families and to involve them in decision making.

Scenario

Gemma, a second-year student nurse, starts her clinical placement on a children's medical ward. She is keen to learn about family-centred care and asks her mentor lots of questions.

PROFESSIONAL CONVERSATION

Helen, a registered children's nurse on part 1 of the nursing and midwifery council's professional register, is Gemma's mentor.

Issues affecting the use of family-centred care theoretical frameworks for nursing practice on different children's wards

I have been qualified for 3 years now. When I worked as a staff nurse on the children's surgical ward we usually asked the families to continue to give 'basic care' to their children in hospital, just like they would at home. I don't think they always wanted to do it but most families would comply, especially when they saw other families doing the care. We wanted them, for example, to feed their children, help with hygiene needs and to play with the children. The families were all treated the same with regard to involving them in caring for their children, except of course if the child was very ill and it was better for the nurse to do all the care then. Sometimes we had to teach the child or the family how to do some of the nursing or medical care to enable them to care for the child on discharge home. This all took time and some of my colleagues used to be rather impatient and judgemental with families who were slower to learn than others.

I started working on the medical ward about 3 months ago. Family-centred care is very different here, because we really do seem to give individual care to the different families. We listen to what the child and different family members have to say and information-giving is a two-way process. After all, the family are the experts on their child. The families still give 'basic care' to their children but we negotiate with them so that they can choose what care they want to participate in and when. We also assess their learning needs and teach them accordingly either to adapt their skills or to learn new ones. In fact, the children and families are much more involved altogether on this ward. The families really do participate in the decision-making process about their children's care and many do work in partnership with us.

Helen is distinguishing between using a functional framework on the children's surgical ward and using a holistic framework on the children's medical ward.

In practice, using a functional framework results in a lack of collaboration between the nurse and family. In other words, families are understood in terms of having a functional value and they become resources to be effectively used and managed by nurses (Darbyshire 1993). The nurse using a functional framework takes on the role of gatekeeper and decides what care the family can participate in (Hutchfield 1999). Families are allowed to continue performing tasks that they would usually perform at home in hospital to help the nurse and to make them feel useful (Darbyshire 1993, Nethercott 1993). Although some families might be involved in more technical aspects of the child's care, that depends on their willingness and ability, as assessed by nurses (Nethercott 1993). The power very much resides with the nurse when this functional approach to family-centred care is used.

The holistic approach to family-centred care had its origins within the framework developed in 1987 by Shelton and colleagues, which identifies a framework of elements all linked together by a strong thread of communication (Shelton & Smith Stepanek 1995). It has a fundamentally different underlying philosophy to the functional approach (Smith et al 2002):

> It is an approach that requires nurses to shift from a professionally centred view of health care to a collaborative model that recognises the family as central to a child's life
>
> (Ahmann 1994, p 113)

The holistic approach is grounded in respect for and cooperation with the family (Hutchfield 1999). It is underpinned by the principle that there should be an exchange of complete and unbiased information between the family and professionals (Shelton & Smith Stepanek 1995). The approach recognises that all families have some strengths. Nurses can help families to recognise these strengths and build on them to participate in the provision of optimum care to their own children. Families are more likely to take the lead in care and to work in partnership with nurses when this approach is used, as opposed to the nurse-led functional approach.

Hierarchical frameworks may also be used to underpin the practice of family-centred care. The evolvement of the concept of family-centred care has seen a move from parental involvement to parental participation through to partnership working and collaborative working, and finally to family-centred care. It could be that one concept has replaced the other during the evolvement of the concept of family-centred care, but Cahill (1996) suggests that there is a hierarchical relationship between the concepts. Hutchfield (1999) proposes that involvement, participation and partnerships are precursors and depicts them at the lower levels of a hierarchy that has family-centred care at the highest level. The differences between the levels of participation are clearly explained. Nurses, through accurate assessment and negotiation with children and families, are able to use the framework to identify the appropriate level of care for individual families and may then facilitate the family engaging in care at this level. Reassessment may result in families staying at the same level or moving up a level on the hierarchy (Darbyshire 1994).

Seminar discussion topic

Advantages and disadvantages of functional, holistic and hierarchical family-centred care theoretical frameworks

There are advantages and disadvantages of using all these theoretical frameworks.

The functional framework may be judged to be appropriate because families with a sick child will prefer nurses to lead the care and to be told what to do. However, families can be disempowered by this approach, in which the power remains with the nurse as the gatekeeper.

Holistic frameworks are positive because the family members are valued and respected as individuals. The family can negotiate its participation in care and is empowered to work in partnership with the nurse. Conversely, some families may feel they have too much responsibility in care and on occasions they could do 'with a break'.

The hierarchical framework is really positive because 'it recognises that families want to participate in the care of their children in hospital at a level of their own choosing' (Smith et al 2002 p 29). Conversely, the hierarchical framework suggests that families move up the hierarchy and that there is not the option to return to a lower level of participation in care.

Another criticism of hierarchical frameworks is that nurses only use them to negotiate levels of care for families and not to find out about family experiences of living with a sick child in hospital (Darbyshire 1994).

To conclude, there are pros and cons to all these frameworks.

Family-centred care: the practice continuum tool

This tool has been developed specifically for use in clinical practice. On the continuum (Fig. 6.1), families are facilitated to move in either direction at any time according to individual family and nursing needs. The practice continuum tool can be used for the delivery of family-centred care in any clinical setting involving families both in hospital and in the community.

The practice continuum tool acknowledges the key elements identified by the literature. Thus it comprises parental/child involvement, participation, partnership and parent/child-led care. 'No involvement' is also included to encompass the full spectrum of care that may be experienced by the child within the context of his or her family. The child/young person has been explicitly identified within the continuum to acknowledge the varying degrees in which they may be active

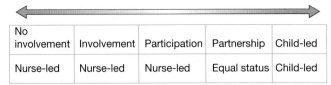

No involvement	Involvement	Participation	Partnership	Child-led
Nurse-led	Nurse-led	Nurse-led	Equal status	Child-led

Fig. 6.1 • Family-centred care: the practice continuum tool (reproduced from Smith et al 2002 with permission of Palgrave Macmillan).

participants in their care including planning, delivery and management.

The practice continuum tool was synthesised from available research and theoretical material, as well as practice experience, and therefore incorporates all the elements of the theoretical frameworks already discussed. Children's nurses should be familiar with the terms contained within the tool but because these terms are sometimes used interchangeably to mean the same thing, and because using the practice continuum tool provides practitioners with a dialogue through which to articulate family-centred care in a meaningful and achievable way, it is important to understand what we mean by the following terms:

- **Nurse-led care, no family involvement**: this may occur in situations where the family is not able or willing to be involved for a particular reason for a period of time. This is still family-centred care because the nurse still uses a family-centred focus in care delivery in the family's absence.
- **Nurse-led care, family/child involvement in care**: this may occur when the family is involved in some basic care, such as feeding, hygiene and/or emotional support. The nurse takes the lead in care management at this stage.
- **Nurse-led, family/child participation in care**: a good rapport is established, which is collaborative in nature, and the family participates in chosen aspects of nursing care following negotiation. The nurse continues to oversee care management and where necessary teaches relevant care skills to the child and/or family.
- **Equal status, family/child partnership in care**: this is exemplified by the change in the nurse's role to becoming more of a supporter and facilitator. As families become more empowered they resume their role as primary care givers and the relationship with the nurse is much more equal in nature.
- **Parent/child-led care, nurse-consulted care**: the family is now expert in all aspects of the child's care. There is a mutual, respectful relationship with the nurse, who is used in a consultative capacity from time to time. Although this is expressed explicitly as parent-led care, the implicit notion is that children are involved in their care and can lead their care in some instances.

No matter where the family is on the practice continuum, it is family-centred care; family-centred care is not only achieved by reaching an 'end stage'. Parents negotiating with the nurse choose where they wish to be on the continuum. For some this may be a progression along the continuum, particularly for those families with a child with an ongoing illness, whereas others may prefer to be involved differently, providing normal childcare and emotional support only.

Research has consistently shown that parents want to be actively involved in their child's care (Espezel & Canam 2003, MacKean et al 2005) and they want their involvement to be negotiated not assumed or expected (Kirk 2001, O'Haire & Blackford 2005). By communicating effectively with families, nurses can focus on their specific needs in relation to family-centred care rather than adopting a blanket approach to it (Smith et al 2002).

The strength of the practice continuum tool is its ability to respond to individual need day by day/shift by shift as the child and family's situation changes. Hence nurses facilitate forward and backward movement along the practice continuum tool as the child's condition changes or as family circumstances dictate. Ongoing evaluation is very much a part of the nurse's caregiving role and therefore incorporating such an explicit approach to family-centred care should not be onerous and will facilitate communication between different nurses caring for the family.

PowerPoint

Access the companion PowerPoint presentation for guidelines on using the practice continuum tool.

Toolkit of skills

To be able to use the practice continuum tool, or any other theoretical family-centred care framework, children's nurses need to have a toolkit of skills to empower families to negotiate their way through the interfaces of different healthcare environments. Good communication and teaching skills are essential for the successful implementation of family-centred care.

Communication skills

Without good communications skills, assumptions may well be made about what families will do for their children in hospital and in the community.

Reflect on your practice

- Think of some examples of good practice in family-centred care that you have observed.
- What communication skills did the nurse use?

You probably mentioned skills like listening, explaining, clarifying, using open-ended questions and negotiating. Communication frameworks that enable skills like these to be used should be chosen to facilitate nurses and families working collaboratively together to care for children. The LEARN model framework (Berlin & Fowkes 1983) promotes interaction between the nurse and family, encouraging active listening by both parties, and acknowledges perceptual differences and similarities with regard to problems and negotiation about the child's care. LEARN is an acronym:

L = Listen
E = Explain
A = Acknowledge
R = Recommend
N = Negotiate.

The Nursing Mutual Participation Model (Curley, cited in Ahmann 1994) requires asking open-ended questions to find out how the child and family feel that they can best participate in care. Families usually know their own child best and therefore professionals should not make independent decisions about involving them in care. Casey (1995) suggests that person-centred nurses are skilled practitioners who are willing to share their knowledge and expertise and to listen to families. Families may well become disempowered if decision making is taken out of their control and they are put in a position where they are expected to undertake aspects of their child's care that they are not competent to do or are not happy about doing.

Empowerment

Reflect on your practice

- Identify a situation in which either a family or yourself was disempowered.
- What were the inner and outer manifestations of this disempowerment?

Disempowerment engenders such feelings as being: out of control, confused, anxious, angry and frustrated over not being heard by healthcare professionals. These are obviously very strong negative feelings, which need to be avoided, and hence there is a need for collaborative working in family-centred care to empower families. Empowerment is a reciprocal social process that helps people to participate with competence (Coleman 1998) and to assert control over factors that affect their lives (Gibson 1991).

PROFESSIONAL CONVERSATION

Helen, a registered children's nurse on part 1 of the nursing and midwifery council's professional register, discusses the empowerment of families with Gemma, a student nurse.

Issues affecting family empowerment on a children's ward

It took me a long while to really understand what empowerment was all about. It wasn't until I started working on this ward that it began to make sense. This was because we are encouraged to get to know the children and their families quite well (even those that are only in a short time) and really build up a trusting relationship with them. This makes it easier to negotiate with them and to agree on their participation in chosen aspects of their child's care. Families also seem more receptive to our teaching and information giving because we have taken time to listen to them and to find out about them as a family unit. We also involve children as much as possible in their own care and decision-making, that does not always have to be about major issues, because it seems to help by enabling them to have some control over the situation. It's really good when the families become competent in doing negotiated aspects of their child's care. The families grow in confidence and then are usually ready to learn to do other aspects of the child's basic or nursing care.

Helen is describing empowerment both as an outcome and a process.

Empowerment outcomes

Children and their families have to take some power and control over their own situation to be able to reach empowerment outcomes. This does not mean having power over others. Instead, it signals that a family has taken some of the power from health professionals so that it can make decisions itself about the child's healthcare and/or give nursing care to the children. In their study of the families of children with middle ear infections, Wuest & Stern (1991) found that empowerment outcomes were domain specific. The families did not achieve an effective management of care outcome and stay there because new events in their child's healthcare journey would result in them moving along the continuum to adopt more passive behaviours until further competencies were developed for empowerment in new domains. However, these families developed an increasing repertoire of management strategies, which they used in different domains of their child's care to achieve empowerment outcomes. This suggests that an empowerment outcome increases family confidence and that it is also a regenerative process. Empowerment outcomes may be achieved in physical, social and/or psychological domains, or an outcome of empowerment may 'simply' mean that children and their families develop a sense of psychological well-being, promoting feelings of being in control of the situation in which they find themselves instead of being powerless or disempowered (Coleman 2002).

The empowerment process

The empowerment process is described as being a four-stage process (Gibson 1995, Kieffer 1984, Tones & Tilford 2001):

- Stage one: the entry stage is triggered by a specific incident, which leads to the discovery of the personal reality of the situation.
- Stage two: critical reflection to search for and identify the root cause of that reality to be able to move forward. Mentor and peer relationships are seen as being important during this stage.
- Stage three: this is a self-development stage, which may involve examining the implications of actions and may result in individuals wanting to 'take charge' of a situation.
- Stage four: this stage involves developing plans of action, gaining participatory competence in care, taking power from professionals and holding on to it.

During the four stages of the empowerment process a caring relationship should evolve between nurse and family, within which there is building of trust, connecting, mutual knowing and creating to promote self-esteem, self-confidence and self-insight (McWilliam et al 1997) to empower children and families.

Conversely, Gibson (1995, 1999) described how mothers of chronically ill children with neurological problems had achieved empowerment outcomes without facilitation from nurses. The mothers in this particular study were empowered in an intrapersonal process to have their voices heard in decision-making and to participate with competence in their children's care. This process was triggered by their frustration on realising that no one was listening to them. A study by Valentine (1998) found that although nurses had the necessary knowledge to empower families, they needed to develop the skills to do it and an empowering environment to practice in.

Activity

Read Gibson (1995) and Valentine (1998).

- How do the findings of these studies relate to your workplace?
- Consider the recommendations of the studies for your workplace.

Scenario

Gemma discusses her written reflective account of a very positive experience of being involved in the empowerment of a child and family with her mentor Helen.

Gemma describes how a child and family achieved empowerment outcomes and the process used to develop competencies. The nursing process was used to provide a systematic framework for practice and three key stages of an empowerment process in children's nursing emerged (Coleman 2002):

1 Relationship building

During the continuing nursing assessment the child and family were listened to and there was a sharing of perceptions and knowledge with the nurse. The nurse explored family strengths, as opposed to weaknesses, to promote self-efficacy beliefs to achieve empowerment outcomes. An assessment was made of issues that the child and the family considered to be problems so that these could be addressed along with the nurse-perceived problems. Using appropriate communication skills, the nurse built up a trusting relationship within which there was respect and valuing of the child and family. This relationship helped the nurse and family to journey together through the four stages of an empowerment process. Contemporary family-centred care policy (DfES 2004) and research (Coyne 2006) recognises that children should be and want to be consulted listened to and involved in decision making and hence should be essential to relationship building.

2 Facilitating participatory experiences to develop competencies

This was a planned process to enable the child and family to develop competence in negotiated aspects of care. Initially, short-term goals were agreed between the nurse and family to promote self-efficacy beliefs. The family was initially helped to adapt the care usually undertaken at home by the parents to the hospital situation, before being taught and facilitated to do some nursing care appropriate to their situation. The participatory experiences had physical, social and psychological dimensions. The child was also offered opportunities for empowerment, by being given choices at an appropriate developmental level about play and who should give him his medicine. Decision making is a complex process though and consistent, structured and robust methods (Baston 2008) and explicit criteria should be used to ensure that children are not pressurised into inappropriate participation (Coyne 2006).

Other children with continuing care needs will also be taught how to do specific physical nursing skills, especially those making the transition to adult services who need to be prepared and empowered for this move. A staged move from a children's to adult outpatients is an example of a planned participatory experience with the young person perhaps attending a joint child/adult clinic prior to attending the adult clinic. Disempowerment can result from lack of a planned transition to adult health services and the Department of Health (2004) identifies that it may be associated with an increased risk if non-adherence to treatment with serious consequences (see RCN 2004 and RCN 2008 for guidance about adolescent transitional care).

3 Information giving to empower families

Information is fundamental to the empowerment of children and families. It is a two-way process with nurses and families sharing information. Information is conveyed to children and families in many different ways including:

- verbal information on an individual basis
- NHS Direct
- written literature including leaflets, books and posters
- other media including videos, television and the internet
- play activities to educate children
- support groups.

A planned approach to information giving is essential to enable children and families to use it to take some control of their situation. Conversely, information may be disempowering if it is given in an ad hoc manner, which for example may result in too much information being given at the wrong time (Coleman 2002). Some healthcare professionals may also be disempowering because, as Dampier et al (2002) found, parents had difficulty in getting professionals to believe that their child was ill and also referred to gatekeepers who made access to care difficult when their children were critically ill. Reeves et al (2006) found that some nurses did not listen to or respect parental opinions hence disempowering them.

Reflect on your practice

Identify one situation when information giving was empowering and another one when information giving was disempowering.

- How did information giving differ in these two situations?

Empowerment in a family-centred care approach is often associated with children with continuing care needs, whose care is parent/child led. However, children and families experiencing day care or acute care may also be empowered to some extent in all the positions identified on the practice continuum tool.

Activity

Discuss in your learning group how participatory experiences to empower children and families may differ according to the following contexts of care:

- day care
- acute care
- continuing care.

Negotiating care with children and families

Negotiation is a recurring theme in the literature on family-centred care. Research in this area repeatedly reminds nurses that negotiation either does not happen or that there is not the willingness or skills for it to happen (Blower & Morgan 2000, Kirk 2001, Reeves 2006).

To facilitate negotiation, nurses need to be equipped not only with the skills to implement it in practice but also a means of incorporating it into everyday practice so that it becomes an everyday part of their role with children and families.

To start this process nurses need to reflect on their current practice and evaluate the extent to which they do currently negotiate care with children and families. Self-awareness and analysis of our own practice enables care delivery to develop and remain dynamic offering the highest possible quality of care to children and their families. For student nurses and qualified nurses reflective practice has become accepted as a way of challenging and preventing routinised practice.

Scenario

'But we're doing it already'

Gemma is attending a study day on family-centred care. In the session the group of child branch students are discussing their experiences of family-centred care. The group discuss how families are involved in the care of their child. A frequent comment was 'We always ask them if they want to be involved and encourage them to participate'.

The lecturer facilitating the study day asks 'Is this negotiated care?'.

You might find it useful to read the research by Callery & Smith (1991).

This scenario highlights a common response to what constitutes how parents become involved in the care of their child. Sometimes parents are not asked and it is just expected they will participate in the care of their child (Roden 2005).

What therefore constitutes negotiation needs to be clarified if nurses are to incorporate the concept into their day-to-day practice. Simply, Gourlay (1987) would see negotiations being about meeting people's needs. In this case not only the nurses' needs but those of the child and family. Expectation and assumption should not therefore play a part in the process, rather it is an acceptable agreement between those involved. This involves a relationship where both parties feel equally able to be involved and have their point of view heard. This can be difficult to achieve, as families often feel at a disadvantage, being in an unfamiliar, potentially stressful environment and needing to be empowered to fully participate. How nurses enable families to overcome these barriers is the key to successful negotiation. Equally, nurses need to feel enabled and empowered to undertake the negotiation.

Encouragement and expectation implies that the involvement is very much on the nurse's terms. Although it might, at face value, seem not unreasonable that a parent would want to be involved in the care of his or her child, non-negotiation does not facilitate different styles of coping and adjustment, the type of support the parents need or informed decision making on which to base their input; neither does it acknowledge that some parents need respite from some of the care demands placed upon them.

The practice continuum tool enables facilitation of the involvement in care by parents or child at a level they have negotiated with the nurse. The following framework, adapted from 'Negotiation of care' (Smith 2002), offers nurses a step-by-step approach to planned negotiation. In following this approach the nurse needs to utilise verbal, non-verbal and written communication skills that are an explicit part of the nurse's role. The LEARN framework (see above) will help.

At the start of any relationship, to minimise the potential for misunderstanding, there needs to be some discussion involving the boundaries and expectations (such as nurses assuming parents will always want to be involved or parents not being sure what their role is or can be). Most clinical areas will have a philosophy or mission statement and information booklet about their ward/unit or department that can be shared to start the negotiation process. This introduces the notion that there are opportunities for involvement that will be discussed.

Assess

In any negotiation process you need to discover each other's needs. The emphasis here is primarily on the family's needs as it adapts to the diagnosis, treatment, prognosis of the child and the demands that will be placed on the different family members. This, coupled with a strange environment, for many make it essential that the nurse uses a range of communication skills with the family (e.g. listening, open-ended questions, silence, paraphrasing to check understanding).

Plan

There needs to be an understanding of what is on offer. In what ways can the family be involved? How can this be facilitated? Everyone needs to be aware of this to avoid differences between staff at changeovers for example. This will also help identify any points that aren't acceptable and reduce the risk of assumptions being made about each other's role.

Record what has been agreed so that everyone is aware of the plan that is being developed. Underpinning planned negotiation is the empowerment of all participants, as discussed earlier in the chapter. As you are planning with the level of involvement at this stage with the family, are you considering the family's information or teaching needs, because these will impact on their decision-making ability and hence their involvement?

Implement

Summarise the agreement and check understanding. How will the agreements be implemented? (Are there any teaching or support requirements to facilitate implementation?) Consider how the negotiated care will be documented.

These issues are important because nurses are responsible and accountable for the care delivered. These are discussed in relation to family-centred care later in the chapter.

Evaluate

Review the agreements. In the same way we evaluate the child's ongoing care, the family's involvement may need to change. Knowing that if something doesn't work it can be changed enhances the trusting relationship between nurse and family. Confidence in the process is more likely to reduce the potential miscommunication between parties and lead to a more positive experience for all.

Using a framework linked to the systematic approach to nursing care that nurse's use on a daily basis should enable negotiated care to become a reality and not just another 'add on' to the day's work that doesn't always happen for many families.

Moving forward with family-centred care also requires this to be a multiprofessional philosophy and as such has become a recurring theme in therapy literature where collaboration between all those involved in the child/young person's care is highlighted (MacKean et al 2005, Titone 2004). Kelly (2007) has devised a model for therapy practice that essentially follows a systematic approach following similar principles to nursing and as such provides pointers to the ease with which interprofessional collaborative practice could be established across all professional groups working with children and families.

Teaching children and families

To participate in family-centred care it is necessary for children and families to learn about the illness/condition and possibly some nursing/medical skills. The position of the family on the Practice Continuum Tool at any given time will signify the teaching and learning that is required. Therefore, nurses require: teaching skills; knowledge of how people learn (social, behavioural, cognitive and humanistic learning theories); what motivates individuals to learn (intrinsic and extrinsic factors); an understanding and ability to assess health beliefs and the implication of role changes for family members, to enable them to take on different care responsibilities and to receive appropriate support.

The challenges of delivering family-centred care

Scenario

Gemma is gaining experience on a children's ward working alongside Helen, her mentor. Gemma has been introduced to the concept of family-centred care in school but linking this theory to ward practice seems less than straightforward to her. She discusses some of her reflections on this issue with Helen at her intermediate interview.

There is potential for family-centred care to be confusing because it can mean different things to children and parents, student and qualified nurses, or other healthcare professionals. The way individuals think of and define things like 'family' or 'care' can vary enormously. Their diverse understanding, assumptions and values may have been shaped by things like personal life experiences thus far and general or professional education. So when it comes to actually practising family-centred care, one of the challenges for children's nurses is to keep abreast of the breadth and depth of the evolving concept through personal commitment to their own continuing development. Unless children's nurses really do internalise and value the concept, in practice it won't be evidenced in what they say and do with children and families (Bradshaw 2002). Also, in the light of current literature, nurses have the extra challenge of teasing out what family-centred care is in terms of their own particular ward or unit, so that they and other healthcare professionals connected to it understand, share and value the philosophy. Then comes the challenge of acquainting children and families with the philosophy and using it to underpin all subsequent interactions with them.

Getting family-centred care theory implemented in practice is not always easy or straightforward. It appears to require a 'bottom-up' approach whereby children's nurses working on the 'shop floor' really believe the concept to be valuable, desire to see it underpinning practice and adjust and align their professional behaviours so that they are congruent with this goal. If such goals are not to be thwarted, then appropriate managerial support is vital. The 'top-down' approach to implementing family-centred care can be equally helpful when nurse managers lead from the front and demonstrate their commitment to it by making clear their expectations that it will be fully implemented and audited in the clinical areas.

Family-centred care involves nurses negotiating choices and desired amounts of involvement or participation in care with children and their families. This involves much skill and sensitivity on the part of the nurse. Nurses have traditionally been seen as the experts who assumed responsibility for orchestrating patient care in line with medical prescriptions and institutional requirements. However, if care is to be truly family-centred, then recognising family expertise in care is vital. When nurse and family meet for the first time, they come together as experts but in different things. The family is often expert on things like getting the child to sleep, knowing what foods to tempt the reluctant eater with, what kind of play captures the child's imagination or distracts him or her, and how best to comfort him or her when upset. The children's nurse is an expert in meeting the ill child's nursing needs. The challenge for children's nurses is to work harmoniously with the family and to engineer pooling of all expertise in order that it may be a powerful force in meeting the child and family's needs.

The way nursing documentation is set out and therefore recorded can itself either hinder or enhance family-centred care. It needs to be developed in such a way that it is a good prompt and makes the elements of family-centred care philosophy overt and an expected requirement.

Activity

Consider your own healthcare trust and find out:

- What commitment to family-centred care does the healthcare trust demonstrate?
- What commitment to family-centred care does the senior nursing management demonstrate?
- What commitment to family-centred care does your ward/unit nursing staff demonstrate?
- What commitment to family-centred care do other members of the multiprofessional team demonstrate?
- How do families – especially those whose first language is not English – become aware of family-centred care and recipients of it?

For each of the above questions, what written, verbal and non-verbal local evidence do you have to support your findings?

Activity

With regard to family-centred care, try to look critically at the nursing documentation on your next new ward before anyone has a chance to explain it to you.

- Who do the documents require you to talk to?
- Whose thoughts and concerns do they require you to record?
- What do they require you to do and for whom?
- Will anyone else be contributing to care and if so what?
- What do the child and family think about care and progress so far? How do you know?
- Are the child and family involved in documentation? What advantages or problems might this raise? (Bradshaw 2002)

Scenario

The staff on Gemma's ward largely seem to value the principles of family-centred care. However, she notices that when other professionals visit children and families on her ward, or when children have to visit other departments, then this doesn't always seem to be the case.

Helen explains that as yet family-centred care is not necessarily a multiprofessional or interprofessional philosophy. From the child and family's point of view, if the professionals that they encounter are not being guided by the same philosophical framework, 'then there is much potential for what families actually receive and the way they receive it to be disjointed and confusing' (Bradshaw et al 2003). As a result, trust relationships between health professionals and families can be damaged and this itself can impinge on the child's therapeutic progress. One strategy developed to help overcome this is interprofessional shared learning, whereby different professionals are exposed to the same evidence-based education, the idea being that the ensuing discussions, critical analysis and interprofessional debate (in this instance on family-centred care) will lead to the different professionals understanding, valuing and practising the philosophy in a corporate, overt way that is therapeutic for children and families.

Current child health policy actively seeks to promote closer working between professional groups to deliver healthcare focused around the needs of the individual patient and family (DoH 2004, DfES 2004). Creating an interprofessional workforce capable of working in partnership and collaboration in care between all of the professional groups and agencies can then become commonplace and embedded in everyday practice. This can only help foster a family-centred approach to care that is interprofessional.

Professional and legal issues

For the nurse, family-centred care creates a range of professional and legal issues that need to be addressed. Nurses undertaking family-centred care owe a specific duty of care not only to the child but also to the parents, siblings and other family members. Negligence results when this duty of care is breached. Nurses delegating care to participating parents should provide them with adequate information and teaching, and ensure that they have the ability to perform the necessary care in a reliable and responsible way (Foxcroft 2002). To discharge the duty of care it is also important to identify when the child is able to make healthcare decisions and participate in care.

Activity

Find out what legal and other guidelines there are to inform you about children's rights and ability to consent, make healthcare decisions and to participate in care.

Nurses should use these guidelines to inform their professional judgement to decide whether a child has sufficient understanding and intelligence to participate in family-centred care, ensuring 'that the child is treated appropriately and that adequate care is provided so that the child does not suffer harm' (Foxcroft 2002 pp 156–157). The nurse also has a duty to supervise family-centred care, ensuring that the family is sufficiently competent to undertake that care before being allowed to act alone.

Nurses are accountable to their employer, to children/families by way of the law and to the Nursing and Midwifery Council (NMC). It has also been established that when discharging his/her duty to patients the nurse owes a duty to act in accordance with a body of responsible medical opinion and in so doing should follow approved professional nursing practice (NMC 2008).

Nurses must adhere to their professional code (NMC 2008) in family-centred care nursing practice. Care plans should be negotiated, agreed and documented with the family so that all concerned are clear as to each person's role in the care of the child. The documentation includes, parental agreement to participation in care, teaching undertaken, parental confidence to do certain tasks and planned review of care dates.

An interactive approach

Read the following scenario. At key points you will be asked to reflect upon the interaction between Imran, his family and the nurse. You will do this by plotting the developing relationship on a series of Practice Continuum Tools. You will be able to review your responses by checking them against those in the Feedback for the scenario questions section.

Scenario

Imran is a 5-year-old boy who is admitted to the children's medical ward following nebulised bronchodilator therapy in A & E for asthma diagnosed today. His past medical history links short-lived, mild wheeziness to common childhood respiratory illnesses but this has never warranted treatment or admission. It is the weekend and he is accompanied by his heavily pregnant mother, father and three older siblings. None of the children have been admitted to hospital before, although they have all visited hospitalised members of their extensive extended family from time to time.

Imran and his family are greeted by his nurse who quickly perceives how bored and restless his boisterous 7- and 8-year-old brothers are following several hours in the accident and emergency department. As Imran's respiratory condition is now stable, his nurse makes him and his parents comfortable by his bedside and meets some of his brothers' play needs by offering them games and the television to watch in the playroom next door where they can still all see each other through the window. Imran's 13-year-old sister chooses to stay with her parents and sits Imran on her knee which he is clearly comfortable with.

Imran's admission is nurse-led because he and his family are unfamiliar with this particular ward environment and what may be required of them. Also they currently lack specialist knowledge and skills in meeting the nursing care needs of a child with asthma. The nurse orientates the family to the ward environment, explains the ward's philosophy of family-centred care and collects data for the assessment of Imran's needs from himself and his family because they are the experts in his usual homecare and have much to offer the current situation. Although his mother appears to understand what is being asked, her answers are monosyllabic and it is largely Imran's sister who supplies the details of his usual activities of living and Imran's father who asks further questions about what the diagnosis of asthma will mean for Imran's future lifestyle. These questions are answered openly and honestly and the nurse supplies supportive literature on asthma together with the ward information leaflet in both English and Urdu (the parent's first language). The nurse and family agree that helping Imran with his breathing, hydration, rest and emotional comfort constitute his priority nursing needs. Imran's mother and sister choose to stay to continue Imran's emotional support and encourage him to drink whilst his nurse monitors his hydration and breathing and administers the required medication.

His father plans to take the brothers to play at their cousin's home before returning to his taxi-driving job.

Question 1

Imagine you are Imran's nurse. It is now time to hand over his care to your colleague on the next shift. State where you think he and his family are positioned on the Practice Continuum Tool at present and give your rationale with reference to the glossary in the family-centred care chapter.

If you wish you can shade the position you think applies. An example of this can be found on the PowerPoint presentation 'Guide to using The Practice Continuum Tool'.

No involvement	Involvement	Participation	Partnership	Parent-led/ child-led
Nurse-led	Nurse-led	Nurse-led	Equal status	Parent-led/ child-led

Ongoing assessment of Imran's progress and evaluation of this plan later in the day reveal it to be satisfactory. Imran's condition is stable and when his father returns later that evening with toilet requisites for his wife she opts to be resident and their daughter goes home with her father. Before they depart, however, Imran's nurse checks that his mother has been orientated to all hospital and ward facilities that she may need and that she is confident and able to make known any changing health needs of her own.

Imran is visited by many of his extended family the following day and they bring his sister to stay with her mother. Evaluation of his condition shows improvements, however he is still quite tired and only minimally interested in play so his nurse has to advocate on his behalf and sensitively renegotiate with his mother and extended family how best to meet his need for therapeutic rest. His father's job proves to be fairly flexible and Imran's nurse negotiates with him to be present at medication times so that he, his wife and daughter can start learning about and administering Imran's medication. Imran does quite well at taking the required bronchodilator and preventative steroid drugs from a metered dose inhaler using a spacer device.

The next day Imran and family are introduced to the asthma nurse specialist who will be continuing to support the family as they make the transition from hospital to home later that day. Imran is now much more playful but continues to cooperate with his parents when they administer his medication under nursing supervision. Before discharge his nurse checks that his parents understand the need for continuing the preventative medication once the bronchodilator therapy stops even though Imran may appear asymptomatic. They are reassured that they may contact the ward or specialist nurse with queries or problems at any time using the telephone numbers supplied in the support literature.

Question 2

Imagine you are the nurse discharging Imran and family into the care of your community colleague. Where will you report their position on the Practice Continuum Tool to be at the time of discharge? Give the rationale for your answer.

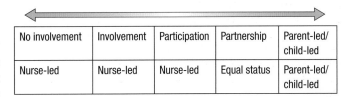

No involvement	Involvement	Participation	Partnership	Parent-led/ child-led
Nurse-led	Nurse-led	Nurse-led	Equal status	Parent-led/ child-led

Two weeks later Imran is admitted from school via the accident and emergency department with an acute exacerbation of his asthma. Yesterday he, his brothers and sister went to stay at their Aunt and Uncle's house when his mother went to the maternity hospital to deliver their new baby sister. This interruption in routine resulted in him missing several doses of his preventative medication. When he became emotional at school due to missing his mother, he became wheezy and his father was contacted to take him to hospital. Several members of Imran's extended family arrive whilst he is being readmitted and it is agreed that a close young adult cousin (his Aunt's eldest daughter) will stay to support Imran emotionally whilst his father returns to visiting his wife and continuing his job. Imran is used to being cared for frequently by his cousin in a family setting and under his nurses direction she encourages him with fluids and engages him in quiet play very effectively. His nurse monitors his condition and administers the prescribed medication.

Question 3

It's handover time again. As Imran's nurse and with reference to the glossary where will you now report him and his family to be on the Practice Continuum Tool and why?

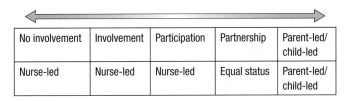

No involvement	Involvement	Participation	Partnership	Parent-led/ child-led
Nurse-led	Nurse-led	Nurse-led	Equal status	Parent-led/ child-led

Imran's breathing is much improved by the following day and his father who has taken time off work spends time discussing his son's medication with his nurse and demonstrates effective administration and supervision of his son taking the inhaled medication. In particular the nurse sensitively re-emphasises the reasons for the preventative medication to be continued when Imran appears asymptomatic. Medically Imran is fit for discharge and whilst Imran is occupied with the nursery nurse in the playroom, his nurse explores this possibility with his father. Knowing that Imran's mother and new baby are to be discharged home that day too, the needs of the whole family and the days practicalities are discussed within the context of negotiating if discharging Imran on the same day would be appropriate. His father is, however, confident to take Imran home with him. Members of the extended family are already there preparing for his wife's return and it is felt that they will be able to support Imran throughout the period when much attention may be focused on the new baby's homecoming.

Question 4

Using the Practice Continuum Tool as a communication tool, plot where you will report Imran and his father to be on it as you again discharge them back into the care of the asthma nurse specialist who will continue his care in the community.

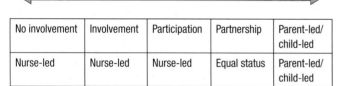

No involvement	Involvement	Participation	Partnership	Parent-led/ child-led
Nurse-led	Nurse-led	Nurse-led	Equal status	Parent-led/ child-led

The asthma nurse specialist continues to build up a trusting relationship with Imran and his family in the community. They consult her quite frequently at first, for example advice is sought when Imran develops an upper respiratory tract infection and some associated wheeziness. Recommencing bronchodilator therapy in this instance until peak flow monitoring indicates that it is safe to discontinue is a situation they then become increasingly confident at assessing, and responding to appropriately themselves. Through continued contact with the asthma nurse specialist in her teaching role, the family are empowered to become knowledgeable, skilful and confident in the management of Imran's asthma. Home visits instigated by the asthma nurse specialist are gradually replaced by mainly telephone contact initiated by the family if they have a query. The mutually respectful relationship that develops between nurse and family is one where each member values what the other can offer the situation. The family become experts in what it means to live with and manage the challenge of Imran's asthma on a daily basis and the asthma nurse specialist retains her broad and specialist children's nursing expertise that is always on offer to the family when they choose to avail themselves of it.

Question 5

Imagine yourself as the asthma nurse specialist. Give your rationale for where would you plot Imran and his family on the Practice Continuum Tool at this point in your relationship with them.

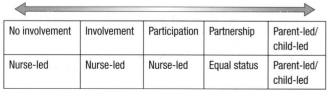

No involvement	Involvement	Participation	Partnership	Parent-led/ child-led
Nurse-led	Nurse-led	Nurse-led	Equal status	Parent-led/ child-led

Feedback for the scenario questions

Question 1 feedback

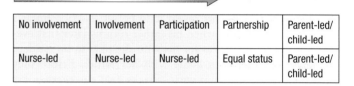

No involvement	Involvement	Participation	Partnership	Parent-led/ child-led
Nurse-led	Nurse-led	Nurse-led	Equal status	Parent-led/ child-led

Imran and his family are currently at the 'Nurse-led, Family Involvement' position on the Practice Continuum Tool. This is because Imran's mother and sister have chosen to continue to be involved with some of his basic care needs that they previously took care of at home. He is comforted by their emotional support and they are the experts at coaxing him to drink what they know to be his favourite fluids. This alone is a very valuable contribution to Imran's care and it helps to minimise potential adverse effects of hospitalisation such as threatened emotional security if children are cared for by strangers in an unfamiliar environment. At this stage it is the nurse with her specialist knowledge and skills in meeting the nursing care needs of asthmatic children who is leading care, care negotiation and being responsible for implementing and evaluating the more specific nursing aspects of Imran's care plan.

Question 2 feedback

No involvement	Involvement	Participation	Partnership	Parent-led/ child-led
Nurse-led	Nurse-led	Nurse-led	Equal status	Parent-led/ child-led

On discharge Imran and his family are at the 'Nurse-led, Family Participation in nursing care' position on the Practice Continuum Tool. In the three days that Imran has been hospitalised, his nurse has taken the lead in firstly negotiating family involvement in things they would normally have done for Imran at home. When this evaluated well, family participation in what was hitherto nursing aspects of care (for example administration of inhaled medication) was then successfully negotiated. Imran's ward-based nurse had begun the teaching of the relevant knowledge and care skills that he and his family would need to continue this care and care evaluation back in the community. Care continued to be nurse-led by the asthma nurse specialist in the community as she continued to facilitate the family's further development of asthma knowledge and management.

Question 3 feedback

No involvement	Involvement	Participation	Partnership	Parent-led/ child-led
Nurse-led	Nurse-led	Nurse-led	Equal status	Parent-led/ child-led

On the first day of readmission Imran and his extended family again settle comfortably at the 'Nurse-led, Family Involvement' position on the Practice Continuum Tool. Although Imran's Aunt is not participating in 'nursing' aspects of care, it is important not to view this as a backwards step, rather it is the family's chosen, negotiated position to be at on that particular day in the context of the whole family's needs and demands. The emotional and hydration support offered by Imran's cousin during this time was a very worthwhile contribution to Imran's care. His nurse continues to lead the nursing aspects of care required.

Question 4 feedback

No involvement	Involvement	Participation	Partnership	Parent-led/ child-led
Nurse-led	Nurse-led	Nurse-led	Equal status	Parent-led/ child-led

When Imran is discharged for the second time, his family are at the 'Nurse-led, Family Participation in nursing care' position on the Practice Continuum Tool. It is still the nurse who is leading negotiations on, for example, if the time is right to discharge Imran back into family care in the community. However the family, in particular his father, are again participating in nursing aspects of care, for example administering and supervising Imran taking his medication effectively.

Question 5 feedback

No involvement	Involvement	Participation	Partnership	Parent-led/ child-led
Nurse-led	Nurse-led	Nurse-led	Equal status	Parent-led/ child-led

Imran and his family are now displaying 'Parent-led/child-led' care. Over time the family has been empowered by the asthma nurse specialist to resume their role as primary care givers in all aspects of Imran's care. As the family become more knowledgeable, skilled, confident and competent in Imran's asthma management, the lead in care is shared in a more equal partnership and as further family expertise develops, the family's ability to take over the lead in care management emerges. This is exemplified by the nurse's role becoming more that of consultant and the family functioning as experts in meeting the challenges of daily asthma management. Nurse specialist expertise and family expertise are demonstrated respectively by both parties in the mutually respectful relationship which has developed and become a powerful force in assisting Imran to master his asthma successfully.

Summary

Contemporary health policy in the 21st century continues to highlight family-centred care as an essential concept for children's nurses. The need to work in partnership with families and involve them in decision making must be supported by children's nurses with the appropriate skills to facilitate this. The practice continuum tool as a framework for the practice of family-centred care will enable nurses to implement this concept in a variety of healthcare settings. Understanding the challenges, the legal and professional implications of family-centred care can only enhance the delivery of quality care.

References

Ahmann, E., 1994. Family-centred care: shifting orientation. Pediatric Nursing 20 (2), 113–116.

Baston, J., 2008. Healthcare decisions: a review of children's involvement. Paediatric Nursing 20 (3), 24–26.

Berlin, E.A., Fowkes, W.C., 1983. A teaching framework for cross-cultural health care. Western Journal of Medicine 139 (6), 934–938.

Blower, K., Morgan, E., 2000. Great expectations? Parental participation in care. Journal of Child Health Care 4 (2), 60–65.

Bradshaw, M., 2002. Implications and challenges for family-centred care. In: Smith, L., Coleman, V., Bradshaw, M. (Eds.), Family-centred care: concept, theory and practice. Palgrave, Basingstoke, pp. 47–61.

Bradshaw, M., Coleman, V., Smith, L., 2003. Interprofessional learning and family-centred care. Paediatric Nursing 15 (7), 30–33.

Bruce, B., Ritchie, J., 1997. Nurses' practices and perceptions of family centred care. Journal of Pediatric Nursing 12 (4), 214–222.

Bruce, B., et al., 2002. A multisite study of health professionals perceptions and practices of family-centered care. Journal of Family Nursing 8 (4), 408–429.

Brunner, L., Suddarth, D., 1986. The Lippincott manual of paediatric nursing, 2nd edn. Harper and Row, London.

Cahill, J., 1996. Patient participation: a concept analysis. Journal of Advanced Nursing 24, 561–571.

Callery, P., 1997. Caring for parents of hospitalised children: a hidden area of nursing work. Journal of Advanced Nursing 26 (5), 992–998.

Callery, P., Smith, L., 1991. A study of role negotiation between nurses and the parents of hospitalised children. Journal of Advanced Nursing 16, 772–781.

Casey, A., 1995. Partnership nursing: influences on involvement of informal carers. Journal of Advanced Nursing 22, 1058–1062.

Coleman, V., 1998. What is the meaning of empowerment and do nurses use it to promote the health of children with a chronic illness. Unpublished Masters dissertation, Sheffield Hallam University.

Coleman, V., 2002. Empowerment: rhetoric, reality and skills. In: Smith, L., Coleman, V., Bradshaw, M. (Eds.), Family-centred care: concept, theory and practice. Palgrave, Basingstoke, pp. 85–113.

Corlett, J., Twycross, A., 2006. Negotiation of parental roles within family-centred care: a review of the literature. Journal of Clinical Nursing 15, 1308–1314.

Coyne, I., 2006. Consultation with children in hospital: children, parents and nurses perspectives. Journal of Clinical Nursing 15, 61–71.

Dampier, S., Campbell, S., Watson, D., 2002. An investigation of the hospital experiences of parents with a child in paediatric intensive care. Nursing Times Research 7 (3), 179–186.

Darbyshire, P., 1993. Parents, nurses and paediatric nursing: a critical review. Journal of Advanced Nursing 18, 1670–1680.

Darbyshire, P., 1994. Living with a sick child in hospital: the experiences of parents and nurses. Chapman and Hall, London.

Department for Education and Skills [DfES], 2004. Every child matters: change for children. Department for Education and Skills Publications, Nottingham.

Department of Health [DoH], 1999. Saving lives: our healthier nation. The Stationery Office, London.

Department of Health [DoH], 2000. The NHS plan, a plan for investment, a plan for reform. DoH, London. Online. Available at: http://www.nhs.uk/nhsplan

Department of Health [DoH], 2003. Getting the right start: national service framework for children: standards for hospital services. DoH, London.

Department of Health [DoH], 2004. National Service Framework for Children, Young People and Maternity Services. DoH, London.

Dunst, C., Trivette, C., 1996. Empowerment, effective help giving practices and family centred care. Pediatric Nursing 22 (4), 334–337.

Espezel, H., Canam, C., 2003. Parent-nurse interactions: care of hospitalized children. Journal of Advanced Nursing 44 (1), 34–41.

Foxcroft, L., 2002. Professional and legal issues. In: Smith, L., Coleman, V., Bradshaw, M. (Eds.), Family-centred care: concept, theory and practice. Palgrave, Basingstoke, pp. 148–170.

Franck, L., Callery, P., 2004. Rethinking family-centred care across the continuum of children's healthcare. Child Care Health and Development 30 (3), 265–277.

Gibson, C., 1991. A concept analysis of empowerment. Journal of Advanced Nursing 16, 354–361.

Gibson, C., 1995. The process of empowerment in mothers of chronically ill children. Journal of Advanced Nursing 21, 1201–1210.

Gibson, C., 1999. Facilitating critical reflection in mothers of chronically ill children. Journal of Clinical Nursing 8 (3), 305–312.

Gourlay, R., 1987. Negotiations for managers. Health Services Manpower review, University of Keele.

Hutchfield, K., 1999. Family centred care: a concept analysis. Journal of Advanced Nursing 29 (5), 1178–118.

Institute of Family Centered Care, 2008. What is patient and family-centered health care? http://www.familycenteredcare.org/faq.htlm (accessed 20.05.08)

Kelly, M.T., 2007. Achieving family-centred care: working on or with stakeholders. Neonatal Paediatric Child Health Nursing 10 (3), 4–11.

Kieffer, C.H., 1984. Citizen empowerment. A developmental perspective. Prevention in Human Services 2 (2/3), 9–36.

Kirk, S., 2001. Negotiating lay and professional roles in the care of children with complex health care needs. Journal of Advanced Nursing 34 (5), 593–602.

Law, M., Hanna, S., King, J., Kestoy, M., Rosenbaum, P., 2003. Factors affecting family-centred service delivery for children with disabilities. Child: Care Health and Development 29 (5), 357–366.

Lee, P., 2007. What does partnership in care mean for children's nurses? Journal of Clinical Nursing 16, 518–526.

Lewis, P., Kelly, M., Wilson, V., Jones, S., 2007. What did they say? How children, families and nurses experience care. Journal of Children's and Young People's Nursing 1 (06), 259–266.

MacKean, G., Thurston, W., Scott, C., 2005. Bridging the divide between families and health professionals' perspectives on family-centred care. Health Expectations 8, 74–85.

McCann, D., Young, J., Waston, K., 2008. Effectiveness of a tool to improve role negotiation and communication between parents and nurses. Paediatric Nursing 20, 14–19.

McWilliam, C., Stewart, M., Brown, J., et al., 1997. Creating empowering meaning; an interactive process of promoting health with chronically older Canadians. Health Promotion International 12 (2), 111–123.

Murphy, M., Fealy, G., (2007). Practices and perceptions of family-centered care among children's nurses in Ireland. Journal of Children's and Young Peoples' Nursing 01 (07), 312–319.

Nethercott, S., 1993. Family centred care: a concept analysis. Professional Nurse September, pp. 794–797.

Nursing and Midwifery Council (NMC), 2008. Nursing and Midwifery Council Code of Professional Conduct. Standards for conduct performance and ethics. NMC, London.

O'Haire, S., Blackford, J., 2005. Nurses' moral agency in negotiating parental participation in care. International Journal of Nursing Practice 11, 250–256.

Reeves, E., Timmins, S., Dampier, S., 2006. Parents experiences of negotiating care for their technology dependent child. Journal of Child Health Care 10 (3), 228–239.

Roden, J., 2005. The involvement of parents and nurses in the care of acutely ill children in non-specialist paediatric setting. Journal of Child Health Care 9 (3), 222–240.

Royal College of Nursing (RCN), 2004. Adolescent Transition Care: Guidance for Nursing Staff. Royal College of Nursing, London.

Royal College of Nursing (RCN), 2008. Lost in Transition: Moving young people between child and adult health services. Royal College of Nursing, London.

Shelton, T., Smith Stepanek, J., 1995. Excerpts from family centred care for children needing health and developmental services. Pediatric Nursing 21 (4), 362–364.

Shields, L., Pratt, J., Hunter, J., 2006. Family centered care: a review of qualitative studies. Journal of Clinical Nursing 15, 1317–1323.

Smith, L., 2002. Negotiation of care. In: Smith, L., Coleman, V., Bradshaw, M. (Eds.), Family-centred care: concept, theory and practice. Palgrave, Basingstoke, pp. 114–130.

Smith, L., Coleman, V., Bradshaw, M. (Eds.), 2002. Family-centred care: concept, theory and practice, Palgrave, Basingstoke.

Titone, J., Russell, C., Sileo, M., Martin, G., 2004. Taking family-centered care to a higher level on the heart and kidney unit. Pediatric Nursing 30, 495–498.

Tones, K., Tilford, S., 2001. Health education: effectiveness, efficiency and equity, 2nd edn. Nelson Thornes, Cheltenham.

Valentine, F., 1998. Empowerment: family centred care. Paediatric Nursing 10 (1), 24–27.

Wuest, J., Stern, P., 1991. Empowerment in primary health care: the challenge for nurses. Qualitative Health Research 11 (1), 80–99.

Ygge, B., Lindholm, C., Arnetz, J., 2006. Hospital staff perceptions of parental involvement in paediatric hospital care. Journal of Advanced Nursing 53 (95), 534–542.

Additional reading

Coleman, V., Smith, L., Bradshaw, M., 2003. Enhancing consumer participation using the practice continuum tool for family-centred care. Paediatric Nursing 15 (8), 28–31.

Smith, L., Coleman, V. (Eds.). In press. Child and family-centred healthcare: concept, theory and practice, 2nd edn. Palgrave Macmillan, Basingstoke.

Useful websites

http://www.actionforsickchildren.org – contains useful information for families and healthcare professionals on major topics in children's healthcare.

http://www.doh.gov.uk/nsf/children/gettingtherightstart – contains the document detailing the National Service Framework for Children setting out the standard for hospital services.

http://www.familycenteredcare.org – American-based institute providing a resource for health professionals through training, information dissemination, policy and research initiatives.

Assessing and planning care in partnership

7

Anne Casey

ABSTRACT

Assessment is the basis for planning and delivering nursing care to children, young people and families. Whether it is a comprehensive, holistic review of a child's health needs and problems, or a rapid, focused check on some aspect of his or her condition, assessment provides the information needed to agree with the child and family what needs to be done, when and by whom. Clinical reasoning skills are required for the nurse to interpret assessment data and identify appropriate actions, using evidence where possible. Information and knowledge management skills are required to support accurate recording and use of information about assessment and care and to enable children, young people and their families to participate fully in the care process.

All aspects of care, from assessment to evaluation, are affected by the context in which the care takes place and in particular by the attitudes and values of the nurse and the care team. Working in partnership requires a specific focus for nursing assessment, planning and evaluation which is different to traditional disease focused models.

LEARNING OUTCOMES

- Appreciate the importance of accurate and detailed observation and assessment (and recording of same).
- Identify and select from a range of assessment approaches for different children and clinical situations.
- Undertake, with supervision, holistic assessment of the infant/child/young person as a basis for planning general nursing care.
- Use assessment data to make initial judgements about the child and family's need for general nursing care, to be validated by an experienced nurse.
- Describe how assessment findings and clinical evidence inter-relate when planning care.
- Incorporate reassessment and evaluation of outcomes in the care plan.
- Recognise the complex nature of clinical reasoning and the roles of the child, family, nurse and multiagency team in assessment, planning and evaluation of care.

The nature of assessment

In any walk of life, assessment is the basis for making decisions about what to do. Unless an action is completely spontaneous, it is usually preceded by the person gathering together relevant facts, thinking about them to make sense of the situation and then weighing up the possible alternatives for what to do next. During and after the action, further thought is given to whether the choice of action was the right one – Is this having the effect I expected it to? What else could I try? Perhaps I jumped to the wrong conclusion about what was wrong?

Assessment is both a process and a result: assessing the level of oil in the engine might give a result of 'its getting low' and a plan to top up next time I'm passing the service station. Of course, if I then notice a patch of oil under the car I revise my initial assessment result to 'there could be a leak' and plan to go straight to a repair centre.

In health care, the process of assessment attempts to answer the question 'What is (probably) going on here?' With some degree of certainty about what is happening, it is possible to make a plan that will address the problem. But there is much more to assessing and planning care than simply discovering the problem and deciding what to do. This chapter explores assessment and care planning in the context of child/family/nurse partnerships to provide insights into these complex interpersonal and clinical processes that are the cornerstones of clinical practice. Recording, communicating and evaluating planned care are also considered, with an emphasis on the clinical and information governance responsibilities of the nurse. The chapter does not cover assessment for the specific purpose of investigating, diagnosing and treating medical conditions; Barnes (2003) is the recommended text for nurse practitioners undertaking what were traditionally medical roles. Assessment of and planning for community and population child health needs are also not covered here (see Chapter 8).

DOI: 10.1016/B978-0-7020-3183-0.10007-4

Assessment and planning in context

The clinical process

When first learning about something as complex as nursing, it helps to use diagrams or models that simplify the situation but demonstrate how things relate and where they fit in the real world of practice. Conceptual models and process models are used in nursing and other disciplines to clarify concepts important to the discipline and define relationships between them. The 'nursing process' was one such model introduced to the UK in the 1970s to help nurses focus on each individual patient and his or her needs, rather than on the medical condition and 'what we always do for patients with *x*'. It is clear that health professionals other than nurses use a similar process and that parents and children follow the same basic steps when managing illness at home. This 'clinical process' as it applies to nursing is outlined in Figure 7.1 to help you visualise the practical steps that are taken in the care and treatment of children and young people.

The first step in the process is prompted by any one of a number of 'triggers': a mother notices a rash on her baby's face, the community nurse visits a sick child at home, the teenager walks into the school drop-in centre, a 4-hourly temperature measurement is due and so on. The steps of assessing, planning, implementing and evaluating can take seconds in an emergency and months or years, for example, in the case of a child who has sustained a severe head injury. Although the model suggests a straight line, where one step neatly follows the one before, the process is anything but linear. Observing a bruise will lead to a plan for further assessment; when teaching a child about his asthma he may reveal concerns about exercise, which will prompt assessment and a different plan; assessment may lead to a decision to take no further action and so on. The three pillars of assessment (listening, observing and measuring) are constant activities throughout the care process. Planned assessments such as hourly monitoring of pain level and ad hoc or opportunistic assessments such as noticing a change in one child while attending to another, become the basis for changes to planned care, new assessments and new plans.

It can be helpful to distinguish between initial or generalised assessment of the kind that would be carried out at a first contact or admission in a non-emergency situation and focused assessment, where attention is directed at a specific state, behaviour, concern or situation. The goals of an initial assessment are to identify:

1. Immediate and ongoing care needs related to the reason for the visit, contact or admission.
2. Other issues/areas of concern.
3. Health promotion needs and opportunities.

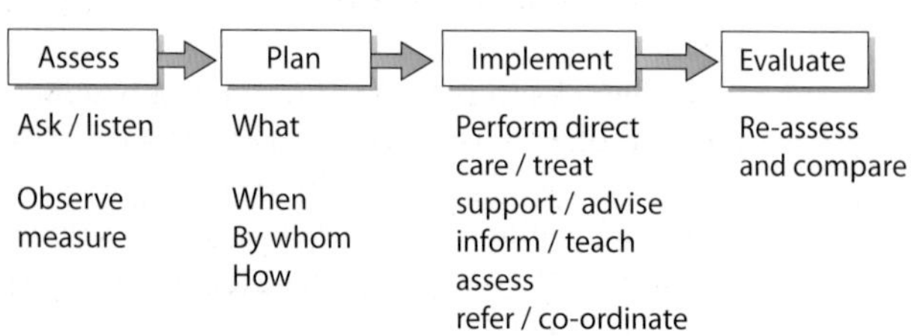

Fig. 7.1 • The clinical process.

It is important to establish a baseline of assessment data that can be used to agree care aims, monitor progress and evaluate outcomes.

Results of initial assessments are used to plan for and to provide care, support, information and education and to communicate with/refer to other professionals. Generalised and focused assessments are discussed later in this chapter after an introduction to clinical reasoning and exploration of the contextual factors that affect both the process and outcome of assessment (and the rest of the care process).

Clinical reasoning

A process model of the kind described above has limitations: one criticism of the nursing process is that it emphasises patient problems (it is sometimes referred to as a 'problem-solving process') and therefore is unsuited to health promotion and 'well person' elements of nursing roles. Although it clearly shows how a nurse could provide individualised, planned care, the process focuses on 'doing' steps, and thus hides the clinical reasoning that is required to sift through the available assessment data and to weigh up the evidence to make good clinical decisions.

Another way of looking at the same process is to consider the cognitive processes that underpin assessment, planning and evaluation, rather than the action steps. 'Clinical reasoning' is a general term covering the cognitive processes of diagnostic reasoning (also known as clinical judgement) and clinical decision making. Higgs (2000) provides an excellent overview of clinical reasoning in the health professions. Knowing about these clinical and cognitive processes can help direct your approach to care and will inform your practice in helping children, young people and families to carry out assessments themselves and make decisions about what actions to take in the light of their own findings.

Activity

Imagine that you woke up this morning with a slight pain in your knee that has worsened during the day. List the things you might ask yourself or do to try to establish what the problem is. What knowledge have you drawn on to inform your 'diagnostic reasoning'?

Figure 7.2 shows how the data that are collected by listening, observing, measuring and communicating with other professionals are sifted and sorted to select what is relevant and then analysed to reach a conclusion on whether the situation is normal for this child, a problem, a risk and so on. If there are insufficient data to reach a conclusion, a further decision is required – what more data do I need? To make good clinical judgements, the person doing the assessment draws on existing knowledge and past experience, and uses cognitive skills such as pattern recognition ('I've seen this kind of thing before') and ruling out by hypothesis testing ('It can't be infection because there's no fever') to reach conclusions. These assessment 'conclusions' are known in some nursing literature and practice as nursing diagnoses.

In the US and many other countries (and to a small extent in the UK) nurses use the concept of nursing diagnosis to describe and communicate to others the primary focus of nursing care. A nursing diagnosis is 'a clinical judgement about individual family or community responses to actual or potential health problems/life processes' (North American Nursing Diagnosis Association (NANDA) 2008). It is usually expressed as a diagnostic statement and reflects some aspect of the child and family's response to a health issue or problem, as distinct from the medical diagnosis of the problem.

One of the benefits of reaching a firm conclusion is that this can be discussed openly. Your initial conclusion about what is making a child cry, for example, could lead you to take certain actions, which might be totally inappropriate unless you confirm your 'diagnosis' with the child. A fully expressed nursing diagnosis contains not only the diagnosis but also the cause or 'related factors' and the assessment data that support your conclusion ('defining characteristics' of the diagnosis) (Carpenito-Moyet 2004). 'Pain in the arm related to the splint rubbing' requires very different action from 'pain in arm related to fracture'.

Deciding what action to take (clinical decision making) uses different knowledge and cognitive skills than judging whether there is a need for action, as Table 7.1 illustrates. Based on the 'diagnosis', and when appropriate, goals or expected outcomes can be discussed and agreed with the child and family so that everyone is clear about what can be expected. Knowledge from research and other evidence (see Chapter 14), and personal experience of what works in this kind of situation, inform cognitive decision-making processes such as narrowing of options and weighing-up pros and cons. Possible actions need to be balanced against available resources to arrive at an agreed plan of what is to be done, by whom and when.

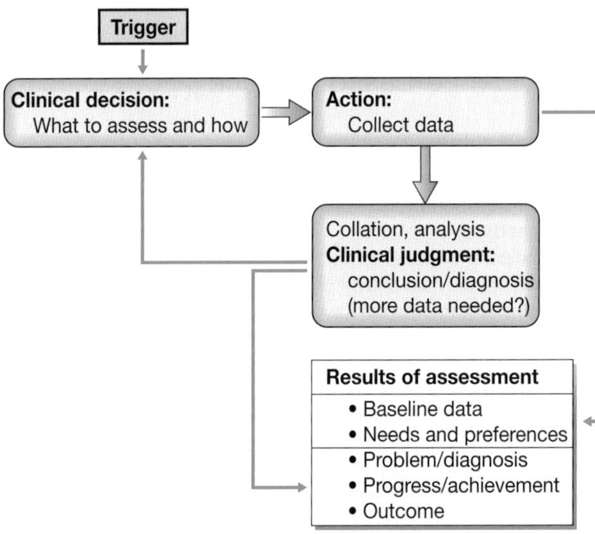

Fig. 7.2 • Clinical reasoning in assessment.

Context for care

Patient care and the clinical process do not take place in isolation. No matter how good the assessment is and how well planned the care, there are many other factors that influence whether the child's and family's expectations of care are achieved and their experience of nursing and health care is a positive one. The context of care, from the interpersonal relationships between family and staff to the prevailing political climate, heavily impact on the quality of the services and care provided. Figure 7.3 illustrates the multitude of factors that have an influence on the care process, many of which are addressed in the chapters in Section 1 of this book. At different times and in different situations the impact of the various factors will be different but four of them are particularly important in nursing:

- Interpersonal: relationships and interactions between and among the child, the family and the clinical team.
- Financial: availability of and ease of access to specific services and resources, e.g. equipment, staff and time.
- Philosophical: the ethos of the team that pervades all aspects of care delivery.
- Ethical: recognition of rights, equity, etc.

Reflect on your practice

Interpersonal context

How could interpersonal relationships between members of a clinical team (an aspect of the interpersonal context) influence the quality of your nursing care? For example, what would happen if the nursing team does not feel able to question medical staff decisions?

Table 7.1 Differences in making clinical judgements and clinical decisions

	Cognitive processes – examples	**Knowledge used**
Making clinical judgements: reaching a conclusion about what is (probably) going on	Collation of data/cues Data analysis Pattern recognition Hypothesis generation and evaluation Dealing with uncertainty	Previous experience of this child or similar situations, patterns, etc. Knowledge of effects of disease, surgery, etc., on child and family Research evidence and patient 'stories' of what it is like to be a child, parent, family member in this situation
Making clinical decisions: deciding what to do – choosing a course of action (in relation to goals)	Critical thinking/weighing up research evidence Identifying and evaluating options Setting priorities and managing constraints: time, resources, crises	Knowledge about what has worked for this child in the past Previous experience of what works in similar situations Evidence, guidelines, protocols for the best approach to take

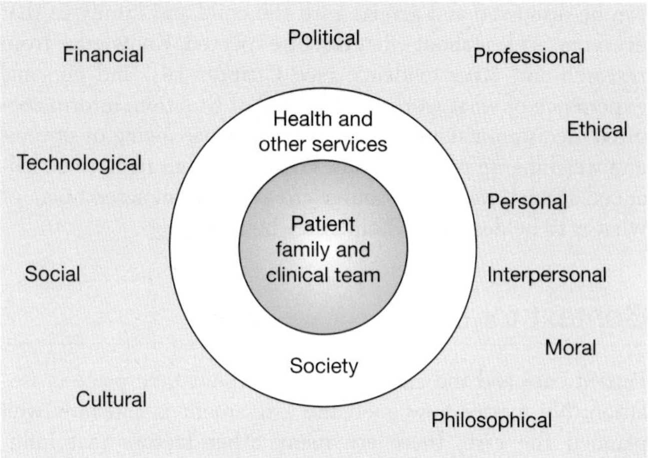

Fig. 7.3 • Context of care: influences on the care process.

Partnership principles applied to assessing and planning care

In Chapter 6, Lynda Smith, Valerie Coleman and Maureen Bradshaw described parental involvement in care as moving along a continuum from nurse led to parent led. Other conceptual models of nursing use similar constructs to help explain aspects of the relationship between nurses and patients, for example, Orem's view of the patient as totally dependent through to self caring (Orem 2001). These kinds of models and terms such as 'nurse led', 'patient centred', 'child friendly' represent particular philosophies: ways of thinking and then acting that directly influence the child's and family's experience of care. Even the language we use implies a particular way of thinking and acting. You might hear the term 'non-compliant' applied in a situation, for example, where a teenager with diabetes is admitted to hospital. 'Non-compliance' suggests that heavy-handed sanctions will be needed to get the patient to manage diet, exercise and insulin properly. If the teenager is described instead as 'making choices that can put her at risk' then the management approach is more likely to be one that reflects an understanding of adolescent needs.

Reflect on your practice

Philosophical context

Nurses often provide information to the child and family about the child's condition or treatment, reflecting a view of children and families as passive recipients of healthcare. What view would you be reflecting if instead of providing information you helped the child to find out where to get information for herself?

The term 'partnership' is widely used in health and social care to represent the ideal or preferred relationship between agencies and between professionals and clients. In the nursing care of children and families it has come to mean a changing, negotiated, shared responsibility for care between child, family and nurse, with support and teaching provided (including teaching of nurses by the child and family). Family involvement in care may be a result of the negotiation of care responsibility but is not necessarily so. Conversely, nursing involvement in care may not be what the child and family want: respite care at home for the child with complex needs may be better provided by a social care assistant with specific training. A key principle of partnership working is that responsibility does not have to be shared equally: the extent to which the child, family member and nurse are ready for and able to contribute to the partnership dictates changes in responsibility – for the child towards independent self-care and for some parents towards leading and delegating care. In some situations, the nursing team may only be able to offer limited services so the burden of care remains with the family.

Partnership complements other constructs valued by nurses caring for children and young people such as 'child-centred care' and respect for children's rights, particularly the right to be informed and to have a say in decision making (see Chapters 10 and 18). There is very little evidence of how children and parents view partnership working (as distinct from research into their views on involvement or participation in care), and little to indicate whether true partnerships are possible in a context where professionals have more power and there are limited resources. In Coyne's (1995) study, parents reported difficulties with lack of information, non-negotiation of roles, and feelings of anxiety and loneliness when caring for their child in hospital.

Evidence-based practice

Negotiated roles

Kirk (2001) investigated whether there was any negotiation of caring roles between professionals and parents of children with complex needs:

From the parents' perspective, their initial assumption of responsibility for the care of their child was not subject to negotiation with professionals. Prior to discharge, feelings of obligation, their strong desire for their child to come home and the absence of alternatives to parental care in the community were key motivating factors in their acceptance of responsibility from professionals (Kirk 2001 p 593).

Professionals had concerns about whether parents were given a choice and the degree of choice they could exercise in the face of professional power. As parents gained experience in caring for their child, and as their relationships with professionals developed, role negotiation started to happen. Kirk concluded that professional expectations of parental involvement probably acted as a barrier to negotiation of roles and that parental choices were initially constrained by their feelings of obligation.

Evidence-based practice

Who knows best?

A study by Waters et al (2003) explored differences between adolescent and parental reports of physical, emotional, mental and social health and well-being. Over 2000 young people (with and without chronic illness) and their parents were involved in the study. All the adolescents were much less optimistic about their health and well-being than their parents. There were significant differences in their reports of general health, mental health, frequency and amount of pain and the impact on the family of their health problems.

CHILD CONVERSATION

Kate aged 11 years with asthma

Kate: *Once I started doing it myself [the asthma diary] I could see much better how I was doing. I could tell the nurse how much Ventolin I'd needed and sometimes we could see what was making it worse. Once we decided for me to try taking Ventolin before going outdoors or for PE when it was cold outside.*

Kate's mum: *She was better at keeping the diary than me, at least at first. Now she only uses it when she's having problems and that helps her see what needs doing.*

Applying a partnership approach to assessment alters the goals that were listed on page 2, which now become:

- With the child and family, to identify:
  - their immediate and ongoing care needs related to the reason for the visit, contact or admission
  - other issues/areas of concern
  - health promotion needs and opportunities
  - their experience and expectations of care and services
  - their readiness and preferences in relation to participation in care and decision making
- To establish a baseline (as before).

Traditional, profession-centred models of care still exist where the mother, not the child or young person, is asked about the child's condition and progress. The clinician interprets the assessment information and informs the parent what needs to happen next. However, in most services it is accepted that the children and young people themselves are the best source of information and that seeking their views and involving them in decision making and self-care are beneficial not just in terms of outcome but in making their whole experience of health care more positive.

Using the communication tools that are most familiar to children and young people, such as mobile phones and the internet, goes some way to improving the child friendliness of services. Although these approaches are still being evaluated, it is possible to envisage young people with diabetes, for example, managing their condition at home with internet-based decision support, e-mail advice and mobile phone text reminders for medication times. But there is still a significant shift needed in the way professionals view the child and young person's world, particularly the child/young person with a chronic condition or disability. More locally delivered services and better use of technology will support moves from a world where the child/young person and the family must adapt their lives to fit around the condition and its management to a world where the condition and its management are adapted to their lifestyles. With more children's nurses as part of the primary care team supporting children and families at home there will hopefully be greater attention focused on assessment and intervention in relation to the safety and suitability of the child's environment, his or her access to community services and the appropriateness of those services. Simple solutions like having appointments outside of college hours seem obvious but there are very few clinics that consider the needs and lifestyles of children and young people.

Table 7.2 Partnership in the care process

Assess	Ask the child, ask the parents/carer
	Invite the child, parents/carer to observe and measure
	Observe and measure
	Confirm your impressions and conclusions with the child and parents/carer, especially their view of the priorities
Plan	Agree appropriate goals with the child and parents/carer
	Discuss possible actions and assist them in making choices
	Agree initial plan for what needs to be done, who will do it, when and how
	Plan for regular shared review of the plan, care responsibilities and teaching and support needs
Implement	Perform direct care as planned (child, parent/carer, nurse)
	Facilitate learning and information sharing
	Provide support and supervision
	Monitor progress and reassess as planned (child, parent/carer, nurse)
	With consent, refer to other professionals and coordinate care
Evaluate	Invite the child, parents/carer to observe and measure outcomes and report their experience of care
	Review and reflect on the care process from child and family perspective and from the professional nursing perspective

Before moving on to the practice of assessment and care planning, it is appropriate to summarise the clinical process as it can look when informed by partnership and other nursing values/philosophies (Table 7.2). Listening to and respecting the child/young person's and family's views and involving them in decision making is not a luxury that only applies in long-term care situations; it is a fundamental right that applies equally in emergencies, in ambulatory and short-stay settings – everywhere that children and young people receive health care.

Assessment and planning in practice

Having considered the process of assessing and planning, the context in which it occurs and the ways in which values and philosophies influence the process, it is now time to address the important question of how to assess and plan care. In this section the focus for nursing assessment is discussed, and assessment approaches and tools introduced. The section concludes with examples of approaches and tools to support evidence-based care planning.

A growing thread throughout health and social care in the UK is the single, shared patient record as a necessary requirement for ensuring continuity in an age when many different disciplines and services may be providing care for one child. This theme will be picked up in the final section of the chapter; recording, communicating and auditing care. A single record suggests a single assessment and one care plan for the child, something that many professionals believe would get rid of many of the communication failures and frustrations that parents and children experience.

The focus of assessment

Even when single, shared patient records are a reality, nurses will still be responsible for the nursing elements of assessment and planning. But what are these, where do you start and how much do you cover? The obvious starting point is to identify those aspects of the health care of children and young people for which nurses are responsible. To some extent these are dictated by Health Service managers through role and job descriptions and can change over time and between settings. But the profession itself, in consultation with the public and other professional groups, defines the core focus of nursing work. The regulatory and professional bodies set standards for practice and education that specify what nurses are educated to do and how they will practice. The Royal College of Nursing (RCN 2003) defines nursing as providing clear directions for assessment and for the way in which care is provided.

PROFESSIONAL CONVERSATION

What is nursing? Extracts from 'Defining nursing' (RCN 2003).

Nursing is ...

- The use of clinical judgement in the provision of care to enable people to improve, maintain, or recover health, to cope with health problems, and to achieve the best possible quality of life.
- The purpose of nursing is to promote health, healing, growth and development, and to prevent disease, illness, injury, and disability. When people become ill or disabled, the purpose of nursing is, in addition, to minimise distress and suffering, and to enable people to understand and cope with their disease or disability, its treatment and its consequences. When death is inevitable, the purpose of nursing is to maintain the best possible quality of life until its end.
- The specific domain of nursing is people's unique responses to and experience of health, illness, frailty, disability and health related life events in whatever environment or circumstances they find themselves.
- The focus of nursing is the whole person and the human response rather than a particular aspect of the person or a particular pathological condition.

Applying and expanding this definition in the client group of children and young people results in a number of different areas of responsibility for nursing, which in some cases could all apply at once:

- protecting
- living with disability
- living healthy lives
- preventing accidents and illness
- managing/living with health problems, including mental health problems.

In this last area, the nursing focus is on the child's/young person's (and family's) experiences of the health problem and its management. Nursing assessment covers the physiological, physical, psychological, social and spiritual effects they may experience, including effects on development and family life. Nursing care is primarily focused not on the disease, injury or disability itself but on the symptoms, limitations, feelings, behaviour, lifestyle changes and so on experienced by the child and the concerns or problems that the family may have in providing care for their child.

Traditional, disease-focused models of nursing assessment are very common and illustrate the need for improved understanding of the unique contribution of nursing. Reductions in medical staff numbers and advances in health technology mean that more and more nurses are taking on what were previously medical roles, from technical tasks to investigation, diagnosis and treatment of disorders. Evidence suggests that with appropriate education and training nurses can provide safe, high-quality clinical services (see Redshaw & Harvey 2002). But the unique contribution that nursing care makes to improving the experiences and quality of life patients and families needs to be recognised so that when nurses do take on new roles overall quality is not compromised.

It is impossible to totally separate the specific focus and contribution of nursing: nurses' work encompasses aspects of many other disciplines from play therapy to prescribing, and often substitutes for parental 'work' – the continual care, protection, comfort, distraction and encouragement that parents provide to their children. However, a clear understanding of those situations that are the primary responsibility of nurses and those that are a collaborative responsibility helps to ensure that nurses meet the requirements of their professional role (Carpenito-Moyet 2004).

Evidence-based practice

Nursing or medicine?

In 1997, Mason & Webb found that nursing records reflected children's medical/physical needs and care but that much practice was focused on psychosocial needs. When nurses were provided with a nursing framework for assessment their clinical judgements were no longer described in terms of the primary medical diagnosis but reflected the family-centred nursing model, including:

- continuity of usual care by parents
- support for family members
- impact of illness and hospitalisation
- participation by parents in nursing and medical care.

As part of their collaborative role with medicine, nurses do include aspects of illness/injury management in their assessments such as:

- assessing any risks for complications of treatment
- monitoring treatment progress
- assessing the child/family ability to carry out treatment plans.

In collaboration with mental health and social care professionals working with children in need and their families, nurses may undertake diagnostic assessments related to development, behaviour, parenting capacity, family functioning and so on (see Hockenberry et al 2003 for examples of physical, developmental and family assessment techniques). As nursing specialist roles expand and more nurse-led services develop, assessments now incorporate tests and investigations relating to the child's medical condition. Combining nursing and medical or other discipline focused assessment is time consuming and complex but marks the difference between the nurse with an expanded role and the nurse as 'doctor substitute'.

Evidence-based practice

Combining nursing and medical roles

Although there is a great deal of research on diabetes care in children, there is a concern that nursing practice may be mostly guided by 'biomedical models'. Marshall et al (2002) argue that 'psychosocial constructs have an important role in the development of self-management of chronic illness in children' and that care in children should focus on family-centred approaches based in the community. They conclude that paediatric diabetes nurse specialists are pivotal in facilitating family-centred care based on personal models of child and family interventions, whilst also addressing the physiological, developmental and treatment issues.

Generalised assessment frameworks

Discussion of the focus of nursing assessment concludes with a very practical question around scope – how wide ranging should your questions be and what observations and measurements should you make? The concept of holism is an important one in nursing: you will not discover how a diagnosis of epilepsy has affected a child's life if your assessment consists of taking the child's temperature, measuring blood pressure and weight and asking when the last fit occurred. However, it will not be appropriate to ask broader questions when the child is already under the care of the epilepsy specialist nurse and you are doing an assessment prior to a CT scan. The breadth and depth of nursing assessments need to be adapted to the child and family situation, the clinical context and – to some extent – the resources available for subsequent action. There would be no point conducting a full assessment of the social and financial impact of weekly hospital treatment if there is no alternative and the family won't be eligible for disability allowances or income support.

Scenario

A child is admitted to the day ward for minor surgery under general anaesthetic. As she had attended the clinic the week before, her height and weight are already noted. After greeting the child and mother and introducing herself, the nurse records the child's temperature, pulse and respirations, asks whether she has had a cough or cold in the previous few days and when she last had something to eat or drink. Having checked that the consent form is signed, the nurse asks whether the mother or child have any questions about the procedure.

This scenario is a good example of the clinical situation alone dictating the assessment. The nurse is using knowledge of what is important for ensuring a safe anaesthetic procedure, but is not using knowledge from nursing theory and research of what the child and the mother might be experiencing or other concerns and needs they may have. This is the crux of good nursing assessment:

- using knowledge from different sources (including from personal experience)
  ↓
- combining it with the results of holistic and focused assessment in order to
  ↓
- apply the knowledge appropriately to the individual child and family in order to
  ↓
- discover (and confirm with them) their care needs.

PROFESSIONAL CONVERSATION

Meena is a third-year children's nursing student.

Theory into practice with caution

We'd been studying Piaget's developmental stages and what they mean in terms of preparing children for surgery. So when I knew I'd be admitting a 4-year-old boy I thought carefully about what his understanding would be at that age about his body and the surgery and being in hospital. I was prepared with simple pictures of tubes going into the tummy and so on but he waved me away and seemed annoyed that I hadn't used the words gastrostomy, abdomen, etc. One of the staff nurses explained he'd been in and out of hospital since birth and had a better understanding of his condition than many of the nurses. It made me realise that, although applying theory in practice was important, I needed to use it to inform what I thought and did for each individual patient, not to make assumptions about what their actual needs were.

The following list summarises the scope of nursing assessment and also suggests a logical prioritisation of assessment topics:

1. Risk to life of child and risk of harm to child.
2. Communication – abilities, means, aids, language, etc.
3. Fears and anxieties – immediate concerns addressed.
4. Systematic and ongoing assessment – generalised, focused, changes, progress.
5. Preferences and needs related to participation in decision making and care.

The first priority must obviously be risks to life and risk of harm. Second, there must be a means of communicating and establishing a relationship with the child/young person and the parents/carer (see Chapter 11). When communication is possible, fears, anxieties and immediate concerns need to be identified and addressed. Appropriate, systematic assessment can then be carried out, including identification of other risks such as potential environmental threats or stress related to family disruption.

Box 7.1

Functional health patterns: a framework for holistic nursing assessment (Gordon 2002)

- Health perception/health management pattern
- Nutrition/metabolic pattern
- Elimination pattern
- Sleep/rest pattern
- Activity/exercise pattern
- Cognitive/perceptual pattern
- Self-perception/self-concept pattern
- Role/relationship pattern
- Sexuality/reproductive pattern
- Coping/stress tolerance pattern
- Value/belief pattern

A number of frameworks are available to help the nurse to decide what topics to cover in generalised assessment, from activities of living (Roper & Tierney 2000) to Gordon's 'functional health patterns' adapted for use with children and young people (Hockenberry et al 2003). Outside the UK, Gordon's (2002) work is one of the most widely used frameworks because it supports comprehensive, patient-centred assessment. The 11 health patterns (Box 7.1) can be used to develop and organise locally developed assessment tools or to test them for holism. A good example of the benefit of such a framework is the issue of complementary and alternative therapies. Assessing activities of living would not usually elicit a family's interest in or use of herbal medicines, for example. Gordon's 'health perception/health management pattern' category directs the nurse to enquire about health beliefs and use of other therapies.

Reflect on your practice

Choose a clinical area that you have worked in and list the topics that you recall being the focus of nursing assessment. Consider your list in the light of Figure 7.4 and the functional patterns in Box 7.1. Would you add anything to your list?

Generalised assessment tools based on this kind of framework give structure to assessments and reinforce the philosophy and values on which they are based. Whatever the clinical context, there will be a core set of items relevant to every child, young person and family such as their understanding of the situation and their special needs. As care needs emerge and a relationship is established, the child and family's preferences and readiness for participation in care and decision making and their information, learning and support needs can be identified.

Depending on the clinical context, specific assessment items will be prioritised, for example, respiration, hydration, skin integrity and pain level in intensive care; self-care, self-image, feeding regime and educational needs in the head injury rehabilitation unit. Some of these areas will be assessed using validated tools like the ones introduced in the next section and in other chapters in this book.

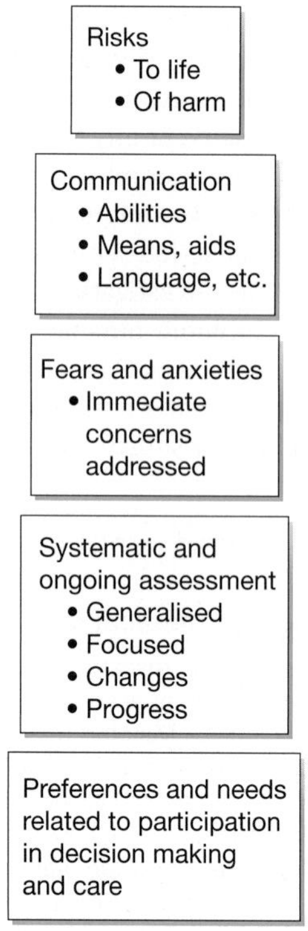

Fig. 7.4 • Nursing assessment: scope and priority.

It would not be possible to publish all possible frameworks that might be appropriate for the many different health and nursing needs of children and young people. However, it is possible to list a set of principles for evaluation of those that are presently available, or to underpin the development of new ones. Most importantly, frameworks for comprehensive nursing assessment of children and young people must support the identification of health issues that require nursing intervention or referral to other team members. They should also:

- be child- and family-centred: consider the child's/young person's rights, responsibilities and relationships within the family and society
- be holistic: covering physiological, physical, social, psychological and spiritual aspects of the developing child/young person
- reflect partnership values: including consideration of child and family preferences related to care, and their involvement in care and decision making
- be practical to use
- be acceptable to children/young people and families
- have a nursing focus: address the effects of the health issue and its management (not the diagnosis and treatment alone).

Although nursing assessment has a specific focus, as with all aspects of children's healthcare, team approaches to assessment should be considered. Many aspects of the child's care are managed by the whole team and joint or shared assessment approaches are becoming the norm. The national (English) standard approach to assessing children in need and their families is one example of an agreed multidisciplinary assessment framework with practice guidance that makes it clear which professionals are responsible for the different aspects of assessment and management (Children's Workforce Development Council 2007). It is important that nursing elements of assessment are included in joint assessment frameworks so that issues related to the child and family experience of the health problem are identified and addressed.

Tools and methods for focused assessment

Unlike generalised frameworks, most assessment tools measure just one aspect of the child's health status. Assessment tools can improve the quality and accuracy of assessments; their usefulness will depend on their purpose, content and practicality. As Harris (2002) points out, the development and evaluation of assessment tools is complex. Any measurement instrument needs to be reliable and valid: it should return consistent results when used repeatedly to measure the same thing and it should measure what it is supposed to be measuring. Signs and symptoms such as raised body temperature, weight loss and ulcerated lips are relatively easy to measure and quantify. However, most aspects of the child and family's responses to health problems and their management (i.e. nursing concerns) are subjective, variable and multifaceted, making them difficult to recognise and even more difficult to 'measure'. Some paediatric and child health assessment instruments have been well researched, notably pain assessment scales (see Chapter 14), quality of life measures (Schmidt et al 2002) and growth and development (Royal College of Paediatrics and Child Health (RCPCH) 2000).

Systematic reviews have been published summarising the best available evidence for use of different measurement tools (e.g. Duce 1996, Eiser & Morse 2001). There are many examples in the literature of tools developed at local level to address clinical problems where assessment is known to be poor, for example, self-harm risk assessment (Marfe 2003) and skin assessment (Rogers 2003). Although clinically relevant, much of this work is still exploratory and unvalidated so should be applied in other contexts with caution.

Taking instruments that have been developed for research and using them in the clinical setting is also problematic, not least because research measurements tend to be at a level of detail that is impractical and unnecessary in the clinical situation. It is possible to adapt tools validated for use with adults, as children's cancer nurses found when they introduced oral assessment scoring (Gibson & Nelson 2000). As a general guide, any tool that is adapted from another setting or client group must first be validated for use with your client group in your clinical setting.

Evidence-based practice

Transferability of assessment tools

Gharaibeh & Abu-Saad (2002) looked at the cultural validity, reliability and children's preferences of three pain assessment tools among Jordanian children. They found that the scales were valid and reliable but that there were gender differences in preference for particular scales, explained by the researchers as part of the socialisation process within the Arab culture.

Box 7.2

Criteria for choosing an assessment tool or device

- Developed for the purpose: the aspect of the child/family's state, behaviour, feelings, etc., that you are wanting to measure/assess.
- Tested and validated in this age group.
- Tested and validated in this clinical context, e.g. in children with same or closely related condition.
- Culturally appropriate.
- Appropriate for and acceptable to the specific child/young person and family, e.g. the child's cognitive level.
  1. Risk to life of child and risk of harm to child.
  2. Communication – abilities, means, aids, language, etc.
  3. Fears and anxieties – immediate concerns addressed.
  4. Systematic and ongoing assessment – generalised, focused, changes, progress.
  5. Preferences and needs related to participation in decision making and care.

Criteria to be considered when choosing an appropriate assessment tool or device are summarised in Box 7.2. Those that do not meet the criteria should be used with caution, as indeed should any measurement tool: the evidence from measurements should be combined with observations and child/parent reports if an accurate assessment is to be made.

Before moving on to planning in partnership, there are several summary points to be made about assessment. First, admitting a patient is not the same as assessing a patient, and assessment is not just a form-filling exercise (Harris 2002). Second, there is no point doing a 'once only' generalised assessment: ongoing review is essential to monitor changes and the success or otherwise of nursing interventions. Finally, without a nursing framework to guide the focus of assessment, care will focus solely on the medical–physical needs of patients (Mason & Webb 1997).

PARENT CONVERSATION

Georgina is the mother of 17-month-old William.

Relying on measurement tools

The nurse in A&E used an ear thermometer and said his temperature was normal. I knew he wasn't well. His temperature had been very high at home; he was pale, his head felt hot but his hands and feet were cold. She didn't seem to hear me saying that his temperature was on the way up again.

Planning care

Whether or not a formal care plan is written down, some level of planning takes place before any action is taken. Based on assessment findings (and on what they are hoping to achieve if goals have been set), the planners identify available options and make decisions about what needs to be done. Chapter 14 goes into detail about how evidence can be used to inform such decisions, not withstanding the influence of resource availability, patient and family choice or other context of care factors. The plan of care is a communication tool and makes clear to all concerned who will be doing what, when and how. It can be as simple as a checklist or as complex as a step-by-step statement of a procedure with timed goals and expected outcomes: the detail and complexity of the plan depends on the communication need. A plan in the child's home that will be used to inform a bank nurse providing respite care will need to be very detailed; a plan for a child seen in A&E with a fever may consist of a standard form with four actions to be ticked by whoever completes them (and space to write additional, individualised actions if required).

Care plans may be based on standard plans or pathways of care. Standard care pathways that have been developed using evidence and expert opinion are one way of implementing evidence-based practice. Care pathways (also known as integrated care pathways) set out detailed steps for the management of patients with a particular problem or undergoing a specific procedure. Ideally, they are developed by the multidisciplinary team and reflect standardised care and treatment as well as expected progress (National Library for Health 2008). To date, care pathways have been mainly implemented in hospitals where care is more predictable but standardised approaches to care in home and school settings may be just as appropriate in some circumstances. As computer records and systems spread throughout the health service, 'e-pathways' will enable evidence-based standards to be better individualised and for individual differences to be analysed to provide improved evidence (de Luc & Todd 2003).

Evidence-based practice

The integrated care pathway as an audit tool

Staff in a paediatric oncology unit aimed to improve care for children with fever and neutropenia by introducing an integrated care pathway. Guidelines for neutropenia were examined and a retrospective analysis of notes undertaken to study what was happening before a pathway was introduced. Following the introduction of the pathway, audit findings revealed variances in practice and identified areas for improvement such as referral to dieticians, types of investigations ordered and time taken to administer the first dose of antibiotics, particularly at night. Evidence from the audit was used to amend the pathway and improve practice (Selwood 2000).

Supporting decision making

Those planning care will be any combination of health professionals, the child/young person and family members. A key role for the nurse working in partnership to plan care is to support decision making by the child/young person and family. The first step is to assess their decision-making preferences, not an easy task but one that acknowledges them as equals and establishes that their experiences and perspectives are valued and will be taken into account.

Activity

Think about your own most recent consultation with a doctor:

- How involved were you in the decision about what action to take?
- How involved would you have preferred to be?
- Having thought about this last question, choose your preference for that particular encounter from the bullet list below:
  - I would prefer to make the decision myself with information only.
  - I would prefer to make the decision myself considering the doctor's view.
  - I would prefer the doctor to make the decision but considering my views.
  - I would prefer the doctor to make the decision.

Having been involved in the decision about what to do, you are more likely to adhere to the course of action than if someone else has decided for you. As long ago as 1977, a doctor writing in the *Lancet* suggested that if doctors 'were willing to let go of the notion that they are responsible for controlling their patients', then patients who wanted to could 'make informed decisions on the basis of their own values' (Slack 1977). Not all parents and children will want to participate in decision making but the danger is in assuming that they do not wish to and ignoring their right to be heard.

Chapter 10 deals with the issue of consent and whether children are really given choices. This question of 'who decides?' applies to all kinds of care decisions, from whether to proceed with a heart–lung transplant to what to have for breakfast. Alderson & Montgomery's (1996) seminal text addresses the challenges of healthcare decision making with children and parents. At the level of day-to-day practice it is the values and attitudes of nurses and other team members that influence whether partnership in decision making is a reality. In addition, healthcare professionals need to have the confidence and be equipped with skills and tools with which to:

- assess preferences (which may change)
- assess competence (which will change)
- provide information without persuasion
- 'teach' decision-making strategies
- record and communicate decisions
- support child and family when they have made their decision (even if you don't agree with it).

Evaluation and outcomes

Evaluation of the effectiveness of care for an individual child (and family) is an important part of nursing care. It needs to take place throughout the care process, with continual reassessment of their responses to interventions so that these can be changed or discontinued if they are ineffective or no longer needed. Initial assessment identifies health problems or issues that need addressing at the beginning of a care programme or episode; outcome evaluation identifies the extent of change in the health problem or achievement of goals related to the health issue.

A number of issues are related to the identification of what have been termed 'nursing sensitive patient outcomes' (those outcomes that are influenced by nursing care). The same difficulties that are faced when assessing less concrete aspects of the child's state, behaviour, feelings, etc., also apply in evaluation. The child and family's own reports of their experience and satisfaction with care are the most important evaluation evidence. However, nurses should supplement this evidence with outcome measures suited to the clinical setting and, where possible, derived from standards or benchmarks. Children and families will not know what should have been done in every case, for example they may accept as normal that the child did not eat during a short stay in hospital. This is an unacceptable outcome when measured against the national (English) benchmark: 'The amount of food patients actually eat is monitored, recorded and leads to action when cause for concern' (NHS Modernisation Agency 2003).

It may be difficult to differentiate the outcomes that are the result of nursing from those that result from interventions by others (including the child and family's own actions). However, it is important to consider 'nursing sensitive patient outcomes' for two main reasons: to monitor and improve effectiveness and to justify resources. Nurses do things for, with and to patients; they act on the results of assessments and decide what is an appropriate course of action. If they don't evaluate the results of their actions (i.e. measure outcomes) they cannot know whether they made the right decision nor learn what works to provide evidence for future practice.

Nursing staff salaries cost a great deal and the more senior the staff the greater the cost. Unless nurses can demonstrate that they contribute to improved outcomes for children and families, their value to health services may not be recognised and posts not funded. Recent evidence that patient safety and outcomes are significantly affected by skill mix of nursing staff show how measures of adverse outcome can be used to justify higher ratios of qualified to unqualified staff (Yang 2003). When new services such as community children's nursing teams or specialist practitioner posts are established, evidence collected about outcomes will be critical for ensuring the long-term viability of these services.

Much of the evidence we have about effectiveness and outcomes can be derived from intervention studies. For example, a study of the efficacy of tepid sponging to reduce fever in children (Sharber 1997) used simple outcome measures of fever reduction and signs of discomfort (crying, shivering, goosebumps). Petryshen et al (1998) used stability of physiological measures such as pulse and respirations as well as length of stay to evaluate the effectiveness of developmental care in very low birth weight babies.

Nursing interventions are directed at a number of child and family's responses to health problems and their management, from symptoms and behaviours through to their feelings and knowledge about their condition and how they cope with self-management at home and school. Table 7.3 lists the kinds of outcome that may be the result of effective nursing interventions with examples of measures that might be useful in outcome evaluation and in audits of quality.

Evidence-based practice

Nurse staffing and patient outcomes

Lower adverse outcome (measured as patient falls, pressure ulcers, respiratory and urinary tract infections, and patient/family complaints) were related to a higher proportion of experienced registered nurses in a study of over 1300 medical-surgical inpatients in Taiwan. Variations in the workload of nurses were found to be the most powerful predictor of nosocomial infections with hours of care provided to the patient the best predictor of adverse patient outcome (Yang 2003).

Table 7.3 Outcomes relevant to nursing and suggested measures

	Measurement
Child/young person: outcome - change in ...	
... symptom, e.g. pain, nausea	Symptom diary Score/scale
... condition/state, e.g. of wound, nutritional state	Description Measurement, e.g. weight
... activity, e.g. mobility, eating, school attendance	Self-report against targets Diary
Child and/or parents/carer: outcome - change in ...	
... behaviour/skill	Self-report Observation
... understanding/attitude, e.g. improved acceptance of ...	Self-report Satisfaction with information giving Observation
... feelings	Self-report Stress and coping measures Anxiety/depression scales
...quality of life/general well-being	Self-report Quality of life measures
Service and child/family/carer outcome	
Reduced length of stay/avoidance of admission	Individual comparisons, e.g. 'managed at home this time' Admission and length of stay statistics
Better provision of equipment/supplies at home	Self-report – satisfaction Monitoring of phone calls
Improved coordination of care	Number of staff visiting

Recording and auditing practice

Information management

As this chapter has shown, the clinical process involves a number of steps and all of these steps generate information about the child's and family's needs and preferences, care decisions that are made, things that are planned and done, and results or outcomes of what was done. Much of this information needs to be communicated and recorded and some of it will need to be used for other purposes such as audit and service planning. Recording, storing, communicating and using information is known as information management. The goal of information management is to ensure relevant information is in the hands of those who need it, at the time they need it, and in a format that they can understand and use. Patients, parents, staff and managers need information so they can make sense of the situation and make decisions about what to do. The child's healthcare record is the main tool for managing this information. Every professional who comes in contact with the patient needs to be able to make timely decisions about what care is needed and how best to deliver that care. If it is to be an effective information tool, the record should support this process of clinical decision making. The Essence of Care benchmark for record keeping, now part of the clinical governance framework for the NHS in England, states that 'all records must be legible, accurate, signed with designation stated, dated, timed, contemporaneous, be able to provide a chronology of events and use only agreed abbreviations' (NHS Modernisation Agency 2003). These 'patient-focused benchmarks' set standards for progress towards single, life-long, patient held records that are secure and support high-quality, evidence-based care.

The purposes of the record dictate its format as well as its content. A key purpose of records is communication between disciplines, which suggests that moves towards a single record, used by all professionals and possibly held by the child or parent, will help to achieve 'fitness for purpose'. Another function is to serve as a secondary source of data: for audit, research and as evidence for legal or other enquiries.

Evidence-based practice

Parent-held records

In the UK, parent-held child health records have been used for many years. In a study of parents' and professionals' views, Charles (1994) found that almost all respondents in both groups liked the record and most professionals believed it improved communication with parents. Parents reported that the record helped them remember important advice and enabled them to play a more active role in their child's health care. The study also showed that over two-thirds of parents had made entries in the parent-held record and the records were more complete than traditional clinic cards.

Content of the record

NMC guidance on record keeping is at a very general level, stating only that the record should 'identify problems that have arisen and action taken to rectify them' and 'provide clear evidence of the care planned, the decisions made, the care delivered and the information shared' (NMC 2007). It is left up to each professional to decide what is appropriate to record and the level of detail that is necessary. In some areas, groups of professionals have reached a consensus on what should be in the record and developed standard formats that at least provide a guide for those using them. One example is the parent-held child health record, which has been used in community settings across the UK for many years. As the NHS moves towards computerised records, the structure and to some extent the content of records will become standardised. Nurses need to be able to identify what it is important to record about nursing care and how that should be structured in electronic records.

WWW

The development of electronic records is an area of rapid change. For information about this topic and on the standards and specifications for nursing content of electronic patient records go to the websites of the health service information departments such as:

- http://www.connectingforhealth.nhs.uk/
- http://www.ehealth.scot.nhs.uk/
- http://www.wales.nhs.uk/IHC

A good way to decide whether the content of your records is adequate is to ask the question: 'Can those coming after me find out from the record what they need to know to continue the care of this child?'. This tests the fitness of the record for the purpose of communication to support continuity of care. A second question that tests the quality of the record for all other purposes is: 'Can those who need to know find out from the record what we found on assessment, what we did and the results of our actions?'. Working in partnership implies that the content of the record will reflect not just the nurse's view but the assessments, plans actions and evaluations of the child/young person, parents and other members of the team.

Data to support audit, management and research can be obtained directly from these records or collected using specific data collection tools. One of the benefits of computerising patient records is that these will provide structured data that can be more easily aggregated and analysed. There will still be a need for other forms of data collection, for example the patient record won't tell you how many staff were available on a particular day or which nurses have specialist qualifications – important information when evaluating the quality of your service.

Information governance

An important part of information management is information governance, a quality framework that brings together legal requirements and professional guidance around record keeping, confidentiality, access to records, data quality, etc. The key principles of information governance are that information is:

H = held securely and confidentially

O = obtained fairly and efficiently

R = recorded accurately and reliably

U = used effectively and ethically

S = shared appropriately and lawfully.

Good practice requires the nurse to ensure that children, young people and parents/carers are informed of what is recorded about them and who has access to that information so that they can choose whether to restrict access to the information in the record or withhold information they do not wish to be shared. This is even more important as electronic records are introduced in all healthcare settings making access easier.

Summary

New skills in information and knowledge management are being developed by nurses concerned to ensure that children and families have control over information and knowledge, that they can make sense of what is happening and participate knowledgeably in decisions. The nurse's role is shifting from one of information provider to one of supporting children, young people and families to access, understand and use information themselves, increasing their independence and their capacity for self care. With these skills and the increasing expectations and skills of the children and young people themselves, true partnerships may become the norm, rather than an ideal that is perhaps seldom achieved.

References

Alderson, P., Montgomery, J., 1996. Health care choices: making decisions with children. Institute of Public Policy Research, London.

Barnes, K. (Ed.), 2003. Paediatrics: a guide for nurse practitioners, Butterworth-Heinemann, Edinburgh.

Carpenito-Moyet, L.J., 2004. Nursing diagnosis: application to clinical practice, 10th edn. Lippincott Williams and Wilkins, Philadelphia.

Charles, R., 1994. An evaluation of parent-held child health records. Health Visitor 67 (8), 270–272.

Coyne, I.T., 1995. Partnership in care: parents' views of participation in their hospitalised child's care. Journal of Clinical Nursing 4 (2), 71–79.

de Luc, K., Todd, J., 2003. E-pathways: computers and the patient's journey through care. Radcliffe Medical, Oxford.

Children's Workforce Development Council (2007) Common Assessment Framework for children and young people: practitioners' guide. Online. Available at: http://www.everychildmatters.gov.uk/resources-and-practice/IG00063/ [accessed 10 November 2008]

Duce, S.J., 1996. A systematic review of the literature to determine optimal methods of temperature measurement in neonates, infants and children. NHS Centre for Reviews and Dissemination 1, 124.

Eiser, C., Morse, R., 2001. Quality-of-life measures in chronic diseases of childhood. Health Technology Assessment 5, 4.

Gharaibeh, M., Abu-Saad, H., 2002. Cultural validation of pediatric pain assessment tools: Jordanian perspective. Journal of Transcultural Nursing 13 (1), 12–18.

Gibson, F., Nelson, W., 2000. Mouth care for children with cancer. Paediatric Nursing 12 (1), 18–22.

Gordon, M., 2002. Manual of nursing diagnosis, 10th edn. Mosby, St Louis.

Harris, R., 2002. Physical assessment of patients: the Byron physical assessment framework. Whurr, London.

Higgs, J., 2000. Clinical reasoning in the health professions, 2nd edn. Butterworth-Heinemann, Oxford.

Hockenberry, M., Wilson, D., Winkenstein, M., et al., 2003. Wong's nursing care of infants and children. Mosby, St Louis.

Kirk, S., 2001. Negotiating lay and professional roles in the care of children with complex health care needs. Journal of Advanced Nursing 34 (5), 593–602.

Marfe, E., 2003. Assessing risk following deliberate self harm. Paediatric Nursing 15 (8), 32–34.

Marshall, M., Fleming, E., Gillibrand, W., et al., 2002. Adaptation and negotiation as an approach to care in paediatric diabetes specialist nursing practice: a critical review. Journal of Clinical Nursing 11 (4), 421–429.

Mason, G., Webb, C., 1997. Researching children's nurses' clinical judgements about assessment data. Clinical Effectiveness in Nursing 1, 47–55.

National Library for Health, 2008. Protocols and care pathways. Online. Available at: http://www.library.nhs.uk/pathways/ [accessed 10 November 2008.

NHS Modernisation Agency, 2003. Essence of Care benchmarks: support for clinical governance. Online. Available at: http://www.cgsupport.nhs. uk/PDFs/articles/Essence_of_Care_2003.pdf [accessed 10 November 2008.

North American Nursing Diagnosis Association (NANDA), 2008. Nursing diagnosis: definitions and classification 2009-2011. NANDA International, Philadelphia.

Nursing and Midwifery Council (NMC) 2007 Record keeping. Online. Available at: http://www.nmc-uk.org/aFrameDisplay.aspx?DocumentID=4008 [accessed 10 November 2008)

Orem, D., 2001. Nursing: concepts of practice. Mosby, St Louis.

Petryshen, P., Stevens, B., Hawkins, J., et al., 1998. Comparing nursing costs for preterm infants receiving conventional vs developmental care. Neonatal Intensive Care 11 (2), 18–24.

Redshaw, M., Harvey, M., 2002. Working together: neonatal nurse practitioners in practice. Acta Paediatrica 91 (2), 178–183.

Rogers, D., 2003. Skin assessment: improving communication and recording. Paediatric Nursing 15 (10), 20–23.

Roper, N., Tierney, A., 2000. The Roper, Logan, Tierney model of nursing based on activities of living. Churchill Livingstone, Edinburgh.

Royal College of Nursing (RCN), 2003. Defining nursing. RCN, London.

Royal College of Paediatrics and Child Health (RCPCH), 2000. Growth reference charts for use in the United Kingdom. RCPCH, London.

Schmidt, L.J., Garratt, A.M., Fitzpatrick, R., 2002. Child/parent-assessed population health outcome measures: a structured review. Child: Care. Health and Development 28 (3), 227–237.

Selwood, K., 2000. Integrated care pathways: an audit tool in paediatric oncology. British Journal of Nursing 9 (1), 34–38.

Sharber, J., 1997. The efficacy of tepid sponge bathing to reduce fever in young children. American Journal of Emergency Medicine 15 (2), 188–192.

Slack, W., 1977. The patient's right to decide. The Lancet 296, 240.

Waters, E., Stewart-Brown, S., Fitzpatrick, R., 2003. Agreement between adolescent self-report and parent reports of health and well-being: results of an epidemiological study. Child: Care. Health and Development 29 (6), 501–509.

Yang, K.P., 2003. Relationships between nurse staffing and patient outcomes. Journal of Nursing Research 11 (3), 149–158.

Public health, primary health care and the development of community children's nursing

8

Mark Whiting

ABSTRACT

This chapter examines the historical development, current arrangements for and possible future provision of primary healthcare nursing services for children in the UK.

LEARNING OUTCOMES

- To develop an awareness of the origins and history of approaches to public health within the United Kingdom
- To develop an knowledge of and insight into the historical development of nursing services for children in non-hospital settings in the United Kingdom
- To develop insight into the range of primary healthcare services provision for children in the United Kingdom
- To develop knowledge in relation to, specifically, the provision of community children's nursing in the United Kingdom

Introduction

Before starting the chapter proper, it is important to provide a brief explanation of the term 'primary health care' as it has been interpreted here. Primary health care can be defined as:

> The provision of health services to individuals and populations within non-hospital settings.

However, this definition is contestable on a number of points. First, although it could be argued that health/illness protection, health promotion and public healthcare are exclusively components of primary health care, the counterargument might be offered that all three of these activities also take place on a very regular basis within hospital settings.

The second area of contention relates to the interface points between hospital and non-hospital services provision, for instance accident and emergency departments, outpatient clinics, short-stay assessment wards, minor injury units, 'walk-in' centres, ambulatory care facilities, hospital-at-home schemes – each of which might arguably be considered to be part of either primary care or secondary care.

This chapter will not specifically set out to provide a clear resolution to these areas of debate, however, when appropriate, discussion within the chapter will incorporate an exploration of both wider public health and health promotion perspectives, and will also consider issues pertaining to the interfaces between in-hospital and out-of-hospital provision.

Historical considerations

The emergence of both primary health care and coordinated approaches to public health in the UK is generally traced to the 19th century, that is, to the second half of the Industrial Revolution. In 1800, around 80% of the British population lived in rural communities, in villages, hamlets and the countryside; within 100 years, almost three-quarters of the population lived in towns and cities (Briggs 1983, Gregg 1976). This had major implications for family life, including significant changes to the care and welfare of children as the nature of rural/village/community existence was transformed. Blair et al (2003) graphically illustrates the consequences of this for the children of the working classes:

> Mothers needed to work up to and straight after childbirth to bring in sufficient income, but the Industrial Revolution had separated the world of work from the world of home, so children were often abandoned to the care of someone else from an early age
>
> (Blair et al 2003 p 88)

This 'someone' was often a young aunt or even an older sibling and, as Lomax (1996 p 2) acknowledges, at that time '…the concept of state or even charitable intervention in family to enhance the welfare of children was frowned upon'. It might be argued that such a view prevails even to the present day! However, Blair and colleagues (2003) suggest that as the 19th century progressed a number of factors came together

DOI: 10.1016/B978-0-7020-3183-0.10008-6

to enable a more coordinated public health response. These included:

- The emergence of philanthropic approaches towards the poor and needy.
- The need for 'self-preservation' for the middle/upper classes as it became widely recognised that diseases such as cholera and smallpox, often endemic in the growing cities, were no respecter of social class.
- Utilitarian approaches to social policy/welfare reform.
- The need for a healthy, well-fed productive workforce.

The mass migration of the population from the countryside into the larger towns and cities led to major problems of overcrowding, and in particular to problems of waste disposal and sanitation. Overcrowded and poor conditions provided the ideal environment for the spread of infectious disease and, during the early part of the 19th century, in response to concerns about potential or actual epidemics, a number of local Boards of Health were established by the Privy Council. Fears of a cholera epidemic lead to the creation of a consultative Board of Health in June 1831 and, later that year, to the establishment of the Central Board of Health under the aegis of the Privy Council. Within the year, nearly 1200 local Boards of Health were established by order of the Council but, just as quickly, as the threat of the cholera epidemic receded, the central and local Boards were dissolved in 1832. However, conditions of public health and, in particular, sanitation remained a concern of the Poor Law Commissioners. Their work, and perhaps most significantly, Edwin Chadwick's 1842 report 'A survey into the sanitary condition of the labouring classes in Great Britain' (with its detailed and graphic accounts of how the insanitary conditions in which the poor were forced to live was a major factor in the spread of disease) led directly to the establishment of The Royal Commission on the Health of Towns.

The Royal Commission set to work immediately, following-up Chadwick's report and undertaking an investigation of sanitary conditions in 50 English towns. The findings of the Royal Commission investigation directly led to the publication of the first Public Health Act in 1848.

WWW

Read a more detailed account of the history leading up to the Public Health Act in the National Archives at:

- http://catalogue.pro.gov.uk/leaflets/ri2180.htm

Perhaps the most widely recognised event from this period of public health history relates to Dr John Snow who, in 1854, plotted the pattern of occurrence of deaths from cholera in the Golden Square area of Soho, London. As a direct result of Snow's work, the spread of disease was linked directly to water supplied from the water pump in Broad Street. Snow himself removed this pump and, within 7 days, the cholera outbreak was officially declared as over. Snow's action demonstrated that the spread of this particular disease could be prevented by replacing a contaminated water supply with an alternative source of clean water.

WWW

Further details of Snow's work can be found on the website of the Royal Institute for Public Health at:

- http://www.riphh.org.uk

Thus the public health movement of the 19th century involved a combination of health services provision (at both local and governmental levels), social reform (at both local and governmental levels) and investigation into the causes, effects and distribution of disease (epidemiology).

A hospital for children

In 1739, over 100 years before the Public Health Act of 1848, Thomas Coram had established the Foundling Hospital in an attempt to provide care for the growing number of babies (often illegitimate children of the poor/working classes) abandoned on London's streets. Coram's initial attempts to secure funding from the government and the Anglican Church were rejected, but with perseverance and the help of charitable funding, he established a hospital that rapidly became overwhelmed with admissions (Franklin 1964, Kosky & Lunnon 1991, Lomax 1996). Government financial support was eventually forthcoming, although Lomax (1996 p 4) suggests that State intervention was, in part, responsible for the discrediting of the hospital, leading to accusations that by agreeing to accept all children arriving at its doors, it encouraged 'irresponsibility and immorality'.

WWW

For a more detailed account of the work of Thomas Coram go to:

- http://www.coram.org.uk/heritage.htm

The Foundling Hospital was primarily concerned with providing protection and education for children. Its support of the medical or healthcare needs of children was somewhat of a secondary consideration. By contrast, the work of Dr John Bunnell Davis, who established a children's dispensary in London in 1816, set out to both treat children (on what would now be described as an outpatient basis) and also 'serve to train parents in the better care of their offspring' (Lomax 1996 p 5). When Davis died in 1824, the work of the dispensary went through a period of decline until the arrival, in 1839, of Dr Charles West, who worked at what was now referred to as the Royal Universal Dispensary for 10 years while simultaneously striving to convert the dispensary into an inpatient hospital. Although this particular aspiration floundered, Charles West is often credited with being almost single-handedly responsible for the establishment of the first Hospital for Sick Children in Great Ormond Street, London, in 1852. West's pioneering endeavour was then followed by a period of 50 years of intense activity in building and establishing children's hospitals throughout the UK. By 1900, there were over 30 children's hospitals and upwards of 50 children's convalescent homes. In addition, many general hospitals had formally dedicated one or more wards exclusively for the care of children (Lomax 1996).

This dramatic growth in the provision of hospital care for children occurred largely as a result of charitable intervention and voluntary funding. Many of the hospitals or wards therein bore the names of the benefactors whose contributions had made the building and staffing of the institutions possible. In addition, 'private' payments for care afforded to children within the hospitals contributed significantly to the hospitals' income and thus to the provision of care to those who could not afford to pay, but who might be considered as 'interesting cases'.

Lomax (1996) suggests that, in addition to providing inpatient and outpatient services, many of the children's hospitals also established private home-nursing services, particularly when they first opened. However, such initiatives were often short-lived, partly because of the expense but also because of resistance from the hospital medical staff and hospital administrators. Charles West, however, considered this to be an essential element of the service provided by Great Ormond Street and, in the mid-1870s, made formal proposals to develop a private domiciliary nursing service to the hospital's management committee:

> Some consideration took place on the reference in Dr West's paper to the training of nurses proposed by the Lady Superintendent in visiting hospital out-patients at their own homes, under the regulations suggested by Dr West and coincided in by the Lady Superintendent. The majority of the Medical Officers were in favour of the plan being made trial of for 6 months, but the lay members of the committee were unanimously opposed to the extension of the work of the hospital beyond the walls
>
> (The Hospital for Sick Children 1874)

WWW

For a more detailed history of the Hospital for Children, Great Ormond Street see:

- http://www.ich.ucl.ac.uk/150/whole_story.html

It was another 14 years before the persistence and persuasion of Dr West and Dame Catherine Wood, the Lady Superintendent of the hospital, led to the establishment of the Great Ormond Street private domiciliary nursing service in 1888 (Whiting 2000). Elsewhere in the country, those children's hospitals that continued to provide a domiciliary outreach service did so on a private, fee-paying basis only.

Nursing children in the community

The provision of non-fee-paying nursing support of children in the community did, however, begin to develop towards the end of the 19th century from two distinct sources: district nursing and in the forerunner of current health visiting service, the Sanitary Reform Associations. In addition, school-nursing services for children began to emerge in the final decade of the century.

District nursing

It is generally accepted that the roots of our present district nursing service lie in the pioneering work of William Rathbone, in Liverpool, who in 1859 engaged the services of a hospital-trained nurse to help care for his dying wife at home. Rathbone was very aware of the appalling living conditions of the over-crowded city of Liverpool and, following his wife's death, he asked the nurse to continue in his employment and provide care to the sick poor people, including children, in the city (Rathbone 1890). By 1874, a National Association for 'Providing Trained Nurses for the Sick and Poor in London and Elsewhere' had been founded (Kratz 1982). In 1887, Queen Victoria's Jubilee Institute for Nurses was established as the first formally organised district nursing scheme. In 1928, this became the Queen's Institute for District Nurses and the institute assumed responsibility for the training of district nurses (Baly 1987).

WWW

Look at the photographic archive of the Queen's Nursing Institute on the Welcome Trust website:

- http://medphoto.wellcome.ac.uk/

During the next 50 years, district nursing services expanded steadily, being organised on a local basis by either voluntary agencies or local authorities (Stocks 1960). The National Health Service Act of 1946 first placed formal responsibility upon local health authorities:

> ...for securing the attendance of nurses on persons who require nursing in their own homes
>
> (NHS Act 1946 part III section 25)

The predominant focus of the work of district nurses was the care of the adult patient. In general, children who required symptom relief/management at home were cared for by their parents with support from the general practitioner, and only occasional input from the district nurse, whereas those who were acutely unwell and whose condition merited closer medical attention were admitted to hospital. In addition, many children with chronic or long-standing illness spent long periods as hospital inpatients, often many miles away from their families in long-stay or rehabilitation facilities.

Successive studies of district nursing practice over the last 40 years have shown that children form only a small part of their caseload (Hockey 1966, McIntosh 1975, OPCS 1982). Jackson (1978), describing the development of a community nursing service aimed specifically at children in Gateshead, commented that, although children had formed a significant part of the early district nursing caseload, the increasing sophistication of paediatric practice meant that more children were admitted to hospital and thus the numbers of children cared for by district nurses diminished steadily. The Court Committee (DHSS 1976 p 81) observed that, although the district nurse syllabus included some detail on the special needs of children and their families, the time allocated was 'inevitably minimal'.

Health visiting

As with district nursing, the history of health visiting can be traced to the middle of second half of the 19th century. The same circumstances that had prompted William Rathbone's philanthropic activities in Liverpool led to the establishment of the Manchester and Salford Sanitary Reform Association in 1852 (Hale et al 1968, While 1985). This was one of a number of initially small-scale efforts that developed in several of the larger cities. Although the Association was founded in 1852, it was not until 1862 that a full-time visitor was first appointed. The role of the visitors was principally one of teaching and counselling, rather than of practical nursing. At this time, no previous nursing experience was deemed necessary for the visitors, whose title changed to 'health visitors' around the turn of the century. The first health visitor training school was established, with considerable guidance from Florence Nightingale, in Buckinghamshire in the 1890s. A requirement for visitors to have previously undergone nurse training was introduced in Manchester at around the time the 'health visitor' title was first introduced.

The Statutory Rules and Orders of the Local Government Act (1929) made provision for a qualification and standard training for health visitors. The National Health Service Act of 1946 required that all health visitors must be qualified as such. As with district nursing, the National Health Service Act placed responsibility on the Local Health Authorities to provide a health visiting service. The Act stated:

> It shall be the duty of every local health authority to make provision in their area for the visiting of persons in their homes by visitors to be called 'health visitors' for the purpose of giving advice as to the care of young children, persons suffering from illness and expectant or nursing mothers, and as to the measures necessary for the spread of infection
>
> (NHS Act 1946 part III section 24 [I])

The work of the health visitor is, however, principally located in the areas of health surveillance and health education, and not in the care of children with discrete nursing needs:

> The professional practice of health visiting consists of planned activities aimed at the promotion of health and the prevention of ill-health
>
> (Council for the Education and Training of Health Visitors (CETHV) 1977)

The Court Committee (DHSS 1976) discussed the role of the various members of the primary healthcare team in caring for the sick child in the community and concluded that although mothers might seek advice on the care of a sick child from the health visitor, only rarely did health visitors undertake any practical nursing care with children. The Committee had recommended the appointment of specialist Child Health Visitors (section 17.25) with joint responsibility for the promotion of health and the management of paediatric nursing problems in the community. However, considerable doubt was expressed at the time (Sartain 1977) – and subsequently (While 1986) – over the wisdom of attempting to combine preventive and curative roles in this fashion, the principal fear being that curative work would take precedence. Health visitors themselves have commented that despite the fact that their work is concentrated in the care of the under-5s, there is a reluctance to take on a more acute, disease-centred role (Jones 1988, Ledger 1988).

School nursing

The contribution of the school nurse to the care of the sick child merits brief consideration at this point. Strehlow (1987) has reviewed the history of the school nursing services in some detail. Although a number of nurses were appointed during the latter years of the 19th century, services were very limited indeed. The first formally organised school nursing services were established in response to the report of the Interdepartmental Committee on Physical Deterioration, published in 1904, which found that 60% of potential army recruits were unfit for military service as a result of a catalogue of health problems, in particular issues concerning undiagnosed/treated chronic illness and the poor nutritional and overall health status of the young men coming forward to enlist for military service.

School nursing services have historically focused predominantly on aspects of child health, including screening and surveillance, and health promotion. The one area of practice that is exceptional to this relates to the field of 'special education', i.e. those settings that have focused their attention on children with particular health problems, such as epilepsy, physical and/or learning disabilities, schools for 'delicate' children and those for children with visual and auditory impairments. The Warnock review of 1978 (Department of Education and Science (DES) 1978) provides a useful review of what is referred to as 'special education for the handicapped'.

Perhaps the two most significant developments in the provision of education for children with health-related problems are, first, the Education Act of 1944, which resulted in the alignment of widely disparate education provision for such children with the new education arrangements for all children within the UK and, second (which followed on from the Warnock Report itself), the integration of children with 'special educational needs' within the mainstream of education provision.

Community children's nursing

District nursing, health visiting and school nursing each provide a piece of the complex historical jigsaw of community nursing provision for children although, as can be seen from the discussion above, none of the these services are specifically configured to provide care for children with nursing needs outside of hospital settings. A children's nurse writing in the *British Medical Journal* in the mid-1980s observed:

> There is an increasing muddle over who does what in the community … but because paediatric community nursing is not apparently regarded as a speciality in its own right, some of the work is being done by district nurses, some by health visitors and some by midwives. This cannot be sensible and perhaps accounts for the fact that often the wrong children are kept at home and the wrong ones admitted to hospital
>
> (Davies 1985 p 547)

This is perhaps not entirely surprising. Throughout the early to middle part of the 20th century, the predominant view of paediatric clinical staff (doctors, nurses and therapists) was that the most appropriate (the best) place to care for the sick child was in hospital. It is interesting to note, that with the introduction of the National Health Service in 1948, the Great Ormond Street Private Community Nursing Service was required by law to disestablish and the service closed in 1949.

At around this time, the pioneering work of John Bowlby (1951), a psychiatrist, and James Robertson (1956), a psychoanalyst and social worker, brought the whole question of hospital care for children into sharp relief. Their work led directly to the realisation that hospitalisation, or other forms of disruption to family/home life, particularly for young children (under the age of 5), for long periods or for repeated episodes of care, had the potential to adversely influence the psychological well-being of the child.

As the 1950s drew to a close, the recommendations of the Ministry of Health Report on the welfare of children in hospital (Ministry of Health 1959: the 'Platt report') heralded a fundamental shift in attitudes to the care of the sick child with its two key recommendations:

1. Greater attention needs to be paid to the emotional and mental needs of the child in hospital, against the background of changes in attitudes towards children, in the hospital's place in the community, and in medical and surgical practice. The authority and responsibility of parents, the individuality of the child, and the importance of mitigating the effects of the break with home should all be more fully recognised (paragraphs 6–14).
2. Children should not be admitted to hospital if it can possibly be avoided (paragraph 17).

In recommending this new approach to caring for children, the Platt Committee identified the need for the care of children outside of hospital to be supported by the development of home nursing schemes for children:

3. Special nursing facilities for looking after sick children at home should be extended (paragraphs 18–19).

The report's authors made specific reference to recently established services in Paddington, Birmingham and Rotherham. However, although the committee's recommendations undoubtedly had an immediate and dramatic effect on the services provided for children and their families within the hospital setting, the impact on the community was almost undetectable. Indeed, it was not for another 10 years after the publication of the report that a single additional paediatric community nursing service was established and, during this period (as noted above), the contribution of district nurses and health visitors to the nursing care of children was very limited indeed.

Those services that had been identified by the Platt Committee were largely concerned with the care of children experiencing acute, episodic illness (Gillett 1954 (Rotherham), Lightwood 1956 (Paddington), Smellie 1956 (Birmingham)). However, in 1969, two new approaches emerged. In Southampton, a paediatric community nursing service was established to support the work of a newly established Day Surgery Unit, with the nurses providing community follow-up for children undergoing a range of surgical procedures (Atwell et al 1973). By contrast, the service established in Edinburgh in the same year was based in the Children's Outpatient Department and concentrated on the outpatient nursing care of children with 'long-term disability' (including diabetes mellitus and coeliac disease) and on those with congenital abnormalities (including cleft lip) (Hunter 1974). In Edinburgh, further developments soon followed both for children who required follow-up of short-term problems and also for those with cystic fibrosis (Hunter 1977).

Some 7 years after the initiatives in Southampton and Edinburgh, the Court report (DHSS 1976), the specific focus of which was community child health services, offered a further endorsement of the Platt report recommendations relating to the development of paediatric community nursing. Once again, these recommendations appeared in large part to fall on deaf ears. Indeed, by 1984 there were still only a smattering of services across the UK and it was not until the late 1980s that there was a significant expansion in what was beginning to be referred to across the UK as 'community children's nursing'.

Activity

Read a more detailed account of the historical emergence of community children's nursing in Whiting (2000).

Further consideration to the current provision of community children's nursing will be provided later in the chapter, but it is important to set that provision within the broader, overall context of child health services and public healthcare provision and it is to those areas that attention will now be directed.

Primary health care and primary healthcare teams

A succession of reorganisations of the NHS during the 1970s resulted in the emergence in the early 1980s of the Primary Health Care Team (PHCT) as the dominant model/focus of community nursing activity. A typical PHCT was based in a health centre, and its work was concentrated on the caseload of one or more general medical practitioners (GPs). The team usually included a GP, district nurse, health visitor and practice nurse, although these were often joined by a community midwife and occasionally by other members of the nursing workforce and a range of allied health professionals.

In 1986, a major review of community nursing was undertaken on behalf of the Department of Health and Social Security by Julia Cumberledge. This review endorsed the by now well-established PHCT model, although neither the specific nursing needs of children nor the emerging practice discipline of community children's nursing featured in any significant part in the review's recommendations.

It was perhaps hardly surprising, therefore, that when the United Kingdom Central Council for Nursing, Midwifery and Health Visiting (UKCC), in part in response to the

Box 8.1

Specialist community health nursing pathways (UKCC 1994)

- General practice nursing
- Community mental health nursing
- Community mental handicap nursing
- Community children's nursing
- Public health nursing – health visiting
- Occupational health nursing
- Nursing in the home – district nursing
- School nursing

Cumberledge recommendations, brought forward proposals for the reform of community nursing education in the early 1990s the nursing needs of children barely merited a mention (UKCC 1991). Two years later, as the proposals for the reform of community nursing education were incorporated into the Council's rather more extensive Post-registration Education Project (UKCC 1993), the needs of children were recognised but were included in a rather intriguing suggestion to develop a new education programme concerned with the '…general nursing care of children which relates to the practice of school nursing and of paediatric nursing' (UKCC 1993 annexe 3 p 1). In the consultation process that followed, school nurses and community children's nurses made strenuous representation to the UKCC. Eventually common sense prevailed and final proposals for the new discipline of specialist community health nursing included separate education pathways leading to qualification as either a school nurse or a community children's nurse as well as for six other community nursing disciplines (UKCC 1994) (Box 8.1).

The programmes of education in specialist community health nursing reflected a growing recognition in the early 1990s of the potential role of all community nurses within the field of public health. The 1994 UKCC report demanded both a clear focus on public health and health promotion within the programmes and required that such themes played a key role within the minimum one-third of the programme that would be based on shared learning across the community nursing disciplines.

This strong emphasis on public health and health promotion had its roots in the World Health Organization's 1978 'Alma Ata' declaration of its goal of 'health for all by the year 2000' and the European review of the global targets, which was published by WHO in 1985.

WWW

Read the 'Alma Ata' document at:

- http://www.who.int/hpr/NPH/docs/declaration_ almaata.pdf

By the time the UKCC recommendations were published, the social policy context in the UK had been set out by the Department of Health (DoH), initially in the publication 'Promoting better health' (DoH 1988), which set out the key philosophical underpinning of the public health agenda, and then in the rather more strategic 'The health of the nation' (DoH 1992), which set the broad policy context for the promotion of health by identifying five key areas of work (Box 8.2) and setting key targets for health improvement within each area.

Box 8.2

Target areas: 'The health of the nation' (DoH 1992)

- Accidents
- Coronary heart disease and strokes
- Mental illness
- Sexual health
- Cancer

In more recent years, this policy has been updated and developed (DoH 1998a, 1999a) with a renewed emphasis upon the need to tackle issues of inequality (DoH 1998b) and, with the Sure Start programme, to make sure that children have a good start in life (DoH 1999b). Nurses have remained at the forefront of this area of health policy, with aspects of children's health being given a high priority in much of the current debate about public health (Her Majesty's Treasury/DoH 2004). Specific concerns relating to obesity, smoking and sexual health in childhood have taken centre stage in much of the current debate.

A public health role for the community children's nurse?

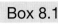

The Cumberledge report (DHSS 1986) recommended that all nurses working in specialist roles outside the hospital setting should be based in the community. However, the justification for such an approach was not made at all clear and was certainly out of step with developments in the provision of community children's nursing (CCN) services. At this time (as before and since), community children's nursing was made up of a heterogeneous mix of services, some based in health centres or community clinics, and some based in hospital children's wards or outpatient departments. A number of teams provided care to children based on traditional medical specialties such as oncology or respiratory care, others took on a more generic role. Much of the work of community children's nurses cut across organisational boundaries between hospital- and community-based services. Indeed, although the recommendation of the Cumberledge report to establish 'neighbourhood nursing teams' based on populations of approximately 25,000 failed to materialise, the late 1980s and early 1990s saw a dramatic expansion in the provision of community children's nursing (Fig. 8.1), with most teams serving a typical District Health Authority based population of around 250,000 (within which there were between 45,000 and 60,000 children) and with many teams working very closely with the one or two children's wards in the local District General Hospital. As more teams were introduced, a range of differing models of service provision began to emerge, including ambulatory care, hospital-at-home care and

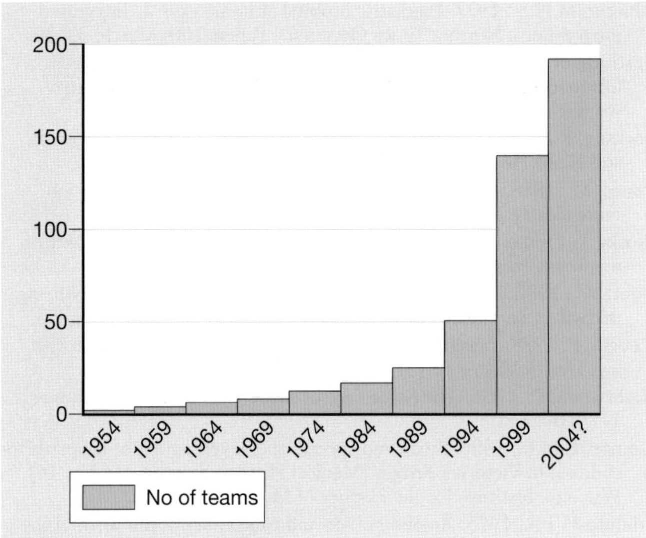

Fig. 8.1 • Growth in the provision of community children's nursing services in the UK (1954–2004).

specialist services based around tertiary centres, each added a new dimension to the complex array of community children's nursing services which featured by the turn of the century.

In general, local teams have developed in response to local demands, and no one model of service provision has yet become clearly established as the preferred model of service delivery. The work of the community children's nursing teams varies, often depending on the needs and/or demands of their local populations. However, there remain very significant variations in the modus operandi of the teams within the UK, as different teams respond to the demands of children/families with a range of nursing need (Box 8.3).

The work of the community children's nurse is very much focused on the needs of individual children and their families. Whereas health visiting and school nursing are population-based services and arguably 'every child has either a named health visitor or a named school nurse', community children's nursing services operate on a referred-child model, so whereas a typical community children's nursing team provides a service to a child population of around 50,000, at any one time only a fraction of that population constitutes part of the community children's nursing caseload.

The scenarios below provide illustrative examples of how the community children's nurse might engage in opportunistic promotion of health at an individual level.

Box 8.3

Range of nursing need for which community children's nursing services might be provided

- Children who are acutely unwell
- Children who have been involved in accidents
- Children who have undergone surgery
- Children with chronic illness
- Children with physical disabilities
- Children with life-threatening/life-limiting illness
- Children who require palliative care
- Children who are learning disabled
- Children with emotional or behavioural disturbance
- Children with mental ill health

Scenarios

David

David, aged 13, has diabetes. Over the course of the last year his weight has increased, moving him from the 75th to the 90th centile. During a home visit, the community children's nurse takes the opportunity to talk to David and his mother about both exercise and diet, and to set these in the context of the possibility of the whole family adopting a more healthy lifestyle.

Assad

Assad is 4 years old and has been referred to the community children's nursing team for removal of sutures from his face following a fall. During the visit, the community children's nurse observes that Assad's 1-year-old brother is beginning to pull himself to a standing position and walk around furniture. There are no stair gates, fire guards or electrical plug socket covers in the house and the nurse is concerned about the generally chaotic nature of the home. She provides Assad's mother with an information leaflet about home safety and successfully engages her in a long conversation about avoiding childhood accidents. She is able to refer the family to the local health/social services accident prevention team, who provides a variety of home safety equipment on a loan/low-cost basis. The nurse makes some summary notes in Assad's Personal Child Health Record and notifies the family health visitor of the outcome of her visit.

Jenny

During a visit to Jenny, a 14-year-old with cystic fibrosis, Jenny's mother expresses concern to the community children's nurse that Jenny is beginning to engage in a sexual relationship with her boyfriend. The nurse knows the family well and has acted as 'key worker' to Jenny for several years. Together, the nurse and mother are able to discuss the situation with Jenny. They provide some initial advice and Jenny agrees to visit the family planning clinic with her mother.

Jack

Jack, aged 3, is about to return to his day nursery following an initial diagnostic admission and treatment for acute lymphoblastic leukaemia. His mother asks the community children's nurse whether she might be able to prepare the staff and children at the nursery for Jack's return. The nurse and mother speak together to all of the staff at the nursery about aspects of infection control and avoidance of possible risk.

As noted above, health visitors and school nurses have a much more wide-reaching role in promoting health within the child population as a whole. Recent public health policy statements (DoH 2004, Her Majesty's Treasury/DoH 2004, Skills for Health 2004) have provided a clear sense of direction for all health professionals working with children, with major policy initiatives focused on sexual health, reduction in teenage pregnancy rates, obesity, smoking, drugs and alcohol. The extent to which the community children's nurse might embrace a wider public health role within such areas remains to be seen. However, CCNs have established a very clear public health role in working with children and young people who are already experiencing health-related problems. Such work should be recognised and valued in the context of the overall public health agenda for children. Clearly, all nurses working with children have a role in health promotion.

References

Atwell, J., Burns, J.M., Dewar, A.K., Freeman, N.V., 1973. Paediatric day case surgery. The Lancet ii, 895–897.

Baly, M., 1987. A history of the Queen's Nursing Institute. Croom Helm, Beckenham, Kent.

Blair, M., Stewart-Brown, S., Waterston, T., Crowther, R., 2003. Child public health. Oxford University Press, Oxford.

Bowlby, J., 1951. Maternal care and mental health. Monograph Series No. 2. World Health Organization, Geneva.

Briggs, A., 1983. A social history of England. Weidenfeld and Nicolson, London.

Chadwick, E., 1842. A survey into the sanitary condition of the labouring classes in Great Britain. Published on behalf of the Poor Law Commissioners. Reproduced in full in Flinn MW (Ed.), 1965 Report on the sanitary condition of the labouring population of Great Britain by Edwin Chadwick. Edinburgh University Press, Edinburgh.

Coram Family 2004 Coram family heritage. Online. Available at: http://www.coram.org.uk/heritage.htm [accessed July 2004].

Council for the Education and Training of Health Visitors (CETHV), 1977. An investigation in the principles and practice of health visiting. CETHV, London.

Davies, A., 1985. Paediatric trained district nurse in the community (letter). British Medical Journal 291, 247.

Department of Education and Science (DES), 1978. Report of the Committee of Enquiry on Special Educational Needs (the Warnock report). HMSO, London.

Department of Health (DoH), 1988. Promoting better health. HMSO, London.

Department of Health (DoH), 1992. The health of the nation. HMSO, London.

Department of Health (DoH), 1998a. Our healthier nation. TSO, London.

Department of Health (DoH), 1998b. Independent inquiry into inequalities in health (Chairman D Acheson). TSO, London.

Department of Health (DoH), 1999a. Saving lives – our healthier nation. TSO, London.

Department of Health (DoH), 1999b. Sure Start. Health Services Circular HSC 199/02. TSO, London.

Department of Health, 2004. Choosing health: making healthier choices easier. TSO, London.

Department of Health and Social Security (DHSS), 1976. Fit for the future. The report of the Committee on Child Health Services (the Court report). HMSO, London.

Department of Health and Social Security (DHSS), 1986. Neighbourhood nursing – a focus for care. Report of the community nursing review (Chairman J Cumberledge). HMSO, London.

Franklin, A.W., 1964. Children's hospitals. In: Poynter, F.N.L. (Ed.), The evolution of hospitals in Britain. Pitman Medical, London.

Gillet, J.A., 1954. Children's nursing unit. British Medical Journal 20th March, 684–685.

Gregg, P., 1976. Black death to industrial revolution: a social and economic history of England. Harrap, London.

Hale, R., Loveland, M.K., Owen, G.M., 1968. The principles and practice of health visiting. Pergamon Press, London.

Harrison, S., 1977. Families in stress. Royal College of Nursing, London.

Her Majesty's Treasury & Department of Health, 2004. Securing good health for the whole population (Chairman D Wanless). TSO, London.

Hockey, E., 1966. Feeling the pulse. Queen's Nursing Institute, London.

Hunter, M.H.S., 1974. A programme of integrated hospital and home nursing care for children. Paper presented to the annual conference of the National Association for the Welfare of Children in Hospital. NAWCH, London.

Hunter, M.H.S., 1977. Paediatric hospital at home care: 1. Integrated programmes. Nursing Times Occasional Papers 10th March, 33–36.

Institute of Child Health 2002 The whole story: the history of Great Ormond Street Hospital for Children. Online. Available at: http://www.ich.ucl.ac.uk/150/whole_story.html.

Jackson, R.H., 1978. Home care for children. The Journal of Maternal and Child Health March: 96 98, 100.

Jones, M., 1988. Health visiting: the time has come to define the job more clearly. Nursing Times 84 (3), 11.

Kosky, J., Lunnon, R.L., 1991. Great Ormond Street and the history of medicine. Hospitals for Sick Children, London.

Kratz, C., 1982. District nursing. In: Allen, P., Jolley, M. (Eds.), Nursing, midwifery and health visiting since 1900. Faber and Faber, London.

Ledger, P., 1988. Feasibility study for weekend and evening health visiting. Health Visitor 61 (3), 71–72.

Lightwood, R., 1956. The home care of sick children. The Practitioner 177, 10–14.

Lomax, E.M.R., 1996. Small and special: the development of hospitals for children in Victorian Britain (Medical History, Supplement No. 16). Welcome Institute for the History of Medicine, London.

McIntosh, J.B., 1975. An observation and time study of the work of district nurses. University of Aberdeen, unpublished PhD thesis, .

Ministry of Health, 1959. The welfare of children in hospital: report of the committee (the Platt report). HMSO, London.

OPCS, 1982. Nurses working in the community. HMSO, London.

Rathbone, W., 1890. Sketch of the history and progress of district nursing from its commencement in 1859 to the present day. Macmillan, London.

Robertson, J., 1958. Young children in hospital. Tavistock, London.

Royal College of Nursing (RCN), 2004. Directory of community children's nursing services. RCN, London.

Royal Institute for Public Health 2004 The John Snow Society. Online. Available at: http://www.riphh.org.uk [accessed July 2004].

Sartain, B.,1977. Views from Hampshire HA. Nursing Times 23rd June, 944–947.

Skills for Health, 2004. National occupational standards for the practice of public health. Skills for Health, Bristol.

Smellie, J.M., 1956. Domiciliary nursing service for infants and children. British Medical Journal 1, 256.

Stocks, B., 1960. A hundred years of district nursing. Allen & Unwin, London.

Strehlow, M.H., 1987. Nursing in educational settings. Harper and Row, London.

The Hospital for Sick Children, 1874 Medical committee minutes, vol 6: special meeting of the joint committee – March 18. Hospital for Sick Children Great Ormond Street, London.

United Kingdom Central Council for Nursing, Midwifery and Health Visiting (UKCC), 1991. Report on proposals for the future of community education and practice. UKCC, London.

United Kingdom Central Council for Nursing, Midwifery and Health Visiting, 1993. (UKCC) Consultation on the Councils proposed standards for post-registration education. UKCC, London.

United Kingdom Central Council for Nursing, Midwifery and Health Visiting, 1994. (UKCC) The future of professional practice – the Council's standards for education and practice following registration. UKCC, London.

While, A.E., 1985. Health visiting and health experience of infants in 3 areas. University of London, unpublished PhD thesis.

While, A.E., 1986. The value of health visitors. Health Visitor 59 (6), 171–173.

Whiting, M., 2000. 1888-1988: 100 years of community children's nursing. In: Muir, J., Sidey, A. (Eds.), Textbook of community children's nursing. Bailliere Tindall, Edinburgh.

World Health Organization (WHO) 1978 Declaration of Alma Ata. WHO, Geneva. Online. Available at: http://www.who.int/hpr/NPH/docs/declaration_almaata.pdf [accessed July 2004].

World Health Organization (WHO), 1985. Targets for health for all. WHO, Copenhagen.

Family responses to ill health and admission to hospital

9

Sarah Dowle   Sally R Siddall

ABSTRACT

Children are admitted to hospital for a variety of reasons. Regardless of reason for admission, the child and family will be apprehensive and feel vulnerable away from their normal environment. This chapter explores why children are admitted to hospital, how the family might have coped up to this point and how a child's ill health can affect both child and family. Social and psychological responses to an admission to hospital are examined and the reader is encouraged to participate actively in the review of this material and application to the clinical environment. Empowerment of the child and family through utilisation of clinical nursing skills and therapeutic communication are reviewed.

LEARNING OUTCOMES

- Discuss the difference between the number of sick children and the number of hospital admissions.
- Detail the various coping strategies commonly utilised by families who have sick children.
- Explore parental reactions/responses to sickness in their child.
- Consider the nature and implications of hospital admissions – planned versus unplanned.

Introduction

Childhood is a journey of new experiences, some good, others not so good. Children cannot be viewed simply as small adults – they have special and changing needs, making varying demands at different stages of their life. Therefore, mere consideration of their age and developmental level is not sufficient in recognising these unique diverse needs. Ill health can be regarded as undesirable and yet also allows the child to develop a coping strategy for being ill. Respect of how a child's life experiences affect his or her ability to cope with illness, and indeed how these experiences ultimately affect the child's future development requires consideration. The experienced illness and the actual event of 'being ill' should be viewed as part of a learning process – the illness can be adapted, fought, accepted or rejected (Douglas 1993). The development of psychological coping mechanisms complements the evidence that illness enhances the maturing immune system to help manage further episodes of ill health (Hall & Elliman 2003).

The child's family, notably the parents, are usually the first to recognise illness and to act on the changing verbal and observational cues gained from knowing their child so well. It is important to remember that the majority of sick children will not require hospitalisation, or even a visit to their own GP, but will be managed by a range of skills and advice gained from previous experience and from others. Recognition of the potential difficulties and coping mechanisms utilised by healthy families and their children requires consideration. The child and family often regard admission to hospital as a serious consequence of ill health, therefore setting the scene for the child and family to be apprehensive, fearful and anxious. Hospitalisation has long been recognised as being a potentially stressful time for children and families alike (Darbyshire 1994). Health professionals on the admitting ward may well consider the child's illness to be relatively 'minor' in terms of morbidity and sometimes fail to anticipate or recognise the family's overwhelming concern. Unfamiliarity with both the situation and the organisational boundaries – the need for compliance, disruption to the family unit and the overall impact these variables have on the family – must be considered throughout.

This chapter seeks to investigate the decision process that leads to a child being admitted to hospital and looks at how the child and family might react in this situation. It will consider both planned and unplanned hospital admissions and consider the socialisation process associated with ill health.

Statistics

Perhaps the most useful activity to set the scene for this chapter is to establish how sick children are managed by the family and by the health services. This will provide an understanding of

DOI: 10.1016/B978-0-7020-3183-0.10009-8

ill-health episodes families experience with their children and also the ratio of primary and secondary care episodes. What will be more difficult to extract is how many children become ill and yet do not see a GP or are referred to the hospital. It will also be useful to see if there are any trends in age groups of children being referred to the GP or hospital:

- In England and Wales children under 16 years comprise 20% of the population (Office for National Statistics Census 2001).
- 19% of consultations with GPs and 15% of practice nurse consultations are with the 16-year and under age group (McCormick et al 1995, Office for National Statistics 2005 (General Household survey 2001/02)).
- The most common childhood system affected is respiratory – accounting for 27.6% of consultations (Health Committee 1997).
- 80% of all episodes of acute childhood illnesses at home are reported to be managed without recourse to health professionals (Department of Health (DoH) 2003).
- One in 10–15 children will be admitted to hospital between birth and the age of 16 (DoH 2003).
- 70–90% of health care takes place within the family – this includes the care of all family members, not just children (Kleinman et al 1978, Scambler 1997).
- A random sample study found that 26% of respondents with at least one severe symptom chose not to consult a doctor (Hannay 1991).
- A subsequent study established that nearly 50% of mothers (sample size 52) identified illness symptoms in their child yet did not seek medical intervention (Cunningham-Burley & Irvine 1991).
- In 2001/02 16% of health service expenditure was spent on children under 16 years of age. On average, £259 is spent on each child aged between 5 and 15 per year, and £1,172 on each child under 5 years of age, including births. This can be compared with £3,315 per year spent on adults over the age of 85 (Office for National Statistics 2005.)

Activity

Consider the statistics outlined above in your learning group:

- What is the most important consideration for nurses in caring for sick children in the community or the hospital setting in terms of age at time of illness?
- Consider the range of nursing skills parents are likely to have as a result of such regular exposure to child ill health.

Coping strategies commonly utilised by families with a sick child

It is suggested there are three inter-related and overlapping arenas in which health care takes place – the 'popular' sector (or family wisdom), the 'folklore' sector (involving cultural and personal beliefs about health care) and the 'professional' sector (Kleinman 1980). It is important for the children's nurse to understand and recognise the importance of these care arenas, as families will usually arrive in the hospital setting with a range of knowledge and interventions taken from the first two sectors that can assist, support and direct the nurse during the admission and planning process. Families are integral to the care and support of their children therefore the impact of any health care intervention must be considered within this context. An understanding of the theories seeking to explain how families cope and interact under stress is essential and several theories have been postulated and subsequently applied to children's nursing (Crawford 2002).

Family wisdom

Much research has been undertaken exploring how parents cope with their sick child, particularly in relation to the provision of care (Helman 1994, Oakley et al 1994). It is important to remember that families have to experience an ill-health situation to learn how to handle the consequences. Advice and help are readily offered and sought from within immediate family and friends. Some of the advice may be sound and 'evidence based' (e.g. the more a child sleeps, the better he or she grows), whereas other help may be more dubious and based on 'old wives tales' (e.g. feed a cold, starve a fever) (Seabrook 1986). Either way, if the child is seen to improve, it is unlikely that external help will be sought such as from the health visitor or GP. This then sets up an 'encyclopaedia' of knowledge that is held by the family and used again as needed.

Helman's work (1995) utilises the 'germ theory', whereby people regard an illness being caused by 'invading germs' and describe the illness in terms of hot/cold and wet/dry symptoms. Once identified in these terms, a visit to the doctor enables the parent to articulate their concern. Research investigating mother's understanding of the causation of illness has revealed significant and useful data for children's nurses to consider. Pill & Stott (1982) found 11 categories of illness causation; five of these were deemed to be external, and therefore out of the parent's control, and the other six were internalised, and therefore within the parent's control (Table 9.1). The factors in the first column perhaps lead the parent to believe that the responsibility for the illness and subsequent management are the responsibility of others, whereas the factors in the second column require an acceptance of responsibility and therefore an agreement to some positive action by the parent to alter the cause of illness.

Activity

- Do you think nurses and doctors work on a similar view in defining the cause of a child's illness so that an effective plan of care, including relevant health promotion/education, can be devised?
- Is there a risk of stereotyping people by using this approach, because of their dress; personal hygiene; personality?

Table 9.1 Categories of illness causation (adapted from Pill & Stott 1982)

External causative factors	Internal causative factors
Environmental: the weather, pollution, pesticides	Type of person you are, e.g. more nervous/unhappy
Heredity and susceptibility	Being 'run down'
Individual susceptibility	'Way of life'
Germs, bugs, viruses, infection	Diet
Stress, worry	Hygiene
	Neglect, not looking after yourself properly

Evidence-based practice

On your own and in your learning group:

- Reflect on methods used within your family to help manage illness.
- Did they work?
- Can you establish if they are evidence based by today's approach to a similar situation?
- Consider the value of the following 'folklore' advice:
- 'Don't wash your hair when you are having a period'
- 'Salt in the bath water helps to heal skin wounds'
- 'Make children sick by getting them to drink salt water if they say they have taken a noxious substance'
- 'Put vinegar on a bee sting, bicarbonate of soda on a wasp sting'

An opposing view is that the development of professional and statutory services has served to erode the need for families to rely on their own family knowledge and skills in caring (Graham 1984). For example, SureStart is an excellent new multiagency (non-statutory) service where parents can seek out a range of advice and guidance and are actively encouraged to do so (Department for Education and Skills and Department for Work and Pensions 2005). The availability and 'free at the point of delivery' health service can serve to reduce the importance of creating the encyclopaedia of family knowledge. The emergence of a 'blame culture' might also have challenged the reliance on family wisdom, resulting in a reduction in the number of parents taking responsibility for healthcare decisions.

Sociological research examining the domestic management of children's healthcare tends to relate to the mother (Broome et al 1998, Pitts & Phillips 1991, Helman 1994). There is further useful analysis of several studies considering the child and family's response to acute illness in children (Youngblut 1998). Nurses need to familiarise themselves with different cultures and how culture can also influence the family's decision to seek its own solution or to utilise health professionals.

Socioeconomic conditions may also influence decision making. Limited access to health centres, chemists and hospitals because of transport and/or cost can serve to delay the decision to seek medical help. The provision of health care within the family is often related to the family income. The mother often acts as housekeeper and carer and therefore recognises the need to provide sufficient resources to meet each role effectively. However, if the 'carer' needs outweigh the 'housekeeper' needs in terms of resources, time and cost, then the family/mother will go without essential provisions. This compromise can lead to conflict within and outside the family (Graham 1984).

Single-parent families invariably have less income than dual-income families, and sometimes less access to other family members and so less emotional and practical support (Blackburn 1991). This can influence the management of a child's illness, with the parent visiting the GP more frequently for reassurance and guidance, or not visiting a GP because of the cost of travel and lack of companionship to share the concerns of the health status of a child. Stereotypes of the 'overconcerned' parent or 'negligent parent' can arise in these instances, and yet there is a sound rationale for why this behaviour might arise.

Activity

- What is meant by 'hot' and 'cold' illnesses as expressed by many Asian cultures? How are each type generally managed?
- Consider the cost, in economic and practical terms, for a parent with three children under the age of 5, living on a farm, to travel to town or health centre to seek advice, equipment and/or treatment for a sick child?

Activity

On your own and subsequently in your learning group:

- Explore your town, supermarket, pharmacist and health centre, and collect a range of available leaflets on helping the sick child. Do they seem to be written for the parent's needs?
- Scan the supermarket shelves to see the range of medicines that are available to families. How are they packaged? Child friendly, colourful, etc. Do they offer easy-to-read instructions, dosage preparations and age restrictions?

Community support

Families have a further range of support to help them in deciding which is the best course of action for their ill child, for example accessing the local pharmacy for advice or just a scan of products that may help (Birchley 2002). Many weekly and monthly family-type magazines contain useful healthcare advice, as do the daily papers. Searching the internet for advice is also done on an increasingly regular basis.

As a result of the explosion in internet usage, many government agencies, in particular the Department of Health (DoH), have set up websites to support the enquiring mind. Several innovative health services have also been created to utilise this latest technology. One such service is NHS Direct. It offers both a telephone service and an internet site (DoH 1997, National Audit Office 2002). Investigate one of these and write up what advice is available for parents to help their sick child and whether the advice is something nurses would undertake in their role in a ward or community setting.

www

Visit the Guardian website and search through the health sections to see the diversity of health advice available:

- http://guardian.com

Visit a common search engine such as Google:

- http://www.google.com

and find out how many hits there are for the medical condition of:

- toothache
- diarrhoea
- conjunctivitis.

Look at the first five English 'hits' for each condition and see how helpful they might be to someone wanting to manage this condition without recourse to a healthcare professional.

Activity

In your learning group: discuss what use any of you have made using NHS Direct.

- Who do you believe it is aimed at?
- Do you know the telephone number?
- Where is your local NHS Direct call centre based?
- Have any of you visited this centre to establish what they do? Would it be useful to ask your course tutor to arrange such a visit?

Read the article by Hall (2003) about the NHS Direct and children's care.

www

Visit the NHS Direct online website and seek out the advice for 'tummyache' in children:

- http://www.nhsdirect.nhs.uk

Seminar discussion topic

In your learning group:

- Discuss how useful a site like NHS Direct is for anxious parents, concerned children and other child carers such as grandparents and child minders.
- Spend 10 minutes exploring the internet to see what other government 'online' support services there are for people, particularly the child and family. Make a list of these and share them with your colleagues for future use.

Seminar discussion topic

In your learning group, select one of the following 'support networks' that you wish to explore in more detail:

- evidence-based home care
- 'folk lore' remedies
- pharmacy support
- available health education leaflets
- NHS Direct.

Primary care support

All children have a right to regular health support and health checks during childhood (Hall & Elliman 2003). The midwife takes a full responsibility for newborn babies up to 28 days and a named health visitor shares and then assumes this responsibility 28 days after birth (Statutory Instrument 1992 No. 635). This health promotion/education role enables parents, and children, to learn about healthy choices and safe ways of dealing with everyday situations, from preventing accidents to managing illnesses. The health visitor will refer health concerns to the family's GP as necessary and make other referrals to other practitioners if felt appropriate; for example social services, speech therapy and child development centres.

Additionally, teams of appropriately qualified nursing staff working in the child's home, school and community settings can provide health care. These teams can consist of school nurses providing health promotion and education within the school setting, offering health interventions, support for children with long-term illnesses and the empowerment of child and family in maintaining the integrity of the family unit.

Likewise, community children's nursing teams (CCNs) provide a link between the secondary and tertiary services and the primary care provision (DoH 1996, Kelly 1998). They typically provide ongoing care interventions for children with known illnesses or following discharge from hospital for routine or emergency health care.

Activity

One of the roles of the midwife following delivery is to help establish the feeding needs of the child with the mother/parents.

- What sort of advice will be given during this time that will provide parents with an insight as to how to cope should they have concerns about their baby's feeding routine in the future?

Activity

A health visitor undertakes a routine hearing check on a 9-month-old baby:

- What teaching and learning is likely to take place for the baby's parent(s) in attendance?
- How is this likely to help the parent(s) at a later time in terms of coping strategies if the child becomes unwell?

Immunisation

Immunisation is the use of a vaccine to protect against a specific disease. Vaccines act on preventing disease in one of three specific ways:

1. Administration of a live bacteria or virus which has been attenuated so it does not cause the disease.
2. Administration of the dead bacteria/virus.
3. Administration of part of the bacteria/virus.

Vaccines also contain substances to enable them to work effectively (DoH 2002).

The fundamental aim of an effective immunisation programme is to reduce the incidence (i.e. the number of people acquiring the disease in the population as a whole) of a specific disease, with the ultimate aim of eradication where possible. It is important, however, to remember that some diseases will never be eradicated either because there is a 'carrier' population (i.e. people who are able to carry a disease but who themselves remain unaffected) or because of the specific mode of transfer/activity (e.g. tetanus is carried in the soil spores). Indeed, despite improvements in hygiene, nutrition, health care and public immunisation programmes, some diseases continue to cause serious complications and fatalities (DoH 2002). Equally, there are dramatic success stories: before the introduction of the measles vaccination in 1988 an average 250,000 cases/year were noted, resulting in 85 deaths. By 1999, a significant reduction to 2438 cases/year, with two deaths, was evident (DoH 2002).

WWW

In view of the media interest in the measles, mumps and rubella (MMR) vaccination visit the following website:

- http://www.mmrthefacts.nhs.uk

Consider the advantages and disadvantages of the vaccination as it is currently offered:

- Identify the knowledge you would require as a parent considering MMR vaccination for your first child.
- As a health professional consider how you would promote the uptake of the immunisation programme.

Activity

Consider, with rationale, the skill mix of children's nurses employed in a community children's nurse team. For example, should there be a member of the team with additional skills and knowledge in adolescent care?

Parson's sick role

There is a well established, although regularly challenged, functionalist theory on how society might expect someone to behave when 'sick' in order to protect the individual and society (Bury 1997). This theory was originally described by Talcott Parson in 1951, and was used by many health practitioners and employers at that time to determine whether the individual was 'sick' or 'ill' (Parson 1951). Medical support and employment support would then be offered according to this analysis.

Activity

- Define the difference between being 'sick' and being 'ill'?

Powerpoint

Access the companion PowerPoint presentation and look at Parson's sick role and then list the two components deemed essential for being 'sick'.

- Can these be easily applied to children?
- How can this theory be supported where children have a permanent disability or are terminally ill?
- Do you see evidence of 'medical dominance' in this theory? If so, what are the implications for such a view?

Scenario

You have woken up this morning with 'bad back' and feel generally unwell. You have taken an anti-inflammatory drug and ring your ward to say you will be unable to come in for your late shift that day.

- Do you think the staff will believe you?
- Do you feel the need to sound weak and ill over the telephone?
- Do you think the nurse receiving your call will ask/expect you to go to see your doctor for further support?

You go to your GP, who offers to sign you 'off sick' for 2 weeks.

- Would you decline the advice because of your need to keep your course theory and practice hours up to date?
- If you do reject the advice, would you expect your GP to be sympathetic or dismissive of your decision? In other words, might your GP subsequently disbelieve your bad back?

Does any of the above fit in with Parson's sick role theory?

Research has established that children are often socialised to deal with an illness relative to the environment they are in (Mayall 1996). At home, parents may actively discourage children from staying home from school and do not let them fulfil the 'sick role' by expecting them to do their homework. This may reflect the parents' coping strategy of hoping the illness is 'make-believe' or not serious, or fulfilling their role as 'constructive agents within the family' (Mayall 1996 p 82). Conversely, at school, children might have to negotiate their illness by seeking help at school breaks and after school. Injuries are more likely to occur in the playground, with the teacher seeing children as 'the objects of their socialisation and curriculum work' (Mayall 1996 p 82). Parents who accept their child's illness will implement the 'sick role' by renegotiating school attendance and workload.

Seminar discussion topic

School children are still heard to refer to the school nurse as the 'nit nurse':

- How far from the truth is this?
- Why do you think children still use this terminology?
- Seek out journal/internet, Nursing and Midwifery Council (NMC) and DoH information about the evolving role of the school nurse.

PROFESSIONAL CONVERSATION

A mother rings the ward to seek advice on her 5-year-old child who was discharged from your ward yesterday following a routine tonsillectomy. She is concerned that her daughter is 'still not wanting to eat'.

Your advice is to try soft foods that her daughter normally likes and to give her plenty of fluids.

The mother states she has tried this to little avail. You ask her if her daughter has any pain and if her prescribed pain relief is effective. The mother says she has not given any because she sees no need – her daughter is not saying she is in pain. You suggest she gives her some anyway. The mother says she can see no need to do this.

You suggest that the mother contacts her own GP or rings the ward back the following day if there is still no improvement. The mother says she does not really think this will be necessary and thanks you for your time and says goodbye.

- What are your thoughts on the mother's behaviour – is her child 'sick' or not?
- Are you tempted to think the daughter cannot be too ill if the mother is reluctant to try out the care you offer?
- Is this 'Parson's non-conforming sick role theory by proxy'?
- What would you do once the call ended?

Doctors are not the only health professionals who expect a degree of conformity to the health advice they give to a child or parent; nurses can also make judgements on parents who perhaps challenge the advice they are given or appear to dismiss it.

The information and activities so far have highlighted how vital it is that children's nurses seek out the knowledge parents and child already hold about the particular illness that necessitates hospital care and, specifically, what management has already been offered. Without these initial enquiries there may be a wide discrepancy between the professional care being offered and how the parent or child perceives this care. Parents might also need to be supported in their own previous understanding so they can also reflect on their skills, knowledge base and application. This may serve to positively reinforce their skills and ability or redirect these. Either way, continued empowerment of the family would result.

Parents, children and the wider family experience many mixed emotions when admission to hospital is decided on. This is in part due to the nature of admission, planned or unplanned (see later). However, most admissions are unplanned and these usually create the greatest upheaval for all concerned (Kendrick et al 2000, Young & McCubbin 2002). The next section explores the range of common emotions experienced by those involved.

Activity

Access the companion PowerPoint presentation Childhood illness and the family and complete the various activities. Share your thoughts with your peer group and ask clinical staff for their views and experiences in some of these areas.

Psychological reactions

Many parents feel both relieved and guilty about their child's imminent admission to hospital. Their relief is based on the reassurance that their child will be cared for by people with the skills and resources to do so effectively; their guilt is because they are anxious that perhaps the care they had offered up to that point was inappropriate or had merely delayed the inevitable admission. They may also feel disappointed or angry because the health advice they might have already sought led them to believe their child was not as ill as they now fear he or she is.

It is imperative that the admitting nurse seeks to establish the nature of the parents' key concerns in these respects. Positive support can then be quickly provided and evaluated. However, appreciation of the parents' role as advocates for their child can mean that the health professional views the parents' concern as paramount, rather than seeking to determine the lived experience of the 'sick' child. This can then restrict the child's own understanding and involvement in decision making if their own perception of what it is like to be ill is unspoken (James 1998).

Scenario

Danny, a 2-year-old boy, is rushed to the local A&E department having suffered a convulsion at home. Both his parents witnessed this and had never seen this before in their son.

On admission, it is established that Danny has a temperature of 40.2°C and the staff plan their care around the likely event that this is a febrile convulsion. This care involves removing the blanket Danny was wrapped in, plus a jacket, jumper, dungarees, a vest and nappy. They quickly explain to parents the importance of letting Danny cool down so as to help prevent a further seizure.

- What do you imagine Danny's parents will think when they see this action and hear the rationale for it?
- Might they feel they are partly responsible for Danny maintaining this high temperature because of the clothes he was dressed in?
- Might they feel inadequate as parents and people?
- How does this parental effort of keeping Danny warm when ill fit with a lay person's views on managing fever?

For further reading on managing a fever, read Harrison (2000).

The adjacent scenario explores the possible effects on child and parents when an acute illness occurs. Health staff need to recognise the limitations of parental knowledge if a particular event has never happened before. It is possible to see how much knowledge can be gained in a very short space of time by the parents witnessing actions and listening to the explanations and rationale for these. Consequently, the majority of parents would be able to recognise and anticipate the changed care approach should a similar situation occur again. This also explains why many childhood illnesses are managed effectively in the community and family home.

Nurses also need to consider how parents manage the continuing ill-health needs of a child with a long-term health problem. Using the above exploration of how parents develop a skill and knowledge base, one might assume the parents of a child with a long-term health need are better equipped and skilled to deal with both minor and major health changes (Kirk 2001). However, it is pertinent to reflect on the nature of many of these conditions and the potential for them to be 'life-limiting' or 'life-threatening'. In these situations, parents often prepare themselves by considering the latest illness as being potentially fatal.

Reflect on your practice

Imagine the feelings of parents of a young boy with cerebral palsy who is admitted with a chest infection for ongoing management. He has been unwell at home now for 5 days, with GP support. His parents are skilled in offering basic suction, chest physiotherapy and adapting his medicine regime to suit his needs.

- How are the parents likely to feel once the GP has decided that hospital care is now the most appropriate way forward?
- How are they, as parents, likely to feel in a physical sense, having been sharing the care between them for such a long time and with broken nights sleep and neglecting their own basic needs?
- Reflect on how often nurses encourage such parents to stay and help because they know the parents can handle their child's physical needs better than they are likely to do. Is it in everyone's best interest to use this strategy of care?
- Dwell on the information parents might have been given when they were first aware of their son's physical disability in terms of:
  - Parents: 'What might cause our son's early death?'
  - Doctor: 'A serious chest infection'.
- How can nurses address this diversity of needs for these parents?

A further issue to be considered was raised in the adjacent 'Reflect on your practice' box. Many families have become adept at utilising medical equipment, pharmacological knowledge and symptom analysis that might easily match or surpass those of the health professionals they come into contact with. These families – and this might include the siblings and the sick child him- or herself – are used to risk assessment and high-level decision-making situations and so feel marginalised if the health professional dealing with the imminent hospital admission uses inappropriate language (e.g. simplifying technical jargon or offering patronising comments that are meant to be supportive). Likewise, the health professional might feel intimidated by the apparent wealth of knowledge and skill being shared and demonstrated by the child and family. The days when the medical world was secret, superior and only accessed by those qualified to do so are gone. Yet paternalism in the health service still exists and can undermine such families and also prevent other families reaching this level of medical/nursing competency if it is not challenged or eliminated (Dickinson & Dignam 2002). Family-centred care must begin at the time of the decision made to admit the child, not when he or she arrives on the ward.

Another important aspect of a sudden, or planned, admission to hospital is how the child's siblings deal with the situation. Seminal work by Eiser explored the effects on siblings when a sick child was admitted to hospital or had a long-term illness (Eiser 1990). It was found that many siblings lost self-esteem, confidence and identity and felt socially isolated. These problems can be expected to be more evident where a sibling has a chronic illness but is not uncommon in a sudden acute illness. Siblings should always be included in the planning of a hospital admission wherever possible and the outpatient clinic is an ideal area for planned preparation to include this type of advice.

Unexpected admissions are different and families often choose to deal with the 'breaking of bad news' at a time they best believe they can support their other children. However, some siblings are left feeling vulnerable and excluded if this is delayed for any length of time, such as waiting for the end of the school day. Nurses have a role in supporting the parent with this type of decision making.

It is important to have useful and easily obtainable information in a variety of formats and languages to help parents in the preparation for hospital care – for themselves, the affected child and his or her siblings. Recent innovations include preparation for hospital by hospital staff visiting children in their own homes before admission, so involving the wider family and answering a range of questions that might be thought of in the safety of the home but lost in the sterility of the hospital environment (Sutherland 2003). The national curriculum also enables some discussion about ill health and the caring professions. This can lead to innovative use of hospital visits or health professionals visiting the classroom. A range of leaflets, videos (e.g. Action for Sick Children) and books (Lansdown 1996) are available in public libraries and from outpatient clinics to further support the needs of the child and family (Adams et al 1991, Carney et al 2003). The internet is another source of useful but not always accurate information, in that it might not reflect the British approach or support the services that are available in other English-speaking countries.

A key aspect, which is of the utmost importance to any children's nurse, is the need to be skilled in understanding and applying the diverse nature of childhood growth and development. Parents are often familiar with how their child's behaviour changes during periods of ill health. There is increasing evidence to suggest even short periods of hospitalisation can result in transitory changes in behaviour (Rennick 1995). However, admission to hospital can further these changes, known as 'regression', and parents may not be skilled or competent at recognising these, sometimes believing their child to be deviant or 'attention seeking'. Regression can be explained as the concentration required by the child to cope with a strange environment and illness, this can be such that it leads to the child adopting everyday practices that they may have 'grown out of'. These include activities such as feeding and drinking using different implements (i.e. a bottle instead of a beaker), a reduction in vocabulary, crawling instead of walking, reverting to wanting a nappy again, or bed wetting. All these and many more activities require little concentration by the child; they are well-learned behaviours whereas the behaviours that replaced them may still require concentration to accomplish them. There is increasing evidence that even short periods of hospitalisation can result in transitory changes in children's behaviour and psychological status (Rennick 1995). Regression is usually self-limiting to the length of the illness or hospital stay but has often been viewed, by family members and health staff, as 'attention seeking' ploys. This view must be rejected and explanations and useful strategies for dealing with these offered as they happen and preferably in anticipation of them occurring.

The following areas are important considerations in the effective management of both child and family when hospital admission is being considered.

Activity

Read Sarah O'Neill's article 'Acute childhood illness at home: the parents' perspective' (O'Neill 2000):

- Make a list of the areas you consider to be important to your developing knowledge base and clinical application.

Activity

Check the health library, public libraries and internet for booklets and leaflets exploring the needs of the child and family when hospital admission is decided upon:

- Do they offer a good insight into how families can be prepared and prepare each other?
- Does your own children's unit offer locally created leaflets? Check these out as well.

WWW

Visit:

- http://www.childrensward.net (click on teddy bear in top left hand corner to enter site)
- http://www.rcseng.ac.uk/services/publications/ publications/pdf/children_hospital.pdf

These are just two sites of many to offer help. However, they were not easy to find and this may be a problem for enquiring parents and family members.

Age of child and developmental status of the child

As we have ascertained, children have special health needs necessitating constant attention and support from their families/carers. Increasing emphasis on child- and family-centred care advocates the involvement of parents in the overall management of their child, impacting on both the quality and role of those delivering care (Audit Commission 1993).

As discussed earlier in this chapter, an essential skill of any children's nurse is the need to be accomplished in understanding and applying knowledge of childhood growth and development. There is much in hospitals that is unfamiliar, perturbing and frightening to a child; the more one can be prepared for an event, to counter the fear of the unknown, the better one copes (Landsdown 1996). Diversity in a child's behaviour can frequently be accounted for by the parents, who will have greater knowledge of how their child reacts in stressful situations and during periods of ill health.

The age and developmental level of children, previous experience of ill health and hospital, and the parents' emotional status are likely to determine the effectiveness of the preparation (Landsdown 1996). When one considers the psychological implications of hospitalisation one must also respect the increasing volume of evidence associating heightened parental anxiety with increased child anxiety (Rennick 1995). Indeed, parent-initiated preparation and interventions to reduce anxiety are reported to influence children's adjustment to and acceptance of medical procedures and hospitalisation (Rennick 1995). Deciding how much children can understand is not easy; one of the reasons this is such a complex skill is the limitation on children's language skills. Even to adults, with complex cognitive skills and understanding, the world can be a bewildering place. Landsdown (1996) suggested that young children use fantasy and magical thinking to reduce tension, resolve conflict and fill gaps in their knowledge. On this basis then, it is suggested younger children are more likely to have misconceptions about the cause of their illness and therefore have less effective coping strategies. The majority of hospital admissions, for either planned or unplanned admissions, involve children under the age of 4.

Activity

- Relate your own experiences of 'regression' while ill to your study group.
- If you left home to start your nursing career, or a previous career; what special items did you want to pack to take with you? Why?
- Do you take any special mascots with you into exams? Why?

Activity

1. Consider the key principles of preparation for, and
2. Identify key areas likely to cause distress in:
   - a preverbal child
   - an adolescent.

A good grasp of child development theories is essential if the child is to have a positive experience within a negative situation.

Nature of hospital admissions – planned versus unplanned

Planned admissions

These can be arranged for medical or, more commonly, surgical needs. Outpatient care will usually have preceded the admission and the waiting list for surgical admissions is considerably shorter than in the adult population. There is often a converse picture of hospital admission in these situations. The healthcarers need to have a healthy child on admission and then proceed to make the child 'clinically ill' by the planned procedure. However, to help offset this, the child and family are aware of the need for admission and can plan ahead, asking relevant questions and so being empowered in advance. A range of services exists to support the imminent admission, so maintaining a degree of control within the family group and hopefully ensuring the integrity of the family dynamics is achieved.

Activity

- Identify the numbers of children admitted as planned and unplanned in your local unit.
- If possible, establish the age ranges for each category of admission.

Use your local hospital's audit officer to assist you in this exercise.

Unplanned admissions

These were considered earlier in the chapter. However, in light of the work undertaken in the above Activity, it becomes apparent how different an unplanned admission is and the likely effects on parents, sick child and siblings can differ. Far more children will experience a hospital stay as a result of an unplanned admission than a planned one. The skills of the nurse lie in determining the likely reactions exhibited by the family and supporting them effectively.

Responses to either type by child/family, including social consequences

Studies done during the last 30 years have identified that the occupational (social) class status of families has a direct link to hospital experiences of children. Work done by Earthrowl & Stacey (1977) indicates that children from social classes C2 to DE would have experienced more emergency admissions than children from AB to C1 (the middle classes), whereas planned admissions saw the reverse of this incidence. This suggests that nurses must therefore have a working understanding of the effects of occupational class in relation to health and the experiences of illness. The Black report (Department of Health and Social Security (DHSS) 1980) and subsequent studies (Davy Smith et al 1994, Townsend et al 1988) suggest that poverty is a key indicator on the likely health status of individuals and families.

Regardless of the occupational class of the family, however, is the knowledge that children are very reliant on their parents for security, direction and approval. An ill child will be even more dependent on such support and cues from the parent. However, the illness in a child will have a major effect on how the parent copes and this may be indicated by distress, anger, denial or relinquishing of normal parenting role. The child may subsequently feel let down by the parent and lose some degree of trust in the decision-making skills previously taken for granted.

Seminar discussion topic

Review Erik Erikson's eight stages of development (Erikson 1950) (these can be found in any good child development text and an overview is given in Chapter 2). Consider the first five stages in light of the above parental reactions when their child needs hospital admission.

The 'trust versus mistrust' stage is a particularly important stage to consider:

- Why do you think this stage is the most important in terms of the child's age and cognitive reasoning skills?
- How can children's nurses use the theory underpinning each of these first five stages to support the child's need to know what is happening?

A 2002 study found differing types of satisfaction/dissatisfaction with information sought as to diagnosis (Starke & Möller 2002). It was established that parents sought information for one of two reasons – to control the professional intervention or to provide sufficient information to others.

Additionally, the publishing of the report investigating the care of babies and children with complex needs at the Bristol Royal Infirmary identified malpractice, by way of a range of individual and system failures, resulting in a drive for reform of the medical profession (DoH 2001). Anachronistic modes of professional practice were identified, with parents having little or no involvement in ongoing discussions about the care of their children (DoH 2001). The prominent role of parents was a distinctive feature of the inquiry: their empowerment throughout this case may also be viewed as contradictory, as arguably their grief was exploited in pursuit of an agenda of reform. The response to the Bristol Inquiry has been remarkable in its unanimity, being welcomed by the government, endorsed by leading medical organisations and approved by representatives of families whose children underwent surgery in the Unit. It would seem the media have broadcast, without reservation, reports demanding that the 'club culture' of the medical profession must be relinquished in favour of a new culture of external regulation with imposed standards and performance indicators (DoH 2001). Consideration of the wider implications of the inquiry, including long-term damaging effects on medical practice, public confidence with the medical profession and relationships between doctors and patients must be sought.

Seminar discussion topic

In your seminar group, read Chapter 17 of the Bristol Royal Infirmary Inquiry (parents' experiences; DoH 2001) and consider how the findings from this chapter can be applied to your own nursing experiences and future care planning.

WWW

Visit:

- http://www.bristol-inquiry.org.uk

This site enables you to see the background to the inquiry and the findings of the report. Although the inquiry was specific to children with complex needs, the findings can be disseminated across all areas where children receive health care.

WWW

Visit:

- http://www.doh.gov.uk/childrenstrusts
- http://www.dh.gov.uk/PolicyAndGuidance/HealthAndSocialCareTopics/ChildrenServicesInformation/fs/en
- http://www.doh.gov.uk/nsf/children/gettingtherightstart (downloadable pdf document)

View these sites and seek out your local NHS Trust's efforts being made to implement the NSF standards.

The release of the Kennedy report (DoH 2001) resulted in early publication of part of the government's 'National Service Framework (NSF) for Children' (DoH 2004). This publication has argued that the fundamental principle is the intention to place patients at the centre of care delivery. Integral to this is the need for quality assurance, including patient safety and children's rights. Identification of clear national standards supported by the National Institute for Clinical Excellence (NICE) and independently monitored by the Commission for Health Audit and Inspection (CHAI; formerly the Commission for Health Improvement (CHI)) are central to delivery of equitable care.

The full 'National Service Framework for Children, Young People and Maternity Services' is now available and supports the need for clear and accessible information being made available to children and their families in health and illness, home and hospital (DoH 2004).

Reflect on your practice

When you need to wash your hands following completion of a procedure, do you typically wash them:

- in the sluice
- at the nurses station
- in view of the parents and children?

Which approach is the most likely to reassure the interested family and onlooker?

Having dwelt on this activity, are you likely to reconsider your usual practice to offer greater confidence to the families in your clinical area?

Choice of ward and informed choice/consent

Nowadays, many NHS Trusts have specific accommodation for young people (National Association for the Welfare of Children in Hospital 1990). However, this is not yet universal and there are various clinical and management approaches to offering adolescent accommodation. The most common is identifying an area within a paediatric unit, although there are some 'stand-alone' units with clinical support from both the paediatric and adult services. There are no specific guidelines as to age group or clinical speciality so a range of protocols exists (National Association for the Welfare of Children in Hospital 1985).

Seminar discussion topic

- An adolescent area within a paediatric ward should receive girls who are seeking to have a termination of pregnancy or to give birth to a baby.
- Adolescent areas should receive all young people who have attempted suicide/parasuicide/self-harm.

Discuss these two statements, offering rationale to support your views. Consider the skill mix of staff in this discussion:

- Explore your local provision to establish the views held in these two specific examples.
- Consider whether other similar situations might prompt moral or ethical consideration.

Evidence-based practice

In your local NHS Trust:

- Find out who provides young people with the information needed to know whether admission to a children's area or an adult area is an option.
- Whose role should it be?
- Is there a medium available to provide such information before admission to hospital?
- Does your local children's unit know of children under the age of 16 being cared for in adult areas?

Summary

In conclusion, it can be seen that there is a diversity of knowledge and skills to be considered when receiving children into hospital. Historical, social, psychological, economic, ethical and moral views are all intertwined and need to be engaged by the admitting nurse, or the community nurse, managing an episode of ill heath in a child. The need for good anticipating skills, an ability to 'stand back' from the immediate needs of the child to establish a dialogue with both child and family is essential if therapeutic communication, sensitive application of the nursing process and a trusting relationship are to develop and survive.

The age of the child, the size of the family, the occupational class and previous family experiences of ill health must all be embraced by the nurse to complement the care already provided and empower the family members to retain and develop, where necessary, skills in the care and management of their child.

References

Adams, J., Gill, S., McDonald, M., 1991. Child health: reducing fear in hospital. Nursing Times 87 (1), 62–64.

Audit Commission, 1993. Children first: a study of children's services. The Stationery Office, London.

Birchley, N., 2002. Parental management of over-the-counter medicines. Paediatric Nursing 14 (9), 24–28.

Blackburn, C., 1991. Poverty and health: working with families. Open University Press, Buckingham.

Broome, M.E., Knafl, K., Pridham, K., Feetcham, S. (Eds.), 1998. Children and families in health and illness. Sage Publications, London.

Bury, M., 1997. Health and illness in a changing society. Routledge, London.

Carney, T., Murphy, S., McClure, J., et al., 2003. Children's views of hospitalization: an exploratory study of data collection. Journal of Child Health 7 (1), 27–40.

Crawford, D.A., 2002. Keep the focus on the family. Journal of Child Health Care 6 (2), 133–146.

Cunningham-Burley, S., Irvine, S., 1991. In: Pitts, M., Phillips, K. (Eds.), The psychology of health: an introduction. Routledge, London.

Darbyshire, P., 1994. Living with a sick child in hospital. Chapman and Hall, London.

Davy Smith, G., Blane, D., Bartley, M., 1994. Explanations for socio-economic differentials in mortality: evidence from Britain and elsewhere. European Journal of Public Health 4, 131–144 Cited in: Field, D., Taylor, S. (Eds.), 1998. Sociological perspectives on health, illness and health care. Blackwell Science, Oxford.

Department for Education and Skills and Department for Work and Pensions 2005 SureStart, www.surestart.gov.uk

Department of Health (DoH), 1996. Child health in the community: a guide to good practice. Stationery Office, London.

Department of Health (DoH), 1997. The new NHS: modern, dependable. Stationery Office, London.

Department of Health (DoH), 2001. The report of the public inquiry into children's heart surgery at the Bristol Royal Infirmary 1984-1995. Learning from Bristol (the Kennedy report). DoH, London.

Department of Health (DoH), 2002. Immunisation: the safest way to protect your child. Stationery Office, London.

Department of Health (DoH), 2003. Getting the Right Start: National Framework for Children's Services Standard for Hospital Services. Stationary Office & www.doh.gov.uk/nsf/children/gettingtherightstart

Department of Health (DoH), 2004. National service framework for children, young people and maternity services. Department of Health, London http://www.dh.gov.uk/PolicyAndGuidance/ HealthAndSocial CareTopics/ChildrenServices/ChildrenServices Information/Children ServicesInformationArticle/fs/en

Department of Health and Social Security (DHSS), 1980. The Black report: inequalities in health. HMSO, London.

Dickinson, A.R., Dignam, D., 2002. Managing it: a mother's perspective of managing a pre-school child's acute asthma episode. Journal of Child Health 6 (1), 7–18.

Douglas, J., 1993. Psychology and nursing children. Macmillan Press, Basingstoke.

Earthrowl, B., Stacey, M., 1977. Social class and children in hospital. Social Science and Medicine 11, 83–88 Cited in: Black, N., Boswell, D., Gray, A., et al., 1984. Health and disease: a reader. Open University Press, Buckingham.

Eiser, C., 1990. Psychological effects of chronic disease. Journal of Child Psychology and Psychiatry 31, 85–98.

Erikson, E.H., 1950. Childhood and society. WW Norton, New York.

Graham, H., 1984. Women, health and the family. Wheatsheaf, Brighton.

Hall, D.M.B., Elliman, E. (Eds.), 2003. Health for all children. Oxford University Press, Oxford.

Hall, K.A., 2003. NHS Direct and children's A&E services: a case review. Paediatric Nursing 15 (5), 36–39.

Hannay, J., 1991. In: Pitts, M., Phillips, K. (Eds.), The psychology of health: an introduction. Routledge, London.

Harrison, M.R., 2000. Nurses' management of fever in children: rituals or evidence based practice? In: Glasper, E.A., Ireland, L. (Eds.), Evidence-based child health care. Macmillan Press, Basingstoke.

Health Committee, 1997. Health services for children and young people in the community: home and school. Third report. The Stationery Office, London.

Helman, C.G., 1978. 'Feed a cold, starve a fever': folk models of infection in an English suburban community and their relation to medical treatment. Culture. Medicine and Psychiatry 2, 107–137.

Helman, C.G., 1994. Culture, health and illness, 3rd edn. Butterworth-Heinemann, Oxford.

James, A., 1998. Children, health and illness. In: Field, D., Taylor, S. (Eds.), 1998 Sociological perspectives on health, illness and health care. Blackwell Science, Oxford.

Kelly, P., 1998. The role of the community children's nurse in enhancing the primary–secondary care interface. In: Glasper, E.A., Lowson, S. (Eds.), Innovations in ambulatory care: a nursing perspective. Macmillan, London.

Kendrick, D., Young, A., Futers, D., 2000. The diagnosis and management of acute childhood illness: is there a role for health visitors? Journal of Advanced Nursing 32 (6), 1492–1498.

Kirk, S., 2001. Negotiating lay and professional roles in the care of children with complex health care needs. Journal of Advanced Nursing 34 (5), 582–592.

Kleinman, A., 1980. Patients and healers in the context of culture. University of California Press, Berkley.

Kleinman, A., Eisenberg, L., Good, B., 1978. In: Helman, C.G. (Ed.), 1994 Culture, health and illness. 3rd edn. Butterworth-Heinemann, Oxford.

Lansdown, R., 1996. Children in hospital: a guide for family and carers. Oxford University Press, Oxford.

McCormick, A., Fleming, D., Charlton, J., 1995. Morbidity statistics from the general practice 1991-2. HMSO, London.

Mayall, B., 1996. Children, health and the social order. Oxford University Press, Buckingham.

National Association for the Welfare of Children in Hospital (NAWCH), 1985. Too young or too old – how and where should adolescents be nursed? NAWCH, London.

National Association for the Welfare of Children in Hospital (NAWCH), 1990. Setting standards for adolescents in hospital. NAWCH, London.

National Audit Office, 2002. NHS Direct in England. The Stationery Office, London.

O'Neill, S.J., 2000. Acute childhood illness at home: the parents' perspective. Journal of Advanced Nursing 31 (4), 821–832.

Oakley, A., Hickey, D., Rigby, A.S., 1994. Love or money? Social support, class inequality and the health of women and children. European Journal of Public Health 4, 265–273.

Office for National Statistics, 2001. Census 2001 www.statistics.gov.uk.

Office for National Statistics, 2005. General household survey (2001/02).

Parson, T., 1951. The social system. Free Press, New York.

Pill, R., Stott, N., 1982. Concepts of illness causation and responsibility: some preliminary data from a sample of working class mothers. Social Science and Medicine 16, 43–52 Cited in: Currer, C., Stacey, M. (Eds.), Concepts of health, illness and disease. Berg, Oxford.

Pitts, M., Phillips, K., 1998. The psychology of health: an introduction. Routledge, London.

Rennick, J.E., 1995. The changing profile of acute childhood illness: a need for the development of family nursing knowledge. Journal of Advanced Nursing 22, 258–266.

Scambler, G. (Ed.), 1997. Sociology as applied to medicine, 4th edn. WB Saunders, London.

Seabrook, J., 1986. The unprivileged. In: Currer, C., Stacey, M. (Eds.), Concepts of health, illness and disease. Berg, Oxford.

Starke, M., Möller, A., 2002. Parent's needs for knowledge concerning the medical diagnosis of their children. Journal of Child Health Care 6 (4), 245–257.

Statutory Instrument 1992 No. 635 The National Health Service (General Medical Services) regulations.

Sutherland, T., 2003. Comparison of hospital and home base preparation for cardiac surgery. Paediatric Nursing 15 (5), 13–16.

Townsend, P., Davidson, N., Whitehead, M., 1988. Inequalities in health. the Black report/the health divide. Penguin, Harmondsworth.

Young, R.T., McCubbin, M., 2002. Family stress, perceived social support and coping following the diagnosis of a child's congenital heart disease. Journal of Advanced Nursing 39 (2), 190–198.

Youngblut, J.M., 1998. Integrative review of assessment models for examining children's and families' responses to acute illness. In: Broome, M.E., Knafl, K., Pridham, K., Feetcham, S. (Eds.), Children and families in health and illness. Sage Publications, London.

Communicating with children and their families

10

Janet Matthews

ABSTRACT

This chapter will enable readers to increase their knowledge and understanding of the impact of communication on child development, daily living and health. The development of communication from conception to adolescence is outlined, highlighting the implications for those who work with children of different ages and their families. Research on communication between health professionals, children and their families is reviewed, taking into account children's rights. Issues which impact on communication with young people who are recipients of long-term health care, and their parents, will be discussed. Guided study activities and reflection on practice will facilitate the development of self-awareness, personal and professional development. Signposts to other chapters and recommended reading as a guide for further study are posted throughout the chapter.

LEARNING OUTCOMES

- Outline the development of communication from birth to adolescence.
- Discuss factors that have an impact on communication with children and families in the context of health care.
- Discuss communication strategies that facilitate family coping when communicating a serious diagnosis.
- Use relevant literature and research to identify good practice when working with children and families when the child has a life-limiting illness or disability and communication barriers.

PowerPoint

Accompanying PowerPoint presentations

Learning outcome 1 relates to presentation Part 1: Child Development and Part 2: Eyesight, speech, language and hearing difficulties, which provides useful website links to valuable information for children, families and health professionals. It also contains information on the role of speech and language therapists.

The remaining learning outcomes relate to Part 3: Communication: the healthcare context.

Introduction

Communication is instinctive from the moment of birth as the infant attempts to communicate with adults (Fig. 10.1), which is essential for development and the communication of need initially at a basic level. To promote child development, health and family integrity, the nurse must learn how children and families communicate but also how to communicate effectively with children of all ages and their families. This chapter will enable the nurse to identify effective communication strategies to ensure children, young people and their parents/carers have the information they need in the appropriate format. Providing clear, understandable information helps the child and family cope with alterations in health by enabling them to maintain control within healthcare contexts. This chapter is designed to help nurses fulfill this role.

Development of communication skills from conception to adolescence

> Beginning life with a rich innate structure, infants begin to change their understanding of persons, themselves and others, being transformed through inter-personal interactions. As infancy comes to an end infants appreciate they are not alone or unique, living as psychological beings, among other psychological beings in the world
>
> (Metzoff & Moore 1998 p 62).

The quality of human interaction at this crucial stage of development impacts on the infant perception of self and how they fit in, a process which begins in utero.

Before we are born

Research by Spence & DeCasper in 1986 indicates that, before birth, babies can hear and recognise their mother's voice. During pregnancy when mothers repeatedly recited stories aloud,

DOI: 10.1016/B978-0-7020-3183-0.10010-4

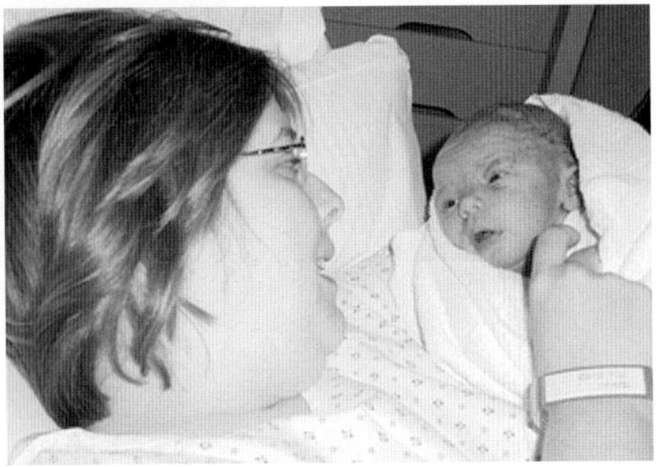

Fig. 10.1 • Engaging with mother 10 minutes after birth.

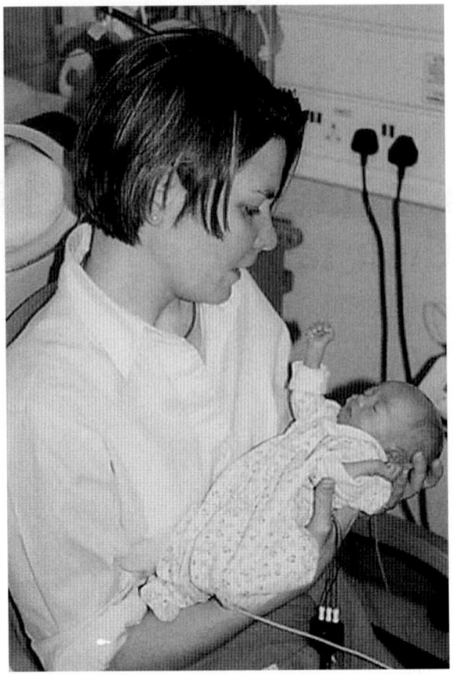

Fig. 10.2 • Face to face.

following birth their neonatal sucking pattern changed on recognition of their mother's voice demonstrating their ability to differentiate their mother's voice from two other story tellers (Zigler & Stevenson 1993).

www

Find out more about DeCasper's Research:

- http://www.uncg.edu/psy/tempfaculty/decasper/intro.html

Neonatal imitation

Several studies in the 1970s demonstrate that neonatal imitation is a 'robust phenomenon' that can be observed from birth (Heimann 1998). This is believed to be due to their innate social motivation to interact, especially in a face-to-face position (Heimann 1998), which takes place within what Kugiumutzakis (1998) describes as the neonatal–maternal 'intersubjective companion space'.

Learning to speak

Between the first and second year of life understanding and production of speech emerge (Zubrick et al 2007). Learning to speak is dependent on exposure to human language and feedback from adult pleasure. This reinforces infant achievements (touch, smiling, play, reciprocal communication, praise) and correction (Bruce 2001, Zigler & Stevenson 1993; Fig. 10.2). Infants are surprisingly sensitive to the quality of communication and seem to understand the significance of different types of communication (Murray 1998). Two-month-old infants demonstrate signs of let-down and disengagement when a happy mother suddenly becomes still and expressionless. Ongoing interactive engagement with an adult is essential to their development.

First sounds

The speed of language acquisition mystifies linguists, who cannot fully explain 'the apparent ease with which almost all babies acquire essential structure of one or more languages in their first three years' (Whitehead 2000 p 1). The real mystery is why it becomes increasingly difficult for a child to develop language skills as they grow older. Unlike animals, children are born with the biological mechanism to enable them to articulate words and the mental processing ability that enables them to isolate speech from other sounds, process and reproduce this information (Zigler & Stevenson 1993). Newborns are particularly receptive to the human voice and, as early as 2 months old, they will respond differently to the mother's voice distinguishing between different sounding words (Zigler & Stevenson 1993). The infant's inner adoration and desire to communicate is reciprocation of the love and adoration communicated by the adult, drawing the infant into the world of language (Matthews 1994, Whitehead 2000). Older siblings also contribute to the development of the young infant (Fig. 10.3).

The immature sound-making skills of the infant constantly change, making it difficult to identify their first word. However, their early sounds are not random – crying begins at birth, cooing by the end of the first month and babbling begins at around 6 months (Oller 1980). It is believed that the repetitiveness of one syllable, e.g. 'ba ba ba', exercises and thus develops the muscles of articulation. Furthermore, the tone and pitch of babbling seems to differ in keeping with the tone and pitch of the language to which the child is exposed (Zigler & Stevenson 1993). Initially babbling can mask deafness but this will diminish if the infant cannot hear feedback. If deafness is not detected early the child will have more difficulty learning to speak. Deaf infants who are signed to from an early age develop sign language at a similar pace to the hearing child

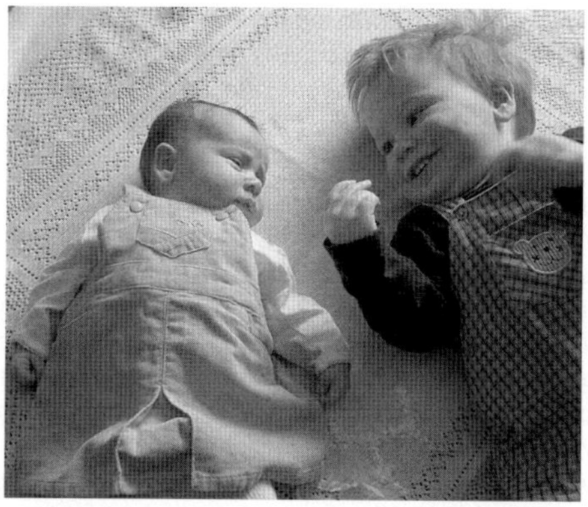

Fig. 10.3 • Older siblings contribute to the development of a young infant.

who is learning to speak. Early assessment and intervention by a speech and language therapist is very important.

PowerPoint

For more information see PowerPoint presentation Part 2: Eyesight, speech, language and hearing difficulties

The speed of language acquisition is variable and individual to each infant and context. Many studies cited by Whitehead (2000) show that a true word (one that is repeated spontaneously in the same context) can be produced from 9 months of life, although this usually takes place between 12 and 18 months. The first early word sounds are personal to the infant and recognised by the carer as a statement of interest or a specific request. Single words (e.g. 'dink' or 'joo') are used to transmit the meaning of a sentence 'give me a drink of juice'. The words are often combined with actions (e.g. banging something), which communicates urgency and determination (Zigler & Stevenson 1993). Parental understanding of the meaning and the context of early words is vital to the child's continuity of development.

Making sense of the world: 1–2 years

The speed and complexity with which infants combine words varies and is generally based on their need to get things done, to involve others or to comment. Emphasis in first sentences is usually placed on the main object requested, e.g. 'book ma ma read'. Communication increasingly becomes a means of exploration and development of personality. Children then use language to share their new experiences with us. Language enables children to think in a symbolic way, which is the principle underpinning learning words using pictures in books and surroundings. Symbolic language is very important for children who have communication difficulties associated with deafness or blindness (Whitehead 2000). Sign language and touch are essentially symbolic, enabling children who are hearing or sight impaired to make sense of their experiences, observations and feelings as they interact socially with others.

Exploring the 'big wide' world: 2–5 years

By the age of two, children have become talkers or signers and communication enables infants to explore who they are (Bruce 2001) and where they fit in the bigger picture. Between 2 and 4 years of age children start to improve their grammar, sorting out singular and pleural differences and past tense by adding 's' and 'ed' (Whitehead 2000, Zigler & Stevenson 1993). Whitehead (2000) states that spontaneous errors created as the child tries to correct early words, e.g. mouses and goed, are evidence of the ability of a child's mind to process and produce the rules of language.

In the preschool years, children start to use joining words ('because', 'and', 'if') as they begin to understand cause and effect, sequencing of events, trial and error (Whitehead 2000). Their increasing ability to use words like 'why', 'how', 'where', 'who' and 'what' is essential to their cognitive development.

Edwards (1998) emphasises that other 'relational motivations', which develop from an early stage, take interaction beyond the boundaries of attachment as the child begins to engage in meaningful reciprocal communication within small groups. The child's vocabulary increases to include words that enable him or her to share feelings and to explore how others are feeling. Dunn (1998) conducted longitudal research, which measured the child's ability to correctly interpret emotions (happiness, anger, fear, sadness) related to various situations. This evidence, outlined below, is vital to the promotion of child and family attachment.

Evidence-based practice

Naturalistic observation longitudinal research Dunn (1998) – 50 2-year-old infants were observed interacting with their mothers and older siblings at home. The results indicated that children had a greater understanding of others at 40 months old if the following observations had been made when they were 24 months old:

- frequently observed talking to family members about their feelings
- engaging in cooperative interaction with their siblings including social pretend play
- exposed to greater emotional intensity, intimacy and frequency of the interaction
- their mothers were more likely to engage in frequent controlling behaviour with older siblings.

The results suggest that personal experience and interest in how parents interact with siblings plays a key role in the development of emotional understanding. Further observation of the children over the next few years revealed that, between 33 and 47 months, talk about feeling to siblings quadrupled while talking to mothers declined. This study reflects the speed at which children develop the capacity to interact with others who, unlike a mother, may not always respond sensitively to them.

Zubrick et al (2007) undertook research to identify factors associated with Late Language Emergence (LLE) beyond 24 months. In a large longitudinal study 1880 (85% of the

2224 participants) returned completed questionnaires providing information on family, maternal, child characteristics and social/economic data. They also answered specific information on the infant's language development. The results suggest the following factors may significantly increase the likelihood of LLE in an infant:

- a family history of LLE
- being born into a larger family
- neonatal low birth weight or born before 37 weeks gestation.

Surprisingly maternal characteristics (age at childbirth, employment, education, smoking, level of stress or depression) or family functioning demonstrated no statistical significance. Zubrick et al (2007) conclude that neurobiological and genetic factors are stronger determinants of LLE than maternal and family psycho-socioeconomic factors.

The primary school years: 5–12 years

Once the child starts school, language development is increasingly influenced by the wider social, cultural experience and literacy. Increasing diversity of experience influences social and moral development characterised by the child's attitude and behaviour towards others. Studies by Braten (1998) support the theory that children who, when distressed, have been recipients of affective care will respond caringly to others in distress. Studies show that children who have been victims of neglect or physical abuse are more likely to demonstrate indifference, fear or aggression (George & Main 1979, Main & George 1985, Klimes-Dogan & Kistner 1990; all cited by Edwards 1998). Childhood influences are not always positive and as a result children learn to use swear words, foul language and give verbal abuse, presenting a challenge to their families, teachers and healthcare providers. A study by Wilson et al (2003) showed that children between 2 and 4 years commonly told lies to cover up wrong-doing or to control another person's behaviour (Wilson et al 2003). Some children lie about their health to avoid going to school or undertaking daily chores. They may lie to conceal an illness or injury due to fear of painful interventions, e.g. tetanus injection, which could have serious implications.

The prevailing characteristics and attitudes in the family become the basis of unwritten rules, which are part of the child's primary socialisation. The child can learn dysfunctional values and ways of communicating with others, which negatively affect the development of all members of the family (Friedman 1992). Dysfunctional communication in families is likely to influence how the child and family communicate with health professionals. Families who have closed dysfunctional patterns of communicating will have more difficulty coping, which may delay psychosocial recovery (Townley & Welton 2000).

Scenario

Brian is a 2nd year student nurse on placement on an acute medical paediatric ward. In his peer reflective group he describes an incident which caused him great concern.

A 5-year-old boy was admitted for investigations of failure to thrive. He seemed to be allergic to so many things. On the handover I was allocated to look after him. I was warned that he was rude and abusive and that his mother and father were also troublesome.

The nurse in charge suggested I speak to them only when spoken to and generally watch my back. I was really anxious when approaching the family but I saw the boy had a book on Manchester United football club so I asked him who his favourite player was and we had a good chat. He was cheeky at times but I discovered that he had a good sense of humour. His mother really appreciated the time I spent talking to her son, which enabled her to go out for a cigarette. Other students also got on well with the family. The mother and child continued to be rude and abusive to the registered nurses and doctors.

Reflect on your practice

Identify and discuss the issues. In a similar situation how would you react?

The 'company-they-keep' hypothesis emphasises that adults who engage with children from an early age must recognise that they play a part in the development of prosocial or antisocial behaviour towards peers, which may continue throughout life (Edwards 1998). Modelling positive behaviour for the developing child is the responsibility of all those who work with children.

The teenager: 13–adulthood

The ongoing development of good communication skills throughout the adolescent years is problematic if the acquisition of language and literacy are not well established at this point. David Bell, Her Majesty's Chief Inspector of Schools, stated:

> Far too many young people reach the end of their compulsory schooling with inadequate basic skills
>
> (Ofsted 2003)

The maturity of the adolescent is closely related to communication. Problems with self-esteem may be the result of a whole range of issues related to schooling and family life. General lack of confidence and unhappiness about the onset of puberty also impacts on the quality of interaction with some teenagers.

Activity

Study Figure 10.4. How is this 12-year-old girl, in her bedroom feeling?

'Just leave me alone please'

'I want to watch my favourite programme without being pestered by my big brother'

'Why does everyone assume I am sad when I just want some space to myself?'

- Consider the danger of observing but not listening to her.

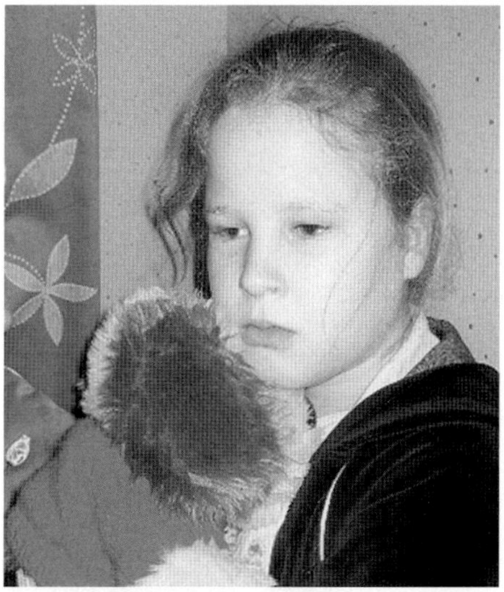

Fig. 10.4 • What is being communicated?

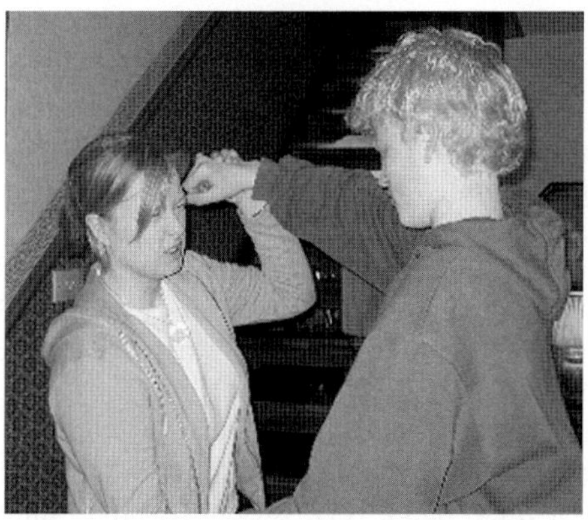

Fig. 10.5 • Teenage sibling fun or fury?

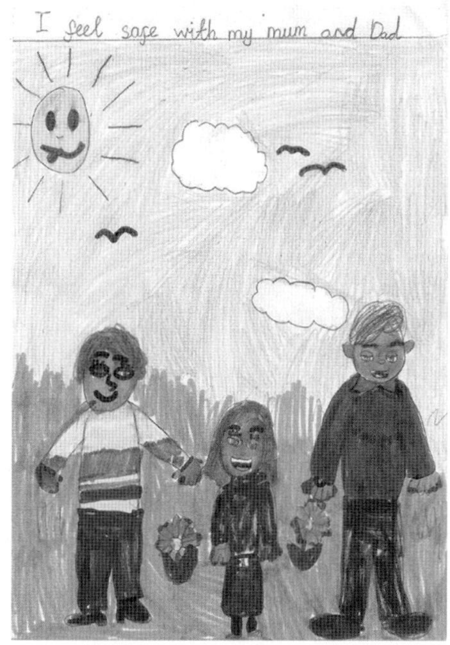

Fig. 10.6 • Expressing feelings through painting.

Family communication patterns will either exacerbate or buffer adolescent stressors (Collins & Russell 1991). Saetermoe et al (1999) refer to several research studies that demonstrate that communication problems within the family affect health and well-being. Aggressive behaviour in children emerged as strongly linked to parental conflict (Davis et al 1998). Lanz et al (1999) conducted a large study that revealed that children from separated or divorced families had more problems communicating with their parents and peer groups than adopted adolescents from intact families. Lanz et al (1999) concluded that male and female adolescent self-esteem is related to how well parents interact with each other. Brown et al's (2007) research findings indicate that parents who talk supportively to their children about parental conflict promote healthy adaptation as the child feels more emotionally secure. According to Morrison & Anders (2001) there is little evidence to support the myth of adolescence as an emotional storm and challenge for parents. Most adolescents maintain close and supportive relations with their parents and 'embody parental values rather than oppose them' (Morrison & Anders 2001 p 69).

It would appear that adults are too quick to label the 'terrible' teenager (Fig. 10.5). If adults consider challenging behaviour in teenage years as the norm can young people be blamed for this? Adolescent transition to adulthood is synonymous with vulnerability and this may present challenges for those who work with young people. The philosophical belief underpinning work with children should be respect for their values, and human rights (Jennings & Hickson 2002). Health professionals need to remember that adolescent physical and emotional transitional stress can be exacerbated by traumatic experiences that impact on the young person's maturity, beliefs, attitudes, health, behaviour and communication. Competent use of age-appropriate communication tools is essential.

The value of play as a communication tool

Children often find it difficult to talk about their fears, frustrations and uncertainty to strangers. Play helps break down barriers with smaller children and enables them to express their feelings (Ellis 2000) and to reduce tension, anger, frustration, conflict and anxiety, which are mainly due to perceived loss of control and self-esteem (Haiait et al 2003). Techniques are used to enable children to project what they want using painting, puppets, drama and story telling (Fig. 10.6). Transferring ownership of emotions and feelings to a character seems to enable children to communicate powerful feelings, which would normally be too difficult to acknowledge due to embarrassment, loyalty or fear (Herpert & Harper-Dorton 2002). When a child is filling the gaps in story telling, caution must be taken in interpreting what is projected from reality and what is based on make believe.

> Sometimes we see the world in fewer dimensions than children and all too often we reduce their imagination, creativity and energy into something that we feel comfortable with
>
> (Carter 2002 p 83)

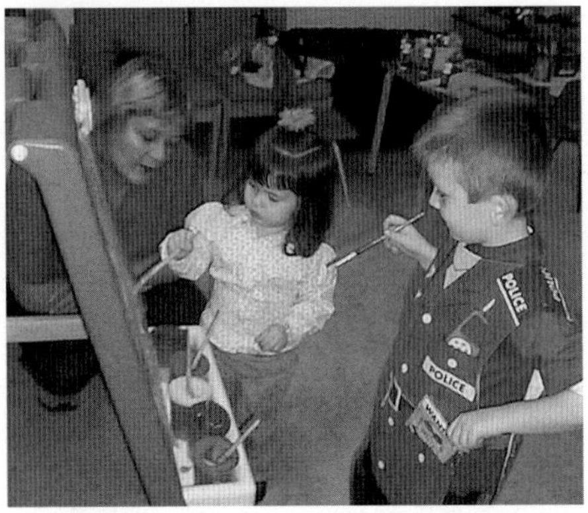

Fig. 10.7 • Painting and communication in hospital.

Play is an effective means of preparing children for admission to hospital and for medical or surgical procedures. Demonstrating interventions on a doll or a teddy enables a child to take part and ask questions. The equipment becomes familiar and misconceptions are dispelled, which can reduce anxiety (Ellis 2000) by increasing their sense of control (Haiait et al 2003). It is within the guided framework of play that children are more likely to paint, write or talk about their emotions and experiences related to their illness, injury, treatment and hospitalisation (Haiait et al 2003) (Fig. 10.7). Play enables nurses, and other health professionals, to connect with child patients and to help them to feel at ease and secure, which is the basis of closeness and trust in a child's relationship (Haiait et al 2003). To communicate effectively with children, taking account of their cognitive development, play must become an essential part of a nurse's toolkit.

Understanding health and illness

In the early 1980s, Bibace & Walsh (1980, 1981) outlined the stages of cognitive development and the relevance to healthcare professionals. It is not until the preoperational stage of development (2–6 years) that children attempt to understand why things happen, often assuming that illness is magically passed through close contact with another sick person. As cognitive development progresses (6–12 years), more concrete operational patterns of thinking enable children to use cause and effect as a basis of their understanding (if you go out in the cold without a coat you will get the cold). Children grasp that the illness is inside their body before they can comprehend how external factors can cause illness internally (Vacik et al 2001). In the formal operational stage, adolescents begin to understand body systems and how physical and psychological processes can result in illness (Vacik et al 2001).

Although Piaget mapped cognitive development into age groups, he repeatedly stressed the importance of sequence over rate. Bibace & Walsh (1980, 1981) point out that a child's understanding is limited because memory, attention, bodily sensations and perception are still in the process of development (see Chapter 11).

Determining an individual child's understanding and perception of illness is critical for effective communication to take place. In the last 30 years, there has been growing evidence of the need for adults to provide clarity when answering children's questions about medical equipment, illness and treatment (Abbot 1990, McGrath & Huff 2001, Pidgeon 1981, Ritchie et al 1984, Tates & Meeuwesen 2002). If age-appropriate strategies are used, children can learn more about their illness, increasing compliance. Children as young as 4 years old have been taught how to effectively manage certain parts of their illness (Vacik et al 2001) (Fig. 10.8).

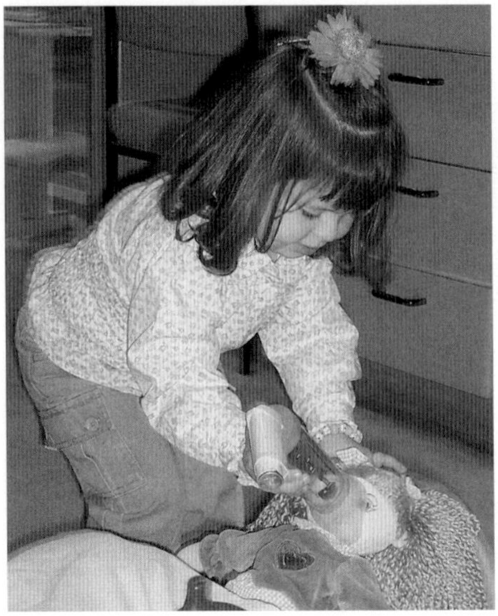

Fig. 10.8 • Two-year-old giving her dolly a nebuliser.

McGrath & Huff (2001) conducted a study of preschool children playing with medical equipment. They discovered that most of them had a very 'unsophisticated' understanding of the use of the equipment but were keen to ask questions and learn. Two children whose older relatives had been in hospital made a good attempt at explaining surgery and the circulatory system:

> ... when the people are asleep. You get a very sharp knife and cut their tummy. That's how they get things out
>
> (McGrath & Huff 2001 p 458)

> ... actually you need blood inside you because it flows around our heart and if we didn't have blood we'd die
>
> (McGrath & Huff 2001 p 458)

Worryingly, the children who did not engage in play had previous experience of hospital (self or sibling) and either did not want to talk about hospital or about a related, unpleasant experience. The 'naive confidence' demonstrated by the other children was replaced by 'fearful descriptions' (McGrath & Huff 2001 p 460). This would suggest that they had developed misconceptions due to lack of understanding of their hospital experience. All of the children in the study demonstrated a readiness to use their imagination to fill the gaps when information was lacking (McGrath & Huff 2001).

Effective communication with children can dispel misconceptions and anxieties, ultimately improving their healthcare experience. Nursing staff must explain to parents that preparing the child for admission to hospital promotes recovery. If a child cannot attend preadmission play clinics where special

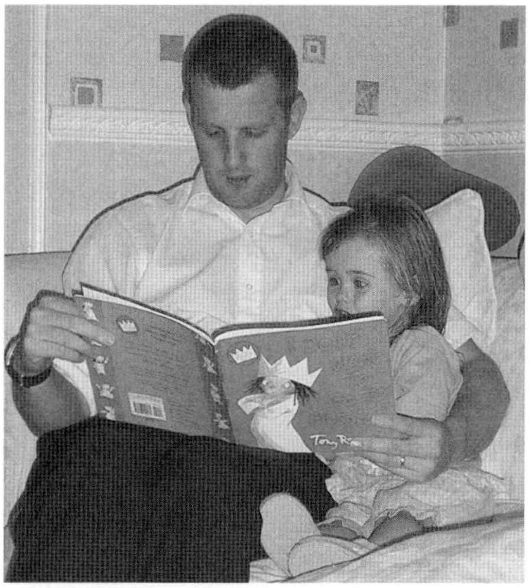

Fig. 10.9 • A father prepares his child at home for admission to hospital.

dolls, storybooks and videos are available, books and videos should be available for preparation at home (Fig. 10.9). However, such techniques may not be appropriate for use with older children (see also Chapter 5).

Communicating with young people in a healthcare context

Bannister & Huntington (2002) highlight the importance of considering young people in local and strategic planning, delivery and evaluation of services. Children express valuable views with as much authenticity and meaning as could be expected from an adult group (Elliot & Watson 2000). Two studies (Elliot & Watson 2000, Tates et al 2002) highlight positive and negative aspects of interaction between health professionals and young people.

Evidence-based practice

Elliot and Watson (2000): 21 semi-structured group interviews involving over 200 children aged between 4 and 16 years on various aspects of health care and the services provided.

- Doctors tended to automatically address parents or other adult carers accompanying them regardless of the child's age.
- Some doctors did not speak to them at all, even during an examination.
- Children doubted a doctor's ability to find out what was wrong with them by asking only their parents who did not know all of their problems.
- When they were allowed to speak some doctors dismissed or trivialised their complaints.
- Doctors used language children could not understand.
- Doctors did not always keep their promises.
- Generally doctors were perceived as important people who had curative powers who were authoritarian and judgemental at times.
- Doctors had a negative image of older children, viewing younger children as small and sweet and not old enough to be trusted.
- Nurses listen more than doctors, are more approachable and perceived as less powerful.
- Children valued the opportunity to talk to a trusted knowledgeable person in confidence about matters they might not be able to discuss with parents and friends.
- Children wanted more information and confidential advice which is relevant for children and young adults.

Tates et al (2002): quantitative analysis of 106 videotaped interactions patterns of communication emerged during GP parent and child interviews.

- Parents generally viewed their child's health as their responsibility so the interview was conducted as if the child was absent.
- Some GPs did take into account the child's age and understanding (the child was asked what the problem was in only 35 out of 104 interviews).
- Some parents restricted child participation by interfering in GP–child interaction.
- Lack of participation on the child's part was not due to lack of understanding.
- Only 5% of children were given information on diagnosis and treatment directly.

The research by Tates et al (2002) corroborates the concerns of the young people highlighted by Elliot & Watson (2000). It is clear that, although some GPs did attempt to consider the child's understanding and engage the child in discussion, this was an exception rather than a rule. Mayall (1996 p 275) states that, from the literature, the child's 'position within medical encounters is doubly dependent on parental and medical staff behaviour'. Therefore, it is the responsibility of the adults in the interaction to provide a developmentally sensitive environment in which children are given the opportunity to be active participants in a healthcare context (Tates et al 2002).

WWW

- http://www.dh.gov.uk/assetRoot/04/06/72/51/04067251.pdf

Take time to consider implications of Department of Health (2003) 'Getting the Right Start: National Service Framework for Children: Standards for Hospital Services'. Pay particular attention to:

- Chapter 2 Standards for hospital services for children: 2.8–2.8; 2.21–2.23 Quality of Setting and Environment
- Chapter 3 Child centred Services: 3.10–3.35 Treating Children and Families with respect
- To what extent are the standards reflected in Scottish Executive (2007) Delivering a Healthy Future: Action Framework for Children and Young People's Health in Scotland?
- http://www.scotland.gov.uk/Resource/Doc/165782/0045104.pdf

Identify key issues from both reports which underpin communicating with children and families in a healthcare context.

Children's rights

In attempts to protect children it is easy to assume that they are incompetent and too foolish to know what is best for them:

> The complexity of this issue can lead clinicians to take the easier option of assuming adults are competent and children are not
>
> (Brook 2000 p 33)

The more pragmatic, balanced approach places the onus on the family and institutions to, on their behalf, ensure children's well-being until they become adults, when they will be able to speak for themselves (Fulton 1996).

WWW

Compare and contrast the Principles in the Declaration of the Rights of the Child 1959.

- http://www.unhchr.ch/html/menu3/b/25.htm

with the Articles in the United Nations Convention on the Rights of the Child 1989

- http://www.unicef.org/photoessays/30048.html

From the photo essay slide show note the change of approach to Children's Rights.

Consider relevance to communication with the child today.

The part adults play in ensuring children's rights are not infringed is clearly documented. Read articles 3, 5, 12 and 13. Consider the implications of each for communicating with the child and family in a healthcare context.

The Convention on Rights of the Child (United Nations General Assembly 1989) precipitated a shift of opinion among academics and professionals, who now believe that children are able and should be encouraged to participate and negotiate in their health care, education and social welfare (Elliot & Watson 2000, Mayall 1996).

Health professionals need to work with each child on an individual basis so that they can determine the level of involvement the child wants and feels comfortable with. However, this takes time, which is often lacking (Brook 2000). The Children Act (DoH 1989) states that parents no longer have rights over their children; instead, parents have responsibilities towards their children and must have regard to their children's views when making any major decision affecting them. Practitioners should ensure that when working with children they listen to each child, provide appropriate information and take account of the child's wishes and feelings (DoH 1989).

WWW

- http://www.hmso.gov.uk/acts/acts1989/Ukpga_19890041_en_1.htm

Take time out to follow links relevant to communication at this website.

How are Children's views considered in the Children Act 1989 and the Children Act Scotland 1995?

- http://www.hmso.gov.uk/acts/acts1995/Ukpga_19950036_en_1.htm

Adults have a legal and moral obligation to ensure children have access to truthful information and the opportunity to share their views in what is still an adult-shaped world in which children are relatively powerless (Elliot & Watson 2000). There is sufficient evidence that when children are involved in this way they are more willing to cooperate and have better healthcare outcomes (Alderson & Montgomery 1996, de Winter et al 1999, Tates et al 2002). This particularly applies to children and adolescents who require long-term health care and, as a result, are more likely to have a clearer understanding of their own health and illness.

Communicating with children and adolescents who have life-limiting illness or disability

PowerPoint

See also PowerPoint presentation Communication: The Health Care Context

From the literature reviewed, recurring issues related to interaction between adolescents who have prolonged healthcare needs and health professionals have emerged (Beresford & Sloper 2003, Couriel 2003, Elliot & Watson 2000, Jacobson & Wilkinson 1994, Lask 2003, Morrison & Anders 2001, Runeson et al 2000). Their collective findings fall into three categories tabled below.

Evidence-based practice

Collective findings from: Beresford & Sloper (2003), Couriel (2003), Morrison & Anders (2001), Lask (2003), Runeson et al (2000), Jacobson & Wilkinson (1994), Elliot & Watson (2000)

Organisational and team issues

- Duration and frequency of contact
- Communications skills of health professionals (HP)
- Lack of consistency in information giving/approach and information overload
- Differing approaches and conflict within a team
- Over-involvement to perceived aloofness confuse adolescents.

Attitude and approach

- Perceived negative attitude of HP
- Ability to understand information is underrated
- Exclusively focusing on the condition
- Different rules of behaviour and expression of feelings and attitudes between adolescent and HP
- Perceived powerfulness of doctor – powerlessness of adolescent
- Wrong assumptions re doctors' and adolescents' knowledge, expectation of treatment, course and outcome of the illness
- Emergence of intense painful emotions (fear, helplessness, anger, despair) which may be reciprocated by HP
- Complete disregard for opinions and feelings of adolescence.

Right to and need for increasing independence

- To be able to choose who is present (parent, medical students)
- Need to be given precedence (over parents)
- Need to be treated respectfully
- HP need to emphasise the adolescent's right to confidentiality
- Respect and showing interest in adolescent interests
- HP make assumptions on needs.

From the collective research findings it is clear that poor organisational skills will impact negatively on the establishment of trust, open communication, professional boundaries and team work. Lack of communication skills, time and continuity will cause confusion and lower confidence in the health professionals. Young people can communicate effectively and have the right to be listened to and make decisions about their care. Health professionals need to respect their rights, communicate effectively with them; they should not be patronised or ignored.

Poor quality of care can lower adolescent self-esteem, understanding of healthcare needs and adherence to treatment regimes – which impacts on the course and outcome of their illness or injury. Health professionals perceived lack of holistic interest in them and their fear of loss of privacy meant that they have difficulty in raising personal or sensitive issues with health professionals (Elliot & Watson 2000) (Fig. 10.10).

There is a widely held view that the limitations of chronic illness and disability affect the behavioural, psychological and social well-being of children and adolescents. However, the results of several studies (comparing children and adolescence with their healthy peers) refute this view. It is important to note that the results of the studies cannot be generalised due to the small sample size, however they do inform health professionals of the possible positive and negative impact of a chronic illness on children and young people.

The conclusion drawn from the largest study reviewed (98 chronically ill adolescents) was that adolescents with chronic illness are socially well-adjusted when compared with a healthy peer group. This is probably because they have developed coping mechanisms during the course of their illness (Meijer et al 2000). It is therefore vital that health professionals do not make assumptions but assess each young person as an individual by engaging them in meaningful interaction (see Chapters 44–47 for further information on caring for children with special needs).

Evidence-based practice

Researchers	Findings
Yarcheskie et al 1987	Adolescents with cystic fibrosis: Did not feel more lonely
Vera et al 1997	Adolescent girls – Insulin dependent diabetes mellitus: No difference in social interaction or social anxiety
Pendley et al 1997	Adolescent cancer survivors: No difference in overall popularity, social anxiety or loneliness
Forero et al 1996	Adolescents with asthma: Reported more feelings of loneliness
Saetermoe et al 1999	When compared to healthy siblings, disabled adolescents had less involvement in family interactions Interactions were less meaningful They had less control in conversation
Noll et al 1993	Adolescents with cancer: Similar levels of self esteem
Meijer et al 2000	Adolescents with a range of chronic illness: Engaged in lower levels of social activities but this could not be contributed to function limitations, although pain was a factor for boys Some girls and boys displayed less adequate social skills

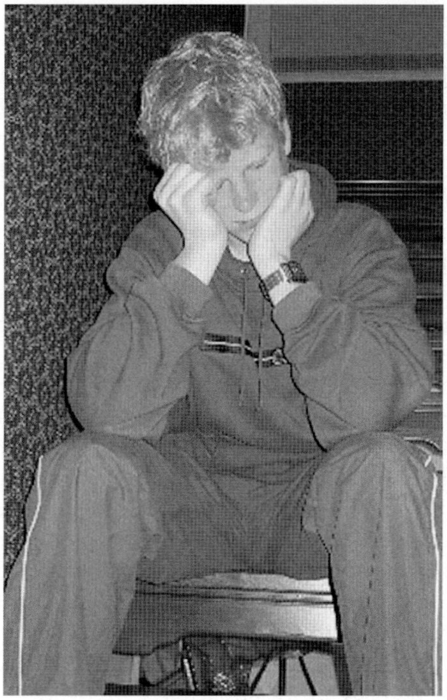

Fig. 10.10 • Can't talk about it.

Communicating with parents

Communicating effectively with parents of sick children is essential because their concerns about their child's health generate stress. Mothers have stated (Neill 2000, Young et al 2002) that when their child is ill they need:

- to be reassured that they have done the right thing for their child
- information on their child's illness and treatment
- to feel respected as recognition of their competence to care for their child.

Instead, parents report dissatisfaction with medical staff who allegedly make them feel stupid and a nuisance for asking too many questions. Cram & Dowd (2008) compared parents' and doctors' understanding of why they were waiting in the emergency room following a non-emergency consultation with the doctor. The researchers, both doctors, reported that of the 200 pairs surveyed 11.5% partially agreed but a significant 21.5% completely disagreed. The likelihood of parents with lower levels of education misunderstanding their reason for waiting was 9% higher than other parents.

Parents with low levels of education are less likely to challenge professional judgements related to the health of their children (Spencer 2000). When doctors dismiss parents' concerns regarding the health of their children, the parents' perceived powerlessness renders them unable to act on their own judgements, which in some cases has resulted in unexpected infant death (Spencer 1984). Mothers' concerns must be taken seriously because they describe their baby's health and happiness in terms of alertness and responsiveness to their environment (Mayall 1996), which are the first assessments undertaken by health professionals in the process of recognition of the sick child.

Parents feel that health professionals are more powerful in the hospital setting (Callery & Smith 1991, Sartain et al 2001). Darbyshire (1994) reports that parents feel frustrated when health professionals in hospital do not hear what they are trying to say. Although nurses strive towards partnership with parents in hospital, a more balanced approach is better achieved in the home (Sartain et al 2001). A study by Kirk (2001) highlighted that, although professionals felt that parents exercised greater parental power in the home, many parents found 'being assertive' difficult in their domestic situation.

Seminar discussion topic

Espezel & Canam (2003, p 34) state:

> *The parent–nurse relationship is considered to be a cornerstone of quality paediatric nursing ... However while family centred care is promoted philosophically by policy makers and nurse leaders ... how is the espoused view enacted in practice?*

Espezel & Canam examine parents' experience of interacting with nurses when their child is in hospital. Critically review the article, discuss with your colleagues. Attempt to answer the question highlighted above.

Communication between parents and healthcare providers may be influenced by their perceptions of who owns the child in hospital. Shields et al (2003) questions whether health professionals are aware of this.

www

Take time to read: Shields et al (2003).

- http://www.blackwell-synergy.com/openurl?genre=article&sid=nlm:pubmed&issn=0309-2402&date=2003&volume=41&issue=3&spage=213

Nurses, who are placed at the communication interface, should urge their colleagues not to take control away from the family. Concerns related to the rights of the child and family could impact on the development of good working relationships, communication skills determining the accuracy, relevance and meaning of information needed by families (Herpert & Harper-Dorton 2002).

Communicating a serious diagnosis

The most difficult time for the parents is when they are facing a diagnosis that informs them that their child is developmentally delayed, has an illness or disability that will place restrictions on one or many aspects of their daily life, or has a life-threatening illness. Although hearing such a diagnosis brings the realisation that their lives as a family are going to change forever, it also brings relief. Parents have reported that being provided with the information enabled them to feel in control again (Fisher 2001), to establish a new type of normality (Bartolo 2002) and to restore order amidst chaos (Starke & Mollier 2002). Studies (Fisher 2001, Starke & Mollier 2002) identified that communication problems generated feelings of uncertainty, which included:

- use of specific medical words or phrases
- being given information too quickly or not quickly enough
- the information was inaccurate or explanations incomprehensible
- overwhelming need to know but difficulty getting answers.

Parents reported having to trap a professional in a room and demand information (Fisher 2001), whereas Starke & Mollier (2002) stated that at times parents needed to limit or modify information received if they felt they could not cope with it. Almost half (23 of the 44 parents) interviewed were satisfied with the information received at the time they were told by the physician that their daughters had Turner syndrome (Starke & Mollier 2002). As a result, parents lacked confidence in the health professional's ability to ensure their child would get the best treatment. Parents (mostly mothers) sought information from the internet or from other agencies (Fisher 2001) so that they could explain the child's problems to others (Starke & Mollier 2002). The quality of information given when communicating a serious diagnosis is crucial because those who are deeply shocked and distressed are unable to take it in (Young et al 2002). Bartolo (2002) emphasises the need for a balancing act because the parents need the professional to be frank and honest but also to show compassion. Switching the focus from negative outcomes to acknowledge positive coping strategies and their child's progress will foster hopefulness.

www

Take time to read: Breaking Bad News Regional Guidelines for Practice

- www.dhsspsni.gov.uk/breaking_bad_news.pdf

(DOH National Council for Hospice and Palliative Care Services Belfast; 2003)

How can these guidelines inform Child Health Care?

Ongoing communication

Communication impacts on the family's ongoing healthcare experience. To understand parental perception of effective communication a small qualitative study (semi structured

Table 10.1 Accommodative behaviours categorised within six communication strategies

Over Accommodative	Accommodative (effective)	Under Accommodative
INTERPRETABILTY		
Over-simplifying, patronising	Clear, direct, succinct explanation where understanding is clarified	Vagueness or inconsistency interaction
DISCOURSE MANAGEMENT		
Speak only when spoken to Always expected to open and lead discussion	Ask questions and seek opinions Open to suggestions, chat	Dominate conversation Not give others space to speak, not listening
INTERPERSONAL CONTROL		
Too personal/familiar Negative talk about others	Treat as equals regardless of status or role	Overstate professional status, being too formal Seen as just another parent
EMOTIONAL EXPRESSION		
Over-sympathise	Reassure parents, True empathy and caring	Hostile or supportive attitude and behaviour
POSITIVE FACE		
Treat like royalty	Be polite, respectful, encouraging Interested in parent as individual	Unconstructive criticism and condescending attitude
NEGATIVE FACE		
Nurses denigrate themselves	Polite, not demanding, not imposing	Demand or order parents, oppressive

interview of 20 mothers and 13 fathers) was undertaken in neonatal intensive care unit (Jones et al 2007). The semi structured interviews were based on Communication Accommodation Theory. The parents were asked to describe an effective and ineffective interaction based on their experience in the unit. Examples of accommodative behaviours are categorised within six communication strategies (Table 10.1; Jones et al 2007).

In the study discourse management and emotional expression emerged as being important, parents valued the opportunity to chat generally and nurses who were warm, caring and reassuring in their approach. Most parents viewed ineffective communication as lack of clarity and vagueness, particularly where questions were not invited or understanding clarified (Jones et al 2007).

When assessing what 'works best' for a family, nurses must maintain 'open and ongoing communication'. Parents need to talk about their child's symptoms but also the 'whole' experience which includes the many 'rough spots' (Woodgate & Degner 2003). Parents need support throughout the entire experience. A collaborative caring and empathic response to psycho-social issues enhances parents' perception of quality of care (Hart et al 2007). This is particularly important as parents, in the early stages, may require to take on more technical roles beyond the normal domain of parenting (Slade 2000). Tasks that seem straightforward to the nurse can be daunting to the parent and should not be rushed. Clear and effective communication is essential so that the parents know exactly what preparation is required for the task, each step of the procedure, and what to do in the event of something going wrong. What they need most is genuine encouragement and feedback on their progress so that growing confidence is based on competence in performing a new skill.

Scenario

Hilary is a 3rd year nursing student on placement on a short stay ward. In her reflective journal she records an incident which took place the week before.

A mother of a child with complex needs told me how upset she was when she was not invited to join the other mum's introductory tour of to the ward facilities. She felt most of the nurses on the ward avoided her. She was horrified to come back from a short break to find her child very distressed as the doctor had attempted and failed to insert an intravenous cannula in her son's arm claiming she was too busy to wait for his Mum.

She is an excellent mother and appears to know far more about her child's disability than any of us, but nobody is taking this into account.

Reflect on your practice

How does Hilary's experience compare with your experiences of caring for children with special needs? How can you prevent similar occurrences happening in your area of work?

As the emphasis on equality and supporting inclusion increases, nurses need to consider their role in meeting the needs of children with special or complex needs and their families.

www

Take time out to explore the role of nurses and other health in promoting health, supporting inclusion at both these government websites.

- http://www.scotland.gov.uk/library5/health/phsi-00.asp
- http://www.scotland.gov.uk/library5/health/phsin-00.asp

The following NSF paper is specifically relevant to communicating with disabled children and their families.

- http://www.dh.gov.uk/assetRoot/04/06/10/47/04061047.pdf

Parents appreciate health professionals who are honest about their professional limitations (Coyne 1997, Fisher 2001, Kirk 2001, Kirk & Glendinning 2002, Stewart et al 1994), especially when the parents are the experts on their children. Professionals who acknowledge and respect parents as experts interact within a different style of doctor–parent relationship (Kirk & Glendinning 2002). Parents needed their expertise to be acknowledged and failing to do so resulted in additional stress (Coyne 1997, Fisher 2001, Kirk 2001, Kirk & Glendinning 2002, Stewart et al 1994). From Fisher's literature review (2001) it is clear that health professionals have the potential to create uncertainty, disrupting normality. They should be aware of the fragility of the parental coping mechanism. There is a consensus that professional interaction should be informed by a sensitive understanding of what parents feel about their role and what they believe to be their needs (Coyne 1997, Fisher 2001, Kirk 2001, Kirk & Glendinning 2002, Stewart et al 1994). They need someone to 'be there' as an easily accessible source of support and information with whom they feel comfortable about sharing their anxieties. They need professional advocates who will help them to obtain the services their child needs (Kirk & Glendinning 2002). From the point of diagnosis, developing and maintaining trust in the health professionals caring for their child was really important to parents (Kirk 2001).

Imparting expert information

Imparting information is essential for parents to make decisions. Alderson (1993) cites several examples of professionals who have communicated information to parents in a sensitive, caring and clear way. Being kept informed of what is happening helps parents adapt a more positive attitude towards staff (Palmer 1993). Dale (1996) presents a list of communication guidelines, taken from an extensive literature review of communication techniques, which were shown to increase understanding and improve doctors' communication skills.

Evidence-based practice

Guidelines for Practice (Dale 1996):

- Start by assessing the parent's emotional state
- Be sympathetic considerate and caring
- Invite the parent to present their own ideas, expectations and questions
- Message should be:
  i. clear, straight forward, direct,
  ii. simplified using shorter words and sentences
- To help recall use:
  iii. primary effects
  iv. explicit categorisation
  v. repetition
- To help understanding:
  vi. where possible avoid technical jargon and include explanation
  vii. help the parent to ask questions about information received
  viii. Use trained translators when working with parents from ethnic minority groups
  ix. write down or give written information
  x. check out understanding at regular intervals and hold a follow-up meeting to check understanding and retention

Dale (1996) believes that one barrier to professional communication is that professionals may believe they have told the parents everything and assume they understand, making no attempt to find out if the message has been heard and understood. Wales et al (2008) as a result of review highlighted that parental satisfaction with communication decreases as more teams are involved in the care process. This is particularly relevant to families off children with complex needs.

Listening

Listening is reported frequently as a key area of weakness (Dale 1996). Parents worry about taking up the professional's valuable time or feel frustrated if the professional cannot offer solutions to problems. Professionals may feel compelled to interject, offer interpretations and solutions when it is not appropriate or find it difficult to gauge what is the appropriate time to respond or be silent. Either party may feel anxious or uncomfortable in silence (Dale 1996). Active listening is achieved by adapting an open posture, maintaining eye contact and an appropriate facial expression. Kagan & Evans (1995) state that, in certain situations, using short verbal/non-verbal responses will be appropriate. In other situations a more active approach is needed – the listener seeks further information by asking appropriate questions, clarifying or paraphrasing, demonstrating empathy and understanding. The timing of questions or reflective statements is very important so that communication is not disrupted inappropriately (Kagan & Evans 1995). Active listeners make sure they do not lose concentration. It is essential that nurses practice active listening skills and use reflection to adapt their skills for different situations. Active listening lets the parent, child and young person know they are important and central to the decision-making process. Listening is a supportive intervention which enables the family to remain in control and participate in partnership with the professional.

Problem solving

Finding solutions to problems can overwhelm the parent who has a child with a life-limiting illness or disability. Dale (1996) states that guided problem solving helps the parent to find the solution to a problem, which is often a personal concern. Negotiated problem solving involves parents and professionals striving towards a joint decision to a problem, which is of concern to both parties. Dale (1996) states that negotiation requires a high level of trust, openness, honesty, assertion and cooperation between the parties involved. There needs to be a willingness to recognise the importance of the other's view point and wishes if agreement is to be reached. It may be necessary for the professional to concede, especially if disagreement occurs early in the relationship-forming process. In the interim, building trust and openness with the family is essential. The ability to compromise is essential for reaching an acceptable middle-ground decision, which is a step in the right direction.

When conflict situations are not recognised, levels of adherence to treatment regimes may fall as an expression of protest or due to lack of appreciation of the benefit (Lask 2003). Acknowledging differences and respecting autonomy validates parents' right to express their opinion and to disagree with others, however wise, senior or powerful they may appear (Lask 2003). Accepting the possibility of conflict within the therapeutic relationship promotes early recognition and resolution (Lask 2003).

Communicating with siblings

Crises emerge throughout the course of a child's life-limiting illness. These can force the parents to put their healthy children on hold, enforcing prolonged periods of separation. Siblings become distressed if they have not been given information that helps explain the change in parental behaviour (Mackenzie 1997), thinking they are in some way responsible (Langton 2000). The siblings of children with chronic illness have an increased risk of developing behavioural or mental health problems, showing signs of attitude change and low self-esteem (Williams et al 2003). It is therefore important that, when communicating with the family, the parents are encouraged to:

- focus on all of their children
- keep in contact and spend time with their other children
- keep siblings informed of what is happening and how their brother or sister is responding to treatment
- involve siblings in decision making
- bring siblings into the hospital and help prepare them for the visit.

At times, the siblings may elect to stay away and not get involved, which may be their way of coping with the crisis. Parents need to be supported in deciding what is the right level of involvement. To do this nurses must work at developing a rapport and trusting relationship with the siblings (Fig. 10.11), particularly if the outcome is likely to be the loss of a brother or sister.

Terminal and bereavement care

Communication regarding end-of-life care is probably the most challenging aspect for health professionals. In hospital the reluctance of senior medical staff to stop aggressive treatment

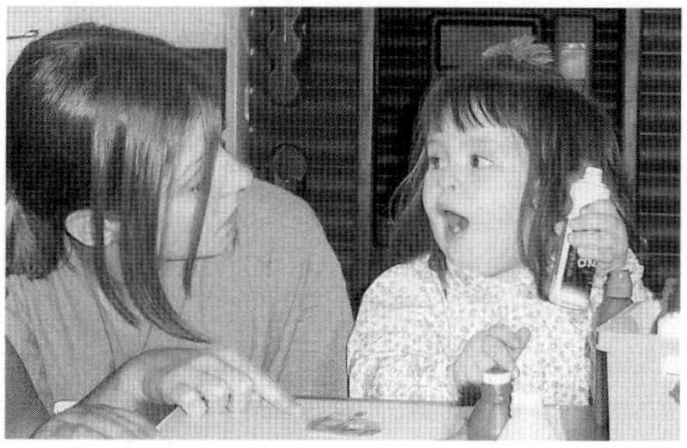

Fig. 10.11 • An intensive care nurse plays with a patient's sibling.

or not wanting to take away hope may delay necessary communication (Hendricks-Ferguson 2007). Lack of confidence or dread of stressful discussion may also be a factor. In a small retrospective study some parents (19 mothers and 9 fathers), having had a child die of cancer 4 years prior to the study, indicated that the information on end-of-life care was needed earlier as opposed to close to their child's death. However, some indicated that information on end-of-life care would not be received well until all possible care options were exhausted (Hendricks-Ferguson 2007). When parents perceived the approach as positive (informative and compassionate) transition and acceptance was easier (Hendricks-Ferguson 2007).

Communicating with families who are facing bereavement is complex as parents often find it difficult to express their feelings and emotions, which may be negative or confusing. In a study by Laakso & Paunonen-Llmonen (2001), many mothers – following the death of their child – did not share their feelings and experiences of grief. They felt that staff did not have the ability to meet their needs and that information was insufficient and ambiguous. It is essential that nurses continue to be accessible and approachable, maintaining open and honest communication (Mackenzie 1997). Professionals are often at a loss as to what to say. Fostering a sense of hope seems inappropriate but is vital and should be based on the family's ability to cope, support each other and come to terms with their loss (Mackenzie 1997). Health professionals need to help parents identify what level of information the dying child and other children can cope with, and help them to work out and rehearse what they want to say:

> We worry that children have neither the emotional maturity to cope nor the breadth of experience to understand about death. We worry that we will not be able to contain our own emotions or find the right words
>
> (Cardranell 1994 p 33)

Cardranell (1994) points out that children as young as four are aware of death and that by the time they are 8 years old children know that we all die. Children will detect emotional tension or anxiety in the non-verbal cues of adults around them, which can be misinterpreted, causing distress. Cardranell (1994) concludes that children have the right to know the truth about what is going to happen to them, especially as older children are able to work it out for themselves. They need to be able to share their thoughts and fears about death, be allowed to ask questions about death and dying, and be involved in making decisions about stopping treatment or dying at home or in hospital. Full involvement of children is good practice but may be too difficult to achieve even with good support. Sometimes children recognise this and in attempting to protect their parents will, if given the opportunity, share their feelings with a nurse who they trust. Confidentiality is a major concern for older children, who may not want their parents to know how they are feeling. However, some parents feel strongly that their child should not be exposed to discussion about prognosis (Goodall 1994). While parental wishes must be respected it is important that all parties are made aware that the nurse cannot lie or collude with attempts to withhold the truth (Goodall 1994).

It is helpful for families to know that nurses and other health professionals are emotionally involved but they must control their grief, avoid intrusion and establish a level of involvement or exclusion that is based on what the child and family needs. Nurses need to enable the family to stay in control, and should commend their ability to cope. Laasko & Paunonen-Llmonen (2001) emphasised the need for education and reflective practice to improve the quality of bereavement care – one of the most challenging roles for health professionals.

Summary

The development of communication from conception to adolescence depends on interaction with the family in the preschool years. As the child's experience extends beyond the boundaries of home, the development of communication and attitude is influenced by children, teachers and other professionals. Child health nurses need a knowledge and understanding of the development of communication to provide best practice. When caring for the child the level of understanding must be assessed so that appropriate communication and play can be used to build trust and help the child to understand their healthcare experience. Nurses play a part ensuring that the rights of the child are not infringed by reminding both parents and other health professionals that they must engage with older children and listen to what they have to say when assessing and planning their care. Poor quality of communication can seriously impact on compliance to treatment regimes, their health experience and outcome. Health professionals who do not take time to listen and respond to the needs of children in the health care context do not safeguard the best interests of children and young people.

Parents' views must be taken seriously because they know their child best and have valid concerns when their child becomes ill. Complete disregard for parental views is dangerous practice and can lead to the death of a child. The parents of a child with long-term healthcare needs are the experts. They need the help of clinical experts who will work in partnership with them using active listening and supportive problem solving, especially in times of crisis. Gaining information by listening to children and their families and providing regular, comprehensible information in a sensitive manner enables the family to stay in control and cope with crisis, even the death of a child. The best teachers are the child and family, if nurses and other health professionals are prepared to listen and learn from them.

References

Abbott, K., 1990. Therapeutic use of play in the psychological preparation of preschool children undergoing cardiac surgery. Issues in Comprehensive Pediatric Nursing 13, 265–277.

Alderson, P., 1993. Children's consent to surgery. Open University Press, Buckingham.

Alderson, P., Montgomery, J., 1996. Health care choices: making decisions with children. Institute for Policy Research, London.

Bannister, A., Huntington, A. (Eds.), 2002. Communicating with Children and Adults. Action for Change, John Kingsley Publishers, London.

Bartolo, P.A., 2002. Communicating a diagnosis of developmental disability to parents: multi-professional negotiation framework. Child: Care, Health and Development 28 (1), 65–71.

Beresford, B.A., Sloper, P., 2003. Chronically ill adolescents' experiences of communicating with doctors: a qualitative study. Journal of Adolescent Health 33, 172–179.

Bibace, R., Walsh, 1980. Development of children's concepts of illness. Psychology and Health 4, 175–185.

Bibace, R., Walsh, M. (Eds.), 1981. Children's concepts of health, illness and bodily function. Jossey-Bass, San Francisco.

Braten, S., 1998. Intersubjective communication and understanding: development and perturbation. In: Braten, S. (Ed.), Intersubjective communication and emotion in early ontogeny, Cambridge University Press, Cambridge.

Brook, G., 2000. Children's competency to consent; a framework for practice paediatric. Nursing 12 (50), 31–35.

Brown, A.M., Fitzgerald, M.M., Shipman, K., Scheidner, R., 2007. Children's expectations of parent-child communication following interparental conflict: do parents talk to children about conflict. Journal of Family Violence 22, 407–412.

Bruce, T., 2001. Learning through play, babies, toddlers and the foundation years. Hodder and Stoughton, London.

Callery, P., Smith, L., 1991. A study of role negotiation between nurses and the parents of hospitalised children. Journal of Advanced Nursing 16 (7), 72–81.

Cardranell, J., 1994. Talking about death – parents and children. In: Hill, L. (Ed.), Caring for dying children and their families, Chapman and Hall, London.

Carter, B., 2002. On 'irafs' and other amazing things… Journal of Child Health Care 6 (2), 82–83.

Collins, W.A., Russell, G., 1991. Mother–child and father–child relationships in middle childhood and adolescence: a developmental analysis. Developmental Psychology 11, 99–136.

Couriel, J., 2003. Asthma in adolescence. Paediatric Respiratory Reviews 4, 47–54.

Coyne, I., 1997. Chronic illness: the importance of support for families caring for a child with cystic fibrosis. Journal of Clinical Nursing 6, 121–129.

Cram, K.J., Dowd, M.D., 2008. What are you waiting for? A study of Resident Physician-Parent Communication in a Pediatric Emergency Department. Annals of Emergency Medicine 51 (4), 361–366.

Dale, N., 1996. Working with families of children with special needs: partnership and practice. Routledge, London.

Darbyshire, P., 1994. Living with a sick child in hospital: the experience of parents and nurses. Chapman and Hall, London.

Davis, B.T., Hops, H., Alperst, A., Sheeber, L., 1998. Child responses to parental conflict and their effect on adjustment: a study of triadic relations. Journal of Family Psychology 12 (2), 163–177.

de Winter, M., Baerveldt, C., Kooistra, J., 1999. Enabling children: participation as a new perspective on child-health promotion. Child: Care, Health, and Development 25, 15–25.

Department of Health (DoH), 1989. The Children Act. HMSO, London. Online. Available at: http://www.hmso.gov.uk/acts/acts1989/Ukpga_19890041_en_1.htm

Department of Health (DoH), 1995. The Children Act Scotland. HMSO, London.

Department of Health (DoH), 2003. Getting the right start: national service framework for children: standards for hospital services. Online. Available at: http://www.dh.gov.uk/assetRoot/04/06/72/51/04067251.pdf

Department of Health & National Council for Hospice and Palliative Care Services Belfast, 2003. Online. Available at www.dhsspsni.gov.uk/breaking_bad_news.pdf

Dunn, J., 1998. Siblings, emotions and the development of understanding. In: Braten, S. (Ed.), Intersubjective communication and emotion in early ontogeny. Cambridge University Press, Cambridge.

Edwards, C.P., 1998. The company children keep: suggestive evidence from cultural studies. In: Braten, S. (Ed.), Intersubjective communication and emotion in early ontogeny. Cambridge University Press, Cambridge.

Elliot, E., Watson, A., 2000. Children's voices in health care planning. In: Glasper, A., Ireland, L. (Eds.), Evidence-based child health care: challenges for practice. Macmillan Press, Basingstoke.

Ellis, J., 2000. Games without frontiers. Nursing Times 96 (26), 32–33.

Espezel, H.J.E., Canam, C.J., 2003. Parent–nurse interaction: care of the hospitalized child. Journal of Advanced Nursing 11 (1), 34–41.

Fisher, H.R., 2001. The needs of parents with chronically sick children: a literature review. Journal of Advanced Nursing 36 (4), 600–607.

Forero, R., Bauman, A., Young, L., Booth Nutbeam, D., 1996. Asthma, health behaviours, social adjustment and psychosomatic symptoms in adolescence. Journal of Asthma 33, 157–164.

Friedman, M.M., 1992. Family nursing theory and practice, 3rd edn. Appleton and Lange, Norwalk, CT.

Fulton, Y., 1996. Children's rights and the role of the nurse. Paediatric Nursing 8 (10), 29–31.

Goodall, J., 1994. Thinking like a child about death and dying. In: Hill, L. (Ed.), Caring for dying children and their families. Chapman & Hall, London.

Haiait, H., Bar-Mor, G., Schobat, M., 2003. The world of the child: a world of play even in hospital. Journal of Pediatric Nursing 18 (3), 209–214.

Hart, C.N., Kelleher, K.J., Drotar, D., Scholle, S.H., 2007. Parent-provider communication and parental satisfaction with care of children with psycho-social problems. Patient Education and Counselling 68, 179–185.

Heimann, M., 1998. Imitation in neonate, in older infants and in children with autism: feedback to theory. In: Braten, S. (Ed.), Intersubjective communication and emotion in early ontogeny, Cambridge University Press, Cambridge.

Hendricks-Ferguson, V.L., 2002. Parental perspective of initial end-of-life care communication. International Journal of Palliative Nursing 2007 13 (11), 522–531.

Herpert, M., Harper-Dorton, K.V., 2002. Working with children, adolescents and their families. Blackwell; London.

Jacobson, L.D., Wilkinson, C.E., 1994. Review of teenage health: time for a new direction. British Journal of General Practice 1994 44, 420–424.

Jennings, S., Hickson, A., 2002. Pause for Thought, Action or Stillness with Young People. In: Bannister A., Huntington, A. (Eds.), Communicating with Children and Adults. Action for Change. John Kingsley Publishers, London.

Jones, L., Woodhouse, D., Rowe, J., 2007. Effective Nurse Parent Communication; A study of parents' perception in the NICU environment. Patient Education and Counselling 69, 206–212.

Kagan, C., Evans, J., 1995. Professional interpersonal skills for nurses. Chapman and Hall, London.

Kirk, S., 2001. Negotiating lay and professional roles in the care of children with complex health care needs. Journal of Advanced Nursing 34 (5), 593–602.

Kirk, S., Glendinning, C., 2002. Supporting expert parents: professional support and families caring for a child with complex health care needs in the community. International Journal of Nursing Studies 39 (6), 625–635.

Kugiumutzakis, G., 1998. Neonatal imitation in the intersubjective companion space. In: Braten, S. (Ed.), Intersubjective communication and emotion in early ontogeny. Cambridge University Press, Cambridge.

Laakso, H., Paunonen-Llmonen, M., 2001. Mothers' grief following the death of a child. Journal of Advanced Nursing 2001 36 (1), 69–77.

Langton, H., 2000. Negotiating care. In: Langton, H. (Ed.), The child with cancer: family-centred care in practice. Baillière Tindall, Edinburgh.

Lanz, M., Iarfrate, R., Rosnati, R., Scabina, E., 1999. Parent–child communication and adolescent self esteem in separated, intercountry adoptive and intact non adoptive families. Journal of Adolescence 22, 758–794.

Lask, B., 2003. Patient–clinician conflict: causes and compromises. Journal of Cystic Fibrosis 2, 42–45.

Mackenzie, H., 1997. The terminally ill child: supporting the family anticipating loss. In: Whyte, D.A. (Ed.), Explorations in family nursing. Routledge, London.

Matthews, J., 1994. Helping children to draw and paint in early childhood. Children and visual representation. Hodder and Stoughton, London.

Mayall, B., 1996. Children, health and the social order. Open University Press, Buckingham.

McGrath, P., Huff, N., 2001. 'What is it'? Findings on a preschoolers' responses to play with medical equipment. Child Care, Health and Development 27 (5), 451–462.

Meijer, S.A., Sinnema, G., Bijstra, J.O., et al., 2000. Peer interaction in adolescents with a chronic illness. Personality and Individual Differences 29 (5), 799–813.

Metzoff, A.N., Moore, K.M., 1998. Infant intersubjectivity: imitation, identity and intention. In: Braten, S. (Ed.), Intersubjective communication and emotion in early ontogeny. Cambridge University Press, Cambridge.

Morrison, J., Anders, T.F., 2001. Interviewing children and adolescents. Skills and strategies for effective DSM-IV diagnosis. The Guilford Press, New York.

Murray, L., 1998. Experimental perturbations of mother–infant communication. In: Braten, S. (Ed.), Intersubjective communication and emotion in early ontogeny. Cambridge University Press, Cambridge.

Neill, S.J., 2000. Acute childhood illness at home: the parents' perspective. Journal of Advanced Nursing 31 (4), 821–832.

Noll, R.B., Bukowski, W.M., Davies, W.H., et al., 1993. adjustment in the peer system of adolescents with cancer: a two year study. Journal of Paediatric Psychology 18, 351–364.

Ofsted 2003 Adult basic skills development hampered by poor quality teaching skills. Online. Available at: http://www.ofsted.gov.uk/publications/index.cfm?fuseaction=pubs.displayfile&id=3410&type=pdf

Oller, D.R., 1980. The emergence of the sounds of speech in infancy. In: Yeni-Komshian, G., Ferguson, C. (Eds.), Child phonology, vol. 1. Academic Press, New York.

Palmer, S.J., 1993. Care of sick children by parents: a meaningful role. Journal of Advanced Nursing 18, 185–191.

Pendley, J.S., Dahlquist, L.M., Dreyer, Z., 1997. Body image and psychosocial adjustment in adolescent cancer survivors. Journal of Pediatric Psychology 22, 29–43.

Pidgeon, V., 1981. Function of preschool children's questions in coping with hospitalization. Research in Nursing and Health 4, 229–235.

Ritchie, J.A., Caty, S., Ellerton, M., 1984. Concerns of acutely ill, chronically ill and healthy preschool children. Research in Nursing and Health 4, 229–235.

Runeson, I., Hermerén, G., Elander, G., Kristensson-Hallström, I., 2000. Children's consent to treatment: using a scale to assess degree of self-determination. Pediatric Nursing 26 (5), 455–458, 515.

Saetermoe, C.L., Farruggia, S.P., Lopez, C., 1999. Differential parental communication with adolescents who are disabled and their healthy siblings. Journal of Adolescent Health 24 (6), 427–432.

Sartain, S.A., Maxwell, M.J., Todd, P.T., et al., 2001. Users views on hospital and home care for acute illness in childhood. Health and Social Care in the Community 9 (2), 108–117.

Scottish Executive, 2007. Delivering a Healthy Future: Action Framework for Children and Young People's Health in Scotland. Edinburgh. Online. Available at: http://www.scotland.gov.uk/Resource/Doc/165782/0045104.pdf

Shields, L.K., Kristensson-Hallström, I., Kristjánsdóttir, G., Hunter, J., 2003. Philosophical and ethical issues: who owns the child in hospital? A preliminary discussion. Journal of Advanced Nursing 41 (3), 213–222.

Slade, A., 2000. Impact of treatment on the family. In: Langton, H. (Ed.), The child with cancer: family-centred care in practice. Baillière Tindall, Edinburgh.

Spence, M.J., DeCasper, A.J., 1986. Prenatal experience with low-frequency maternal speech sounds influences newborns' perception of female voices. International Conference on Infant Studies. Los Angeles. April.

Spencer, N., 2000. Poverty and child health, 2nd edn. Radcliffe Medical, Oxford.

Spencer, N.H., 1984. Parents' identification of the ill child. In: MacFarlane, J.A. (Ed.), Progress in child health. Churchill Livingstone, Edinburgh.

Starke, M., Mollier, A., 2002. Parents' need for knowledge concerning the medical diagnosis of their children. Journal of Child Health Care 6 (4), 245–257.

Stewart, M.J., Ritchie, J.A., McGrath, P., Thompson, D., Bruce, B., 1994. Mothers of children with chronic conditions: supportive and stressful interactions with partners and professionals regarding caregiving burdens. Canadian Journal of Nursing Research 26 (4), 61–82.

Tates, K., Meeuwesen, L., 2002. Bensing J 'I've come for his throat': roles and identities in doctor–parent–child communication. Child: Care, Health and Development 28 (1), 109–116.

Townley, M., Welton, S., 2000. In: Langton, H. (Ed.), The child with cancer: family-centred care in practice. Baillière Tindall, Edinburgh.

UNICEF 1989 United Nations General Assembly: United Nations Convention on the Rights of the Child, Geneva. Online. Available at: http://www.unicef.org/photoessays/30048.html

UNICEF 1959 United Nations General Assembly Declaration of the rights of the child, Geneva, 1959. Online. Available at: http://www.unhchr.ch/html/menu3/b/25.htm

Vacik, H.D., Nagy, M.C., Jessee, P.O., 2001. Children's understanding of illness: student's assessments. Journal of Pediatric Nursing 16, 6.

Vera, L., Nollet-Clémencon, C., Vila, G., et al., 1997. Social anxiety in insulin-dependent girls. European Psychiatry 12, 58–63.

Wales, S., Crisp, J., Moran, P., Perrin, M., Scott, E., 2008. Assessing communication between health professionals, children and families. Journal of Children's and Young People's Nursing 2 (2), 77–83.

Whitehead, M., 2000. The development of language and literacy. Hodder and Stoughton, London.

Williams, P.D.W., Williams, A.R., Graff, J.C., et al., 2003. A community-based intervention for siblings and parents of children with chronic illness or disability: the ISEE study. Journal of Pediatrics 142 (3), 386–393.

Wilson, A.E., Smith, M.D., Ross, H.S., 2003. The nature and effects of young children's lies. Social Development 12 (1), 21–44.

Woodgate, R.L., Degner, L.F., 2003. A substantive theory of keeping the spirit alive: the spirit within children with cancer and their families. Journal of Paediatric Oncology Nursing 20 (3), 103–119.

Yarcheskie, A., Mahon, N.E., Kraynyak-Luise, B., Baker, C.D., 1987. Testing the validity of categories in a theoretical perspective on chronic illness. International Journal of Nursing Studies 24, 249–260.

Young, B., Dixon Woods, M., Findlay, M., Henry, D., 2002. Parenting in a crisis: conceptualising mothers of children with cancer. Social Science Medicine 33, 1835–1847.

Zigler, E.F., Stevenson, M.F., 1993. Children in a changing world. Development and social issues, 2nd edn. Brooks/Cole Publishing, Pacific Grove.

Zubrick, S.R., 2007. Taylor, C.L., Rice, B.L., Slegers, D.W., Late Language Emergence at 24 months: An Epidemiological Study of Prevalence, Predictors and Covariates. Journal of Speech. Language and Hearing Research 50, 1562–1952.

The dynamic child: children's psychological development and its application to the delivery of care

11

Helen E Rushforth

ABSTRACT

This chapter offers an overview of psychological developmental theory and its application to children's nursing practice. Particular emphasis is placed on cognitive development. The work of Jean Piaget, Lev Vygotsky and other contributors to the field is critically appraised. Implications for children's nursing practice are articulated by exploring the application of the different psychological developmental theories to children's understanding of health and illness concepts. The chapter then considers language development and personality development, again exploring the implications of these theories within children's nursing.

LEARNING OUTCOMES

- Recognise the importance of an understanding of the role of cognitive developmental theory within children's nursing.
- Gain enhanced insight into the ways in which children conceptualise health, illness and their internal bodies, and be able to use this information to offer enhanced explanations to children and families.
- Gain an appreciation of children's language and personality development, and be able to articulate the ways in which these theories can also contribute to the care given by the children's nurse.
- Develop insight into the critical appraisal of psychological theory and its application to care delivery.

Introduction

The purpose of this chapter is to offer readers an overview of key theories in children's psychological development, and to consider these in terms of their relevance to children's nursing practice. Particular emphasis is placed on cognitive developmental theory, as this appears to have the most direct relevance for care delivery. To illustrate this, an exploration of the ways in which children conceptualise health and illness is offered as a key example of the application of theory to practice. Consideration is also given to the related areas of language and personality development, which also have important implications for the delivery of child health care.

A range of developmental theories is explored within this chapter, and readers are encouraged to critically consider the appropriateness of each as a tool to guide their future professional development. Perhaps the most important guiding principle in selecting an appropriate theory to underpin practice is to consider the congruence of the theories offered with other contemporary notions of childhood, children's rights, and child healthcare delivery. Increasingly, recognition is being made of children's potential to be 'active participants' in their health care, rather than passive recipients. Thus it is particularly appropriate to question the continued dominance of many theories, particularly in cognitive development, which cast children in a primarily dependent role. If developmental psychology is to continue to have meaning for the healthcare practitioners of the 21st century, then it must reflect contemporary views of childhood in other domains.

The nature–nurture debate

For any student considering developmental psychology, the nature–nurture debate is a key concept that underpins the work of almost all the major contributors. Thus an understanding of the nature–nurture concept is a useful starting point. Santrock (1999 p 21) defines nature as 'an organism's biological inheritance' and nurture as 'environmental experiences'. Therefore, the nature perspective would argue that a personality characteristic, e.g. moral behaviour, will develop naturally over time irrespective of external influences. By contrast, the nurture perspective would take the position that morality is a phenomenon that is learned, and thus is dependent on external stimuli.

In reality, of course, there are few who would argue that any aspect of child psychological development is entirely attributable to one or the other perspective, and it is increasingly

DOI: 10.1016/B978-0-7020-3183-0.10011-6

acknowledged that the acquisition of any human characteristic is inevitably a synthesis of both inherited and environmental influences. So when a particular psychologist is described as being a nativist (nature, e.g. Piaget) or empiricist (nurture, e.g. Carey), this does not mean the psychologist believes the characteristic is entirely attributable to nature or nurture, but rather that he or she believes one or the other to be the dominant influence within that area of child development. Thus it is helpful to see nature–nurture not as an either/or concept but rather as a continuum. And indeed, although some theorists come very much from one or other end of the continuum, others sit far closer to the midline (and are often referred to as the interactionists or constructivists, e.g. Vygotsky). These psychologists suggest a more equal contribution of both nature and nurture to a particular aspect of development.

Cognitive development

Although developmental psychology considers a variety of important domains, there is little doubt that the topic with the greatest influence for the child healthcare practitioner is that of cognitive development. From the outset it is important to acknowledge the dominance within this field of Jean Piaget (1896–1980); his profound influence on our understanding of childhood cannot be overestimated. However, although Piaget's invaluable contribution to developmental psychology is both acknowledged and valued, it is important to question the appropriateness of the domination of some of his assertions within the theory and practice of child healthcare delivery. Consequently, this chapter balances the Piagetian perspective with the views of other cognitive developmental psychologists, particularly Lev Vygotsky (1896–1934), thereby offering alternative tools to guide practice, which may be more congruent with other contemporary views of childhood.

Piagetian perspectives

Piaget was a prolific author whose worked spanned most of his very long and active life as a psychological theorist. Most students with some insight into Piaget's work will be familiar with his four stages of cognitive development, a summary of which is offered below (derived from Bee & Boyd 2008, Daly et al 2006, Meadows 2006, Piaget 1929, 1930, Piaget & Inhelder 1969, Santrock 1999, 2009, Taylor et al 1999).

Sensory motor stage: from birth to around 2 years

Piaget identifies this first stage as characterised by the links formed between the infant and the environment as the infant comes to understand the relationship between actions, sensation and movement. Piaget divided the stage into six subsections (for more detail see Piaget & Inhelder 1969 pp 4–12). These stages characterise the infant's development from being primarily reflexive/reactive (stage 1) through processes of trial and error, experiment and reinforcement (stages 2–5), to finally being able to actively understand and manipulate aspects of his or her world (stage 6). In other words, the infant has a gradually increasing awareness of the relationship between action and effect.

Piaget saw a key concept within this stage as something he called 'object permanence'. This means that for the younger infant 'out of sight' is also 'out of mind'. In contrast, older infants (Piaget argued from around 8 months) realise that an object exists even when it cannot be seen. Also, throughout this first stage the child is described as egocentric, i.e. 'the child's initial universe is entirely centred on his [sic] own body' (Piaget & Inhelder 1969 p 13).

Preoperational stage: from around 2 years to around 7 years

Piaget viewed the next two stages as a vital period of transition. At the beginning of this second stage, Piaget argued that the child's behaviour is characterised by actions; by its end the child will have reached the level of operations, summarised by Santrock (1999 p 203) as 'internalised sets of actions that allow the child to do mentally what was done physically before'. Piaget regarded achieving this as of pivotal importance and saw the preoperational period as dominated by organisation and preparation towards becoming 'operational' (Piaget & Inhelder 1969 p 96). Consequently, the stage tends to be characterised negatively, by what children are not yet able to do, rather than what they can. Examples include their perceived inability to classify objects into groups, to think logically and to engage in moral reasoning. A key skill not yet achieved is that of conservation, i.e. the ability to realise that something might 'stay the same' despite a change in appearance. For example, a preoperational child would think the amount of juice in a short, fat glass becomes 'more' when poured into a tall, thin glass (see also Channel 4 Television 2001, Santrock 2009).

Also within this stage is a continued focus on the child's egocentricity, characterised particularly by the inability to be able to see the world from another's point of view or to distinguish another's point of view from their own (both visually and intellectually). Closely linked to this is Piaget's belief that these children could not conceptualise a world beyond their direct experience, i.e. what he or she had actually seen or experienced. Practically applied, it can be seen how such beliefs can limit perceptions of the preoperational child's abilities in a whole variety of conceptual domains. Piaget also noted that these children display animism, the attribution of 'life' to non-live objects.

Concrete operational stage: from around 7 years to around 11 years

Piaget saw this stage as characterised by children becoming 'operational', and thus being able to do many of the activities that they were working towards in the preoperational stage. He argued that operational children are capable of logical, systematic thought, and able to 'conserve' concepts such as number, mass, length, weight and volume. They are also able to classify and seriate objects/items, and to understand logical relationships between them. However, Piaget felt at this 'concrete' stage that children could only understand problems related to direct experience; they are not seen as capable of abstract or hypothetical thought, or the manipulation of variables.

Formal operational stage: from around 12 years onwards

Piaget used the term 'propositional operations' to describe this final stage. He regarded these skills as congruent with preparation for adolescence, with the child able to think in abstract terms and capable of 'the handling of hypotheses and reasoning with regard to propositions removed from concrete and present operation' (Piaget & Inhelder 1969 p 131). Thus young people are able systematically to explore the solutions to an abstract or hypothetical problem, including everything from algebra to decisions concerning their future! An important extension of this is described as 'reflective abstraction' – self-awareness in relation to one's own strategies and thoughts.

Other key concepts in Piaget's work

These four stages are the centre-piece of Piaget's theories of childhood but many other important concepts also exist within his works. Those with particular relevance for child health practitioners can be summarised as follows:

- The way in which children think is fundamentally different from the way in which adults think.
- Development is fundamentally reliant on the concept of maturation, i.e. developmental pace is predetermined, and the teacher cannot accelerate this process.
- The child's understanding derives from self-directed actions upon the physical world. Thus, the teacher's role is limited to constructing learning opportunities, and it is primarily through the child's independent interaction with the world that learning takes place.
- The child develops in a series of 'discrete stages' like 'caterpillar, chrysalis, butterfly', as opposed to a continuous development such as 'kitten to cat'.

(See also Bee & Boyd 2008, Santrock 2009, Taylor et al 1999.)

Within Piaget's theories three additional key concepts underpin a child's emergent understanding of the world (derived from Meadows 2006, Piaget 1929, 1930, Piaget & Inhelder 1969, Santrock 2009, Vacik et al 2001):

- **Scheme or schema**: the cognitive structure whereby the child organises his or her understanding of a particular concept.
- **Assimilation**: new information is incorporated into the child's existing schema, i.e. that which the child already knows.
- **Accommodation**: existing understanding ceases to be sufficient to make sense of the world. The schema is reorganised to understand the world in a new way.

To illustrate these somewhat abstract concepts, it might be helpful to consider an example. Imagine for a moment the child seeing a picture of a zebra for the first time.

- If the child already has a **schema** for horses, he or she might very well suppose that the zebra is another type of horse.
- This then would be **assimilation**: the child has taken the new information and incorporated it into his or her existing schema.
- However, through education and/or experience, the child will learn that the new animal is not a horse but actually something rather different, i.e. a zebra. Therefore the child develops a new schema for the zebra (and perhaps a wider schema for African animals). Thus a change in the child's understanding of the world has taken place, i.e. **accommodation**.
- Successful accommodation was viewed as essential to ongoing cognitive development, and enabled the child to achieve what Piaget called **equilibrium**.
- However, the risks inherent within the process are that from time to time **misunderstanding** will occur, e.g. instead of accommodation, the child happily goes on to describe an animal as a 'stripy horse'.

Reflect on your practice

Before reading further, think about the following situation. Suppose you are admitting Jack, a 5-year-old child, to hospital for a course of intravenous antibiotics due to pneumonia:

- Consider Piaget's views on cognitive development. In what ways might your care of Jack be influenced if you assumed all of Piaget's assertions to be true?
- Think particularly about what explanations you might give to Jack regarding the treatment and care he will receive?
- Do you feel entirely comfortable with the approach you would take, or is there some conflict with your current experience and understanding of hospitalised children?

Influences of Piagetian theory on contemporary practice

Piagetian theories influenced the delivery of child health care throughout much of the latter half of the 20th century and many of his views continue to be profoundly influential. For example, in the care of infants, Piaget's theory of 'object permanence' suggests that under about 8 months a child does not realise an object still exists when it cannot be seen, a theory applied not only to inanimate objects but also to people. Thus it has been argued in some centres that younger infants will not be unduly distressed when separated from their parents. So although unrestricted parental visiting is now more or less universally accepted within child health care, the parents of infants continue to be excluded in some care settings from anaesthetic rooms, recovery rooms and a variety of other procedures, on the grounds that this age group of children won't be unduly distressed by parental absence.

For the 'pre-operational' child, assumptions are often made about what the child is or is not able to understand about an illness, procedure or investigation. A Piagetian perspective would assume that children under the age of about seven were incapable of conceptualising their internal anatomy, and thus suggests that it may be pointless to attempt any realistic explanation of an internal procedure. As will be discussed in detail later, such guidelines were heavily influential during the 1970s and 1980s. A Piagetian stance would also contend that other misconceptions are inevitable and cannot be overcome until a child reaches a certain point of maturation. Examples include 'immanent justice' (Santrock 2009), which is the belief that pain or injury is a punishment, and 'overgeneralising contagion', e.g. believing cancer is 'catching'.

Even as the child becomes 'operational', assumptions continue to be made. As Piaget asserts that the concrete operational child cannot hypothesise, look meaningfully into the future or make decisions based on abstract concepts, it is often suggested that, until mid to late adolescence, a child cannot make an informed decision about what might be in his or her 'best interests'. Such beliefs have historically limited children being offered any meaningful involvement in decisions regarding their care – a situation which continues to exist in some care settings even today.

Thus it can be seen how important it is to gain an accurate picture of the extent to which Piaget's beliefs represent 'truth'. If there are doubts about some aspects of his theory, then such doubts must inevitably be extended to the application of Piagetian principles to care delivery. It is therefore important both to review the literature that takes a more critical view of Piaget's work and also to consider different theoretical perspectives that might offer alternative tools to guide contemporary practice.

Critiquing Piaget

The 1970s and 1980s were characterised by a series of challenges to Piaget's perspective on child development, with a whole range of authors suggesting that Piagetian theory unreasonably limited our beliefs in children's abilities and that, in reality, children were capable of far more than Piaget gave them credit for.

In respect of the preoperational child, various studies have demonstrated the ability of young infants to visually recognise their parents and distinguish them from strangers (see Taylor et al 1999 pp 25–26). Similarly, Santrock (1999, 2009) and Bee & Boyd (2008) describe studies where infants demonstrate learning at just a few weeks old, far younger than Piaget would have accepted that these infants could proactively manipulate their environment. In one example, Santrock (1999 p 153) cites the work of Rovee-Colyer (1987), who took infants at just a few months old and tied their foot to a ribbon that moved a mobile. Weeks later, when placed under the mobile, the infants will once again kick in an attempt to move the mobile, despite no ribbon being in place.

Similar critiques of Piagetian theory are found in respect of the preoperational child. For example, in his study of egocentricity, Piaget devised a test known as the 'three mountains experiment' (Piaget & Inhelder 1956). The child was shown a three-dimensional model of three differently coloured mountains, positioned so that clearly different views of the mountains were visible from each of the four sides of the model (see Piaget & Inhelder 1969 or Santrock 1999 p 205 for more detail). The child was given a series of four two-dimensional drawings representing the view from each side of the model, and asked to 'work out' which drawing represented the view of a doll positioned on the opposite side of the model to the child. The fact that most children aged under 7 were unable to do this was central to Piaget's persistent belief in their egocentricity; their inability to see the world from another's point of view.

Yet in contrast, Donaldson (1978), one of Piaget's foremost critics, constructed another experiment where children were far more successful, using an intersection of two walls in a 'cross shape' (see Donaldson 1978 pp 21–22 or Taylor et al 1999 p 58 for more detail). Two policeman models were positioned in such a way that they could see behind most of the walls but not all. In this study, children who got the three-mountain test wrong were frequently able to position a naughty doll so that the policemen were unable to see her; clearly they had to understand what the world looked like from the policemen's perspective to do this. Perhaps the key difference, Donaldson suggests, is that this experiment 'made sense' to the child and so was more readily understood. Clearly if children below 7 years are able to see another's point of view there are major implications for beliefs regarding their egocentricity.

Activity

Gaining evidence of children's ability to see the world from another's perspective may be simpler even than Donaldson suggests:

- Take a favourite toy belonging to a child as young as 3 and position it facing the wall. Ask the child what the toy can see?
- Now move the toy to face in different directions in the room, and ask the same question.

Many 3- and 4-year-old children will happily tell you what the toy can or can't see. Yet these children are up to 4 years younger than those Piaget claimed were still egocentric.

In another of her critiques of Piaget's work, Donaldson also challenged some of his conservation experiments. For example, Piaget had conducted a study where children are asked to view two identical rows of sweets and say whether the rows are the same. The experimenter then repositions the sweets in one row so they are further apart, but leaves the same number. When re-questioned in Piaget's study, many children under seven insisted the row where the sweets have been moved now contained 'more'. Yet when Donaldson (1978) replicated the study using a 'naughty teddy' to move the sweets, significantly fewer children got the answer wrong than in a control group where, like in Piaget's original study, the researcher moved the sweets. Donaldson argued this was because the answer 'still being the same' now 'made sense', unlike the Piagetian version in which many children assumed the answer must now be different. Indeed, central to Donaldson's (1978) theories about Piaget was a recurrent theme that his experiments were designed in such a way that the children were often set up to fail, and that as a consequence children's abilities at a given age/stage were at significant risk of being underestimated.

For the concrete operational child, again, numerous studies challenge Piaget's perspectives. One particular study with clear healthcare implications is by Alderson (1993). She interviewed 120 children, many of whom fell into Piaget's concrete operational age group, and demonstrated the ability of several of these children to make carefully considered and informed choices about non-essential surgery.

It is beyond the scope of this chapter to illuminate the dozens of similar examples of experiments that call into question many of Piaget's findings (see Bee & Boyd 2008, Berger 2008, Berk 2006, 2008, Donaldson 1978, Santrock 2009 for more details). It is important to stress, however, that it is not Piaget's fundamental assertions about the systematic way in which children develop cognitively that are necessarily being challenged; his model continues to offer extremely valuable insight into the sequential ways in which children develop. Rather it is the nativist domination in his theories that has become the key focus of his critics, i.e. the:

- inevitability of constraints imposed by age and maturation
- protracted timescale taken to reach each developmental stage
- impossibility of accelerating the developmental process by education
- minimal credence given to the influences of experience, society and culture
- fact that, translated into practical terms, such beliefs have the potential to limit opportunities – given to younger children in particular – to understand their world and make sense of their experiences.

However, if these critiques of Piaget's work cast doubt on his theories in this way, then there are also inevitably important implications for many of the traditional applications of his theory to care delivery. Thus it may no longer be safe to assume that a 4-month-old baby can go for surgery alone and not be adversely affected by parental separation before he or she is asleep. Similarly, it might be unsafe to assume that a 4-year-old cannot understand an explanation of his or her heart surgery, or that a 9-year-old is unable to contribute meaningfully to a decision to undergo leg lengthening. It is therefore vital that such assumptions are carefully considered in light of the research that casts doubt on aspects of Piagetian theory, and also in the light of the views of alternative theorists, who may offer a more positive interpretation of younger children's cognitive development.

Carey: 'novice to expert shift' theory

One of the key theorists who offers a very different view to that of Piaget is Carey (1985). In her 'novice to expert shift' theory, Carey – writing from an empirical perspective – argued that there is nothing fundamentally different about the way in which children and adults think and come to an understanding of the world. She argued that it is knowledge, not maturation, that is the key. Where only a little knowledge of a topic exists, thinking is 'novice', and thus it is likely that a concept will be misinterpreted or only partially understood. In contrast, the expert thinker has a great deal of knowledge of a topic, and thus sophisticated understanding exists. Crucially though, Carey argued that both children and adults are capable of 'novice' and 'expert' levels of understanding simultaneously, depending on how much they know about a particular topic.

For example, Carey cites 3-year-old dinosaur 'experts' who can tell you not only the names of all the dinosaurs but their eating habits, habitat, chronology and relative size. She similarly recognises young computer experts and chess players. Equally possible is novice thinking by adults when learning about a new topic for the first time, as evidenced for example by game-show contestants attempting to draw their internal anatomy! Thus, Carey argues that whilst children are far more likely to be 'novice' thinkers on a range of topics because their overall knowledge level is inevitably less, there is nothing about childhood thinking per se that limits children's understanding. Consequently a child as young as three may well be able to develop a sophisticated understanding of a topic provided the knowledge is imparted at an accessible level and pace.

What emerges when comparing Piaget's nativist perspective and Carey's empirical perspective is a polarity between their two views, which regard either maturation or learning as very much the dominant forces in child development. It is the interactionist perspective, however, that offers the possibility of bridging this nature–nurture gap. Thus the theories of Lev Vygotsky (1896–1934) perhaps offer the most useful tool for healthcare practitioners in seeking developmental theory to underpin their practice (Daly et al 2008, Holaday et al 1994, Rushforth 1999, Shayer 2003).

Vygotsky and the 'zone of proximal development'

Vygotsky (1978) was working in Russia at a similar time to Piaget, but his early death (aged just 38) and delayed translation of his work hindered his wider recognition for many years. Importantly, unlike Carey, his views were not in opposition to those of Piaget, and, indeed, more recent authors have argued that there are rather more similarities than differences in their work (Shayer 2003). Like Piaget, Vygotsky believed in the importance of maturation and biological processes but he saw the interplay between these processes and the child's social world as being of prime importance. He saw thought processes as uniquely human and derived from children's early exposure to language, and from social and cultural influences conveyed to the child by both family and teachers. Indeed, the nature of the role of 'the teacher' is perhaps one of the key differences between Piagetian and Vygotiskian perspectives.

Central to Vygotsky's work was his notion of the 'zone of proximal development', which he defined as:

> The distance between the actual developmental level as determined by independent problem solving and the level of potential development as determined through problem solving under adult guidance or in collaboration with more capable peers
>
> (Vygotsky 1978 p 86)

In other words, he saw the actual developmental level as the point of maturation that the child has already reached, but also recognised that at any given point in time the child had the potential for additional knowledge and understanding to be gained in that particular area of development. Thus the zone of proximal development looks at development 'prospectively', taking what the child knows as a starting point and using this to discern what the child is capable of achieving in the immediate future. Thus Vygotsky argued that you cannot determine any child's cognitive level without observing both what they already know and how they respond to instruction, hence the role of the teacher being so crucial (for more detail see Daly 2008, Holaday et al 1994, Rushforth 1999, Santrock 2009, Shayer 2003, Taylor & Woods 2005).

Translating Vygotskian perspectives into practice

The significance of Vygotsky's perspective in contrast to Piaget's is considerable because it offers the possibility of enhancing and accelerating the child's development by teaching. Unlike Carey, Vygotsky felt there were maturational limits on how far a child's understanding could develop at a given point in time. However, although these limits are in many ways congruent with the stages Piaget describes, in Vygotsky's theories the child can achieve understanding at a far earlier age than Piaget would suggest. Thus Vygotsky's theory offers teachers and health practitioners the possibility of considerably enhancing children's understanding through education.

Thus if a Vygotskian perspective rather than a Piagetian perspective influences our healthcare practice, the key difference is that a child's developmental potential is not persistently viewed in negative terms but rather in positive ones. Piagetian 'tools to guide practice' are framed in terms of what children are unable to understand (e.g. Taylor et al 1999 p 64). By contrast, a Vygotskian perspective encourages the practitioner to find out what the child already knows and then to use this as a basis for working with the child and family to help the child to reach an enhanced level of understanding (Gaffney 2000, Holaday et al 1994, Rushforth 1999).

Vygotsky's work was further developed by Bruner (1972), who used the analogous term 'scaffolding' to describe the role of teachers (both professionals and parents) within the 'zone of proximal development'. Bruner saw this human scaffolding as a 'supportive mechanism', which was gradually withdrawn as the child strengthens in his or her own knowledge and understanding. Bruner believed that any topic could be meaningfully conveyed at some level to any child, provided it was appropriately individualised and congruent with what the child already knew and understood.

Reflect on your practice

Case study: Vygotskian perspectives

Consider again Jack, the 5-year-old child admitted to hospital described earlier. Now reconsider his care from a Vygotskian perspective:

- What differences emerge when compared with the earlier Piagetian perspective?
- Which approach to Jack's care are you more comfortable with and why?

Children's conceptualisation of health, illness and their internal bodies

One example of applying cognitive developmental theory to practice is consideration of the ways in which children conceptualise health and illness concepts. The ways in which we interpret children's abilities in this domain has considerable potential to influence the quality of care they receive, their understanding of their illness and treatment, and the extent to which they can be actively involved in decisions pertaining to their care. A summary is offered here; for a more detailed consideration of this area see Bibace & Walsh (1981), Rushforth (1999) and Siegal & Peterson (1999).

Since the middle part of the 20th century, numerous authors have researched children's ability to understand the concepts of health, illness and their internal bodies. The early 1960s through to the mid-1980s saw the publication of numerous studies suggesting that children's understanding of these concepts increased with age. Many studies also offered clear links with Piagetian theory, arguing the inevitability of the many misconceptions displayed by the younger children within the studies. However, the seminal work within the field was arguably that of Bibace & Walsh (1980, 1981), who offered a stage theory of children's conceptualisation of illness that was very closely aligned to Piaget's earlier described stage theory of cognitive development. Thus preoperational children (aged 2–7) were seen as having an illogical or magical understanding of illness, and concrete operational children (aged 7–11) were seen as having a limited and largely external understanding with little awareness of internal biological processes. It was only the formal operational child (aged 11+) who was viewed as likely to have any detailed understanding of illness physiology (see Vacik et al 2001 for a fuller summary).

A similar stage theory was also published by Perrin & Gerrity (1981). The title of this study, 'There's a demon in my belly' (actually the child had been told he had oedema) clearly conveyed the typical misconceptions of younger children. Like Bibace & Walsh (1980, 1981) before them, Perrin & Gerrity (1981) argued that such misunderstandings are an inevitably consequence of cognitive immaturity.

However, the later 1980s and 1990s saw a gradual turning point within the literature. A growing body of authors recognised that such studies, although offering useful tools in terms of understanding the way in which children conceptualise health and illness, were also misrepresenting younger children's potential to gain enhanced understanding of these health and illness concepts.

As early as 1980, and many years ahead of their peers, Kister & Patterson (1980) noticed that children who better understood 'contagion' were less likely to display 'imminent justice explanations' (the belief that illness was a punishment). Thus for the first time they acknowledged that enhancing understanding had the potential to reduce children's fears and misconceptions.

Also of interest at this time was the work of Burbach & Peterson (1986), who offered the first systematic review of the earlier literature, and again criticised the Piagetian dominance within the earlier work. Similarly Eiser (1989), a prominent UK researcher in the field, challenged the Piagetian dominance in her own earlier work and suggested the earlier discussed theory of Carey (1985) as an important alternative perspective.

One of the most important studies at this time was the work of Vessey (1988), who tested children's knowledge of their internal anatomy before and after instruction. She was thus the first author to clearly demonstrate the potential for children to achieve enhanced understanding of their internal bodies in response to instruction. Many other authors from this era also carried out studies that demonstrated children's greater understanding of health and illness concepts. These included Bird & Podmore (1990), Hergenrather & Rabinowitz (1991) and Longsdon (1991). It is important to state that these authors did not dismiss Piaget's theories outright, but they certainly challenged his assertions that children's potential to understand was limited by their maturation. All offered evidence of children demonstrating far more sophisticated levels of understanding than Piaget had previously given them credit for.

In reviewing these more recent studies, it is easy to see the parallels with Vygotsky's work, although it was only in Holaday et al's 1994 paper that this link was first explored explicitly. Subsequently, around the turn of the century, many authors offered studies that demonstrate considerable understanding of health, illness and internal anatomy by even very young children (Elliott & Watson 2000, Gaffney 2000, Gaudion 1997, McEwing 1996, McGrath & Huff 2001, Schmidt 2001, Williams & Binnie 2002, Yoos 1994). However, what is interesting in many of these more recent papers is the balanced viewpoint often taken in recognising the contribution of the key theorists as complementary rather than in opposition. Thus, although Piaget's negativity in respect of younger children's understanding of the world is repeatedly challenged, the contribution of his stage theory to our understanding of childhood and cognitive development is readily acknowledged. Yet alongside this, the Vygotskian perspective that acknowledges children's potential to achieve enhanced understanding with careful teaching is also increasingly recognised. However, readers should be aware that some authors from this period (e.g. Betz et al 2000, Taylor et al 1999, Twycross 1998, Williams 1995) continued to offer guidelines for practice that frame younger children's potential understanding in negative Piagetian terms. Whilst the evidence base to support any particular theorist is far from conclusive, any guideline for practice that suggests that certain groups of children cannot or will not understand particular health and illness concepts should be viewed with caution.

Most recent research continues to recognise children's potential to understand far more than earlier researchers gave them credit for. It also increasingly seeks to understand some of the complex ways in which children construct their understanding of the world by exploring understanding of quite specific illness concepts. Many such papers offer insights with useful application to child health nursing practice on a variety of subjects including Fox et al (2008), Franck et al (2008), McDonald & Rushforth (2006), Myant & Williams (2005-2008) and Piko & Bak (2006).

It is also important to acknowledge the fundamental importance of recognising children as individuals, thereby emphasising the importance of basing any explanation to a child on an understanding of what he or she already knows. This is particularly important in respect of the care of children with chronic illness, where there may be assumptions that knowledge levels are good because of previous experience. Yet various studies (e.g. Burbach & Peterson 1986, Crisp et al 1996, Veldtman et al 2000) have repeatedly failed to demonstrate a clear link between illness experience and understanding of health and illness concepts. To make such assumptions therefore places the child at considerable risk, leading Ireland (1997) to advocate the 'gather, give, gather' model of explanation giving. In other words, find out what the child already knows, give the explanation and then (because we know how readily misunderstandings can occur despite good explanation) recheck the child's understanding to ensure that the explanation has been safely received.

As stated earlier, despite these recent studies, the evidence base is still far from perfect. In particular, researchers continue to study what children already know and to make assumptions about what they are capable of knowing. This view fundamentally opposes Vygotsky's assertion of the need to explore a child's response to instruction to recognise what he or she is capable of understanding. Thus, far more research like that of Vessey (1988) or Williams & Binnie (2002) is needed to address this deficit. This would help to create an evidence base that effectively guides future practitioners on the best ways of conveying information regarding health and illness concepts to the children in their care.

Reflect on your practice

Case study: children's concepts of Illness

Suppose Chloe, a 4-year-old girl, tells you after her appendicectomy that the reason her tummy hurts is 'because I have been naughty':

- What might be the reasons for her beliefs?
- How can you help her to realise this is not the case, and understand the real reasons for what has happened and why?
- What theories are influencing your explanation giving?

Concepts of health and illness: application to care delivery

Application: concepts of illness

The potential to enhance children's understanding through information giving has relevance both for the acutely ill child admitted to hospital and also for the care of children with chronic illnesses. For the child undergoing a planned admission, this body of literature has considerable potential to greatly enhance hospital-based preparation programmes (for more detail on these, see Chapter 9). Even for emergency admissions, readily understandable explanations of illnesses and procedures are a crucially important aspect of care delivery.

Appropriate education for chronically ill children is central to helping those with conditions such as asthma, eczema, cystic fibrosis and diabetes become active participants in their care from an early age. Not only can it empower them to take control of their illness, it also enables them to make informed decisions about aspects of their treatment, as well as increasing their safety when they are among adults who have limited familiarity with their condition.

The Vygotskian (1962) principles of gathering information to find out what the child knows before any informative intervention takes place, as discussed above, cannot be overemphasised. As the school curriculum gradually introduces different approaches to biological and health education, knowledge levels within similar age groups are likely to be greater, but potentially more diverse, than ever. This arguably also further limits the usefulness of age-dependent stage theories. Furthermore, it is likely that within a class of up to 35 children, at least some will have misunderstood aspects of the teaching. Thus whilst giving an explanation to a child it may be necessary for misconceptions to be corrected before new knowledge can be explored. Despite children's clear potential to gain understanding at an enhanced level with appropriate instruction, misconceptions are, as noted earlier in discussion of Piagetian schemas, a very real risk within new learning. Thus children might be distressed by misunderstanding concepts we might take for granted, for example:

- **balloons**: analogous for bladders, lungs and stomachs, but children know that balloons can 'burst'
- **dye**: as in various radiographic investigations, but clearly having a potentially very different meaning
- **test**: a term widely used but again with a negative connotation for most children
- **bugs**: a term sometimes used by health staff to denote infection but which again is potentially frightening in a child's conception of sinister creatures
- **put to sleep**: if used to describe an anaesthetic could readily be misunderstood by a child whose pet has been 'put to sleep' by the vet; the concept of a 'special sleep' and an emphasis on waking up when the procedure is over is clearly vital.

(See also Barnes 2003, Taylor et al 1999.)

Activity

Hannah, aged 3, has come home from playschool having had a talk about hospitals, and has announced to her mother that:

> *'When we go to playschool tomorrow we are going to have our tonsils out and you can bring them home in a box'.*

Considering the theories discussed so far, how did Hannah end up with this misconception, and in what way could this talk have been better organised to avoid this potential problem.

Application: concepts of health

The implications of the children's concepts literature for the ways in which children conceptualise health are important. Given that contemporary health policy suggests that infant and junior school children need to be taught about key concepts such drug abuse, sexual health and relationships, it is vital that we consider ways of conveying messages to children about these complex concepts in ways that they can understand. An approach that emphasises the typical 5-year-old's limited preoperational understanding is of little value here, and it is the work of authors such as Carey (1985) and Vygotsky (1978) that arguably offers better tools to guide both nurses, and those in schools who engage in personal, social and health education (PSHE) with this age group.

Even for older age groups of children the challenges of constructing effective health promotion campaigns can be considerable, and in particular conveying the longer-term adverse consequences of unhealthy behaviours to children and young people is extremely difficult (Oakley et al 1995). Indeed, Piaget's caution about the challenges even adolescents have in appreciating the longer-term consequences of actions might well be relevant here, although others would argue this is more to do with adolescent 'denial' than an inability to understand (see Santrock 2009). Nevertheless, it is arguably important that health promoters focus on the positive and short-term benefits of healthy choices within any health promotion campaign (such as weight loss increasing attractiveness to potential partners, for example) rather than the longer-term risks (such as death from heart disease 50 years hence).

Wider application of the children's concepts of health and illness literature to care delivery

Detailed consideration of how all aspects of the literature pertaining to children's conceptualisation of health and illness can be applied to practice is beyond the scope of this chapter. Specific areas that the reader might wish to further consider include the study of children's perceptions of pain (Franck et al 2008, Gaffney 2000, Harbech & Peterson 1992, Rushforth 1999), children's competence to consent (Alderson 1993, Alderson & Montgomery 1996, Rushforth 1999) and children's understanding of death (Bluebond-Langer 1989, Smith & McSherry 2004).

Finally, it has been suggested in recent years that healthcare practitioners often have an inadequate understanding of how children conceptualise health and illness (Rushforth 1996, Vacik et al 2001). Although there is a lack of contemporary research in this area, if the situation is the same today, it is possible that such a lack of understanding might in turn inhibit the quality of communication and information-giving undertaken by children's nurses and other healthcare practitioners. Ensuring clear coverage of this domain of practice in health professional education therefore remains of vital importance in curriculum design.

Language development

Many texts offer detailed accounts of the ways in which children develop language, often breaking it down into the complex processes of phonology, morphology, semantics and pragmatics.

The importance of these processes in helping children with specific problems cannot be overestimated but the greater priority for most healthcare practitioners working with children is an understanding of the psychological processes underpinning language development, and the extent to which these can be influenced by a period of illness or hospitalisation. Alongside this is the importantce of students having a sufficient understanding of what constitutes normal language development if they are to be able to access expert opinion and help for a child whose linguistic development appears to be delayed.

The empiricist perspective

Skinner (1957) took a view of language development that is congruent with the empiricist perspective. He believed that children's earliest language development was shaped from their meaningless infant 'babbling', through a process of reinforcement. This involves parents praising, reiterating and thereby reinforcing sounds that most closely approximate to actual words (e.g. 'ma ma ma', 'da da da'). This is seen alongside the process of 'imitation', suggesting that children's verbatim copying of words, phrases and sentences uttered by adults enables them to construct sentences themselves.

This view of language development, sometimes referred to as the behaviourist perspective, sees children very much as a 'blank slate', on whom language is imposed. However, as Berk (2008) points out, the 3- or 4-year-old child typically has a vocabulary of around 14,000 words, which he or she can use correctly to construct sophisticated and grammatically correct, or near correct, sentences. Thus, if the behaviourist perspective alone was responsible for language development, it would rely on parents and others engaging in the equivalent of extremely intensive language tuition processes. Many contemporary psychologists agree that the empiricist perspective alone is insufficient to explain young children's sophisticated language development.

The nativist perspective

Interestingly, published in the same year as Skinner's work, another seminal text (Chomsky 1957) proposed an opposing view of language development. Chomsky viewed children as far more active participants in the process of language acquisition. Although exposure to adult language was clearly important, he argued that they were effectively 'pre-programmed' to learn language via what he referred to as the language acquisition device (LAD). He saw this as a mental 'apparatus', which innately enables children to actively construct their vocabulary into grammatically sound sentence constructions (see also Daly et al 2008).

Chomsky drew on the evidence of when children get things wrong to support his theory. For example, children who say they 'ridded' their bike, 'didded up' their shoes or 'maked a picture for Mummy' are using words they are unlikely to have been taught or even heard in that context. Rather, it appears that children have actively constructed the words by mistakenly interpreting or overgeneralising their grammatical understanding. For Chomsky, this was supportive of his view that a maturational process was primarily responsible for what he viewed as the unique human ability to construct language.

Perhaps one of the most persuasive arguments in support of Chomsky's perspective is the ease with which younger children can assimilate a new language or learn two languages simultaneously. However, critics of Chomsky's perspective have questioned whether it is realistic to suggest that children have an innate grammatical structure (Berk 2008), and argue that it would be unsafe to underplay the role of both parents and teachers in the development of meaningful language and purposeful communication.

The interactionist perspective

These views have led to a third, interactionist, perspective on language development. This viewpoint recognises both the inherent linguistic abilities of young children and the importance of education and social experience in informing and shaping these inherent processes. The perspective is supported by the work of Bruner (1983), who believes that a rich social environment is central to language acquisition, while at the same time acknowledging the importance of innate determinants of both linguistic and social behaviour. As an extension of this perspective, Vygotsky (1962) also argued that play is intrinsically linked to the language development process.

Vygotsky also acknowledged the fundamentally important contribution of both innate and social processes to language development. He further believed language was central to development of children's thought processes, with social exposure and language learning being gradually internalised by the child to become the human thought processes central to cognitive development. Thus, for Vygotsky, the acceleration of language learning was linked implicitly to accelerating cognitive developmental processes and children's abilities in a whole variety of other domains (Holaday et al 1994).

It is important that beliefs regarding links between linguistic and cognitive ability are not applied universally. There are significant numbers of children with little or no verbal language but highly sophisticated cognitive development (e.g. some children with cerebral palsy). This can be at least partly explained by the observation that children's development of language comprehension occurs more rapidly than their ability to produce language (Berk 2008); the latter requiring additional cognitive and neuromuscular skills. However, there are also clear indications that children with delayed language development can struggle with a whole range of cognitive processes. For these children there appears to be a link between language and reasoning, and thus enhancing a child's language development through the provision of speech and language therapy can be the key that 'unlocks' other aspects of their cognitive development (Wood 1988). Furthermore, acceleration of language development, both comprehension and articulation, can enable many children to 'keep up' with their peers in mainstream education, when they would otherwise have lagged impossibly far behind.

Practical applications

In considering these perspectives on language development, a number of important considerations emerge for practitioners caring for younger children, particularly in hospital settings. These include the following two key perspectives:

- The importance of providing a **stimulating environment**, which maintains the child's exposure to social language. This is particularly important for children whose parents cannot be resident, for those requiring long-term admission and those requiring isolation. Infants with complex problems who spend many months in hospital, often in an incubator, are particularly vulnerable. Parents can be supported and encouraged in this provision of social language stimulation, and helped to understand the positive contribution they can make to their child's ongoing development. There is growing belief in the value of even 6-month-old infants being read to daily, in terms of potential benefits to their cognitive and linguistic development.
- The importance of knowing **normal developmental milestones** well enough to recognise a child whose language development may require additional support and intervention. More detail on this can be found in a range of texts on physical development and/or child assessment (e.g. Barnes 2003). Many children are helped enormously by speech and language therapy but a nurse might well be the first health professional to recognise that a child could benefit from such support, particularly if the family has had minimal contact with other health professionals. In the first instance, follow-up of such concerns are best made via the named health visitor (in the UK), who will know of current interventions. It is also useful to recognise that unless specific problems can be predicted due to a pre-existing condition, speech and language therapy does not normally commence until 3 years of age.

Reflect on your practice

Sian, aged 3 years and 6 months, is admitted to your ward for routine surgery. She is the youngest of four children. During the admission process you observe that Sian is speaking only in single words, and also that these words are quite difficult for you to understand. You explore this concern with Sian's mother during the admission process but Sian's mother seeks to reassure you, saying:

> *'Oh, I'm not worried, I think it's just that her older brothers do all the talking and translating for her – she'll get there in the end.'*

When you ask whether Sian's health visitor is concerned her mother says:

> *'Oh, I haven't seen her since Sian was about 12 months. If I don't know what I'm doing after four of them, then I never will!'*

- Based on your experience and on your knowledge of speech and language development, are the mother's assumptions about Sian's language development correct?
- What actions should you take to ensure that your concerns are followed up?

Personality development

As with other aspects of psychological development, the development of personality has been linked very strongly to the nature–nurture debate, focusing on the extent to which personality is innately inherited and predestined, and the extent to which it is shaped by society and environmental influences. Ultimately, here also one is left to conclude that both factors play a part. Innate determinants are clearly influential, as attested by studies of twins reared apart who display markedly similar personality traits (see Santrock 2008 for examples). However, experience undoubtedly also shapes personality, and two important theorists have contributed to these dimensions of our understanding of personality development, Erikson (1902–1994) and Freud (1856–1939). Although in many ways their work currently receives less recognition than that of the cognitive developmental theorists, they offer perspectives that greatly influence our understanding of many phenomena, such as infant attachment, child-rearing practices, moral development and sex role identification. There are consequently clear implications for child healthcare delivery.

Erik Erikson

Erikson, like Piaget, offered a stage theory of development (Erikson 1950). Erikson's theories are fully summarised in Chapter 2 by Hemphill & Dearmun, but are discussed briefly here so that their place within developmental theory can be fully appreciated. Importantly, when compared with Piaget, Erikson's theories offer a far more holistic view of the individual. Furthermore, his stages were not restricted to childhood but rather reflected ongoing development throughout the lifespan, a psychological perspective that particularly gained popularity throughout the 1990s and remains popular today (e.g. Bee & Boyd 2008, Berger 2008, Berk 2006, Santrock 2008). Such a perspective is very important for practitioners who care for adults as well as children, and can even help child health practitioners' understanding of the parents and grandparents with whom they work.

Also in contrast to Piaget, Erikson's theory is readily accessible. It was published within a single volume 'Childhood and Society' (Erikson 1950), and later became available in a 'popular' paperback edition (Erikson 1965), which gave wide access to the lay public as well as the professional readership. The core of Erikson's work is his 'eight stages of man' (Erikson 1965; see also Table 2.1), which he sees as a series of conflicts thorough which the developing individual needs to pass. At any point in the process, a developmental conflict can have a negative effect on personality and future development. Importantly though, Erikson's stages cannot be seen as sequential. Although the age groups indicated are likely to represent the earliest point at which that stage becomes significant, the importance of each of the earlier stages is maintained to some extent throughout the lifespan, and is thus vulnerable at any point to deviation into the alternative path.

Activity

Turn to Chapter 2 (**pp 22–23**) and read Hemphill & Dearmun's summary of Erikson's stage theory before reading the rest of this chapter.

Links between Erikson's work, other developmental theories and care delivery

1. Trust versus mistrust

As Hemphill & Dearmun describe in Chapter 2, trust is seen as the essential norm of babies' early experience, in the presence of food, sleep and other essential bodily functions. The infant's first real act of trust is 'to let the mother out of sight without undue anxiety or rage' (Erikson 1965 p 239), arguably based on a certainty that she will always be there to meet his or her needs. This may explain why the younger infant seems to derive positive comfort from parental presence, but not to protest strongly in its absence, in opposition to Piaget's notion of 'object permanence' – 'out of sight' and therefore 'out of mind'. Thus trust is seen to depend on the quality of the maternal relationship (later theorists would include the father and significant others). Although it is part of normal development to recognise the possibility that these support figures may not always be present (hence the protest on separation made by the older infant), prolonged parental separation can be seen to be intrinsically linked to development of 'mistrust', which Erikson would argue can even perpetuate into adulthood. It can thus be seen how closely Erikson's perspective links with Bowlby's (1969) notion of 'attachment' and the need for the infant to have a close and continuous relationship with a 'mother figure' and significant others. It also links with the extensive work surrounding the harmful effects of hospitalisation by Robertson (1952) and others (see Chapter 5 or Taylor et al 1999 for a summary). The widespread belief in the importance of parental presence with children in hospital is testament to the value placed on these theories, and beliefs in the harmful effects of separation.

2. Autonomy versus shame and doubt

As Hemphill & Dearmun explain in Chapter 2, the development of control within aspects of the younger child's world is seen as central to the development of autonomy. 'Shame and doubt' are seen as negative outcomes of this process. To use Erikson's own words:

> For if denied the gradual and well-guided experience of the autonomy of free choice (or if, indeed, weakened by an initial loss of trust) the child will turn against himself …
>
> (Erikson 1965 p 244)

From a nursing care perspective the negative consequences of lack of autonomy for the child will be inappropriate endeavours to gain control in any way possible. Examples could include such phenomena as inappropriate toileting behaviour (e.g. soiling or constipation) or, in an older child, more proactive processes of rebellion and even self-harm. Appropriate levels of autonomy are therefore vital for a child's healthy development, and these principles should be readily reflected in the care of sick or hospitalised children. Although many processes are essential to the child's well-being, choices such as 'which arm is used for a blood test', 'which parent accompanies them for a procedure' or 'whether something happens before or after breakfast', can all help to restore a sense of control for the child in what is often a very threatening and 'controlling' environment. The potential value of such choices to the child's well-being cannot be overestimated.

Reflect on your practice

Consider Sanjay, a 4-year-old boy admitted to hospital following a fractured femur. He must stay on bed rest, on traction, for 5 weeks:

- What are some of the threats to Sanjay's autonomy that exist as a result of this experience?
- What are the realistic choices Sanjay can be given within his treatment and care delivery that can help to minimise the threats to his autonomy?

3. Initiative versus guilt

'Initiative' links in many ways to the notion of autonomy, and characterises development of understanding and the child's active construction of the world, concepts congruent with Vygotskian theory. Erikson sees initiative as fundamental to all learning processes. The child is seen as deriving pleasure from actively setting out to achieve certain goals, and indeed doing so. Key aspects of this stage, as detailed in Chapter 2 by Hemphill & Dearmun, are issues pertaining to psychosexual development. Here, important links with Freudian theory (which Erikson readily identified as influencing his work) can be seen; these will be discussed more fully in the next section.

'Guilt' is closely linked with initiative, in that the child will frequently overstep boundaries. He or she will encounter a range of negative emotions as a result of external, and increasingly internal, regulation of his or her inappropriate behaviour. This stage can thus also be very closely linked to the child's moral development (Santrock 2009). Erikson (1965 p 248) sees the consequence of these processes as the child becoming 'divided in himself' with internalised 'infantile' and 'parental' sets of guidelines emerging in parallel and influencing future aspects of behaviour. In the most extreme cases, children who encounter problems at this stage can require support from experts in child mental health. In contrast, however, most children show a more balanced adherence to 'both selves', requiring regular guidance, but gradually achieving a sense of individual responsibility and 'self-regulation' as they progress through childhood.

4. Industry versus inferiority

This stage is seen as concurrent with the school age child and, as Hemphill & Dearmun describe in more detail in Chapter 2, reflects a central focus on learning and social development. These theories also have implications within the healthcare arena.

For many children, educational processes are continued in hospital settings and individualised programmes of learning are essential to ensure a child's self-esteem is not harmed by this different educational encounter. Also, some procedures that a child undergoes, such as 'bat ear repair', 'birth mark removal', 'hypospadias repair' or 'leg lengthening' will often have primarily social functions, including acceptance of children by their peers. Whereas some would justifiably debate the importance of changing 'societal acceptance of individual differences' rather than changing 'the individual who is different', the potential harm caused to children by teasing and bullying should not be under-estimated. Thus although education of all children in accepting diversity is clearly vital, it is also important that in a fiscally dominated healthcare environment such seemingly 'non-essential' procedures are not lost to the private sector.

5. Identity versus role confusion

This fifth (and final childhood) stage is characteristic of the adolescent and with the development of self-identity. As Hemphill & Dearmun explain in Chapter 2, adolescence represents a particularly turbulent time for the child. Although the reality is that most adolescents 'make it', the potential negative outcome is 'role confusion', which can arise from any number of factors, e.g. uncertainty regarding sexual identity or orientation, uncertainty about future career paths, or coping with delayed physical development. In extreme cases such situations can have a profoundly negative effect on the individual's personality development. However, most adolescents normally experience some elements of 'role confusion', responding by what Erikson (1965 p 253) describes as 'overidentification, to the point of apparent complete loss of identity'. Such overidentification and associated peer pressure might be important influential factors in experimentation with drugs, smoking, alcohol and sexual activity. Thus the need for carefully targeted and insightful health promotion is paramount.

For adolescents who are sick, this can be a particularly difficult time to cope with illness. For many chronically ill children, social and physical development can lag behind that of their well peers, leading to teasing and feelings of alienation. Altered body image (e.g. hair loss in cancer) can also be particularly difficult for this age group to cope with. Even a brief hospital stay can be extremely traumatic, threatening privacy and dignity, new-found autonomy and the fragile sense of self-identity. Adolescent units are widely regarded as the ideal environment for this age group but, to date, most adolescents continue to be cared for in either paediatric or adult environments. Careful consideration must be given by healthcare practitioners to the psychological effects of hospitalisation in either setting and every effort made to minimise such harmful effects (see Taylor et al 1999).

Reflect on your practice

Consider Ania, an adolescent girl aged 13, recently diagnosed with leukaemia. She will require repeated hospital admissions and an extensive programme of chemotherapy:

- What might be some of the psychological challenges and risks Ania faces during her period of illness?
- How can both hospital- and community-based practitioners help Ania to minimise these risks and to emerge from her illness experience with a sense of 'identity' as opposed to 'role confusion'?

Activity

Smith & McSherry (2004) have published a concept analysis of children's understanding of spirituality, which is an important but often under-recognised aspect of children's care delivery. They use Erikson's first five stages to frame their exploration of children's spiritual development.

- Based on what you now know about Erikson's theory, consider the different stages and how each might influence children's spiritual development. Then read the article and compare your thoughts and ideas with those offered by Smith & McSherry.

Sigmund Freud's theory of personality development

Freud (1856–1939) belonged to a school of thought that is often referred to as psychoanalytic, in that it sought to explain individual differences in personality. Erikson represented the same school and his theories are more usually reported in texts after the earlier theories of Freud. Furthermore, Erikson regularly referred to Freudian theory in support of his own hypotheses about human development. However, whereas Erikson's holistic perspective remains widely respected, Freudian theory is often regarded as being somewhat eccentric and 'off beam', largely because of his beliefs around the domination of sexuality on personality development. Yet by relating Freudian theory to the previous consideration of Erikson's work, it can perhaps be seen that Freud's theory does retain some useful practical application for students of child development.

The id, ego and superego

Freud (1938/1973, 1923/1974) (see also Berk 2008, Santrock 2009) recognised three facets of personality: the id, the ego and the superego:

- The id is the inherited component, biologically influenced and desiring immediate gratification of need.
- The ego is an emergent component, influenced by the environment. It regulates the id's desire for immediate gratification into socially acceptable channels.
- The superego is the final component, governing 'conscience'. It is therefore potentially in conflict with the desires of the id.

Parallels can thus already be seen with Erikson's notion of conflict within the different stages of development, which expand Freud's fundamental notions of the relationship between id, ego and superego in mediating individual desires.

Freudian stages of personality development

Freud (1938/1973) further argued that there were five key stages of personality development (see also Berk 2008, Erikson 1965, Santrock 2009, Taylor et al 1999):

1. The oral stage (birth to 1 year)

This stage is dominated by the id, with the gratification of hunger being the primary drive that is satisfied by sucking to take in nutrition. For Freud, lack of gratification of oral urges led to nail biting and thumbsucking, which he regarded as deviant behaviours. Lack of oral gratification has also been used to explain cigarette smoking and excessive eating by older children and adults.

However, 'non-nutritive sucking' of either a dummy/pacifier or fingers is seen as normal within infant development. Indeed, for an infant unable to feed orally, a pacifier is regarded as essential to maintain the sucking reflex. Furthermore, infants clearly derive a great comfort from sucking, which often extends well into childhood. It can be argued that denying the infant the opportunity to suck may be a contributor to the child developing parental 'mistrust' in Eriksonian terms, with consequent problems in the child's future personality development.

The importance of such beliefs is evidenced, for example, in the practice of 'sham feeding'. This historically allowed a child with a long-term gastrointestinal problem, which contraindicated oral feeding (such as tracheo-oesophageal fistula), to take in milk via the mouth and then collect it via an upper oesophageal stoma situated in the neck. This procedure is currently rare because it can be quite distressing for both child and parents, although it is still occasionally seen. But the fact that it exists at all is testimony to the importance placed on oral stimulation in infant development.

2. The anal stage (1–3 years)

In this stage Freud argued that pleasure was primarily gained from the processes of passing urine or having a bowel action. He argued that the role of the ego was to learn that the pleasure had to be appropriately channelled in time or place via the process of 'toilet training'. Thus for Freud a child 'potty trained' too soon may later develop obsession with order and cleanliness (hence the expression 'anally retentive'), whereas a child not properly trained at all is likely to demonstrate untidiness and an acceptance of mess and squalor.

Criticisms of Freudian theory include a rejection of his singular acceptance of the domination of anal pleasure at this point in life. Certainly, it would appear not only that oral pleasures continue but also that many other factors influence the child's experience of pleasure and his or her future personality development. However, in terms of Erikson's notion of autonomy, it can be seen that bladder and bowel function offers children powerful modes of exerting control over their parents or carers. Within normal development this might include the toddler who regularly 'needs a wee' in the middle of dinner (unless it is something he or she especially likes!) but it can also have more extreme manifestations. At a conscious or subconscious level constipation is seen as having significant psychological components for many children, and is frequently linked to other behavioural problems (Smith & Ward 2003). In terms of seeking attention, inappropriate passing of urine or faeces is also a good way for the desired attention to be achieved; remember a child who receives inadequate attention will often choose chastisement in preference to no attention at all.

3. The phallic stage (3–6 years)

This stage is perhaps the one that caused the greatest controversy when Freud's theories were first published. He argued that pleasure is now derived from genitally focused desires. He suggested that boys feel sexual desire for their mother but fear their father's disapproval. Consequently they end up identifying with the father and adopting the father's personality characteristics, behaviours and beliefs. For girls the reverse situation exists, i.e. paternal desire and maternal identification. Freud refers to these phases respectively as the oedipal phase and the Electra complex, and saw the resolution of this conflict as effectively the development of the superego and the individual's personality.

These theories have been widely and controversially used to describe a whole range of phenomena, including promiscuity, frigidity and deviant sexual behaviour. Evidence to support such beliefs remains minimal but many psychologists nevertheless retain some respect for aspects of Freudian theory. Links can be seen between the Eriksonian notion of 'guilt' and Freudian beliefs that morality and the conscience were products of the child's resolution of his or her desires for the opposite sex parent. However, although such extreme beliefs remain controversial, it would appear probable that, at some level, parental attitudes, behaviours and indeed relationships influence children's sexual development (Lips 1997).

For boys, Freud also described an important additional phenomenon he referred to as castration anxiety, which he saw as a fear of genital mutilation based on a belief that girls might have once had a penis that had been 'cut off' as a punishment. This theory is particularly pertinent for child health practitioners caring for boys who require procedures such as circumcision or hypospadias repair (hypospadias being a urethral opening not at the end of the penis; Atwell 1997). Boys with hypospadias, for example, often require repeated operations, and the psychological consequences of such experiences perhaps remain both under-recognised and under-researched.

4. The latency period (6 years to puberty)

For Freud, this stage was one in which sexual desire and instinct were repressed, hence the preference for friends of the same sex. Curiously, as the title 'latency' suggests, Freud believed little of importance would happen in the absence of sexual development. For Erikson, by contrast, this latency was put to good use in the notion of 'industry' as the child focuses on the processes of academic learning and ongoing social development.

5. The genital stage (puberty onwards)

This stage is characterised by the emergence of adult sexual desire, and all the repressed sexual desires of childhood can now be appropriately channelled into sexual relationships with

Reflect on your practice

Imagine you are caring for Matthew, a 4-year-old child who has been admitted with a history of severe constipation and soiling, which requires intervention under anaesthesia as well as laxative drug therapy. No physiological cause for the problem has been identified. His older brother, Jacob, has severe Down syndrome and his parents are currently considering separating:

- How might you consider Matthew's problems in Freudian and Eriksonian terms?
- What advice and support might his parents be given to help overcome the problem?

partners. This forms an important part of Erikson's views of the adolescent's search for identity, although for Erikson it was balanced by recognition of other important factors in adolescent development. Nevertheless, sexual identity is recognised as a vital part of adolescent development and the perceived appropriateness or inappropriateness of various sexual activities would appear to be an ongoing and cyclic process within different cultures and generations. Currently, within Western society, views on sexual behaviour have been greatly influenced by the existence of effective contraception, and also more recently by the emergence of human immunodeficiency virus (HIV) (Lips 1997). Thus, although recent decades have seen relaxation in attitudes towards sexual behaviour, there is an important need to convey responsibility around sexual health, and the risks of both teenage pregnancy and virus transmission. Child health professionals and schoolteachers are seen as having a pivotal role in the education of children and adolescents in these domains, hence the emergent concept of PSHE.

Some important observations about 'truth' and 'understanding' in developmental psychology

When studying developmental psychology, including the range of seminal theories considered here, there are important observations to be made with regard to the difference between primary and secondary sources; recognition of these factors is important for any student of the subject. For example, when considering the work of Piaget it is usual for authors constructing a portrayal of his theory to use a whole range of secondary sources. The reason for this is that, for a significant proportion of his life, Piaget published virtually a book a year, and thus it is only at doctorate level that the student of Piaget can hope to comprehensively study his original work and synthesise from it an overview of his perspectives on child development. Even then they are likely to be reliant on someone else's translation of French into English!

Furthermore, as Piaget grew older, his views and perspectives changed, and thus his assertions in the 1920s tend to differ somewhat from his perspective when he was still writing in the 1970s. But reliance on secondary sources is inevitably accompanied by a degree of risk in terms of the extent to which they truly represent what Piaget said; indeed it is probable that many texts have themselves used earlier secondary sources, and so on ad infinitum. (If you doubt this, one key original Piaget text borrowed for this chapter from a major university library had last been borrowed 13 years ago!) Consequently, the theory portrayed might have strayed somewhat from the original; distorted in the telling like a childhood game of 'Chinese whispers'. Thus the 'Piagetian perspective' on child development may be attributable as much to the speculation of others as to the work of Piaget himself.

In seeking to illustrate this point, the student seeking clear elucidation of the 'four stages of cognitive development', for example, is likely to have a long and difficult search through Piaget's original work. What one finds repeatedly is a range of developing ideas and debates (e.g. as in his 1929 'Children's conceptualisation of the world'). However, although Piaget (1929) is frequently cited as the source of the 'four stages' so widely quoted, these are at best implicitly contained within a series of observations he made of different children and their responses to various abstract questions. Even Piaget & Inhelder (1969), offered as a summary of Piaget's work 'so far', appears nearer to, but still someway off, the neat 'four-stage' theory with which we are familiar. By contrast, the student of Erikson's work will have no such challenges, being able to read the 'eight stages of man' within a single chapter of his original work (Erikson 1965).

What is important, then, is that all who cite the work of developmental psychologists – especially the seminal authors – must be sure always to acknowledge their sources, whether primary or secondary, and always try to use primary sources wherever possible. The importance of this is not only in seeking to minimise the 'Chinese whisper' effect but also in being able to openly acknowledge the inherent biases that different students of developmental psychology inevitably have. The author of this chapter, for example, openly acknowledges and articulates her doubts about the appropriateness of many Piagetian theories to contemporary child health practice. But other authors will argue from a far more pro-Piagetian stance and in contrast might be much more critical of the work of Vygotsky or Erikson, for example.

Ultimately, then, it is up to each reader to make up his or her own mind based on the available information, opinion and evidence. The plea therefore within this chapter, is not for you to adopt 'wholesale' the theories and perspectives offered. Rather, it is that you read as widely and critically as possible, engage in debate with peers and professional colleagues, and take every opportunity to reflect upon the extent to which the different theories are borne out by current best evidence and practice experience. Only in this way can you make a fully informed decision about these theoretical perspectives and their practical application, and make judgements regarding which theories best inform contemporary healthcare practice and have the greatest potential to enhance care delivery.

Summary

This chapter has offered the reader a review of seminal and contemporary theories pertaining to children's psychological development. Particular emphasis has been placed on the importance of cognitive development, language development and personality development, as it is these aspects of psychological development that are seen as having particular relevance to the health care of children and families provided by the child healthcare practitioner.

In reviewing these theories, clear links can be seen throughout with the care that children and families receive. In particular, understanding of psychological theory can be seen as influencing communication with children, the quality of explanation giving, the quality of preparation and a minimising of the harmful effects of hospitalisation.

However, what the chapter has hopefully also offered the reader is an opportunity to reflect on the contrasting theories and theoretical perspectives that influence how psychologists, educators and healthcare practitioners view child development. In contrast to some aspects of care delivery, where best available evidence clearly supports a particular approach to treatment, aspects of psychological care are often subject to differences in opinion and ongoing debate. Thus, although few would debate the importance of minimising the potentially harmful effects of parent/child separation for example, other aspects of psychological care remain a matter of opinion. Thus there is arguably an ongoing need for much more in the way of focused, applied research into many of the aspects of care delivery debated within this chapter.

This being said, it is hoped that the insight gained from studying this chapter will offer the student of children's nursing a useful guide to some of the key child developmental theories, and their potential application to children's nursing practice. Although physical care is infinitely more measurable than psychological care, the latter is arguably no less important in all but the most critically ill child. Thus if this chapter leads the reader to pause and consider the importance of these psychological perspectives within care delivery, then there is a very real chance that the insight gained could make a considerable difference to the quality of care which children and families receive.

References

Alderson, P., 1993. Children's consent to surgery. Open University Press, Buckingham.

Alderson, P., Montgomery, J., 1996. Children's services. What about me? Health Service Journal 106 (5498), 22–24.

Atwell, J., 1997. Paediatric surgery. Arnold, London.

Barnes, K., 2003. Paediatrics: a clinical guide for nurse practitioners. Butterworth Heinemann, Edinburgh.

Bee, H., Boyd, D., 2008. Lifespan development. Pearson Education, New Jersey.

Berger, K., 2008. The developing person through the lifespan, 7th revised edn. Worth Publishers, New York.

Berk, L., 2006. Development through the lifespan, 4th Edn. Pearson Education, New Jersey.

Berk, L., 2008. Child development, 8th edn. Pearson Education, New Jersey.

Betz, C., 2000. California healthy and ready to work transition health guidelines: developmental guidelines for teaching health care self care skills to children. Issues in Comprehensive Pediatric Nursing 23 (4), 203–244.

Bibace, R., Walsh, M., 1980. Development of children's concepts of illness. Pediatrics 66 (6), 912–917.

Bibace, R., Walsh, M. (Eds.), 1981. Children's concepts of health, illness and bodily function, Jossey-Bass, San Francisco.

Bird, J., Podmore, V., 1990. Children's understanding of health and illness. Psychology and Health 4, 175–185.

Bluebond-Langer, M., 1989. Worlds of dying children and their well siblings. Death Studies 13, 1–16.

Bowlby, J., 1969. Attachment and loss. Hogarth Press, London vol. 1.

Bruner, J.S., 1972. The relevance of education. Allen and Unwin, London.

Bruner, J.S., 1983. Child's talk: learning to use language. WW Norton, New York.

Burbach, D., Peterson, L., 1986. Children's concepts of physical illness: a review and critique of the cognitive developmental literature. Health Psychology 5, 307–325.

Carey, S., 1985. Conceptual change in childhood. MIT Press, Cambridge, MA.

Channel 4 Television, 2001. The child as thinker. Part 4 of the 6-part series The child's world. Broadcast 10 January 2001. Channel Four Television, London.

Chomsky, N., 1957. Systematic structures. Mouton, The Hague.

Crisp, J., Ungerer, J., Goodnow, J., 1996. The impact of experience on children's understanding of illness. Journal of Pediatric Psychology 21 (1), 57–72.

Daly, M., Byers, E., Taylor, W., 2006. Understanding early years theory in practice: an accessible overview of early years theory. Heinemann. Oxford.

Donaldson, M., 1978. Children's minds. Fontana Press, Glasgow.

Eiser, C., 1989. Children's concepts of illness: towards an alternative to the stage approach. Psychology and Health 3, 93–101.

Elliott, E., Watson, A., 2000. Children's voices in health care planning. In: Glasper, E.A., Ireland, L. (Eds.), Evidence-based child health care. Macmillan, Basingstoke.

Erikson, E., 1950. Childhood and society. WW Norton, New York.

Erikson, E., 1965. Childhood and society, revised edn. Penguin, London.

Fox, C., Buchanan-Barrow, E., Barrett, M., 2008. Children's understanding of mental illness: an exploratory study. Childcare. Health and Development 34 (1), 10–18.

Franck, L., Sheikh, A., Oulton, K., 2008. What helps when it hurts: children's views on pain relief. Childcare. Health and Development 34 (4), 430–438.

Freud, S., 1973. An outline of psychoanalysis. Hogarth Press, London (original work published 1938).

Freud, S., 1974. The ego and the id. Hogarth Press, London (original work published 1923).

Gaffney, A., 2000. Pain and Piaget: qualitative change with age in the content area about children's ideas of pain. The Irish Journal of Psychology 21 (3-4), 194–202.

Gaudion, C., 1997. Children's knowledge of their internal anatomy. Paediatric Nursing 9 (5), 14–17.

Harbech, C., Peterson, L., 1992. Elephants dancing on my head: a developmental approach to children's concepts of specific pains. Child Development 63, 138–149.

Hergenrather, J., Rabinowitz, M., 1991. Age-related differences in the organisation of children's knowledge of illness. Developmental Psychology 27 (6), 952–959.

Holaday, B., LaMontagne, L., Marciel, J., 1994. Vygotsky's zone of proximal development: implications for nurse assistance of children's learning. Issues in Comprehensive Paediatric Nursing 17, 15–27.

Ireland, L.M., 1997. Children's perceptions of asthma: establishing normality. British Journal of Nursing 6 (18), 1059–1064.

Kister, M., Patterson, C., 1980. Children's conceptions of the causes of illness: understanding contagion and use of imminent justice. Child Development 51, 839–846.

Lips, H., 1997. Sex and gender: an introduction, 3rd edn. Mayfield Publishing, Mountain View, CA.

Longsdon, D., 1991. Conceptions of health and health behaviours of preschool children. Journal of Paediatric Nursing 6 (6), 396–406.

McDonald, H., Rushforth, H., 2006. Children's views of nursing and Medical roles: implications for advanced nursing practice. Paediatric Nursing 18 (5), 32–36.

McEwing, G., 1996. Children's understanding of their internal body parts. British Journal of Nursing 5 (7), 423–429.

McGrath, P., Huff, N., 2001. What is it? Findings of pre-schoolers responses to play with medical equipment. Child Care. Health and Development 27 (5), 451–462.

Meadows, S., The child as thinker. 2nd edn. Routledge, London.

Myant, K., Williams, J., 2008. What do children learn about biology from factual information? A comparison of interventions to improve understanding of contagious illnesses. British Journal of Educational Psychology 78 (2), 223–244.

Myant, K., Williams, J., 2005. Children's concepts of health and illness: understanding of contagious illness, non-contagious illness and injuries. Journal of Health Psychology 10 (6), 805–819.

Oakley, A., Bendelow, G., Barnes, J., et al., 1995. Health and cancer prevention: knowledge and beliefs of children and young people. British Medical Journal 310, 1029–1033.

Perrin, E., Gerrity, P.S., 1981. There's a demon in your belly: children's understanding of illness. Pediatrics 67 (6), 841–849.

Piaget, J., 1929. The child's conception of the world. Routledge and Kegan Paul, London.

Piaget, J., 1930. The child's conception on physical causality. Kegan Paul, Trench, Trubner and Co, New York.

Piaget, J., Inhelder, B., 1956. The child's conception of space. Routledge and Kegan Paul, London.

Piaget, J., Inhelder, B., 1969. The psychology of the child. Routledge and Kegan Paul, London.

Piko, B., Bak, J., 2006. Children's perceptions of health and illness: images and lay concepts in pre-adolescence. Health Education Research 21 (5), 643–653.

Robertson, J., 1952. A two-year-old goes to hospital (film). In: Taylor, J. (Ed.), 1999 Nursing children: psychology, research and practice, 3rd edn. Stanley Thornes, Cheltenham.

Rovee-Colyer C 1987 Learning and memory in children. In: Osofsky JD (ed.) Handbook of infant development, 2nd edn. Wiley, New York. Cited by: Santrock J 1999 Life-span development, 7th edn. McGraw Hill College, Boston

Rushforth, H., 1996. Nurses' knowledge of how children view health and illness. Paediatric Nursing 8 (9), 23–27.

Rushforth, H., 1999. Practitioner review: communicating with hospitalised children. Journal of Child Psychology and Psychiatry 40 (5), 683–691.

Santrock, J., 1999. Life-span development, 7th edn. McGraw Hill College, Boston.

Santrock, J., 2009. Life-span development, 12th edn. McGraw Hill College, Boston.

Schmidt, C., 2001. Development of children's body knowledge using lungs as an exemplar. Issues in Comprehensive Pediatric Nursing 24 (3), 177–191.

Shayer, M., 2003. Not just Piaget, not just Vygotsky, and certainly not Vygotsky as an alternative to Piaget. Learning and Instruction 13 (5), 465–485.

Siegal, M., Peterson, C., 1999. Children's understanding of biology and health. Cambridge University Press, Cambridge.

Skinner, B.F., 1957. Verbal behaviour. Appleton Century Crofts, New York.

Smith, J., McSherry, W., 2004. Spirituality and child development: a concept analysis. Journal of Advanced Nursing 45 (3), 307–315.

Smith, L., Ward, C., 2003. Childhood constipation and encopresis. In: Barnes, K. (Ed.), Paediatrics: a clinical guide for nurse practitioners. Butterworth Heinemann, Edinburgh.

Taylor, J., Woods, M., 2005. Early childhood studies, 2nd edn. Hodder Arnold, London.

Taylor, J., Muller, D., Wattley, L., Harris, P., 1999. Nursing children: psychology, research and practice, 3rd edn. Stanley Thornes, Cheltenham.

Twycross, A., 1998. Children's cognitive level and perception of pain. Paediatric Nursing 14 (1), 35–37.

Vacik, H.W., Nagy, C.M., Jessee, P.O., 2001. Children's understanding of illness: students' assessments. Journal of Pediatric Nursing 16 (6), 429–437.

Veldtman, G., Matley, S., Kendall, L., Quirk, J., Gibbs, J., Parsons, J., Hewison, J., 2000. Illnesss understanding in children and adolescents with heart disease. Heart 84, (4), 395–397.

Vessey, J., 1988. Comparison of two teaching methods on children's knowledge of their internal bodies. Nursing Research 37, 262–267.

Vygotsky, L.S., 1962. Thought and language. MIT Press, Cambridge, MA.

Vygotsky, L.S., 1978. Mind in society. Harvard University Press, Cambridge, MA.

Williams, C., 1995. Children's understanding of treatment in the A&E department. British Journal of Nursing 4 (7), 385–387.

Williams, J., Binnie, L., 2002. Children's concepts of illness: an intervention to improve knowledge. British Journal of Health Psychology 7 (2), 129–148.

Wood, D., 1988. How children think and learn. Blackwell, Oxford.

Yoos, H.L., 1994. Children's illness concepts: old and new paradigms. Pediatric Nursing (US) 20 (2), 134–140.

Physical growth and development in children

12

Janet Kelsey Gill McEwing

ABSTRACT

This chapter will give the reader a broad understanding of the growth and development of children. Physical growth will be defined and methods of measurement discussed. Normal stages of child development are described and activities suggested to encourage the reader to make links with practice.

LEARNING OUTCOMES

- Define growth and development and understand how they can be assessed.
- Demonstrate an understanding of the anatomy and physiology of the newborn baby.
- Gain an overview of the development of the child from birth to adolescence.
- Be aware of the importance of assessing child development and the detection of deviations from normal.

Introduction

The physical development of the child is only one aspect of its whole development, which includes cognitive, social and emotional elements. Inherited attributes and environmental factors will affect physical development. These factors interact to cause effects on the child's development from conception to adulthood.

Babies and children vary considerably in exactly when and in what way they progress in all areas of development. It is not always appropriate to assign exact ages in months and years to stages of development, although an approximate age range is possible.

Activity

- Write down what you think is meant by the terms 'growth' and 'development'.
- Why might it be important to you as a nurse to have some understanding of the growth and development of children?

Factors affecting growth and development

- Genetic/chromosomal factors: inherited rate of growth and individual differences
- Racial factors
- Endocrine system
- Drugs
- Illness: children grow more slowly during periods of illness but there might be increased growth to catch up after recovery
- Nutrition: poorly nourished children grow more slowly and do not reach their full potential size; malnutrition can have a permanent effect on some parts of the brain and nervous system
- Environment: the ability to practise skills, e.g. crawling, walking.

Other factors also govern growth and physical changes. Hormones are the most important of these (Table 12.1).

Physical growth

Physical growth and maturation is important for child development. Maturation is the:

> ... universal sequence of biological events occurring in the body and the brain that permits psychological function to appear, provided that the infant is healthy and lives in an environment containing people and objects
>
> (Mussen et al 1990)

Growth is defined as an increase in the size of and number of cells that results in an increase in size and weight of the whole, or any of its parts. In clinical practice, growth of the infant is generally measured by estimating the weight, length, head circumference and, in certain circumstances, skin-fold thickness.

DOI: 10.1016/B978-0-7020-3183-0.10012-8

Table 12.1 The hormones involved in growth and physical development

Gland	Hormone	Aspects of growth
Thyroid	Thyroxine	Normal brain development and overall rate of growth
Adrenal	Adrenal androgen	Involved in some changes at puberty, particularly the development of secondary sex characteristics in girls
Testes	Testosterone	Formation of male genitals before birth. Also triggers the sequence of changes in primary and secondary sex characteristics at puberty in the male
Ovaries	Oestradiol	Development of the menstrual cycle and breasts in girls. Less important than testosterone for secondary sex characteristics in boys
Pituitary	Growth hormone activating hormone	Rate of physical maturation. Signals other glands to secrete hormones

Pattern of growth

The most obvious thing about children's physical development is that they get bigger as they get older. Growth proceeds in a continuous pattern but is not smooth; the most rapid growth takes place in utero, the first 2 years of life and during adolescence (Fig. 12.1). However, acceleration and deceleration occur in response to illness and changes in nutrition or environment. As Figure 12.1 shows, infants grow very quickly in the first year of life, adding 25–30 cm to their height.

Children gain weight at an equally rapid rate, doubling birth weight by the age of 5–6 months and tripling it by the end of the first year. The birth size of a normal infant is determined by the mother. Inherited factors, however, are one of the greatest influences affecting the final stature of the child. Although children tend to attain a stature between those of their parents, some children take after one parent, a grandparent or even a more remote member of the family.

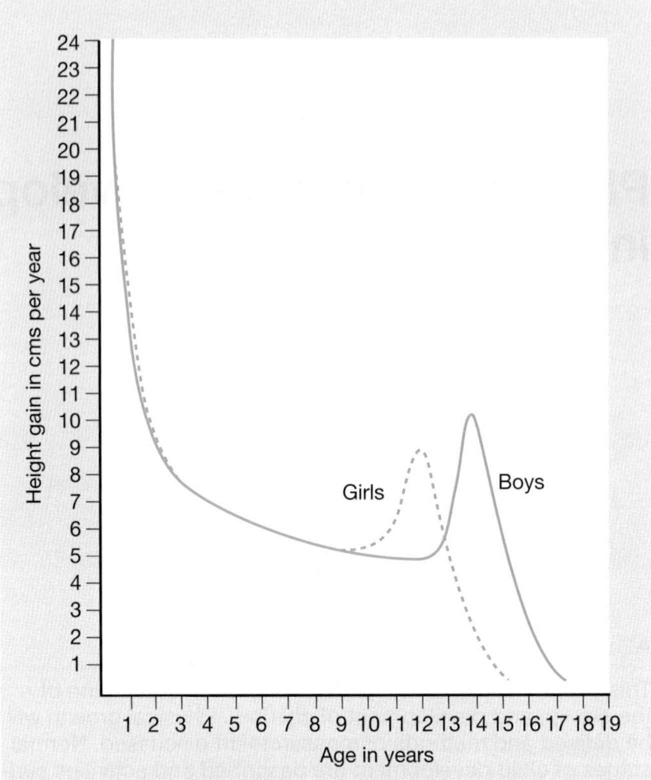

Fig. 12.1 • Rates of growth (adapted from Bee 1997).

Measuring growth

Length/height

An infant's recumbent length is measured supine on a measuring board, placing the head firmly at the top of the board and the heels of the feet at the foot-board (Figs 12.2 and 12.3).

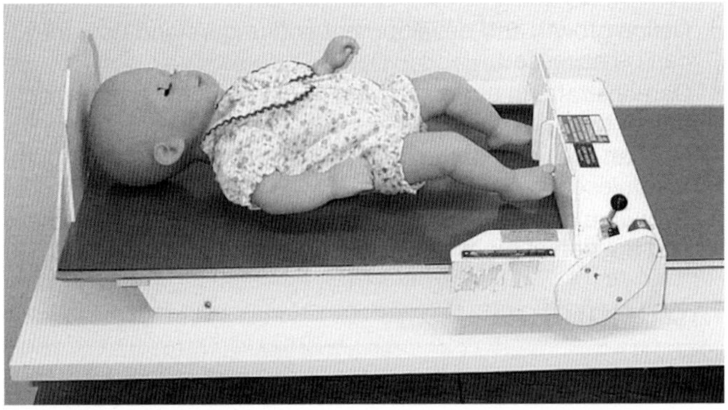

Fig. 12.2 • Infant length.

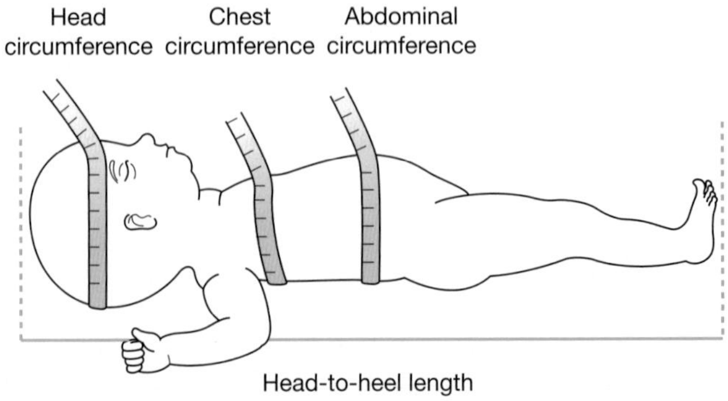

Fig. 12.3 • Measurement of the head, chest, abdominal circumference and the recumbent length.

Classic clues: height

The height of an infant increases by around 12 cm during the first 6 months of life. By the age of 1 year, the height has increased by almost 50% and by the age of 2 years an infant is about half as tall as he or she will be as an adult (Bee 1997). There is a rapid increase in size during the first 2 years, which then settles down to a slower and steadier rate: 5–7.5 cm in height per year and 3 kg in weight per year. Adolescence then brings a 'growth spurt', following which height and weight are slowly gained until adult size is achieved.

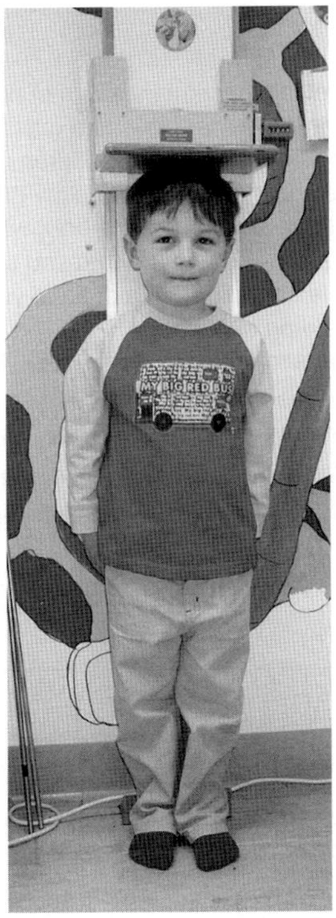

Fig. 12.4 • Child height.

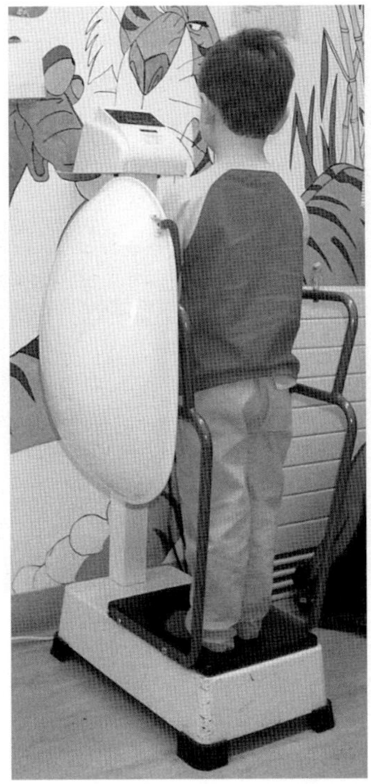

Fig. 12.5 • Child weight.

Height is the measurement taken when children are measured upright. Shoes should be removed and the child should stand as tall and straight as possible with the head in mid-line and the line of vision parallel to the floor. The most accurate measurement of height is gained by using a wall-mounted stadiometer (Fig. 12.4). It might be useful to remember that the height will be less when measured in the afternoon than in the morning. This effect can be reduced by applying modest upward pressure under the jaw or mastoid process.

Classic clues: weight

On average an infant gains 600–800 g in weight per month. An infant's weight at 6 months will therefore be almost double the birth weight. By the first year of life, weight has tripled.

Weight

Infants should be weighed naked and preferably at the same time of the day. Older children can be weighed in light clothing without their shoes (Fig. 12.5).

Head circumference

This measurement is important because the size of the skull is closely related to the size of the brain. It is usually recorded in children who are under 3 years of age or in cases where the growth of the brain/skull is under observation. It is advisable to use a paper disposable tape measure for this measurement as linen tape measures stretch and produce inaccurate results (Hockenberry et al 2003). The head should be measured around the point of greatest circumference, this is usually slightly above the eyebrows and pinna of the ears and around the occipital prominence at the back of the skull.

Classic clues: head circumference

The head growth of an infant is rapid. In the first 6 months the circumference increases by between 8 and 9 cm. By the first year there is an increase of 33% in the overall size of the head.

Surface area

The child's surface area can be calculated once the height and weight of the child is known using the body surface area nomogram. This measurement is important for the prescription of some drugs.

Activity

Find a copy of the body surface area nomogram and calculate the body surface area for:

- a newborn weighing 3 kg and 50 cm in length
- a 6-year-old child weighing 20 kg and with a height of 115 cm.

Skinfold thickness

Skinfold thickness is a quick and easy method of measuring subcutaneous fat that allows for the estimation of an individual's body fat. The most common site for measuring skinfold thickness is the triceps; others include the subscapula, suprailiac, abdomen and upper thigh. The measurement is made by pinching the skin between two fingers and measuring the skinfold thickness using specially designed callipers (Fig. 12.6).

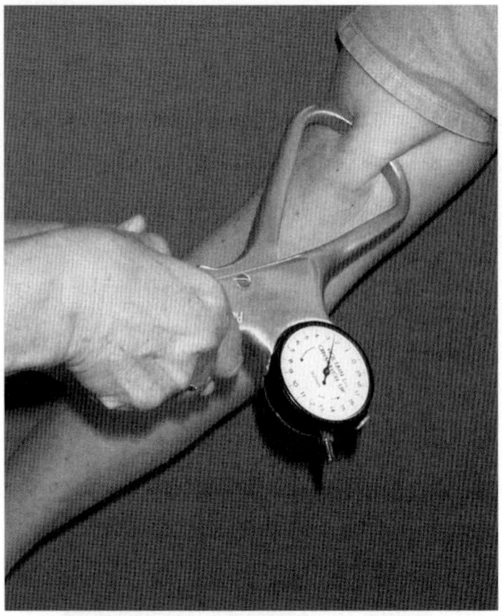

Fig. 12.6 • Skinfold thickness.

Bone age

Bone age is a method of measuring skeletal maturity; the appearance of the epiphyseal centres is compared with standard charts. This is best achieved using the child's left wrist and hand, where the 20 bones can be judged against that recognised as the normal pattern of development.

Activity

Two groups of factors that strongly influence normal growth and development are heredity and environment. From your observations of children, give two examples from each group.

WWW

Go to:

- http://www.nelh.shef.ac.uk

Search for and read the growth reference charts, paying attention to the recommendations of the expert consensus group on the use of growth reference charts in the UK.

Assessment of growth

Centile charts have been developed using statistics of children's growth patterns. They give estimations of expected height, weight and head circumference for boys and girls at different ages. An infant usually has a similar centile at birth for head circumference and weight. Children of large parents tend to be towards the 90th centile and those of small parents tend towards the 10th, most will remain on these centiles for the rest of their lives. A common problem in the paediatric outpatient department is short parents who think that their child is not growing as expected because he or she is not as big as their peers. Plotting growth measurements confirms that the child's growth is normal and that the child's final size will be similar to that of the parents.

Activity

Percentile charts provide a useful measure of normal growth. Different charts are available for boys and girls, for different age groups and for different cultures. Children may need to be assessed if they are above the 97th or below the 3rd centile. Some show height and weight measurements only, whereas others also show head circumference. To ensure that you understand the format of a percentile chart, look at a chart in your practice area and answer the following questions:

- What sex, age and measurements does it cover?
- Which percentiles does it show?
- Where on the chart would you find a child of abnormal growth?
- If Helen is 3.5 years and 98 cm tall, which percentile is she on?
- How many children fall below the 50th centile and how many above?
- John is on the 90th centile. Is he above or below the average for his age?

Activity

Plot the following weight, height/length and head circumferences on to growth charts from your practice area.

John (male)

Age	*Weight (kg)*	*Head (cm)*	*Length (cm)*
Birth (40 weeks)	3.5	34	51
6 weeks	5	38	56
20 weeks	7.25	42	66
36 weeks	9.75	46	72

Rebecca (female)

Age	*Weight (kg)*	*Head (cm)*	*Length (cm)*
Birth (37 weeks)	2.6	34	50
4 weeks	4	36	52
12 weeks	6.25	41	61
40 weeks	9.25	44.25	68

Some children resemble one parent more than the other in final size. If only their weights are recorded, they may appear to have faltering growth if father is small, or gaining weight excessively if father is tall. If weight is plotted against head circumference then they can be seen to be running in parallel, i.e. the whole of the child's size is approaching that of a particular parent.

Growth charts give an early warning of some problems, such as obesity, which will be indicated by the child's weight starting to deviate upwards even though the head circumference remains on the same centile.

Changes in shape and proportion

After 2 years, the rate of growth slows down and the child gains approximately 2.7 kg in weight each year until adolescence. Changes in proportion and shape take place at the same time. An adult's head is an eighth of his total height but in a 2-year-old the head is a quarter of the total body length. In addition to this, a 2-year-old has a large body and shorter legs in proportion to that of an adult (Bee 1997).

If a child is growing and his or her shape is altering then there must be changes occurring in the child's bones, muscles and fat. Bones increase in number, become longer and grow harder. Although bones are not all formed at birth, the newborn baby has virtually all the muscle fibres that will ever be needed. As a child grows, the muscle fibres get longer, thicker and less watery.

Development

According to the Penguin dictionary (Allan 2001), the definition of development is 'to bring out the possibilities of something, to acquire gradually'. It is the sequence of organic changes by which the fertilised ovum becomes the mature human being. An increase in complexity of the individual involves structure and function; the emerging of an individual's capacities through learning, growth and maturation. Maturation can be defined as an increase in competence and adaptability; a change in the complexity of a structure that makes it possible for that structure to work. Many of the debates about child development have centred on the nature versus nurture controversy. The former believe that human behaviour is guided by inborn factors and argues that differences are a result of heredity. Those who err towards nurture stress the importance of acknowledging the influence of a child's physical and social environment. According to them, individual differences are a result of the child's life experiences. The reality is probably somewhere in between. What is certain is that development is a complex process in which many variables play a part. We as nurses need to assess each child on an individual basis.

Measuring development

Development is measured using developmental scales. It is divided into four major areas:

1. Physical: growth, vision, hearing, locomotion, coordination.
2. Cognitive: language and understanding.
3. Psychosocial: adapting to the society and culture to which the child belongs.
4. Emotional: control of feelings and emotions.

As with growth we need to have some idea of what is the norm. The charts by Sheridan (1997) and Frankenburg & Dodds (1967) (the Denver Developmental Screening Test) were developed to show what can be expected at key stages of development. Sheridan (1997) is a little didactic, she herself suggested that her charts should be used only by experienced professionals. The Denver scale is a little more flexible, allowing the assessor to accommodate the individuality of the child, although it is suggested that the user should be trained in the use of the scale.

Differences in rate

There may be individual differences in the rate and timing of developmental progress, e.g. three perfectly normal infants may sit unaided at 5, 6 or 9 months. However, the sequence of developmental progress is always the same. A child may be consistently early, average or slow in development, e.g. a child whose bone development is slower probably walks later and eventually reaches puberty later.

The development of walking can be used to illustrate the factors that influence growth and development (Bee 1997):

- Newborn infants held with the sole of the foot on a table move their legs in a reflex walking action.
- By 8 weeks: infants briefly hold their head up if held in a standing posture.
- At 36 weeks: infants pull themselves up and remain standing by grasping furniture.
- At 48 weeks: infants walk forwards if both hands are held, or sideways if holding furniture.
- By 52 weeks: infants walk forwards if held by one hand.
- At 13 months: infants walk without help.

Factors required for the development of walking

A complex set of changes occurs in the muscles, bones, and nervous system:

- Nutrition: for growth
- Environment: in which to practice walking
- Genetics: were the parents early walkers?

The child's ability to walk (or not) will also affect other areas of development such as social, emotional and intellectual.

Activity

From your experience of your own childhood, can you think of areas where the rate and timing of the development for certain skills was different between yourself and others. Make some notes about your ideas.

Developmental assessment

In the main, developmental assessments are performed by the child's health visitor and GP, although there might be occasions when a paediatrician will also perform them. These assessments include the evaluation of:

- locomotion or gross motor development referring to large muscle skills
- fine motor or manipulation skills: referring to small muscle skills
- hearing and speech
- vision
- social development, e.g. feeding, dressing and social behaviour.

To assess deviations from normal, it is first necessary to know about normal development. The development of a child between the ages of 0 and 18 months is very complex. These are the major milestones and their approximate age of appearance:

- smile: 1–2 months
- laugh: 6 months
- sits (with support): 6 months

Table 12.2 Interlinked aspects of development

Skill	Information	Activity	Next stage
Drawing	Holding pencil	Drawing	Writing
Running	Spatial awareness	Running	Football, dancing

- sits (without support): 8–9 months
- crawls: 8–9 months
- stands/walks: 12 months
- pincer grip: 12 months
- delicate pincer: 18 months
- walks backwards: 18 months.

Activity

Watch a video showing different aspects of child development, find one at your university library or your local health promotion centre.

All aspects of development are interlinked. Skills are acquired sequentially; an example of this is the sequence of development of motor skills, which is often described as cephalocaudal, i.e. head (cephalo) to toe via the spine (caudal). So, initially, head control is developed before the baby is able to sit independently; this is followed by crawling and finally by control of the lower limbs for standing and walking. Each new skill usually appears at the most appropriate time to make use of information coming in to carry out activities to prepare for the next stage (Table 12.2).

It is important to know about child development to:

- teach and advise parents
- have reasonable expectations of the child
- be able to plan suitable activities and play
- be able to identify limits and capabilities
- be able to recognise deviations from the norm and be alert to regression (behaviour from an earlier stage of development), disability and abnormality.

Transition from intrauterine to extrauterine life

This demands considerable effective physiological changes by the baby to ensure survival. Simultaneously, he or she has to make major adjustments in his or her respiratory and circulatory systems, as well as gaining control of his or her body temperature. The baby emerges to encounter, light, noise, cool air, gravity and tactile stimuli. Adaptation to extrauterine life involves the onset of respiration, circulatory changes and thermal adaptation.

Onset of respiration

Regular respirations begin 60–90 seconds after complete expulsion from the mother as a result of both chemical and thermal stimulation. Thermal stimulation is caused by the sudden cooling of the infant leaving the warm environment of the uterus (37.7°C) and entering the cold atmosphere of the outside environment (approximately 21°C). This cooling excites sensory impulses in the skin that are transmitted to the respiratory centre. In addition, low levels of oxygen, high levels of carbon dioxide and low pH initiate impulses that excite the respiratory centre. At term, approximately 100 mL lung fluid is present within the respiratory tract. Some fluid is expelled through the mouth, assisted by the pressure on the thorax during vaginal delivery; the remainder is absorbed via the pulmonary lymphatics during the first 24 hours of life. The first breath requires a large pressure to open the terminal airways and overcome the initial stiffness of the lungs.

Table 12.3 Newborn measurements

	Girls	Boys
Weight on 50th centile	3.4 kg	3.5 kg
Length on 50th centile	50 cm	51 cm
Occipitofrontal circumference on 50th centile	34.5 cm	35 cm

Circulatory changes

Separated from the placenta, the infant must make major adjustments within the circulatory system to divert deoxygenated blood to the lungs for reoxygenation. The transition from fetal to postnatal circulation involves the closure of the foramen ovale, the ductus arteriosus and the ductus venosus.

Fetal blood pressure (BP) is low as a result of low vascular resistance in the placental circuit. A systolic BP of around 76 mmHg is found at birth; this level rises to 96 mmHg by 4 weeks. Coughing, crying and straining raise the BP.

The newborn baby

Measurements

The average measurements at the 50th centile are shown in Table 12.3. The weight of the infant at birth also correlates with the incidence of perinatal morbidity and mortality. At birth, head circumference head is usually 2–3 cm greater than the circumference of the chest.

Appearance

- Head: one-quarter the body size (Fig. 12.7).
- Plump.
- Prominent abdomen.
- Lies in an attitude of flexion.
- Lusty cry used to evoke a response from attendants with a view to controlling environment.

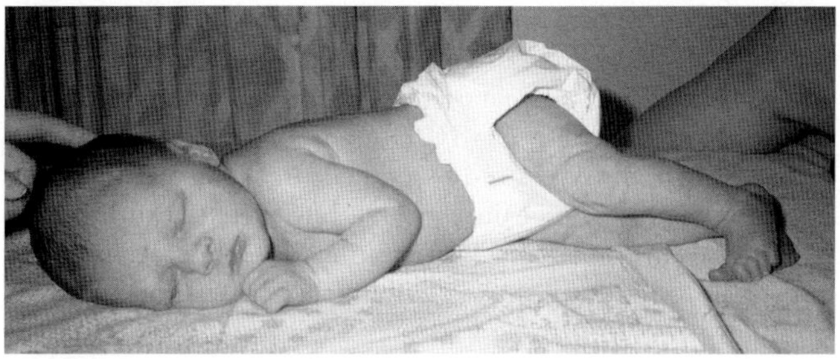

Fig. 12.7 • The newborn baby.

The skin

The skin has a film of vernix caseosa – a white sticky substance that is absorbed within a few hours and thought to have a protective function. The skin is thin and delicate; it is prone to blistering, infection and excoriation. Lanugo (downy hair) covers the skin and is plentiful over the shoulders, upper arms and thighs. Colour depends on ethnic origin.

Sebaceous glands are active late in fetal life and early infancy because of the high levels of maternal androgens. Plugging of the sebaceous glands causes milia. The epidermis and dermis are loosely bound to each other and very thin; friction such as removing sticky tape can separate the layers and cause blistering. The eccrine sweat glands (found mainly on the palms of the hands and the soles of the feet and forehead) are functional at birth and respond to heat and emotional stimulus. By the age of 43 weeks, palmar sweating can be used in pain assessment. The mature baby has many skin creases on its palms and soles; the nails are fully formed and adhere to the fingertips. Melanin levels are low at birth therefore the skin of the newborn is lighter than that it will be as a child, which means that young babies are more susceptible to the harmful effects of the sun. The hair is soft and silky; there may be lots or nearly none. The same is true for the eyebrows. The cartilage of the ears is well formed. The cord stump necroses and falls off within the first 10 days of life.

Genitalia and breasts

In both sexes the breasts may be enlarged in the period immediately after birth. They may also discharge clear fluid. This is due to the stimulation caused by maternal hormones; these effects subside in the first few weeks of extrauterine life (MacGregor 2000). There are nodules of breast tissue around the nipple. The testes are descended and the scrotum has plenty of rugae, the prepuce is adherent to the glans penis. The labia majora cover the labia minora.

Thermoregulation

Heat regulation is critical to the newborn baby's survival. The baby's capacity for heat production is adequate but several factors predispose to excessive heat loss. The newborn's large surface area increases the possibility of heat loss to the environment, although this is normally partially compensated for by their position flexion, which effectively decreases the amount of surface area exposed to the environment. The subcutaneous fat layer is thin, giving poor insulation. This also allows transfer of core heat to the environment and cooling of blood. The hypothalamus in the brain has the capacity to promote heat production in response to stimuli received to thermoreceptors. Babies cannot shiver, nor are they able to voluntarily increase muscle activity to generate heat. Infants do produce heat by non-shivering thermogenesis and that generated by the heart, liver, brain and skeletal muscles.

Noradrenaline (norephinephrine) is secreted by the sympathetic nerve endings in response to chilling and stimulates fat metabolism in brown adipose tissue (BAT); this is unique to the newborn baby. BAT has a greater capacity for heat production through intensified metabolic activity than ordinary adipose tissue. BAT is situated between the scapulae, around the neck, in the axilla, behind the sternum, and around the kidneys, trachea, oesophagus, adrenal glands and some arteries. However, this process does require energy, so the infant's oxygen requirement will increase. The regeneration of this tissue also requires good nutrition; a poor calorie intake will mean that the brown fat is not replaced and the infant will be less able to maintain body heat in a cool environment. Healthy, clothed infants will maintain their temperature provided the environmental temperature is maintained between 18°C and 20°C, nutrition is adequate and movements are not restricted. The temperature of the newborn is 37.5°C and by the age of 13 years it has reduced to 36.6°C; this is because infants produce more heat per kilogram body weight than older children. The temperature regulatory system is immature in the newborn infant, rendering infants and small children susceptible to temperature fluctuations. Factors such as environmental temperature, increased activity, crying or infection can cause a rapid increase in body temperature in the infant.

Eyes

At birth, the eyeball is too short for its lens therefore babies focus best at approximately 20 cm (Fig. 12.8). As the eyeball continues to grow, distance vision is achieved. The ciliary muscles are immature, limiting the ability of the eyes to accommodate and fixate for any length of time. Babies have been shown to demonstrate visual preferences for some colours rather than others. No tears are present and eyes are easily infected. Corneal, papillary and blink reflexes are present.

Hearing

Once the amniotic fluid is drained from the external ear canal the acuity is similar to that of an adult. Babies can detect pitch, loudness and timbre of sound in addition to location and changes in complex sounds. The internal and middle ear is larger in proportion at birth and the external canal small. The mastoid process and the bony part of the external canal have not yet developed. The tympanic membrane and facial nerve are close to the surface and easily damaged.

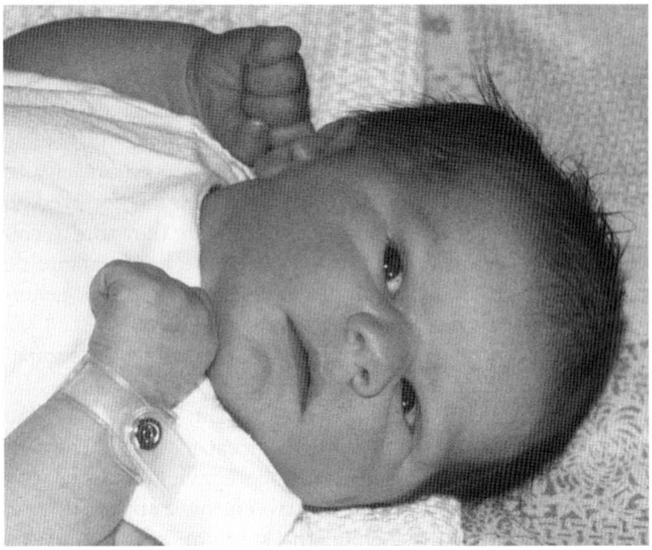

Fig. 12.8 • The eyes.

Respiratory system

The respiratory system is developmentally incomplete. The lungs mature after birth and new alveoli continue to grow for many years. There are 20 million alveoli at birth, increasing to 300 million alveoli in the fully formed lungs of the adult (Meadow & Newell 2002). This means that infants and young children have a relatively small alveolar surface area for gaseous exchange. Airway resistance in children is high due to the small diameter of the respiratory tree. The lumen of the peripheral airways is narrow, which predisposes the infant to airway obstruction. The infant's breathing is mainly abdominal: the abdomen distends, the diaphragm contracts and the thorax expands. The chest wall is very compliant and therefore easily distorted, which can increase the work of respiration.

Babies are obligatory nose breathers and do not convert automatically to mouth breathing when nasal obstruction occurs. Respiratory rate is 30–60 per minute. Respirations are shallow and the pattern alters during sleeping and waking. Many term babies have periods of rapid breathing alternating with periods of breathing at a slower rate, or they may not breathe for periods of up to 15 seconds – this is normal as long as the colour and heart rate do not change significantly and the infant then begins to breathe again spontaneously (MacGregor 2000). Periods of apnoea, when breathing ceases for more than 20 seconds, are only common in babies under 32 weeks' gestation unless there is an underlying condition.

Cardiovascular system

The heart rate is roughly 120–160 beats per minute and fluctuates with respiratory function, activity and sleep. It reaches a maximum at month, after which there is a gradual slowing until adult levels at 12–16 years of age. Peripheral circulation is sluggish and there may be mild cyanosis of hands and feet with mottling of skin when exposed.

Normal blood pressure ranges between 50/25 and 70/40 mmHg. The amount of total circulating blood is 80 mL/kg or approximately 300 mL at birth. Haemoglobin (Hb) = 15–20 g/dL; 70% is fetal Hb, which is replaced by adult Hb in the first 2 years of life. Mean cell volume (MCV)/100 L = 135 femtolitres = 10^{-12} g.

Breakdown of excess red blood cells in the liver and spleen predisposes to jaundice in the first few weeks. Prothrombin levels are low due to a lack of vitamin K. Colonisation of the intestine promotes synthesis of vitamin K. The white cell count is initially 18×10^9/L and reduces rapidly. Cardiac output is related to the heart rate and the stroke volume; as children have smaller hearts the stroke volume is reduced. The heart then needs to beat faster in order to oxygenate their body tissues.

Renal system

The newborn baby's kidneys weigh 23 g; this will have doubled by 6 months and trebled by the end of the first year (Sinclair 1991, cited in MacGregor 2000). The renal system is functional before birth but the workload is minimal. The infant is not able to concentrate or dilute urine very well in response to variations in fluid intake, and cannot compensate well for high or low solutes in blood. The ability to excrete drugs is also limited. However, the newborn can excrete amino acids and conserve sodium and glucose. The glomeruli are immature; they are resistant to aldosterone, which results in limited ability to concentrate the urine. This lack of ability to conserve or excrete water makes the baby vulnerable to dehydration. The glomerular filtration rate is 30 mL/min/m^2 at birth, 100 mL/min/m^2 at 9 months, and reaches adult values at year (Davenport 1996, cited in MacGregor 2000). Dehydration, hypotension and hypoxaemia all produce a fall in glomerular filtration rate, so renal function becomes compromised very quickly in a crisis. Urine is voided by reflex emptying of the bladder. The first urine is passed either at birth or during the first 24 hours and then increases in frequency as the fluid intake increases. The specific gravity should be 1.020. After birth, the kidneys increase in size in proportion to body length, the weight doubling in the first 10 months as a result of tubular growth.

Endocrine system

The endocrine system produces limited quantities of antidiuretic hormone from the posterior pituitary gland, thus making the infant more susceptible to dehydration. The effect of maternal hormones may cause the labia to be hypertrophied and the breasts engorged.

Gastrointestinal system

This system is structurally complete but functionally immature. The teeth are usually still buried in the gums. Sucking pads in the cheeks give them a full appearance. Sucking and swallowing reflexes are coordinated.

The stomach's capacity at birth is approximately 10–20 mL, although this increases rapidly in the first few weeks of life up to 150 mL by 1 month. The cardiac sphincter is weak, making the baby prone to regurgitation or possiting and gastric emptying time is 2.5–3 hours. Hydrochloric acid is present in the stomach at birth but, due to swallowing of amniotic fluid, the pH is nearly neutral. Acid secretion commences within 8 hours of birth and digestion in the stomach is then reliant on the action of hydrochloric acid and rennin to cause the formation of curds by coagulating the casein in milk. Human milk contains e-fructose, a bacterium that raises the acidity of the gut inhibiting the growth of *Escherichia coli* bacteria. Adult levels of acid secretion are reached by the age of 10 years.

Intestine

The breakdown of most food occurs in the intestine. In the young infant the colon has a small volume and therefore results in frequent bowel movements. Food reaches the caecum in about 4 hours. The breakdown of protein into large polypeptides is brought about by pepsin and hydrochloric acid. Subsequent breakdown into amino acids occurs by the action of the pancreatic enzymes, trypsin, chymotrypsin and polypeptides, and by enzymes derived from the small intestinal mucosa, such as enterokinase. Hence enzymes are available to catalyse proteins and simple carbohydrates but deficient production of pancreatic amylase impairs utilisation of complex carbohydrates. A deficiency of pancreatic lipase until 4–5 months of age reduces the infant's capacity to convert fat into fatty acids and glycerol. The gastrocolic reflex opens the ileocaecal valve so that feeding is often accompanied by emptying of the bowel and meconium, which is present in the large colon from 16 weeks' gestation, is normally passed within 24 hours and totally excreted within 48–72 hours. Meconium is blackish in colour, tenacious and contains bile, fatty acids, mucous and epithelial cells. Following passage of the meconium, the stools change to brownish yellow, their frequency and consistency depending on the method of feeding. Breastfed babies' stools are loose, bright yellow and inoffensive. Bottle-fed babies stools are paler, semi-formed and have a sharper odour; there is an increased tendency to constipation.

The liver occupies 40% of the peritoneal cavity at birth (MacGregor 2000). There is decreased activity of the enzyme glucuronyl transferase, which is needed to conjugate bilirubin resulting in physiological jaundice of the newborn. The liver also stores less glycogen, leaving the infant susceptible to hypoglycaemia.

Absorption of minerals and vitamins

Vitamin B is absorbed from the terminal ileum. Iron, calcium, magnesium, sodium, potassium, ascorbic acid, folic acid and water-soluble vitamins are absorbed from the proximal small intestine.

Activity

Find out what advice is given to the parents of newborns regarding feeding. How does this relate to the absorption capabilities of the infant's stomach and intestines?

Reflect on your practice

- Explain to a junior nurse or parent why newborn babies are at risk of jaundice.
- How do babies digest cows milk?

Immunological adaptations

There are three main immunoglobulins: G (IgG), A (IgA) and M (IgM). Infants are unable to produce their own immunoglobulins until 5 weeks old. IgG can cross the placenta so that at birth the baby's level is as high as the mother's. Breast milk, and especially colostrum, provide the infant with additional IgG. This gives passive immunity for the first few months of life, which gives the infant protection against most of the major childhood illnesses such as diphtheria, measles, poliomyelitis and rubella for about 12 weeks, provided the mother has antibodies to these diseases. The fetus can manufacture IgM and IgA but it takes 2 years to achieve adult levels. IgA protects against infections of the respiratory and gastrointestinal tract and eyes. The thymus gland, where lymphocytes are produced, is relatively large at birth and continues to grow until 8 years of age.

Reproductive system

Spermatogenesis does not occur until puberty. The total complement of primordial follicles containing primitive ova is present in the ovaries at birth.

Skeletomuscular system

All muscles are present at birth, although the muscle tissue is 35% water. The long bones are incompletely ossified allowing for growth at the epiphyses. The bones of the skull are incompletely ossified essential for growth of the brain and moulding during labour. Moulding is resolved within a few days of birth. The posterior fontanelle closes within 6 weeks and the anterior fontanelle remains open for up to 18 months. This allows assessment of intracranial pressure by palpation.

In ventral suspension the head droops below the plane of the body (Fig. 12.9) and when the infant is pulled to sit there is marked head lag (Figs 12.10 and 12.11).

Neurological system

Compared with other systems this is very immature both anatomically and physiologically at birth. The most fully developed parts of the brain are the medulla (or hindbrain) and the midbrain. The least developed part is the cortex. This is no surprise when you consider the function of these areas of the brain and the abilities of the newborn/older child:

- The medulla is in the lower part of the skull and regulates sucking, breathing, heart rate, body temperature and muscle tone.

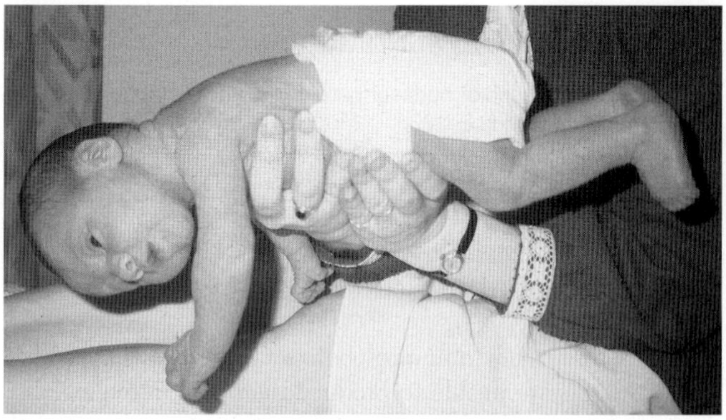

Fig. 12.9 • In ventral suspension, the head droops below the plane of the body.

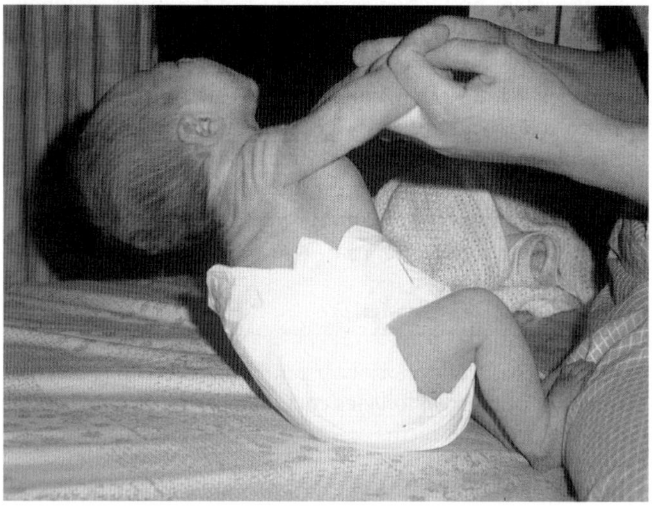

Fig 12.10 • Pulled to sit, there is a marked head lag.

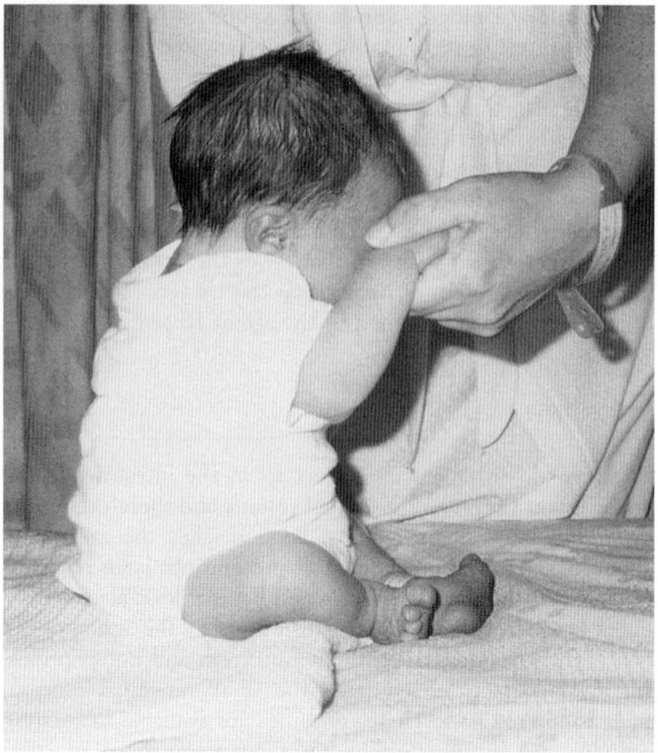

Fig 12.11 • Pulled to sit, there is a marked head lag.

- The midbrain governs attention, sleeping, eating and eliminating. This part of the brain is similar to the brain of lower animals, i.e. the primitive reflexes are in control.
- The cortex governs perception, body movements, complex thinking and language. It follows that development of certain areas of the cortex sets limits on the development of the child's motor and perceptional skills.

The nerve cells or neurons of the brain are present at birth but the neurons of the cortex are not well connected. Over the first 2 years of life, the number and density of the dendrites, and speed of the synapses, increase rapidly, along with the size of individual neurons and the total weight of the brain (Bee 1997). At birth the spinal cord is not fully myelinated. Fibres that are not myelinated conduct slowly and inefficiently. Myelination of the nerves leading to and from the brain is almost complete by the time the child is 2 years old. Myelination and growth of connective tissue continues until adolescence. After birth, brain growth is rapid, requiring constant and adequate supplies of oxygen and glucose. The immaturity of the brain renders it particularly vulnerable to hypoxia, biochemical imbalance, infection and haemorrhage. Temperature instability and uncoordinated muscle movement reflect the incomplete state of brain development and incomplete myelination of the nerves.

A neonate is equipped with many reflexes, the presence of which indicates normality and integrity of the neurological and skeletomuscular system. Reflexes are automatic physical responses triggered involuntarily by a specific stimulus. Many of these reflexes are still present in adults (e.g. the knee jerk, automatic eye blink when a puff of air hits the eye, and the involuntary narrowing of the pupil when exposed to a bright light).

The newborn infant also has a set of 'primitive' reflexes. These are controlled by the more primitive parts of the brain: the medulla and the midbrain. By about 6 months, when the portion of the brain governing more complex activities such as perception, body movement, thinking and language has developed more fully, these primitive reflexes begin to disappear, as if superseded by the higher-level brain functions.

Some primitive reflexes are essential for survival, such as the breathing reflex and the reflexes involved in eating. Infants who are touched on the cheek will automatically turn towards the touch and search for something to suck on; this is the rooting reflex (Fig. 12.12). The suck reflex is demonstrated when infants locate a suitable object that fits in the mouth and automatically begin to suck and swallow.

There are other primitive reflexes that do not have an obvious use. Infants who are confronted with a loud noise or some kind of physical shock will throw their arms outward and arch their back; this is the startle reflex. The Moro reflex occurs when the baby suffers a change in equilibrium or sudden jarring, which causes tension and abduction of the extremities and fanning of the fingers, followed by flexion and adduction of

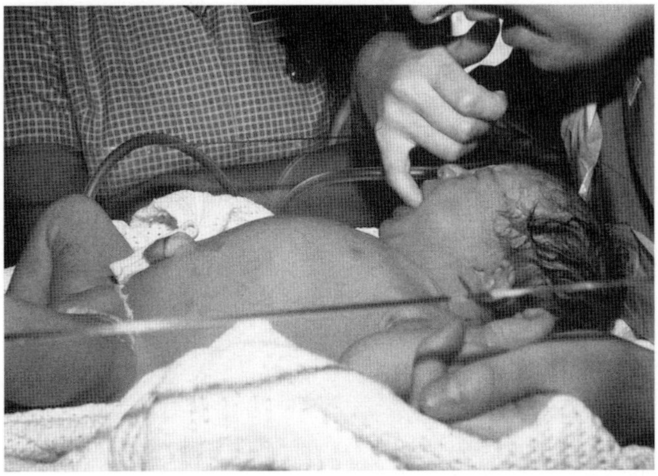

Fig 12.12 • The rooting reflex.

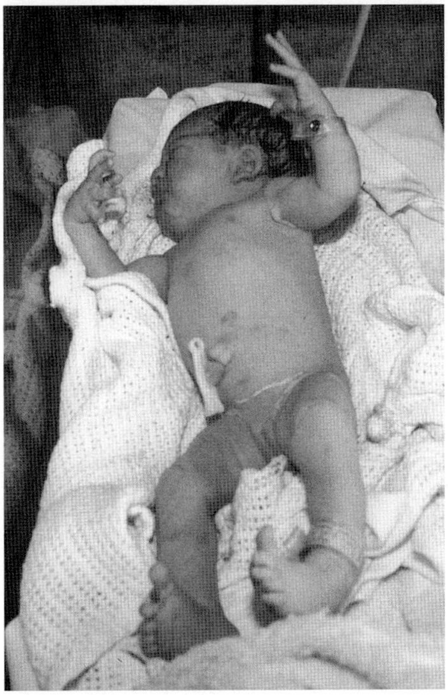

Fig. 12.13 • Moro reflex.

the extremities and the infant may cry (Fig. 12.13). The step reflex can be demonstrated by holding the baby so the sole of the foot touches a hard surface, this causes a reciprocal flexion and extension of the leg simulating walking (Fig. 12.14). If you touch an infant on the bottom of the foot, the Babinski reflex will be demonstrated when the toes are first splayed out and then curled in. If you touch an infant on the palm of the hand, his or her fingers will curl around your hand and hold on tightly, this is called the grasp reflex.

These reflex patterns are interesting not only because they may be remnants from our evolutionary past but because their presence past the age of roughly 6 months may signal the existence of some kind of neurological problem. The Babinski reflex is used as a diagnostic tool by neurologists who suspect the existence of some dysfunction.

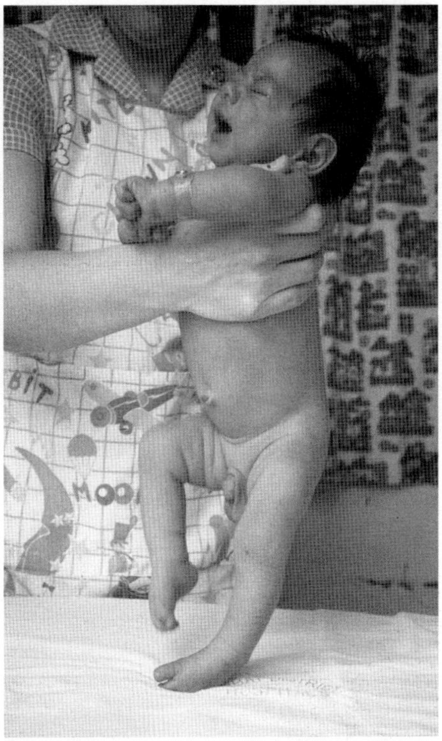

Fig. 12.14 • The step reflex.

1 Month to 2 years

Aged 1 month

After birth, the rate of weight gain and growth in length accelerates to reach a maximum velocity between 4 and 6 weeks. The velocity of growth then declines rapidly until 4–5 years. Weight has a similar growth curve to height. Other organs show variations in their growth curve.

Posture and large movement

When the baby is pulled to sit, the head lags until the body is vertical (Fig 12.15) when the head is held momentarily erect before falling forward.

When held sitting, the back is one complete curve (Fig. 12.16).

In ventral suspension, the head is in line with the body and the hips are semi-extended (Fig. 12.17).

Vision and fine movement

- Pupils react to light.
- Turns head and eyes to light source.
- Follows pen torch briefly with eyes at 25 cm.
- Shuts eyes tightly when light is shone in them.
- Fixes and follows.
- Watches mother's nearby face when she feeds or talks to him with increasingly alert facial expression.

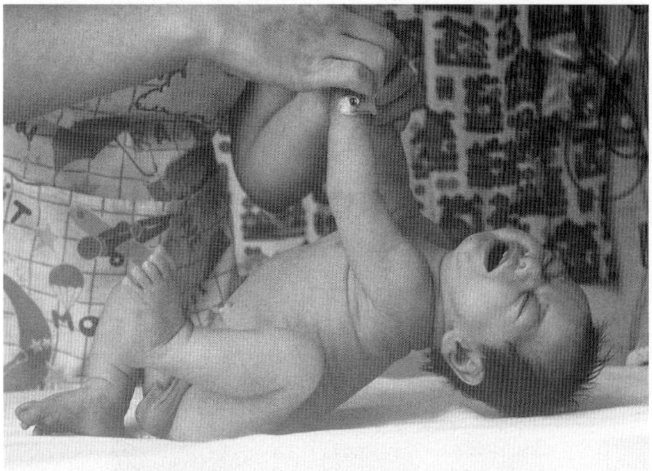

Fig 12.15 • When pulled to sit, the head lags until the body is vertical.

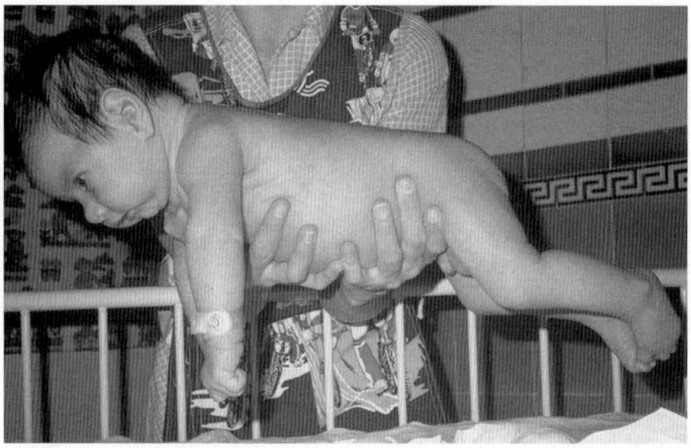

Fig. 12.17 • In ventral suspension the head is in line with the body and the hips are semi-extended.

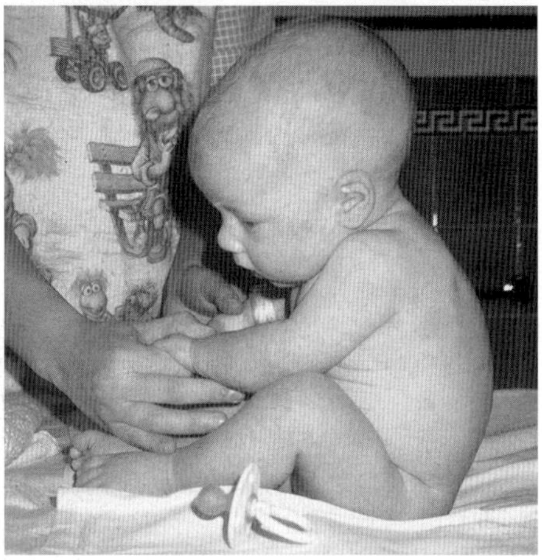

Fig. 12.16 • When held sitting, the back is one complete curve.

Hearing and speech

- Startled by sudden noise.
- Stops whimpering and (usually) turns towards sound of nearby soothing voice, but not when screaming or feeding.
- Cries lustily when hungry or uncomfortable.
- Guttural noises when content.
- Coos responsively to mother's talk from 5 to 6 weeks.

Social behaviour and play

- Sucks well.
- Sleeps most of the time when not being fed or handled.
- Expression still vague: more alert later, progressing to social smile and responsive vocalisations at 5–6 weeks. Hands are normally closed but fingers are grasped when palm is touched.
- Stops crying when picked up and spoken to. Turns to regard nearby speaker's face. Needs head support when being carried, dressed or bathed. Passive acceptance of bath and dressing routines gradually changes to an increasing awareness and response.

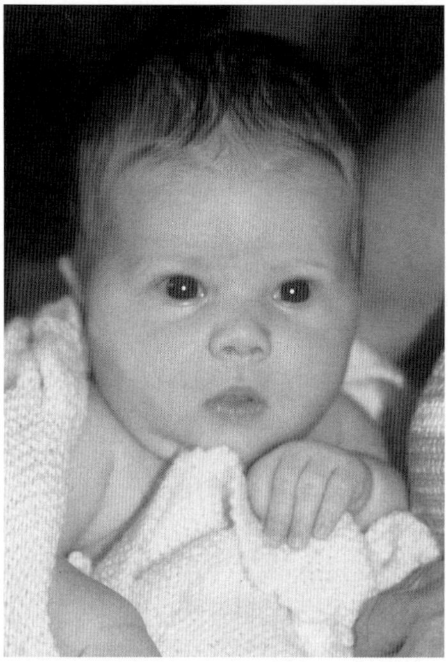

Fig. 12.18 • Aged 6 weeks.

Infant assessment

Hearing is usually assessed soon after birth or within 4 weeks if a hospital-based programme or 5 weeks if community-based in response to the Newborn Hearing Screening Programme (Healthy child programme – pregnancy and the first five years of life, DoH, 2009).

At 6–8 weeks a physical examination and a general assessment of alertness, vision and motor function should take place.

Vision

The infant turns to regard the speaker's face (Fig. 12.18). The infant holds gaze and follows to 90° – failure to do so is not normal but may be due to distraction. Infants who do not follow should be rechecked.

Motor function

When placed prone, infant will lift their head for a few seconds. Infants who normally sleep prone are more advanced at this than others. Infants who fail this test should be retested 2 weeks later.

Other assessments

- Testes (boys)
- Assessed for developmental dysplasia of the lips
- The heart rate and sound
- Any matters of concern raised by parents or professionals.

Age 6 weeks upwards

Sleep

At 3–7 months infants sleep through the night with two or three short naps during the day. Rapid eye movement (REM) sleep is less frequent by 6 months and levels off at 25–30% total sleep time. There are four stages to sleep:

1. Drowsiness
2. Sleeping: easily wakened
3. Sleep becomes increasingly deeper: heart rate stable, muscles relaxed, brain waves slow
4. Deepest: difficult to rouse from.

A single night-time sleep contains all four stages arranged in cycles. The length of the sleep cycle gradually increases with age.

Skeletal system

The growth and development of bone consists of two processes, which occur at the same time: the creation of new cells and tissue and the consolidation of these tissues into a permanent form. The number of bones increases in the hand, wrist, ankle and foot. New centres of ossification in bones of hand and wrist are present at 5–6 months. These are useful for determining skeletal age. The length of the bones, particularly the long bones of the arms and legs, also increases to attain increase in height. Infant bones contain much more water than those of the adult, which makes them softer and more malleable (this ability to bend enabled the fetus to curl up inside the uterus). The bones of the skull are joined together as the fontanelles fill with bone; this process is usually complete by the age of 2 years. The ossification process takes place throughout infancy to adulthood. Girls mature faster than boys. At birth, girls are 5–6 weeks ahead in level of skeletal maturity.

3 Months

Posture and large movement

- Supine: prefers to lie with head in midline, limb movements smooth (Fig. 12.19).
- Pulled to sit: little or no head lag (Fig. 12.20).

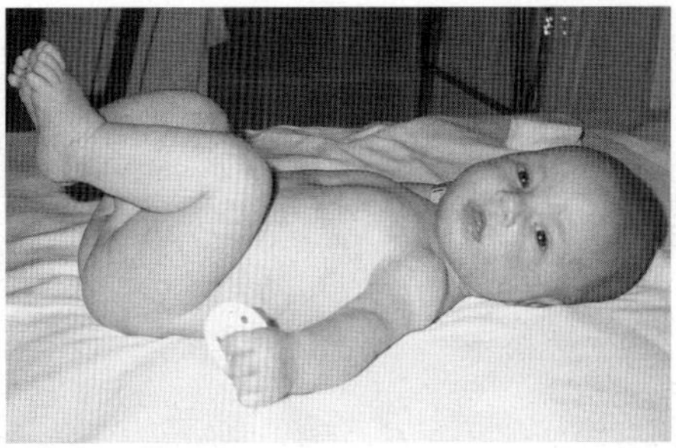

Fig. 12.19 • When supine, prefers to lie with head in midline, limb movements smoother.

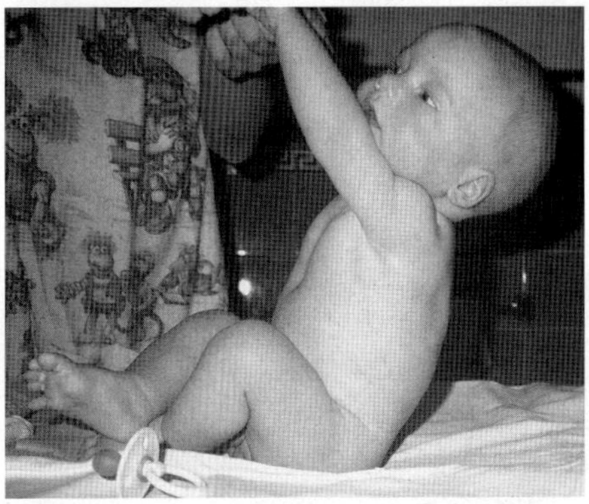

Fig. 12.20 • Pulled to sit, there is little or no head lag.

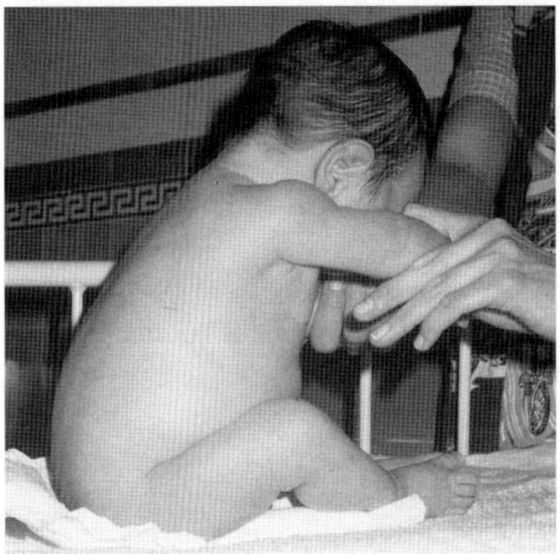

Fig. 12.21 • Held sitting, the back is straight except for the lumbar region.

- Held sitting: the back is straight except for lumbar region (Fig. 12.21).
- In ventral suspension: head held well above line of body (Fig. 12.22).
- Prone: lifts head and upper chest, uses forearms for support, buttocks flat (Fig. 12.23).

Vision and fine movement

- Visually alert, responds to nearby human face.
- Turns head deliberately to look around.
- Follows hanging ball at 30 cm through 180°.
- Watches movements of own hands and demonstrates finger play.

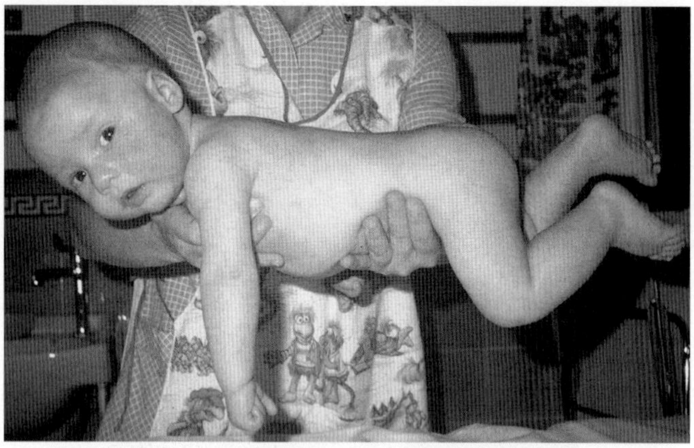

Fig. 12.22 • In ventral suspension, the head is held well above the line of the body.

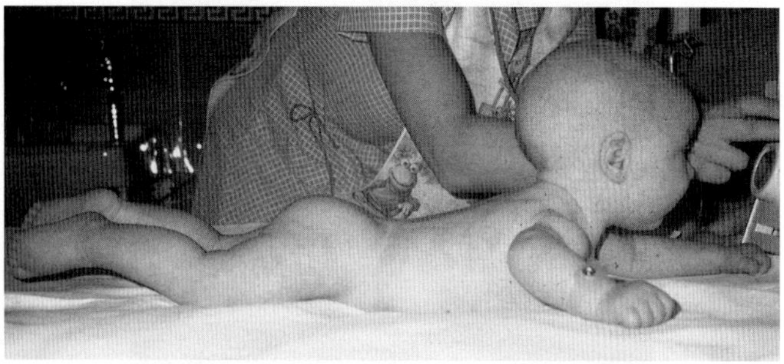

Fig. 12.23 • When prone, lifts head and upper chest and uses forearms for support; the buttocks are flat.

- Recognises feeding bottle and makes eager movements as it approaches.
- Defensive blink present.
- Holds rattle for a few seconds but doesn't look at it at the same time.

Hearing and speech

- Sudden loud noises still cause distress, eyes close tightly and the infant cries.
- Definite quietening or smiling in response to mother's voice.
- Vocalises happily when spoken to, can also vocalise when playing alone.
- Cries when uncomfortable or angry.
- Sometimes sucks or licks lips when food is being prepared.
- Demonstrates excitement when hears people approaching.

Social behaviour and play

- Intense gaze at mother's face when being fed.
- Reacts to familiar situations by showing excitement.
- Enjoys bathing.
- Responds with obvious pleasure when played with.

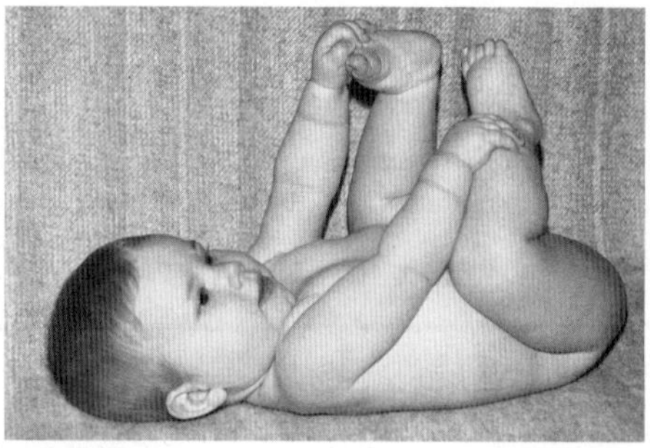

Fig. 12.24 • When supine, raises the head to look at the feet, lifts legs into the vertical and grasps the feet.

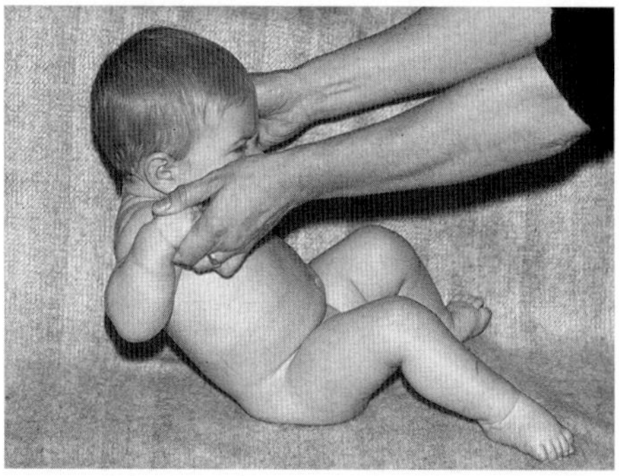

Fig. 12.25 • When the hands are held, braces shoulders and pulls self to sit.

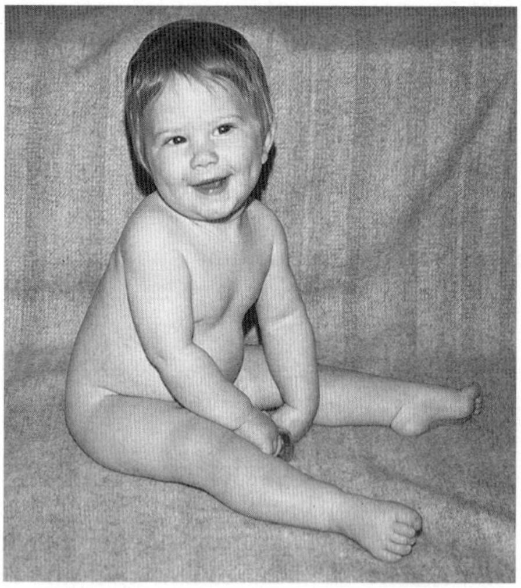

Fig. 12.26 • Held sitting, the head is firmly erect and the back is straight. Can sit momentarily alone.

6 Months

Posture and large movement

- Supine: raises head to look at feet, lifts legs into vertical and grasps feet (Fig. 12.24).
- When hands are held: braces shoulders and pulls self to sit (Fig. 12.25).
- Held sitting: head firmly erect, back straight. Can sit momentarily alone (Fig. 12.26).

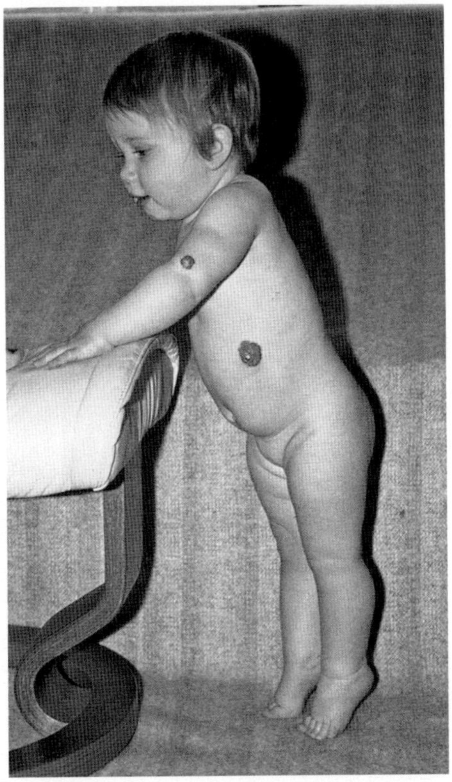

Fig. 12.27 • When held standing, bears weight on feet and bounces up and down. Can stand momentarily holding on to furniture.

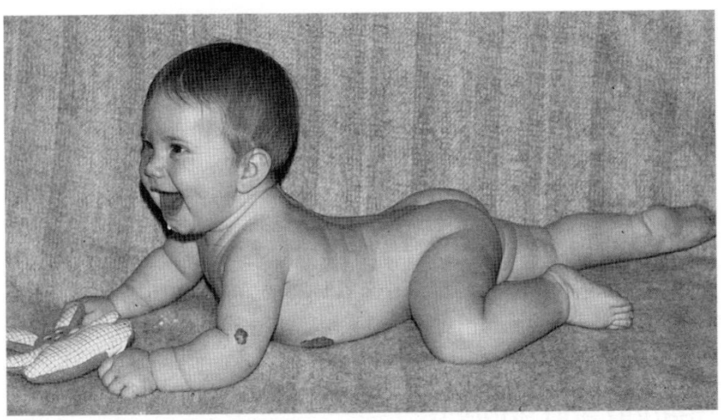

Fig. 12.28 • When placed prone, lifts head and chest well up, supporting self on extended arms

- Held standing: bears weight on feet and bounces up and down.
- Can stand momentarily when holding on to furniture (Fig. 12.27).
- When placed prone: lifts head and chest well up, supporting him- or herself on extended arms (Fig. 12.28).

Vision and fine movement

- Visually insatiable, moves head and eyes eagerly when attention attracted.
- Shows interest and watches adult movements at a distance.
- Eyes move in unison.
- Immediate fixation on interesting small objects at 30 cm.

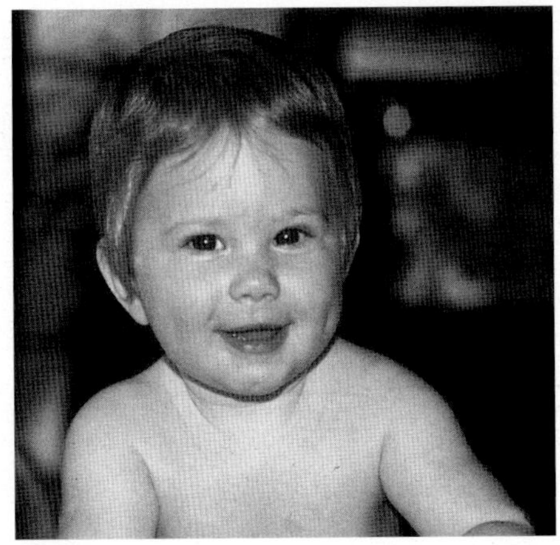

Fig. 12.29 • Aged 8 months.

- Uses whole hand to palmar grasp and passes object from one hand to the other.
- When toys fall outside visual field: does not follow them.

Hearing and speech

- Turns immediately to mother's voice.
- Vocalises tunefully to self and others
- Using single or double syllables: 'adah', 'goo', 'aroo'.
- Laughs and chuckles.
- Screams with annoyance.
- Demonstrates different responses to mother's tone of voice.

Social behaviour and play

- Reaches out and grasps small toys.
- Takes everything to mouth.
- Plays with feet and hands.
- Puts hands around bottle and pats it.
- Shakes rattle deliberately to make sound.
- Manipulates objects attentively passing from hand to hand.
- Friendly with strangers but does show some anxiety if approached too quickly.

8 Months (Fig. 12.29)

Mothers are asked if there have been any problems or illnesses since the last check. They are asked if the infant is making sounds and for details of the diet, including whether the infant is chewing solids. Alertness and interest, weight and length are checked.

Vision

Near vision should demonstrate that the infant can see a small pellet about 20 cm away and he or she usually reaches out for it.

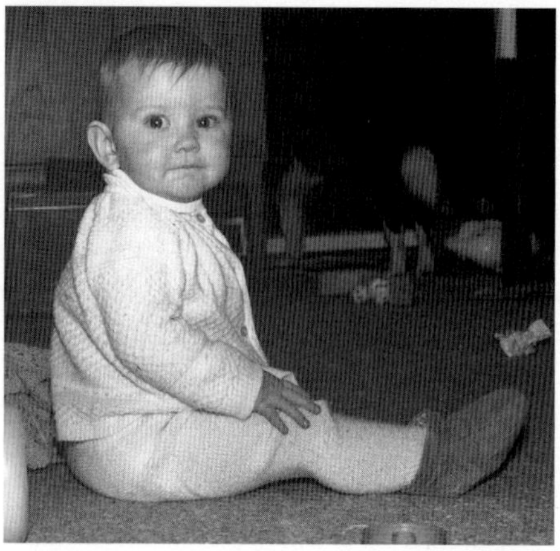

Fig. 12.30 • An 8-month infant can sit without being held.

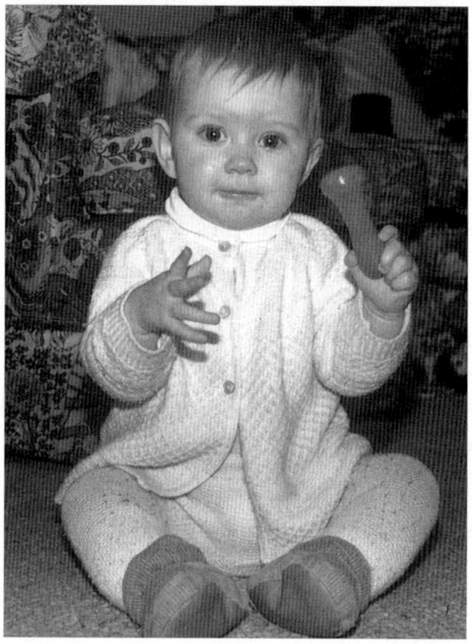

Fig. 12.31 • An 8-month infant picks up and explores objects presented to them.

Motor function

- From the prone position: infants should get up on their wrists.
- When pulled from supine: they should be able to sit spontaneously for a minute or two.
- Children can normally sit without help at 8 months (Fig. 12.30); they should be able to take their weight on their legs when they are held standing.
- If a cube is placed in front of them, infants should grab it with their whole hand (Fig. 12.31). Infants should transfer objects from one hand to the other.

Hearing

The distraction method is the hearing test used at this age. The distracter holds the infant's attention while the tester produces a sound. Careful attention to detail is essential to produce reliable results. The most common reasons for failure to respond to sound are tiredness, lack of interest, distraction, ear wax, otitis media and lack of familiarity with the test sounds. Infants who fail this test should be retested 2 months later. At 8 months, infants normally respond to their own name.

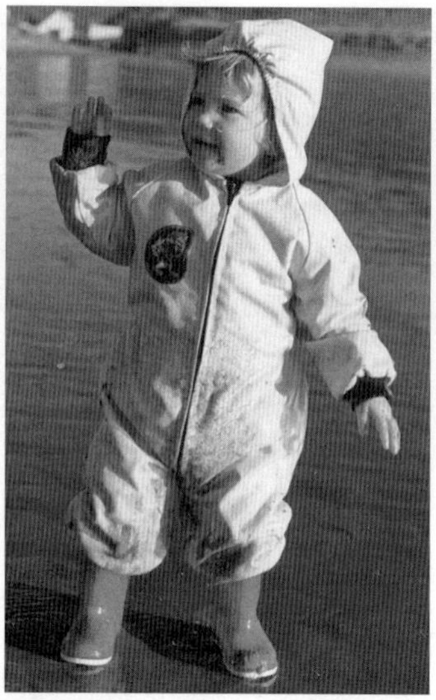

Fig. 12.32 • Aged 1 year.

1 Year (Fig. 12.32)

Posture and large movement

- Crawls on hands and knees, shuffles on buttocks or bear walks.
- Usually able to stand alone, may walk.

Vision and fine movement

- Looks in correct place for toys dropped out of sight.
- Recognises familiar people at 7 m distance.

Hearing and speech

- Turns immediately to own name.
- Comprehends simple instructions associated with gesture, e.g. 'come to mummy'.

Social behaviour and play

- Drinks from a cup.
- Waves 'bye-bye', plays 'pat-a-cake'.
- Helps with dressing, e.g. holding out arm for sleeve.

18 Months

Posture and large movement

- Walks competently, starts and stops safely.
- Walks upstairs with hand held.

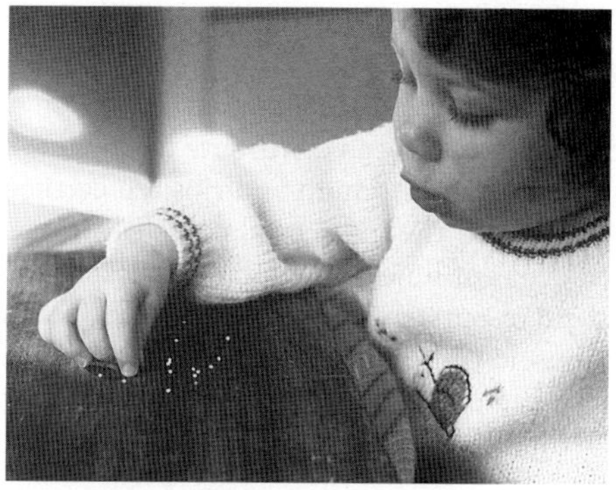

Fig. 12.33 • Aged 18 months.

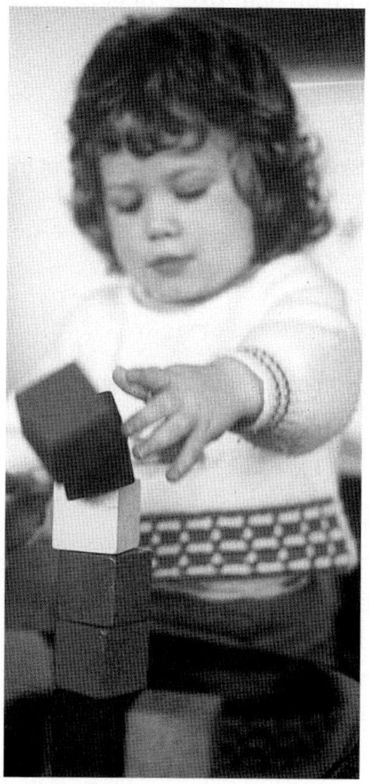

Fig. 12.34 • Vision and fine movement.

Vision and fine movement

- Picks up small sweets, beads, etc., with delicate pincer grasp (Fig. 12.33).
- Beginning to show a preference for using one hand.
- Enjoys simple picture books, recognises objects.
- Builds tower of three cubes (Fig. 12.34), knocks it down.

Hearing and speech

- Uses 6–20 words and understands more.
- Attempts to sing.

Social behaviour and play

- Holds spoon, gets food safely to mouth (Fig. 12.35).
- Takes off clothes but unable to dress self.

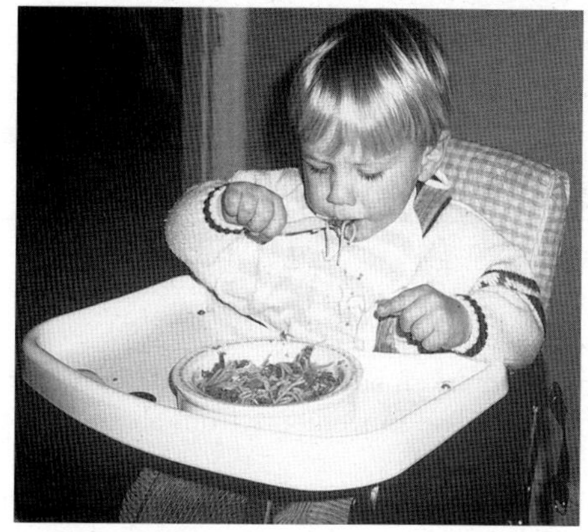

Fig. 12.35 • Social behaviour and play.

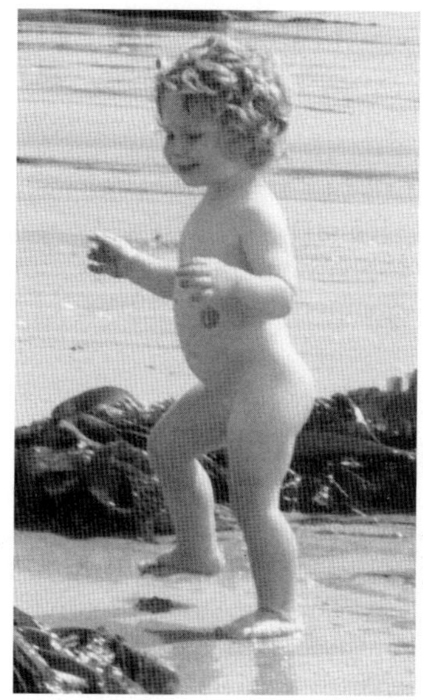

Fig. 12.36 • Physical appearance.

The physiological changes of a toddler

The physical appearance is squat with a pot-belly and slightly bowed legs (Fig. 12.36); by preschool children become more slender and graceful.

The rate of increase of head circumference slows with head and chest having roughly the same circumference by 1–2 years of age. In the second year the increase in head circumference is 2.5 cm. By 5 years the rate of increase has reduced to 1.25 cm a year. Between 12 and 18 months the anterior fontanelle closes (Hockenberry et al 2003).

Myelinisation of the spinal cord is almost complete by 2 years of age and brain growth is 75% complete. As specific areas of the brain develop, the child progresses developmentally, e.g. as the cortex develops then better control of the arms, legs and feet is gained.

During infancy, the capacity of the stomach increases to allow digestion of three meals a day and milk in the evening. Bowel movements have reduced to one or two a day, although bowel irregularity is common as the infant changes from a bland simple weaning diet to that of the family. Young children cannot control their bowel until they develop central nervous system control, although the tendency to defaecate after

Table 12.4 Recommended daily requirements of calories and protein

	Energy allowance (kcal/kg)	Protein (g)
0–6 months	108	13
6 months to year	98	14

breakfast is often taken advantage of. Children have daytime control of their bowel movements from about 24–30 months old (MacGregor 2000).

The skin matures during early childhood, with the epidermis and the dermis becoming more tightly bound together, thus the effectiveness of the skin as a barrier to infection and against fluid loss is improved.

The child's ability to maintain body temperature improves, with the capillaries constricting and dilating in response to cold and heat and shivering as an effective means of thermogenesis.

The volume of the respiratory tract increases but the internal structures of the ear and throat continue to be short and straight with the lymphoid tissue of the tonsils and adenoids large, which predisposes the young child to otitis media, tonsillitis and upper respiratory tract infections.

Metabolism

This is affected by an assortment of intrinsic and extrinsic factors. The basal metabolic rate (BMR) is highest in newborns. BMR closely relates to the proportion of surface area (SA) to the body mass, which decreases with maturity. The rate of metabolism determines caloric and protein requirements (Table 12.4) – during illness, needs can be high.

There is an increased metabolic rate (about twice that of an adult) and an increased respiratory demand for oxygen consumption and carbon dioxide elimination. The proportion of energy intake used to build and maintain tissue changes as the child grows:

- Birth: 40%
- 3 months: 40%
- 1–2 years: 20%
- 9–11 years: 4–10%.

Respiratory system

Overall lung growth has been measured in children using annual radiographs. Lung width and length follows a similar growth curve to overall height, with an adolescent growth spurt. Boys are on an average larger than girls in all lung dimensions.

The number of alveoli increases after birth reaching 90% at age 4 years. By the age of about 10 the increase in alveoli ceases and is followed by an increase in size. The total capacity of a child's lungs increases from 1.4 L in the 5-year-old child to 4.5 L at the time of puberty (MacGregor 2000). The ribs lie more horizontally in infants and contribute less to chest expansion. This results in infants and young children breathing diaphragmatically and respiration rate therefore is observed by watching abdominal movement rather than the movement of the chest.

The muscles are more likely to fatigue than those of adults and young children are more prone to respiratory failure. Anything that impedes diaphragm contraction or movement, e.g. abdominal distension, can contribute to the development of respiratory failure. The sternum and ribs are cartilaginous, the chest wall is soft and the intercostal muscles are poorly developed. In the event of illness, the infant's chest wall may move inwards instead of outwards during inspiration (retractions).

Smooth muscle is present throughout the lungs at birth and bronchospasm can occur even in the very young infant.

Lymphatics: B and T cell systems

The total amount of lymphoid tissue in the body (thymus, lymph nodes and lymphoid tissue of gut) increases throughout childhood.

Activity

What childhood illness is a particular indicator of this growth and what common surgery is carried out?

Activity

Think of the implications of malnutrition and understimulation on a young infant.

Dental eruption

Deciduous teeth begin to appear at the following ages (Fig. 12.37):

- Incisors: 6–9 months
- Canines: 16–19 months
- 1st molars: 10–15 months
- 2nd molars: 16–27 months.

Salivary glands

These start to function at 2–3 months; hence this is when babies start drooling.

Normal observations

Respiration

- 1–11 months: 30/min.

Heart rate: 3 months to 2 years

- Resting awake: 80–150 bpm.
- Sleeping: 70–120 bpm.
- Exercise or fever: up to 220 bpm.

Temperature

- 37.5°C.

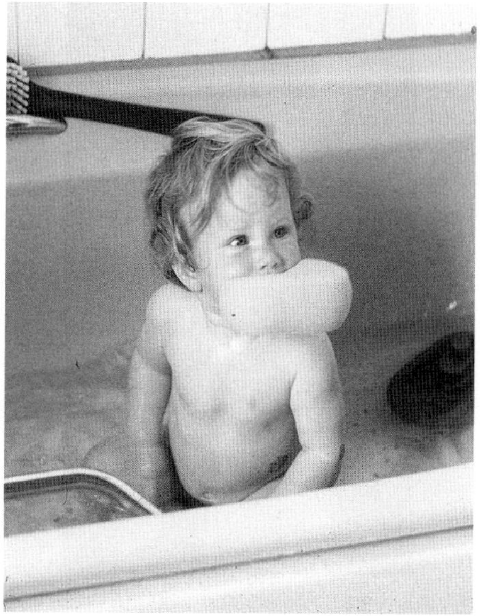

Fig. 12.37 • The pain and irritation of teething is relieved by biting.

Table 12.5 Blood pressure (mmHg) by age

Age	Girls	Boys
3 months	89/51	91/50
6 months	91/53	90/53
12 months	91/54	90/56

Blood pressure

Table 12.5 shows blood pressure by age.

General trends in height and weight gain during childhood

Weight gain

Table 12.6 shows weight gain by age.

Height

Table 12.7 shows height gain by age.

The preschool child

During this period the child grows 6–8 cm and gains 2 kg each year. The child has 20 deciduous teeth at 2.5 years.

The 2-year-old

- Walks, runs, stops and starts to avoid collisions.
- Squats to play and rise again (Fig. 12.38).

Table 12.6 Weight gain by age

Age	Weight gain
Birth to 6 months	Weekly 140–200 g
	Doubles by end of 4–7 months
6–12 months	Weekly 85–140 g
	Triples by end of first year
Toddlers	Yearly 2–3 kg
	Quadruples age 2.5 years
Preschoolers	Yearly 2–3 kg

Table 12.7 Height gain by age

Age	Height gain
Birth to 6 months	Monthly 2.5 cm
6–12 months	Monthly 1–5 cm
Toddlers	By age 2 years 50% adult
Preschoolers	Yearly gain 7.5 cm
	Birth length is doubled by 4 years

- Climbs on furniture to look out window or open door.
- Attempts to throw and kick a ball.
- Operates a sit-and-ride toy.
- Has difficulty with spatial awareness.
- Has strong sense of identity. Will resist things being done to them.
- Temper tantrums common.
- Holds a pencil like a rod and copies straight lines.
- Usually dry by day.
- Spontaneously engages in make-believe play (Fig. 12.39).

The 3-year-old

- Speech is well developed (girls better than boys).
- Understands sharing, turn taking.
- Is nimble and can judge distances.
- Jumps, stands briefly on one leg.
- Rides a tricycle and other toys (Fig. 12.40).
- Motor skills well established, can climb stairs with alternate feet (coming down puts both feet on the same step).
- Is clean and dry and can self-feed.
- Can build a tower of eight or nine cubes.
- Holds a pencil using almost a mature grasp, copies circles, cuts with scissors.
- Can attempt to dress self, can pull on clothes over head, pull up pants but needs help with buttons (Fig. 12.41).
- Joins in active make-believe play (Figs 12.42–12.44).

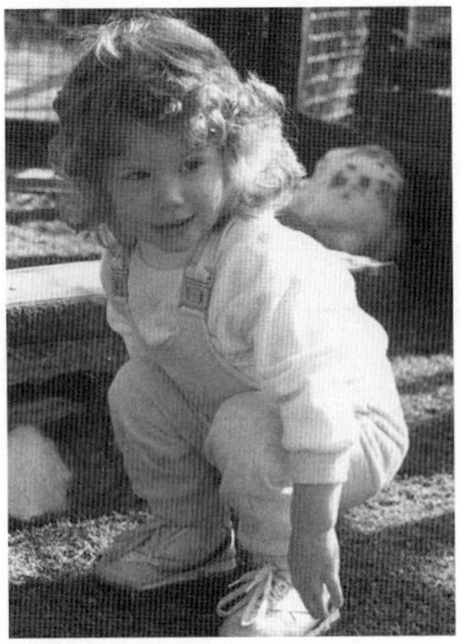

Fig. 12.38 • The 2-year-old.

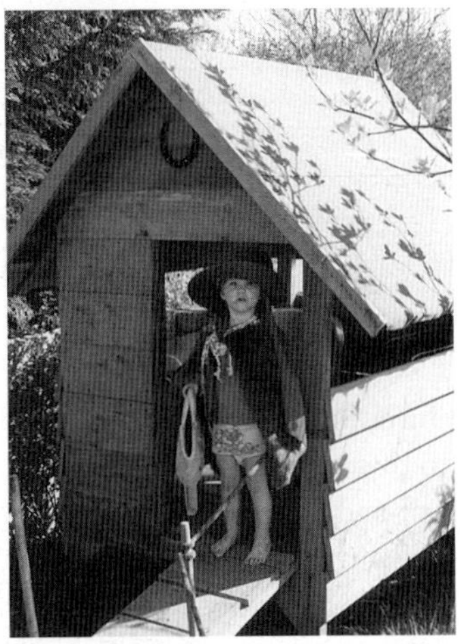

Fig. 12.39 • Spontaneously engages in make-believe play.

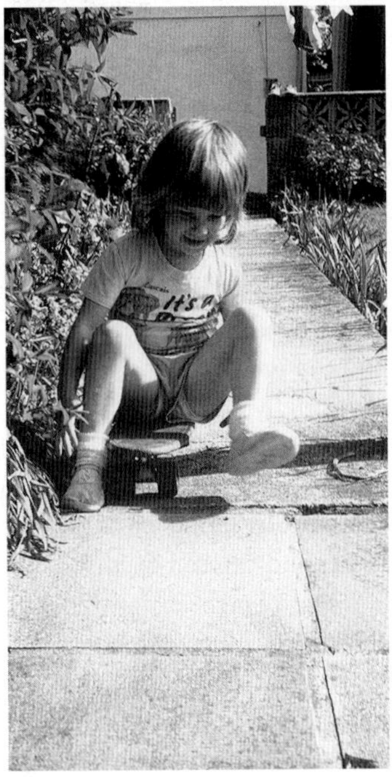

Fig. 12.40 • A 3-year-old enjoys riding on toys.

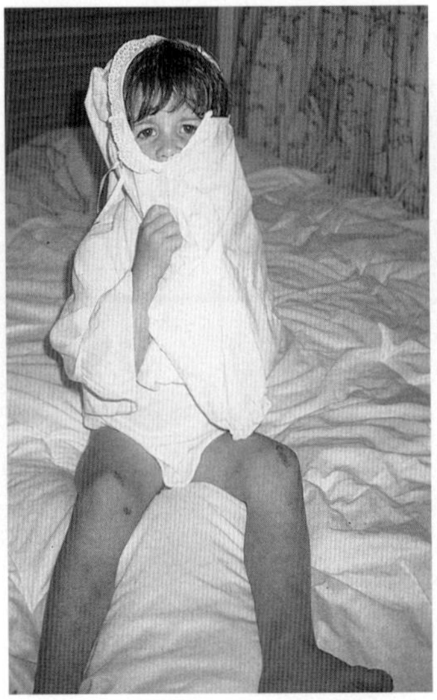

Fig. 12.41 • At 3 years, children start trying to dress themselves.

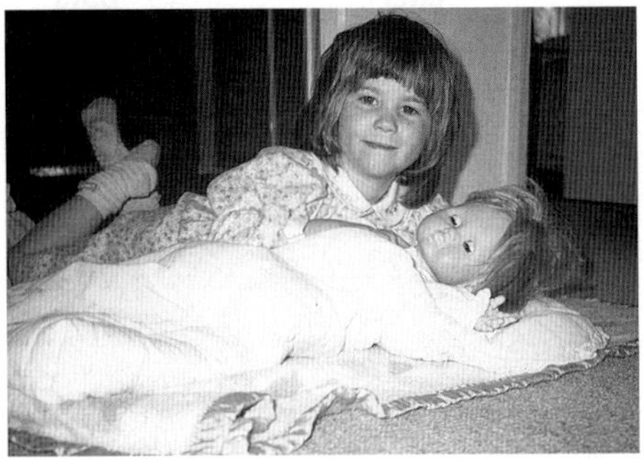

Fig. 12.42 • Joins in make-believe play.

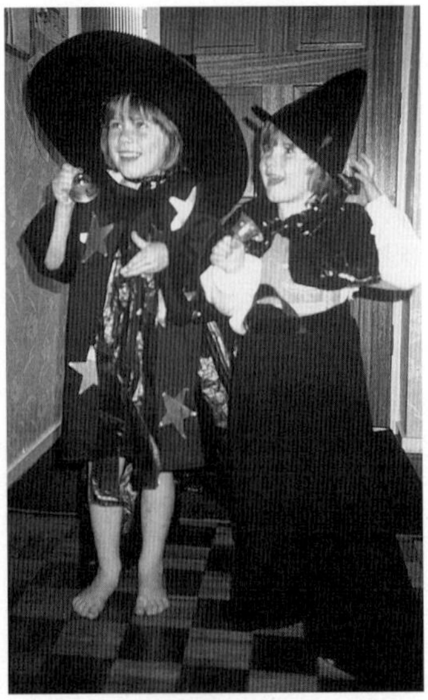

Fig. 12.43 • Joins in make-believe play.

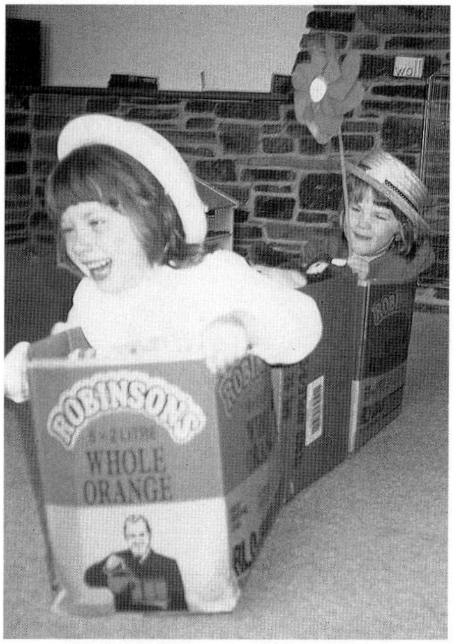

Fig. 12.44 • Joins in make-believe play.

The 4-year-old

- Self-care skills are developing, is willing to attempt to brush own hair (Fig. 12.45) and brush own teeth (Fig. 12.46).
- Holds a pencil in a mature grasp (Fig. 12.47) and copies circles and crosses as well as drawing an accurate body shape.
- Matches and names four primary colours.
- Gives full name, home address and sometimes age.
- Enjoys jokes, knows several nursery rhymes.
- Walks and runs skillfully and negotiates objects at speed without running into them.
- Can balance (Fig. 12.48), hop and climb up and down stairs.
- Enjoys the company of and is aware of the feelings of other children.
- Looks forward to treats and has some concept of time.
- 'Lordosis' (pot belly) disappears.

Activity

The child's need for sleep varies at different ages:

- Find out how much sleep you would expect a 1-year-old and a 4-year-old to require?

Activity

Between the ages of 1 and 5 years growth slows considerably compared with the first year of life:

- What would be considered an average weight gain per year?
- What would be considered an average height gain?
- Birth weight is quadrupled by what age?
- Adult height is twice the child's height at what age?
- Brain growth is what percentage complete by 2 years?
- At what age should myelination of the spinal cord be complete?
- What age should the anterior fontanelle close?
- At what age would you expect a child to be:
  dry by day?
  dry by night?
- What energy (k/cal/g) and protein (g) requirements are needed for a 1–3-year-old daily?
- What would you expect the normal pulse, respirations and BP to be of a 4-year-old?
- At what ages would you expect to see a growth spurt in children?

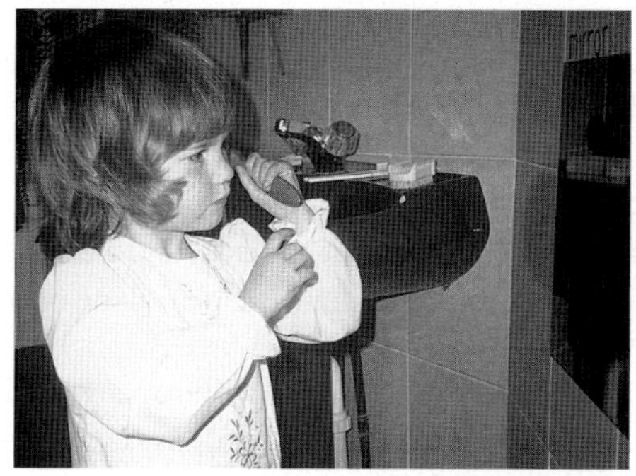

Fig. 12.45 • A 4-year-old learning to brush her hair.

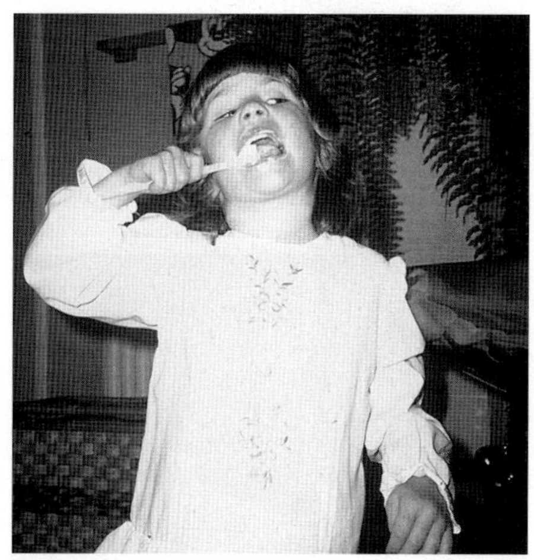

Fig. 12.46 • Learning to clean her teeth.

Child assessment completed before 5 years

Assessments of hearing and vision should be completed either before or soon after starting school.

A pre-school hearing screen should be performed with follow-up by the audiology services if there are any concerns. All children should also be screened for visual impairment between 4 and 5 years of age by an orthoptist-led service.

Physical growth from 5 years to adolescence

Physical changes are less obvious than 0–5 years. Children grow taller, change shape and acquire new skills. By the age of 5 years the child's height and weight are increasing steadily at the rate of 5 cm and 2–3 kg/year. Boys are on average 2.5 cm taller and 1 kg heavier than girls during early school years, however by 12 years of age girls are both taller and heavier than boys in their peer group.

- The 5-year-old is able to:
  - draw a recognisable person or house, and write his or her own name
  - hop, skip, swing, jump, balance, climb, dance and throw a ball (Figs 12.49–12.51)
  - ride a two-wheel bicycle
  - choose friends
  - undress and dress, except for laces and ties (Fig. 12.52)
  - perform domestic and dramatic play alone or with friends (Figs 12.53 and 12.54).
- Age 6: swings by arms and skips with rope (Fig. 12.55).
- Age 7: 'walks the plank' (Fig. 12.56), uses a bat and ball (Fig. 12.57).
- Age 8–10: hopscotch, skipping games.

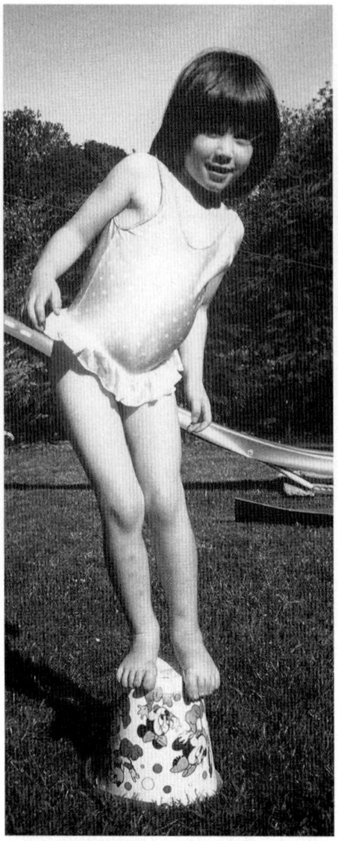

Fig. 12.48 • Demonstrating balance.

Skeletal growth

The growth of the trunk and extremities exceeds that of the head.

The centre of gravity lowers and body proportions become slimmer. Growth hormone stimulates longitudinal growth in a dose-dependent manner, however other influences on growth

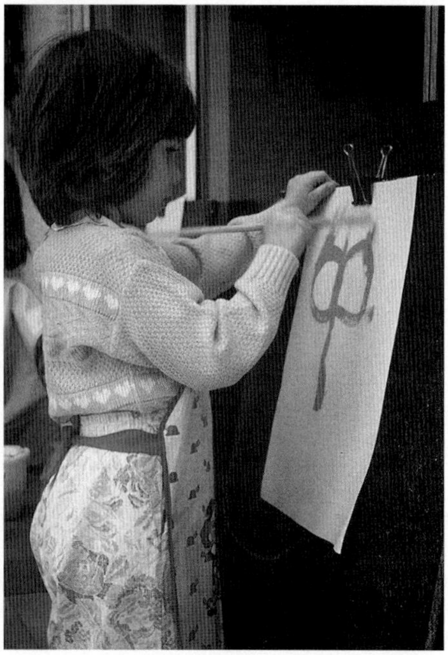

Fig. 12.47 • Demonstrating a mature grip.

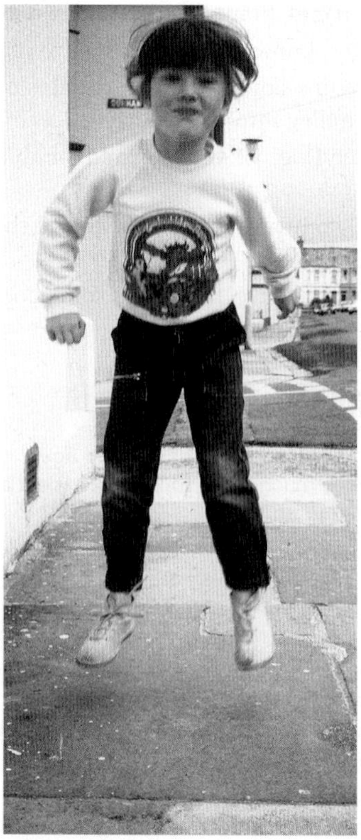

Fig. 12.49 • A 5-year-old learning sophisticated motor skills.

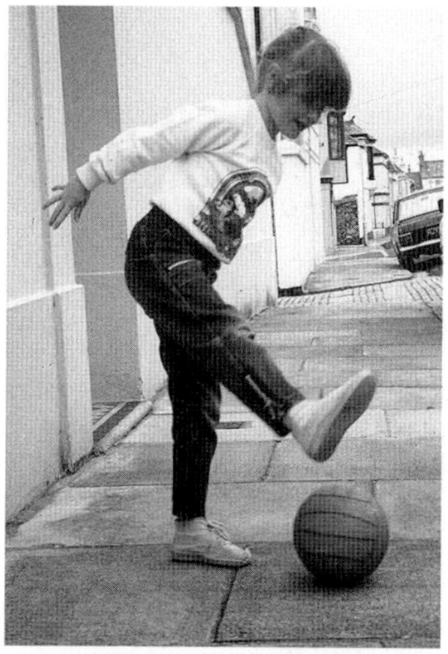

Fig. 12.50 • A 5-year-old learning sophisticated motor skills.

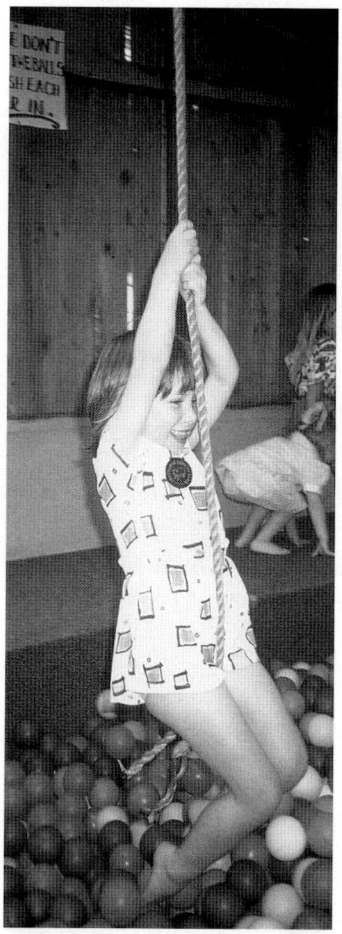

Fig. 12.51 • A 5-year-old learning sophisticated motor skills.

are socioeconomic, emotional and genetic factors. Problems are caused by ill-fitting shoes, chairs of the wrong height and carrying heavy loads, such as school bags.

The muscles are also immature and susceptible to damage.

Growth is reflected in limb length. Girls stop growing sooner than boys because of epiphyseal unity, which is under the control of oestrogen secretion. Boys' longer growth is reflected in

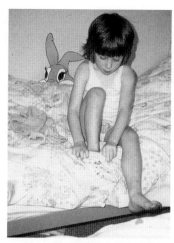

Fig. 12.52 • Dress and undress except for laces and ties.

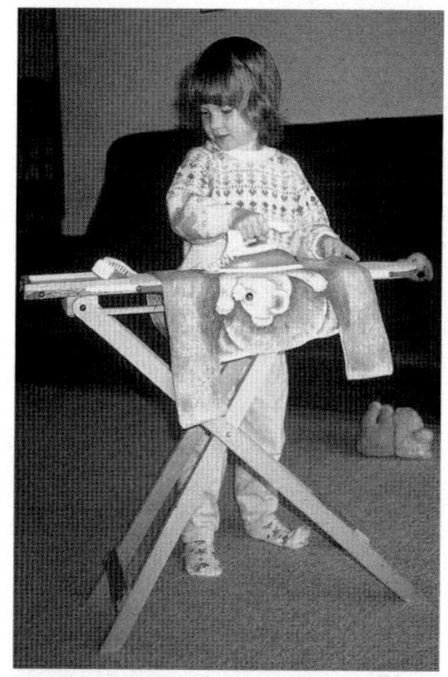

Fig. 12.53 • Performs domestic and dramatic play alone or with friends.

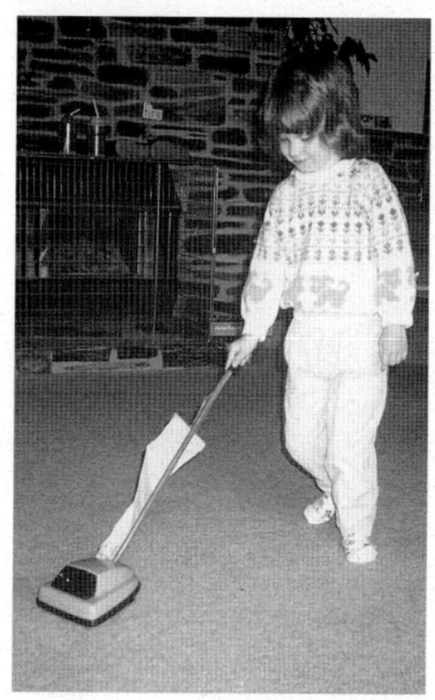

Fig. 12.54 • Performs domestic and dramatic play alone or with friends.

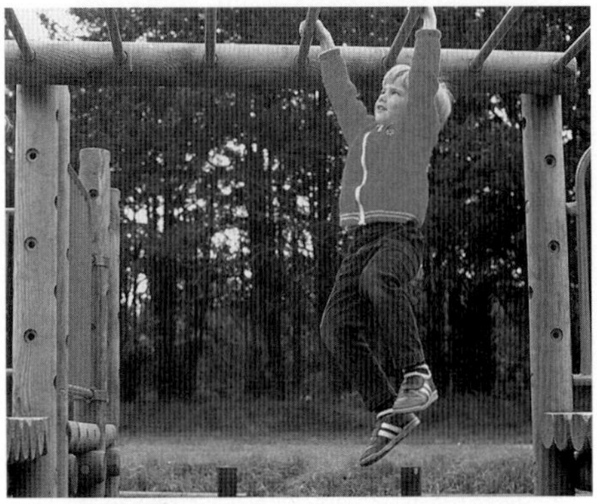

Fig. 12.55 • Aged 6, swings by the arms and skips with a rope.

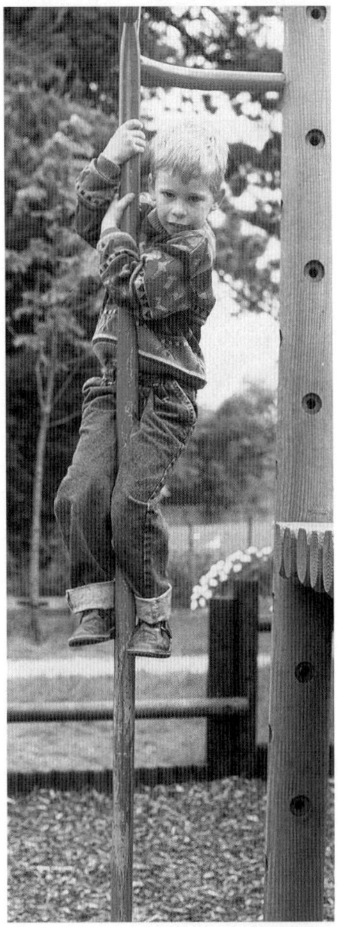

Fig. 12.56 • Aged 7, greater strength and body control.

their greater height and longer arms and legs. The extremities grow first, followed by neck, hip, chest, shoulder, trunk and depth of chest, hence the long-legged, gangly appearance of teenage boys with trousers and jumpers that never fit the limbs as well as the body.

Activity

Assessment of growth: go to the web site of the Royal College of Paediatrics and Child Health and search for growth charts for the latest information

Teeth

Children start to lose their deciduous teeth and permanent teeth appear at about the rate of four per year between the ages of 7 and 14 years.

Activity

Find out the sequence of teeth eruption for permanent dentition from a recommended textbook.

Head

- 6 months (Fig. 12.58).
- 5 years (Fig. 12.59).
- 10 years (Fig. 12.60).
- 13 years (Fig. 12.61).
- 16 years (Fig. 12.62).

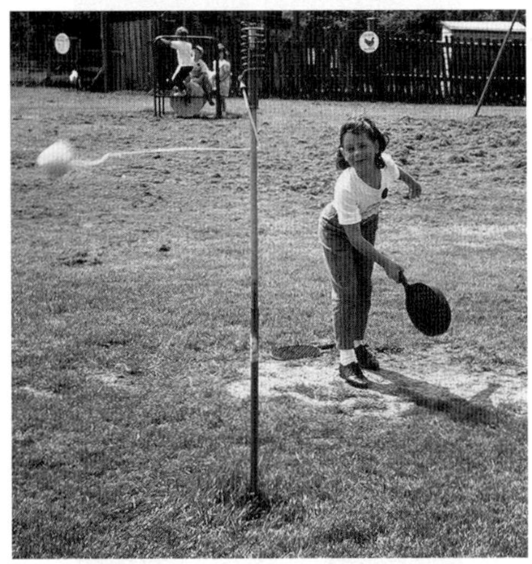

Fig. 12.57 • Aged 8–10, uses a bat and ball.

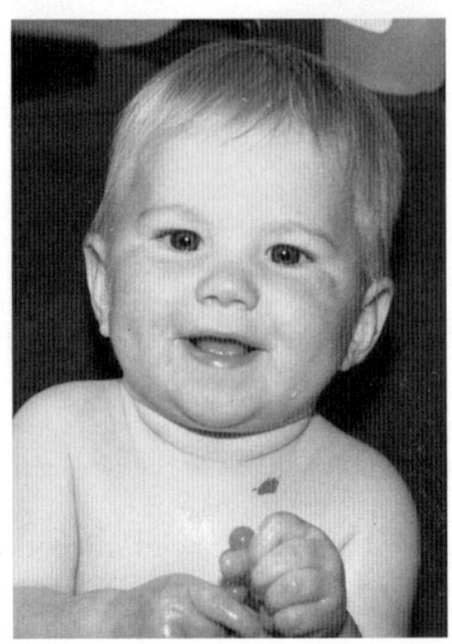

Fig. 12.58 • Aged 6 months.

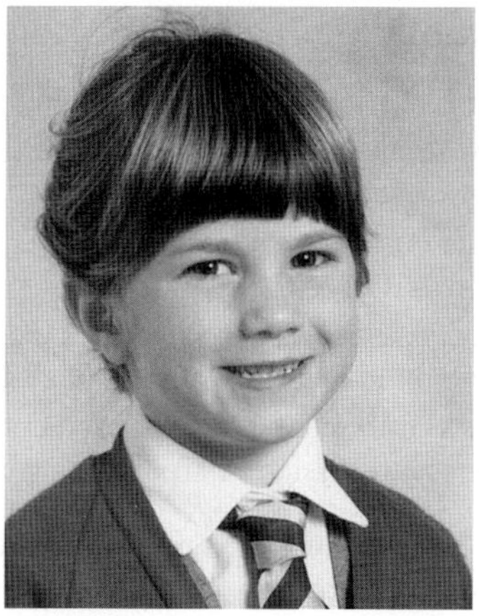

Fig. 12.59 • Aged 5 years.

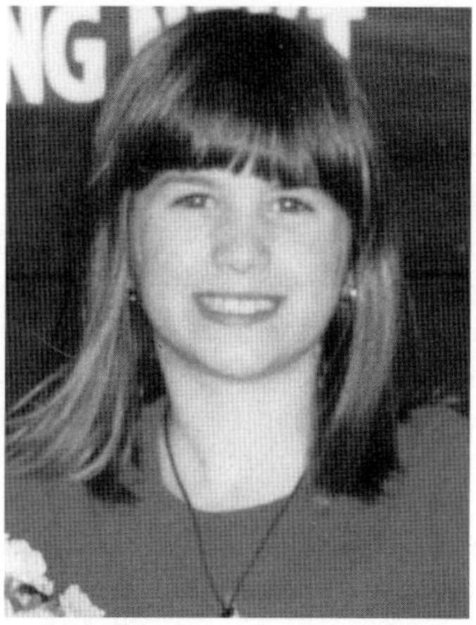

Fig. 12.60 • Aged 10 years.

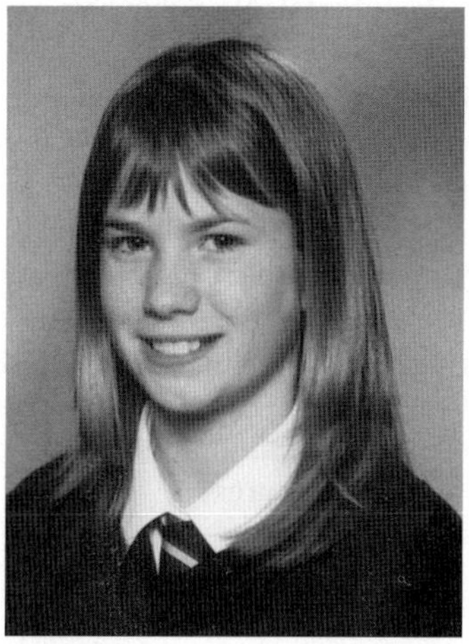

Fig. 12.61 • Aged 13 years.

The shape of the child's face changes from infancy to adulthood. Facial proportions change and the face grows faster in relation to the cranium. The frontal sinuses become visible on X-ray. When the permanent teeth erupt they force the shape of the jaw to change to accommodate them. In adolescence, both the jaw and the forehead alter, the jaw grows forward and the forehead becomes more prominent. This changes the overall shape of the face from a rounded appearance to one that is longer and more angular. The head and eyes are extra large in children; by the age of 8 years the child's head is 90% of its adult size. As facial remodelling continues and the jaw reaches adult size, there is hypertrophy of the laryngeal mucosa and enlargement of the larynx and vocal cords.

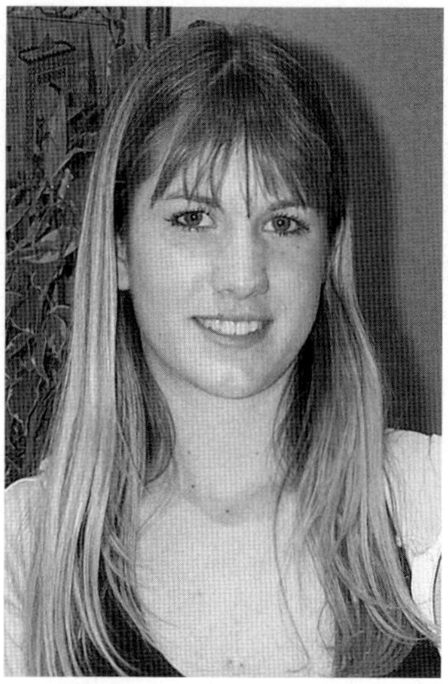

Fig. 12.62 • Aged 16 years.

Body mass

Muscle growth follows that of bone and is therefore greater in boys.

Cardiovascular system

This participates in the muscular growth spurt – its weight nearly doubles (this is more pronounced in boys). The systolic BP rises at an accelerated rate during puberty, and pulse rate decreases. Blood volume, Hb, and red blood cell count rise more in boys than girls; by adulthood, women have one million fewer red cells per mL than men.

Respiratory system

The size and capacity increase; the respiratory rate decreases. Boys take in more air at one breath than girls, due to the increased chest and shoulder size.

Peak flow rate measures the maximum flow achieved in expiration after a maximum inspiration. Normal ranges of peak flow rates are:

- 5 years: 150 L/min.
- 10 years: 240 L/min.
- 15 years: 400 L/min.

Skin

Oestrogen causes the skin of the female to develop a soft smooth, thicker texture. The sebaceous glands are particularly active and the eccrine and apocrine sweat glands become fully functional. Body hair takes on the characteristic distribution patterns and the texture changes.

Adolescence

Puberty is triggered by a chain of hormonal effects that bring on visible physical changes. The biology of puberty is triggered by hormonal influences and is controlled by the anterior pituitary in response to a stimulus from the hypothalamus (Fig. 12.63).

Sexual maturation of girls

The average age for appearance of breast buds is 10–11 years, with a range between 9 and 11.5 years. The appearance of pubic hair usually follows breast development by about 2–6 months, although in about one-third of girls the appearance of pubic hair may occur first. There is often an increase in normal vaginal discharge associated with uterine development. Menarche usually occurs 2 years after the appearance of breast buds with a critical weight of 45 kg or 17% body fat required before menarche begins.

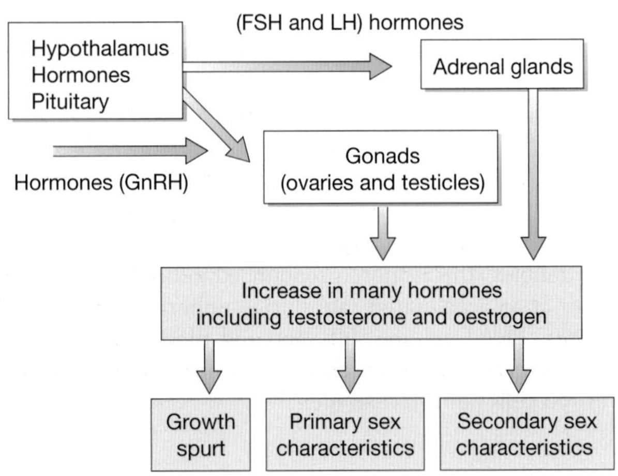

Fig. 12.63 • The hormones produced in adolescence.

Development of the breasts (Fig. 12.64)

- Stage one: Elevation of papilla.
- Stage two: Small area of elevation around papilla, enlargement of areolar diameter.
- Stage three: Further development of breast and areola with no separation of their contours.
- Stage four: Projection of areola and papilla to form a secondary mound (may not appear in all girls).
- Stage five: Mature configuration, projection of papilla only caused by recession of areola into general contour.

Growth of pubic hair follows the same pattern as for boys, with stage one having no pubic hair, through stages two and three when the hair goes from sparse and downy to more coarse and curly, and stages four and five when the hair becomes denser, curled and finally adult in quality, with spread of hair to the thighs. Figure 12.65 shows the pubertal changes for girls.

Sexual maturation of boys

Maturation begins in boys with an increase in the rate of growth of the testes and scrotum at about age 12 years of age. There is slow growth of pubic hair at about the same time and, approximately year later, accelerated growth of the penis. Ejaculation occurs about 1.5 years after the accelerated growth of the penis begins. Body and facial hair usually appear about 2 years after the beginning of pubic hair growth. The lowering of the voice occurs quite late in puberty. Some changes also occur to the male breast this includes an enlargement of the areola; there may also be some enlargement but this usually disappears within a year or so.

Marshall & Tanner (1969) describe the developmental stages of genital development in boys as:

- Stage one: Prepubertal. No pubic hair – essentially the same as in childhood.
- Stage two: Pubertal. Initial enlargement of the scrotum and testes with reddening of the scrotal skin.
- Stage three: Penile lengthening, thinning of the scrotal skin, testicular enlargement which begins between 10.5 and 14.5 years with pubic hair spread sparsely over the entire pubis.
- Stage four: Glans enlargement, penile broadening, testicular enlargement, scrotal increase in size and deepening of pigmentation with more abundant pubic hair but restricted to the pubic area.

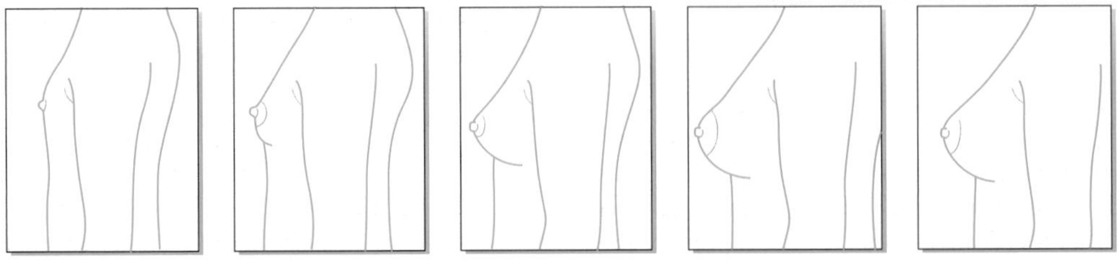

Fig. 12.64 • Development of the breasts.

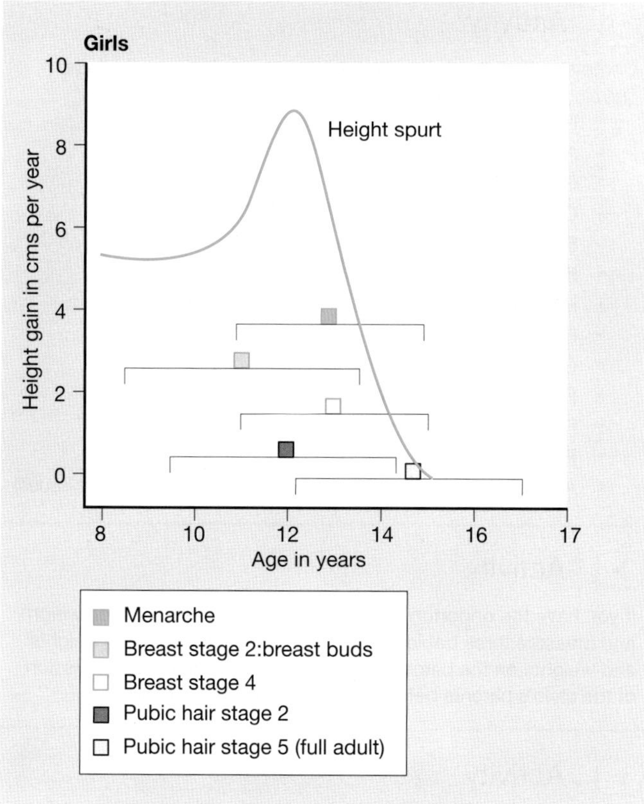

Fig. 12.65 • The pubertal changes for girls (Chimlea 1982 (cited in Bee 1997), Garn 1980, Tanner 1962).

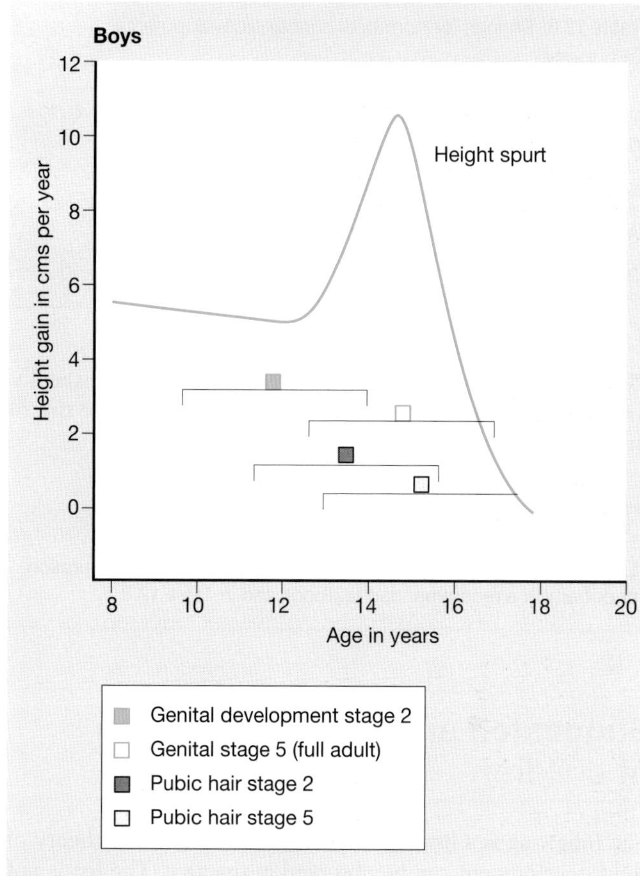

Fig. 12.66 • The pubertal changes for boys (Chimlea 1982 (cited in Bee 1997), Garn 1980, Tanner 1962).

- Stage five: Adult size and shape with spread of hair to inner thighs.

Spermatogenesis is active from the time of penile growth; and ejaculate can be produced from 1 year after its onset. Figure 12.66 shows the pubertal changes for boys.

Activity

Look up www.cua.edu and serch for pubertal processes

The adolescent growth spurt

The internal organs grow, including the lungs and heart, which increases physical endurance.

The lymphoid system, including the tonsils and adenoids, decreases in size, improving asthma, in some teenagers.

The growth of the skeletal system is reflected in limb growth. Boys' longer growth is reflected in their greater height and longer arms and legs.

Muscle mass increases in boys and girls. For girls, this peaks at menarche then slows; for boys it continues, resulting in a higher lean body mass in boys.

Adolescence is a time of continued brain growth. There is no actual increase in number of neurons but growth of the myelin sheath continues until at least puberty, thus enabling faster neural processing, which corresponds with the development of cognitive abilities.

The rate of growth may double during the pubertal growth spurt. The final 20–25% of linear growth is achieved; this can be as much as 12.5 cm in a peak year. Girls gain an average of 5–20 cm in height and 7–25 kg in weight; boys gain 10–30 cm in height and 7–30 kg in weight.

Both the growth spurt and onset of menstruation are occurring earlier now than they used to. Since 1850, the age at which menarche occurs has been declining in Western countries, probably the result of better nutrition, fewer diseases and good medical care. For example, in the US, girls first menstruated at 13–15 years; this is now 11–13 years. This means that girls are reaching the 'critical weight' of 45 kg, which must be attained before menstruation can begin, earlier than in former times.

Activity

What size do you think the knights of yesteryear were?

They were actually about the size of today's 12-year-old. A more recent example can be seen at La Scala opera house, which was built between 1776 and 1778 with seats that were 33 cm wide; this means of course that this must have been the average size of the bottom! In 1975 aircraft seats were 60 cm

Table 12.8 Timings for hormonal changes/developments at puberty

	Boy	Girl
Begins as early as	10.5 years	7.5 years
Begins as late as	16 years	11.5 years
Average onset	12 years	10 years
Peaks	14 years	12 years

wide. (Do you know how wide they are today? Watch the TV commercials to find out.) What does this say about the size of our bottoms?

Activity

Look up the hormonal changes and sequence of sexual maturation at puberty in a recommended textbook and in Table 12.8

Suggested areas for observation of children

The following is a list of placement areas where the theory of child development can be observed in practice. The list is not exclusive and you may visit other areas where you can observe children:

- Child health clinics
- Developmental screening
- Home visits with health visitor
- School health checks
- Practice nurses
- Family centres
- Mother and toddler groups
- Play groups
- Nurseries
- Schools
- Youth centres/organisations, e.g. Cub Scouts, Girl Guides, youth centres
- Voluntary-sector child-oriented organisations, e.g. riding for the disabled, youth enquiry service, play centres, toy libraries.

When observing and interacting with children, consider their developmental progress using a developmental screening chart as a framework. Please use it simply as a guide to your observation, do not feel you have to test the child or check every item. Do not attempt any of the specific screening tests, such as hearing, physical examinations of the hips and testicles and checking of reflexes. Do not record any information that might compromise the confidentiality of the child (Nursing and Midwifery Council 2009), e.g. name, address.

The following three activities can help to focus your findings when observing children.

Activity

Complete the following worksheet as a record of your findings.
Developmental observation exercise

- Practice area
- Age of child
- Gender
- Context of observation
- Background of child (if applicable)
- Social behaviour and play
- Hearing and speech
- Fine motor and vision
- Gross motor
- Feeding and nutrition (if applicable)
- Physical appearance
- Personality and demeanour
- Additional comments (e.g. reasons for any developmental issues)

Activity

If you have the opportunity, when out with the health visitor, weigh and measure three babies or young children and plot their heights and weights on the percentile chart. Be sure to ask the permission of the child's parents before you undertake this exercise.

Activity

The ways in which family life affects development are many. Through daily incidents and decisions parents affect their child's development in both positive and negative ways. Think of some examples in which parents can affect their child's development:

- Sean is 5 months old and cannot sit unaided
- Sue is 2 years old and screams when her mother dresses her but she cannot cope on her own
- John is 6 and is slow in beginning to read
- Gill has just begun her periods and her body is changing
- Gary is 16 with no qualifications, out every night and surly

References

Allen, R., 2001. The Penguin English dictionary. Penguin Books, London.

Bee, H., 1997. The developing child, 8th edn. Harper Collins, London.

Frankenburg, W.K., Dodds, J.B., 1967. The Denver developmental screening test. Journal of Pediatrics 71, 181–191.

Garn, S.M., 1980. Continuities and change in maturational timing. Constancy and change in human development. Harvard University Press, Cambridge, Mass.

Hockenberry, M.J., Wilson, D., Winkelstein, M.L., Kline, N.E., 2003. Wong's nursing care of infants and children, 7th edn. Mosby, St Louis.

MacGregor, J., 2000. Introduction to the anatomy and physiology of children. Routledge, London.

Marshall, W.A., Tanner, J.H., 1969. Variations in pattern of pubertal changes in girls. Archives of Diseases in Childhood 44, 291.

Meadow, R., Newell, S., 2002. Lecture notes in paediatrics, 7th edn. Blackwell Science, Oxford.

Mussen, P.H., 1990. Child development and personality, 7th edn. HarperCollins College Division Row, New York.

Nursing and Midwifery Council (NMC), 2009. Confidentiality advice sheet. NMC, London.

Sheridan, M., 1997. From birth to five years, children's developmental progress. Revised and updated by Marion Frost and Dr Ajay Sharma. Routledge, Cornwall.

Tanner, J.M., , 1962. Growth at adolescence. Blackwell Scientific Publications, Oxford.

Preparing the family for stressful life events

Child life and the role of therapeutic play

13

Gary Mountain Sue Fallon Barbara Wood

ABSTRACT

Gaining a critical appreciation and understanding of the life world of children and their families within the health-illness experience is a central tenet of family-based health care. The intent of this chapter is to help readers develop their knowledge and understanding of how individual children, young people and their families perceive and adjust to the various life stressor(s) they experience along the health-illness continuum. Being in tune with how families perceive the stressor(s) they are experiencing provides for early recognition and the planning of interventions that monopolise on the resources and strengths available and promote family empowerment.

LEARNING OUTCOMES

- Identify the major categories of stress in children and young people.
- Discuss the aetiological processes of stress in children/young people and their family.
- Debate the short- and long-term impact of adverse life events on the child, young person and the family.
- Evaluate the effectiveness of some of the assessment models and/or frameworks available, which claim to predict the implications of adverse events on the family.
- Understand the roles and responsibilities of the children's nurse in providing structured psychosocial-emotional preparation and support for children/young people and their family.
- Appreciate the role of therapeutic play as a tool in helping children/young people understand and deal with particular stressful life events.

Introduction

Although stress in adults has been well researched, the existence and reactions of children and young people to life stressors – despite the accumulating evidence that they are frequently some of the most affected subsections of our society – have not been investigated. Accepting this point, it can be seen that in attempting to understand this complex topic we also need to take account of the interdependence of the individual within the family, the family system and the environment (Friedman 1998) and therefore individuals are best understood in the context of their family.

Stress is a constant aspect of daily living and is initiated by both positive and negative life events. Some form of stress is accepted as commonplace in our lives and perhaps ceases only at the time of death (Selye 1978). A number of suppositions are central to the theme of stress in children, young people and their families (Box 13.1).

At a simple level, the analysis of the impact of stress on children, young people and their families involves close examination of the following key elements: (a) the stressor(s) involved and the stress responses invoked; (b) the resources available to individuals and groups when faced with stressful events; (c) the coping strategies that may or may not be called on to deal with the stress response; and (d) the outcomes. Other broader conceptual models may refer to some of the above as 'mediators' and 'moderators' of the relation between stress and outcomes, as well as of the reciprocal and dynamic relationships between these variables (Grant 2003). However, although this simplistic interpretation may seem plausible, a number of general issues and questions need to be considered.

First, children and their families can experience an infinite variety of categories, or even clusters of categories, of life stressors along a continuum ranging from ordinary 'hassles' to adverse and severe events or crises. There are events that many children would consider as unusually stressful. These might include:

- death of a parent or grandparent
- abuse
- disturbed family relationships
- birth of a sibling
- illness or accident involving the child or their parent
- parental unemployment
- change of school, in particular starting secondary school (Sharman 1997).

DOI: 10.1016/B978-0-7020-3183-0.10013-X

Box 13.1

Summary of life's stressors in children and families

- Stress in it numerous variations can be perceived as normal; it is the individual's and family's perceptions that are important
- Stress sometimes places extraordinary demands on individuals and their families
- Most individuals and their families adapt reasonably well to life's stressors
- If individuals/families do not adapt reasonably well, negative outcomes (which can be short or long term) can follow

Further lists of acute stressful life events and their impact on children are available, e.g. those detailed in Coddington's (1972) life events scales (cited in Clunn 1991). However, in a broad review of the literature findings, it is apparent that the most stressful events all appear to centre on tangible loss or circumstances that threaten loss (Hobfoll 1988).

Second, there is an array of related measurement problems. A critical review of the mass of available evidence-based literature found that research designs have adopted a wide variety of methodologies. Many of the designs make serious attempts to disaggregate a large number of stressful events and determine how they might be combined (reduced) into meaningful and useable subscales to try and predict cause and effect relationships. The stressor measures used in research studies have been found to combine neutral, negative and positive items; this could produce misleading findings. Aggregating stressors that are different in nature into a single measure could mask the impact of the different stressors on the individual. For example, economic deprivation would be associated with a range of additional specific stressful experiences, including conflict (exposure to abuse, marital conflict) and loss-based stressors (e.g. loss of role, death). However, studying each stressor individually demands complex statistical modelling techniques that would involve an array of parameters and a fragmented approach.

The number of potential outcome variables can be exceedingly large. It is necessary to study multiple outcome variables because they may be related not only to the nature of the stressor but also to its sequelae. Possible consequences are complex, which again makes measurement and prediction difficult. To complicate matters even further, sources of stress are closely related to an array of possible psychological and physical outcomes that are mediated by a mass of possible intervening factors such as age, gender, developmental level and the environmental context. Outcome measures can be further confounded or masked when the use of measures is eclectic. Thus it is easy to detect, even at this early stage, that studies will need to draw on sophisticated statistical modelling techniques when trying to disentangle cause and effect relationships.

Third, various factors might increase children's and young people's likelihood of exposure to stress or may moderate the effects of stress. The transition into adolescence is frequently cited as being characterised by an accumulation of stressful events and psychological challenges (Ge et al 1994). The salience and impact of certain social contexts such as the family, peers and school have a tendency to be singled out as having a significant influence on children and young people. Nevertheless we must remember that children are not simply passive recipients but also make an active contribution to their social worlds (Rudolph & Hammen 1999), and the processes of growth, maturation and expansion of environmental influences that occur with increasing age will inevitably change the nature of stressful experiences (Berk 2001).

Finally, just as there are an infinite number of stresses, so there is an array of coping strategies. Although these are likely to be less sophisticated than those used by adults, because of a relative lack of life experiences, they are perhaps just as resource intensive.

It is only possible here to start critically examining a small selection of the key life stressors children and young people experience and their underlying aetiological processes in the hope that the reader may be motivated to seek out further studies.

Life stressors, social responses and coping/adaptive strategies

Stressors are said to be the initiating or precipitating agents that activate the stress process and stress is the response or state of tension produced by the stressor(s) or by the actual/perceived demands that remains unmanaged (Friedman 1998 p 437). In reality, stress is a normal part of a child's or young person's life trajectory and encompasses common, developmental stressors of everyday life for which there may be fairly well-defined coping mechanisms (Santrock 2001) as well as unusual adverse events or crises. Apart from the well-known categories of major stressors or major life events, such as poverty, family instability, life-threatening illness and child abuse, it is crucial that we do not lose sight of the social context of modern everyday life that children and young people experience. It is within this context that children and young people may experience life's 'hassles'. These might be managed well or they might accumulate to such an extent that they present a significant threat to the child and/or family.

A useful model for understanding stress responses in children and young people is that presented by Moos (2002). This offers an 'integrated stress and coping framework' that can help the reader begin to understand the complex interplay between children and young people's acute and chronic life stressors and the variety of coping and adaptation strategies available. The framework comprises five main elements:

- The first (environmental system) reflects key life domains. These should be relatively stable conditions that include the family climate, ongoing life stressors and social resources.
- The second element is classified as the personal system, which includes the person's biogenetic characteristics and such personal resources as cognitive and intellectual abilities, social competence, self-confidence, self-esteem and personality.
- Element three includes the transitory conditions that children and young people may face, such as novel life events, which might in turn offer either new opportunities for learning and personal development or conversely dysfunction.

Moos (2002) states that these three sets of factors shape and indeed are almost precursors to, the child/young person's cognitive appraisal and coping skills (element 4) and, in turn, the child's/young person's health and well-being (element 5) (for a full explanation of this model, see Moos 2002).

The school environment as a potential major stressor

From a very early age, the school environment is where a child or young person can directly and indirectly experience stress. The impact of the pressures and expectations within the school environment are certainly among the most frequently reported stressors by adolescents (de Anda et al 2000). Relevant stressors include fear of success or failure, test or performance anxiety and fears associated with the unrelenting academic pressure often imposed in today's school environment. In a study by de Anda (2000), apart from concerns about future goals, school-related items show the highest recorded frequency in high school students. The pressure of time, achievement and expectations in the form of tests, grades, homework and pressures from parents were reported as being stress factors that were felt 'often' to 'very often' on a daily and weekly basis by adolescent respondents.

When the school environment imposes a significant continuing source of stress, children tend to avoid school altogether. These children almost become school phobic and appear to experience relatively significant emotional and physical effects even at the very thought of going to school. Unfortunately, such children can inadvertently become categorised as persistent truants and labelled as exhibiting behavioural problems.

Children can face other types of stress at school apart from those associated with scholarly activities. Bullying has become a significant social problem in contemporary school life. Kidscape (http://www.kidscape.org.uk) is a national charity that supplies sensitive advice for bullied children as well as providing individuals and organisations with the practical skills and resources necessary to keep children safe from harm. Kidscape (2009) feels that this kind of work is vital given the frightening statistics that:

- Each year 10–14 youth suicides are directly attributed to bullying.
- Bullied children are six times more likely to contemplate suicide than their non-bullied counterparts.
- One in 12 children are badly bullied to the point that it affects their education, relationships and even their prospects for work in later life.
- Kidscape maintain a website with current information for all purposes and free, downloadable literature. Downloads include anti-bullying activity sheets which are truly child-centred in their approach to encouraging young children to share their experience of bullying.

The loss of a parent

The loss of parent, either through death or through separation/divorce, is a devastating loss that permanently changes the family dynamics. Although some children are well cared for when facing such stressors, other longitudinal studies show that even among adults who claim to have coped with the loss of a parent in childhood, certain life cycle events, such as marriage, can sometimes trigger a surge of maturational grief responses (Moos 1986). It is also now acknowledged that children whose parents divorce are exposed to multiple losses and adversities that may have a negative impact on the child's health, well-being and achievement in life many years later (Papalia et al 1999).

Separation and divorce – and the consequent single parenthood – inevitably bring changes in financial circumstances. Compared with children in 'intact' families, children in one-parent families are more likely to experience sibling conflict, family disruption and less support. They are also more likely to have household responsibilities, more contact with siblings, less family cohesion, and less support, control or discipline (Papalia et al 1999). Children suffering the loss of a parent (whatever the cause) may suffer higher rates of enuresis, delinquency, a range of illnesses including hypertension and mental health problems, and are more likely to leave school at an earlier age (Burges 1994, Jenkins & Urstrun 1998, Papalia et al 1999). Longitudinal studies following-up children who have experienced the loss of a parent have found that some of them are still experiencing problems 10 or more years later (Koenen et al 2007, Papalia et al 1999).

Parental psychopathology and child abuse

Differences in what is termed the 'emotional tone' of the family can have profound effects on children (Mountain 2008). In particular, children who live in situations of neglect or abuse are more likely to experience disorganised/disorientated attachments to their parents, have negative, ill-conceived self-concepts, find it difficult to engage in social interactions and consequently have difficulty forming social relationships. These children may develop particular characteristics and personality traits that in turn make them less well liked. For example, there is an abundance of evidence to suggest a link between abuse and children's low self-esteem, emotional maladjustment, dependency, underachievement, depression, faltering growth, deliberate self-harm and other psychological distress in later life (Papalia et al 1999).

Many forms of mental health problem in parents have a direct impact on the quality and nature of parenting. Therefore nearly all types of mental health problems in parents have been linked to an increased likelihood of behavioural and emotional problems in children and young people (Graham et al 1999). Research on the children of depressed parents signals a clear causal relationship between depression in parents and problems of adjustment and depression in their children. Similarly, toddlers of depressed parents are more likely to exhibit emotional and behavioural disturbances, delayed language and cognitive developments (Steinhausen & Verhulst 1999).

Adolescent life stressors

The period of adolescence (whenever this is said to commence) has traditionally been described as a particularly critical period of physical, psychological and social change for young people, often characterised by emotional and psychological stress and, indeed, clusters of crises. However, although contemporary studies concur with some of these claims in some cases, they are not always generalisable to all adolescents. Indeed, in most cases adolescents are remarkably level-headed and well equipped to resolve many of the problems they encounter during this transitional period (Erwin 1998).

Nevertheless with the continuing rise of reported mental illness episodes and suicidal behaviours in adolescence (Stoleb & Chiribogo 1988), along with clear associations between stress and psychological symptoms (Jenson et al 1991), one can logically and safely conclude that for some individuals within this relatively large section of society certain life stressors can appear to have a significant and dramatic effect on their lives. According to Lau (2002), this can be partly explained by the fact that negative life events, especially if cumulative in nature, negatively affect adolescents' adjustment in various ways. Similarly, it must be remembered that the foundation for adolescence begins to be laid during early childhood (Jackson & Rodriguez-Tome 1995).

As well as exposure to violence, abuse and divorce, which we have already noted, other examples of adolescent life stressors include disciplinary action taken against them, incidence of rejection/humiliation by others, moves to new environments, terminations of friendships or relationships, and conflict with relatives or peers. Across the various stressors the various research studies have chosen to study, there is little evidence to detect patterns of specificity in any of them apart from the broad outcomes associated with sexual abuse (McMahon et al 2003). As noted earlier, it is well recognised that the nature of the family climate or environment is a key context that sets the stage for adolescent development and affects adolescent's reactions to life stressors (Moos 2002). In particular, the family and peers provide a source of social support that helps the young person facing life stressors to maintain his or her coping efforts. The quality of social support and peer relations (rather than the number of social supports) has been demonstrated to be associated with favourable mental health outcomes. A growing sense of group membership also appears to play a key protective role in negating the effects of life crises in adolescents (D'Attilio et al 1992, Morano et al 1993).

Given the centrality of the family environment, it may come of no surprise to learn that 50% of suicidal adolescents are found to come from broken homes – family environments characterised by divorces or single-parent structures. Adolescents who have experienced violence or sexual abuse are also at higher risk of negative mental health outcomes. Parents of suicidal adolescents tend to be more depressed, consume more alcohol, and have lower self-esteem and increased anxiety.

Gender differences have been found to exist. There is a tendency for female adolescents to report more sensitivity than boys to interpersonal stressors and to those related to peer values regarding dress and appearance (Coleman 1990). There is a dearth of research on the links between ethnic differences and life stressors. However, a few studies indicate that issues surrounding identity, including the impact of prejudice and stereotypes are additional stressors for young people from different cultural groups (Phinney & Alipuria 1990).

The notion of 'family stress' will now be examined briefly before moving on to explore the social resources and coping responses children, young people and family members may utilise to manage life stressors.

Family stress

Boss (1988 p 704) claims that the family, as a group, is not coping if even one member manifests stress-related symptoms. If this stringent criterion is adopted then family stress can be seen as a natural and logical extension of individual stress applied to the family domain and, importantly, both the individual and family are of equal importance when examining the impact of life's stressors.

To paraphrase Hobfoll & Spielberger (1992), family stress is the state in which both family members and the family as a unit are challenged by the environment in a way that overtakes the individual or collective resources and threatens the well-being of individuals within the family, or the family as a whole.

Whereas Moos' (2002) framework has a tendency to be directed to individual stress, McCubbin & McCubbin's (1993) resiliency model is family-centred and focuses not only on the factors that produce crisis/non-crisis in families but also how family members adjust and how the family adapts during and after crisis.

A focus on stressors is key in virtually all theories of family stress but different theorists envisage different conceptions of the nature of those stressors. Traditionally, research has tended to focus on stressors being caused by pressures for change on the family system or the accumulation of demands for change. According to Hill (cited in Health Advisory Service 1995), a stressor consists of those life events or occurrences that are sufficient magnitude to bring about change in the family system.

Family stressors can derive from interpersonal, environmental, economic or sociocultural events or experiences (Friedman 1998) and they can be acute, chronic, major, minor and/or ongoing (Hobfoll & Spielberger 1992). The perception and interpretation of stressors is highly subjective and individual to each family unit. For example, what one family may perceive as challenging opportunities may be perceived as threatening and overwhelming by another.

Like stress responses in the individual, family life stressors can be accumulative or 'pile up' (McCubbin & Patterson 1983). Likewise, a family stressor event is only a stimulus that holds the potential for beginning the process of change of stress. Whether it does or does not depends on the family's response to the stressor (Boss 1988). According to Boss, family crisis differs from, but precedes, stress when stress is so significant that the family's resources are no longer adequate to maintain the structure. In families who face adversity, boundaries are not maintained, customary roles and tasks are no longer performed and individual members may no longer function at optimal levels. However, it should be noted that crises could result in families redefining themselves. A positive outcome arising from, say, the admission of a child to a paediatric intensive care unit, may result in a higher level of family functioning after recovering from the crisis event.

Coping

'Stress' and 'coping' are terms used ubiquitously in the literature without specific definition and consensus as to the meanings of the concepts. A useful definition of coping comes from Cohen & Lazarus (1979), who view coping as:

> … a wide range of problem-solving efforts both externally orientated and intra-psychic used to manage, master, tolerate, reduce or minimise the environmental and internal demands and conflicts between them or exceed an individual's resources.

Analysis of the processes involved and resources available to individuals and their families has found coping to comprise individual, family and/or socially based strategies. We must also remember that a multicultural perspective on the subject is vital and that, cross-culturally, individual, family and socially based coping strategies are not only sometimes different but can often be in direct conflict with each other.

To achieve the goals of coping the child/young person needs to engage in a number of activities or tasks. However, just as there are an infinite number of life stressors so there are an infinite number of coping strategies and responses. Nevertheless, a number of protective factors seem to increase a child's capacity to cope with stress, these include (Spender et al, cited in Townley 2002):

- an easy temperament, e.g. some children make friends easily whereas others struggle with establishing relationships
- higher intelligence
- support from parents
- support from peers
- a sense of humour
- positive experiences at school
- support from other adults outside the immediate family
- religious faith
- a tendency to plan and set goals for life decisions
- positive experiences that help to neutralise the effects of adverse factors
- taking extra responsibility, which can lead to increase in self-esteem
- cognitive processing of experiences, i.e. the ability to find meaning in life experiences and learn from them.

Years of research appear to have failed to identify either higher-order or core categories of specific coping responses. Almost every activity can be considered to be a way of coping and each one has its body of research. These can be behavioural, cognitive or emotional in nature and include problem solving, information seeking, planning, negotiation, compliance, self and other blame, help seeking, social support, opposition, venting, selecting optimisation, compensation, rumination, disclosure and discussion, primary and secondary control, optimism and positive illusions to name but a few.

Additionally, individual predisposing factors influence a child's or young person's capacity to cope. These include age, gender, temperament, arousal, imagery and/or coping response styles, which in turn may influence both the perception of the problem and the ability to motivate resources or engage the support of others. Current research into coping tends to favour longitudinal designs, repeating measures over a short time or over several years, often including markers of the progress of stressful events. The criteria for measuring the outcomes of the coping process usually focus on the psychosocial, physical and functional status of the child or young person at a given single or multiple points.

Two points are worth noting at this stage. First, whereas some of the aforementioned coping strategies may be effective in dealing with stress in the short term, we also need to examine the predicted longer-term consequences of these strategies. Second, whereas it is hoped that many of the coping strategies children and young people employ are adaptive, maladaptive ways of coping exist, including catastrophising and panic, social isolation, blame of others, denial, withdrawal confrontation, aggressive behaviour and even substance misuse (de Anda et al 2000).

The family environment

Family support and structure are key influencing factors associated with children's and young people's ability to cope and adapt to life's stressors. Numerous research studies point to a strong correlation between parental functioning and competence and the family environment generally, and how children succeed or not with many life stressors. In a chapter of this kind it is therefore important that we at least make some reference to the notion of family coping as opposed to individual coping. Boss defined family coping as 'the management of a stressful event by the family and by each individual in the family'. She goes on to assert that it is the cognitive and affective process by which individuals and their family system adjust to, rather than eradicate stress (Boss 1988).

In his Conservation of Resources Theory, Hobfoll (1988) claims that the role of resources is pivotal for families trying to cope with stressors. He defines resources as those things that people (or this case families) value or that act as a means of obtaining or protecting that which they value. The theory suggests four principal resource categories:

1. Object resources (e.g. transport and housing)
2. Condition resources (e.g. good marital relationships)
3. Personal resources (e.g. self-esteem)
4. Energy resources (e.g. money and time).

The theory states that stress occurs with resource loss even if total resources available are not outstripped. Furthermore, loss of resources makes families more vulnerable because they have fewer resources available to deal with future stressors. Loss of resources can be cumulative, whereby resource loss sets up an adverse reaction where further loss is likely. Hence the family becomes less resilient and more vulnerable. Conversely, future gains are more likely to follow after resource gain, i.e. by successfully meeting the challenges of some life stressors, the family gains confidence and competence to address more stressful challenges heading its way.

A number of family resources have been identified as especially important in coping with stressful life events. Among these are:

- flexibility/adaptability versus rigidity
- cohesion versus separateness
- communication versus privacy
- boundary clarity versus boundary ambiguity.

A full explanation of each of these can be found in Hobfoll & Spielberger (1992 p 103). An additional key resource the family has available outside of, but yet interconnected with, the family system is that of social support. Again, a review of the literature helps identify three major sources:

- support network resources
- supportive behaviour
- the subjective appraisal of support.

All three aspects of social support are important and have different causes and influences.

The short- and long-term impact of stress caused by life events

If a child's mental health needs are not met, or are only partially met, when the child faces a stressful situation this might result in a particular physical or psychological problem or disorder. In a review of the literature on the association of environmental stressors on the psychological and physical health of children, Grey (1993) cited many studies that seem to suggest that there is a link between stress and the development of symptoms of a particular disorder or disease. For example she cites two small studies that suggest that major psychological stress may be one of the precipitating factors in the onset of leukaemia symptoms (Green & Swisher 1969, Miller 1982). The onset and exacerbation of diabetes and diabetic ketoacidosis have been associated with stressful life events in the year before their diagnosis and in the triggering of acute ketoacidosis in children (Fallon 1995, Johnson 1982, Stein & Charles 1971). There is also evidence to suggest that life stressors are also associated with the exacerbation of asthma (Johnson 1982). Recurrent abdominal pain has also been found to relate directly to increased stress levels (Wilson-Sharrer & Ryan-Wenger 1991).

Other studies also cited by Grey (1993) suggest a link between stressful life events and psychological problems, such as low self-esteem, poor school performance (Bedell 1977), maladaptive behaviour (Sandler & Block 1979), suicidal behaviour (Pfeffer et al 1979), teenage pregnancy (Coddington 1979), drug addiction (Duncan 1977) and psychiatric hospitalisation (Vincent & Rosenstock 1979). Buchanan & Tenbrink (1997) add that in adulthood the consequences of unmet mental health needs associated with stressful life events in childhood may result in poorer relationships with partners and own children, mental health problems and possible serious physical illnesses.

Sharman (1997) suggests that if parents are aware that stress can precipitate the onset of asthmatic or diabetic symptoms they may be able to prevent this by ensuring that the need for extra emotional support is anticipated and that the support is given. This is good preventive advice but, as further research has shown, stress alone is not the one single precipitator to illness and thus parents should not be made to feel guilty if a child develops symptoms or an illness that does have a tenuous link with increased stress. This point leads onto Grey's (1993) observation of the flaws of much of the research she reviewed. Her major criticisms were that there is difficulty in describing, and thus estimating, the magnitude of various stressful life events and that there is a glaring lack of data on intervening and mediating variables that may modify the impact of stress on the development of illness. This observation is supported by McMahon et al's (2003) review of the literature, which concludes that apart from the major stressor of child sexual abuse there is very little evidence to uniquely link specific stressful life events to the onset of specific physical or mental illnesses or diseases.

McMahon et al (2003) suggest that many different avenues of stressful experience can lead to the same outcome (equifinality) or that similar stressful conditions can lead to multiple outcomes (multifinality). They add that the outcomes of stressful situations depend on many systems that moderate or mediate the effect on a child's behaviour, such as family variables, larger contextual variables, environmental stressors and biological vulnerability.

Assessment and appraisal of stress in children and families within the healthcare context

Given the knowledge that hospitalisation and illness are major stressors for children and young people, how do we assess how stressed they actually are? Townley (2002) suggests that before any assessment the nurse must have an understanding of the normal developmental stages and mental health needs of children and young people. Hill (cited in Health Advisory Service 1995) suggests that mental health in children and young people is indicated by:

- the capacity to enter into and sustain mutually satisfying personal relationships.
- continuing progression of psychological development.
- an ability to play and learn so that achievements are appropriate for age and intellectual level.
- a developing sense of right and wrong.
- the degree of psychological distress and maladaptive behaviour that is within the normal limits for the child's age and context.

There is a wide range of standardised inventories designed to measure individual child life stressors. Due to the number and diversity of potential life stressors in children and young people, as well as the wide range of contexts healthcare professional may find themselves in, it is difficult to recommend any one particular assessment scale. However, before assessment it would be useful for a children's nurse to be familiar with Coddington's (1972) work, if only to be aware of some of the most common social acute stressors, both positive and negative, that children might experience in addition to the stress that hospitalisation and illness may bring. Similarly the Stress Impact Scale (SIS) by Hutton and Roberts, reviewed by

Drummond & Meier (1995), claims to measure the occurrence and effect of 70 potentially stressful events on adolescents.

Following on from the above, it is also important that the children's nurse is aware of some of the mental health risk factors, such as those related to home, family, school and peers, that may make a child more susceptible to develop mental health problems as a result of stress. The Mental Health Foundation (1999) suggests that these include:

- Risk factors in the child:
  - Genetic influences
  - Low IQ and learning disability
  - Specific developmental delay
  - Communication difficulty
  - Difficult temperament
  - Physical illness, especially if chronic/or neurological
  - Academic failure
  - Low self-esteem.
- Risk factors in the family:
  - Overt parental conflict
  - Family breakdown
  - Inconsistent or unclear discipline
  - Hostile and rejecting relationships
  - Failure to adapt to child's changing needs
  - Physical, sexual and/or emotional abuse
  - Parental psychiatric illness
  - Parental criminality, alcoholism or personality disorder
  - Death and loss, including loss of friendship.
- Risk factors in the community:
  - Socioeconomic disadvantage
  - Homelessness
  - Disaster
  - Discrimination
  - Other significant life events.

Finally, the other baseline information the children's nurse must acquire prior to assessment relates to the stressors children experience that are specific to hospitalisation. Melamed et al (1988) details the common (most reported) features of hospital-related stressors in children.

Activity

Taking each of the components mentioned above, how might a 2-year-old respond to hospitalisation/illness and how might you help a 2-year-old overcome his or her responses?

WWW

Click on the following hyperlinks for useful good practice ideas in relation to preparing children for hospitalisation:

- http://www.actionforsickchildren.org/sitemap.asp
- http://childrenfirst.nhs.uk/kids/index.html
- http://www.kidshealth.org/parent/system/index.html

Not every child will experience all these stressors or respond to a stressor in the same way. The response will depend on the child's previous experience with the same or similar procedures, and on the parents' ability to prepare the child for the impending event and their skill to communicate effectively what this will involve. The practitioner's ability to prepare the child for the event in advance is essential. Also, instructions given to children should be appropriate to their level of understanding and ability to carry out those instructions (Melamed 1993).

Assessment tools

When assessing psychological stress levels in children, nurses depend largely on their observation skills and the child's self report (Grey & Hayman 1987). Both methods are useful but both are also prone to major subjectivity. Observation of the child's behaviour can be limited by observer bias, the timing of the observation and where the observation takes place. Similarly, the child's self report can also be affected by a number of factors, such as the child's willingness and/or ability to communicate and cooperate, and how the child actually recalls and reports a particular stressful event. This indicates the value of and need for a multidisciplinary approach with assessment, utilising observation and self-report taking place over a period of time and in different situations before conclusions about a child's level of stress/anxiety are made.

Townley (2002) points out that for most nurses working in general children's wards it is inappropriate and impractical to carry out lengthy and detailed assessments of a child's full mental health status. He suggests that a quick assessment tool/framework for use in general ward situations would be more useful. The aim of this aspect of assessment is to establish the extent of the anxiety, unhappiness or distress that the stressor of illness and/or hospitalisation is causing the child. The nurse competently facilitating the expression of the reasons behind the child's feelings could achieve this. The nurse must not force the child to express his or her thoughts and feelings but must go at the child's pace. This process requires time, sensitivity and creativity.

Children often find it easier to communicate through play and art. Sharman (1997) suggests a wide range of play strategies to establish a therapeutic relationship with a child. These in turn would enable children to feel comfortable to then express their thoughts and feelings of what it is that actually worries them or makes them feel tense or stressed. This information will form the key basis of the information required for assessment.

All nurses working with children must also be able to work with their families. Increasingly, nursing research is pointing to the importance of child-centred care and family nursing (Friedman 1998, McCubbin & McCubbin 1993), whereby the sick child is assessed but within the context of the whole family (Mountain 2007). Thus assessment and understanding of how the parents and other family members perceive and cope with stressors (i.e. the child's hospitalisation) is key to the understanding of how the child will behave and cope in that situation.

Activity

There is a wide range of family assessment tools with varying complexity and sophistication:

- Search the literature to find an example of a family assessment tool.
- Consider how this tool may possibly be adapted for application to your practice area.
- Consider the skills the practitioner may need and the adaptations that may need to be made to use this or similar assessment tools in your area of practice.

The items outlined above offer the practitioner a number of areas to consider when approaching an assessment of the older child's stressors and her/his capacity to cope (Spender et al, cited in Townley 2002).

Illness and hospitalisation as a major source of stress in children

Success and a sense of competence in mastering challenging life experiences such as illness and hospitalisation contribute to a child's evolving self-concept (Harter 1983). To enable children and parents to cope with a situation that may be fully outside their experience, planning and rehearsing coping strategies congruent with their individual styles, beliefs and developmental capacities can be used. Indeed, successful coping with one stressful event increases a child's coping repertoire and confidence to address subsequent stressors (Lutz 1986). It has long been recognised that children and young people benefit tremendously from preparation and support before hospitalisation (Eisner 1990, Glasper & Thompson 1993, Robertson 1995, While 1994). This recognition is supported in a number of studies (Adams et al 1991, Bielby 1984), which demonstrate that children who receive some type of preadmission preparation cope much better with hospitalisation, have fewer behavioural problems after discharge, spend less time as an inpatient and return to school more quickly than their counterparts.

For a child, more than for an adult, the prospect of a hospital admission can be very distressing and frightening. When admission is an emergency, time for preparation is extremely limited as the following conversation reveals. It is highly likely that these traumatic memories and behaviours will be carried into future similar situations (Solnit 1984), and may persist well into adulthood (Sugar 1992).

CHILD CONVERSATION

C J Wood, aged 12 years.

8.15 a.m. Saturday 28 July my whole world turned upside down. As I lay floating on top of the water the paramedics told me that they had to get me out of the pool and to hospital as quickly as possible. They kept telling me not to move, and my mum kept saying the same and telling me she loved me. As all of this was going on all I could think about was am I going to live? I was absolutely terrified.

As the paramedics lifted me onto the stretcher they told me that I must not move my head! As I was lying there I couldn't feel or move my arms or legs. The paramedics wrapped me in foil to keep me warm as we made our way to the ambulance.

I had never been in an ambulance before so I was a bit scared! I had to have an oxygen mask over my mouth. I kept complaining about my arms and legs because I couldn't move and there was so much pain. The paramedics didn't give me any information on what was going to happen in the accident and emergency department and although I didn't know what to expect, I thought something really bad was going to happen as everyone around me was whispering and my mum was crying but trying to be calm at the same time.

The paramedics rushed me into the accident and emergency department and I heard someone shout 'straight into resus'. I was lifted off the stretcher and on to a very hard, cold table. There were loads of doctors and a mass of faces looking down at me telling me not to move and that I was going to be OK.

The doctors didn't tell me that they were going to put a few injections into my arms, hands, feet and legs: they just went on and did it! I was very frightened, I mean I didn't know what the injections were going to do to me or what they were for! I wasn't used to any of this. The doctors never told me. That was what I was worried about the most. I didn't have a clue what was happening or what to think! The doctors kept telling me I was going to be OK but I didn't know what to believe.

My mum and dad came into the room. I wish they had been with me I wanted them beside me; they would believe me about the pain! I don't think they had been allowed in at first. I remember my dad was a dreadful colour and my mum was trying to be brave but was so upset. She obviously knew one of the nurses in the room as they were hugging each other.

After about 2 hours in the department I started to get feeling back into my legs. I thought to myself after all I'm going to be OK! But still nothing in my arms or hands. Overall I was in the department for 3½ hours. It felt like a lot longer.

My mum tried to explain things to me about what was happening, as the doctors seemed to have forgotten I was still there. They only spoke to mum and dad. I know I had a lot of pain but it was me who was hurting. Why wouldn't they talk to me?

Activity

As a children's nurse:

- What key issues is the child in the conversation above trying to communicate?
- What lessons can be learnt from this scenario for your future nursing practice?

WWW

Visit the following website for further children's accounts regarding their experiences in hospital:

- http://www.bch.org.uk

The appointment of Ministers for Children, Children's Commissioners, together with the Children's National Service Frameworks highlight the seriousness and importance of the rights of the child. These rights have been acknowledged within the last decade, but there are elements that remain solely within the domain of adults. Children's participation in healthcare decisions is well supported by Alderson & Montgomery (1996). Cohen & Emmanuel (1999) suggest that the need to involve and consult young people places a duty on governments and professionals to seek, and take full account of, the views of young people in the planning and delivery of services. Consultation with children is crucial. As Article 12 of the United Nations Convention on the Rights of the Child (UNCRC) states:

> Parties shall assure to the child who is capable of forming his or her own views the right to express those views freely in all matters affecting the child, the views of the child being given due weight in accordance with age and maturity of the child
>
> (DoH 1999)

The process by which children are consulted must reflect a commitment by the healthcare team to respect the dignity, welfare and views at all times of that child (Balen et al 2000). Children being prepared for admission to hospital must be empowered to express their views, and they should expect due notice to be taken of those views. Parents and carers are tuned into their child's ability to express their views from birth. As healthcare workers, we must liaise closely with the parents/carers to ensure the child's views are acknowledged. In some instances, children are not able to speak for themselves in situations that may have an impact on their short- or long-term future, therefore as advocates for children we must have the opportunity to speak for them. As children's nurses, we are authentic representatives who should value the individuality and diversity of the child.

Activity

What are the first thoughts that enter your head when you hear 'consultation with children'? It is quite common for people to dismiss this as a right of children, and see it in an adult domain. What do you think might have influenced the way in which you answered this question? Now consider the various ways you may approach this in your practice area.

Findings by Eisner (1990) suggest that children from 2 years of age, have well-ordered ideas about what hospital is like and what happens there; information that is presumably gained from such sources as television, books and other people's accounts. Yet, despite this children are infrequently involved in choices about their care and treatments. Flatman (2002) suggests there are various ways of consulting with children, but considerations should include:

- Communication: age-appropriate methods
- Checking comprehension: using both visual and verbal clues
- Motivation: value placed on interaction should be made clear, be meaningful for the child and offer tangible rewards
- Accuracy of representation of children's views
- Confidentiality
- Parental concerns: informed about nature and intention of consultation and consent sought.

Whether a planned admission or an emergency admission, children respond better when they are supplied with basic information about what is going to happen to them (Ivory 1998). A report published by Rennick (2002) supports what children's nurses have known for a long time, namely that children who are admitted to hospital unprepared may have lingering psychological problems months after they return home:

> Children who were younger, more severely ill, and who endured more invasive procedures had significantly more medical fears, a lower sense of control over their health, and on-going post-traumatic stress responses for six months
>
> (Rennick 2002 p 133)

Effective communication, which is jargon-free and appropriate to all involved, is essential for ensuring clarity with regard to who is providing what care and how they intend to do it (Heywood 2002). Marks (1994) suggests that aspects of care are generally discussed and planned separately, which leads to the increased risk of a fragmented view of the care pathway. If care is organised separately, children and carers could receive a disjointed care experience. However, if each element of care is planned as part of the whole, and the child and family are involved in all aspects of planning, then there is a greater chance of their perceived needs being met. Children and carers need clear information so that their choices and options can be increased. Kitson (1999 p 42), states:

> Understanding the support network around patients, and their carers' capacity to cope both in the short and long term, are dimensions of care that need to be considered within the remit of continuity of care.

Active participation by children in preparation for hospital admission is a good way to reduce anxiety and increase compliance during any medical and nursing procedures. Useful pointers include:

- Tell children where they are going, what is going to happen to them and why.
- Be honest with children. Too much information can be overwhelming, stick to the essentials.
- Don't start preparing too soon, a few days is usually adequate.
- Use simple language and give clear explanations appropriate to the child's age.
- Encourage children to ask questions.
- Give child something to look forward to after their treatment.
- Let the children know it is OK to feel scared and encourage them to talk about their feelings.
- Let the children pack their own bag to instill a sense of involvement.

Each child will react differently to hospital admission. The following highlights a number of stress responses exhibited by children to hospitalisation:

- Separation anxiety: some children feel secure and safe as long as their parents are there, but this is not always possible and some children can react badly to the absence of a parent or carer. Regression in their behaviour may be noticeable, e.g. bed wetting, tantrums, refusal to eat, withdrawn, crying a lot.

- Older children may fear a loss of new skills, separation from friends/school, loss of privacy. They may even blame their parents and see hospitalisation as a form of punishment.
- Young adults may feel embarrassment over loss of privacy and independence, threatened, anxious over their separation from their peers and anxious about their illness.

Activity

Think of the times when you have felt low or anxious, or wanted to be alone, or perhaps when you have felt angry:

- Identify the factors in your life around that time that might have influenced the way you responded.
- Consider the children and young adults you come into contact with in your practice area. What are the factors they are exposed to that might lead to such responses?

Written and illustrated information is effective in relieving stresses associated with hospitalisation. Stone (1994) designed a leaflet ('Preparing your child for hospital: a parents' guide') to educate parents on how to prepare their child for hospital admission. The parental survey demonstrated that the leaflet did help parents to prepare children for elective admission to hospital. Written information comes in many formats, from leaflets and books written specifically for children (e.g. 'Topsy and Tim') to excellent pages on the internet. Visual/audio material in the form of videotapes and children's hospital programmes are a good preparation.

Perhaps one of the most effective forms of preparation is play therapy. Play is an essential element in every child's life. It enables them to communicate and develop many other life skills and, as well as being fun, it can also be an emotionally balancing activity for the child (Barry 2000). Play is fundamental for a healthy childhood, but for a child who is being admitted to hospital or is in hospital it serves the further purpose of helping the child to adjust to its new circumstances. Children who are experiencing illness express their needs differently to adults and viewed as a language, play becomes a crucial tool in helping a child adjust to a period of time in hospital.

Play facilities aim to (GOSH/ICH, 2002):

- provide a normal, reassuring experience and increase each individual child's ability to regain confidence, independence and self-esteem
- promote normal child development and help children regain skills lost through regression and the effects of illness and hospitalisation
- aid diagnosis and help the child understand illness and treatments, and participate in decision-making
- encourage families to be involved in the child's care and play and to relieve anxiety and anger by providing a creative outlet
- encourage and enable other members of staff to be involved in the child's play
- ensure the play environment is safe, stimulating and well maintained
- promote the value of play in hospital through training and education
- provide fun!

Activity

Having read through the aims of play, give some thought to play activities that could promote well-being in a child to be admitted to hospital or for a child already on your ward:

- Which of the activities do you feel that you currently engage in?
- Consider how you might extend these activities to assist other children.

www

There are some excellent examples of good practice in relation to the provision of play in the health care context at:

- http://www.addenbrookes.org.uk.html

Activity

Consider the many issues that have been discussed in this section and write a list of those about which it might be useful to have more information available for children and young people, parents and carers. Over the next few weeks, collect resources such as booklets and websites, which will help to increase the resources in your practice area.

Summary

This chapter set out to draw together contemporary authoritative sources, reflection, case study material and experiences to help advance the readers understanding of a complex and vast topic. It is worth noting that, despite rigorous and strategically planned literature reviews being undertaken, there is a definite absence of systematic reviews of the evidence on this theme, which can be used to inform our thinking.

Although stress in adults has been well researched and documented, much less is known about the existence and reactions of children and young people to life's stressors. Hopefully, what should have become apparent is that numerous methodological limitations abound that not only hamper generalisation of research findings but also could be cited as one of the main reasons for the relative dearth of studies focusing specifically on the subject. The problem is further compounded when attempts are made to broaden the critique to include the interdependence between the child, her/his family and the environment.

Children are subject to an array of stressors throughout their lives, from ordinary to severe, and, as with adults, those who are unable to develop appropriate coping or adaptation strategies are at greater risk of falling ill. The results of various studies point to an overarching theme; that particular stressors cannot be related to particular internal/external outcomes. Among the various stressors examined, the only consistent evidence for specificity focuses on the impact of sexual abuse. Even then, the outcomes of such studies must be interpreted with caution. This chapter focused on a limited selection of the key life stressors children and young people have been deemed to experience and, while avoiding pathologising the phenomenon, some of the underlying aetiological processes were offered for critical examination. It has been argued that it is almost impossible to compile a hierarchical order of stress categories or clusters. Nevertheless, it is clear that the most stressful events, regardless of the impetus appear to centre on loss or the threat of loss.

The overriding theme in terms of helping children cope/adapt to stressors points to the necessity of a stable, loving, supportive family unit. Longitudinal research is needed to evaluate the longer-term consequences of stress and coping on the child and family and the effectiveness of new and existing interventions for helping children and young people facing stress.

Family assessment is pivotal to family nursing. Just as an array of instruments is available to the healthcare professional to assess family needs, so too are there standardised inventories designed to measure individual life stressors. Instruments that are easy to administer and score will most likely be preferred and adopted by healthcare staff and family members. It is strongly recommended that readers gain a working knowledge of some of the instruments so that they can critically assess their reliability, validity and utility for practice. Unfortunately, most of the instruments critiqued may not be easily administered nor scored.

Children and young people are susceptible to the negative impact of acute/critical illness and hospitalisation. Real-life reflective accounts included in this chapter have hopefully served to illustrate the impact of associated stressors on the cognitive, affective and emotional domains of family functioning in such contexts. As well as requiring complex and comprehensive assessment, healthcare professionals need to know how the family uses existing support mechanisms, how family members clarify what they need and expect from each other – as well as from the health and social care system – and apply effective and appropriate interventions that help them cope with or at least adjust to the stress invoked reactions. Individual responses may vary tremendously, depending on a range of factors such as the quality and strength of the family relationships. Responses by individuals are complex entities with no single element that can explain the whole. Helping those children and families experiencing stress represents a major challenge to healthcare professionals. Some of the key features, it could be argued, include assessing the needs of the child and her/his family, detecting any adverse responses to stressors and assisting the child and family with the use of appropriate interventions. Allowing for cultural diversity when assessing and meeting the needs of children and families facing stress is a crucial way of demonstrating sensitivity and personalised care.

References

Adams, J., Gill, S., McDonald, M., 1991. Reducing fears in hospital. Nursing Times 87 (1), 624.

Alderson, P., Montgomery, J., 1996. Health care choices – making decisions with children. Institute for Public Policy Research, London.

Balen, R., Holroyd, C., Mountain, G., Wood, B., 2000. Giving children a voice: methodological and practical implications of research involving children. Paediatric Nursing 12, 24–29.

Barry, P., 2000. I go to the hospital to play, oh, and while I'm there I see the doctor. Online. Available at: http://www.nahps.org.uk/ playprep.htm [accessed 24 September 2003].

Berk, L.E., 2001. Child development. McGraw Hill, Boston.

Bedell, J.R., 1977. Life stress and the psychological and medical adjustment of chronically ill children. Journal of Psychosomatic Research 21, 237–242.

Bielby, E., 1984. A childish concept. Nursing Mirror 159 (18), 268.

Boss, P., 1988. Family stress management. Sage, CA.

Buchanan, A., Tenbrink, J.A., 1997. Recovery from emotional and behavioural problems. NHS Executive. Anglia & University of Oxford, Oxford.

Burges, L., 1994. The developing person through the life span. Worth, New York.

Clunn, P., 1991. Child psychiatric nursing. Mosby, St Louis pp 110-111.

Codddington, R.D., 1972. The significance of life events as etiologic factors in the diseases of children. II. A study of a normal population. Journal of Psychosomatic Research 16, 205–213.

Coddington, R.D., 1979. Life events associated with adolescent pregnancies. Journal of Clinical Psychiatry 40, 180–185.

Cohen, J., Emmanuel, J., 1999. Positive participation: consulting and involving young people in health related work: a planning and training resource. Health Education Authority, London.

Cohen, F., Lazarus, R.S., 1979. Coping with the stresses of illness. In: Stone, G.C., Cohen, F., Adler, N.S. (Eds.), Health psychology. Jossey-Bass, San Francisco.

Coleman, J.C., 1990. The nature of adolescence. Routledge, New York.

D'Attilio, J.P., Campbell, B.M., Lubold, P., et al., 1992. Social support and suicide potential: preliminary findings for adolescent populations. Psychological Reports 70, 76–78.

de Anda, D., Baroni, S., Boskin, L., et al., 2000. Stress, stressors and coping among high school students. Children and Young Services Review 6, 441–463.

Department of Health (DoH), 1999. Convention on the rights of the child. Second report to the United Nations committee on the rights of the child by the United Kingdom. Executive summary. The Stationery Office, London.

Drummond, R.J., Meieir, S.T., 1995. Review of the Stress Index Scale. In: Conoley, J.C., Impara, J.C. (Eds.), Mental measurements year book, 12th edn. University of Nebraska Press, Lincoln, NE, pp. 994–995.

Duncan, D.F., 1977. Life stress as a precursor to adolescent drug dependence. International Journal of the Addictions 12, 1047–1056.

Eisner, C., 1990. Chronic childhood disease: an introduction to psychological theory and research. Cambridge University Press, Cambridge.

Erwin, P., 1998. Friendship in childhood and adolescence. Routledge, London.

Fallon, S., 1995. Hospital nursing care. In: Kelner, C.J.H. (Ed.), Childhood and adolescent diabetes. Chapman & Hall, London.

Flatman, D., 2002. Consulting children: are we listening? Paediatric Nursing 14 (7), 28.

Friedman, M.M., 1998. Family nursing: research, theory & practice, 4th edn. Appleton & Lange, Stamford.

Ge, X., Lorenz, F.O., Conger, R.D., et al., 1994. Trajectories of stressful life events and depressive symptoms during adolescence. Developmental Psychology 30, 467–483.

Glasper, E.A., Thompson, M., 1993. Preparing children for hospital. In: Glasper, E.A., Tucker, A. (Eds.), Advances in child health nursing. Scutari Press, London.

GOSH/ICH, 2002. The play service fact sheet. Great Ormond Street Hospital, London.

Graham, P., Turk, J., Verhulst, F., 1999. Child psychiatry. Oxford University Press, Oxford.

Grant, K.E., 2003. Stressors and child/adolescent psychopathology: moving from markers to mechanisms of risk. In: McMahon, S.D., Grant, K.E., Compas, B.E., et al (Eds.), Stress and psychopathology in children and adolescents: is there evidence of specificity? Journal of Child Psychology and Psychiatry 44 (1), 107–133.

Green, W.A., Swisher, S.N., 1969. Psychologic and somatic variables associated with the development and course of monozygotic twins discordant for leukaemia. Annals of the New York Academy of Science 164, 394–408.

Grey, M., 1993. Stressors and children's health. Journal of Pediatric Nursing 8 (2), 85–91.

Grey, M., Hayman, L.L., 1987. Assessing stress in children: research and clinical implications. Journal of Pediatric Nursing 2 (5), 316–327.

Harter, S., 1983. Developmental perspectives on the self esteem. In: Mussen, P. (Ed.), Handbook of child psychology, 4th edn. Wiley, New York.

Health Advisory Service, 1995. Health Advisory Service child and adolescent mental health services: together we stand. HMSO, London.

Heywood, J., 2002. Enhancing seamless care: a review. Paediatric Nursing 14 (5), 18–20.

Hobfoll, S.E., 1988. The ecology of stress. Hemisphere, Washington, DC.

Hobfoll, S.E., Spielberger, C.D., 1992. Family stress: integrating theory and measurement. Journal of Family Psychology 6 (2), 99–112.

Ivory, P., 1998. Taking the scare out of hospital care for your child. Quest 5 (3), 1–6.

Jackson, S., Rodriguez-Tome, H., 1995. Adolescence and its social worlds. Lawrence Erlbaum, Hove.

Jenkins, R., Urstrun, T.B., 1998. Preventing mental illness: mental health promotion in primary care. Wiley, Chichester.

Jenson, P.S., Richters, J., Ussery, T., et al., 1991. Child psychopathology and emotional influences: discrete life events versus ongoing adversity. Journal of American Academy of Child and Adolescent Psychiatry 30, 303–309.

Johnson J II, , 1982. Life events as stressors in childhood and adolescence. In: Lahey, B.B., Kazdin, A.E. (Eds.), Advances in clinical child psychology. Plenum, New York.

Kidscape 2009 Online. Available at: http://www.kidscape.org.uk

Kitson, A., 1999. The essence of nursing. Nursing Standard 13 (23), 42–46.

Koenen, K.C., Moffitt, T.E., Paulton, R., et al., 2007. Early childhood factors associated with the development of post-traumatic stress disorder: results from a longitudinal birth cohort. Psychological Medicine 37(2), 181–192.

Lau, B.W.K., 2002. Does the stress in childhood and adolescence matter? A psychological perspective. The Journal of the Society for the Promotion of Health 122 (4), 238–244.

Lutz, W., 1986. Helping hospitalised children and their parents cope with painful procedures. Journal of Pediatric Nursing 1, 24–32.

Marks, L., 1994. Seamless care or patchwork quilt? Discharging patients from acute hospital care. Kings Fund Institute, London.

McCubbin, M.A., McCubbin, H.I., 1993. Families coping with illness: the resiliency model of family stress, adjustment and adaptation. In: Danielson, C., Hamel-Bissell, B., Winstead-Fry, P. (Eds.), Families, health, and illness: perspectives on coping and intervention. Mosby, St Louis, pp. 21–63.

McCubbin, M.A., Patterson, C., 1983. Family stress and adaptation to crises: a double ABCX model of family behaviour. In: Olson, D., Miller, B. (Eds.), Family studies review yearbook. Sage, Beverly Hills, CA, pp. 125–135.

McMahon, S.D., Grant, K., Compas, B.E., et al., 2003. Stress and psychopathology in children and adolescents: is there evidence of specificity? Journal of Child Psychology and Psychiatry 44 (1), 107–133.

Melamed, B.G., 1993. Putting the family back in the child. Behavioural Research Theory 31 (3), 239–247.

Melamed, B.G., Siegel, L.J., Ridley-Johnson, R., 1988. Coping behaviours in children facing medical stress. In: Field, T., Schneiderman, N., McCabe, P. (Eds.), Stress and coping. Lawrence Erlbaum, Hillsdale, NJ.

Mental Health Foundation, 1999. Bright futures: promoting children and young people's mental health. Mental Health Foundation, London.

Miller, M.S., 1982. Child's stress: understanding and answering of stress signals of infants, children and teenagers. Doubleday, Garden City, NY.

Moos, R.H., 1986. Coping with life crises. Plenum, New York.

Moos, R.H., 2002. Life stressors, social resources, and coping skills in youth: applications to adolescents with chronic disorders. Journal of Adolescent Health 30, 22–29.

Morano, C.D., Cisler, B.A., Lemerond, J., 1993. Risk factors for adolescent suicide behaviour: loss, insufficient familial support, and hopelessness. Adolescence 28, 112.

Mountain, G., 2007. Family nursing. In: Glasper, A., McEwing, G., Richardson, J. (Eds.), The Oxford handbook of children's and young people's nursing. Oxford University Press, Oxford.

Mountain, G., 2008. Parenting in society: a critical review. In: Smith, L., Coleman, V. (Eds.), Child and family centred healthcare, 2nd edn. Palgrave, Basingstoke.

Papalia, D.E., Olds, S.W., Feldman, R.D., 1999. A child's world: infancy through adolescence. McGraw-Hill, New York.

Pfeffer, S.R., Conte, I.I.R., Plutchick, R., Jerrett, I., 1979. Suicidal behaviour in latency-age children: an empirical study. Journal of the American Academy of Child Psychiatry 18, 679–692.

Phinney, J.S., Alipuria, L.L., 1990. Ethnic identity in college students from four ethnic groups. Journal of Adolescence 13, 171–183.

Rennick, J., 2002. Children's psychological responses after critical illness and exposure to invasive technology. Journal of Developmental and Behavioural Paediatrics 23 (3), 133–144.

Robertson, L., 1995. The giving of information is the key to family empowerment. British Journal of Nursing 4 (12), 692.

Rudolph, K.D., Hammen, C., 1999. Age and gender as determinants of stress exposure, generation, and reactions in youngsters: a transactional perspective. Child Development 70 (3), 660–667.

Sandler, I.N., Block, M., 1979. Life stress and the maladaptation of children. American Journal of Community Psychology (7), 425–440.

Santrock, J.W., 2001. Child development. McGraw-Hill, New York.

Selye, H., 1978. The stress of life. McGraw-Hill, New York.

Sharman, W., 1997. Children and adolescents with mental health problems. Baillière Tindall, London.

Solnit, A., 1984. Preparing. Psychoanalytic Study of the Child 39, 613–632.

Stein, S.P., Charles, E., 1971. Emotional factors in juvenile diabetes mellitus: a study of early life experiences. American Journal of Psychiatry 128, 56–60.

Steinhausen, H., Verhulst, F., 1999. Risk and outcomes in developmental psychology. Oxford University Press, New York.

Stoleb, M., Chiriboga, J., 1998. A process model for assessing adolescent risk for suicide. Journal of Adolescence 21, 359–370.

Stone, K., 1994. Preparing your child for hospital: a parents' guide. Child Health 2 (4), 165.

Sugar, N.F., 1992. Toddlers' traumatic memories. Infant Mental Health Journal 16 (4), 259–270.

Townley, M., 2002. Mental health needs of young people. Nursing Standard 16 (30), 38–45.

Vincent, K.R., Rosenstock, H.A., 1979. The relationship between stressful life events and hospitalised adolescent patients. Journal of Clinical Psychiatry 40, 262–264.

While, A., 1994. Day case surgery. Maternal Child Health 19 (6):1846.

Wilson-Sharrer, V., Ryan-Wenger, N.M., 1991. Measurements of stress and coping amongst school aged children with and without recurrent abdominal pain. Journal of School Health 61 (2), 86–91.

The evidence base for children's nursing practice

14

Peter Callery Sarah Neill

ABSTRACT

Children's nurses are now expected to be able to provide the evidence base that underpins their clinical practice. This simple statement hides the complex nature of the processes involved in bringing together such evidence, given the vast wealth of published resources. The first part of this chapter aims to explore the sources of evidence available to children's nurses and how they can be used to develop the evidence base for a particular area of practice. Every good research textbook includes general guidance on critiquing research evidence but these texts do not generally explore issues specific to research involving children. These are explored in some depth in the next section of the chapter. Finally, the historical context of children's nursing research is discussed, from which some of the emerging themes for future research are outlined.

LEARNING OUTCOMES

- Describe the sources of evidence that can contribute to development of interventions in children's nursing.
- Describe a hierarchy of evidence for interventions in children's nursing.
- Describe evidence required in implementation of interventions.
- Describe critical appraisal issues specific to research with children.
- Describe emerging themes in children's nursing research.

Introduction

The volume of research publications is daunting. Asthma, as the most common illness of childhood and involving children's nurses in community and hospital settings, can illustrate the volume and types of evidence used in children's nursing practice. Ovid Medline lists 7091 papers in English indexed under 'Asthma' 'limited to child (0–18 years)' in the period 1996 to July 2003. A systematic approach is therefore required if research is to be used to inform decisions about care. The evidence-based medicine movement has developed principles and procedures for searching and assessing research literature. Nurses can use the approach to base their own practice on evidence provided that there is recognition of the special features of children's nursing.

Formulating questions

It is important to define the question that evidence is required to answer. The more clearly focused the question, the more likely that it will be possible to identify the most appropriate evidence available for the answer. Questions can be expressed in terms of four elements, using the PICO framework:

P = patient
I = intervention
C = comparison
O = outcome (Sackett et al 1997).

Craig (2002) illustrated how this framework can be used to identify and answer questions arising from practice in nursing. Her first example was a child who had developed a pressure ulcer on the back of her head when recovering from open heart surgery (Craig 2002). The question about the individual child: 'How can I prevent further pressure ulcers from developing in this child?' can be developed into a question to be answered by systematic review of randomised, controlled trials: 'In critically ill children, are constant low-pressure beds more effective than high specification foam mattresses in preventing pressure ulcers (defined here as constant discolouration of the skin, or partial or full thickness skin loss)?' (Craig 2002). This type of question is well suited to the PICO framework because it is concerned with a nursing action (the choice between a constant low-pressure bed and a foam mattress) that can be clearly associated with one consequence, formation of pressure ulcers. The direct link between cause and effect makes possible the use of experimental designs, including the randomised, controlled trial.

DOI: 10.1016/B978-0-7020-3183-0.10014-1

Evidence-based principles might suggest that all practice should be based on experimental research. However, even though experimental methods are well suited to pharmaceutical therapy, many drugs are not tested and therefore not specifically licensed for use in children (Conroy et al 2000). The limitations of the evidence base for treatment of children and young people is highlighted by the few studies that provide the basis for treating 40,000 people under the age of 18 years with major depressive disorder (Ramchandani 2004). Experiments to compare different treatments have not been conducted in children for various reasons. Some treatments are given to small numbers of children, which makes large-scale trials difficult to arrange or expensive. Ethical considerations can present difficulties in establishing trials to compare different treatments, particularly when alternative treatments are not available.

Not everything that nurses do can be tested by an experiment. Limitations of the PICO framework are illustrated by another of Craig's examples: a health visitor wants to understand why mothers feed infants with formula milk rather than breast feeding. The question is concerned with identifying information that could lead to an intervention to promote breast feeding. Craig (2002) suggested the question be formulated using the Patient and Outcome elements of the framework, excluding the Intervention and Comparison elements: 'What are the factors identified by mothers who live in deprived inner city areas that influence them to breast feed or to bottle feed using infant milk formula?'; a qualitative design would be required.

'Why?' questions such as this can be answered by understanding the world from the viewpoint of the people concerned. It is therefore best to take an open-ended approach, avoiding assumptions that may not be shared by the people who are to be studied. The types of question that are most appropriately asked would therefore be concerned with how mothers make decisions about feeding their infants. There is a risk that the prior definition of patient (or, in this case, population) and outcome is based on assumptions about common characteristics of mothers and the definition of breast feeding as an outcome. The formulation of the question therefore requires reference to a theory of why mothers in deprived areas will have similar concerns about breast feeding.

The application of the PICO framework in children's nursing can be complicated by tensions between children's and parents' perspectives and interests. Children and parents may have different understandings of health problems and different goals for care. Questions about care may need to reflect differences between parents' and children's concerns and goals.

Activity

Think about your day-to-day practice and identify a problem that you need evidence to solve (e.g. 'What will prevent development of pressure ulcers in critically ill children?'):

- Try to turn your identified problem into a question that follows the PICO framework.
- What sort of evidence could provide the answer that you need?
- Is there a clear link between cause and effect and could an experiment be performed?

Complex interventions

Nursing interventions in children's health care are often 'complex interventions':

> Complex interventions in health care, whether therapeutic or preventative, comprise a number of separate elements which seem essential to the proper functioning of the intervention although the 'active ingredient' of the intervention that is effective is difficult to specify. If we were to consider a randomised controlled trial of a drug vs. a placebo as being at the simplest end of the spectrum, then we might see a comparison of a stroke unit to traditional care as being at the most complex end of the spectrum. The greater the difficulty in defining precisely what, exactly, are the 'active ingredients' of an intervention and how they relate to each other, the greater the likelihood that you are dealing with a complex intervention
>
> (MRC Health Services and Public Health Research Board 2000)

WWW

The full MRC document can be downloaded from the web as (you will need to download the free Acrobat Reader software to read it):

- http://www.mrc.ac.uk/pdf-mrc_cpr.pdf

Health visitors wishing to promote breast feeding will develop complex interventions. They might devise educational programmes whose 'active ingredients' include the quality of continuing relationships with mothers, information about the benefits of breast feeding and the method of communication, whether in groups or through individual contact.

Similar complexity can be seen in many nursing interventions. In hospital, nurses help children to cooperate with delivery of drug therapy by nebuliser, which requires the child to wear a mask. Community nurses explain how to use medication to control asthma at home. In each case the 'active ingredient' is difficult to identify: the manner in which the nurse forms a relationship with child and family, the content of the nurse's explanations, and the time and place at which the information is provided could all have important effects.

Identification and measurement of outcomes presents particular difficulties in children's nursing. Some outcomes are clear-cut, e.g. the formation of pressure ulcers, whereas others can be assessed only in relation to children's development, e.g. satisfactory growth, or require assessment by children themselves, e.g. assessment of quality of life.

Activity

Identify a complex intervention from your area of practice. List the possible 'active ingredients'.

Types of evidence

Once the question has been identified, the next task is to identify the best evidence that will contribute to the answer. A systematic approach to literature searching is required to ensure that important evidence is not missed. A hierarchy of the different forms of evidence available can be used to identify the best evidence that is available. For example, studies can be organised in order of the strength of their design (Muir Gray 1997):

- I. Strong evidence from at least one systematic review of multiple, well-designed, randomised controlled trials.
- II. Strong evidence from at least one properly designed randomised, controlled trial of appropriate size.
- III. Strong evidence from well-designed trials without randomisation, single group, cohort, time series or matched case-control studies.
- IV. Evidence from well-designed, non-experimental studies from more than one centre or research group.
- V. Opinions of respected authorities based on clinical evidence, descriptive studies or reports of expert committees.

Categorisation of evidence usually follows the principle that the best evidence is to be found in studies that have minimised bias through design, for example by randomly allocating subjects to intervention and control groups to enable comparison of the effects of treatments. However, the design of a study does not guarantee the quality of the evidence (Wilson et al 1995).

www

More detailed categorisation of studies is presented and explained at the website of the Centre for Evidence-based Medicine:

- http://www.cebm.net/levels_of_evidence.asp#levels

Nursing interventions in asthma illustrate the use of evidence from studies of various designs and the contribution of qualitative research to the evidence base for children's nursing practice.

Systematic reviews

A systematic review of randomised, controlled trials of education in asthma concluded that:

> Educational programmes for the self management of asthma in children and adolescents improve lung function and feelings of self control, reduce absenteeism from school, number of days with restricted activity, number of visits to an emergency department, and possibly number of disturbed nights. Educational programmes should be considered a part of the routine care of young people with asthma
>
> (Guevara et al 2003)

The review used a systematic method of searching the literature. The search terms used for Medline (1966–98), Embase (1980–98), and CINAHL (1982–98) were:

asthma OR wheez*

AND education* OR self management OR self-management

AND placebo* OR trial* OR random* OR double-blind OR double blind OR single-blind OR single blind OR controlled study OR comparative study.

Other databases and journals were also searched and 318 studies were identified. The quality of studies was assessed on the basis of the design, including whether allocation to the intervention or to the control group was known before each subject was included in the study. This criterion for quality was therefore concerned with potential bias: whether all the children in the population to be studied had an equal chance of being included in the sample. Once these criteria were applied, 45 of 318 identified studies were potentially eligible. However, 13 were excluded when other quality criteria were applied, leaving 32 trials totalling 3706 children and adolescents with asthma.

The stricter the criteria used for selecting studies eligible for inclusion in a systematic review, the fewer studies that will be included, so judgements about the criteria to be applied are important in designing such reviews. Guevara et al (2003) summarised the studies they reviewed:

> Most were relatively small randomised controlled trials and enrolled children with severe asthma. Fifteen trials enrolled adolescents aged 13 to 18 years, and 12 enrolled children aged 2 to 5 years; no study stratified data on age. The educational programmes were diverse and targeted children, parents, or both. Most had programmes with multiple sessions and symptom based strategies.

The conclusions that could be reached by the review were therefore limited by the characteristics of the studies that were included. Guevara et al's review could make limited comments about: non-severe asthma, interventions at different ages, the types of education that is most effective and whether education should be directed at children, parents or both. The conclusion that education should be incorporated into the routine care of children with asthma is welcome but somewhat limited.

Guevara et al recommend further research, and here they are more specific. They suggest that:

> Future studies should test alternative components directly to determine their relative effectiveness, for example, studies should focus on morbidity measurements and quality of life and directly compare strategies based on peak flow with those based on symptoms and compare strategies aimed at the individual with those aimed at the group.

These suggestions highlight the importance of understanding the intervention thoroughly. Guevara et al are essentially asking what might be the 'active ingredient' of education: is it directed at preventing the occurrence of acute episodes of illness or at improving quality of life? Is the active ingredient individualised education or education provided for groups? Their other question, 'Should education be based on symptoms or on peak flow measurement?' can be answered by another study from lower in the hierarchy of study designs. Forty asthmatic children (5–16 years) were asked to:

> … perform peak flow measurements twice daily for 4 weeks by means of an electronic peak flow meter and to record values in a written diary. Patients and parents were unaware that the device stored the peak flow values on a microchip. Data in the written diary (reported data) were compared with those from the electronic diary (actual data)
>
> (Kamps et al 2001)

The authors reported that children's peak flow results were so unreliable that they should not be trusted:

> The percentage of correct peak flow entries decreased from 56% to <50% from the first to the last study week ($p < 0.04$), mainly as a result of an increase in self-invented peak flow entries … Peak flow

> diaries kept by asthmatic children are unreliable. Electronic peak flow meters should be used if peak flow monitoring is required in children with asthma
>
> (Kamps et al 2001)

This illustrates how descriptive studies that add to understanding of how people behave in health care can make important contributions to developing evidence-based practice. (The '*p*' value reported by Kamps refers to the probability that the difference was caused by chance, in most studies it is accepted that a result is statistically significant if there was a less than 5% (1 in 20) likelihood that the differences between two values could have been caused by chance.)

Randomised controlled trials

Randomised controlled trials (RCTs) have shown that nurses can make important differences to the health of children with asthma by educating them about self-management of their condition:

> A prospective randomised control study of an asthma home management training programme was performed in children aged two years or over admitted with acute asthma. Two hundred and one children were randomised at admission to either an intervention group ($n = 96$), which received the teaching programme, or a control group ($n = 105$). A nurse-led teaching programme used the current attack as a model for the management of future attacks and included discussion, written information, subsequent follow up and telephone advice aimed at developing and reinforcing individualised asthma management plans. Parents were also provided with a course of oral steroids and guidance on when to start them … Subsequent readmissions were significantly reduced in the intervention group from 25% to 8% in individual follow up periods that ranged from two to 14 months
>
> (Madge et al 1997)

Madge et al's study demonstrated both the value and limitations of RCTs. The study showed that children educated by a nurse fared better, with less need for readmission and reduction in asthma symptoms. However, the problem of deciding what the 'active ingredient' is evident. One nurse delivered the education – would other nurses have been as effective? The education was delivered as children were discharged from hospital. The authors followed-up children to assess the duration of the effect of education but this analysis was limited by the variation in the period of follow-up from 2–14 months. There is evidence that asthma attacks affect receptiveness to information in adults with asthma:

> strong cognitive/affective responses to attacks may motivate improved self-care and this represents a window of opportunity for self-care interventions
>
> (Greaves et al 2002)

Was the education effective in Madge et al's study because it was delivered while the children were being discharged from hospital? In a qualitative study of parents' and children's perspectives on asthma it was reported that parents gave more emphasis to acute attacks than children and that they accepted some symptoms as tolerable provided that they did not result in an acute attack (Callery et al 2003). Could education at the time of an attack reinforce parental focus on acute attacks and hospitalisations rather than drawing parents' attention to controlling low-level symptoms that might affect children's quality of life? In addition to the educational intervention, the authors reported that parents were given oral steroids and instructions about their use. Were oral steroids one of the 'active ingredients' that resulted in improved outcomes for the intervention group? These questions arise because of the difficulty of separating different effects, or confounding variables, on the outcomes. The questions also indicate the importance of a thorough understanding of interventions and how they are seen by those involved, including children as well as parents and health professionals. Therefore descriptive studies, including qualitative studies, are required to complement experimental studies in the development and evaluation of complex interventions.

Activity

Find research paper(s) that explore a problem relevant to your nursing practice:

- What type of evidence has been used to study the problem?
- What other types of design could be used to study this problem?

Researching complex interventions

Phases of development may be required to test complex interventions (MRC Health Services and Public Health Research Board 2000).

The first phase is preclinical and is concerned with developing the underlying theory for the intervention. Studies of educational interventions in asthma have been criticised for neglecting this phase, so that educational programmes have been developed without first identifying the theory that will guide practice (Clark & Gong 2000).

- Phase I – in which the components of the intervention are identified and assessed – commences once the theoretical framework has been identified. This phase is concerned with identifying the active ingredients.
- Phase II is an exploratory trial, or pilot study, that checks that an experimental study can be conducted.
- Phase III is the full trial.
- The final phase, IV, is concerned with long-term implementation: can others produce similar results with the intervention and maintain them over time?

The need for detailed developmental work before trialling interventions was highlighted in a report on diabetes education in childhood:

> This review recommends that a phase of programme development be undertaken involving a consultation process with adolescents with type 1 diabetes, their families, doctors, nurses, health economists and health psychologists. This consultation exercise would enable the establishment of possible interventions that are seen as plausible and potentially effective by patients and their parents, feasible and practical in the context of the NHS diabetes services and understood and accepted by doctors and nurses as key and integral parts of diabetes care. The interventions would also need to have the potential to be cost-effective and be based on sound behavioural principles.

> Such interventions, if subsequently demonstrated by commissioned research to be effective, would he much more likely to be implemented than ones developed without such a process
>
> (Hampson et al 2001)

Therefore a range of designs, including descriptive studies and qualitative studies, is required at different stages in the development of nursing interventions. Whereas this is true in all healthcare practice, it is particularly important in children's nursing. Studies must be designed to reflect the needs of children and not merely to apply concepts from adult health care to children. Evidence is required about children's perspectives, as well as the perspectives of adults involved in their care.

The evidence for children's nursing practice can therefore be complex and require skilled interpretation. Knowledge of both quantitative and qualitative research methods is required to assess evidence, particularly about complex interventions.

WWW

You can keep up to date with the evidence base for practice by reading a good evidence-based journal such as *Evidence Based Nursing*, which uses rigorous procedures to identify and summarise the practice implications of new research publications. The website is:

- http://ebn.bmjjournals.com/

Box 14.1

Definitions (from Broome & Stieglitz 1992)

- **Informed consent:** an interactive process between subject and researcher involving disclosure, discussion and a complete understanding of a proposed research activity, and which culminates in the individual freely expressing a desire to participate.
- **Parental consent:** all of the components of informed consent and should include consideration of the implications of research involvement for the child.
- **Assent:** an interactive process between a child and researcher involving disclosure, discussion and a limited understanding of a proposed research activity, wherein the child freely expresses a preference for participation but has insufficient maturity to make a fully informed and autonomous decision.
- **Dissent:** an interactive process between a child and researcher involving disclosure, discussion and a limited understanding of the proposed research activity, wherein the child freely expresses an objection to the participation but has insufficient maturity to make a fully informed and autonomous decision.

Critical appraisal issues specific to research with children: ethical and methodological issues

Critical appraisal of research involves consideration of the ethical conduct of research as well as the rigour of the methodological process. When the subjects of the research are children, specific ethical and methodological issues need to be considered. In Western societies, children continue to be viewed as 'becoming' rather than 'being' a social person, an idea that results in notions of children as vulnerable, incompetent and dependent on adults (Christensen 1998). The resulting power differential between children and adults presents a range of different ethical issues that need to be considered in the critical appraisal process.

This section of the chapter will explore the ethics of conducting research with children including: guidelines for the ethical conduct of research with children, researcher role conflict for healthcare professionals, children as researchers, and the psychological impact of the research on child participants, with the intention of highlighting issues specific to researching with children for appraisers and planners of research.

Ethics of conducting research with children

The protective approach to children might initially provoke a reaction that excludes children from involvement in research, thereby protecting them from any potentially harmful effects – physical or psychological. This approach would result in less knowledge about children, excluding them from the benefits of research (Morrow & Richards 1996). Not to conduct research with children would therefore be unethical (Darbyshire 2000, Royal College of Paediatrics and Child Health: Ethics Advisory Committee (RCPCH) 2000).

It is therefore important to conduct research with and for children but to do so in such a way as to ensure their voluntary participation. Children, as well as adults, need to be able to make an uncoerced, informed decision before consenting to their participation in research. Even when children are not 'Gillick competent', i.e. of sufficient understanding and intelligence to understand fully what is proposed, opportunities need to be provided with sufficient appropriately formatted information to enable them to assent or dissent to their involvement (see Box 14.1 for definitions of consent, assent and dissent). Critical appraisal of research with children should therefore include consideration of how consent or assent was sought from children and their parents or guardians. For further discussion on the assessment of a child's competence to consent to research, readers are referred to Alderson & Morrow (2004), and to Chapter 3.

It should be noted that ensuring uncoerced consent is particularly important, because coercion has serious possible effects on the validity of data gathered. This applies most particularly to qualitative research, which might result in children giving the responses they feel are wanted, but also in quantitative research where physiological measures of anxiety are used – as when participation in research is not voluntary, the participation itself may increase anxiety rather than any intervention being measured.

Activity

Find a research study involving children and identify:

- The procedures used to obtain consent to participation in the research from children and/or their parents.
- The extent to which children's competence to consent has been assessed prior to seeking consent.
- How the process for seeking consent could have been improved for your chosen research study.

Guidelines on research with children

A number of published guidelines can be used as standards against which to measure an individual research project. However, the only guidelines written specifically for child health research in the UK to date are those from the RCPCH (2000), to which the Department of Health (DoH 2005) research governance document also refers. These guidelines provide some direction for researchers (and those assessing research proposals for research ethics committees (RECs)) concerning the consent process and include consideration of acceptable areas to research with children. Guidance is available for researchers on writing information sheets and consent forms for research involving children from the National Research Ethics Service (2007). It should be noted, in accordance with the DoH (2005) guidance, that REC approval is required for all child health research projects. Any research critique should include consideration of whether the project was ethical to conduct with children as a sample or whether comparable research could have been conducted on adults instead. The RCPCH guidelines focus quite clearly on quantitative research, as they state that research is only worthwhile if the project:

> involves a statistically appropriate number of subjects.

Further guidance for qualitative research needs to be sought elsewhere. The reader is referred to the National Children's Bureau's (2006) guidelines for research, which provides detailed practical advice for researchers and therefore is also useful for those critiquing such research. For a review of guidelines for research with children up to 2004 see Neill (2005).

WWW

Read the Royal College of Paediatrics and Child Health's guidelines (RCPCH 2000) online via the *Archives of Disease in Childhood* website:

- http://adc.bmjjournals.com/cgi/content/full/archdischild;82/2/177

WWW

Read the Department of Health's research governance document online:

- http://www.dh.gov.uk/en/publicationsandstatistics/publications/publicationspolicyandguidance/dh_4108962

WWW

Read the National Children's Bureau's guidelines for research online:

- http://www.ncb.org.uk/dotpdf/open%20access%20-%20phase%201%20only/research_guidelines_200604.pdf

Activity

Find a research study with a sample of children and analyse it using both the Royal College of Paediatrics and Child Health's guidelines and those from the NCB.

- How effective did you find each set of guidelines?
- What, if any, different issues did you identify from using one set of guidelines or the other?

Researcher role conflict

Readers of research, and researchers themselves, also need to be aware of the potential for role conflict – when the researcher is a healthcare professional – between his/her role as a researcher who is present only to gather data from the child, and his/her role as a healthcare professional when issues concerning the child's ongoing health care emerge. For example, a child may tell the researcher during an interview about their dissatisfaction with their current treatment. The researcher may know about more effective treatment available or that the child's current treatment is no longer recommended practice. To ignore the needs of the child and continue with the interview would be unethical and would also indicate a lack of concern for the child that could damage the relationship between the researcher and the child and therefore reduce the extent, and validity of, the data collected.

Child protection and confidentiality

Whenever healthcare professionals are involved with children child protection must be considered. This is no less the case when the activity concerned is research, presenting the researcher with a further role conflict. Researchers would normally offer guarantees of confidentiality and inform participants that their identity will not be disclosed in any research reports or to anyone other than the researchers involved. Yet where the respondent is a child, the NCB (2006) state clearly that confidentiality must be limited because:

> Where a child or young person divulges that they or others are at risk of significant harm, or where the researcher observes or receives evidence of incidents likely to cause serious harm, the researcher has a duty to take steps to protect the child or other children.

Projects involving children should include consideration of the way in which children are informed of these limitations.

Activity

- Identify two other situations that might result in researcher role conflict.
- Discuss with your peer group how such conflict could be managed without undermining the ethical conduct of the research.

Children as researchers

Children are increasingly becoming involved in research as a part of the research team, including acting as interviewers, partly following the trend towards user involvement in research and partly to reduce the power imbalance that exists between an adult interviewer and a child. Traditionally, in adult qualitative research attempts are made to match interviewer and interviewee for age, social position, gender and ethnicity (Hood et al 1996, Mahon et al 1996) to avoid any power imbalance between researcher and subject. More recently, even in the adult research methods literature, it has been recognised that this is not always possible. Instead honesty about the nature of the differences has been advocated (Mallory 2001). This provides a possible approach with children – to discuss with them the differences between themselves as researchers and/or as research participants and the coercive effect such power imbalances may have.

Increasingly participatory research methods are being used with children which engage children in the research process (Coad & Evans 2008, Kirby 1999). Children from middle childhood upwards have participated in projects as researchers (Alderson & Morrow 2004, Coad & Evans 2008). Coad & Evans (2008) describe five levels of children's participation in research from simple participation as research respondents to child/young person led research teams with adults facilitating the process. Readers are referred to their original publication for a detailed discussion on this topic. Whenever children are involved as researchers, ethical problems must be addressed, in particular, around the child protection issues mentioned above – should child researchers be placed in a position where they may receive disturbing information from another child? Such research projects need to be assessed carefully on the basis of the appropriateness of the focus of the research, the methods used and the skills required of the researcher (Mahon et al 1996). Research reports should provide information on how such young interviewers are prepared for, supported through, and debriefed after the research.

Protecting the child from harm

Monitoring the impact on the child

The RCPCH (2000) guidelines are very clear about the need to protect the child from unnecessary physical harm. They state that the decision concerning whether the research is allowed to take place should be based on an assessment of the balance of potential benefit against potential harm. In research involving physical procedures the degree of 'harm' involved is relatively predictable. The psychological impact on the child is less predictable, but it is well recognised that it may occur at the time or at a later date (Mahon et al 1996, National Children's Bureau 2006). Research projects involving children should include strategies for the emotional support for children immediately after data collection and the provision of information about sources of help for the future. Throughout the research process, researchers need to monitor the child's non-verbal signs for any indication of unwillingness to take part or to continue with the research (Alderson & Morrow 2004).

The child's comfort with the research process

The child's comfort with the whole process is likely to affect the consent process and the quality of the data collected. Children need to feel emotionally safe with any individual to be able to talk about their views or experiences or to submit to physical investigations. Appraisers of research should consider how children were put at their ease, for example through the use of ice-breaking techniques (Borland et al 1998). Children's understanding of what is involved in a project is affected by the way in which information is presented in terms of the content and the pace of information giving (Ireland & Holloway 1996).

Methodological considerations when children are involved in research

Qualitative research should also be critiqued for the flexibility provided in terms of the methods used to gather data. Whereas some children are content to talk enabling the use of interviews for data collection, others might feel more comfortable drawing or taking pictures of relevant objects and places (Coad 2007, Coyne 1998, Matthews et al 1998). Children are then encouraged to talk about the resulting images. Researchers, initially in the social science field (Boyden & Ennew 1997, Matthews & Tucker 2000) and now in the field of child health (Coad 2007, Coad & Lewis 2004), emphasise the importance of using methods which interest and therefore engage children and which are within the child's ability. A wide range of data collection methods have been used from drawings and photographs (referred to above) to poetry, drama, role play and video (Kirby 1999). When children's and young people's interest in the research process, as well as the topic, is engaged the resulting data will be much richer, providing greater insights into the world of children and young people.

Historical overview of children's nursing research: the context for the emerging themes of the future

Research in children's nursing and child health care is a relatively new field of enquiry. Alderson (1993) points out that research involving children only began seriously in the latter part of the 20th century. Traditionally, children have been seen as subjects to be acted upon by others (Christensen 1998) rather than individuals to be asked to participate in research in their own right. This should not be surprising given the social construction of childhood that has largely prevailed throughout the 20th and into the 21st centuries, which sees childhood as the precursor to adulthood rather than as a stage of life to be valued in its own right. However, as will be discussed below, ideas about children are changing and this is influencing the way in which research is conducted in children's nursing and child health care.

During the 20th century children were studied using mostly experimental, observational and standard measurement techniques. This research generally took no account of the research subject's (child's) viewpoint (Alderson 1993). When research did focus on the child's experiences, this was primarily conducted through proxies, in research about rather than with children. Included here is much of the research on parent participation (for example: Algren 1985, Darbyshire 1994, Neill 1996a, 1996b) or on partnership (for example: Casey 1995, Cleary 1992, Coyne 1995) within which adults set themselves up as the interpreters of children's behaviour. Although much was learnt about adults' perceptions of childhood experiences through this research, nothing was learnt about the child's own experiences, from which knowledge services could be developed more in tune with the child's wants and needs.

Social perceptions of childhood are changing, albeit slowly. Children are gradually being given the opportunity to be listened to, not just heard. Hearing is merely the perception of sound whereas listening involves paying attention to what is being said. The United Nations Convention on the Rights of the Child (United Nations General Assembly 1989) includes two articles that focus specifically on children's rights to have their views taken into account:

- Article 12: Parties shall assure to the child who is capable of forming his or her own views the right to express those views freely in all matters affecting the child, the views of the child being given due weight in accordance with the age and maturity of the child.
- Article 13: The child shall have the right to freedom of expression; this right shall include freedom to seek, receive and impart information and ideas of all kinds, regardless of frontiers, either orally, in writing or in print, in the form of art, or through any other media of the child's choice.

WWW

The full text of the UN Convention on the Rights of the Child (1989) can be viewed online at:

- http://www.unicef.org/crc/crc.htm

It has taken some time to see these rights being operationalised at a national level in England:

- The Department of Health (2002) produced an action plan to guide the involvement of children and young people in the NHS entitled 'Listening, hearing and responding'.
- A Children and Young People's Unit (2001) was created to support cross-government work on child poverty and youth disadvantage.
- Consultation with children underpinned the development of the National Service Framework for Children (Department of Health and Department for Education and Skills 2004).

These initiatives reflect the emergence of the agenda for service user involvement in health care. It is clear that children should have the right to contribute to research themselves, rather than through others and that changes in society are taking place which should support such research.

Research is emerging that does reflect both the changes in society's perception of children and the changes within children's nursing itself where the emphasis has moved from parent participation and partnership with parents to listening to children first and foremost. Research conducted with children as active research participants, which seeks their views on health and health care, has been increasing rapidly since the 1990s (for example: Action for Sick Children 1998, Alderson 1993, Coad & Coad 2008, Coyne 1998, Lewis et al. 2004, Pridmore & Bendelow 1995). Children have also begun to get involved as researchers, either as a member of the research planning team, as interviewers, data analysts, and/or as members of child/young people led research teams (Alderson & Morrow 2004, Coad & Evans 2008). There are now a range of books also devoted to the subject of researching with children which provide extensive guidance on how to engage with children in the research process (Alderson & Morrow 2004, Christensen & James 2007, Farrel 2005, Fraser et al 2004, Greene & Hogan 2005, Greig et al 2007, Kirby 1999, Lewis & Lindsay 2000, Lewis et al 2004).

Further research is still needed to continue to develop the evidence base for practice grounded in children's perspectives on child health/health services. It is also to be hoped that in focusing on the child, researchers will not forget that children live in families and that there is a need to explore the interrelationships between the adults and the children in families with respect to their influence on children and families' health and their perspectives on healthcare services. Finally, it should be remembered that whereas the discussion here has focused largely on qualitative approaches to research to generate a knowledge of children's perspectives, it should not be forgotten that such research will lay the foundations for more large-scale quantitative research. Quantitative approaches are also needed to test many treatment modalities. Little work has so far been conducted here, leaving practice based on custom and practice rather than a sound evidence base. This situation should be remedied in future research.

Summary

Guidance on research involving children indicates a general agreement that not to undertake research with children would be unethical because there would then be no evidence on which to develop relevant and effective services. Appraisal of research with children should include methods used to put the child at ease with the researcher as well as an assessment of methods used to obtain consent. Consent should be obtained from both the child and the parent or guardian. Where the child does not have sufficient understanding of what is involved and the implications of such involvement, the assent of the child should be sought. Strategies in place to manage the potential role conflict between the researcher as health professional and the researcher as data collector should be identified. Research involving interviews with children should be assessed against the NCB (2006) guidance concerning the limitations on confidentially for child protection issues. Appraisers also need to consider whether the potential impact of the child, physically and psychologically has been addressed. Finally, in reviewing the methodologies chosen in qualitative research with children, appraisers should be able to identify flexibility in the range of options provided for children to share their knowledge, views and experiences.

WWW

Visit the Children and Young People's Unit website and find out about activities in progress and consider their relevance to your practice area:

- http://www.cypu.gov.uk

Visit the National Service Framework's website to find out about the latest progress in implementing the NSF:

- http://www.doh.gov.uk/nsf/children.htm

What are you doing in your practice area towards the implementation of the NSF?

References

Action for Sick Children, 1998. Pictures of healthcare. A child's eye view. Action for Sick Children, London.

Alderson, P., 1993. Children's Consent to Surgery. Open University Press, Buckingham.

Alderson, P., Morrow, V., 2004. Ethics, social research and consulting children and young people. Ilford, Barnardo's.

Algren, C.L., 1985. Role perception of mothers who have hospitalised children. Children's Health Care 14, 6–9.

Borland, M., Laybourn, A., Hill, M., Brown, J., 1998. Middle Childhood. The Perspectives of Children and Parents. Jessica Kingsley, London.

Boyden, J., Ennew, J., 1997. Children in Focus: a manual for participatory research with children. Radda Barnen (Swedish Save the Children), Stockholm.

Broome, M.E., Stieglitz, K.A., 1992. The consent process and children. Research in Nursing and Health 15, 147–152.

Callery, P., Milnes, L., Couriel, J., Verduyn, C., 2003. Qualitative study of children's and parents' beliefs about childhood asthma. British Journal of General Practice 53, 185–190.

Casey, A., 1995. Partnership nursing: influences on involvement of informal carers. Journal of Advanced Nursing 22, 1058–1062.

Children and Young People's Unit, 2001. Learning to Listen. Core Principles for the Involvement of Children and Young People. Department for Education and Skills, Annesley, Nottinghamshire.

Christensen, P.H., 1998. Difference and similarity: How children's competence is constructed in illness and its treatment. Children & Social Competence: Arenas of Action. Hutchby, I and Moran-Ellis. Falmer, London.

Christensen, P.H., James, A. (Eds.), 2007. Research with children. Perspectives and practices, 2nd edn. Routledge, London.

Clark, N.M., Gong, M., 2000. Management of chronic disease by practitioners and patients: are we teaching the wrong things? British Medical Journal 320, 572–575.

Cleary, J., 1992. Caring for children in hospital. Parents and nurses in partnership. Scutari Press, London.

Coad, J., 2007. Using art-based techniques in engaging children and young people in health care consultations and/or research. Journal of Research in Nursing 12 (5), 487–497.

Coad, J., Coad, N., 2008. Children and young people's preference of thematic design and colour for their hospital environment. Journal of Child Health Care 12 (1), 33–48.

Coad, J., Evans, R., 2008. Reflections on practical approaches to involving children and young people in the data analysis process. Children & Society 22, 41–52.

Coad, J., Lewis, A., 2004. Engaging children and young people in research. Literature review for The National Evaluation of the Children's Fund (NECF). National Evaluation of the Children's Fund & University of Birmingham, Birmingham.

Conroy, S., Choonara, I., Impicciatore, P., et al., 2000. Survey of unlicensed and off label drug use in paediatric wards in European countries. British Medical Journal 320 (7227), 79–82.

Coyne, I., 1995. Partnership in care: parents' views of participating in their hospitalized child's care. Journal of Clinical Nursing 4, 71–79.

Coyne, I.T., 1998. Researching children: some methodological and ethical considerations. Journal of Clinical Nursing 7 (5), 409–416.

Craig, J.V., 2002. Skills for evidence-based practice: how to ask the right question. In: Craig, J.V., Smyth, R.L. (Eds.), The evidence-based practice manual for nurses. Churchill Livingstone, Edinburgh.

Darbyshire, P., 1994. Living with a sick child in hospital. The experiences of parents and nurses. Chapman & Hall, London.

Darbyshire, P., 2000. Guest editorial. From research on children to research with children. Neonatal, Paediatric and Child Health Nursing 3 (1), 2–3.

Department of Health (DoH), 2002. Listening, hearing and responding. Department of Health Action Plan: core principles for the involvement of children and young people. Department of Health, London.

Department of Health (DoH), 2005. Research governance for health and social care, 2nd edn. Department of Health, London.

Department of Health and Department for Education and Skills (DfES), 2004. National Service Framework for children, young people and maternity services. Department of Health & Department for Education and Skills, London.

Farrel, A. (Ed.), 2005. Ethical research with children. Open University Press, Maidenhead.

Fraser, S., Lewis, V., Ding, S., Kellet, M., Robinson, C. (Eds.), 2004. Doing research with children and young people. Sage (in association with The Open University), London.

Greaves, C.J., Eiser, C., Seamark, D., Halpin, D.M.G., 2002. Attack context: an important mediator of the relationship between psychological status and asthma outcomes. Thorax 57, 217–221.

Greene, S., Hogan, D. (Eds.), 2005. Researching children's experience. Approaches and methods. Sage, London.

Greig, A., Taylor, J., MacKay, T., 2007. Doing research with children, 2nd edn. Sage, London.

Guevara, J.P., Wolf, F.M., Grum, C.M., Clark, N.M., 2003. Effects of educational interventions for self management of asthma in children and adolescents: systematic review and meta-analysis. British Medical Journal 326, 1308–1309.

Hampson, S., Skinner, T., Hart, J., et al., 2001. Effect of educational and psychosocial interventions for adolescents with diabetes mellitus: a systematic review. Health Technology Assessment 5 (10), 1–79.

Hood, S., Kelley, P., Mayall, B., 1996. Children as research subjects: a risky enterprise. Children & Society 10, 117–128.

Ireland, L., Holloway, I., 1996. Qualitative health research with children. Children & Society 10 (2), 155–164.

Kamps, A.W., Roorda, R.J., Brand, P.L., 2001. Peak flow diaries in childhood asthma are unreliable. Thorax 56, 180–182.

Kirby, P., 1999. Involving young researchers: How to enable young people to design and conduct research. Joseph Rowntree Foundation, London.

Lewis, A., Lindsay, G. (Eds.), 2000. Researching children's perspectives. Open University Press, Buckingham.

Lewis, V., Kellet, M., Robinson, C., Fraser, S., Ding, S. (Eds.), 2004. The reality of research with children and young people. Sage (in association with The Open University), London.

Madge, P., McColl, J., Paton, J., 1997. Impact of a nurse-led management programme in children admitted to hospital with acute asthma: a randomised controlled study. Thorax 52 (3), 223–228.

Mahon, A., Glendinning, C., Clarke, K., Craig, G., 1996. Researching children: methods and ethics. Children & Society 10, 145–154.

Mallory, C., 2001. Examining the difference between researcher and participant: an intrinsic element of grounded theory. In: Schreiber, R.S., Stern, P.N. (Eds.), Using grounded theory in nursing. Springer Publishing Company, New York, pp. 97–112.

Matthews, H., Limb, M., Taylor, M., 1998. The geography of children: some ethical and methodological considerations for project and dissertations work. Journal of Geography in Higher Education 22 (3), 311–324.

Matthews, H., Tucker, F., 2000. Consulting children. Directions JGHE Study Guide. Journal of Geography in Higher Education 24 (2), 299–310.

Morrow, V., Richards, M., 1996. The ethics of social research with children: an overview. Children & Society 10, 90–105.

MRC Health Services and Public Health Research Board, 2000. A framework for development and evaluation of RCTs for complex interventions to improve health. Medical Research Council, London.

Muir Gray, J.A., 1997. Evidence-based healthcare. How to make health policy and management decisions. Churchill Livingstone, Edinburgh.

National Children's Bureau, 2006. Guidelines for research. National Children's Bureau, London.

National Research Ethics Service, 2007. Information Sheets & Consent Forms. Guidance for Researchers & Reviewers. NHS National Patient Safety Agency, Version 3.2 London.

Neill, S.J., 1996a. Parent participation 1: literature review and methodology. British Journal of Nursing 5 (1), 34–40.

Neill, S.J., 1996b. Parent participation 2: findings and their implications for practice. British Journal of Nursing 5 (2), 110–117.

Neill, S.J., 2005. Research with children: a critical review of the guidelines. Child Health Care 9 (1), 46–58.

Pridmore, P., Bendelow, G., 1995. Images of health: exploring beliefs of children using the 'draw-and-write' technique. Health Education Journal 54 (4), 473–488.

Ramchandani, P., 2004. Treatment of major depressive disorder in children and adolescents. British Medical Journal 328, 3–4.

Royal College of Paediatrics and Child Health: Ethics Advisory Committee, 2000. Guidelines for the ethical conduct of medical research involving children. Archives of Disease in Childhood 82, 117–182.

Sackett, D., Richardson, W., Rosenburg, W., Haynes, R., 1997. Evidence-based medicine. Churchill Livingstone, Edinburgh.

Wilson, M.C., Hayward, R.S.A., Tunis, S.R., Bass, E.B., Guyatt, G., 1995. How to use clinical guidelines: what are the recommendations and will they help you in caring for your patients? Journal of the American Medical Association 274 (20), 1630–1633.

Involving children in healthcare research

15

Jennifer Allison   Rosemary King   E Alan Glasper

ABSTRACT

The aim of this chapter and its companion PowerPoint presentation is to explore the research process and investigate the various issues involved when children participate in clinical research.

LEARNING OUTCOMES

- Recognise that conducting research with children is different.
- Examine elements of informed consent and assent.
- Appreciate the need for conducting research with children.
- Understand how research is conducted with children.
- Explore methods of actively involving children as researchers.

Introduction: children are not small adults

Nurses, and indeed any professional wishing to be involved in research with children, must have a basic understanding of the fundamental differences between adults and children. Children are not small adults, so having an appreciation of what children really are will increase the likelihood of a successful outcome. Rates of physical and psychological change throughout childhood are so great that simply discussing 'the child' as one would 'the adult' is not sufficient. Further subgroups are necessary to describe childhood fully. Common divisions of childhood include infant, child and teenager. These can be divided more finely and have been discussed in other chapters (see Chapter 11).

The legal definition of a child in England, Wales and Northern Ireland is simply anyone under the age of 18 years (Department of Health (DoH) 2001a); in Scotland it is under 16 years (Age of Legal Capacity (Scotland) Act 1991). But the characteristics and diversity of childhood creates a far more complex picture. Children's unique qualities will impact upon every aspect of the research project and ultimately determine its success or failure. Most importantly, infants, children and teenagers are distinctive individuals and the nurse involved in research with children must continually assess and meet the needs of these young volunteers.

Physical and physiological differences

There are physical differences between children and adults both in terms of size and proportion. In relation to the rest of their bodies, newborns' heads are much larger than those of adults. Their brains and nervous systems are not fully grown or formed. There is rapid growth of the infant brain during the first year of life and even the structure of the infant skull changes, e.g. initial presence and then closure of fontanelles. Children's abdomens look large and distended, their arms and legs small. These differences in proportions result in higher body surface area in relation to height and higher basal metabolic rate (BMR). This in turn results in higher energy requirements. Growth is a unique facet of childhood and requires energy. Infants also need more calories per kilogram than adults to maintain normal function (MacGregor 2001).

Children have faster heart rates, breathe faster and have lower blood pressure. Young children also suffer from illnesses that do not exist in the adult population: respiratory distress syndrome, bronchiolitis, croup and necrotising enterocolitis are just a few (Behrman & Kliegman 1998). The developing organ systems of children can respond to drugs very differently from fully developed adults. Adverse events may not be obvious initially. Long-term effects on growth and development become apparent only as the child grows (International Conference on Harmonisation (ICH) 2000).

Unless exposed to teratogens in utero, infants are born as a 'clean slate'. They have not damaged their lungs with cigarette smoke or pollution. Their livers have not been subjected to

DOI: 10.1016/B978-0-7020-3183-0.10015-3

abuse by alcohol; their arteries are not clogged with cholesterol plaques. Children metabolise most drugs at a much faster rate than adults and the potential for accidental damage is much greater. In addition, it is not uncommon for initial or phase I paediatric drug studies to produce recommended doses much higher than adult doses (Morland 2003).

Physical and physiological changes are numerous and continuous throughout childhood. These changes impact on all relationships. Knowledge and understanding of this dynamic process will allow the research nurse to have meaningful interaction with the child or young person based on age-appropriate expectations.

WWW

Visit the European Medicines website for access to International Conference on Harmonisation (ICH) documents and EU regulations:

- http://www.emea.eu.int

Developmental differences

Developmental changes occur alongside physical maturation. This is an ongoing, ever-changing process. It is accepted theory that children move along a continuum in an expected and orderly fashion, but the exact timing is unique for each child. Piaget, Erikson and Freud devised established theories of development. Each examined children's development but from different perspectives (Behrman & Kliegman 1998). Table 15.1 provides the basic components of their theories. For further information see Chapter 11.

Table 15.1 Summaries of the different theories of child development

Age	Piaget	Erikson	Freud
Birth–18 months		Trust versus mistrust	Oral stage
Birth–2 years	Sensorimotor		
18 months–2 years		Autonomy versus shame and doubt	Anal stage
2–6 or 7 years	Preoperational		
3–6 years		Initiative versus guilt	Phallic stage
6 or 7–11 years	Concrete operations		
6–12 years		Industry versus inferiority	Latency stage
12 years–adult	Formal operations		
Adult		Identity versus role confusion	Genital stage

Adapted from Behrman & Kleigman 1998 pp 18–19.

Developmental stages will help determine the way a child responds and behaves. Young research volunteers can be expected to react in certain ways depending on these stages. Therefore, it is possible for the research nurse to anticipate the reaction prior to approaching the child. However, these stages of development should serve only as a guideline – it is also imperative to assess each child as an individual. Children of the same age can differ greatly and are constantly changing and developing. Being equipped to interact appropriately with children at all stages is vital to establishing a successful relationship with each child.

Alderson & Montgomery (1996) question traditional theories that used the obvious physical growth of children as a metaphor for maturation of mental and emotional abilities, resulting in a gradual increase in ability while assuming younger children remain unable to participate in decisions. They argue that the experience of the child has greater impact on ability than age. However, this view and traditional theories agree that children mature at uneven rates. Therefore, researchers must continually evaluate the individual and changing needs of young volunteers.

Scenario

Julia is a third year child branch student on placement in a Clinical Research Facility (CRF). Three-year-old Amanda arrives with her parents for a bronchoscopy. She requires this diagnostic procedure and will be part of a research study, as bronchial wash samples will also be taken. She requires anaesthetic cream for a cannula. Julia asks her if she would like to sit on the treatment table or in the chair on mummy's lap. Amanda points to the treatment table with a brightly coloured toy on the pillow. Why did Julia give her a choice? Would this have been different if Amanda was 6 months old, or 12 years old?

Social differences

An appreciation of the unique social environment of children further enhances the creation of a successful relationship with a young volunteer. The family unit is the socially accepted and identifiable model of childcare and socialisation (DoH 2003a). It is rarely permissible to involve children in research without involving the child's family. Building a trusting relationship with a child volunteer requires an equally strong relationship with the family. As is made clear later in this chapter regarding issues of consent, without parental consent it is impossible to proceed with the research project (DoH 2001a). Studies have shown that parental attitudes are most influential in a child or young person's decision-making process. As decisions become more complex, younger children appear more susceptible to parental influence (Broome & Richards 2003). Young children are totally dependant within the family unit, a situation rarely seen within other patient groups. The UK National Service Framework (NSF) for Children (DoH 2003a) recognises this and mandates 'children and young people should receive care that is integrated and coordinated around their particular needs, and the needs of their family'.

www

Search for the UK National Service Framework for Children online at the Department of Health website

- http://www.dh.gov.uk

Powerpoint

Access the companion PowerPoint presentation and look at examples of child-friendly information leaflets used in the Wellcome Trust Clinical Research Facility.
How do these compare with information you have used on placements?

Communication

Information is the cornerstone of the research process and is basic to the concept of informed consent, which will be discussed in detail later.

It is the duty of the research nurse to provide the necessary information to the family and the child. This can be achieved in a number of ways including printed materials, audiovisual format and discussions. Regardless of the method used, all information must be age appropriate and formatted in a way easily understood by the child and family, so that informed decisions can be made. Issues of age and development will impact on the types of information given to children. Creative use of drawings, play, puppets and dolls can aid in the information process (DoH 2001a). Communication with children will require very different techniques depending on age and developmental needs. Once again it is not good enough to say 'this is the way to communicate with a child' because infants will require very different methods to preschoolers or teenagers. The ability to judge a situation and intervene appropriately with individual children cannot be overestimated.

www

Visit the UNICEF website at:

- http://www.unicef.org

The full document The United Nations Convention on the Rights of the Child can be found at:

- http://www.unicef.org/crc/fulltext.htm

Child protection issues

Children participating in research have the same rights to protection offered all research volunteers by the declaration of Helsinki (World Medical Association (WMA) 2000). These issues will be discussed later in this chapter. In addition there is further protection from the Children Act (DoH 1989) and the NSF for Children (DoH 2003a), which stipulate requirements regarding the specific needs of children. This includes a Draft Standard on Child Protection stating:

> Children have the right to be protected, and adults a responsibility to protect them from harm.
>
> (DoH 2003a)

Families have a right to expect separate facilities, properly staffed by paediatricians, sick children's nurses and play therapists. Television, well-equipped playrooms and age-appropriate food are just some of the requirements. Collaboration between agencies is necessary, with multidisciplinary development of child protection guidelines, policies and involvement in Serious Case Reviews. All staff must have child protection training and those who have direct contact with children require pre-employment police checks (DoH 2003a). For further information on child protection, see Chapter 19.

Activity

Look at the Child Protection policies when on different placements.

- How do they compare?
- How do they ensure that staff are properly trained in child protection?
- Have you had a police check?

Vulnerability and autonomy

The lack of autonomy allowed children by society increases the vulnerability of young research volunteers. The amount of independence afforded to children is a matter of choice for society. It has been argued that children are unable to exercise choice due to cultural constraints rather than biological necessity. When children are not given the opportunity or permission to exercise their autonomy, it is often mistakenly assumed that they do not have the capacity to do so (Alderson & Montgomery 1996).

Activity

Discuss the following questions with your colleagues.

- How does the lack of autonomy increase the vulnerability of children?
- Have you seen examples of highly capable youngsters being prevented from participating fully in their health care?

The United Nations (UN) Convention on the Rights of the Child, Article 12 (UN General Assembly 1989) sets no minimum age for involvement in decisions and refers to children's 'evolving capacity', with adult members of society expected to foster participation.

Under UK law, children lack complete autonomy and are unable to make some decisions independently. Although they always have the right to assent or agree to participate, their parents usually make legal decisions and consent on their behalf (DoH 2001a). Issues of Gillick competency, consent and assent will be discussed later, as will involving children actively in the research process. The NSF for Children mandates the delivery of child-centred care and staff to support children 'to be active partners in decision making' (DoH 2003a). The child must come first and his or her needs are paramount within any research project.

At the basis of the research process is the trusting relationship between volunteer and researcher. It is critical that the research nurse prepares the child properly, taking into account the unique needs of each child with respect to age, development and social/family considerations. Research professionals must also put the needs and best interests of their volunteers first, ahead of research aspirations (DoH 2005). Using age- and developmentally appropriate interactions and information, research nurses can be strong, dependable advocates for their young patients. Theories of growth and development, combined with an understanding of physical differences and needs of children, provide guidelines for researchers working with children and young people. However, assessing each child as a unique individual will increase the likelihood of successful interactions and research. Alderson & Montgomery (1996) warn there is a risk of holding on to outdated misconceptions that can result in the infantalisation of highly capable children and young people. Balancing the amount and types of support given to children can be difficult to judge and adults are often overcautious in assessing children's capabilities. Research nurses must ensure young volunteers are looked after in an appropriate and safe manner. Investing time to build a relationship will allow informed dialogue so that children are given the protection they need and the choices they deserve.

Issues of informed consent and assent

Consent is a legal contract entered into by an adult or individual with parental responsibility; assent is the voluntary permission of an individual without legal status (Lamprill 2002).

How do you obtain consent from children?

In the document 'Seeking consent: working with children' (DoH 2001a), the DoH stipulates that for consent to be considered valid, the person giving consent must be:

- competent: capable of making the decision
- acting voluntarily
- informed by the researcher to enable a decision to be made.

In the UK, children and young people acquire the right to give or withhold consent for treatment in stages. At 18 years of age, young people in England, Wales and Northern Ireland become legal adults with the absolute right to give or refuse consent (DoH 2001a). Under Scottish law, young people achieve this right at 16 (Age of Legal Capacity (Scotland) Act 1991). No one can consent on behalf of another competent adult. In the rest of the UK, 16–17-year-olds are presumed competent to give consent for treatment. However, this becomes complicated when the child refuses consent, because the parents can override the wishes of their dissenting 16- or 17-year-old child. Under-16s are not legally competent unless they are deemed to be 'Gillick competent', i.e. if they have sufficient understanding and intelligence to enable them to understand fully what is proposed. Therefore, there is no specific age when a child becomes competent; it depends on the individual child and complexity of treatment (DoH 2001a).

For a young or non-Gillick competent child, consent must be given by a parent or person with 'parental responsibility', someone with legal responsibility for the child as stated in the Children Act (DoH 1989). It is important to note that unmarried fathers and stepfathers might not have this legal right unless afforded so by a court of law or by a Parental Responsibility Agreement with the mother. Therefore professionals must ensure that consent is obtained from an adult with this right of parental responsibility (DoH 2001a).

What does the NMC say regarding consent?

The NMC in 'The Code: standards for conduct, performance and ethics for nurses and midwives' (NMC 2008a) states that consent must be obtained 'before any treatment or care.' This new version of the code has been changed and lacks previous statements such as:

> You are personally accountable for ensuring that you promote and protect the interests and dignity of patients and clients, irrespective of gender, age ...

No-one has the right to give consent on behalf of another competent adult. In relation to obtaining consent for a child, the involvement of those with parental responsibility in consent procedure is usually necessary, but will depend on the age and understanding of the child. If the child is under the age of 16 in England and Wales, 12 in Scotland and 17 in Northern Ireland, you must be aware of legislation and local protocols relating to consent (NMC 2002).

Following the implementation of The Code, the NMC developed a document specifically for nurses working with children and young people. 'Advice for nurses working with children and young people' is meant to aid interpretation of The Code in a complex setting where tension might exist between the rights and needs of children and those of their parents. Specific guidance is given regarding consent:

> Empower children and young people and their parents through providing information and giving them time to make decisions ...
> help children make decisions using play and other appropriate means of communication.
>
> (NMC 2008b)

WWW

For more information on Gillick competency and the landmark court case go to:

- http://www.confidential.oxfordradcliffe.net/gillick

What is competency?

The issue of competency can be complicated but the DoH (2001a) has given some guidelines. Someone is deemed competent if they:

> Comprehend and retain information material to the decision, especially as to the consequences of having or not having the intervention in question ...
>
> Use and weigh this information in the decision-making process
>
> (DoH 2001a)

Children's competency is not an issue when they agree to treatment – it is when they refuse that questions of competency are raised (Alderson 1995). Until the youngster is 16 in Scotland, or 18 in the rest of the UK, parents have the legal authority to reverse the wishes of their child and give consent for treatment even if the youngster withholds consent (Age of Legal Capacity (Scotland) Act 1991, DoH 2001a). This creates a double standard for consent, with young people under the age of 18 free to agree and give consent but not able to disagree and withhold consent (Alderson 1995). The 'NSF for Children' (DoH 2003a) states that:

> Consent policies should include what to do when there is disagreement between a competent young person and their parent.

Therefore it is advisable to check local policies regarding consent. In extreme cases of disagreement, the courts can decide whether or not treatment is given (DoH 2001a).

WWW

Visit the Department of Health website to review consent guidance:

- http://www.dh.gov/consent

The full Declaration of Helsinki document can be found at the World Medical Association website:

- http://www.wma.net/e/policy/b3.htm

Activity

Read the consent policies on your ward placement; look at the consent forms:

- How often do you see 16-year-olds sign their own forms?
- Do you observe younger Gillick competent children signing consent for procedures?

What makes consent informed?

The 'DoH Research Governance Framework' (2005) states that 'informed consent is at the heart of ethical research'. That is to say that information must be given so that consent is based on sufficient knowledge of what is planned and any possible risks involved. Extensive patient information sheets are required for each study and are ethically approved as part of formal research protocols. When children are involved in studies, special age-appropriate information sheets are needed (Robinson 2001). As stated in part 22 of The Declaration of Helsinki (WMA 2000), there is clear stipulation as to the type of information researchers are mandated to provide. This includes information regarding:

> Aims, methods, sources of funding, any possible conflicts of interest, institutional affiliations of the researcher, the anticipated benefits and potential risks of the study and the discomfort it may entail.

The DoH (2001a) clearly states that children should be involved in decision making and suggests the use of toys, pictures and play and to ensure that written information is given in age-appropriate language. Prospective volunteers should be given this information in advance of their participation, ideally at least 24 hours prior to the signing of consent forms. This enables them to consult with their family, GP or any person with whom they choose to discuss the study and possible concerns. It also allows time to formulate questions for the researcher prior to participation (Alderson 1995). The person obtaining consent must also 'check the child's understanding' (DoH 2001a). This can be achieved by including a simple quiz, which can be kept as a record of comprehension with other study forms (Lamprill 2002).

What about research?

Participation in research is not mandatory. Participants in research studies are called 'volunteers'. That word describes an individual who freely takes part in the research process. Protection and care of the research subject is enshrined in internationally accepted guidelines.

The first international standard was written in 1947 as a reaction to the atrocities of the Second World War, and later became known as the Nuremberg Code. The ten principles have become the basis for ethical research practice involving humans. These principles include freely given consent, capacity to consent, freedom from coercion, comprehension of the risks and benefits, minimisation of risk and harm with a favourable risk/benefit ratio, the presence of qualified investigators using appropriate research designs and freedom for the subject to withdraw at any time. Children were excluded from participating in research by the stipulation of informed, voluntary consent free of coercion (Burns 2003).

The WMA Declaration of Helsinki, adopted in 1964 and then regularly amended (WMA 2000), has since allowed the participation of children in research as long as there is consent from a parent or 'legally authorised individual in accordance with applicable law'. It also states that when the subject is a 'minor child' and 'able to give assent to decisions about participation in research, the investigator must obtain that assent in addition to the consent from a legally authorised representative'. This document distinguishes between therapeutic research, described as 'research combined with medical care', and non-therapeutic research involving 'healthy volunteers'.

The principles of the Declaration of Helsinki (WMA 2000) led to the creation of an international standard for clinical trials involving human subjects. The International Conference on Harmonisation guideline for good clinical practice (ICH GCP) came into effect in 1997 with the objective of providing a 'unified standard for the European Union, Japan and the United States to facilitate the mutual acceptance of clinical data by the regulatory authorities in these jurisdictions'. The principles established in ICH GCP guidelines 'may also be applied to other clinical investigations that may have an impact on the safety and well-being of human subjects', not just clinical trials (ICH 2002).

In the UK, the DoH has developed the Research Governance Framework for Health and Social Care (DoH 2005) to set standards and improve research quality by promoting good practice. In section 1.1, it recognises the need for health and social research while ensuring public confidence through 'high scientific, ethical and financial standards, transparent decision-making processes, clear allocation of responsibilities and robust monitoring arrangements' (DoH 2005).

www

The Department of Health Research Governance Framework can be found at the DoH research and development website:

- http://www.dh.gov.uk/research

Risk versus benefit

The DoH (2001a) states that children may participate in therapeutic research based on new treatment that may be as effective or more effective than standard treatment. Participation in non-therapeutic research is possible if doing so is 'not against the interests of the child and imposes only a minimal burden'. In both cases it is stipulated that sufficient information must be given prior to participation. Minimal burden is not clearly defined and it is left to the researcher to assess each child and gives the examples of bone marrow donations and more simple injections. The bone marrow would require a therapeutic benefit to the child but an injection would not. However, as there is considerable variation in response to injections researchers must bear in mind the individual reaction of young volunteers. Some children might not consider an injection a 'minimal burden'.

The risk/benefit ratio first mentioned in the Nuremberg Code remains a source of debate. Alderson (1995) argues that 'risk' is vague and refers to both possible and definite harms, whereas 'benefits' implies there will be definite good. She states that 'risk and hoped-for benefits' is a more balanced phrase. These terms can be misleading depending on their context, with clarity needed regarding who is at risk and who will benefit. There is potential for great benefit to society at the great expense of a few volunteers. However, the Declaration of Helsinki (WMA 2000) states 'the considerations related to the well-being of the human subject should take precedence over the interests of society'. This ethical stance is reaffirmed in the DoH Research Governance Framework, which mandates 'The dignity, rights, safety and well being of participants must be the primary consideration in any research study' (DoH 2005).

Is your volunteer acting voluntarily?

Assent, Gillick and the right to refuse

Wherever possible assent or agreement to participate should be obtained from all children and young people. Researchers must take time to prepare parents to provide consent and pre-Gillick competent children to provide assent. Importantly, the DoH (2001a) states that even when the parent has given consent for participation in 'non-therapeutic research', if a child of any age disagrees then the research should not go ahead. It is interesting to note that this does not include 'therapeutic' research. So it would seem that the child once again has the right to consent but not the complete right to dissent. In the case of participation in a research study, it would be foolish to include a child in a study against his or her parents' wishes (Lamprill 2002). Whereas a competent child may consent for participation without parental approval, this would be highly unrealistic and impractical (Robinson 2001). Best practice would dictate that with proper preparation a trusting relationship between the child, family and research team would prevent the occurrence of such extreme situations. The research nurse must be an advocate for the young volunteer and support them to have a voice in the research process.

Assessing Gillick competency for research consent requires determining the youngsters' understanding of research protocols. This includes complicated concepts such as placebos and their use in randomised controlled trials. Montgomery (2001) suggests that all projects need Gillick assessment and that a child may have sufficient understanding of one study but not of another. This creates a situation where a child is Gillick competent for one research project but not necessarily for all studies. Therefore it is imperative that children and young people are properly assessed for each study in which they participate.

Another fundamental component of consent for research is the right for the volunteer or parent to change their minds. This was first stated in the Nuremberg Code, and reaffirmed in the Declaration of Helsinki (WMA 2000):

> The subject should be informed of the right to abstain from participation in the study or to withdraw consent to participate at any time without reprisal.

Consent forms and patient information sheets must state that participation is optional (Lamprill 2002). Children and young people need to understand this right and researchers must be certain that young volunteers and their parents feel able to stop at any time during the study without it affecting their care.

Scenario

Ten-year-old Aidan and Leo, his 16-year-old brother, attend a CRF as part of a research study investigating the genetics of phenylketonuria (PKU). Jane, a second year Child Branch student nurse is assisting Research Nurse Sylvia. Ross, the boys' father, is very abrupt with the nurses as Sylvia goes over the patient information sheets and consent forms with him and the boys. 'This isn't necessary just give them to me and I'll sign them. I must get back to work.' Sylvia tries to explain she must be certain the boys understand and agree and she also asks Leo for his consent. 'Don't be ridiculous, he's just a boy and of course they agree' What should Sylvia say? What would you do?

Advocacy and best interest

The International Conference on Harmonisation (ICH) Document E11 (ICH 2000) gives clear guidelines regarding the need to balance the protection of young, potentially very vulnerable research volunteers with the benefits to be gained from participation in research. Research nurses must be the advocates for their young volunteers and empower them to make decisions free of any coercion. Recruitment must be free from inappropriate inducements to the parent or child and while reimbursement for expenses is allowed, it must be included in the protocol and approved by the ethics committee (ICH 2000).

The UN Convention on the Rights of The Child, Article 12 (United Nations General Assembly 1989) states that children have a right to participate in the decision-making process that may be relevant to their lives. Adults are also expected to promote and empower children so that they may express their views and influence decisions. Standards for healthcare professionals in the NSF for Children (DoH 2003a) include the need to provide a child-centred service, with the needs of the child put first. Choices should be offered to all children and young people regarding aspects of treatment. Young people must 'never feel that decisions are being made over their heads' (DoH 2001a). This should be the ethos of the multidisciplinary research team. In 'Advocating for children', the Royal College of Paediatrics and Child Health (RCPCH 2000) has adopted as an overall aim 'To advocate the rights of children and young people in society and to promote their health needs and services'. It refers to the concept of 'best interest' enshrined in the UN Convention on the Rights of The Child, and expects 'all members to act within the framework'. This clear guidance for all professionals working with children, combined with the mandate of the NMC (2008b), requires the research nurse to advocate for the best interests of young volunteers. This includes working with the research team and family to facilitate the child's participation as a partner in the research process. Providing information, choices and support for young volunteers will allow the continued development of safe, accurate and successful research.

PROFESSIONAL CONVERSATION

Jane is a student nurse on placement with her mentor Sylvia, a research nurse.

Issues regarding children's assent and parental consent for participation in research

I have been on placement in the clinical research facility for 3 weeks. My mentor Sylvia and I had a difficult morning with a family participating in a genetic study. During lunch we chatted about the issues of consent and assent, and how to include competent children in the consenting process. I understand that young people must be involved and sometimes nurses must be advocates for youngsters – even if that means disagreeing with their parents.

How research is conducted with children

Involving children in research requires the same child-centred approach as caring for sick children in a ward setting (DoH 2003a). Successful completion of any research project involving children demands careful planning, organisation, implementation and evaluation.

Researchers have to find ways of engaging children using negotiation rather than imposition (Barker & Weller 2003). To be successful, researchers need to think about how children will perceive them (Balen et al 2001). Children like to meet a person they can trust and someone who is fun to be around, therefore researchers need to make an effort to ensure they are creative (Curtin 2000) and provide an age-appropriate approach. Instead of employing existing adult methodologies, child-led methodologies have been developed to enable children to communicate using qualitative methods, e.g. drawing, dairies and photography (Avery 2003, Balen et al 2001). Such methods aim to build a rapport, trust and confidence, allowing children to clearly articulate their views and opinions. Hence by giving information in a child-centred way the researcher can empower young people, gain their trust and cooperation and obtain their assent to be active participants in research.

When designing information sheets, consent forms and constructing quantitative research tools such as questionnaires, child-centred researchers should be aware of the significance children and young people place on language. It is also important to consult with children about the development of appropriate research methods. Researchers should not impose their own interpretations, made up of adult feelings and presumptions, which can suppress or misrepresent the voices of children (Barker & Weller 2003).

WWW

Visit this website for access to programmes that help to ensure the language used is reading age appropriate:

- http://www. usingenglish.com/glossary/fog-index.html

Activity

When conducting a study with many components, consider how best to facilitate the young child's coping ability. For example, the use of star charts enables a child to plot their progress and at the same time provide a simple reward.

Construct a star chart for use in your working environment that would help children in your care cope with procedures.

Research methodology and design that is suitable for use with children

Research methods can be divided into two main approaches, quantitative and qualitative:

- Quantitative research is structured, usually experimental and employs standard methods, e.g. randomised controlled trials. It produces data amenable to statistical analysis.
- Qualitative research methods are holistic, observational, unstructured or semi-structured, and the data are presented in the form of quotations or descriptions, though some basic statistics may be presented. Increasingly the two approaches (triangulation) are combined within one research project (Scanlon 2003).

Before deciding on which method to use the researcher needs to be satisfied that they have chosen the most appropriate design, which provides suitable answers to the following questions (Edwards & Talbot 1994):

- Is this method going to provide the kind of information required?
- Is this method going to build up as accurate a picture of the events as possible?
- Is this the most suitable design for the children concerned and can it be done in the time available?

By combining a range of research methods within one study, known as triangulation, a picture can be built up of the phenomenon under investigation from a range of perspectives (Morrow 2001). For example, in their pilot study, Avery et al (2003) used a 'quality of life' questionnaire and the children took photographs of how their lives were affected by their illness and then wrote about their feelings when they took their photographs.

A pilot study can be described as a 'dummy-run' and enables the researcher to see whether the methods chosen do indeed collect the data needed to answer the chosen research question. This also provides an opportunity to get feedback from children themselves on the chosen methodology and their experience of participation (Balen et al 2001).

Research with children is carried out for many different reasons, and therefore different child-centred methods are required to elicit information.

Activity

- Is there an aspect of nursing care for children you are involved in that you would like to investigate further?
- Discuss with your colleagues what approach you might use for conducting this investigation.

Health-related quality of life studies

What is quality of life?

The World Health Organization (1996) has defined quality of life as:

> An individual's perception of their position in life in the context of the culture and value systems in which they live and in relation to their goals, expectations, standards and concerns. It is a broad ranging concept affected in a complex way by the person's physical health, psychological state, level of independence, social relationships and their relationship to salient features of the environment.

www

Read the article by Camilleri-Brennan & Steele 1999:

- http://www.rcsed.ac.uk/journal/vol44_4/4440010.htm

Children can be reliable informants, presenting accurate accounts of their experiences. However, engaging children in research and ensuring their voices are heard requires a specific non-adult approach (Curtin 2000). By involving children in research, we can learn about children's perspectives on their worlds, and the personal meanings children attribute to events and actions. By actively participating in research children can be given a voice and children can have practice in making life decisions.

Quality of life can be determined by the extent to which hopes and ambitions are matched by experience. Participating in a study can clarify a child's perceptions of their position in life, in relation to their goals, expectations, standards and concerns within the surroundings of their culture and value systems. Such quality of life studies can be used both to establish things children regard as important in their lives and to evaluate a child's current state against some ideal. The use of quality of life measures in clinical practice can help to ensure that treatment and evaluation focus on the child rather than the disease (Higginson & Carr 2001).

Other ways of assessing the quality of life from the perspective of children and adolescents include self-reporting questionnaires, interviews and computer-assisted forms. The researcher may want to obtain a complete family-centred analysis and should consider the quality of life of the children's families. By asking the parents and, if possible, siblings for their perception of a sick child's quality of life as well as their rating of their own quality of life, a fuller picture can be obtained (Bullinger et al 2002).

Illness, especially chronic illness and its consequences, affects the lives of children but little is known about the effects of ill health or medical interventions on children's development and how they adjust or compensate for the negative effects of hospitalisation, intrusive medical procedures and the uncertainty of survival. To understand these effects it is important to fully assess children's quality of life. There have been various definitions of health-related quality of life, however researchers agree that quality of life is a multidimensional, subjective and dynamic concept (Camilleri-Brennan & Steele 1999).

Activity

Go to your local nursing library, access and read Avery et al (2003). Discuss with colleagues what aspects of your nursing care given to a cohort of children could similarly be investigated.

Discuss what insight this would give you into the quality of life of the children and their families, and how you could then change your practice to improve the children's quality of life.

When adults wish to communicate with children it is important that they develop strategies that recognise children's age-specific cognitive development, attention span and language. Like adults, children make sense of their worlds and define meanings using previous experience. Unlike adults they have limited past experiences to make sense of new events (Fleitas 1998). Children are continually developing and changing with age so assessing quality of life in children differs from quality of life in adults. Children's quality of life should be looked at within four categories:

1. Children's physical development.
2. Children's developing concepts of quality of life.
3. Children's cognitive development: the researcher should be aware that children's understanding of various spheres, including health, appear to be more related to experience than age or level of cognitive development.

4. Content of the questionnaire: as quality of life is usually measured by a questionnaire, the content of questionnaires should be suitably child-centred for the group being investigated (Bradding & Horstman 1999, Vincent & Higginson 2003).

Such quality of life questionnaires can be used to gather relatively straightforward information and can be employed to study groups or children with a particular problem. This allows comparisons with other groups. When developing or using a validated questionnaire it is important to ensure it will produce the type of information sought (Hinds 2000). However, using questionnaires with children can produce misleading information. A child may not be able to recall the necessary information, may not have sufficient language skills to understand the meaning of the question or may lack the written skills to produce a comprehensible response. The resourceful researcher can be creative in the production of questionnaires, placing importance on both the visual presentation and the order in which the questions are presented. Questions should gradually shift from least to most sensitive, general to detailed, concrete to abstract. Children find it easier to answer questions about the present and events they have just experienced than about the past.

It is important to use appropriate vocabulary to suit the age and literary ability of the children concerned (Curtin 2000, Oppenheim 2002). To produce valid responses clear instructions should be given for the use of scaled responses to questions, e.g. with a rating of 1 for 'not at all' to 6 for 'very much'. Or the researcher may consider the use of pictures instead of words: six simply drawn faces numbered 0 to 5 with various degrees from smiling through neutral to misery (iconic Likert scale). The child is asked to indicate how much he or she likes or dislikes a statement. Alternatively the researcher can use linear scales (visual analogue scale) based on a horizontal line with a mark at one end indicating the most positive aspect and a mark at the other end indicating the worst aspect (Dockerell 2000).

PowerPoint

Access the companion PowerPoint presentation to view an iconic Likert scale and a visual analogue scale.

www

Visit the 'Wong on web' website for examples of rating scales:

- http://www3.us.elsevierhealth.com/WOW/faces.html

www

For an interactive online version of the Quality of Life Research Unit, University of Toronto Adult Quality of Life Profile, and descriptions of a variety of studies involving children, adolescents and families, visit:

- www.utoronto.ca/qol

Conducting research interviews with children and young people

When seeking children's views and opinions, researchers act as facilitators. An alternative technique they can employ is the interview. Interviews should be conducted in child-friendly surroundings, where the child is made to feel safe and comfortable; this might be in their home, or school or suitable playroom within the hospital setting. The researcher should be constantly aware of the children's perspective, develop innovative approaches and ensure the environment is child-centred. Before asking questions in an interview, the researcher should inform children that there are no right or wrong answers and that it is all right if they do not have an answer. The interviewer should use open-ended questions when asking children to report directly on their beliefs or knowledge as such questions allow children themselves to structure the type and extent of their responses (Curtin 2000, Dockerell 2000).

Williamson & Butler (1995) suggest children and young people can attempt to conceal the problems of their worlds from adults to avoid 'being humiliated by misunderstanding, misrepresentation and misplaced responses'. This concealment can be a considerable barrier to adults involved in gathering data from children. The answers given may not reflect the child's true opinion but be what they think the adult wants to hear. Rather than impose a series of questions, the creative researcher can encourage children to talk more by using activities that most children enjoy:

- Brainstorming: spider diagrams, mind maps
- Sentence completion: e.g. 'Having a peanut allergy affects my life at school because …
- Prompt cards: single cards with pictures or words.
- Pictorial vignettes: a series of pictures
- Ranking exercises: pictures or sentences on cards which children are asked to put in order of importance
- Play: encouraging the child to describe his or her ideas, thoughts or emotions through a third person, e.g. teddy
- Role-play: generating ideas, thoughts and emotions about a scenario the child acts out.

These methods can give children their own voice and ensure their ideas and explanations are heard and understood. Sorensen (1989) suggests the use of children's diaries or journals for data collection in research. The researcher must ensure the child understands what is required, by giving clear instructions, yet keeping the layout as open as possible. They may then discover the child's viewpoints of daily life, unhampered by observer presence or other formal data collection methods. Diaries give children freedom of thought and expression, by the use of their own language and drawings.

Activity

Go to your local nursing library, access and read Kennedy et al 2003 on the use of interactive data collection (IDC) software for collecting research data with school age children.

- Discuss this approach with your colleagues.

The write and draw method

Young children and those with lesser abilities are under-represented in research studies. These groups can find the non-verbal approach an easier way to express themselves because they can find it hard to convey feelings verbally, especially with adults they do not know well. The use of play, painting or drawing can enable children to express themselves clearly. Practically all school-aged children are familiar with producing drawings and writing about them. The write and draw method involves children being invited to draw pictures related to aspects of health or ill health and to write about what is happening in their pictures (Backett-Milburn & McKie 1999). This is considered to be child-friendly, non-threatening and facilitating the expression of views by children. It does not necessitate the adult being continually involved in the process, so the children are free to concentrate and think about their own ideas but they are able to ask for adult help to communicate their thoughts in writing when they wish (Bradding & Horstman 1999).

When a child asks the researcher to scribe draw-and-talk, the researcher should do so verbatim, without prompting or influencing the child's thoughts and emotions. Different approaches can be used: draw and write, as previously described, and draw and label, when children choose to draw pictures and label them to show aspects of the theme, e.g. health or ill-health. The write only method, which Pridmore & Lansdown (1997) suggest, is a quick way of identifying major categories of information. The researcher can expand on the issues identified by using more enjoyable activities such as drawing and dialogue. These methods have been used successfully with individuals as well as in larger groups of children.

WWW

Visit the web site:

- http://her.oupjournals.org/cgi/content/ful/14/3/387

Read the full text of Backett-Milburn & McKie (1999) for a critique of the 'write and draw' method.

Using focus groups

Focus group research involves a planned conversation with a selected group of children or young people to gain information about their views and experiences about a subject. Children participating in research need to feel safe. Children generally find safety in numbers so focus groups can provide a comfortable way of interaction between children; a well-chosen group of five or six children provide social support to each other. This methodology can be used to gain information relating to how children think, what their views are and capture their experiences by obtaining several perspectives about the same topic and the ways in which others influence individuals in a group situation (Gibbs 1997). This approach allows children to explain their perceptions of an event, an idea or an experience. Such groups are useful when there is a need for more insight and understanding of the child's experience and when seeking the perspective of children (Hinds 2000). In such a forum children need to fully understand what is expected of them. It is therefore essential that the questions be posed clearly, concisely and unambiguously in child-led language (Balen et al 2001). The moderator or facilitator needs to help the children feel at ease and facilitate interaction between all the children in the group by asking open questions, at times probing for more detail, keeping the session focused by steering the conversation back on course and ensuring everyone participates and has a chance to speak (Gibbs 1997).

Activity

Ask children about the quality of care they receive and in what ways they think the nursing care they receive could be improved:

- How best could you do this?
- Discuss this with your colleagues.

Randomised controlled trials

A randomised controlled trial (RCT) is the gold standard of research (Glasper & Ireland 2000). This method is the favoured design used to find out the effectiveness and safety of new clinical treatments including drug trials and explore different approaches to disease management. Patients are randomly assigned to a treatment (intervention) group or control (comparison) groups, sometimes blindly (i.e. the patient and family do not know which group they are in). Additionally, many studies use double blinding (neither the patient nor researcher know who is in which group). Only during analysis is the blinding removed.

Randomisation helps to minimise bias and ensures that children are allocated to either arm of the trial in the fairest way possible, taking into account all the risks and benefits. The active group receives the new treatment under investigation and the control group receives a placebo, or the best historically known treatment to date (Forman & Ladd 1995). At the end of the trial the results are collected and unblinded when necessary. Everyone then knows who was on which arm of the trial and the outcomes of the treatment from the children in both groups. Both groups are followed up over a period of time to see if there are any differences in the outcome.

RCTs are often run by commercial companies and are conducted over a period of time, from different sites (hospitals), and in different countries. This ensures that the findings are not unique to one setting and gives extra validity to the results (Swage 2000).

Conducting such a clinical trial with adults is one thing but to do so with children is even more challenging (Robinson 2002). It is only feasible with the cooperation and collaboration of all those involved. This includes groups of people, i.e. children, parents, investigators, research nurses, pharmaceutical sponsors and ethics committees, all of whom have varying roles to play, with different perceptions. This can lead to conflicting priorities. Lamprill (2003) calls for pharmaceutical sponsors to adopt a more child-friendly approach to their studies, taking child and family needs into account when planning protocols.

Although parents do have altruistic motives for consenting to their children taking part in research studies, Rothmier et al (2003) suggest that most parents give consent to learn more about their child's disease. Similarly, Lamprill (2003) suggests that parents will not allow their children to be exposed to more than minimal risk or suffering. However, they may accept higher risk if there is a chance the child could benefit significantly from taking part in the study.

Pharmaceutical sponsors should remember that families live in the 'real world', so when the unexpected occurs – as it often does – this can hinder the smooth running of a paediatric trial. Lamprill (2003) describes a child who dropped his inhaler down the lavatory, a dog who ate a large pot of study medication, and a courier who arrived before the blood sample was prepared! Paediatric adverse events can be non-specific; children are often described as 'off food' or 'off colour'. As children's nurses are aware, there may be no specific symptoms but children can feel generally unwell and cannot express themselves, this is difficult to record in the formality of a drug trial.

Whatever the problems that arise during paediatric clinical trials, researchers should never lose sight of their purpose. In many instances this is to ensure that medication used to treat children is properly adapted for use in the growing child, and to establish appropriate safe doses that achieve maximum effect with minimal side effects.

This section has provided a brief overview of how research is conducted with children; other research methods can equally well be employed. Whatever methodology is used, the thoughtful, sensitive and responsible child researcher must be mindful of adapting the method to the age and capacity of the children concerned, and to leave the child, of whatever age, enriched for having participated in the research process and feeling good about her or his contribution (Brown & Haylor 1989).

PowerPoint

Access the companion PowerPoint presentation for examples of other research methods.

For further information on research methods suitable for use in research with children see:

Greig A, Taylor J (1999) Doing research with children. Sage Publications, London

Lewis A, Lindsay G (2000) Researching children's perspectives. Open University Press, Buckingham.

Why is it necessary to undertake research with children?

Children have a right to benefit from relevant research. Historically, health professionals have been reluctant to include children in research studies and clinical trials due to their vulnerability and their inability to give informed consent (Rosato 2000). It can no doubt be argued that they have been doing the childhood population a great disservice by denying them the most appropriate medicines and treatments. Children have a right to be given medication and treatments that are safe and effective whatever the age of the child. The Children's National Service Framework (NSF) (DoH 2003a) states that the use of medicines in children should be guided by the best available evidence of clinical effectiveness, cost effectiveness and safety, ideally derived from clinical trials conducted with children. When including this vulnerable population in clinical trials it is vital that the research nurse is familiar with issues surrounding informed consent and children's assent. There should be a proper balance between the need to recruit children to clinical trials and research studies and the need to protect their rights as human subjects (Meaux & Bell 2001).

As mentioned earlier, children are not simply small adults: their bodies are constantly growing and developing and metabolic rates change with age. In many cases data based on studies performed on adults cannot be directly applied to children. This is because on a pharmacological and pharmacokinetic level a child does not behave in the same way as an adult, yet many medicines prescribed for children have never been studied in children (Vasmant 2003). Children require treatments that are disease specific to them. A medicine may not be metabolised at the same speed in a child as in an adult, a child may not absorb a cream applied to the skin in the same way as an adult and an aerosol inhaler may not be dispersed in the lungs of a child as in an adult (ICH 2000). Therefore it is necessary to study these differences and to improve our knowledge of medicines used to treat children. This will enable professionals to make informed decisions when prescribing drugs for children.

Unlicensed and 'off-label' medicines and therapies

Children need to be protected from use of unlicensed and 'off-label' medicines and therapies:

- Unlicensed medicine: has no product licence for use in the UK.
- 'Off-label' use of medicines: a drug has a UK licence but is being used outside the licence for a purpose or with a population for which it has not been approved, e.g. dose, suitable formulation, route of administration or age group (RCPCH 1999).

Too few drugs are licensed for use with children and hence some children are denied treatment (Wilson 1996). Good practice also includes using medicines for which there is a sound theoretical basis for believing they are effective in children. Therefore, many medicines prescribed for children in the UK are prescribed outside of licensed indications, i.e. 'off-label' or unlicensed. The use of such medicines is necessary in paediatric practice when there is no suitable alternative. The RCPCH and The Neonatal and Paediatric Pharmacists Group statement (1999) clearly states that 'such uses are informed and guided by a respectable and responsible body of professional opinion'.

It can be argued that the use of unlicensed and 'off-label' drugs to treat children has resulted in children being used as research subjects but without the controlled supervision of a clinical trial or systematic commitment to learn how to use the drug (Rosato 2000). When a child becomes sick, the paediatrician or GP must decide whether to prescribe a drug, considering the risk versus benefit. If a drug is not licensed for children in the UK, a doctor prescribing it for a child needs to extrapolate from the adult dose a suitable dose for that child, which may lead to inaccuracies. However, failing to prescribe the drug 'off-label' may deny the child the most effective intervention available.

The Children's NSF (DoH 2003a) acknowledges that the use of 'off-label' and unlicensed medicine has particular implications for clinical governance and in 2003 an NSF Working Group was set up to work towards improving medication safety, particularly in babies and young children. Standard 10 of the NSF – Medicines for Children and Young People provides further and more detailed guidance (DoH 2004).

American and European perspectives

Over the past decade in the USA, research into medicines for children has been encouraged (Meaux & Bell 2001). The National Institutes for Health (NIH) maintain a policy that children (i.e. individuals under the age of 21) must be included in all human subjects research conducted or supported by the NIH, unless there are scientific and ethical reasons not to include them (NIH 1998). The European Commission (EC) has introduced a similar approach to the USA (Vasmant 2003). The European Health Council's Resolution on Paediatric Medicinal Products in December 2000 stated that children have their own varying characteristics and cannot be treated like adults, and called on the EC to make appropriate proposals to develop clinical research and development into medicines for children. While the ICH Guideline for good clinical practice, first operational in 1997, provides crucial, basic standards for research practice (ICH 2002), ICH E11 (2000) looks specifically at children's participation in medicinal product research. Issues regarding preterm neonates through to young adults are examined with guidance to minimise risk. With the potential for accidental or deliberate harm so great, the international community has created these guidelines for professionals who involve children and young people as research volunteers. This guidance has led to new European Union Regulation: EC No 1901/2006. Known as the Paediatric Regulation, it came into force in September 2007 with the objective to better protect children while improving their health through development of high-quality medicines (EMEA 2008).

Activity

Access the American NIH Policy and Guidelines on the Inclusion of Children as Participants in Research Involving Human Subjects:

- http://grants.nih.gov/grants/guide/notice-files/not 98-024.html

Discuss with your colleagues the importance of conducting clinical trials in medicines used with children. Is this in the best interest of the individual child or children as a population?

Developments in the UK clinical research infrastructure

While the regulatory environment was evolving, work was underway to ensure the continued excellence of clinical research undertaken in the UK. The Research for Patient Benefit Working Party led by Dr Mark Walport, Director of the Wellcome Trust, was set up to address the concerns raised by a range of interested groups including the NHS, pharmaceutical industry, research councils, charities, academia and patients. They advised on steps required to ensure the UK remained a leader in clinical research. This unique partnership resulted in the creation of the United Kingdom Clinical Research Collaboration (UKCRC):

> A partnership working to establish the UK as a world leader in clinical research, by harnessing the power of the NHS

Key activities of the UKCRC include developing:

- infrastructure in the NHS
- research workforce
- incentives for research
- coordination of research funding
- streamlined systems for regulation and governance.

Developing the research infrastructure included creation of Networks to coordinate and support research across the UK under the direction of the United Kingdom Clinical Research Network (UKCRN) (DoH 2007). Topic Specific Clinical Research Networks include:

- National Cancer Research Network (NCRN) (http://www.ncrn.org.uk/)
- Dementias and Neurodegenerative Disease Research Network (DeNDRoN) (http://www.dendron.org.uk/)
- Diabetes Research Network (DRN) (http://www.ukdrn.org/)
- Mental Health Research Network (MHRN) (http://www.ukmhrn.info/index.html)
- Primary Care Research Network (PCRN) (http://www.ukcrn.org.uk)
- Stroke Research Network (SRN) (http://www.uksrn.ac.uk/)
- Medicines for Children Research Network (MCRN) (http://www.mcrn.org.uk).

The aim of the MCRN is:

> to facilitate the conduct of randomised prospective trials and other well-designed studies of medicines for children, including those for prevention, diagnosis and treatment.

This commitment by the UK government, industry, academia and charities should address many of the long-standing concerns regarding the involvement of children in research. In particular it is hoped to improve the care of children and their families, improve the coordination, speed and integration of research, while maintaining and enhancing the quality of research and widening participation of children (MCRN 2007).

How research provides a foundation for evidence-based practice

Children's nurses strive for excellence in planning the care of individual children and their families. The UK government's framework of clinical governance makes clinical nurses, doctors and managers accountable for the care they deliver. Child health nursing practice is required to develop clinical nursing protocols and interventions based on sound evidence-based research, rather than a nursing practice based on 'custom and practice', 'myths and rituals' (Glasper & Ireland 2000). The Children's NSF (DoH 2003a) expects clinical practice to follow the best available research evidence. By using evidence-based protocols and guidelines, professionals can achieve high standards of care for children and young people in all areas in which they are cared for.

Evidence-based nursing care is on the basis of partnership and multidisciplinary collaboration. Nurses are able to learn from the work and experience of nursing, medical and allied professional colleagues who undertake child health research, which can then be applied to clinical practice (Glasper & Ireland 2000). The evidence showing the effectiveness of interventions is reported, i.e. published, in research papers and is known as primary research, which is either quantitative or qualitative and directly focuses on patients. An increasing, enormous, base of primary research is available (Swage 2000). To view the broad picture, systematic reviews are used to search and filter out the good quality from the lesser quality primary research, to gather reliable evidence that is scientifically robust enough for decisions to be made on what care to provide for children and their families (Casey 2000).

To carry out a systematic review, a researcher needs to perform a literature search, i.e. collect and review primary papers on the chosen subject, then to critically appraise the research articles and summarise the evidence presented according to standard criteria (Swage 2000). Finally, by using professional judgement, the researcher can interpret and evaluate the evidence and make an informed decision about using the findings in their evidenced-based clinical practice.

Activity

From your nursing library access this well-documented example of a systematic review, which has led to a change in practice:

- Creery D, Mikrogianakis A 2003 Sudden infant death syndrome: what are the effects of intervention to reduce the risk of sudden infant death syndrome? Clinical evidence. BMJ Publishing Group, London

This is available online at:

- http://www.clinicalevidence.com

How to critique a research paper

Nurses do not have to be researchers to practise evidence-based nursing, however they do need to be able first to assess research outcomes in a critical way, and second to separate insignificant and unsound research findings from significant studies that are worthy of interest. The critiquing process is about systematically reviewing and questioning each stage of the research process (Crombie 1996).

When reading a research paper it is useful to use a formal approach using a framework of questions that deal with all the aspects of the research process; the following is adapted from Bayea & Nicoll (1997):

1. What is the research question?
2. What is the basis for the research question?
3. Why is the research question important?
4. How was the research question studied?
5. Does the study method make sense?
6. Were the correct subjects selected for the study?
7. Was the research question answered?
8. Does the answer make sense?
9. What is the implication for practice?
10. What is next?

WWW

Visit the Critical Appraisal Skill Programme (CASP) and Evidence-based Practice website for further guidance on how to critique qualitative and quantitative research papers:

- http://www.phru.nhs.uk/Pages/PHD/CASP.htm

You will need to use your judgement and experience to evaluate the appropriateness of the research study. Consider the strengths and weaknesses of the study design, methodology, data analysis and interpretation of the findings. You should indicate reasons for your judgements and the findings should be as objective as possible.

Activity

Before critiquing a research paper, read: Chapter 25 (Evaluating research reports) in Polit DF, Hungler BP (1995) Nursing research: principles and methods, 6th edn. Lippincott, Philadelphia.

- Select a topic of interest to you and find a research article, which you can critique.

How to conduct a literature review/search

- Visit your local nursing/medical library where you can access nursing and medical journals
- Conduct on line searches using MEDLINE, EMBASE, CINAHL, NICE
- Access search engines on the internet:
  - www.cochrane.org
  - www.infotrieve.com
  - www.pubmed.com.

How research studies are beginning to identify the origins of disease and contribute to its prevention in later life

Adults are grown up children and carry the legacy of their childhood with them throughout their lives (DoH 2003a). Research aiming to help prevent disease throughout life is focusing more on the search for the inborn determinants of disease. Parents and their children are being studied as both genes and the environment influence a child's development during fetal and early life. Research has shown this to have a long-term impact on an individual's health throughout life. The 'fetal origins' hypothesis proposed that alterations in fetal nutrition and endocrine status result in developmental adaptations that permanently change structure, physiology and metabolism, thereby predisposing to disease in adult life (Godfrey & Barker 2001).

Activity

Visit your local nursing library, access and read: Godfrey KM, Barker DJP 2001 Fetal programming and adult health. Public Health and Nutrition 4(2B):611–624.

- Discuss this article with your colleagues.

In fetal life, the tissues and organs of the body go through critical periods of development. Humans are 'plastic' in their early life and are moulded by the environment. The growth of a fetus is influenced by its genes; this can be influenced by the environment, in particular the nutrients and oxygen received by the mother. 'Programming' describes the process that occurs during pregnancy whereby a stimulus or insult during a critical period of development has lasting or lifelong effects (Godfrey & Barker 2001). Research suggests that alterations in maternal nutrition can have long-term effects on the offspring in later life. It has been shown that coronary heart disease, hypertension and type 2 diabetes originate in impaired intrauterine growth and development (Godfrey & Barker 2000).

Paediatric research groups in various countries throughout the world are searching for reasons and answers to the increased prevalence of allergic disorders, such as eczema, asthma, hay fever and food allergy. Studies have been following children from the fetal period or from birth onwards. It has been found that allergic disease results from an extremely complex interaction of genetic traits and environmental influences (programming), such as the exposure to allergens, infections and variations in nutrient intake (Warner et al 2000a, b). A more comprehensive understanding of these events is required before researchers are able to prevent the onset of such diseases. Until such time, they require the help of children and their parents with research studies. Research into allergy and coronary heart disease are two examples of how research with children can show genetic and early environmental factors that influence the development of both paediatric and adult disease.

What about children and young people as researchers?

With support, children and young people are able to organise and conduct research studies. Engaging with children and young people directly results in services better able to meet their needs (DoH 2003a). The DoH document 'Strengthening accountability, involving patients and the public' (DoH 2003b) states that 'the single most important piece of advice is to talk to the target group about the best way to consult and involve them'. However, children and young people are included in Section 9 of this document, 'Involving specific groups that the NHS has traditionally found hard to reach' and states that additional support may be required for such groups (DoH 2003b).

Attitudes that continue to marginalise children highlight the need for those who work with this 'hard to reach' group to make the investment of time and resources, to engage them so they are given a voice. It is this marginalisation of children that increases the need for their involvement. From a very early age children are able to express their views and they must be listened to (DoH 2001c). This is mandated by Article 13 of The United Convention on the Rights of the Child (UN General Assembly 1989): 'the child shall have the right to freedom of expression; this right shall include freedom to seek, receive and impart information and ideas of all kinds'.

As is detailed elsewhere in this chapter, research can result in life-changing, life-prolonging results for the individual and others, and research will be more relevant if young people are involved in identifying the topics studied. Reaching the target group, in this case children and young people, can prove difficult for adults; young researchers are better able to access their peers. Youngsters often create a less formal, relaxed environment conducive to open and honest dialogue. In addition, their involvement can have an impact on professionals by exposure to young people's lives and concerns while providing valuable personal development for the young researchers (Kirby 1999).

WWW

Visit the following website to see how The Children's Trust is involved in head injury and disability research:

- http://www.thechildrenstrust.org.uk

How can young patients and volunteers be involved?

Guidance for involving the public as active partners in research is given in the Research Governance Framework (DoH 2005). It states that participants should be involved in the design, conduct, analysis and reporting of research.

The NSF for Children (DoH 2003a) states that children and young people should be 'involved in the planning and improvement of services'. Methods for involvement might include:

- compliment and complaint boxes
- surveys and questionnaires

- consultation exercises: large or small groups
- creative consultations using drama, music, games
- facilitate young people to provide a service: take part in staff development and recruitment, provide mentor advice
- establish advisory groups (DoH 2001b).

Patient and volunteer involvement can encompass a variety of methods. Within Hospital Trusts, corporate and directorate leads work to meet national and local clinical governance key performance standards (KPS). The new confusingly named patient and public involvement forums (PPIFs) are statutory, independent bodies, different from the existing groups, also known as patient and public involvement (PPI) or user's groups, set up to meet clinical governance KPS (DoH 2003c). One important KPS requires active PPI groups in each directorate, including child health and other areas that treat children such as outpatients and emergency departments. Members of PPI groups are patients or carers who meet and address areas of concern they have, giving a voice to patients and volunteers, including children (DoH 2003b). Activities should be group led, but might include a review of patient information leaflets using a DoH toolkit. This allows direct input into the design and content of patient information and helps to ensure they are clear, attractive and understood by the people who use them, with children reviewing child-oriented information (DoH 2003d).

WWW

Search for the complete DoH toolkit at:

- http://www.dh.gov.uk

Activity

Go to Chapter 37 for more on patient information leaflets:

- Read information leaflets on your ward placements.
- Are there separate ones for children and teenagers?

Models of involvement

INVOLVE (formerly Consumers in NHS Research) is an organisation that promotes NHS, public health and social care research. It has clearly identified three levels of public participation in the research process:

- The first level has been defined as **consultation**: information is given to the public by a group of healthcare providers or researchers.
- The next step is **collaboration**: there is a partnership between the two groups and a sharing of ideas.
- The highest level of participation would be **user control**: when the public takes charge and manages the research study (Hanley et al 2000).

WWW

Visit the following website to see how a small group of children and parents have set up and run a foundation to fund research into familial dysautonomia, a rare (less than 600 patients worldwide) genetic disease. Their participation has led to improved treatments and discovery of the gene:

- http://www.familialdysautonomia.org

Another model is the public involvement continuum, which ranges from minimum to maximum involvement and is described in DoH 2003b. This document offers advice and practical ideas to put PPI into practice. It gives the following categories with many examples of activities:

- Giving information: exhibitions, leaflets, the press
- Getting information: public panels, radio phone-ins, questionnaires, interviews
- Forums for debate: focus groups, patient/carer groups, seminars
- Participation: expert patients, health panels, shadowing, story telling
- Partnership: community development, large group processes.

All the above methods can be used with children. Specific advice includes:

- Develop links with schools and youth groups.
- Ensure information is in appropriate language, style and format.
- Speak directly with and involve children and young people – not just their parents.
- Consider using video, interactive material and the internet (DoH 2003b).

Facilitating involvement of young researchers

Participation early in the research process is recommended, ideally at the first step of deciding what topic should be researched, as greater influence can be achieved with early involvement (Joseph Rowntree Foundation 2000). Ideally, topics for research would be determined by children and young people, and not imposed by medical or scientific researchers (Kirby 1999). This requires support for the young people, who probably will not have experience of research or engaging with others in this way. As with older 'non-professional' researchers, training in research methods such as interviewing skills, questionnaire completion and data recording, will be necessary, as will clear guidelines for confidentiality and data protection issues (Kirby 1999). Young people as researchers – a learning resource pack (Worrall 2000) – includes exercises and handouts for use with novice researchers. Its aim is to 'provide materials for workers training young people in participatory research' and gives practical advice for engaging young researchers in projects.

INVOLVE also provides in depth briefing notes for researchers through the NHS Research Support Unit (Hanley et al 2000).

These notes illustrate various aspects of involvement and practical guidelines that can be utilised. By breaking down the research process into stages it is possible to see how each step leads to the next. With support, young researchers can participate at any stage.

WWW

Visit the INVOLVE website for more information on involving your patients as active partners in research, and the full text of their briefing notes for researchers:

- http://www.invo.org.uk

Activity

- How might you involve youngsters in hospital?
- How could you determine which topics are important to them?
- What techniques might work best with children who can't read?

Difficulties involving children and young people as researchers

Young researchers can experience many of the same difficulties that adult or professionals encounter. These youngsters have reported a shift in perception during interviews from being a peer to authoritative figure, with the subjects becoming defensive. Young researchers might also be reluctant to probe for details. In addition, recruiting volunteers through a peer group might be successful but will not yield a suitably diverse group. It might be difficult for some young people to approach others whom they do not know. They can also face problems accessing youngsters through recruitment routes such as schools (Kirby 1999).

Young people researching adults rather than peers will face other issues. Young researchers might intimidate some adults, or adults might use jargon or words the youngster does not understand, which could lead to intimidation of the young person. Young people will require support, especially if interviews reveal sensitive or upsetting information. Child protection issues must be considered so that young researchers and subjects are safe. Working in pairs, interviewing in public areas such as schools or cafes, providing mobile phones, ID cards, and submitting daily plans of activity are possible strategies to safeguard involved children (Kirby 1999).

Scenario

David and Jonathan are 15 years old and have volunteered for training as young researchers on a study being set up at a local youth group. They will be interviewing children and their parents about the ways they travel to and from school.

What kind of training and support might they need? What are some of the problems they might encounter in the community?

How is the government supporting public involvement in healthcare and research?

A framework for quality improvement was outlined in 'A first class service: quality in the new NHS' (DoH 1998). This included the development of national service frameworks underpinned by clinical governance frameworks that assure the quality of clinical services. Hospital Trust directorates are mandated to meet the agendas of clinical governance frameworks in seven key areas. The patient and public involvement (PPI) section ensures patient and public participation at all levels of healthcare delivery. At the same time, the independent Commission for Health Improvement (CHI, which has since become the Commission for Health Audit and Inspection (CHAI)) was developed to monitor quality and progress and initiate a continuing programme of national patient surveys, addressing various issues that impact on patient care and satisfaction (DoH 1998).

This commitment to provide a patient-centred healthcare service was reaffirmed in the NHS Plan (DoH 2000). The Commission for Patient and Public Involvement in Health (CPPIH) was founded in January 2003 to fund, establish and manage Patient and Public Forums (PPIFs) in every trust and PCT. These forums are a resource for the public, promoting their involvement and monitor Patient Advice and Liaison Service (PALS). PALS provide information about health services and about independent complaints advocacy services (ICAS). PPIFs will have legal powers to inspect, report and make recommendations based on patient views and experiences, with the aim to have a PPIF member on every NHS Trust Board (DoH 2003c). INVOLVE promotes public involvement in the NHS, public health and social care research, and recommends the principle of public representatives in NHS research and development programmes (DoH 2005). A commitment to public involvement is now firmly in practice and extends to healthy research volunteers, including child volunteers and their families.

How involved are children and young people?

In the 'Learning to listen' action plan published by the Children's and Young People's Unit (DoH 2001b), the DoH set out the following core principles regarding the participation of youngsters:

- A visible commitment to involving children and young people
- That their involvement be valued
- Equal opportunity to get involved
- That standards for participation are provided, evaluated and improved.

Therefore, the onus is on the health professionals to ensure that these principles are met. The subsequent report (DoH 2003e) describes many examples of good involvement by children and young people. It mentions the CPPIH and its role to ensure 'children's and young people's views are represented on patient forums' and also states that children should be supported as forum members, with the use of child-friendly information.

In addition, it gives details of the 'Building a culture of participation' research project to illustrate the benefits of involvement. This project aimed to give an indication of participation, provide information and advice on involvement, and report on the creation of a 'participatory culture'. This research project found:

- There is no single way to involve children, but depends on many factors.
- Listening must lead to change to ensure all the current activity actually makes a difference.
- There are real benefits from listening and acting on children's views, including improved service development as well as support for children and personal development.
- However, too little attention is given to studying outcomes of participation and support is needed at all levels of management to create participatory organisations.

The report concludes that challenges remain and more resources are needed. Monitoring methods, sharing information and widening involvement into more government work will help to develop necessary standards that can be applied to a range of organisations. Providing a forum for expression and participation will help children and young people play an active part in society (DoH 2003e).

Seminar discussion topic

Select an area of clinical practice from your current clinical placement. Conduct a full review of the research literature. Is there a strong enough evidence base to warrant its continued application?

Summary

The unique and specific qualities of children make child-oriented research an absolute necessity. Child-friendly methodologies allow youngsters to freely give their assent for participation as research volunteers. With proper training and support it is also possible to actively involve them as researchers. Regardless of how, or why, they are involved, the interests of each individual child are paramount. It is essential that professionals involving children in healthcare research follow the broad principles of good clinical practice with the highest scientific and ethical standards. Children's nurses are the guardians of good research practice.

Acknowledgements

The authors would like to thank the Wellcome Trust Clinical Research Facility (WTCRF) at Southampton University Hospitals Trust for permission for use of printed materials and photographs for the PowerPoint presentation, and colleagues there for their support. They would also like to acknowledge the initial contribution of Julie Mitton, former Education and Development Coordinator at the WTCRF.

References

Age of Legal Capacity (Scotland) Act, 1991. HMSO, London.

Alderson, P., 1995. Listening to children. Barnardo's, Ilford, 21, 23, 55, 56.

Alderson, P., Montgomery, J., 1996. Health care choices: making decisions with children. Institute for Public Policy and Research, London pp 6, 10–12, 18.

Avery, N.J., King, R.M., Knight, S., Hourihane, JO'B, 2003. Assessment of quality of life in children with peanut allergy. Pediatric Allergy and Immunology 14, 378–382.

Backett-Milburn, K., McKie, L., 1999. A critical appraisal of the draw and write technique. Health Education Research 14 (3), 387–398.

Balen, R., Holroyd, C., Mountain, G., Wood, B., 2001. Giving children a voice: methodological and practical implications of research involving children. Paediatric Nursing 12, 10.

Barker, J., Weller, S., 2003. 'Is it fun?' Developing children centred research methods. International Journal of Sociology and Social Policy 23, 1–2.

Bayea, S.C., Nicoll, L.H., 1997. Ten questions that will get you through any research report. AORN Online 65 (5), 978–979.

Behrman, R., Kleigman, R. (Eds.), 1998, Nelson's essentials of paediatrics. 3rd edn. WB Saunders, Philadelphia pp 4-9, 192, 213 482, 483.

Bradding, A., Horstman, M., 1999. Using the write and draw technique with children. European Journal of Oncology Nursing 3 (3), 170–175.

Broome, M.E., Richards, D.J., 2003. The influence of relationships on children's and adolescent's participation in research. Nursing Research 52 (3), 191–197.

Brown, M.S., Haylor, M., 1989. Nursing research with preoperational age children: the use of standardized tests. Journal of Paediatric Nursing 4, 1.

Bullinger, M., Schmidt, S., Petersen, C. Disabkids Group, 2002. Assessing quality of life of children with chronic health conditions and disabilities: a European approach. International Journal of Rehabilitation Research 25, 197–205.

Burns, J., 2003. Research in children. Critical Care Medicine 31 (suppl 3), S131–S136.

Camilleri-Brennan, J., Steele, R.J.C., 1999. Measurement of quality of life in surgery. Journal of the Royal College of Surgeons Edinburgh 44, 252–259.

Casey, A., 2000. The role of professional journals in promoting evidence-based care. In: Glasper, E.A., Ireland, L. (Eds.), Evidence-based child health care challenges for practice. Palgrave, Basingstoke.

Creery, D., Mikrogianakis, A., 2003. Sudden infant death syndrome: what are the effects of intervention to reduce the risk of sudden infant death syndrome? Clinical evidence. BMJ Publishing Group, London.

Crombie, I.K., 1996. The pocket guide to critical appraisal. BMJ Publishing Group, London.

Curtin, C., 2000. Eliciting children's voices in qualitative research. The American Journal of Occupational Therapy 55, 3.

Department of Health (DoH), 1989. The Children Act. HMSO, London.

Department of Health (DoH), 1998. A first class service: quality in the new NHS. HMSO, London.

Department of Health (DoH), 2000. NHS plan. HMSO, London.

Department of Health (DoH), 2001a. Seeking consent: working with children. HMSO, London.

Department of Health (DoH), 2001b. Learning to listen – core principles for the involvement of children and young people. HMSO, London.

Department of Health (DoH), 2003a. Getting the right start: National Service Framework for Children Standard for Hospital Services. HMSO, London.

Department of Health (DoH), 2003b. Strengthening accountability, involving patients and the public: practice guidance of the Health and Social Care Act. HMSO, London.

Department of Health (DoH), 2003c. Advice note, patient and public forums. 4 December 2003. DoH, London.

Department of Health (DoH), 2003d. Toolkit for producing patient information, ver 2. HMSO, London.

Department of Health (DoH), 2003e. The learning to listen report. HMSO, London.

Department of Health (DoH), 2004. National Service Framework for Children, Young People and Maternity Services: medicines for children and young people. HMSO, London.

Department of Health (DoH), 2005. Research governance framework for health and social care, 2nd edn. HMSO, London.

Department of Health (DoH), 2007. Research for Patient Benefit Working Party – final report. HMSO, London.

Dockerell, J., 2000. Researching children's perspectives: a psychological dimension. In: Lewis, A., Lindsay, G. (Eds.), Researching children's perspectives. Open University Press, Buckingham.

Edwards, A., Talbot, R., 1994. The hard-pressed researcher. A research handbook for the caring professions. Longman, London.

European Medicines Agency (EMEA), 2008. Better medicines for children. EMEA, London.

Fleitas, J., 1998. Spinning tales from the world wide web: qualitative research in an electronic environment. Qualitative Health Research 8 (2), 283–292.

Forman, E.N., Ladd, R.E., 1995. Ethical dilemmas in pediatrics, a case study approach. University Press of America, London.

Hanley, B., Bradburn, J., Gorin, S., et al., 2000. Involving consumers in research and development in the NHS: briefing notes for researchers. Consumers in NHS Research Support Unit, Eastleigh.

Higginson, J., Carr, A.J., 2001. Measuring quality of life: using quality of life measures in the clinical setting. British Medical Journal 322 (7297), 1297–1300.

Hinds, D., 2000. Research instruments. In: Wilkinson, D. (Ed.), The researcher's toolkit. The complete guide to practitioner research. Routledge Farmer, London.

Gibbs, A., 1997. Focus groups. Social research update. Online. Available at: http://www.soc.surrey.ac.uk/sru/SRU19html

Glasper, E.A., Ireland, L., 2000. Evidence-based child health care. Palgrave, Basingstoke.

Godfrey, K.M., Barker, D.J.P., 2000. Fetal nutrition and adult disease. American Journal of Clinical Nutrition 71 (5 Suppl), 1344S–1352S.

Godfrey, K.M., Barker, D.J.P., 2001. Fetal programming and adult health. Public Health and Nutrition 4 (2B), 611–624.

International Conference on Harmonisation (ICH), 2000. Topic E11 Clinical investigation of medicinal products in the paediatric population. EMEA, London.

International Conference on Harmonisation (ICH), 2002. Guideline for good clinical practice. EMEA, London.

Joseph Rowntree Foundation, 2000. Involving young people in research projects. Joseph Rowntree Foundation, York.

Kennedy, C., Charlesworth, A., Chen, J., 2003. Interactive data collection benefits of integrating new media into pediatric research. Computers, Informatics. Nursing 21 (3), 120–127.

Kirby, P., 1999. Involving young researchers. Joseph Rowntree Foundation, York pp 14, 16–19, 21, 26, 39, 64, 125.

Lamprill, J., 2002. Asking for children's assent to take part in clinical research. Good Clinical Practice Journal 9 (8), 9–12.

Lamprill, J., 2003. Prioritise and plan for children's needs. Good Clinical Practice Journal 10 (8), 17–19.

MacGregor, J., 2001. Introduction to the anatomy and physiology of children. Routledge, London pp 21, 30, 42, 113.

Meaux, J.B., Bell, P.L., 2001. Balancing recruitment and protection: children as research subjects. Comprehensive Pediatric Nursing 24, 241–251.

Medicines for Children Research Network (MCRN), 2007. Medicines for children research network. MCRN Coordinating Centre, Liverpool.

Montgomery, J., 2001. Informed consent and clinical research with children. In: Doyal, L., Tobias, S. (Eds.), Informed consent in medical research. BMJ Publishing Group, London. p178.

Morland, B., 2003. Why children with cancer benefit from phase 1 studies. Good Clinical Practice Journal 10 (8), 11–14.

Morrow, V., 2001. Using qualitative methods to elicit young people's perspectives on their environments: some ideas for community health initiatives. Health Education Research 16 (3), 255–268.

National Institutes of Health (NIH) 1998 Policy and guidelines on the inclusion of children as participants in research involving human subjects. Online. Available at: http://grants.nih.gov/grants/guide/notice-files/not98-024.html

The Nursing and Midwifery Council (NMC), 2002. Code of professional conduct. NMC, London.

The Nursing and Midwifery Council (NMC), 2008a. The Code: standards for conduct, performance and ethics for nurses and midwives. NMC, London.

The Nursing and Midwifery Council (NMC), 2008b. Advice for nurses working with children and young people. NMC, London.

Oppenheim, A.N., 2002. Questionnaire design, interviewing and attitude measurement. Continuum International Publishing Group, London.

Polit, D.F., Hungler, B.P., 1995. Nursing research: principles and methods, 6th edn. Lippincott, Philadelphia.

Pridmore, P.J., Lansdown, R.G., 1997. Exploring children's perceptions of health: does drawing really break down barriers? Health Education Journal 56, 219–230.

Robinson, S., 2001. Informed consent in children. Good Clinical Practice Journal 8 (8), 5–6.

Robinson, S., 2002. Child-friendly concerns. Good Clinical Practice Journal 9 (8), 15.

Rosato, J., 2000. The ethics of clinical trials: a child's view. The Journal of Law, Medicine and Ethics 28 (4), 362–378.

Rothmier, J.D., Lasley, M.V., Shapiro, G.C., 2003. Factors influencing parental consent in pediatric clinical research. Pediatrics 111 (5), 1037–1041.

Royal College of Paediatrics and Child Health (RCPCH), 2000. Advocating for children. RCPCH, London.

Royal College of Paediatrics and Child Health (RCPCH) and The Neonatal and Paediatric Pharmacists Group, 1999. The use of unlicensed medicines or licensed medicines for unlicensed application in paediatric practice. Policy statement. RCPCH, London.

Scanlon, M., 2003. Issues in research. In: Wilkinson, D. (Ed.), The researcher's toolkit the complete guide to practitioner research. Routledge Farmer, London.

Sorensen, E.S., 1989. Using children's diaries as a research instrument. Journal of Pediatric Nursing 4, 6.

Swage, T., 2000. Clinical governance in health care practice. Butterworth Heinemann, Oxford.

United Nations General Assembly, 1989. Convention on the rights of the child. UNICEF, Geneva.

Vasmant, D., 2003. Europe grows impatient over delays in paediatric initiatives (guest editorial). Good Clinical Practice Journal, August:1–3.

Vincent, K.A., Higginson, I.J., 2003. Assessing quality of life in children. In: Carr, A.J., Higginson, J., Robinson, S. (Eds.), Quality of life. BMJ Publishing, London.

Warner, J.A., Jones, C.A., Jones, A.C., Warner, J.O., 2000a. Prenatal origins of allergic disease. Journal of Allergy and Clinical Immunology 105 (2), 493–496.

Warner, J.O., Jones, C.A., Kilburn, A.S., Vance, G.H.S., 2000b. Prenatal sensitization in humans. Pediatric Allergy and Immunology Suppl 13, 6–8.

Williamson, H., Butler, I., 1995. Children speak: perspectives on their social worlds. In: Brannon, J., O'Brien, M. (Eds.), Children and parenthood. Proceedings of the International Sociological Association Committee for Family Research Practice, 1994, London. Institute of Education, University of London, London, pp. 294–330.

Wilson, J.T., 1996. Strategies for pediatric drug evaluation: a view from the trenches. Drug Information Journal 30, 1149–1162.

Wong, D.L., Baker, C.M., 1988. Pain in children: comparison of assessment scales. Pediatric Nursing 14, 9–17.

World Health Organisation Quality of life Group, 1996. What quality of life? World Health Organisation Quality of life assessment. World Health Forum 17:354–6.

World Medical Association (WMA), 2000. 52nd General Assembly: Declaration of Helsinki. WMA, Edinburgh.

Worrall, S., 2000. Young people as researchers, a learning resource pack. Joseph Rowntree Foundation and Save the Children, London pp 2–7.

Ensuring quality and the role of clinical audit

16

Janice Watson Cathryn Battrick

ABSTRACT

The aim of this chapter and the companion PowerPoint presentation is to introduce key quality issues that arise during the provision of services and care to children and their families. Current government initiatives and key policy documents are identified and their impact on the provision of quality services explored. In particular, the central importance of clinical audit is discussed and the key stages of the audit cycle described.

LEARNING OUTCOMES

- Discuss clinical governance, with reference to the key elements, activities and processes associated with the clinical governance framework.
- Consider what quality means in a health care context.
- Explore recent government policy on quality in the NHS.
- Review key quality tools and their use in providing quality services.
- Demonstrate a sound understanding of the audit process and its importance to the quality agenda.
- Examine the role of key agencies in assuring quality improvements in health care.

Introduction

In 1983, the World Health Organization (WHO) stated that by 1990 all member states should have built effective mechanisms for ensuring the quality of patient care within their health care system, thus clearly identifying the global, central importance of quality in health care.

Arguably, quality in health care was first recognised by Florence Nightingale, who was a pioneer of systematic observation, standard setting and improvement of care and who clearly advocated the importance of quality in health care as early as the 19th century. During the Crimean War, Nightingale realised that admission to a battle hospital actually increased a soldier's chances of death, so she set standards against which she measured practice. This process led to a drastic reduction in the rates of hospital-acquired infection and dramatically cut the mortality rate. Furthermore, Nightingale (1863) reiterated the need to collect data and measure outcomes in health care:

> In attempting to arrive at the truth, I have applied everywhere for information, but in scarcely an instance have I been able to obtain hospital records fit for any purpose of comparison … They would show subscribers how their money was being spent, what amount of good was really being done with it or whether the money was doing mischief rather than good.

In 1959, the publication of the Platt Report, entitled 'Welfare of Children in Hospital Report' (Ministry of Health 1959), was an early attempt to raise standards in the care of sick children in hospital, although the aspirations of this report went largely unfulfilled. For several decades the wise words of Nightingale and the key features of the Platt Report went relatively unheeded, although voluntary organisations maintained an impetus for the need to improve quality of care. In particular, the work of Action for Sick Children, previously known as the National Association for the Welfare of Children in Hospital (NAWCH) made important contributions to the quality of care afforded children in hospital and introduced a 'Charter for Children in Hospital' in 1984. This charter encouraged nurse managers to monitor standards of care in children's departments.

In general, the nursing profession had an interest in quality care, which grew with the development of the Royal College of Nursing and the RCN Standards of Care Project (Parsley & Corrigan 1999). From this work, nursing embraced the dynamic standards-setting system based on the Donabedian (1966) structure–process–outcome framework, but three main factors have resulted in an upsurge of interest in quality in recent years:

- Public expectations
- The sheer complexity of health care organisations and interventions

DOI: 10.1016/B978-0-7020-3183-0.10016-5

- Recognition of the opportunities for improvement through good practice, but also following the rising rate of litigation and high-profile cases of major failures in the NHS, such as the Bristol Royal Infirmary heart surgery tragedy.

In response to these factors, the UK government introduced a significant set of reforms in the NHS, which shifted the focus towards quality of care and formed one of the main principles underpinning the incoming Labour government's agenda for the NHS. In the White Paper 'The New NHS: Modern Dependable' (Department of Health (DoH) 1997), the government declared that the new NHS would have quality at its heart; quality was to be the driving force for decision making at every level of the service and the agenda for quality was set in the White Paper 'A First Class Service' (DoH 1998). This paper identified three main components for ensuring high-quality care:

- The setting of clear standards and the introduction of the National Institute for Clinical Excellence (NICE) and the National Service Frameworks (NSFs).
- Delivering these standards at local level: clinical governance.
- Monitoring of standards: to be done by the Care Quality Commission: previously the Commission for Audit and Inspection (CHAI; previously the Commission for Health Improvement (CHI)), the NHS Performance Assessment Framework and the National Patient and User Surveys (Brocklehurst & Walshe 1999).

Figure 16.1 shows the relationship between these components; clinical governance being pivotal to this model.

Defining quality in health care has been fraught with difficulties, with many examples of attempts to describe in detail what good quality is in any service. The work of Donabedian (1966) highlights the inherent dangers in this, stating that the criteria of quality are nothing more than value judgements. Basically, quality can be almost anything to anyone, based on their own values, beliefs and goals within both health care and society in general.

Quality as a concept is important in so far as we want to be able to measure it to improve it, and the identification of components of quality are one way in which this has been attempted. One such example is Maxwell's six dimensions of quality (1984), which are:

- access to service
- relevance to need
- effectiveness
- equity
- social acceptability
- efficiency and economy.

Importantly, the information gained from such performance measures is only meaningful if it is used to bring about improvement. It is therefore more useful to consider quality as a cycle of improvement (Fig. 16.2).

PROFESSIONAL CONVERSATION

Student nurse Kelly Jones has read in her local paper that her local hospital has been awarded only two stars. She asks her assessor how these ratings are awarded.

Maxwell's (1984) six dimensions of quality are reflected in the NHS Performance Assessment Framework, a set of performance indicators, or measures, that allow the performance of health authorities and NHS Trusts to be compared; some have been published in the form of league tables (Swage 2000). Individual trusts are assessed against these indicators and, depending on their score, a star rating is awarded, with five stars being the highest any Trust can achieve. These dimensions are:

- Health improvement and reducing health inequalities.
- Fair access irrespective of geography, socioeconomic group, ethnicity, age or gender.
- Effective delivery of appropriate health care that complies with agreed standards.
- Efficiency and the achievement of value for money.
- Patient/carer experience by assessing the way in which patients/carers view the quality of care they receive to ensure the NHS is sensitive to individual needs.
- Health outcomes of NHS care to assess the direct contribution of NHS care to improvement in overall health closing the loop back to the goal of health improvement (Pickering & Thompson 2003, Scally & Donaldson 1998, Swage 2000).

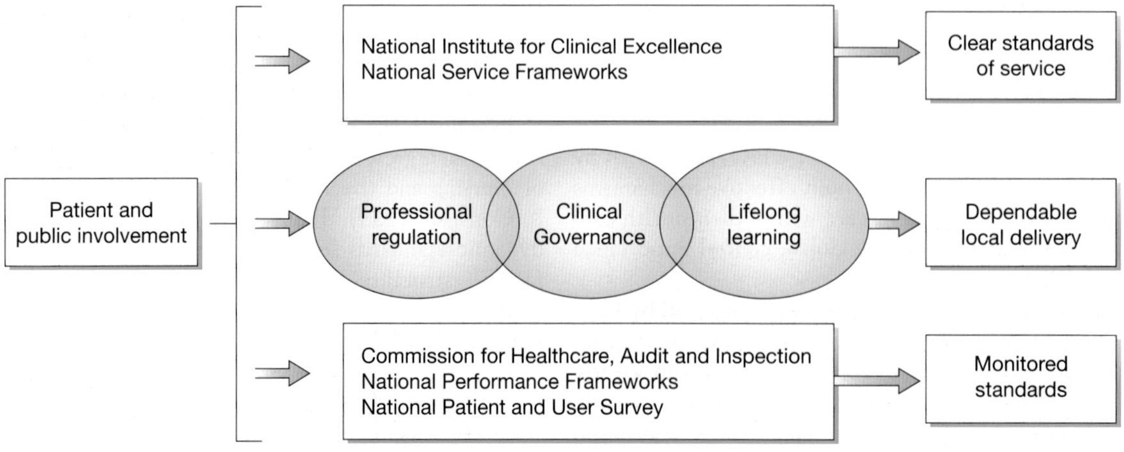

Fig. 16.1 • The NHS quality framework.

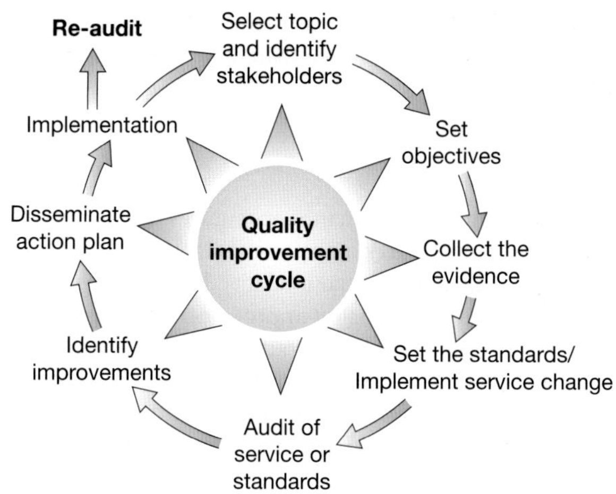
Re-audit
Select topic and identify stakeholders
Set objectives
Collect the evidence
Set the standards/ Implement service change
Audit of service or standards
Identify improvements
Disseminate action plan
Implementation
Quality improvement cycle

Fig. 16.2 • The quality improvement cycle.

Activity

The value of hospital league tables has been hotly debated in the media. Go to:

- http://www.chi.nhs.uk/ratings

and choose the England ratings and Acute Trust indicators in the left hand menu. In particular, review the ratings for Great Ormond Street Children's Hospital and Birmingham Children's Hospital:

- What were their star ratings and do you think these are a fair way to represent the performance of any Trust?
- Do you feel the indicators give a snapshot of the true activity of the hospital and the quality of the services they provide?
- Do you feel these ratings help families make an informed choice about the quality of care they can expect to receive from any given Trust?

Quality is therefore represented as being a continuous process, which is an organisation-wide endeavour. Two such organisational approaches, which have been adopted within the NHS, are total quality management (TQM) and continuous quality improvement (CQI). CQI aims at embedding continuous quality improvement at all levels and across all services with the goal of achieving changes in practice that improve patient outcomes. Within the NHS, TQM and CQI are often used synonymously and interchangeably.

Total quality management

TQM is a business philosophy that was first introduced by Deming and Juran in the USA. It is a method of managing quality issues throughout every aspect of an organisation. Deming (one of the proponents of TQM) advocated a systematic approach to problem solving and promoted the PDCA cycle: Plan, Do, Check and Act. Juran, who is considered the father of quality, established a theory of quality management which evolved during the 1940s, 1950s and 1960s (Parsley & Corrigan 1999) and involves everyone and everything that happens in an organisation. Quality is therefore a continuous process expanding across departments and professional boundaries; it is:

> ... an integrated, corporately led programme of organisational change designed to engender and sustain a culture of continuous improvement based on customer orientated definitions of quality
>
> (Joss & Kogan 1995 p 13)

Key TQM processes

- Focus on the needs and expectations of the market and consumers (i.e. health care and its patients).
- Achieve top quality performance in all areas of activity.
- Install whatever operating procedures – simple or complex – are necessary to achieve top quality performance.
- Critically and continuously examine the processes to reduce and remove non-productive activities, inefficiencies and waste.
- Develop and monitor measures of performance, set standards against which this performance is measured and identify required improvements.
- Understand the need for, and develop, an effective communication strategy.
- Develop a non-hierarchical team approach to problem solving and delegate responsibility for change.
- Develop good procedures for communication and feedback to staff at any level of good work.
- Continuously review the above processes to develop a culture for never-ending improvement.

The aim is to 'get it right first time every time'.

PROFESSIONAL CONVERSATION

Student nurse Jones has been reading an article in a nursing magazine, which has referred to TQM. She asks her assessor how TQM works in the NHS.

Clinical governance is an example within the NHS which reflects the TQM philosophy of managing quality issues. The key processes identified with TQM can be directly related to systems and processes associated with clinical governance. These include quality improvement activities like audit, data collection, and record keeping; clear lines of responsibility and accountability, risk management policies, procedures for identifying poor performance, and public and user involvement. So, you see, TQM is very relevant to the NMS.

Activity

Spend 20 minutes reflecting on your clinical experience and see if you can identify any quality processes that are or were evident in your day-to-day practice.

The rise of clinical governance

For health care to become more patient focused, and if quality improvements are to be made, then health care professionals need to embrace the wider aspects of care, which include:

- recognising the contribution of other colleagues from other disciplines
- organisational behaviour and change
- clinical audit
- working in teams.

A substantial shift in the culture of the NHS was required so that quality improvement became central to the work of the NHS, with an emphasis on collaboration rather than competition. To achieve this cultural shift the government determined that clinical governance would be used as a framework, with the patient–professional partnership at the pinnacle of a temple model supported by seven pillars (Scally & Donaldson 1998) (Fig. 16.3).

Each pillar represents professional and managerial processes integral to quality improvement. Clinical governance acts like an umbrella under which all aspects of quality can be gathered and monitored and the WHO's description of quality as being composed of four elements forms the basis for the development of clinical governance. These four elements are:

1. professional performance: technical quality
2. resource use: economic efficiency
3. risk management
4. patient satisfaction (Buetow & Roland 1999).

Clinical governance is defined as:

> A framework through which NHS organisations are accountable for continuously improving the quality of their services and safeguarding high standards of care by creating an environment in which clinical care will flourish
>
> (DoH 1998)

Clinical governance is to be the framework used to bring about a new culture, which places quality as central to the work of all in the NHS. It covers the organisation's systems and processes for monitoring and improving services. This culture will be manifest in the ten C's of clinical governance (Heard et al 2001):

- clinical performance
- clinical leadership
- clinical audit
- clinical risk management
- complaints
- continuing health needs assessments
- changing practice through evidence
- continuing education
- culture of excellence
- clear accountability.

Importantly, clinical governance encourages health care professionals to take control and demonstrate their ability to self-regulate and maintain public service accountability. Health care professionals are to take the lead in quality improvement strategies within a structure of increased external accountability. Clinical governance is part of a strategy for quality improvement in the context of a nationally coordinated programme of clinical guideline development with a nominated individual in each organisation responsible for clinical governance. Clinical governance is quality at a local level and focuses on processes of care, which include clinical decision making, appropriateness, clinical effectiveness and evidence-based practice (Pickering & Thompson 2003, Swage 2000). The key features of clinical governance (Scally & Donaldson 1998) are:

- clear lines of responsibility and accountability for quality
- programme of quality improvement activities
- clear risk reduction policies
- procedures for identifying and addressing poor performance
- public and user involvement.

Figure 16.4 is a mind map of the key activities associated with clinical governance.

Activity

Put yourself at the centre of a mind map like the one in Figure 16.4 and then identify how you can contribute to the clinical governance agenda. You might want to include things like:

- clinical supervision
- reflection
- education and training
- involvement in ward meetings.

In July 2004 the Department of Health issued 'Health and Social Care Standards and Planning Framework 2005/06–2007/08'. This document outlined priorities for the NHS as follows:

- Health and well-being of the whole population
- Good management of people who have long-term conditions, such as MS

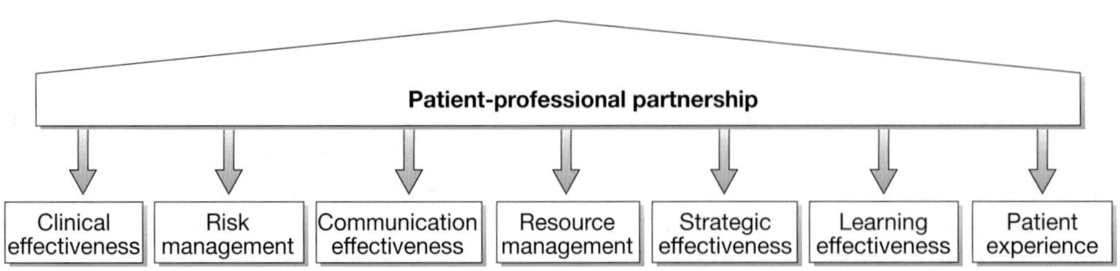

Fig. 16.3 • The temple model of clinical governance.

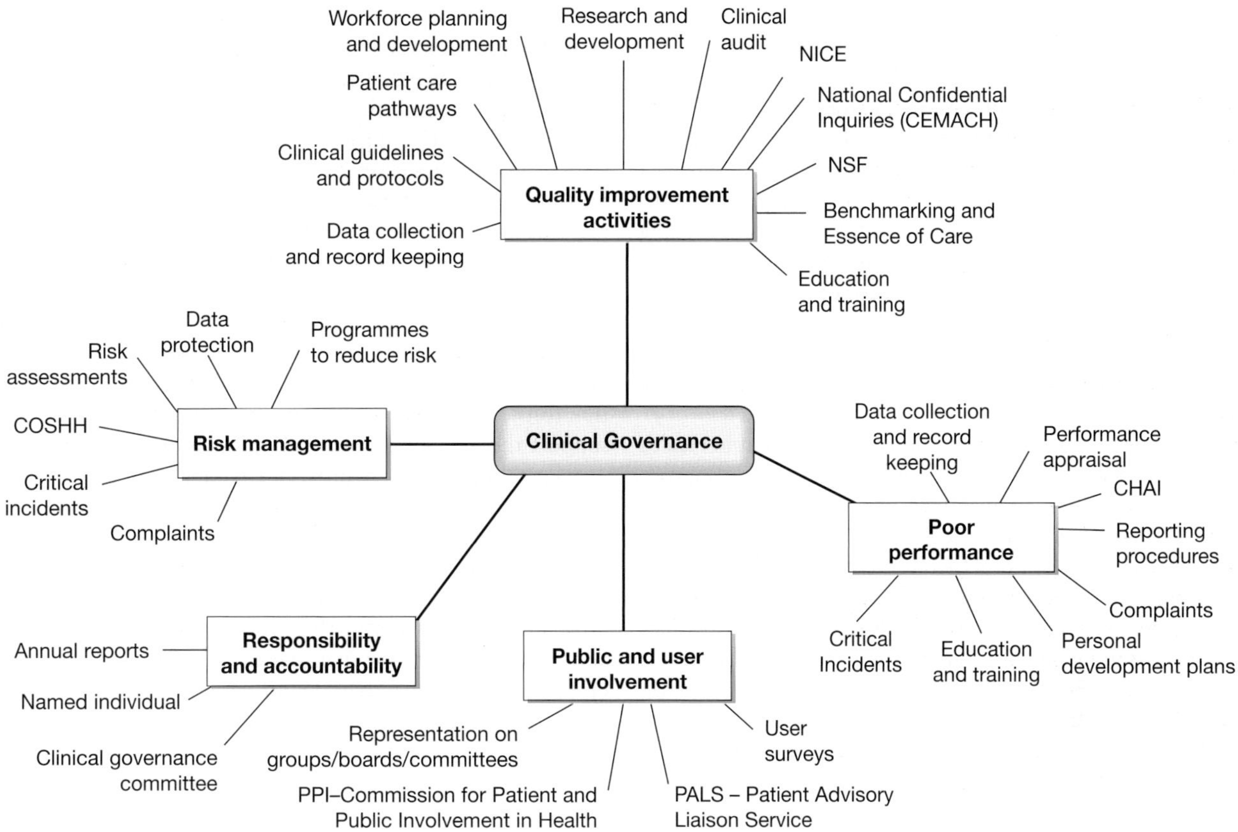

Fig. 16.4 • Mind map of the key activities associated with clinical governance.

- Improving access to services
- Putting the patient/user experience at the centre of health service care.

Two other major changes were announced in this document:

- Standards for Better Health (DoH 2004). This documented a move away from targets, such as waiting times for operations, to a number of high quality national standards which all hospitals and other health care providers will have to meet. This set out the framework for all NHS organisations and social service authorities to use in planning over the next 3 financial years
- Payment by Results. This is a scheme that provides a national tariff of fees that hospitals may charge for specific interventions, so there is a standard set price for e.g. consultation with a neurologist. In theory, therefore, patients may have more choice about where to access treatment as the money travels with the patient, rather than doctors setting up a contract with a specific hospital.

High Quality Care for All – the Lord Darzi final review

Lord Darzi's final review, 'High Quality Care for All', was published in June 2008. It was highly relevant to planners and commissioners across health and social economies and those providers forging closer partnerships so as to deliver care closer to home. The review concludes a series of reports, consultations and recommendations for a 10-year vision for a world class NHS that is fair, personal, effective and safe. It was based on extensive consultation with 60,000 staff, patients and stakeholder groups (including 2000 clinicians).

An overarching outcome from the review was the focus on bringing about change at the local level, based on sound evidence and in partnership with patients and staff. The vision is that there is 'an NHS that gives patients and the public more information and choice, works in partnership and has quality of care at its heart. Quality is defined as 'clinically effective, personal and safe'. The first major priority identified is to tackle the 'significant variations' in the quality of care provided across the country. However, it is acknowledged within the review that local flexibility to respond to specific contexts was important, with statements such as: 'The NHS should be universal, but that does not mean that it should be uniform.'

User involvement

The involvement of service users is an important tenet to the implementation of clinical governance. This presents a challenge to those who are involved in the provision of health care services to children. Although children can be reliable informants who are able to accurately reflect their own lived experiences of being a patient in hospital, it is often assumed that they are not competent to offer a legitimate viewpoint on their experience of health care services (Glasper 2004, Woodfield 2001).

Since the publication of the Bristol Inquiry and the Children's National Service Framework, government recommendations have been quite strident in their call for greater patient and public involvement. The Commission for Patient and Public Involvement in Health (PPI) is tasked with giving the public a voice in decisions that affect their health and is operationalised through the Patient Advisory Liaison Service (PALS) at individual Trust level. Importantly, an innovative audit tool is being developed for CHAI to access Trusts against the Children's NSF based on a model already in use by Essence of care (NHS Modernisation Agency 2003), which will allow individual organisations to benchmark themselves against the NSF standards. It is hoped that this will help to raise the voice of children and truly involve them in their own health care services.

The Commission for Patient and Public Involvement in Health (CPPIH) was established in January 2003 to set up and support Patients' Forums. This independent, non-departmental public body (NDPB) was abolished on the 31 March 2008 when Patients' Forums were replaced by Local Involvement Networks (LINks).

LINks aim to give citizens a stronger voice in how their health and social care services are delivered. Run by local individuals and groups and independently supported – the role of LINks is to find out what people want, monitor local services and to use their powers to hold them to account. Sometimes the people who use services don't feel they have a strong enough voice to change aspects of their health or social care. The introduction of LINks is part of a wider process to help the community have a stronger local voice. A LINks role once it is up and running is to:

- Ask local people what they think about local health care services and provide a chance to suggest ideas to help improve services.
- Investigate specific issues of concern to the community.
- Use its powers to hold services to account and get results.
- Ask for information and get an answer in a specified amount of time.
- Be able to carry out spot-checks to see if services are working well (carried out under safeguards).
- Make reports and recommendations and receive a response.
- Refer issues to the local 'Overview and Scrutiny Committee'.

Picker Institute Europe works with patients, professionals and policy makers to promote understanding of the patient's perspective at all levels of health care policy and practice. Their results form part of the core quality standards set out by the Care quality commission (www.cqc.org.uk). Their national surveys help them find out about patients' and service users' experiences of health care.

Benchmarking

Benchmarking is not new in paediatrics. The North-West Paediatric Benchmarking Project was established in 1994 and today includes in its membership a large number of NHS and academic staff, although the origins of benchmarks are in fact in industry. Benchmarking provides a structured approach to the sharing of best practice utilising all levels of evidence in identifying standards of excellence (Ellis 2000).

Clinical practice benchmarking focuses on practice in which practitioners identify the structures and processes that contribute to good practice, provides a scoring system to measure the structures and processes and comments on the actual practice. Furthermore, an external review panel reviews the benchmarking statements. The comparison of scores enables sharing, which leads to development and innovation. The scoring system aims to be as objective as possible to maximise reliability and validity, although it is recognised that, due to the nature of the evidence on which the scores are based, there will always be some element of subjectivity. The comments made in relation to the scores are therefore very important and are used to support the development of action plans (Ellis 2000).

Clinical practice benchmarking is identified as being a valuable quality improvement initiative with several groups established in a variety of specialities throughout the UK. Repetition of effort is eliminated and vital time and resources saved, making it a cost-effective system for ensuring quality care. By involving practitioners in the process motivation is increased and an environment for change established with practice development an ongoing activity (Stark et al 2002).

Essence of care

The NHS Plan (DoH 2000) reinforced the need to get back to basics and get them right. It provides a tool to help practitioners take a patient-focused approach and a structure to sharing and comparing practice. Furthermore, it is an across the age continuum tool. 'Essence of care' (NHS Modernisation Agency 2003) has resulted in the identification of benchmarks covering nine fundamental aspects of care, which are:

- communication
- food and nutrition
- privacy and dignity
- continence and bladder and bowel care
- personal and oral hygiene
- pressure ulcers
- record keeping
- safety of clients with mental health needs in acute mental health and general hospital settings
- principles of self-care.

Of particular relevance are the benchmarks for communication between patients, carers and health care personnel, and in particular coordination of care, which requires that the wishes of patients and/or carers are listened to, considered and acted on appropriately, and that patients and/or carers are involved in person-centred planning, the single assessment process and discharge planning (NHS Modernisation Agency 2003). If benchmarking is used in the spirit for which it is intended then the voices of the children should be heard as we strive to improve the quality of care afforded to this client group. The benefits of 'Essence of care' are that it:

- improves quality of care
- involves patients, users and carers

- has a structured approach to sharing and comparing practice
- requires the development of action plans to remedy poor practice
- is integral to the clinical governance agenda.

National service frameworks

The National Service Frameworks (NSFs) were set up as a rolling programme in 1998 to improve the quality of statutory services (NHS and the Social and Education services). They were established to tackle variations in care by setting national guidelines. The aim of an NSF is to:

- set national standards for a defined service or care group
- put in place strategies to support the implementation of these standards
- establish milestones against which progress will be measured.

Each NSF concentrates on a different area, with one having been specifically set up for children. The Children's NSF was established in February 2001 and is focused on developing new national standards for children across the NHS and in Social Services and the Education system. Most importantly, the Children's NSF is about putting children and young people, and their families, at the centre of their care and building services around all their needs. The Children's NSF has three main aims (DoH 2003):

- Improving services
- Tackling inequalities
- Enhancing partnerships.

Within the children's NSF there are individual external working groups (EWGs). These groups work together to ensure all children are receiving high-quality services; they concentrate on (CHI 2004):

- the health of all children
- maternity services
- child and adolescent mental health services
- children in special circumstances
- hospital and acute services
- use of medicines in children
- disabled children.

Clinical audit

The primary principle of clinical audit has always been to develop health care practice, something that practitioners have been attempting to do for generations. Clinical audit is a key quality improvement activity and NHS Trusts are now mandated through government legislation (DoH 2000) to have a comprehensive programme of quality improvement activity that includes clinicians participating fully in clinical audit. Clinical audit is taking a leading role in ensuring quality improvement activity is done collaboratively and systematically, influenced by the publication of numerous NHS policy statements (DoH 1997, 1998, 1999, 2000).

Health care systems need to find ways to ensure health care professionals are able to provide patients with the highest possible, and affordable, standards of care. Rawlins (1999) states that there is an abundance of evidence that the clinical care given to patients too often departs from best practice.

As a result of the 1998 public inquiry into paediatric cardiac surgical services at Bristol Royal Infirmary (DoH 2001), subsequent recommendations regarding audit were fully accepted by the government. In particular, the inquiry recommended that audit should be at the core of a system of local monitoring of performance and be fully supported by Trusts, to ensure that health care professionals have access to the necessary time, facilities and advice. All Trusts should have a central audit office to coordinate audit activity, provide advice and support and bring together the results of audit. Finally, clinical audit should be compulsory for all professionals providing clinical care and the requirement to participate should be included as part of the contract of employment.

In 1993 the NHS Executive (Mann 1996) set out the fundamental principles associated with clinical audit. These state that clinical audit should:

- be professionally led
- be seen as an educational process
- form a part of routine clinical practice
- be based on the setting of standards
- generate results that can be used to improve outcome of quality care
- involve management in both process and outcome of audit
- be confidential at the individual patient/clinician level
- be informed by the views of patients/clients.

The developing role of evidence-based medicine and clinical effectiveness has led to more recent policy statements by the NHS Executive, which have focused on the role that clinical audit has to play in clinical effectiveness by getting research into practice (Thomas 1999). Mann (1996) reported that clinical audit is, and should remain, a clinically led initiative that seeks to improve the quality and outcome of patient care through clinicians examining and modifying their practices according to standards of what could be achieved, based on the best evidence available.

The need for high-quality audit has been driven forward over recent years, within the NHS, primarily through the introduction of clinical governance. This was introduced into the NHS to indicate integration of clinical quality improvement with organisational and service performance at all levels. Scally & Donaldson (1998) highlighted that clinical quality, through clinical governance, would enable it to be integrated with financial control and service performance, at all levels of organisations, providing health care that will be managed well.

Clinical audit therefore plays a central role in this process. It is firmly placed in professional practice and is an essential pillar of clinical governance. This was confirmed by Johnson et al (2000), who state that well-planned audit is in a good position to be applied effectively to improve both clinical decisions and organisational efficiency. However, they stressed, to ensure clinicians play a pivotal role in this, greater attention needs to be made on the factors that have been shown to allow audit to flourish and those that have been shown to impede its progress.

An important point to note is that much of the local clinical audit activity that takes place in the UK is not published and therefore important and valuable information is not being shared.

A particular challenge to healthcare providers is how to involve children as service users in clinical audit. Children can provide rich and meaningful information regarding their experiences and opinions as consumers of health care (Woodfield 2001). It is important to use creative and imaginative methods in order to elicit children's views. Woodfield (2001) argues in order to improve the quality of care provided to children through clinical audit, children themselves should be involved in the process.

Scenario

Student nurse Kelly Jones has been asked to participate in an audit of family satisfaction by giving families a discharge questionnaire. She asks her assessor 'What is a clinical audit?' and 'How is it undertaken?'

What is clinical audit?

Clinical audit is a systematic review of care against explicit criteria, which seeks to improve patient care and outcomes through the implementation of change. For audit to succeed there needs to be a supportive organisational environment, with staff who are well prepared and fully understand the methods to be used (NICE 2002). The environment refers to both the structure and culture, and it is structure that provides the link back to the business of clinical governance, professional regulation and life-long learning. Culture, on the other hand, refers to an environment that encourages openness and creativity, and where errors and failures can be reported and investigated with no fear of blame (Morrell & Harvey 1999, NICE 2002).

Clinical audit can be described as having five principal stages (NICE 2002):

1. Preparing for audit
2. Selecting criteria
3. Measuring performance
4. Making improvements
5. Sustaining improvements.

A variety of methods may be used at each of these stages requiring the use of a broad range of methods from a number of disciplines. These include organisational development, statistics and information management. Individual health care staff or groups of professionals in single or multidisciplinary teams, usually supported by clinical audit staff, undertake clinical audit, which may be a project involving all services in a region or country. Effective systems for managing audit and implementing change are important and this might mean that more time is spent on creating the right environment than on the method itself (Dixon 1996).

Conducting a clinical audit

Stage one: preparing for audit (NICE 2002)

Good preparation is essential to ensure a successful audit project and requires:

- Project management: consisting of topic selection, planning and resources, communication.
- Project methodology: project design, data issues, how the project will be implemented, stakeholders to be involved and the level of support for local improvement.

There are five key elements to address when preparing for audit:

1. *Involvement of users and sources of user information*. The involvement of users in decisions about their care and health care services is central to government strategy. Their voice can be heard through, for example:
   - the Patient Advisory Liaison Service (PALS)
   - patient stories or focus groups.
2. *Topic selection*. This will be based on an organisation's individual local priority, reflecting national targets, NICE guidelines and the implementation of National Service Frameworks. Or it might be as a result of:
   - letters of comment or complaint
   - critical incident reports
   - direct observation of care
   - direct conversations
   - following a clinical governance review
   - through benchmarking
   - appraisal of new or existing evidence.
3. *Purpose of the audit*. The need for clear objectives is fundamental to successful audit and enables the identification of suitable audit methods (Morrell & Harvey 1999). The aims of an audit may be couched in some of the following terms:
   - to improve …
   - to change …
   - to enhance …
   - to ensure …
4. *Provision of necessary structures for the conduct of a successful audit*. Such as:
   - time
   - funding
   - meetings.
5. *A skilled audit team*. This is needed to ensure that the audit is valid and robustly conducted; these skills include:
   - project leadership, organisation management
   - clinical, managerial leadership
   - audit method skills
   - change management skills
   - facilitation and negotiation skills.

Stage two: selecting criteria (NICE 2002)

Criteria are used to access the quality of care provided by an individual, team or organisation; they are also commonly stated as standards. Criteria refer to a level of performance and can be classified into three groups:

1. Structure: staffing, skill mix, equipment.
2. Process: actions and decisions taken, e.g. communication, assessment, documentation, discharge planning.
3. Outcomes of care: physical or behavioural responses to an intervention, e.g. drug therapies.

The selection of valid criteria is essential if improvements are to be made in care. Valid criteria are measurable and based on the best available evidence (Parsley & Corrigan 1999).

External sources of valid criteria

- NICE: National Institute for Clinical Effectiveness.
- SIGN: Scottish Intercollegiate Guidelines Network.
- Systematic reviews: Cochrane Library.
- Benchmarking: 'Essence of care' (NHS Modernisation Agency 2003).

Internal sources of valid criteria

Following the systematic review of relevant literature:

- patient care pathways
- local protocols
- local guidelines.

Importantly, there needs to be an external peer review process of internally developed criteria with service user involvement through, for example, focused groups. The process used to obtain criteria for audit from evidence should be methodical, relate to important aspects of care and it should be measurable. Also, if the standards are incomplete or based on views of professionals or groups, formal consensus methods are preferred.

Stage three: measuring performance (NICE 2002)

Methods of data collection should be carefully considered and, where possible, the use of existing data should be used. The audit group needs to consider who will collect data, and must ensure that they are capable, acceptable and non-threatening to patients and staff. Morrell & Harvey (1999) highlight the need to consider the consent of patients and staff before data collection begins and stress that guidance (e.g. the General Medical Council's 2004 'Confidentiality: protecting and providing information') needs to be followed to address issues of confidentiality.

Activity

Access the guidance on 'Confidentiality: protecting and providing information' at:

- http://www.gmc_uk.org/standards

Write down the key points from this guidance and why this is important to our practice.

Four key areas should be addressed when measuring levels of performance:

1. Planning data collection:
   - User groups need to be identified (e.g. all premature infants between 32 weeks' and 36 weeks' gestation receiving care within the neonatal intensive care unit) and exceptions noted.
   - Which health care professionals are involved in the users care.
   - The time period over which the criteria apply.
2. Selecting the sample:
   - How big a sample do you need to be confident in the findings?
   - Resource constraints: time, access, costs.
3. Data collection: this is generally done retrospectively, after the care has been provided, although it can be collected concurrently to provide almost immediate feedback. As information technology becomes more advanced, concurrent audit becomes a more viable option. A tool is developed; this is usually a form, which identifies the precise information that is to be obtained. Any data collection tool should be piloted before use to ensure it captures the information required and to check that there is no ambiguity in the interpretation of the form by those who will collect the data. The form needs to be user friendly to ensure full data collection. Data can be collected using computerised programmes specifically designed for audit.
4. Data analysis:
   - How the data are analysed influences what and how the information is collected and should be identified at an early stage.
   - Data can be qualitative, qualitative or a combination of both. Findings from an audit can be a simple percentage representation of the data, tables and graphs through to full qualitative description.

Stage four: making improvements (NICE 2002)

This is vital for effecting change. Practitioners frequently recognise the need to complete the audit cycle but may not have the skills, time, patience, authority or resources needed to improve the quality of care. Changes in practice may be achieved more effectively if a strategy involving several different types of action is used (Malby 1995). Related factors that may also influence the likelihood of change include what the implication of the change is to service users, the effectiveness of teamwork, and the organisational environment. All these may therefore need to be considered when implementing change (Fig. 16.5).

Stage five: sustaining improvement (NICE 2002)

Although improving performance is the primary goal of audit, sustaining that improvement is also essential. Any systematic approach to changing professional practice should include plans to monitor and evaluate change and ways to maintain and reinforce that change (NHS Centre for Review and Dissemination 1999). Leadership plays a vital role in this, with

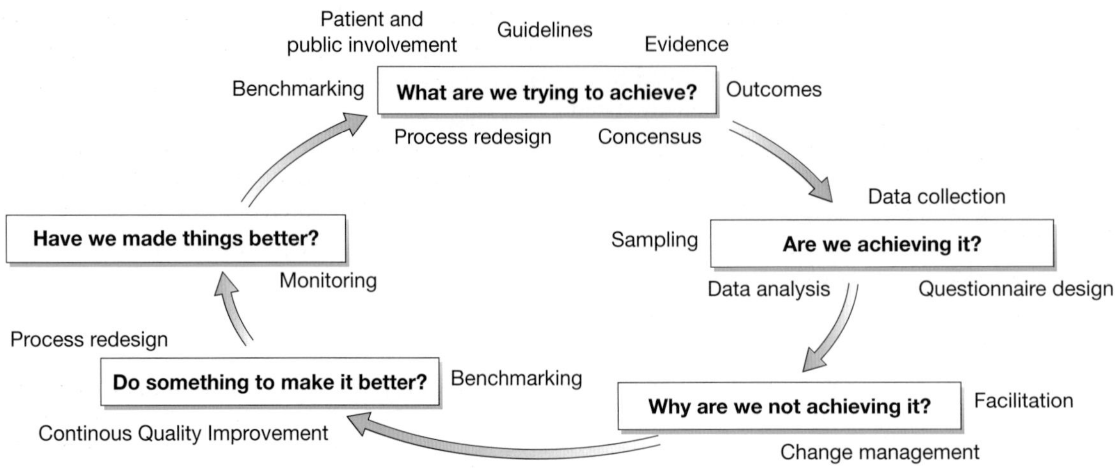

Fig. 16.5 • The clinical audit cycle (NICE 2002).

quality improvement embedded in all aspects of an organisation's work, sustained through monitoring and re-audit (NICE 2002).

New health technologies are sometimes adopted into everyday clinical practice without adequate evidence of their clinical effectiveness and cost effectiveness. Conversely, clinicians can be too slow to introduce new methods of practice even when they have been shown to be effective and give value for money. Clinicians do not have the time and expertise to evaluate each and every possible new intervention but, when this is done for them, the resulting guidelines or guidance are too often of an inadequate or indeterminate quality, and are indigestible or inaccessible. It was for these reasons that the National Institute for Clinical Excellence (NICE) was established.

Examples of improving care through audit

Evidence-based practice

Implementing a children's day assessment unit in a district general hospital (from Beverley et al 1997)

The implementation of a paediatric day assessment unit to a district general hospital was as a result of increasing numbers of children being referred for admission over the previous decade and questioning of the appropriateness of the referral and admission of these children. The implementation of short-stay assessment facilities has been used in Australia and found to be an effective patient–management strategy. Within this district hospital, issues were identified that required a review of the paediatric service. These issues included large peaks and troughs in patient activity exacerbated by uncoordinated admission procedures, with 20 different consultant surgeons from five different surgical specialties admitting children for elective surgery, which occasionally resulted in cancellations due to a lack of beds. Furthermore, there was the desire to meet the Audit Commission's recommendation for there to be two children's trained nurses on duty at all times on the children's wards.

In planning for the introduction of a day assessment unit, representatives from the surgical and primary care teams were included in the project team and analysis of historic paediatric patient activity undertaken. Operational protocols were developed and key facilities secured for the assessment unit, e.g. a play-room, treatment areas. Furthermore, families discharged home from the assessment unit were given a contact telephone number in case they required further advice or support once at home.

An audit of the first year's activity demonstrated a fall in the number of children admitted overnight as an emergency, 658 children were assessed as an emergency but did not require admission to the inpatient ward, and a fall in staff nurse costs.

Evidence-based practice

Telephone follow-up after paediatric day surgery (from Higson & Bolland 2000)

Following a review of the literature it was clearly identified that telephone follow-up calls are an effective tool in providing support and advice to families following discharge from hospital. Together with geographical, financial and staff resource considerations, day surgical units within a children's teaching hospital worked together to produce standards of care for telephone follow-up. To measure the effectiveness of the introduction of telephone call follow-up an audit tool was developed so the process of the telephone call follow-up could be evaluated. This was completed every 6 months. Concerns identified were with regard to pain management following certain surgical procedures, which resulted in children being prescribed stronger analgesia to take home with them following surgery. Patient information was also addressed and evidence-based information leaflets were developed using the information gained from the follow-up telephone calls, which were given to the children and their families during their admission.

Evidence-based practice

Integrated care pathway for infants with bronchiolitis (Peter & Fazakerley 2004)

Integrated care pathways are structured multidisciplinary care plans detailing essential steps in the care of a patient with a specified condition. They are regarded as a means by which local protocols and evidenced-based clinical guidelines can be combined, incorporating the means by which to evaluate the outcomes through the utilisation of variance analysis. There is, however, a recognised lack of empirical evidence of their effectiveness in clinical care therefore the audit process was used to evaluate the effectiveness of the introduction of a clinical pathway for infants with bronchiolitis.

A retrospective review of a number of case notes was undertaken over a 3-year period, 70 prior to implementation of the pathway, 70 following introduction of the pathway and a further 70 following revision of the pathway. Aspects audited included hospital admission criteria, oxygen therapy, hydration, investigations and drug therapy. Staff knowledge of bronchiolitis and satisfaction was also assessed before and after implementation. Improvements identified were increased staff knowledge and satisfaction, less inappropriate chest radiographs, less unnecessary antibiotic administration and improved A&E triage assessment.

Activity

To familiarise yourself with the audit process, contact your local clinical audit office and ask if you can see a completed audit relevant to your area of specialty. Ask yourself the following questions:

- Why was the topic chosen?
- Who were involved and was there user involvement?
- What was the purpose of the audit?
- What criteria did they use and what was the evidence base for these criteria – were they internal or external?
- How were the data collected and was any tool used? If so, was the tool user friendly?
- Were the data collected retrospectively or prospectively?
- How was confidentiality addressed?
- Who was the user group for the audit and was it specific?
- How was the sample size chosen?
- Were the data collected over a specified time period?
- How were the data analysed and were they easy to understand?
- What was the outcome of this audit – did it result in a change in practice?
- Was there an action plan for the implementation of any change?
- What have you gained by completing this activity?

The role of the national institute for clinical effectiveness

NICE has been charged with providing NHS staff with robust, authoritative and reliable guidance on current 'best practice'. Guidance from NICE covers individual technologies as well as the management of a wide range of conditions. NICE will also advise on appropriate methods of clinical audit in those areas where it has provided guidance. It has been established as a Special Health Authority with its own corporate and legal identity and has direct responsibility to the Secretary of State for Health (NICE 2002). NICE currently provides three kinds of guidance:

1. Appraisal and guidance on new and existing health technologies, e.g. newer drugs for epilepsy in children, juvenile idiopathic arthritis (etanercept).
2. To develop clinical guidelines for practice through a variety of national collaborating centres, e.g. National Collaboration Centre for Women's and Child Health. Developing clinical guidelines on the diagnosis and management of type 1 diabetes in children and young people.
3. Interventional procedures: makes recommendations about whether interventional procedures used for diagnosis or treatment are safe enough and work well enough for routine use.

Activity

Go to http://www.nice.org.uk/cms/ipsearch.aspx, insert paediatrics in the relevant speciality and identify interventional procedures that are specific to paediatrics – one example is Coblation tonsillectomy:

- Do you think this kind of guidance is helpful?
- How do you think this might improve the quality of care children might receive from health care services?

NICE has developed guidance for the NHS on clinical audit and coordinates the results from the National Confidential Enquiries. Although the guidance it provides to health authorities, NHS Trusts, primary care groups and health professionals is in the form of advice and, as a whole, is not mandatory, there is an expectation that its recommendations will be universally accepted. Although it is widely acknowledged that strict adherence to clinical guidelines is not in the best interests of some patients, health professionals are wise to record their reasons for non-compliance in patients' medical records.

The four National Confidential Enquiries are also encompassed within NICE to ensure greater clarity and coherence to their findings, and to inform the Institute on areas for which guidance is needed. The Confidential Enquiry into Maternal and Child Health (CEMACH) was launched in April 2003. CEMACH incorporates the Confidential Enquiry into Maternal Deaths (CEMD) and the Confidential Enquiry into Stillbirths and Deaths in Infancy (CESDI) covering the period from 22 weeks' gestation to 28 days, but will also be extending its remit to encompass morbidity and a new national enquiry into child health (NICE 2002). This, however, is due to change and responsibility for the National Confidential Enquiries will be transferring from NICE to the National Patient Safety Authority (NPSA).

To ensure transparent public and user involvement in the work of NICE, a citizens' council has been established. This is a 30-member group involving representatives from all sections of society who are able to have their say on the wider issues and have their judgements considered by NICE when they are issuing guidance to the health care sector (NICE 2002).

Ensuring Trusts have robust audit programmes in place to monitor the implementation of these guidelines is now the role of the Care Quality Commission, whose previous legal name was the Commission for Health care, Audit and Inspection (CHAI); it was previously known as the Commission for Health care Improvement (CHI)).

The role of the care quality commission (CQC)

The Care Quality Commission was formed on 31 March 2009 under the Health and Social Care Act 2008. It replaces :

- the Commission for Health Improvement (CHI)
- the National Care Standards Commission
- the Audit Commission.
- The Heath Commission – The Commission for Health care Audit and Inspection

Activity

To familiarise yourself with clinical governance reviews, go to:

- http://www.chi.nhs.uk/eng/organisations/west_mid/ brm_childrens/2002/brm_childrens.pdf
- What are the key areas of action the trust needs to address?
- What were CHI's conclusions at Birmingham Children's Hospital?

CQC has a wide range of enforcement powers including warning letters, temporary suspension and fines. The ultimate remit is to drive up quality of health and social care. The Care Quality Commission has a wide range of functions, the main ones being to:

- independently assess the performance of the health service from patients' perspectives
- coordinate NHS inspections with a range of other health care organisations: clinical governance reviews
- identify how effectively public funds are used within health care
- develop an independent second stage for complaints about the NHS that cannot be resolved locally
- investigate serious failures
- publish regular ratings of NHS hospitals and Trusts and provide an annual report on health care in England and Wales
- report on key issues, such as coronary heart disease
- publish data on staff and patient surveys
- manage the clinical audit programme
- report to the Secretary of State any serious concerns about the quality of public services or how they are run.

The Care Quality Commission will use core standards to establish the quality of care patients can currently expect and develop standards, which represent the aspirations for the future. Seven domains are identified for the proposed standards, which take account of the NSFs and guidance issued by NICE, these are:

1. safety
2. clinical and cost effectiveness
3. governance
4. patient focus
5. accessible and responsible care
6. care environment and amenities
7. public health.

By visiting the CQC website (http://www.cqc.org.uk) health care professionals and the public can gain access to the work undertaken. In particular, information for service providers falls into seven key areas:

1. Reviews and inspections
2. Performance ratings
3. Standards and criteria
4. NHS surveys
5. Self-assessment
6. Guidance for the NHS: an example being ward staffing guidance
7. National clinical audit: new/current and proposed.

By publicly identifying where improvement is required and sharing good practice within the service, the Care Quality Commission aims to help the NHS raise standards of patient care. In March 2009, the Health care Commission also took over the functions of the Mental Health Act Commission and became the new health and social watchdog for England.

Activity

Having appraised yourself of a clinical governance review go to:

- http://www.chi.nhs.uk/eng/organisations/london/gosh/2003/gosh/pdf.

Identify the key issues evident in this review. Now go to:

- www.chi.nhs.uk/eng/organisations/london/gosh/ 2003/gosh_action_plan.pdf

You should have found the action plan to address the issues raised from this review.

- Do you think this action plan demonstrates clearly what is to be achieved, by whom and within what time frame?
- What do you think could affect the implementation of this action plan?

Summary

The importance of providing high-quality health care services is key to current government policy, with several important national directives and policy documents promoting a culture of quality in health care. Several support agencies and national bodies have been appointed to help embed quality in the NHS, with clinical governance being a central framework to drive the required changes at local Trust level. Importantly, quality is promoted as an individual enterprise, which is to be encouraged across all health care professionals and the central role of clinical audit is widely acknowledged as a key tool in providing quality services. All health care professionals, at whatever level, need to be familiar with key quality activities and recognise the centrality of providing quality care, thereby ensuring a quality service to children and their families.

References

Beverley, D.W., Ball, R.J., Smith, R.A., et al., 1997. Planning for the future: the experience of implementing a children's day assessment unit in a district general hospital. Archives of Disease in Childhood 77, 287–293.

Brocklehurst, N., Walshe, K., 1999. Quality in the new NHS. Nursing Standard 13 (51), 46–53.

Buetow, S.A., Roland, M., 1999. Clinical governance: bridging the gap between managerial and clinical approaches to quality of care. Quality in Health Care 8, 184–190.

Commission for Health Improvement (CHI), 2004. Getting the right start: national service framework for children, young people and maternity services, published part 1: standards for hospital services. CHI, London.

Darzi, A., 2008. High quality care for all. NHS Next Stage Review final report, Department of Health. HMSO, London.

Department of Health (DoH), 1997. The new NHS: modern dependable. HMSO, London.

Department of Health (DoH), 1998. A first class service: quality in the new NHS. HMSO, London.

Department of Health (DoH), 1999. Making a difference. HMSO, London.

Department of Health (DoH), 2000. The NHS plan. HMSO, London.

Department of Health (DoH), 2001. Learning from Bristol: the report of the public inquiry into children's heart surgery at the Bristol Royal Infirmary 1984-1985. Cmd 5363. HMSO, London.

Department of Health (DoH), 2003. Children's National Service Framework. HMSO, London.

Department of Health (DoH), 2004. Standards for better health: health care standards for services under the NHS, HMSO, London.

Dixon, N., 1996. Good practice in clinical audit. A summary of selected literature to support criteria for clinical audit. National Centre for Clinical Audit, London.

Donabedian, A., 1966. Evaluating the quality of medical care. Milbank Memorial Fund Quarterly 44 (3), 166–206.

Ellis, J., 2000. Sharing the evidence: clinical practice benchmarking to improve continuously the quality of care. Journal of Advanced Nursing 32 (1), 215–225.

Glasper, E.A., 2004. Preserving and enhancing standards of care in the NHS. British Medical Journal 13 (6), 293.

Harvey, G., 1996. Relating quality assessment and audit to the research process in nursing. Nurse Researcher 3 (3), 35–46.

Heard, S.R., Schiller, C., Aitken, M., et al., 2001. Continuous quality improvement: educating towards a culture of clinical governance. Quality in Health Care 10 (Suppl II), ii70–ii80.

Higson, J., Bolland, R., 2000. Telephone follow-up after paediatric day surgery. Paediatric Nursing 12, 30–32.

Johnson, G., Crombie, I.K., Davies, H.T.O., et al., 2000. Reviewing audit: barriers and facilitating factors for effective clinical audit. Quality in Health Care 9, 23–36.

Joss, R., Kogan, M., 1995. Advancing quality: total quality management in the National Health Service. Open University, Buckingham.

Malby, B., 1995. Clinical audit for nurses and therapists. Scutari Press, Middlesex.

Mann, T., 1996. Clinical audit in the NHS. Using clinical audit in the NHS: a position statement. NHS Executive, Leeds p 36.

Maxwell, R.J., 1984. Quality assessment in health. British Medical Journal 288, 1470–1472.

Ministry of Health, 1959. Committee of the Central Health Services Council. Report of the Committee on the Welfare of Children in Hospital. Ministry of Health, London.

Morrell, C., Harvey, G., 1999. The clinical audit handbook. Baillière Tindall, London.

National Institute for Clinical Effectiveness (NICE), 2002. Principles for best practice in clinical audit. Radcliffe Medical Press, Oxford.

NHS Centre for Review and Dissemination, 1999. Getting evidence into practice. Effective Health Care 5. University of York, York.

NHS Modernisation Agency, 2003. Essence of care. NHS Modernisation Agency, London.

Nightingale, F., 1863. Notes on hospitals, 3rd edn. Longmans, Roberts and Green, London.

Parsley, K., Corrigan, P., 1999. Quality improvement in health care: putting evidence into practice, 2nd edn. Stanley Thornes, Cheltenham

Peter, S., Fazakerley, M., 2004. Clinical effectiveness of an ICP for infants with bronchiolitis. Paediatric Nursing 16 (1), 30–35.

Pickering, S., Thompson, J., 2003. Clinical governance and best value. Churchill Livingstone, London.

Rawlins, M., 1999. NHS: in pursuit of quality: the NICE. Lancet 353 (9158), 1079–1082.

Scally, G., Donaldson, L., 1998. Clinical governance and the drive for quality improvement in the NHS in England. British Medical Journal 317, 297–298.

Stark, S., MacHale, A., Lennon, E., Shaw, L., 2002. Benchmarking: implementing the process in practice. Nursing Standard 16 (35), 39–42.

Swage, T., 2000. Clinical governance in health care practice. Butterworth Heinemann, Oxford.

Thomas, B., 1999. Research and audit in effective health services. Nursing Standard 13 (33), 40–42.

Woodfield, T., 2001. Involving children in clinical audit. Paediatric Nursing 13 (30), 12–16.

World Health Organization (WHO), 1983. The principles of quality assurance: report on a WHO meeting. WHO, Geneva.

Useful Websites

http://www.nice.org.uk
http://www.chi.org.uk
http://www.york.ac.uk
http://www.health carecommision.org.uk
http://www.gmc-uk.org/standards
http://www.cqc.org.uk
http://www.pickereurope.org

17

The management of pain in children

Alison Twycross Joanna Smith Jennifer Stinson

ABSTRACT

The aim of this chapter and its companion PowerPoint presentation is to outline current best practice in relation to the management of acute and chronic pain in children. Part 1 focuses on the management of acute pain and Part 2 concentrates on chronic pain. Effective assessment is an integral part of pain management and is the first step in successful pain management, and therefore will be explored in depth. General pain management strategies are discussed for both acute and chronic pain.

LEARNING OUTCOMES (ACUTE PAIN)

- Recognise the importance of effective pain management for every child.
- Understand current best practice guidelines relating to managing acute pain in children and the steps needed to manage pain effectively.
- Identify appropriate pain assessment tools for children of different ages.
- Be aware of the different types of analgesic drugs that can be used to relieve acute pain in children.
- Identify non-drug methods of pain relief that can be used to manage acute pain in children.

LEARNING OUTCOMES (CHRONIC PAIN)

- Be able to discuss the differences between acute and chronic pain.
- Describe the main types of chronic pain experienced by children and the prevalence of chronic pain among children.
- Understand current best practice guidelines relating to managing pain in children and the steps needed to manage pain effectively.
- Be aware of the different treatment methods that are used to manage chronic pain in children.
- Recognise the importance of the multi-disciplinary team in managing chronic pain.

DOI: 10.1016/B978-0-7020-3183-0.10017-7

Part 1: The management of acute pain in children

Alison Twycross Joanna Smith

Introduction

Children experience acute pain for a range of reasons, from minor trauma as a result of every day play and activities to the pain that occurs as a result of the physiological consequences of disease processes or major trauma. In hospital, surgical procedures and medical investigation are the most common reasons children experience acute pain. This chapter begins by defining pain and summarising the physiology of acute pain. The gate control theory will be used to explain individual variations in the perception of pain. The evidence supporting the fact that children feel as much pain as adults is summarised and the reasons why pain needs managing effectively are identified. Children's perceptions of their postoperative pain management are discussed and an outline of how children's perception of pain develops as they mature cognitively is provided. Recommendations from clinical guidelines relating to pain in children will be drawn upon to outline the steps nurses need to take to manage children's pain effectively.

What is acute pain?

Pain is a complex multifaceted phenomenon. The definition of pain given by the International Association for the Study of Pain (IASP) acknowledges this and explains how the many facets of pain interrelate and affect pain perception:

> Pain is an unpleasant sensory and emotional experience associated with actual or potential tissue damage, or described in terms of such damage
>
> (IASP 1979 p 249)

However, although supporting the concept of pain as a subjective phenomenon, this definition falls short in relation to those unable to communicate verbally, including neonates and young children. Pain perception is an inherent part of life present in the early stages of development and serves as a signalling system for tissue damage. The IASP definition has been amended to incorporate this aspect:

> The inability to communicate in no way negates the possibility that an individual is experiencing pain and is in need of appropriate pain relieving treatment
>
> (IASP 2001 p 2)

www

Find out more information about the IASP definition of pain and other pain-related terminology at:

- http://www.iasp-pain.org/AM/Template.cfm?Section=General_Resource_Links&Template =/CM/HTMLDisplay.cfm&ContentID=3058

The anatomy and physiology of pain

Pain can be broadly divided into two groups: protective pain sensations (acute pain) and abnormal non-protective pain sensations (chronic pain) (Cervero & Laird 1991). Acute pain is sometimes referred to as normal, sensory or nociceptive pain. Acute pain is typically of short duration, and has a defined course with a direct causal link to a disease, injury, surgery or a medical procedure (Ready & Edwards 1992). This reflects the basic understanding that this type of pain is a normal response to the sensory stimulation of sensory nerve endings located in the skin, muscle, glands and internal organs, known as nociceptors. Being sensitive to both painful and tissue damaging stimuli and responding appropriately are essential to prevent or minimise further injury. If nociceptors are stimulated sufficiently, for example, following injury or tissue damage, a nerve impulse is generated and conveyed by neuronal pathways to the brain, where the stimulus is interpreted as pain. There are many sites that can potentially enhance or inhibit the progression of the impulse. This results in a unique and specific experience for each individual, explaining why pain is a bio-psycho-social phenomenon.

Activity

Read Twycross (2009a) for more information about the factors affecting children's perceptions of pain.

Various theories have been postulated to explain the physiological and psychological processes involved in the pain experience and the modulation of neuronal pathways. Several decades after it was first proposed by Melzack and Wall in 1965 the *gate control theory* still commands universal support (Weisenberg 2000). The gate control theory provides the most likely physiological explanation for the complexity of the processes involved in the perception of pain. The gate control pain theory will now be discussed in relation to the modulation of pain. The gate control theory of pain proposes that there is a *gating* mechanism in the dorsal horn of the spinal cord through which peripheral information passes (Wall & Melzack 1989) (Fig. 17.1). The degree to which the *gate* is opened or closed determines the degree of the pain perception.

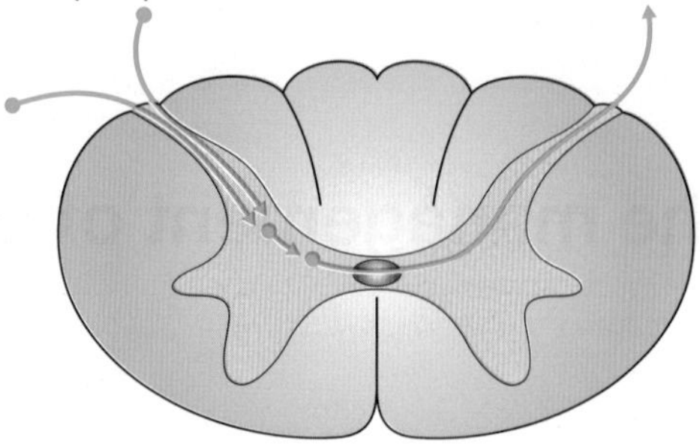
Descending nerve fibres from the brain connect with interneurons modulating the pain process
Nerve fibres cross the spinal cord and ascend towards the thalamus
Impulses from nociceptors arriving at the spinal cord link with ascending and descending tracts via interneurons

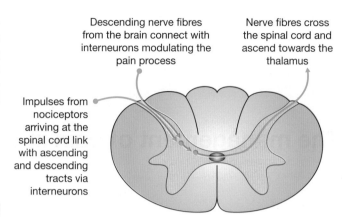

Fig. 17.1 • Spinal cord pathways.

Two interactive systems influence the *gating* mechanism. The first is competitive peripheral input, where in certain situations the 'gate' can remain closed despite stimulation by a nerve impulse originating from a noiceceptor (Wall & Melzack 1989). The classic example of this competitive nerve input explains the pain inhibition that occurs when *mummy rubs it better*. A kick on the knee would activate noiceceptors and if the stimulus was large enough a nerve impulse would be initiated, the *gate* would open and allow interconnections to be made via the spinal cord to the brain. The brain would interpret the sensation as pain. However, if the knee is rubbed vigorously, non-painful sensory fibres would also be activated, competing with the nociceptor stimulation. The stronger impulse would dominate.

The second type of modulation occurs as a result of descending nerves from the brain interacting with the *gating mechanism* in the dorsal horn of the spinal cord (Wall & Melzack 1989). Descending nerves, depending on the type of neurotransmitter released, have the potential to stimulate SG cells which *close* the gate or the T cells which *opens* the gate. Thus impulses arriving at the dorsal horn are either inhibited or if allowed to proceed to the brain the initial stimulus is perceived as pain.

Activity

Read Smith (2009) for more information about the anatomy and physiology of pain.

Does pain in children differ from pain in adults?

The neurophysiological mechanisms that produce pain sensation appear to work in the same way in children as in adults. Despite this, some healthcare professionals still believe that, in a similar situation, children do not feel as much pain as adults. Such beliefs possibly stem from the fact that children in pain often behave differently from adults. Evidence shows that children experience as much pain as adults (Table 17.1).

PROFESSIONAL CONVERSATION

Ian is 11 years old and has had repeated orthopaedic surgery throughout his life. He is extremely anxious about experiencing pain postoperatively. He had been involved in planning postoperative pain methods with the staff and it has been decided to use a patient-controlled analgesic system postoperatively. Ian has been reviewing the pain assessment tool and familiarising himself with the equipment.

Ian's dad is his main carer. He has approached James a mature student and expressed anxieties about 'Ian injecting himself' with morphine and feels that Ian is at a vulnerable age and needs to be 'warned about the danger of drugs not encouraged to use them'.

Issues affecting the relationship between Ian, his father and the staff

James is undertaking his first placement within child branch and has built up a good working relationship with Ian. He is concerned about Ian's dad's attitude and feels Ian is able to make his own choices:

- What issues do you think are important for James to discuss with his mentor in relation to Ian and his family?

Activity

Think about why it is important to manage children's pain effectively.

Why do we need to manage pain effectively?

Painful experiences are part of life for every child (McGrath & Hillier 2003, Perquin et al 2000). Pain has an important purpose, serving as a warning or protective mechanism and

Table 17.1 Key misconceptions about pain in children

Misconception	Evidence
Infants do not feel as much pain as adults	• Myelin does not influence the generation of a nerve impulse; the presence of myelin increases the speed of the impulse (Fitzgerald & Howard 2003). • The process of myelination begins at about 22 weeks' gestation (Fitzgerald & Howard 2003). • Pain pathways (although immature) are present at birth and pain impulses are able to travel to and from the pain centres in the brain (Coskun & Anand 2000, Fitzgerald 2000, Wolf 1999). • Neonates exhibit behavioural, physiological and hormonal responses to pain (Abu-Saad et al 1998, Carter 1997, Franck 1986, Hogan & Choonara 1996, Stevens 1999).
Infants cannot feel pain because of an immature nervous system	• Complete myelination is not necessary for pain to be felt (Volpe 1981) • Painful stimuli are transmitted by both myelinated and unmyelinated fibres (Volpe 1981, Craig & Grunau 1993). • Incomplete myelination implies only a slower conduction speed in the nerves, which is offset by the shorter distances the impulse has to travel (Volpe 1981, Anand & Hickey 1987). • Noxious stimuli have been shown to produce a cortical pain response in preterm babies (Bartocci et al 2006, Slater et al 2006).
Pain pathways in young infants are not developed sufficiently for them to experience pain	• Neural pathways are in place in utero and maturation continues into adulthood, consequently pain responses exist even in the very premature neonate (Fitzgerald & Howard 2003). • Immature synapses within the spinal cord may cause activation of nerve impulses below the normal threshold increasing the pain response (Fitzgerald & Howard 2003). • Immature *gating mechanisms* in the neonate result in an inability to distinguish between some types of stimuli, which may result in an exaggerated pain response (Fitzgerald & Howard 2003).
A young child's lack of previous experiences limits their ability to experience pain	• Emotional processing and cognitive abilities develop over time, which may influence pain coping mechanisms (Fitzgerald & Howard 2003). • Infants and young children have not yet developed these coping strategies and therefore they express pain differently (Fitzgerald and Howard 2003).
Young children cannot indicate where pain is located	• Children as young as 4 years old can demonstrate on a body chart where they hurt without knowing the names of body parts (Van Cleve & Savedra 1993). • Children are able to report the intensity of pain by the age of 3–4 years (Harbeck & Peterson 1991).
Active children are not in pain	• Increased activity is often a sign of pain (Eland 1985).
A child engaged in playing activities cannot be in pain	• Children are particularly gifted in the use of distraction and use play as a diversion and as a coping mechanism (Eland 1985, McCaffery & Beebe 1989).
Sleeping children cannot be in pain	• Sleep may be the result of exhaustion because of persistent pain (Hawley 1984).

people who are unable to feel pain often suffer extensive tissue damage (Melzack & Wall 1996). However, unrelieved pain has a number of undesirable physical and psychological consequences. Twycross (2009b) summarises these as follows:

Physical effects:

- Rapid, shallow, splinted breathing, which can lead to hypoxaemia and alkalosis.
- Inadequate expansion of lungs and poor cough, which can lead to secretion retention and atelectasis.
- Increased heart rate, blood pressure and myocardial oxygen requirements, which can lead to cardiac morbidity and ischaemia.
- Increased stress hormones (e.g. cortisol, adrenaline, catecholamines), which in turn increase the metabolic rate, impede healing and decrease immune function.
- Slowing or stasis of gut and urinary systems, which leads to nausea, vomiting, ileus and urinary retention.
- Muscle tension, spasm and fatigue, which leads to reluctance to move spontaneously and refusal to ambulate, further delaying recovery.

Psychological effects:

- Behavioural disturbances – fear, anxiety, distress, sleep disturbance, reduced coping, developmental regression.

Poor pain management in early life can affect children when older (Grunau et al 1998, Rennick et al 2002, Saxe et al 2001, Taddio et al 1997, Taddio et al 2002). When the consequences of unrelieved pain are considered the need to manage children's pain effectively is clear.

Activity

Find out more about the long-term consequences of pain in neonates by reading Grunau (2000) and Goldschneider & Anand (2003).

Find out more about the effects of poorly managed pain on older children in McGrath & Hillier (2003).

Children's views about how well pain is managed in practice

Activity

In your learning groups consider how well you think children's pain is managed in the clinical area?

Children's perceptions of how well their postoperative pain is managed have been examined in several studies (Alex & Ritchie 1992, Doorbar & McClarey 1999, Polkki et al 2003, Woodgate & Kristjanson 1996). Children suggested that nurses need to take a more active role in pain management. More specifically, children indicated that:

- pain is managed poorly in hospital
- nurses need to communicate with them about their pain and to listen to what they were saying about their pain
- nurses should ask them about their pain on an hourly basis
- children wished nurses had given them more or stronger analgesic drugs when they asked for them.

Other studies have found that children continue to experience unrelieved moderate to severe pain postoperatively (Johnston et al 2005, Vincent & Denyes 2004), suggesting that current guidelines are not being implemented effectively into practice.

Seminar discussion topic

Children continue to experience moderate to severe unrelieved postoperative pain (Johnston et al 2005, Polkki et al 2003, Vincent & Denyes 2004). This is despite the evidence to guide practice (both clinical guidelines and research evidence) being readily available:

- Discuss what steps children's nurses can take to ensure that postoperative pain is managed effectively.

Cognitive development and perception of pain

When managing pain in children it is important to understand how children develop concepts relating to pain. This will enhance the quality of care that nurses provide and enable nurses to:

- provide appropriate explanations of illness and hospitalisation
- provide sensitive reassurance for children
- gain greater understanding of what children are saying to them
- gain insight into how children interpret all the strange occurrences that can accompany illnesses.

Activity

Think about your interactions with children of different ages:

- How do you think a child's perception of pain changes as they mature cognitively?

The impact of a child's level of cognitive development on their perception of pain has been explored in a number of studies over the past 30 years (Crow 1997, Gaffney 1993, Hurley & Whelan 1988, Jeans & Gordon 1981, Ross & Ross 1984, Scott & Huskisson 1978). The results of these studies indicate that children's perception about the cause and effect of pain develops in line with Piaget's Stages of Cognitive Development (Table 17.2). The implications for nursing practice are highlighted in Table 17.2.

It is important to note that a child's experiences of illness and hospitalisation may influence their perception of and their ability to cope with pain, for example, they may regress to an

Table 17.2 Age specific perceptions of pain in children and implications for practice (adapted from Gaffney et al 2003, Twycross 2009b)

Piaget's stage of development	Perception/presentation of pain	Implications for practice
Sensorimotor (0–2 years)	• Pain is a physical experience primarily expressed by changes in behaviours such as restlessness, irritability, tension, abnormal crying/grizzling/screaming, abnormal posture/movements.	• Understanding the normal activities and behaviours for each child and comparing these to those presented during illness is paramount. • Excellent observations skills are necessary, particularly in relation to interpreting verbal sounds/words, facial expression and body language.
Preoperational (2–7 years)	• Pain is primarily perceived as a physical experience, with an inability to distinguish between the cause of pain and its effect. • Pain is often perceived as a result of their own behaviour, for example as a punishment for a wrongdoing. • Pain may also be perceived as the responsibility of someone else and the child may believe magical acts can remove the pain. • Increased ability to verbalise needs will correlate to language skills developments.	• Carers must be aware that the child may be aggressive when offered help and will not understand the connection between treatment and pain relief. • Allowing the child to express their feelings is important; encourage the child to describe the pain in their own language. • Much reassurance is needed to explain pain is not a punishment. • Family input is vital, however parents may not have experienced their child in pain and not understand change in behaviours. • Guidance relating to comforting their child and distraction techniques will be necessary.
Concrete operational (7–12 years)	• There is more understanding of the physical properties of pain and can relate pain to body parts. • Fears about the consequence of pain and damage to the body are great, vivid imagination can lead to fears of total body destruction. • Towards the end of this period some rational thinking develops. • Pain concepts beginning to form and can describe effects that influence pain, the 'if' and 'when' scenarios.	• The child needs clear explanations about cause of pain and treatments and opportunity to discuss fears and believes and reassurance relating to body destruction.
Formal operational (12 years and older)	• There is the beginnings of depth of understanding, but may not be consistent due to limited life experiences and therefore may imagine sinister consequences of the pain.	• Adolescents need clear explanations about cause of pain and treatments and opportunity to discuss fears and beliefs about the potential impact of the pain.

Activity

How do you think recurrent pain/painful procedures affect a child's perception of pain?

earlier stage of development. Conversely, children with chronic illness, often develop an understanding of concepts associated with a later stage of development.

How should pain in children be managed?

In the context of nursing, pain management equates well to the stages of the nursing process (Yura & Walsh 1988) – assessment, planning, implementation and evaluation – to the treatment of pain. What this means in practice is outlined in the *evidence based practice* box below. The steps that need to be taken to manage acute pain effectively are outlined in Figure 17.2.

Evidence-based practice

A review of clinical guidelines relating to the management of pain in children indicates that effective management of pain requires nurses to:

1. take a pain experience history from child and parent on admission
2. assess children's pain using a valid and reliable, age-appropriate pain assessment tool
3. take into account children's behavioural cues and physiological indicators of pain when assessing pain
4. administer appropriate analgesic drugs
5. use non-drug methods of pain relief
6. involve parents in their child's pain management
7. adopt a multidisciplinary approach
8. document pain scores and interventions
9. reassess pain having given time for pain-relieving interventions to take affect and, if necessary, alter the plan of care
10. communicate with children and their parents about all aspects of pain management

(Developed from: American Pain Society 2001, ANZCA 2007, Howard et al 2008)

www

Pain standards and guidelines related to managing acute pain in children available online include:

American Academy of Pediatrics and American Pain Society (2001) The assessment and management of acute pain in infants, children and adolescents, Pediatrics, 108(3): 793-797. Available from: http://www.ampainsoc.org/advocacy/pediatric2.htm

Association of Paediatric Anaesthetists of Great Britain and Ireland: Howard R, Carter B, Curry J, Morton N, Rivett K, Rose M, Tyrrell J, Walker S and Williams G (2008) Good Practice in Postoperative and Procedural Pain Management, Pediatric Anesthesia, 18: 1-81. http://www.blackwell-synergy.com/toc/pan/18/s1

Australian and New Zealand College of Anaesthetists and Faculty of Pain Medicine (2007) Acute Pain Management: Scientific Evidence, Updated 2nd edition, Australian and New Zealand College of Anaesthetists, Melbourne. Available from: http://www.anzca.edu.au/resources/books-and-publications/acutepain_update.pdf

NHS Quality Improvement Scotland (2004) Best Practice Statement: Postoperative Pain Management, NHS Quality Improvement Scotland, Edinburgh. (Children's postoperative pain addressed in Section 11). Available from: http://www.nhshealthquality.org/nhsqis/files/Post_Pain_COMPLETE.pdf

Royal College of Nursing (2000a) The recognition and assessment of acute pain in children: update of full guideline, RCN Publishing, London. Available from: http://www.rcn.org.uk/data/assets/pdf_file/0004/269185/003542

Reflect on your practice

Think about your pain management practices:

- Do your pain management practices always conform to this best practice checklist and/or to the postoperative pain management algorithm (Fig. 17.2)?

Assessing pain in children

Pain assessment is the first step in the management of pain. To treat pain effectively, ongoing assessment of the presence and severity of pain and the child's response to treatment is essential. Pain assessment poses many challenges in infants and children including (McCaffery & Pasero 1999):

- the subjective and complex nature of pain
- developmental and language limitations that preclude comprehension and self-report
- dependence on others to infer pain from behavioural and physiological indicators.

When assessing pain in children there are three key steps:

- *Step 1*: Take and document a pain history
- *Step 2*: Assess the child's pain using a developmentally appropriate pain assessment tool

Severe 7–10	IV opioid Paracetamol ± NSAID consider IV if NBM (**OR** bolus LA infusion)	Continue IV opioid Add adjuvants (e.g. tramadol, ketamine, diazepam, clonidine, amitryptiline, gabapentin) Continue paracetamol ± NSAID (**OR** adjust LA infusion)	Continue IV opioid ± boluses Continue regular adjuvants ± boluses Monitor bolus requirements Continue regular paracetamol ± NSAID (**OR** adjust LA infusion)	Decrease IV opioid/adjuvants once pain ≤ 7 and < 2 boluses per 12 hours (Consider converting to oral opioid/adjuvant) Continue regular paracetamol ±NSAID (Sease LA infusion by DAY 5)
Moderate 4–6	Oral opioid Paracetamol ± NSAID (**OR** bolus LA infusion)	Additional oral opioid dose Consider IV opioid bolus Add adjuvant (e.g. tramadol, diazepam) Continue paracetamol ± NSAID (**OR** adjust LA infusion)	Continue regular oral opioid Continue regular adjuvant Monitor number of rescue doses Continue regular paracetamol ± NSAID	Decrease/cease opioid once pain ≤ 4 and < 2 rescues in 24 hours Decrease adjuvant frequency to PRN if pain ≤ 4 Continue paracetamol ± NSAID (Cease LA infusion by day 5)
Nil–mild 0–3	Oral paracetamol	Paracetamol regularly	Continue regular or PRN paracetamol	Cease paracetamol once less than 2 doses per day If previous moderate–severe pain: Cease PRN adjuvants once < 2 doses per day Cease NSAID once < 2 doses per day

Fig. 17.2 • A decision-making algorithm for postoperative pain management in children.

- *Step 3*: Reassess pain having allowed time for pain relieving interventions to work.

Parents and significant family members know their child best and can recognise subtle changes in manner or behaviour. They have a particularly important role in pain assessment and should be involved at all three steps.

Step 1: taking a pain history

Activity

What do you think should be included in a pain history?

How will this information help you manage a child's pain more effectively?

A pain experience history has been identified as an important element of pain management (Hester & Barcus 1986, Hester et al 1998, RCN 1999). A pain experience history provides information about the child's likely response to pain and could be invaluable in deciding on effective treatments for pain. An outline of questions to include in a pain experience history is provided in Table 17.3.

Table 17.3 Pain history for children with acute pain (adapted from Hester & Barcus 1986, Hester et al 1998)

Child's questions	Parent's questions
Tell me what pain is	What word(s) does your child use in regard to pain?
Tell me about the hurt you have had before	Describe the pain experiences your child has had before
Do you tell others when you hurt? If yes, who?	Does your child tell you or others when he or she is hurting?
What do you want to do for yourself when you are hurting?	How do you know when your child is in pain?
What do you want others to do for you when you are hurt?	How does your child usually react to pain?
What don't you want others to do for you when you hurt?	What do you do for your child when he or she is hurting?
What helps the most to take your hurt away?	What does your child do for him- or herself when he or she is hurting?
Is there anything special that you want me to know about when you hurt? (If yes, have child describe)	What works best to decrease or take away your child's pain?
	Is there anything special that you would like me to know about your child and pain? (If yes, describe).

Step 2: assessing the child's pain using a developmentally appropriate pain assessment tool

Reflect on your practice

What methods do you use to assess pain in children?

The three approaches to measuring pain are:

- self-report (that is, what the child says)
- behavioural (that is, how the child behaves)
- physiological indicators (that is, how the child's body reacts).

(Stinson et al 2006)

These measures are used separately or in combination in a range of pain assessment tools that are available to use in practice. Self-report measures are considered the *gold standard* and should be used with children who are:

- old enough to understand and use self-report scale (for example, 3 years of age and older)
- not overtly distressed.

With infants, toddlers, preverbal, cognitively impaired and sedated children behavioural pain assessment tools should be used (von Baeyer & Spagrud 2007). If the child is overtly distressed, for example due to pain, anxiety or some other stressor, no meaningful self-report can be obtained at that point in time. The child's pain can be estimated using a behavioural pain assessment tools until such time as the child is less distressed for example, following the administration of analgesic drugs (Stinson 2009).

Self-report tools

Several self-report pain assessment tools have been designed for use with school-aged children. These are outlined in Table 17.4.

Activity

Further information about self-report tools in children can be found in von Baeyer (2006) and Stinson (2009).

Behavioural (observational) tools

Activity

In your learning groups consider when you think behavioural cues may be a useful way of establishing whether a child is in pain.

The tools developed to assess pain in infants and young children generally use behavioural indicators of pain. A wide range of specific, expressive, behaviours have been identified in infants and young children that are indicative of pain:

- Individual behaviours (for example, crying and facial expression)

Table 17.4 Self-report tools (adapted from Stinson 2009)

Tool	Description
Verbal Rating Scales (VRS)	Consist of a list of simple word descriptors or phases to denote varying degrees or intensities of pain. • Each word or phrase has an associated number. • Children are asked to select a single word or phrase that best represents their level of pain intensity and the score is the number associated with the chosen word. • One example of a VRS is using word descriptors of *not at all* = 0, *a little bit* = 1, *quite a lot* = 2 and *most hurt possible* = 3 (Goodenough et al 1997).
Faces Pain Scales	Faces pain scales present the child with drawings or photographs of facial expressions representing increasing levels of pain intensity. • The child is asked to select the picture of a face that best represents their pain intensity and their score is the number (rank order) of the expression chosen. • Faces scales have been well validated for use in children aged 5–12 years (Champion et al 1998, Stinson et al 2006). • There are two types of faces scales – line drawings (for example, Faces Pain Scale – Revised, Fig. 17.3) and photographs (for example, Oucher, available from: http://www.oucher.org/the_scales.html). • Faces pain scales with a happy and smiling *no pain* face or faces with tears for *most pain possible* have been found to affect the pain scores recorded. For example, the smiling lower anchor of the Wong-Baker FACES Pain Scale has been found to produce higher pain ratings than those with neutral faced anchors (Chambers & Craig 1998). Therefore, faces pain scales with neutral expressions for *no pain* such as that developed by Hicks et al (2001) are generally recommended.
Numerical Pain Scales (NRS)	Consists of a range of numbers (for example, 0–10 or 0–100) that can be represented in verbal or graphical format. • Children are told that the lowest number represents *no pain* and the highest number represents *the most pain possible*. The child is instructed to circle, record or state the number that best represents their level of pain intensity. • Verbal NRS tend to be the most frequently used pain intensity measure with children over 8 years of age in clinical practice. • They have the advantage that they can be verbally administered without a print copy and are easy to score. They do require numeracy skills and, therefore, should be used in older school-aged children and adolescents. • While there is evidence of their reliability and validity in adults, verbal NRS have undergone very little testing in children. • An example of a well validated scale incorporating a graphic NRS is the Oucher (Beyer 1984). The Oucher comprises two separate scales; the photographic faces scale and a 0–10 vertical NRS. Older school-aged children and adolescents usually use the NRS.
Graphic Rating Scales	The most commonly used graphic rating scale is *The Pieces of Hurt Tool* (Hester 1979). • This tool consists of four red poker chips, representing *a little hurt* to *the most hurt you could ever have*. • The child is asked to select the chip that represents his/her pain intensity and the tool is scored from 0 to 4. • The Pieces of Hurt Tool has been well validated for acute procedural and hospital-based pains and is recommended for use in young pre-school children (Stinson et al 2006). • The Pieces of Hurt Tool is easy to use and score and the instructions have been translated into several languages including Arabic, Thai and Spanish. • Drawbacks to its use include cleaning the chips between patient use and the potential for losing chips.
Visual Analogue Scales (VAS)	• Require the child to select a point on a vertical or horizontal line where the ends of the line are defined as the extreme limits of pain intensity. • The child is asked to make a mark along the line to indicate the intensity of their pain. There are many versions of VAS for use with children. • Have been extensively researched and have been recommended for most children aged 8 years and older (Stinson et al 2006). • While VAS are easy to reproduce, photocopying may alter length of line and they require the extra step of measuring the line which increases the burden and likelihood for errors.

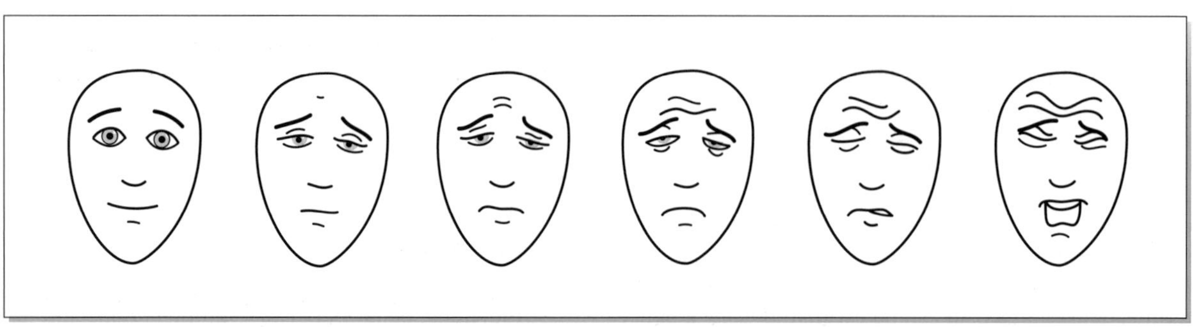

Fig. 17.3 • The faces pain scale (reproduced from Hicks et al 2001 with permission from the International Association for the Study of Pain).

Table 17.5 Behavioural indicators of pain in children

General behaviours	Specific behaviours
Changed behaviour	Banging head
Irritability	Pulling ear
Flat effect	Curling up on side
Unusual posture	Refusal to move limbs
Screaming	Constantly rubbing specific region
Reluctance to move	
Aggressiveness	
Increased clinging	
Unusual quietness	
Loss of appetite	
Restlessness	
Whimpering	
Sobbing	
Lying 'scared stiff'	
Lethargy	
Disturbed sleep pattern	

- Large movements (for example, withdrawal of the affected limb, touching the affected area, and the movement or tensing of limbs and torso)
- Changes in social behaviour or appetite
- Changes in sleep/wake state or cognitive functions.

Evidence-based practice

Observational tools are indicated for children who are:

- too young to understand and use self-report scales (for example, less than 4 years old)
- too distressed to use self-report scales
- impaired in their cognitive or communicative abilities
- very restricted by bandages, surgical tape, mechanical ventilation or paralysing drugs
- considered to have self-report ratings that are exaggerated, minimised or unrealistic due to cognitive, emotional or situational factors

(von Baeyer & Spagrud 2007)

Some of the behavioural indicators of pain are listed in Table 17.5. An example of a tool used for preverbal children is the FLACC (Merkel et al 1997) (Table 17.6). When using the FLACC it is important to remember that:

- It is intended for use in children 2 months to 8 years of age but has been used in children 0–18 years
- It has been validated for procedural and postoperative pain
- Each category is scored on a 0–2 scale, which results in a total score between 0 and 10

Table 17.6 The FLACC pain assessment tool (Merkel et al 1997)

Categories	Behaviours	Scoring
Face	No particular expression or smile	0
	Occasional grimace or frown, withdrawn, disinterested	1
	Frequent to constant quivering chin, clenched jaw	2
Legs	Normal position or relaxed	0
	Uneasy, restless, tense	1
	Kicking or legs drawn up	2
Activity	Lying quietly, normal position, moves easily	0
	Squirming, shifting back and forth, tense	1
	Arched, rigid or jerking	2
Cry	No cry (awake or asleep)	0
	Moans or whimpers, occasional complaints	1
	Crying steadily or sobs, frequent complaints	2
Consolability	Content, relaxed	0
	Reassured by occasional touching, hugging to being talked to, distractable	1
	Difficult to console or comfort	2

Neonates and children clearly display metabolic, hormonal, and physiological responses to pain. These physiological reactions all indicate the activation of the sympathetic nervous system, which is part of the autonomic nervous system, and is responsible for the *fight or flight* response associated with stress (Sweet & McGrath 1998). Physiological parameters that can indicate that a child is in pain are outlined in Table 17.7. Other physiological indicators of pain include sweating and dilated pupils.

Table 17.7 Physiological signs used to assess pain (adapted from Sweet & McGrath 1998)

Observation	Change Indicating Pain
Heart rate	Increases when in pain (after an initial decrease)
Respiratory rate and pattern	There is conflicting evidence about whether this increases or decreases, but there is a significant shift from baseline. Breathing may become rapid and/or shallow
Blood pressure	Increases when a child is in acute pain
Oxygen saturation	Decreases when a child is in acute pain

- It cannot be used in intubated or paralysed patients
- Consolability requires (a) an attempt to console, and (b) a subjective rating of response to that intervention, which complicates the scoring.

(Stinson 2009)

Activity

Read von Baeyer & Spagrud's (2007) article for further information about behavioural tools for assessing pain in children.

Physiological indicators

Activity

In your learning groups consider which physiological indicators may be a useful way of establishing whether a child is in pain.

Evidence-based practice

On their own, physiological indicators do not constitute a valid clinical pain measure for children; a multidimensional or composite measure that incorporates physiological and behavioural indicators, as well as self-report is, therefore, preferred whenever possible (Franck et al 2000, von Baeyer & Spagrud 2007).

PROFESSIONAL CONVERSATION

Joe is 6 months old and had a cleft lip and palate repaired 3 days ago. Claire, the student nurse looking after him has noticed that he is not drinking much orally, and that every time Joe smiles he bursts into tears. She overhears Joe's mother on the phone saying that 'he doesn't seem himself today. I thought he might be in pain but the nurses say that he isn't.'

Claire begins to wonder whether Joe may be in pain and decides to speak to her mentor about this.

Pain assessment in cognitively impaired children

Activity

In your learning groups discuss the challenges of assessing pain in cognitively impaired children.

Infants and children with cognitive impairment or developmental delay who are unable to report pain may be at greater risk for under-treatment of pain (McGrath 1998). These include children with cerebral palsy, neuro-developmental disorders, severe developmental delay and children with pervasive developmental disorders. Pain experienced by these children is particularly difficult to assess accurately (Stinson 2009). While these children are generally unable to report pain, credible assessment can usually be obtained from the parent or another person who knows the child well (Breau et al 2002, Hunt et al 2004, 2007). However, proxy judgements have been shown to underestimate the pain experience of others (Chambers & Craig 1998, Kelly et al 2002, St Laurent-Gagnon et al 1999).

Factors to consider in the assessment of pain in children with a significant cognitive impairment include:

- underlying neurological condition/process
- developmental level (for example, cognition, communication, motor function)
- usual behaviour and health condition (for example, baseline condition)
- usual means of communication (for example, verbal, non-verbal)
- caregiver's views
- impact of concurrent illnesses
- differential diagnosis (for example, consider all sources of distress and pain).

(Oberlander et al 1999)

Parents and caregivers tend to report a diversity of behavioural responses to pain but the categories outlined above are common to almost all children and provide cues to caregivers that their child might be experiencing pain. This underlines the importance of obtaining a thorough baseline history from caregivers of children with cognitive impairments (Stinson 2009). While there are several pain assessment tools for these children, the most well validated measure is the Non-Communicating Children's Pain Checklist (Fig. 17.4) (Breau et al 2002). The paediatric pain profile has also been developed for use with this group of children (Hunt et al 2004, 2007) (see http://www.ppprofile.org.uk/).

Activity

Read Oberlander & Symons (2006) for further information about the assessment of pain in cognitively impaired children.

Step 3: reassessing pain

How often should pain be assessed?

Effective pain management depends on regular assessment of the presence and severity of pain and the patient's response to pain management interventions. Every patient should have their pain assessed:

- on admission to hospital
- when they visit an emergency department or an ambulatory clinic
- at least once per shift (if they are an inpatient)
- before, during and after an invasive procedure.

(Stinson 2009)

Pain should be assessed regularly following surgery and/or if the patient has a known painful medical condition (Stinson 2009). Pain should be assessed hourly for the first 6 hours. After this, if the pain is well controlled, it can be assessed less frequently (for example, every 4 hours). If the pain is fluctuating, regular assessment should continue for 48–72 hours, after this the pain intensity will normally have peaked and be starting to subside (Stinson 2009).

Reflect on your practice

How often do you evaluate the effectiveness of the pain-relieving interventions you have used?

How often do you assess a child's pain postoperatively?

Please indicate below how often this person shows the signs of Subscales I to IV in the **last 5 minites. If an item does not apply to this person (for example, this person does not eat solid food or cannot reach with his/her hands), then indicate 'not applicable' for that item.**

0 = not at all **1 = just a little** **2 = fairly often** **3 = very often** **NA = not applicable**

1. Vocal					
1. Moaning, whining, whimpering (fairly soft)	0	1	2	3	NA
2. Crying (moderately loud)	0	1	2	3	NA
3. Screaming/yelling (very loud)	0	1	2	3	NA
4. A specific sound or word for pain (e.g. a word, cry or type of laugh)	0	1	2	3	NA
II. Social					
5. Not cooperating, cranky, irritable, unhappy	0	1	2	3	NA
6. Less interaction with others, withdrawn	0	1	2	3	NA
7. Seeking comfort or physical closeness	0	1	2	3	NA
8. Being difficult to distract, not able to satisfy or pacify	0	1	2	3	NA
III. Facial					
9. A furrowed brow	0	1	2	3	NA
10. A change in eyes, including: squinting of eyes, eyes opened wide, eyes frowning	0	1	2	3	NA
11. Turning down of mouth, not smiling	0	1	2	3	NA
12. Lips puckering up, tight, pouting, or quivering	0	1	2	3	NA
13. Clenching or grinding teeth, chewing or thrusting tongue out	0	1	2	3	NA
IV. Activity					
14. Not moving, less active, quiet	0	1	2	3	NA
15. Jumping around, agitated, fidgety	0	1	2	3	NA
V. Body and limbs					
16. Floppy	0	1	2	3	NA
17. Stiff, spastic, tense, rigid	0	1	2	3	NA
18. Gesturing to or touching part of the body that hurts	0	1	2	3	NA
19. Protecting, favouring or guarding part of the body that hurts	0	1	2	3	NA
20. Flinching or moving the body part away, being sensitive to touch	0	1	2	3	NA
21. Moving the body in a specific way to show pain (e.g. head back, arms down, curls up, etc.)	0	1	2	3	NA
VI. Physiological					
22. Shivering	0	1	2	3	NA
23. Change in colour, pallor	0	1	2	3	NA
24. Sweating, perspiring	0	1	2	3	NA
25. Tears	0	1	2	3	NA
26. Sharp intake of breath, gasping	0	1	2	3	NA
27. Breath holding	0	1	2	3	NA

Score summary

Category	**I**	**II**	**III**	**IV**	**V**	**VI**	**TOTAL**
Score							

Fig. 17.4 • Non-communicating children's pain check list (Breau et al 2002).

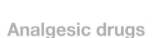

WWW

Additional web-based information about pain assessment can be found at:

- Great Ormond Street Hospital for Children NHS Trust (GOSH) and UCL Institute of Child Health (ICH): http://www.ich.ucl.ac.uk/gosh/clinicalservices/Pain_control_service/Custom%20Menu_02

(Provides information on RCN pain assessment guidelines and recommended pain assessment tools in children.)

- Partners Against Pain: http://www.partnersagainstpain.com/index-mp.aspx?sid=3

  Provides printable PDFs of commonly used paediatric pain scales.
- Ped-IMMPACT: http://www.immpact.org

(Recommendations for the design, execution and interpretation of paediatric pain clinical trials including PDFs of systematic reviews of self-report and observational pain tools for 3–18 years.)

Analgesic drugs

Appropriate analgesic drugs should be administered based on the pain assessment. Analgesic drugs should be given regularly to control pain and be appropriate for the severity of the pain (Fig. 17.5). A lower dose of analgesia can be effective if it is given before the pain becomes unbearable (McCaffery & Pasero 1999).

Three main types of drug are used to manage pain in children: paracetamol, non-steroidal anti-inflammatory drugs (NSAIDs) and opioids. An analgesic ladder simplifies and guides the prescription of analgesia but should be flexible and sensitive enough to meet a child's individual needs (World Health Organization 1998). An example of an analgesic ladder is provided in Figure 17.5. Information about each drug type and its action is outlined in Table 17.8.

Analgesic techniques

Analgesic drugs can be administered using several routes (for example oral, rectal, intravenous, subcutaneous) and by a variety of techniques (continuous infusion, patient-controlled analgesia (PCA), by nurse-controlled analgesia (NCA)). The choice of route and method of administration will depend on many factors, including the:

- cause of pain and predicted duration of acute pain intensity score
- child's cognitive abilities: this is particularly important when considering PCA systems
- child's physical status: e.g. oral medication is not suitable if a child is vomiting or has impaired gut motility, subcutaneous administration may not be suitable if there is poor tissue perfusion and intravenous administration may not be appropriate if venous access is problematic
- ability to monitor the child
- time available to prepare the child and family: this is particularly important when using PCA
- support available from anaesthetic and/or pain service
- local practice, policies and guidelines.

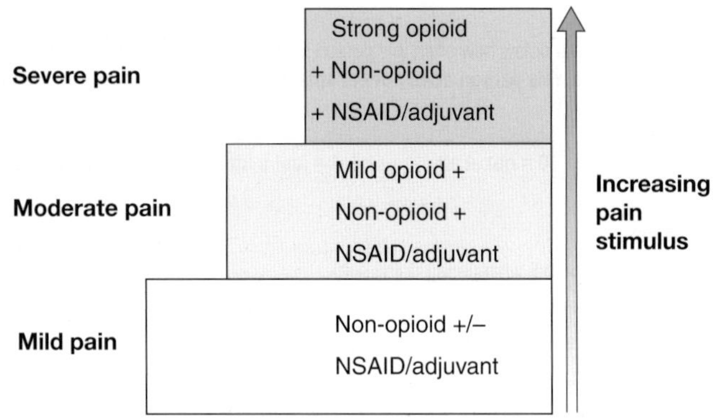

Fig. 17.5 • WHO analgesic ladder (adapted from WHO 1996).

Advanced analgesia systems are an important part of acute pain management. Several of these will now be described.

Intravenous infusion of opioid drugs

Intramuscular injections are unpopular with children because of their fear of needles. In addition drugs administered intermittently result in peaks and troughs in the level of analgesia for the child. Continuous intravenous morphine infusions have been used in the management of postoperative pain following major surgery in children since the early 1980s (Bray 1983, Bray et al 1986) because of their ability to produce more consistent analgesia levels and the facility to add bolus doses as required. The infusion is administered by an infusion pump with the infusion rate adjusted according to the child's response and needs. Opioid infusions are usually commenced intraoperatively and the most common opioid used is morphine. The side effects of opioids must be quickly identified through accurate hourly observations of pulse rate, respiratory rate, volume delivered, oxygen saturation, pain score, sedation score and nausea and vomiting should be recorded. It may be necessary to adjust the rate of the infusion to maintain the child in a pain free state and minimise side effects. This is best accomplished by the prescription being written as a sliding scale. All patients receiving an opioid infusion should have an opioid antagonist pre-prescribed which should be administered if opioid-induced respiratory depression occurs.

Patient-controlled analgesia

Patient-controlled analgesia (PCA) has become the gold-standard for acute pain management since its introduction into paediatric medicine in the early 1990s (Lehmann 2005, McDonald & Cooper 2001). PCA uses a programmable infusion pump that enables the child to self-administer a small intravenous bolus dose of an opioid drug. PCA is used for the management of moderate to severe pain in children over 5 years. In some instances children as young as 4 years can manage PCA, but this is uncommon (McDonald & Cooper 2001). PCA is safe, effective and viewed as a highly satisfactory method of analgesia delivery by staff, patient and families. Adverse effects are rare and can be reduced by the addition of opioid-sparing analgesics (for example, paracetamol) (Ellis

Table 17.8 Analgesic drugs: Information and action (adapted from Dowden 2009a)

Drug type	Information	Action
Paracetamol	• Is the most commonly used analgesic drug for children. • Has antipyretic (fever reducing) activity, but minimal anti-inflammatory effects (unlike NSAIDs). • Is highly effective as a sole analgesic for mild to moderate pain. • Enhances analgesia when used in combination with NSAIDs or tramadol (Remy et al 2006). • Also has opioid sparing effects (reduces the amount of opioid required) of up to 20% in adults when given in combination with opioids (Remy et al 2006). • Is probably underused in patients with moderate to severe pain, when many clinicians rely heavily on opioids (Harrop 2007).	• Paracetamol selectively inhibits prostaglandin synthesis (probably by inhibiting cyclo-oxygenase-3 [COX-3]) in the central nervous system. • This is why it has antipyretic and analgesic effects but no anti-inflammatory effects or unwanted gastrointestinal effects (Chandrasekharan et al 2002, Harrop 2007, Morton 2007, Remy et al 2006). • Normal gastrointestinal function is required for oral paracetamol administration, thus if the child has an ileus the intravenous or rectal routes are more efficacious.
Nonsteroidal anti-inflammatory drugs (NSAIDs) e.g. ibuprofen, diclofenac	• Used to treat mild to moderate pain, especially inflammatory-mediated conditions. • Used mainly in the postoperative setting, following trauma or for home-based pain and fever management. • Have antipyretic activity as well as anti-inflammatory and analgesic activity. • Have a significant opioid sparing effect and may reduce morphine requirements by up to 30–40% (Morton 2007).	• NSAIDs act by inhibiting the synthesis of prostaglandins by inhibiting the production of (cyclo-oxygenase-1) COX-1 and (cyclo-oxygenase-2) COX-2 enzymes. • This reduces inflammatory pain-inducing chemicals and thus decreases the response of peripheral and central pain receptors. • NSAIDs should be avoided or used with caution in patients with bleeding disorders or at risk of haemorrhage; renal impairment; dehydration or hypovolaemia; moderate to severe asthma with nasal polyp disease; known aspirin or NSAID allergy; or history of gastrointestinal ulceration or bleeding
Opioids, e.g. codeine, morphine	• Used for treating moderate to severe pain. Come in different levels of potency and efficacy, referred to as weak opioids (for example, codeine) or strong opioids (for example, morphine, hydromorphone). • Can be given in reduced doses without loss of analgesic effect when used in combination with non-opioids such as paracetamol and NSAIDs. • Have no ceiling dose for severe pain with dosing only limited by adverse effects. • For acute pain management, one opioid is not superior over others but some opioids are better tolerated by some patients thus they may benefit from changing to another opioid if they have adverse effects (ANZCA 2005).	• All opioids bind to opioid receptors located in the peripheral nervous system, central nervous system and spinal cord. • Opioid receptors are distributed variably in the CNS with higher concentrations of receptors in areas most involved with nociception, for example, the cerebral cortex, amygdala, thalamus and spinal cord. • Opioids have the following side effects: respiratory depression; sedation; nausea and vomiting; constipation; miosis (pupil constriction); euphoria; dysphoria; pruritus; and urinary retention.

et al 1999, McDonald & Cooper 2001, Australian and New Zealand College of Anaesthetists and Faculty of Pain Medicine (ANZCA) 2005).

Children require a detailed explanation on how the lockout system works, which is a built-in safety device designed to prevent children from receiving an overdose of opioid when using PCA. PCA is usually commenced intraoperatively and the most common opioid used is morphine. PCA can be used in combination with a background infusion of the opioid to improve the analgesia in children with high opioid requirements. Children receiving PCA should be monitored closely and have hourly observations of (Dowden 2009b):

- pulse rate
- respiratory rate
- the volume delivered
- oxygen saturation
- pain score
- sedation score
- incidents of nausea and vomiting.

It is important that the child's parents also understand the concept of PCA, so they can support their child in its use and understand that they must not press the button for the child.

Activity

Read Dowden (2009b) for more information about dosing regimens for PCAs.

Nurse-controlled analgesia

Nurse-controlled analgesia (NCA) can be used in children's settings and is essentially a morphine infusion with the ability to administer controlled boluses of the drug at times of increased pain. To prevent an overdose of morphine, a longer lockout time is employed than when using PCA. Nurses should consult the child and parents about the need for extra analgesia but it is the responsibility of the nurse to press the button to administer the drug. The same observations are carried out as when using PCA.

Epidural anaesthesia/analgesia

Epidural analgesia is produced by injecting or infusing a local anaesthetic agent and/or an opioid into the epidural space. The effect of the epidural is related to the drugs infused – local anaesthetic agents (commonly bupivacaine) block nerve function at the site of the catheter which usually corresponds to the wound site, and opioid analgesics (commonly fentanyl or morphine) block opioid receptor sites within the spiral horn (Ochsenreither 1997). Local anaesthetic agents may be given alone, usually as a single dose, typically into the caudal epidural space in theatre following surgical procedures below the umbilical region in children (Howard 2003). Following major surgery a continuous infusion of a local anaesthetic agent and an opioid is an excellent method for ensuring effective pain relief. The combination of local anaesthetic agents and opioids has a synergistic effect, enabling a reduction in drug dosages and concentrations resulting in minimal side effects while achieving a good level of analgesia (Al-Shaikh 1997, Jacques 1994, Ochsenreither 1997). However, epidural analgesia is not without risks and the child's care must be managed by suitably skilled and experienced staff. Table 17.9 outlines the hourly observations required when caring for a child with an epidural.

Seminar discussion topic

Heidi is a third year nursing student undertaking a specialist placement on a high-dependency surgical ward. She is enjoying her placement and has been learning to care for children with complex surgical needs, particularly enhancing her practical skills in relation to managing acute pain in children and the use of complex analgesia systems.

Heidi has been caring for Luke, 9 months old, who has undergone major bowel resection for Hirschsprung's disease. Luke had initial complications due to a delayed paralytic ileus and abdominal distension.

Heidi felt able to care for Luke in relation to ensuring all physical needs were met and manage his epidural analgesia. However she found it difficult to assess Luke's pain and often felt that because he had an epidural infusion of morphine that staff felt this was dealing adequately with any pain experienced:

- What issues do you think are important to discuss in relation to this scenario within Heidi's learning set?

Subcutaneous analgesia

When it is not possible to use PCA or epidurals, a catheter can be inserted subcutaneously at the time of the operation, enabling intermittent boluses of opioid analgesia to be administered without having to give an intramuscular injection. It is important to check the needle site regularly for signs of infection or displacement.

Table 17.9 Hourly observations required when a child has an epidural infusion

Observation	Rationale
Pain intensity	To ensure effective pain relief is being provided
Pulse	May increase if child's pain is not adequately controlled
Respiratory rate and oxygen saturation levels	To detect respiratory depression (potential problem with opioids) To detect rostral spread of local anaesthetic which would cause respiratory failure
Temperature	Epidural catheters pose a potential infection risk
Blood pressure	Opioids and local anaesthetics can potentially cause vasodilatation and hypotension – this is uncommon in children younger than 8 years
Level of block	To ensure the block is not unilateral or too high An ice cube can be used to assess the level and extent of the motor block by detecting loss of cold sensation The point at which the child perceives cold sensation is the level of the block
Sensation	Indicates the level of the block
Motor movement	Tested alongside the level of the block
Pressure areas	Indicates any problems with mobility Motor paralysis indicates excessive local anaesthetic
Site of epidural	To check for leakage and inflammation
Sedation	A possible side effect of opioids
Side effects of drugs	Nausea and vomiting Pruritis Urine retention Local anaesthetic toxicity – oral tingling followed by a rapid decrease in blood pressure, confusion and fitting
Volume infused (used)	To ensure that the epidural infusion is running as prescribed
Patency of IV cannula	To ensure intravenous access is available to give antidote if required

Discontinuing advanced analgesia systems

The reduction of advanced analgesia methods and transition to oral medication must be carefully planned. It is important to ensure that oral pain relief is prescribed and administered before the effective of the intravenous/subcutaneous medication has worn off. The aim of pain management is to maintain children in a pain-free state rather than waiting for them to be in pain before administering analgesia.

Misconceptions relating to analgesic drugs

Several misconceptions about pain in children exist; there are many and varied reasons for this. Some of these are due to a lack of knowledge, inaccurate education or a poor understanding of the similarities and differences between children and adults (Dowden 2009a). The key misconceptions about the use of analgesic drugs for children are outlined in Table 17.10.

Addiction, dependence and tolerance

Confusion exists among many nurses about tolerance and physical dependence and the terminology relating to substance abuse (ANZCA 2005, Charlton 2005). Unfortunately this misinformation is passed on to colleagues, patients and their families, leading to further confusion, unnecessary anxiety and sub-optimal pain management (ANZCA 2005). To diminish confusion and encourage uniformity of practice a number of lead clinical organisations including the American Pain Society, the American Academy of Pain Medicine and the American Society of Addiction Medicine developed consensus statements and agreed definitions. ANZCA (2005) outlines a summary of these statements and definitions (Table 17.11).

Fears of addiction related to the use of opioids for severe and short-term pain are unsupported with the incidence of addiction considered to be very low (<1%) (Ballantyne & LaForge 2007, Bryant et al 2003, Jovey et al 2003). However, signs of both tolerance and physical dependence can occur in patients following administration of opioids and other drugs (for example, benzodiazepines and other sedative agents) for more than 5–10 days (Yaster et al 1997).

WWW

The American Pain Society has also defined addiction see:

- www.ampainsoc.org/advocacy/opioids2.htm

Table 17.10 Misconceptions about the use of analgesic drugs for children (Charlton 2005)

Misconception	Facts
All children are sensitive to analgesic drugs	Infants and children require the same categories of analgesic drugs as adults, however age-appropriate dosing must be considered
Children are at greater risk (than adults) of addiction from opioids	The fear of opioid addiction in children has been greatly exaggerated with the incidence <1%
Opioids are not safe to use for infants and children	Opioids are no more dangerous to infants and children than they are to adults The risk of respiratory depression is no greater for infants and children provided the dose is appropriate

Table 17.11 Definitions of opioid terminology (ANZCA 2005)

Tolerance	Decreased effectiveness of a drug over time, thus a higher dose of the drug is needed to achieve the same effect. Tolerance develops to desired (*analgesia*) and undesired (*sedation, itch, etc.*) effects of opioids at different rates.
Physical dependence	A physiological response to the abrupt discontinuation (or dose reduction or reversal) of a drug that leads to a withdrawal (abstinence) syndrome.
Addiction	Psychological dependence on drugs with drug seeking and drug using behaviour that is characterised by cravings, compulsion, loss of control and lack of concern for social or health consequences.
Withdrawal syndrome	A cluster of physiological signs and symptoms that occur following the abrupt discontinuation of an opioid.

Non-drug methods

Activity

Which non-drug methods of pain relief do you use/have you seen used?

With reference to the gate control theory explain how these pain relief methods work.

Several non-drug pain-relieving strategies are available and should be used in conjunction with analgesic drugs. Table 17.12 summarises the research regarding some of the non-drug methods used to manage acute pain in children. The skills of the multidisciplinary team are important; play therapists and clinical psychologists, in particular, have an important role when using non-drug methods.

Parents can identify their children's pain behaviours (Chambers et al 1996, Finley et al 1996, Reid et al 1995, Watt-Watson et al 1990, Wilson & Doyle 1996). However, many parents believe that nurses will also know if their child is in pain and therefore leave pain management to them (Woodgate & Kristjanson 1996). Twycross (2007) also found little evidence of nurses engaging parents in their child's pain management.

Parents can help with a number of distraction activities but may need guidance from healthcare professionals as to how they can best help their child. Children describe parental presence as being excellent distracters from *things which hurt* (Polkki et al 2003, Woodgate & Kristjanson 1996). The results of several studies indicate that when parents are taught how to distract their child during a painful procedure children experience less anxiety and pain (Greenberg et al 1999, Kleiber et al 2001, Manimala et al 2000, Walker et al 2006). Teaching parents distraction techniques for their child has a two-fold effect – it reduces parental feelings of helplessness and benefits the child by reducing their distress. Parents need to be helped to select a distraction technique that is appropriate for their child.

Table 17.12 Non-drug methods pain-relief for acute pain in children: summary of research evidence

Method	Comments
Distraction	Distraction appears to be useful tool for reducing children's pain (Dahlquist et al 2002a, b, Sinha et al 2006, Tanabe et al 2002, Vessey et al 1994)
	A Cochrane review of both cognitive-behavioural and cognitive interventions for the management of needle-related pain found distraction to be particularly effective (Uman et al 2006)
Heat and cold	In Ebner's (1996) study cold therapy was not found to be significant in reducing procedural pain
	A Cochrane review included nine studies, and found that heat wraps can reduce back pain in adults, but that the evidence for cold treatment is sparse. There is moderate evidence that heat provides a short-term reduction in pain, but there are no good data showing whether or not cold therapy has any effect (French et al 2006)
	Anecdotal evidence suggests that the use of heat and cold are useful:
	• McCarthy et al (2003) state that the application of superficial cold or heat is used as part of physiotherapy when pain is present. Cold is recommended within the first 24–48 hours of the injury to prevent swelling while heat is usually used after the first 24–48 hours
	• Dampier & Shapiro (2003) also state that heat packs and hot baths are helpful for sickle cell disease pain but that cold usually makes the pain associated with sickle cell disease worse
Hypnosis (Imagery)	Hypnosis has been found to reduce:
	• Pain associated with bone marrow aspirations and lumbar punctures in children with cancer than non-hypnotic techniques (Zeltzer & LeBaron 1982)
	• Postoperative pain (Lambert 1996, Huth et al 2004)
	• Recurrent abdominal pain (Ball et al 2003, Weydert et al 2006)
	• Distress behaviours demonstrated during the cardiac catheterisation (Pederson 1995)
	A systematic review of eight studies ($n = 313$) by Richardson et al (2006) compared hypnosis with other cognitive and cognitive behavioural interventions for the management of procedural pain in children with cancer. There was some evidence of effectiveness
	A systematic review carried out by Uman et al (2006) examining psychological interventions for the management of needle-related pain in children found hypnosis to be an effective method
Relaxation	Relaxation appears to be an effective pain relieving intervention for recurrent migraine and tension headaches (Holden et al 1999, Larsson et al 2005, Eccleston et al 2006)
	Relaxation also appears to be effective in reducing the pain associated with venepuncture (Powers 1999)
Transcutaneous Electric Nerve Stimulation (TENS)	Only one study has examined the use of TENS to relieve children's pain; TENS was found to be effective for venepuncture pain in a blinded placebo controlled trial of school children ($n = 514$) aged 5–17 years (Lander & Fowler-Kerry 1993)

Parents also need information about managing their child's pain at home following discharge (Howard 2003, RCN 2009). This should include:

- the site and intensity of the pain
- the expected duration of the pain
- how much analgesia to give and when
- that they can give more than one analgesic drug
- possible side effects of analgesia prescribed
- how to obtain further advice or help.

Activity

Read Twycross (2009c) for a review of the research that has been undertaken in relation to using non-drug methods to relieve pain in children.

Communication

Communicating with the child and their parent is an essential part of pain management. Despite this Twycross (2007) found that nurses rarely initiated communications about pain with parents and children. Ineffective communication results in children's pain not being managed effectively and affects the quality of their child's pain relief. A child's self-report of pain is considered the gold standard. Nurses should therefore communicate with the child about their pain whenever possible.

Reflect on your practice

How often do you discuss children's pain management with their parents?

Do you prepare parents for managing their child's pain after discharge?

Reflect on your practice

How often do you communicate with children about their pain and how it can/will be management?

Documentation

Regular assessment and documentation facilitates effective treatment and communication among members of the healthcare team, patient and family (Stinson 2009). Pain is considered to be the *fifth vital sign* and, therefore, should be assessed and documented along with the other vital signs. Putting mechanisms in place that make documentation of pain easy for clinicians helps ensure consistent documentation. Standardised forms/tools for the documentation of pain allow for the initial assessment and ongoing re-assessment (for example, admission assessment forms, vital signs chart). They can also be used for the documentation of the efficacy of pain relieving interventions. Including pain intensity as part of the vital signs record allows for pain to be assessed, documented and taken as seriously as other vital signs (Stinson 2009).

Reflect on your practice

Think about the documentation about pain management you have seen in the clinical area.

- How thorough is it?
- What is included?

Pain management: an ethical imperative

The United Nations, in its Declaration on the Rights of the Child, states that:

> children should in all circumstances be among the first to receive protection and relief, and should be protected from all forms of neglect, cruelty and exploitation
>
> (United Nations 1989)

This principle can be applied to the management of pain, particularly as good practice guidelines are available (American Pain Society 2001, ANZCA 2007, Howard et al 2008). Further the UNICEF Child Friendly Hospital Initiative highlights the importance of pain management, stating that:

> A team will be established in the hospital whose remit is to establish standards and guidance in the control of pain and discomfort (psychological as well as physical) in children
>
> (UNICEF 1999 p. 8)

Part 2: The management of chronic pain in children

Alison Twycross Jennifer Stinson

Introduction

This section provides an overview of chronic pain in children. It defines and describes the main types of chronic pain experienced by children and discusses the impact of this on the child and family. Key factors that have been found to influence the development of chronic pain are outlined. The principles of treatment are outlined and the role of the multidisciplinary team in the management of children's chronic pain is described.

What is chronic pain?

Chronic pain is a term used to describe persistent or recurrent pain. Chronic pain in children and adolescents is commonly defined as any prolonged pain that lasts a minimum of 3 months, or any recurrent pain that occurs at least three times throughout a minimum period of 3 months (Van Der Kerkhof & van Dijk 2006). The differences between acute and chronic pain are set out in Table 17.13.

www

Go to:

- http://www.iasp-pain.org/AM/Template.cfm?Section=General_Resource_Links&Template=/CM/HTMLDisplay.cfm&ContentID=3058

Look up the definitions of the following terms:

- Neuropathic pain
- Allodynia
- Dysesthesia
- Hyperalgesia
- Hyperpathia
- Paresthesia

How common is chronic pain in children?

Activity 18

In your learning groups think about how common you think chronic pain is in children and young people.

Once you have thought about this read Van Der Kerkhof & van Dijk's (2006) paper and make some notes about the findings of the study.

Little is known about the epidemiology of chronic pain in children (McGrath 1999, Van Den Kerkhof & van Dijk 2006). Chronic pain has been reported in children as young as 3 years, but is most prevalent in early teens and is more commonly

Table 17.13 Differences between acute and chronic pain

Characteristic	Acute pain	Chronic pain
Cause	Usually single obvious cause (e.g. tissue damage due to surgery)	Usually multiple causative or triggering factors Neuronal or CNS abnormality (plasticity, sensitisation)
Type	Nociceptive and or neuropathic	Nociceptive, neuropathic or mixed; psychosocial factors
Purpose	Protective; activation of sympathetic nervous system	No protective function; rarely accompanied by signs of activation of sympathetic nervous system
Duration	Short-lived (days to weeks)	Long lasting (> 3 months) or recurring beyond time of normal healing, may be associated with chronic disease
Pain intensity	Usually proportionate to severity of injury	Often out of proportion to objective physical findings
Treatment	Usually easy to treat with single modalities (pharmacological or physical)	More difficult to treat, requiring multidisciplinary, multi-modal treatment approach
Outcome	Expected to resolve with healing	Pain persists in significant proportion (30–62%); with smaller proportion developing pain associated disability syndrome

reported by girls (Lynch et al 2007, Perquin et al 2000, Wilder et al 1992).

Causes of chronic pain

WWW

A Position Statement from the American Pain Society on Paediatric Chronic Pain can be found at:

- http://www.ampainsoc.org/advocacy/pediatric.htm

Activity

In your learning groups consider what may cause chronic pain.

Chronic pain may be part of a chronic medical condition, develop following surgery, illness or injury, or have no obvious cause (Table 17.14). Chronic pain conditions can be nociceptive, neuropathic, or mixed (combination of nociceptive and neuropathic) in nature and/or associated with psychological factors.

Table 17.14 Types of chronic pain in children (Stinson & Bruce 2009)

Category/Aetiology	Examples
Disease-related pain	Sickle cell disease Haemophilia Epidermolysis bullosa Osteogenesis imperfecta Rheumatological conditions Post-viral (e.g. herpes) Cancer and treatment-related pain (e.g. chemotherapy, radiotherapy)
Injury-related pain	Burns Sprains, fractures Post-surgery (e.g. phantom-limb pain, scar tissue, nerve damage) Complex regional pain syndrome (e.g. post-fracture or sprain)
Non-specific (unexplained/ chronic benign pain)	Headache Recurrent abdominal pain Complex regional pain syndrome Low back pain Widespread chronic pain Chronic fatigue syndrome
Somatoform disorders	Pain disorder Conversion disorder

Common chronic pain conditions in children and adolescents

The common chronic pain conditions are outlined in Table 17.15. The lack of an obvious cause for abdominal pain can result in considerable distress for the child and family and it is essential that children are not subjected to unnecessary tests. The signs and symptoms that may indicate underlying pathology and thus the need for further investigation include:

- weight loss
- pain that wakes the child at night
- abdominal pain that is not near the umbilicus
- fever
- dysuria
- abnormal stools
- abnormal blood test results.

(Scharff et al 2003)

WWW

Headaches have been classified by the International Headache Society:

- http://216.25.100.131/ihscommon/guidelines/pdfs/ihc_II_main_no_print.pdf

Table 17.15 Chronic pain conditions in children and young people

Chronic pain condition	Description
Headache	• The most common types in children are migraine with and without aura and tension-type headaches. Migraine headaches may transform into tension-type headaches and vice versa; and these two types may co-exist in the early phases (Grazzi 2004). • Chronic daily headache is a relatively new diagnostic category to categorise those individuals who do not meet the criteria for episodic tension or migraine headaches. It is defined as an almost continual headache (>15 days per month) in the absence of a serious underlying medical condition (McGrath 2006). • Headaches are the most commonly reported chronic pain in children. For the most common types of headaches in children, the actual causes are not known. It is important to rule out serious neurological or neurosurgical causes for the headaches (for example, cerebral haemorrhage, shunt malfunction) prior to implementing chronic pain management strategies (Stinson & Bruce 2009).
Chronic abdominal pain	• Defined as three or more bouts of abdominal pain and associated gastrointestinal symptoms over a period of at least 3 months that are severe enough to interfere with normal activities. • Chronic abdominal pain is common in childhood, usually affecting children 5–15 years of age. • Females appear to be affected slightly more than males. • The majority of children with chronic abdominal pain have no obvious underlying cause for their pain and therefore are classified as having functional abdominal pain (Jones & Walker 2006).
Functional abdominal pain (FAP)	• Defined as abdominal pain without obvious pathology and includes functional dyspepsia (indigestion), irritable bowel syndrome, abdominal migraine and functional abdominal pain syndrome (Subcommittee on Chronic Abdominal Pain 2005). • Until recently the term recurrent abdominal pain (RAP) was used to describe this condition, but is now considered outdated.
Musculoskeletal pain	• Includes complex regional pain syndrome, juvenile primary fibromyalgia, idiopathic chronic limp (growing pains) and back pain syndromes (Connelly & Schanberg 2006, El-Metwally et al 2005). • Juvenile primary fibromyalgia syndrome (JPFS) is characterised by diffuse chronic musculoskeletal pain with numerous tender points on palpation in the absence of an underlying condition. Aetiology is unknown and it is more common in females during adolescence. Other common symptoms include sleep disturbances, chronic anxiety and/or tension, fatigue and abdominal pain (Anthony & Schanberg 2001). • Idiopathic chronic limb pain in children is often referred to as growing pains. Growing pains typically present as recurrent bilateral non-articular pain in the lower extremities that occur late in the day or at night. In severe cases, pain can occur daily and have a significant impact on the child and family (Connelly & Schanberg 2006). • Chronic low back pain in children was thought to be relatively uncommon. However, recent epidemiological evidence suggests that it is an important (that is, has a marked impact on daily activities) and increasing problem in school-age children and adolescents (Bejia et al 2005, Watson et al 2002).

Neuropathic pain (see Table 17.16 for additional definitions of key terms related to neuropathic pain)	• Neuropathic pain is often described as burning, stabbing or shooting and may be spontaneous or evoked (that is, having a trigger factor such as touch or change in temperature).
	• Neuropathic pain conditions may also be characterised by sensory disturbances such as allodynia, dysaesthesia, hyperalgesia, hyperpathia and paraesthesia.
	• There may also be motor abnormalities such as tremor, spasms, atrophy, dystonia and weakness and autonomic disturbances such as cyanosis, erythema, mottling, increased sweating, swelling and poor capillary refill (Berde et al 2003, Johnson 2004).
	• Examples of neuropathic pain in children include:
	  • complex regional pain syndrome (CRPS)
	  • phantom-limb pain
	• Children with cancer also experience neuropathic pain, which may either be due to the cancer treatment (for example, chemotherapy or radiotherapy) or the underlying cancer itself (for example, due to the tumour impinging on a spinal nerve root).
	• Common types of neuropathic pain conditions are described below.

Activity

Read Stinson & Bruce (2009) for more information about the types of paediatric migraine.

Activity

Read Stinson & Bruce (2009) for more information about the different types of functional abdominal pain.

Common types of neuropathic pain conditions

Complex regional pain syndrome

WWW

- For a definition of CRPS go to: http://www.ninds.nih.gov/disorders/reflex_sympathetic_dystrophy/reflex_sympathetic_dystrophy.htm

Table 17.16 Key terms related to neuropathic pain

Term	Definition
Allodynia	Severe pain triggered by innocuous (non-harmful) stimuli such as stroking, the touch of clothing on the affected area, or changes in temperature.
Dysaesthesia	An unpleasant abnormal sensation, which may be spontaneous or evoked (e.g. shooting, tingling sensations).
Hyperalgesia	A reduced threshold to pain.
Hyperpathia	Increased pain from stimuli which are normally painful (e.g. increased sharpness from a pin prick).
Paraesthesia	An abnormal sensation, which may be spontaneous or evoked (e.g. pins and needles).

Complex regional pain syndrome (CRPS) is a syndrome of chronic neuropathic pain associated with dysfunction of the autonomic nervous system. CRPS is further classified into two types:

- Type 1 manifests following injury without a definable nerve lesion
- Type 2 occurs following damage to an identifiable nerve.

The pathophysiology of CRPS is not well understood, however it is believed to be a systemic disease involving both the central and peripheral nervous systems (Jäing & Baron 2004). Both types of CRPS are also known by other names; CRPS I is referred to as reflex sympathetic dystrophy (RSD), while CRPS II is referred to as causalgia.

The incidence of CRPS in children is not known but it is more common in females in later childhood and adolescence. CRPS in children is seen more commonly in the lower limbs and often follows a minor injury or traumatic event (Wilder et al 1992, Dangel 1998, Low et al 2007). The pain is persistent and is disproportionate to the initiating injury (Connelly & Schanberg 2006).

Children with CRPS have a better prognosis than adults (Berde et al 2003). Most children will have complete resolution of symptoms with non-invasive treatment, however a small proportion will continue to have pain or relapse (20%) (Low et al 2007). Early recognition and treatment are associated with the best chance of good outcomes.

Evidence-based practice

A clinical diagnosis of CRPS requires:

- the report of at least two symptoms of persistent neuropathic pain for example:
  - burning
  - dysesthesia
  - paresthesia
  - mechanical allodynia
  - hyperalgesia to cold
- at least two physical signs of autonomic nervous system dysfunction, for example:
  - cyanosis
  - mottling
  - oedema
  - cooling of the affected area
  - hyperhydrosis (excessive sweating)

(Low et al 2007)

Phantom-limb pain

Congenital or traumatic (accidental or surgical) loss of a limb can result in sensations in the missing limb, some that are painful (*phantom-limb pain*, described as burning, cramping, shooting) and some that are not (*phantom-limb sensation*, described as tingling or itchy). In addition, there can also be pain in the stump (*stump pain*). These sensations tend to begin within days of the amputation and they usually decrease in frequency and duration over time and are more common in children who have experienced traumatic amputations (Wilkins et al 1998).

Factors triggering and maintaining chronic pain

There are many factors that influence a child's perception of and ways they behave when in pain. Many studies have provided evidence that a few biological, physical, psychological, family and social factors play an important role in chronic pain in children (Fig. 17.6). However, little is known about which factors or combination of factors predispose children to chronic pain and disability.

The *coping styles* of the child, parents and family have a huge influence on chronic pain. Maladaptive or ineffective coping styles have been linked to anxiety, depression and functional disability in children with chronic pain (Eccleston et al 2004, Kashikar-Zuck et al 2001, 2002). Pain catastrophising, or characterisations of pain as awful, horrible and unbearable, is recognised as an important factor in chronic pain in children and adults (Sullivan & Adams 2006). Pain catastrophising is a multidimensional construct that includes:

- rumination (excessive focus on pain sensations)
- magnification (exaggerating the threat value of pain sensations)
- helplessness (perceiving oneself as unable to cope with pain symptoms).

Studies have found associations between catastrophising and increased pain, disability, depression and emotional distress in children and adolescents with chronic pain (Crombez et al 2003, Kashikar-Zuck 2001, Lynch et al 2007, Merlijn 2006, Vervoort et al 2006). Education of the child and family is essential to reduce fear and misconceptions related to chronic pain and to teach appropriate coping strategies (relaxation and cognitive restructuring).

Gender differences are apparent in relation to chronic pain in older school age children and adolescents. Chronic pain is more common in girls, who also report more intense, more frequent and more prolonged pain than boys (Hunfield et al 2001, Martin et al 2007 Perquin et al 2000). Differences in coping styles also exist, with girls using more emotional coping styles such as catastrophising (Keogh & Eccleston 2006, Lynch et al 2007). Differences in self-reported trigger factors are also present between boys and girls (Roth-Isigkeit et al 2005).

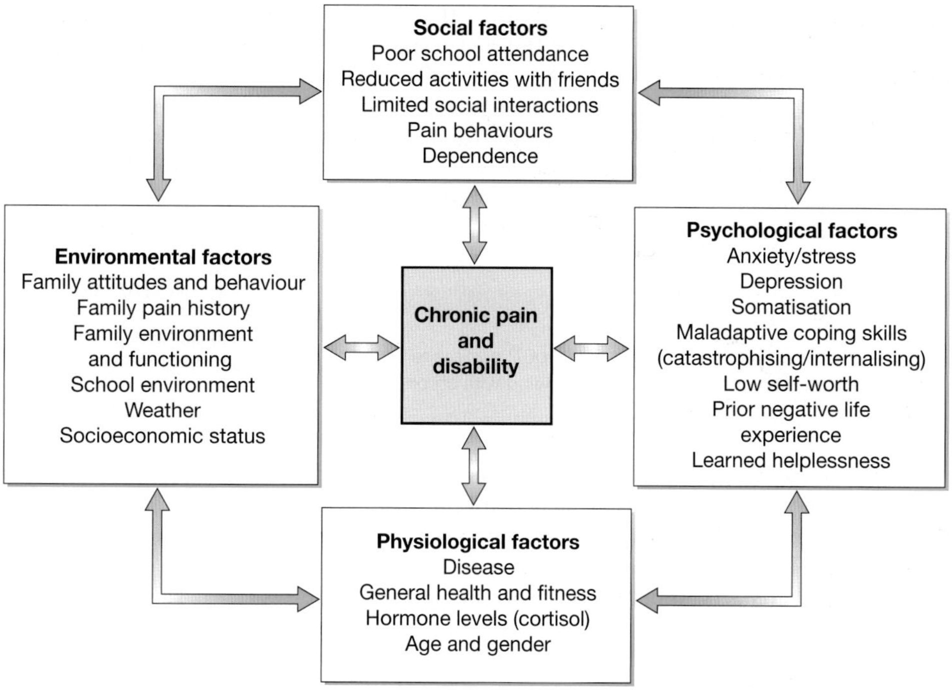

Fig. 17.6 • Factors associated with children's chronic pain (Stinson & Bruce 2009).

Due to lack of knowledge of the psychosocial aspects and complexity of chronic pain, children with unexplained or persistent chronic pain are sometimes viewed as malingerers or attention seekers, or made to feel that the problem is *all in their head*. This can further exacerbate the pain and increases the family's distrust of health professionals and leads them to doubt healthcare professionals' ability to diagnose and treat the pain.

Once serious or treatable physical causes are ruled out, most children and parents need and are willing to accept an explanation based on both physical (sensitisation of pain receptors) and psychological (stress or worry) factors. This helps prevent or reduce the continued search for the cause of the pain (von Baeyer 2006).

Pain-related disability

Activity

What percentage of children with chronic pain do you think are disabled by it?

What factors might contribute to the level of disability experienced?

Many children and adolescents experience persistent or recurrent pain; 30–40% of children with chronic pain develop pain-related disability (Gauntlett-Gilbert & Eccleston 2007, Scharff et al 2005). Scharff et al (2005) identified three levels of disability in children and adolescents with chronic pain:

- 30% of the sample were classified as highly distressed (high anxiety, depression and escape/avoidance) and disabled
- 18% were in the moderately distressed/disabled group
- 52% of the sample were comparatively well functioning and not distressed.

Biological, psychological, social, cultural and developmental factors can impact pain-related functioning (Bursch et al 2006b). Miró et al (2007) explored the factors that predict pain-related disability in children and found that the factors that had the greatest influence on long-term disability were:

- children's self-concept as being disabled
- a hesitance to perform exercise because of fear of potential injury
- children's catastrophising.

A recent study suggests that higher levels of functional disability are associated with greater pain intensity and depression (Gauntlett-Gibert & Eccleston 2007). Perceptions of self-worth seem to be important in reducing the relationship between pain and functional disability in children with chronic pain (Guite et al 2007).

Reflect on your practice

What can nurses do to prevent the development of pain-related disability in children?

The impact of chronic pain on the child and family

Activity

Think about the effect experiencing chronic pain would have on a child's life and on their family.

Chronic pain negatively impacts all aspects of the child's life (Hunfield et al 2001, Merlijn et al 2006) and results in frequent use of healthcare services (Perquin et al 2001, Sleed et al 2005). It is associated with significant levels of functional impairment in areas such as academic performance and school attendance, emotional functioning, sleep disturbance, peer and social functioning, and parental burden (parenting stress and dysfunctional family roles).

Activity

Read Carter et al (2002) and Castle et al (2007) and make notes about how children and families describe living with chronic pain.

In Roth-Isigkeit et al's (2005) study more than two-thirds of the sample reported restrictions in activities of daily living due to pain and 30–40% reported moderate effects of their pain on school attendance, participation in hobbies, maintenance of social contacts, appetite and sleep, and increased use of healthcare services due to pain. Further, in Konijnenberg et al's (2005) study 72% of children suffered impairment in sport activities, 51% had school absenteeism, 40% experienced restrictions in social functioning, and 34% had problems with sleep. Depression, emotional distress and anxiety are common in children with chronic pain (Kashikar-Zuck et al 2001, Konijnenberg et al 2006, Merlijn et al 2003).

Chronic pain also has an effect on families. Hunfield et al (2002) found that the pain had a mild impact on children and their families. However, pain showed a negative impact on family life in terms of restrictions in social activities and personal strain. Hunfield et al (2001) also found that pain had a negative impact on quality of life (physical and psychological functioning) and negatively impacted family life (restrictions in mother's social life). Family functioning can be affected and parents report a life dominated by uncertainty, fear, distress and loss (Eccelston 2005, Jordan et al 2007). Parents report marital and financial problems and experience feelings of helplessness, despair and depression (Eccleston et al 2004, Hunfield et al 2001).

Activity

See Twycross (2009a) for more information about the factors that affect children's perception of pain.

Management of chronic pain

Pain assessment

Activity

Think about what needs to be considered when managing chronic pain in children and what strategies can be used to manage pain.

The first stage of managing chronic pain is to do a thorough pain history. The questions you need to consider asking are outlined in Table 17.17. Pain diaries are another way to track pain in children with recurrent or chronic pain. While paper-based diaries have been used in clinical and research practice for decades, they are prone to recall biases and poor compliance. More recently, real-time data collection methods using electronic hand-held diaries have been developed for children with recurrent and chronic pain (Palermo et al 2004, Stinson et al 2005, 2008).

Activity

Read Stinson (2009) for more information about validated pain assessment tools available for use with children.

Pain-relieving interventions

The treatment of chronic pain involves the use of a range of psychological, physical and pharmacological interventions (Table 17.18). Pain is a bio-psycho-social phenomenon and hence a multidisciplinary, multimodal approach that incorporates the 3 P's (physical, psychological and pharmacological interventions) is likely to be most effective. Treatment should also address pain-related disability with the goal of maximising functioning and improving quality of life. This approach includes specific treatment targeting possible underlying pain mechanisms, as well as symptom-focused management addressing pain, sleep disturbance, anxiety, or depressive feelings.

The main goal of treatment is to return the child to a functional state that will enable them to participate in daily activities and return to school, rather than focusing solely on reducing or controlling the pain. The general goals of treatment are:

1. increasing independent function in terms of activities of daily living, school, social and physical activities
2. facilitating adaptive problem solving, communication and coping skills
3. reducing specific symptoms, deficits, or problems revealed in a comprehensive bio-psycho-social assessment (for example, anxiety, depression, poor sleep)
4. helping children and their families to understand the nature of pain, the pain condition, and its treatment from a holistic perspective.

(Stinson 2006)

A child's initial consultation includes either a joint interview and physical examination or separate interviews with each healthcare professional. Comprehensive physical and psychosocial assessments may last a few hours to a full day, depending on the child's previous diagnostic tests and the assessment measures used (for example, standardised sensory testing, questionnaires). The team then meets to formulate the child's treatment plan (Fig. 17.7).

Decisions regarding the most appropriate treatments should be individualised and based on the assessment of the child. Interventions should be aimed at treating any trigger factors, as well as the underlying cause(s) of the pain wherever possible. Many children and adolescents with chronic

Table 17.17 Pain history questions for children with chronic pain and their parents/carers (Stinson & Bruce 2009)

Description of pain	**Type of pain** – Is the pain acute (e.g. medical procedures, postoperative pain, accidental injury), recurrent (e.g. headaches) or chronic (e.g. juvenile idiopathic arthritis)? **Onset of pain** – When did the pain begin? What were you doing before the pain began? Was there any initiating injury, trauma or stressors? **Duration** – How long has the pain been present (e.g. hours/days/weeks/months)? **Frequency** – How often is pain present? Is the pain always there or is it intermittent? Does it come and go? **Location** • Where is the pain located? Can you point to the part of the body that hurts? (Body outlines can be used to help children indicate where they hurt) • Children greater than 3 to 4 years of age can mark an 'X' to indicate painful areas, shade in with crayons areas of pain or choose different colours to represent varying degrees of pain intensity • Does the pain go anywhere else (e.g. radiates up or down from the site that hurts)? Pain radiation can also be indicated on body diagrams **Intensity** • What is your pain intensity at rest? What is your pain intensity with activity? (Use an appropriate pain assessment tool) • Over the past week what is the least pain you have had? What is the worst pain you have had? • What is your usual level of pain? **Quality of pain** • School-age children can communicate about pain in more abstract terms • Describe the quality of your pain (e.g. word descriptors such as sharp, dull, achy, stabbing, burning, shooting or throbbing)? • Word descriptors can provide information on whether the pain is nociceptive or neuropathic in nature or a combination of both
Associated symptoms	• Are there any other symptoms that go along with or occur just before or immediately after the pain (e.g. nausea, vomiting, light-headedness, tiredness, diarrhoea, or difficulty ambulating)? • Are there any changes in the colour or temperature of the affected extremity or painful area? (These changes most often occur in children with conditions such as complex regional pain syndromes)
Temporal or seasonal variations	• Is the pain affected by changes in seasons or weather? • Does the pain occur at certain times of the day (e.g. after eating or going to the toilet)?
Impact on daily living	• Has the pain led to changes in daily activities and/or behaviours (e.g. sleep disturbances, change in appetite, decreased physical activity, change in mood, or a decrease in social interactions or school attendance)? • What level would the pain need to be so that you could do all your normal activities (e.g. tolerability)? What level would the pain need to be so that you won't be bothered by it? (Rated on similar scale as pain intensity) • What brings on the pain or makes the pain worse (e.g. movement, deep breathing and coughing, stress etc.)?
Pain relief measures	• What has helped to make the pain better? • What medication have you taken to relieve your pain? If so what was the medication and did it help? Where there any side effects? • It is important to also ask about the use of physical, psychological and complementary and alternative treatments tried and how effective these methods were in relieving pain (See Chapter 5) • The degree of pain relief or intensity of pain after a pain relieving treatment/intervention should be determined.

pain can be managed effectively by their family doctor. However, referral to a multidisciplinary paediatric pain programme should be considered for children with complex or ongoing chronic pain.

Evidence-based practice

Key points in the management of chronic pain are implementing:

- a multidisciplinary approach
- a rehabilitation approach
- using multimodal treatments
- early treatment associated with best outcomes

(APS Position Statement on Chronic Pain, Kashikar-Zuck 2006, Stinson 2006)

Non-drug methods of pain relief

Pharmacological strategies are often insufficient in alleviating pain and increasing functioning. Several non-drug pain-relieving strategies are available. Table 17.19 summarises the research regarding some of the non-drug methods used to manage chronic pain in children. The skills of the multidisciplinary team are important; play therapists and clinical psychologists, in particular, have an important role when using non-drug methods.

Activity

Read Twycross (2009b) for a review of the research that has been undertaken in relation to using non-drug methods to relieve pain in children.

Table 17.18 An overview of interventions for chronic pain management in children (Stinson & Bruce 2009)

Pharmacological interventions	Physical interventions	Psychological interventions
Simple analgesics	Exercise	Education (about pain experience and pain problem)
Opioid analgesics	Thermal stimulation (heat, cold, desensitisation)	Sleep hygiene
Anticonvulsants	Physiotherapy	Relaxation
Antidepressants	Occupational therapy	Biofeedback
Antiarrhythmics (alpha-adrenergic blockers)	Massage	Behavioural therapies
Anxiolytics	TENS	Cognitive therapies
Hypnotics	Acupuncture	Cognitive behavioural therapy (CBT)
Anaesthetic agents	Nerve blocks	Acceptance and commitment therapy (ACT)
Cannabinoids		Family therapies
		Psychotherapy

Evaluate child with chronic pain

Assess sensory characteristics
Conduct medical examination and approriate dignostic tests
Evaluate possible involvement of nococeptive and neuropathic mechanisms
Appraise situational factors contributing to child's pain

Diagnose the primary and secondary causes

Current nociceptive and neuropathis components
Attenuating physical symptoms
Relevance of key cognitive, behavioural and emotional factors

Select appropriate therapies

Drugs
Analgesics
Adjunct analgesics
Anaesthetics

Non-drugs
Psychological
Physical
Behavioural

Implement pain management plan

Provide feedback on causes and contributing factors
Provide rationale for integrated treatment programme
Develop mutually agreed treatment goals
Measure child's pain and functional improvement regularly
Evaluate effectiveness of treatment plan
Revise plan as necessary

Fig. 17.7 • Treatment algorithm for children with chronic pain (adapted from Brown 2006).

Physiotherapy

Chronic pain often leads children to avoid physical activities due to fear of re-injury or because it exacerbates the pain. Lack of muscle use leads to loss of muscle strength, flexibility, endurance and overall de-conditioning. Therefore, physiotherapy is an integral component, and in certain instances (for example, with CRPS) it is the cornerstone of treatment for children with chronic pain (Engel & O'Rourke 2006). Physiotherapy is usually administered on an outpatient basis with the ultimate goal of teaching the child to continue the programme at home. Regular exercise (for example, 20 minutes three times per week) can also help improve sleep, mood, self-esteem and energy levels (McCarthy et al 2003, Engel & O'Rourke 2006, Stinson 2006).

Psychological therapies

There are many psychological therapies available to treat chronic pain in children (Table 17.19). Often these therapies are integrated into a comprehensive cognitive-behavioural therapy (CBT) programme that is directed at identifying and ameliorating trigger factors that affect the child's pain and disability. Such programmes usually include:

- education about the pain
- learning cognitive behavioural pain coping skills (for example, imagery, distraction and relaxation)
- stress management (for example, identifying and coping with stressful situations, using thought stopping, cognitive restructuring, assertiveness and problem solving)
- relapse prevention.

(Hermann 2006)

All patients and their families should be provided with developmentally appropriate information about the nature of pain (i.e. difference between acute and chronic), their specific pain condition, and its treatment from a holistic perspective (pharmacological, physical and psychological strategies). There are several trustworthy websites about chronic pain in children that patients can be directed to (e.g. http://www.aboutkidshealth.ca pain resource centre) as well as books.

A systematic review documented the efficacy of CBT for chronic headache and abdominal pain in children (Eccleston et al 2003b). There is strong evidence that these psychological therapies can be administered without a therapist being physically present (Elgar & McGrath 2003), using alternative models of service delivery such as the Internet (Stinson 2008) or on computer disks (CD-ROMs) (Connelly et al 2006). Biofeedback has also been found to be effective for the treatment

Table 17.19 Non-drug methods pain-relief for chronic pain in children

Method	Comments
Acupuncture	• Acupuncture is a system of ancient medicine, healing and Eastern philosophy originating in China. Acupuncture is based on the theory that energy (Chi) flows through the body along channels known as meridians, which are connected by acupuncture points. If the flow of energy is obstructed, pain results (Kemper & Gardiner 2003, Rusy & Weisman 2000). The energy flow is restored by inserting needles at acupuncture points along the meridians involved, which eliminates or reduces pain (Kemper & Gardiner 2003, Rusy & Weisman 2000) • Acupuncture has been shown to be effective in treating chronic pain in children (Kemper et al 2000, Lin et al 2002, Pintov et al 1997, Zeltzer et al 2002) • A review of the use of acupuncture as a pain relieving intervention for children has been undertaken by Kundu & Berman (2007)
Biofeedback	• Biofeedback involves measuring physiological indicators such as blood pressure, heart rate, skin temperature, sweating and muscle tension and conveying such information to the person to raise awareness and conscious control of the related physiological activities. Types of biofeedback include finger temperature, a-electroencephalography (EEG) biofeedback, muscle electromyography (EMG) and temporal pulse biofeedback (McGrath et al 2003). Each of these methods is used to alert the patient to muscle tension, which allows them to recognise the early signs of tension and implement relaxation techniques • Biofeedback has been shown to be particularly effective in the treatment of headaches (Arndorfer & Allen 2001, Hermann & Blanchard 2002, Scharff et al 2002) • Biofeedback has also been used with children with juvenile rheumatoid arthritis (Lavigne et al 1992) and children with sickle cell disease, who participated (Cozzi et al 1987)
Cognitive behavioural therapy	• Cognitive behavioural therapy aims to improve the way that an individual manages and copes with their pain. The child is taught to use techniques such as distraction, relaxation and biofeedback to help them manage their pain • Several studies have explored the effectiveness of cognitive behavioural therapy (CBT) in the management of children's pain and found it to be effective (Dahlquist et al 1985, Eccleston et al 2003, Jay et al 1987, Jay et al 1991, Liossi & Hatira 1999, Surjala et al 1995) • A Cochrane review exploring the effectiveness of psychological interventions for the management of sickle cell disease pain included three studies. Some evidence for the effectiveness of cognitive behavioural therapy was found. Further research is needed (Anie & Green 2000)
Hypnosis (and guided imagery)*	• Hypnosis involves helping children to focus their attention away from the feared components of a procedure and to focus on an imaginative experience that is viewed as comforting, safe, fun or intriguing (Zeltzer et al 1997) • Hypnosis was found to be significantly better at reducing pain associated with bone marrow aspirations and lumbar punctures in children with cancer than non-hypnotic techniques ($p < 0.05$) (Zeltzer & LeBaron 1982) • Hypnosis has been found to decrease postoperative pain (Lambert 1996, Huth et al 2004) and to reduce anxiety during cardiac catheterisation (Pederson 1995) • A significant reduction in pain was found among children with recurrent abdominal pain who were trained in relaxation and hypnosis (Ball et al 2003, Weydert et al 2006) • A systematic review of eight studies ($n = 313$) by Richardson et al (2006) compared hypnosis with other cognitive and cognitive behavioural interventions for the management of procedural pain in children with cancer. There was some evidence of effectiveness • A systematic review carried out by Uman et al (2006) examining psychological interventions for the management of needle-related pain in children found hypnosis to be an effective method
Massage	• Massage therapy involves manipulation of the body by combining tactile and kinaesthetic stimulation performed in purposeful sequential application (Tsao et al 2006). The precise mechanism of action is not known (Ireland & Olson 2000) • Massage has found to be effective for relieving pain in children with juvenile rheumatoid arthritis (Field et al 1997) and for children with severe burns (Hernandez-Reif et al 2001) An overview about the use of massage therapy in children can be found in Beider et al (2007)
Physiotherapy	• See p. 26–27
Relaxation	• Relaxation appears to be an effective pain relieving intervention for recurrent migraine and tension headaches (Eccleston et al 2006, Holden et al 1999, Larsson et al 2005).

*The terms hypnosis and guided imagery are often used inter-changeably but the methods used within research papers are not always comparable. The reader is advised to check the original papers for the actual method used.

of headaches in children (Hermann & Blanchard 2002) (see Table 17.17).

More recently, acceptance and commitment therapy (ACT) is being adopted as a treatment approach in chronic pain programmes (Wicksell 2007). This approach emphasises the acceptance of or willingness to experience pain and other interfering experiences (fear of pain with activities) rather than trying to control or reduce symptoms. The goal is to achieve functionality even in the presence of interfering pain and distress. There is early evidence of the effectiveness of this approach in children with chronic pain (Wicksell et al 2005, 2007).

Sleep hygiene

Sleep disturbances are common in children with chronic pain (Lewin & Dahl 1999, Palermo & Kiska 2005). Pain can interfere with the quality and quantity of sleep and insufficient sleep can cause daytime sequelae (behavioural and emotional changes) that undermine the coping skills necessary for effective pain management. Therefore, efforts should be directed towards improving the sleep hygiene (good sleep habits) of children with chronic pain.

www

For specific strategies to improve sleep hygiene see the National Sleep Foundation at:

- http://www.sleepfoundation.org

Pharmacological interventions

Pharmacological interventions are of benefit for certain types of chronic pain, although research involving children is extremely limited. Few medications are specifically created or licensed for use in children, especially for the treatment of chronic pain (Grégoire & Finley 2007). The clinical use of these medications in children is extrapolated from the research evidence in adults with chronic pain. The types of drug used include:

- anticonvulsants
- antispasmodic drugs or muscle relaxants
- bisphosphonates (e.g. pamidronate)
- cannabinoids (e.g. nabilone)
- opioids
- simple analgesics
- serotonin selective reuptake inhibitors (SSRIs)
- lignocaine (lidocaine)
- tricyclic antidepressants (TCAs).

Activity

For more information about the evidence base for the pharmacological interventions used to manage chronic pain read Stinson & Bruce (2009).

Invasive therapies

Non-invasive therapies are the mainstay of treatment of paediatric chronic pain conditions. However, intravenous regional analgesia (single regional blocks or continuous lumbar sympathetic blocks) can be a useful adjunct in children with CRPS who do not respond to treatment with non-invasive therapies (Dangel 1998). More recently, spinal cord stimulation has been reported to be effective in a case series of seven female adolescents with severe, incapacitating and therapy resistant CRPS type I (Olsson et al 2008).

Multidisciplinary approach

The key to the success of chronic pain management in children is adopting a multidisciplinary, multimodal rehabilitation approach (Kashikar-Zuck 2006). Because of the complexity of chronic pain, no single discipline has the expertise to assess and manage it independently. While not all children require a multidisciplinary approach, the services provided by multidisciplinary pain treatment programmes (chronic pain clinics) are considered the optimal therapeutic model for the management of chronic pain in children (Peng et al 2007).

Chronic pain clinics

Specialised interdisciplinary chronic pain teams are now the standard of care for children with complex chronic pain conditions (Stinson 2006). Chronic pain teams for children generally include specialist physicians (for example, anaesthetists, neurologists and psychiatrists), nurses and allied health professionals (for example, psychologists, occupational therapists and physiotherapists) (Peng et al 2007). More recently, teams may also include complementary and alternative therapists (for example, acupuncturists and/or massage therapists). The specific team members involved in any one case depend on the individual needs of the child and family (Stinson 2006).

There are a limited number of chronic pain services for children (Peng et al 2007). For example, a recent survey found only five multidisciplinary chronic pain programmes in Canada and all were located in large urban centres (Peng et al 2007). Children's chronic pain services typically offer outpatient programmes, however some centres offer inpatient, day or residential treatment programmes (Berde & Solodiuk 2003). The Bath Pain Management Unit provides a residential programme of pain management based on the principles of cognitive behavioural therapy. Three months after attending the programme, adolescents report reduced anxiety, pain and depression and many had returned to normal activities and had improved school attendance (Eccleston et al 2003a, 2006b).

www

For more information about the Bath Pain Management Unit go to:

- www.bath.ac.uk/pain-management/

Ongoing assessment and re-evaluation of the treatment plan is essential. One way to monitor children with chronic pain is through the use of electronic pain diaries. Diaries can be used to obtain a better understanding of the impact of pain on their daily lives and activities as well as the pain intensity (Stinson et al 2008). Diaries can also be a useful way to help children and adolescents keep track of improvements in their physical, social and psychological functioning.

Long-term outcomes

Little research has been conducted on long-term outcomes of children treated for chronic pain conditions. While clinic waiting lists for children are less than that for adults with chronic pain, some children may wait up to 9 months to be seen in a multidisciplinary clinic (Peng et al 2007). One study found that for 65% of patients attending a chronic pain clinic outcomes were good with significant improvement reported in school attendance, sleep and participation in sports (Chalkiadis 2001). Conversely, Martin et al (2007) interviewed children with chronic pain 3 years following their last visit at a large metropolitan multidisciplinary paediatric pain clinic and 62% were found to still have pain and the frequency of pain episodes increased with age.

Seminar discussion topics

1. Multidisciplinary chronic pain clinics are recommended for children with complex chronic pain problems. However, the majority of children with chronic pain can be managed effectively in the community.
2. Discuss what roles children's nurses can play to optimise community-based care for children with chronic pain and their families.

References

Abu-Saad, H.H., Bours, G.J., Stevens, B., Hamers, J.P., 1998. Assessment of pain in the neonate. Seminars in Perinatology 22 (5), 402–416.

Alex, J.A., Ritchie, M.R., 1992. School-aged children's interpretation of their experience with acute surgical pain. Journal of Pediatric Nursing 7 (3), 171–180.

Al-Shaikh, B., 1997. Epidural analgesia in ICU. Care of the Critically Ill 13 (3), 20–24.

American Academy of Pediatrics, American Pain Society, 2001. The assessment and management of acute pain in infants, children and adolescents. Pediatrics 108 (3), 793–797.

Anand, K.J.S., Hickey, P.R., 1987. Pain and its effects in the human neonate and fetus. New England Journal of Medicine 317, 1321–1329.

Anie, K.A., Green, J., 2000. Psychological therapies for sickle cell disease and pain. Cochrane Database of Systematic Reviews Issue 3 Art. No.: CD001916.

Anthony, K.K., Schanberg, L.E., 2001. Juvenile primary fibromyalgia syndrome. Current Rheumatology Reports 3, 165–171.

Arndorfer, R.E., Allen, K.D., 2001. Extending the efficacy of a thermal biofeedback treatment package to the management of tension-type headaches in children. Headache 41, 183–192.

Australian and New Zealand College of Anaesthetists (ANZA), 2007. Acute pain management: scientific evidence, 2nd edn. ANZA, Melbourne.

Australian and New Zealand College of Anaesthetists and Faculty of Pain Medicine [ANZCA], 2005. Acute pain management: scientific evidence, 2nd edn. Australian and New Zealand College of Anaesthetists, Melbourne.

Ball, T.M., Shapiro, D.E., Monhelm, C.J., Weydert, J.A., 2003. A pilot study of the use of guided imagery for the treatment of recurrent abdominal pain in children. Clinical Pediatrics 42 (6), 527–532.

Ballantyne, J.C., LaForge, K.S., 2007. Opioid dependence and addiction during opioid treatment of chronic pain. Pain 129, 235–255.

Bartocci, M., Bergqvist, L.L., Longercrantz, H., Anand, K.J.S., 2006. Pain activates cortical areas in the preterm newborn brain. Pain 122, 109–117.

Beider, S., Mahrer, N.E., Gold, J.I., 2007. Pediatric massage therapy: An overview for clinicians. Pediatrics Clinics of North America 54, 1025–1041.

Bejia, I., Abid, N., Ben Salem, K., et al., 2005. Low back pain in a cohort of 622 Tunisian school children and adolescents: an epidemiological study. European Spine Journal 14, 331–336.

Berde, C.B., Lebel, A.A., Olsson, G., 2003. Neuropathic pain in children. In: Schechter, N.L., Berde, C.B., Yaster, M. (Eds.), Pain in infants, children and adolescents, 2nd edn. Lippincott, Williams and Wilkins, Baltimore, pp. 620–641.

Berde, C.B., Solodiuk, J., 2003. Multidisciplinary programs for management of acute and chronic pain in children. In: Schechter, N.L., Berde, C.B., Yaster, M. (Eds.), Pain in infants, children and adolescents. Lippincott Williams and Wilkins, Baltimore, pp. 471–486.

Beyer, J.E., 1984. The Oucher: A user's manual and technical report. Hospital Play Equipment. Illinois, Evanston.

Bray, R.J., 1983. Post-operative analgesia provided by morphine infusion in children. Anaesthesia 38, 1075–1078.

Bray, R.J., Woodhams, A.M., Vallis, C.J., et al., 1986. A double blind comparison of morphine infusion and patient controlled analgesia in children. Paediatric Anaesthesiology 6, 121–127.

Breau, L.M., McGrath, P.J., Camfield, C., Finley, G.A., 2002. Psychometric properties of the Non-communicating Children's Pain Checklist-Revised. Pain 99, 349–357.

Brown, S.C., 2006. Cancer pain: Palliative care in children. In: Schmidt, R.F., Willis, W.D. (Eds.), Encyclopaedia reference of pain. Springer-Verlag, Heidelberg, pp. 220–224.

Bryant, B., Knights, K., Salerno, E., 2003. Pharmacology for Health Professionals. Elsevier (Australia) Pty Ltd, Sydney.

Bursch, B., Tsao, J.C., Meldrum, M., Zeltzer, L.K., 2006. Preliminary validation of a self-efficacy scale for child functioning despite chronic pain (child and parent versions). Pain 125 (1-2), 35–42.

Carter, B., 1997. Pantomimes of pain, distress, repose and lability: the world of the preterm baby. Journal of Child Health Care 1 (1), 17–23.

Carter, B., Lambrenos, K., Thursfield, J., 2002. A pain workshop: An approach to eliciting the views of young people with chronic pain. Journal of Clinical Nursing 11 (6), 753–762.

Castle, K., Imms, C., Howie, L., 2007. Being in pain: a phenomenological study of young people with cerebral palsy. Developmental Medicine and Child Neurology 49 (6), 445–449.

Cervero, F., Laird, J., 1991. One pain or many pains? A new look at pain mechanisms. News in Physiological Sciences 6, 268–273.

Chalkiadis, G.A., 2001. Management of chronic pain in children. Medical Journal of Australia 175, 476–479.

Chambers, C.T., Craig, K.D., 1998. An intrusive impact of anchors in children's faces pain scales. Pain 78 (1), 27–37.

Chambers, C.T., Reid, G.J., McGrath, P.J., Finley, G.A., 1996. Development and preliminary validation of a postoperative pain measure for parents. Pain 68, 307–313.

Champion, G.D., Goodenough, B., von Baeyer, C.L., Thomas, W., 1998. In: Finley, G.A., McGrath, P.J. (Eds.), Measurement of pain in infants and children. Progress in pain research and management, measurement of pain by self-report, Vol. 10IASP Press, Seattle, pp. 123–160.

Chandrasekharan, N.V., Dai, H., Roos, K.L., Evanson, N.K., Tomsik, J., Elton, T.S., Simmons, D.L., 2002. COX-3, a cyclooxygenase-1 variant inhibited by acetaminophen and other analgesic/antipyretic drugs: cloning, structure, and expression. Proceedings of the National Academy of Sciences of the United States of America 99 (21), 13926–13931.

Charlton, J.E. (Ed.), 2005. Core curriculum for professional education in pain, 3rd edn. IASP Task Force on Professional Education, IASP Publications, Seattle.

Connelly, M., Rapoff, M.A., Thompson, N., Connelly, W., 2006. Headstrong: a pilot study of a CD-ROM intervention for recurrent pediatric headache. Journal of Pediatric Psychology 31, 737–747.

Connelly, M., Schanberg, L., 2006. Latest developments in the assessment and management of chronic musculoskeletal pain syndromes in children. Current Opinion in Rheumatology 18 (5), 496–502.

Coskun, V., Anand, K.J.S., 2000. Development of supraspinal pain processing. In: Anand, K.J.S., Stevens, B.J., McGrath, P.J. (Eds.), Pain in neonates, 2nd edn. Elsevier, Amsterdam, pp. 23–54.

Cozzi, L., Tryon, W.W., Sedlacek, K., 1987. The effectiveness of biofeedback-assisted relaxation in modifying sickle cell crisis. Biofeedback Self Regulation 12, 51–61.

Craig, K.D., Grunau, R.V.E., 1993. Neonatal pain perception and behavioural measurement. In: Anand, K.J.S., Stevens, B.J., McGrath, P.J. (Eds.), Pain in neonates. Elsevier, Amsterdam, pp. 67–105.

Crombez, G., Bijttebier, P., Eccleston, C., et al., 2003. The child version of the pain catastrophizing scale (PCS-C): A preliminary validation. Pain 104 (3) 639–446.

Crow, C.S., 1997. Children's pain perspectives inventory (CPPI): developmental assessment. Pain 72, 33–40.

Dahlquist, L.M., Busby, S.M., Slifer, K.J., et al., 2002b. Distraction for children of different ages who undergo repeated needle sticks. Journal of Pediatric Oncology Nursing 19 (1), 22–34.

Dahlquist, L.M., Gil, K.M., Armstrong, F.D., Ginsberg, A., Jones, B., 1985. Behavioral management of children's distress during chemotherapy. Journal of Behavior Therapy and Experimental Psychiatry 16 (4), 325–329.

Dahlquist, L.M., Pendley, J.S., Landthrip, D.S., Jones, C.L., Streber, C.P., 2002a. Distraction intervention for preschoolers undergoing intramuscular injections and subcutaneous port access. Health Psychology 21 (1), 94–99.

Dampier, C., Shapiro, B.S., 2003. Management of pain in sickle cell disease. In: Schechter, N.L., Berde, C.B., Yaster, M. (Eds.), Pain in infants, children and adolescents, 2nd edn. Lippincott, Williams and Wilkins, Baltimore, pp. 489–516.

Dangel, T., 1998. Chronic pain management in children. Part II: Reflex sympathetic dystrophy. Paediatric Anaesthesia 8, 105–112.

Doorbar, P., McClarey, M., 1999. Ouch! Sort it out: children's experiences of pain. RCN Publishing, London.

Dowden, S.J., 2009a. Pharmacology of Analgesic Drugs. In: Twycross, A., Dowden, S.J., Bruce, L. (Eds.), Pain management in children: a clinical manual, Wiley-Blackwell, Oxford.

Dowden, S.J., 2009b. Managing Acute Pain in Children. In: Twycross, A., Dowden, S.J., Bruce, L. (Eds.), Pain management in children: a clinical manual, Wiley-Blackwell, Oxford.

Ebner, C.A., 1996. Cold therapy and its effect on procedural pain in children. Issues in Comprehensive Pediatric Nursing 19 (3), 197–208.

Eccleston, C., 2005. Managing chronic pain in children: the challenge of delivering chronic care in a 'modernising' health care system. Archives of Disease in Childhood 90, 332–333.

Eccleston, C., Crombez, G., Scotford, A., Clinch, J., Connell, H., 2004. Adolescent chronic pain: patterns and predictors of emotional distress in adolescents with chronic pain and their parents. Pain 108 (3), 207–208.

Eccleston, C., Jordan, A.L., Crombez., G., 2006. The impact of chronic pain on adolescents: a review of previously used measures. Journal of Pediatric Psychology 31 (7), 684–697.

Eccleston, C., Malleson, P.N., Clinch, J., Connell, H., Sourbut, C., 2003a. Chronic pain in adolescents: evaluation of a programme of interdisciplinary cognitive behaviour therapy. Archives of Disease in Childhood 88, 881–885.

Eccleston, C., Yorke, L., Morley, S., Williams, A.C., Mastroyannopoulou, K., 2003b. Psychological therapies for the management of chronic and recurrent pain in children and adolescents. Cochrane Database Systematic Reviews CD003968.

Eland, J., 1985. The child who is hurting. Seminars in Oncology Nursing 1 (2), 116–122.

Elgar, F.J., McGrath, P.J., 2003. Self-administered psychosocial treatments for children and families. Journal of Clinical Psychology 59, 321–339.

Ellis, J.A., Blouin, R., Locket, J., 1999. Patient-controlled analgesia; optimising the experience. Clinical Nursing Research 8 (3), 283–294.

El-Metwally, A., Salminen, J.J., Auvinen, A., Kautiainen, H., Mikkelsson, M., 2005. Lower limb pain in a preadolescent population: prognosis and risk factors for chronicity – a prospective 1- and 4-year follow-up study. Pediatrics 116, 673–681.

Engel, J.M., O'Rouke, D.A., 2006. Chronic pain in children, physical medicine and rehabilitation. In: Schmidt, R.F., Willis, W.D. (Eds.), Encyclopaedia reference of pain, Springer-Verlag, Heidelberg, pp. 368–371.

Field, T., Hernandez-Reif, M., Seligman, S., et al., 1997. Juvenile rheumatoid arthritis: benefits from massage therapy. Journal of Pediatric Psychology 22 (5), 607–617.

Finley, G.A., McGrath, P.J., Forward, S.P., et al., 1996. Parents' management of children's pain following 'minor' surgery. Pain 64, 83–87.

Fitzgerald, M., 2000. Development of the peripheral and spinal pain system. In: Anand, K.J.S., Stevens, B.J., McGrath, P.J. (Eds.), Pain in neonates, 2nd edn. Elsevier, Amsterdam, pp. 9–22.

Fitzgerald, M., Howard, R.F.M., 2003. The neurobiologic basis of pediatric pain. In: Schechter, N.L., Berde, C.B., Yester, M. (Eds.), Pain in infants, children and adolescents, 2nd edn. Lippincott, Williams and Wilkins, Philadelphia, pp. 19–42.

Franck, L., 1986. A new method to quantitatively describe pain behavior in infants. Nursing Research 35 (1), 28–31.

Franck, L.S., 1998. The ethical imperative to treat pain in infants: are we doing the best we can? Neonatal Intensive Care 11 (5), 28–34.

Franck, L.S., Greenberg, C.S., Stevens, B., 2000. Pain assessment in infants and young children. Pediatric Clinics of North America 43 (3), 487–512.

French, S.D., Cameron, M., Walker, B.F., Reggars, J.W., Esterman, A.J., 2006. Superficial heat or cold for low back pain. Cochrane Database of Systematic Reviews (Issue 1) Art. No.: CD004750.

Gaffney, A., 1993. Cognitive Development Aspects of Pain In School-Age Children. In: Schechter, N.L., Berde, C.B., Yaster, M. (Eds.), Pain in infants, children and adolescents. Williams and Wilkins, Baltimore, pp. 75–86.

Gaffney, A., McGrath, P.J., Dick, B., 2003. Measuring pain in children: developmental and instrument issues. In: Schechter, N.L., Berde, C.B., Yester, M. (Eds.), Pain in infants, children and adolescents. 2nd edn. Lippincott Williams and Wilkins, Philadelphia.

Gauntlett-Gilbert, J., Eccleston, C., 2007. Disability in adolescents with chronic pain: patterns and predictors across different domains of functioning. Pain 131, 132–141.

Goldschneider, K.R., Anand, K.J.S., 2003. Long-term consequences of pain in neonates. In: Schechter, N.L., Berde, C.B., Yaster, M. (Eds.), Pain in infants, children and adolescents, 2nd edn. Lippincott Williams and Wilkins, Baltimore, pp. 58–70.

Goodenough, B., Thomas, W., Champion, G., McInerney, M., Young, B., Juniper, K., Ziegler, J.B., 1997. Pain in 4 to 6 year-old children receiving intramuscular injections: a comparison of the faces pain scale with Oucher self-report and behavioural measures. Clinical Journal of Pain 13 (1), 60–73.

Grazzi, L., 2004. Headache in children and adolescents: conventional and unconventional approaches to treatment. Neurological Science 25, S223–S225.

Greenberg, R.S., Billett, C., Zahurak, M., Yaster, M., 1999. Videotape increase parental knowledge about paediatric pain. Pediatric Anaesthesia 89, 899–903.

Grégoire, M.C., Finley, G.A., 2007. Why were we abandoned? Orphan drugs in pediatric pain. Paediatrics and Child Health 12, 95–96.

Grunau, R.E., 2000. Long-term consequences of pain in human neonates. In: Anand, K.J.S., Stevens, B.J., McGrath, P.J. (Eds.), Pain in neonates, 2nd edn. Elsevier, Amsterdam, pp. 55–76.

Grunau, R.V.E., Whitfield, M.F., Petrie, J., 1998. Children's judgements about pain at aged 8-10 years: Do extremely low birthweight children differ from their full birthweight peers. Journal of Child Psychology and Psychiatry 39 (4), 587–594.

Guite, J.W., Logan, D.E., Sherry, D.D., Rose, J.B., 2007. Adolescent self-perception: associations with chronic musculoskeletal pain and functional disability. Journal of Pain 8 (5), 379–386.

Harbeck, C., Pederson, L., 1992. Elephants dancing in my head: a developmental approach to children's concepts of specific pains. Child Development 63, 138–149.

Harrop, J.E., 2007. Management of pain in children. Archives of Disease in Childhood: Education and Practice Edition 92, ep101–ep108.

Hawley, D., 1984. Postoperative pain in children: misconceptions, descriptions and interventions. Pediatric Nursing 10 (1), 20–23.

Hawthorn, J., Redmond, K., 1998. Pain causes and management. Blackwell Science, Oxford.

Hermann, C., 2006. Psychological treatment of pain in children. In: Schmidt, R.F., Willis, W.D. (Eds.), Encyclopaedia reference of pain, Springer-Verlag, Heidelberg, pp. 2037–2039.

Hermann, C., Blanchard, E.B., 2002. Biofeedback in the treatment of headache and other childhood pain. Applied Psychophysiology & Biofeedback 27 (2), 143–162.

Hernandez-Reif, M., Field, T., Largie, S., et al., 2001. Childrens' distress during burn treatment is reduced by massage therapy. Journal of Burn Care and Rehabilitation 22 (2), 191–195.

Hester, N., 1979. The preoperational child's reaction to immunization. Nursing Research 28 (4), 250–255.

Hestor, N.O., Barcus, C.S., 1986. Assessment and management of pain in children. Pediatrics: Nursing Update 1 (14), 1–8.

Hestor, N.O., Foster, R.L., Jordan-Marsh, M., et al., 1998. Putting pain measurement into clinical practice. In: Finley, G.A., McGrath, P.J. (Eds.), Measurement of pain in infants and children. IASP Press, Seattle, pp. 179–198.

Hicks, C.L., von Baeyer, C.L., Spafford, P.A., et al., 2001. The faces pain scale revised: toward a common metric in pediatric pain measurement. Pain 93 (2), 173–183.

Hogan, M., Choonara, I., 1996. Measuring pain in neonates: an objective score. Paediatric Nursing 8 (10), 24–27.

Holden, E.W., Deichmann, M.M., Levy, J.D., 1999. Empirically supported treatments in pediatric psychology: recurrent pediatric headache. Journal of Pediatric Psychology 24, 91–109.

Holden, E.W., Deichmann, M.M., Levy, J.D., 1999. Empirically supported treatments in pediatric psychology: recurrent pediatric headache. Journal of Pediatric Psychology 24, 91–109.

Howard, R., 2003. Acute pain management in children. In: Rowbotham, D.J., MacIntyre, P.E. (Eds.), Clinical pain management: acute pain. Arnold, London, pp. 437–462.

Howard, R., Carter, B., Curry, J., Morton, N., Rivett, K., Rose, M., Tyrrell, J., Walker, S., Williams, G., 2008. Good practice in postoperative and procedural pain management. Pediatric Anesthesia 18, 1–81.

Hunfield, J.A.M., Perquin, C.W., Bertina, W., et al., 2002. Stability of pain parameters and pain-related quality of life in adolescents with persistent pain: a three year follow-up. Clinical Journal of Pain 18, 99–106.

Hunfield, J.A.M., Perquin, C.W., Duivenvoorden, H.J., et al., 2001. Chronic pain and its impact on quality of life in adolescents and their families. Journal of Pediatric Psychology 26, 145–153.

Hunt, A., Goldman, A., Seers, K., Crichton, N., Mastroyannopoulou, K., Moffat, V., Oulton, K., Brady, M., 2004. Clinical validation of the paediatric pain profile. Developmental Medicine and Child Neurology 46 (1), 9–18.

Hunt, A., Wisbeach, A., Seers, K., et al., 2007. Development of the paediatric pain profile: role of video analysis and saliva cortisol in validating a tool to assess pain in children with severe neurological disability. Journal of Pain and Symptom Management 33 (3), 276–289.

Hurley, A., Whelan, E.G., 1988. Cognitive development and children's perception of pain. Pediatric Nursing 14 (1), 21–24.

Huth, M.M., Broome, M.E., Good, M., 2004. Imagery reduces children's post-operative pain. Pain 110, 439–448.

International Association for the Study of Pain (IASP), 1979. Pain terms: a list with definitions and notes on usage. Pain 6, 249–252.

International Association for the Study of Pain (IASP), 2001. IASP definition of pain. IASP Newsletter 2, 2.

Ireland, M., Olson, M., 2000. Massage therapy and therapeutic touch in children: state of the science. Alternative Therapies in Health and Medicine 6 (5), 54–63.

Jacques, A., 1994. Epidural analgesia. British Journal of Nursing 3 (14), 734–738.

Jäing, W., Baron, R., 2004. Experimental approach to CRPS. Pain 108, 3–7.

Jay, S., Elliott, C.H., Fitzgibbons, I., Woody, P., Siegel, S., 1985. A comparative study of cognitive behavior therapy versus general anesthesia for painful medical precedures in children. Pain 62 (1), 3–9.

Jay, S.M., Elliott, C.H., Woody, P.D., Siegel, S., 1991. An investigation of cognitive-behavior therapy combined with oral valium for children undergoing painful medical procedures. Health Psychology 10 (5), 317–322.

Jeans, M.E., Gordan, D., 1981. Developmental characteristics of the concept of pain, Paper presented at the 3rd world congress on pain. Scotland, Edinburgh.

Johnson, L., 2004. The nursing role in recognizing and assessing neuropathic pain. British Journal of Nursing 13 (18), 1092–1097.

Johnston, C.C., Gagnon, A.J., Pepler, C.J., Bourgault, P., 2005. Pain in the emergency department with one-week follow-up of pain resolution. Pain Research and Management 10 (2), 67–70.

Jones, D.S., Walker, L.S., 2006. Recurrent abdominal pain in children. In: Schmidt, R.F., Willis, W.D. (Eds.), Encyclopaedia reference of pain, Springer-Verlag, Heidelberg, pp. 359–363.

Jordan, A.L., Eccleston, C., Osborn, M., 2007. Being a parent of the adolescent with complex chronic pain: an interpretative phenomenological analysis. European Journal of Pain 11 (1), 49–56.

Jovey, R.D., Ennis, J., Gardner-Nix, J., Goldman, B., Hays, H., Lynch, M., Moulin, D., 2003. Use of opioid analgesics for the treatment of chronic non-cancer pain – A consensus statement and guidelines from the Canadian Pain Society, 2002. Pain Research and Management 8 (Suppl A), 3A–14A.

Kachoyeanos, M., Zollo, M., 1995. Ethics in pain management of infants and children. American Journal of Maternal/Child Nursing 20, 142–147.

Kashikar-Zuck, S., 2006. Treatment of children with unexplained chronic pain. Lancet 367, 380–382.

Kashikar-Zuck, S., Goldschneider, K.R., Powers, S.W., Vaught, M.H., Hershey, A.D., 2001. Depression and functional disability in chronic pediatric pain. Clinical Journal of Pain 17, 341–349.

Kashikar-Zuck, S., Vaught, M.H., Goldschneider, K.R., Graham, T.B., Miller, J.C., 2002. Depression, coping, and functional disability in juvenile primary fibromyalgia syndrome. Journal of Pain 3 (5), 412–419.

Kelly, A.M., Powell, C.V., Williams, A., 2002. Parent visual analogue scale ratings of children's pain do not reliably reflect pain reported by child. Pediatric Emergency Care 18 (3), 159–162.

Kemper, K.J., Gardiner, P., 2003. Complementary and alternative medical therapies in pediatric pain treatment. In: Schechter, N.L., Berde, C.B., Yaster, M. (Eds.), Pain in infants, children and adolescents, 2nd edn. Lippincott, Williams and Wilkins, Baltimore, pp. 449–461.

Kemper, K.J., Sarah, R., Silver-Highfield, E., et al., 2000. On pins and needles? Pediatric pain patients' experience with acupuncture. Pediatrics 105 (4), 941–947.

Keogh, E., Eccleston, C., 2006. Sex differences in adolescent chronic pain and pain-related coping. Pain 123 (3), 275–284.

Kleiber, C., Croft-Rosenberg, M., Harper, D.C., 2001. Parents as distraction coaches during IV insertion: a randomised study. Journal of Pain and Symptom Management 22 (4), 851–861.

Konijnenberg, A.Y., Uiterwaal, C.S., Kimpen, J.L., van der Hoeven, J., Buitelaar, J.K., de Graeff-Meeder, E.R., 2005. Children with unexplained chronic pain: substantial impairment in everyday life. Archives of Disease in Childhood 90 (7), 680–686.

Kundu, A., Berman, B., 2007. Acupuncture for pediatric pain and symptom management. Pediatric Clinics of North America 54, 885–899.

Lambert, S.A., 1996. The effects of hypnosis/guided imagery on the postoperative course of children. Developmental and Behavioral Pediatrics 17 (5), 307–310.

Lander, J., Fowler-Kerry, S., 1993. TENS for children's procedural pain. Pain 52, 209–216.

Larsson, B., Carlsson, J., Fichtel, A., Melin, L., 2005. Relaxation treatment of adolescent headache sufferers: Results from a school-based replication series. Headache 45, 692–704.

Lavigne, J.V., Ross, C.K., Berry, S.L., Hayford, J.R., Pachman, L.M., 1992. Evaluation of a psychological package for treating pain in juvenile rheumatoid arthritis. Arthritis Care and Research 5, 101–110.

Lehmann, K.A., 2005. Recent developments in patient-controlled analgesia. Journal of Pain and Symptom Management 29 (5), S72–S89.

Lewin, D.S., Dahl, R.E., 1999. Importance of sleep in the management of pediatric pain. Journal of Developmental and Behavioural Pediatrics 20, 244–252.

Lin, Y., Bioteau, A., Lee, A., 2002. Acupuncture for the treatment of pediatric pain: a pilot study. Medical Acupuncture 14 (1), 45–46.

Liossi, C., Hatira, P., 1999. Clinical hypnosis versus cognitive behavioral training for pain management with pediatric cancer patients undergoing bone marrow aspirations. International Journal of Clinical & Experimental Hypnosis 47 (2), 104–116.

Low, A.K., Ward, K., Wines, A.P., 2007. Pediatric complex regional pain syndrome. Journal of Pediatric Orthopedics 27, 567–572.

Lynch, A.M., Kashikar-Zuck, S., Goldschneider, K.R., Jones, B.A., 2007. Sex and age differences in coping styles among children with chronic pain. Journal of Pain and Symptom Management 33 (2), 208–216.

Manimala, M.R., Blount, R.L., Cohen, L.L., 2000. The effects of parental reassurance versus distraction on child distress and coping during immunizations. Children's Health Care 29 (3), 161–177.

Martin, A.L., McGrath, P.A., Brown, S.C., Katz, J., 2007. Children with chronic pain: impact of sex and age on long-term outcomes. Pain 128, 13–19.

McCaffery, M., Beebe, A.B., 1989. Pain: clinical manual for nursing practice. CV Mosby, St Louis.

McCaffery, M., Pasero, C., 1999. Pain: clinical manual, 2nd edn. Mosby, St Louis.

McCarthy, C.F., Shea, A.M., Sullivan, P., 2003. Physical therapy management of pain in children. In: Schechter, N.L., Berde, C.B., Yaster, M. (Eds.), Pain in infants, children and adolescents, 2nd edn. Lippincott, Williams and Wilkins, Baltimore, pp. 434–448.

McDonald, A.J., Cooper, M.G., 2001. Patient-controlled analgesia. An appropriate method of pain control in children. Paediatric Drugs 3 (4), 273–284.

McGrath, P.A., 1999. Chronic Pain in Children. In: Crombie, I.K. (Ed.), Epidemiology of pain, IASP Press, Seattle, pp. 81–101.

McGrath, P.A., 2006. Chronic daily headache in children. In: Schmidt, R.F., Willis, W.D. (Eds.), Encyclopaedia reference of pain, Springer-Verlag, Heidelberg, pp. 359–363.

McGrath, P.A., Hillier, L.M., 2003. Modifying the psychological factors that intensify children's pain and prolong disability. In: Schechter, N.L., Berde, C.B., Yaster, M. (Eds.), Pain in infants, children and adolescents, 2nd edn. Lippincott, Williams and Wilkins, Baltimore, pp. 85–104.

McGrath, P.J., Hetherington, R., Finley, G.A., 2003. Chronic Pain in Children. In: Jensen, T.S., Wilson, P.R., Rice, A.S.C. (Eds.), Clinical pain management: chronic pain/practical applications & procedures. Arnold Publishing, London, pp. 637–646.

McGrath, P.J., Rosmus, C., Campbell, M.A., Hennigar, A., 1998. Behaviours caregivers use to determine pain in non-verbal, cognitively impaired individuals. Developmental Medicine and Child Neurology 40, 340–343.

Melzack, R., Wall, P., 1996. The challenge of pain, updated 2nd edn. Penguin, London.

Merkel, S., Voepel-Lewis, T., Shayevitz, J.R., Malviya, S., 1997. The FLACC: a behavioral scale for scoring post-operative pain in young children. Pediatric Nursing 23 (3), 293–297.

Merlijn, V.P., Hunfield, J.A., van der Wouden, J.C., Hazebroek-Kampschreur, A.A., Koes, B.W., Passchier, J., 2003. Psychosocial factors associated with chronic pain in adolescents. Pain 101 (1-2), 33–43.

Merlijn, V.P.B.M., Hunfield, J.A.M., van der Wouden, J.C., Hazebroek-Kamschreur, A.A.J.M., Passchier, J., Koes, B.W., 2006. Factors related to quality of life in adolescents with chronic pain. Clinical Journal of Pain 22, 306–315.

Miró, J., Huguet, A., Nieto, R., 2007. Predictive factors of chronic pediatric pain and disability. The Journal of Pain 8, 774–792.

Morton, N.S., 2007. Management of postoperative pain in children. Archives of Disease in Childhood, Education in Practice Edition 92, ep14–ep19.

Oberlander, T.F., O'Donnell, M.E., Montgomery, C.J., 1999. Pain in children with significant neurological impairment. Developmental and Behavioral Pediatrics 20 (4), 235–243.

Oberlander, T.F., Symons, F., 2006. Pain in children and adults with developmental disabilities, Paul H. Brookes Publishing Company, Baltimore.

Ochsenreither, J.M., 1997. Analgesia in infants. Neonatal Network 16 (6), 79–83.

Olsson, G.L., Meyerson, B.A., Linderoth, B., 2008. Spinal cord stimulation in adolescents with complex regional pain syndrome type 1 (CRPS-I. European Journal of Pain 12, 53–59.

Palermo, T.M., Kiska, R., 2005. Subjective sleep disturbances in adolescents with chronic pain: relationship to daily functioning and quality of life. Journal of Pain 6, 201–207.

Pederson, C., 1995. Effect of imagery on children's pain and anxiety during cardiac catheterization. Journal of Pediatric Nursing 10 (6), 365–374.

Pederson, C., Harbaugh, B.L., 1995. Nurses' use of nonpharmacologic techniques with hospitalised children. Issues in Comprehensive Pediatric Nursing 18, 91–109.

Peng, P., Stinson, J., Choiniere, M.STOP PAIN Investigator Group, et al., 2007. Dedicated multidisciplinary pain management centres for children in Canada: the current status. Canadian Journal of Anesthesia 54, 963–968.

Perquin, C.W., Hazebroek-Kampschreur, A.A.J.M., Hunfield, J.A.M., et al., 2000. Pain in children and adolescents: a common experience. Pain 87, 51–58.

Perquin, C.W., Hazebroek-Kampscheur, A.A.J.M., Hunfield, J.A.M., van Suijlekom-Smit, L.W.A., Passchier, J., van der Wouden, J.C., 2001. Chronic pain among children and adolescents: physician consultation and medication use. Clinical Journal of Pain 16, 229–235.

Pintov, S., Lahat, E., Alstein, M., Vogel, Z., Barg, J., 1997. Acupuncture and the opioid system: Implications in the management of migraine. Pediatric Neurology 17, 129–133.

Polkki, T., Pietila, A.-M., Vehvilamen-Julkunen, K., 2003. Hospitalized children's descriptions of their experiences with postsurgical pain relieving methods. International Journal of Nursing Studies 40, 33–44.

Powers, S.W., 1999. Empirically supported treatments in pediatric psychology: procedure-related pain. Journal of Pediatric Psychology 24, 131–145.

Ready, L.B., Edwards, W.T., 1992. Management of acute pain: a Practical Guide, Task Force on Acute Pain, International Association for the Study of Pain. IASP Publications, Seattle.

Reid, G.J., Hebb, J.P.O., McGrath, P.J., Forward, S.P., 1995. Cues parents use to assess postoperative pain in children. Clinical Journal of Pain 11 (3), 229–235.

Remy, C., Marret, E., Bonnet, F., 2006. State of the art of paracetamol in acute pain therapy. Current Opinion in Anesthesiology 19, 562–565.

Rennick, J.E., Johnston, C.C., Dougherty, G., Platt, R., Ritchie, J.A., 2002. Children's psychological responses after critical illness and exposure to invasive technology. Journal of Developmental & Behavioral Pediatrics 23 (3), 133–144.

Rich, B.A., 2000. An ethical analysis of the barriers to effective pain management. Cambridge Quarterly of Healthcare Ethics 9, 54–70.

Richardson, J., Smith, J.E., McCall, G., Pilkington, K., 2006. Hypnosis for procedure-related pain and distress in pediatric cancer patients: a systematic review of effectiveness and methodology related to hypnosis interventions. Journal of Pain and Symptom Management 31 (1), 70–84.

Ross, D., Ross, S., 1984. Childhood pain: the school-aged child's viewpoint. Pain 20 (2), 179–191.

Roth-Isigkeit, A., Thyen, U., Stoven, H., Schwarzenberger, J., Schumaker, P., 2005. Pain among children and adolescents: Restrictions in daily living and triggering factors. Pediatrics 115 (2), 152–162.

Royal College of Nursing (RCN), 1999. Clinical guidelines for the recognition and assessment of acute pain in children: recommendations. RCN Publishing, London.

Royal College of Nursing (RCN), 2000. The recognition and assessment of acute pain in children: technical report. RCN Publishing, London.

Rusy, L.M., Weisman, S.J., 2000. Complementary therapies for acute pediatric pain management. Pediatric Clinics of North America 47 (3), 589–599.

Saxe, G., Stoddard, F., Courtney, D., et al., 2001. Relationship between acute morphine and the course of PTSD in children with burns. Journal of the American Academy of Child & Adolescent Psychiatry 40 (8), 915–921.

Scharff, L., Langan, N., Rotter, N., et al., 2005. Psychological, behavioural and family characteristics of pediatric patients with chronic pain. A 1-year retrospective study and cluster analysis. Clinical Journal of Pain 21, 432–438.

Scharff, L., Leichtner, A.M., Rappaport, L.A., 2003. Recurrent Abdominal Pain. In: Schechter, N.L., Berde, C.B., Yaster, M. (Eds.), Pain in infants, children and adolescents, 2nd edn. Lippincott, Williams and Wilkins, Baltimore, pp. 719–731.

Scharff, L., Marcus, D.A., Masek, B.J., 2002. A controlled study of minimal-contact thermal biofeedback treatment in children with migraine. Journal of Pediatric Psychology 27 (2), 109–119.

Scott, J., Huskisson, E.C., 1979. Graphic representation of pain. Pain 2, 175–184.

Sinha, M., Christopher, N.C., Fenn, R., Reeves, L., 2006. Evaluation of nonpharmacologic methods of pain and anxiety management for laceration repair in the pediatric emergency department. Pediatrics 117 (4), 1162–1168.

Slater, R., Cantarella, A., Gallela, S., Worley, A., Boyd, S., Meek, J., Fitzgerald, M., 2006. Cortical pain response in human infant. Journal of Neurosciences 26 (14), 3662–3666.

Sleed, M., Eccleston, C., Beecham, J., Knapp, M., Jordan, A., 2005. The economic impact of chronic pain in adolescence: Methodologocal considerations and a preliminary costs-of-illness study.,. Pain 199 (1–3), 183–190.

Smith, J., 2009. Anatomy and Physiology of Pain. In: Twycross, A., Dowden, S.J., Bruce, L. (Eds.), Pain management in children: a clinical manual. Wiley-Blackwell, Oxford.

St. Laurent-Gagnon, T., Bernard-Bonnin, A.C., Villeneuve, E., 1999. Pain evaluation in preschool children and by their parents. Acta Paediatrica 88 (4), 422–427.

Stevens, B., 1999. Pain in infants. In: McCaffery, M., Pasero, C. (Eds.), Pain: clinical manual, 2nd edn. Mosby, St Louis.

Stinson, J.N., 2006. Complex chronic pain in children, interdisciplinary treatment. In: Schmidt, R.F., Willis, W.D. (Eds.), Encyclopaedia reference of pain. Springer-Verlag, Heidelberg, pp. 431–434.

Stinson, J., 2009. Pain assessment in children. In: Twycross, A., Dowden, S.J., Bruce, L. (Eds.), Pain management in children: a clinical manual. Wiley-Blackwell, Oxford.

Stinson, J., Stevens, B.J., Feldman, B., et al., 2008. Construct validity of a multidimensional electronic pain diary for adolescents with arthritis. Pain 136, 281–292.

Stinson, J., Stevens, J., Feldman, B., Streiner, D., McGrath, P., Dupuis, A., Gill, N., Petroz, G., 2008. Construct validity of a multidimensional electronic pain diary for adolescents with arthritis. Pain 136 (3), 281–292.

Stinson, J., Wilson, R., Gill, N., Yamada, J., Holt, J., 2005. A systematic review of internet-based self-management interventions for youth with health conditions. Journal of Padiatric Psychology 34 (5), 495–510.

Stinson, J., Yamada, J., Kavanagh, T., Gill, N., Stevens, B., 2006. Systematic review of the psychometric properties and feasibility of self-report pain measures for use in clinical trials in children and adolescents. Pain 125 (1-2), 143–157.

Subcommittee on Chronic Abdominal Pain, 2005. Chronic abdominal pain in children. Pediatrics 115 (3), 812–815.

Sullivan, M.J.L., Adams, H., 2006. Castrophizing. In: Schmidt, R.F., Willis, W.D. (Eds.), Encyclopaedia reference of pain. Springer-Verlag, Heidelberg, pp. 297–298.

Surjala, K.L., Donaldson, G.W., Davis, M.W., Kippes, M.E., Carr, J.E., 1995. Relaxation imagery and cognitive-behavioral training reduce pain during cancer treatment: a controlled clinical trial. Pain 63, 189–198.

Sweet, S.D., McGrath, P.J., 1998. Physiological measures of pain. In: Finley, G.A., McGrath, P.J. (Eds.), Measurements of pain in infants and children. IASP Press, Seattle, pp. 59–81.

Taddio, A., Goldbach, M., Ipp, M., Stevens, B., Koren, G., 1995. Effect of neonatal circumcision on pain responses during vaccination in boys. The Lancet 345, 291–292.

Taddio, A., Katz, J., Ilersich, A.l., Koren, G., 1997. Effect of neonatal circumcision on pain response during subsequent routine vaccination. The Lancet 349, 599–603.

Taddio, A., Shah, V., Gilbert-MacLeod, C., Katz, J., 2002. Conditioning and hyperalgesia in newborns exposing to repeated heel lances. Journal of the American Medical Association 288 (7), 857–861.

Tanabe, P., Ferket, K., Thomas, R., Paice, J., Marcantonio, R., 2002. The effect of standard care, ibuprofen, and distraction on pain relief and patient satisfaction in children with musculoskeletal trauma. Journal of Emergency Medicine 28 (2), 118–125.

Tsao, J.C.I., Meldrum, M., Zeltzer, L.K., 2006. Efficacy of complementary and alternative medicine approaches for pediatric pain: state of the science. In: Finley, G.A., McGrath, P.J., Chamber, C.T. (Eds.), Bringing pain relief to children: treatment approaches. Humana Press, Totowa, pp. 131–158.

Twycross, A., 2007. Children's nurses' post-operative pain management practices: An observational study. International Journal of Nursing Studies 44 (6), 869–881.

Twycross, A., 2009a. Pain: A bio-psycho-social phenomenon. In: Twycross, A., Dowden, S.J., Bruce, L. (Eds.). Pain management in children: a clinical manual. Wiley-Blackwell, Oxford.

Twycross, A., 2009b. Why managing pain in children matters. In: Twycross, A., Dowden, S.J., Bruce, L. (Eds.). Pain management in children: a clinical manual. Wiley-Blackwell, Oxford.

Twycross, A., 2009c. Non-drug methods of pain-relief. In: Twycross, A., Dowden, S.J., Bruce, L. (Eds.). Pain management in children: a clinical manual. Wiley-Blackwell, Oxford.

Uman, L.S., Chambers, C.T., McGrath, P.J., Kisely, S., 2006. Psychological interventions for needle-related procedural pain and distress in children and adolescents. Cochrane Reviews 18 (4), CD005179.

UNICEF, 1999. Global millennium targets: UNICEF child-friendly hospital initiative. Paediatric Nursing 11 (10), 7–8.

United Nations General Assembly, 1989. Convention on the rights of the child. United Nations, New York.

Van Cleve, L.J., Savedra, M.C., 1993. Pain location: validity and reliability of body outline markings by 4 to 7 year old children who are hospitalized. Pediatric Nursing 19 (3), 217–220.

Van Der Kerkhof, E., van Dijk, A., 2006. Prevalence of chronic pain disorders in children. In: Schmidt, R.F., Willis, W.D. (Eds.), Encyclopaedia reference of pain. Springer-Verlag, Heidelberg, pp. 1972–1974.

Vervoort, T., Goubet, L., Eccleston, C., Bijttebier, P., Crombez, G., 2006. Catastrophic thinking about pain is independently associated with pain severity, disability and somatic complaints in school children and children with chronic pain. Journal of Pediatric Psychology 31, 674–683.

Vessey, J.A., Carlson, K.L., McGill, J., 1994. Use of distraction with children during a painful procedure. Nursing Research 43 (6), 369–372.

Vincent, C.V.H., Denyes, M.J., 2004. Relieving children's pain: Nurses' abilities and analgesic administration practices. Journal of Pediatric Nursing 19 (1), 40–50.

Volpe, J., 1981. Neurology of the newborn. Saunders, Philadelphia.

von Baeyer, C., 2006. Understanding and managing children's recurrent pain in primary care; A biopsychosocial perspective. Paediatrics and Child Health 12, 121–125.

von Baeyer, C.L., 2006. Children's self-reports of pain intensity: Scale selection, limitations and interpretation. Pain Research and Management 11 (3), 157–162.

von Baeyer, C.L., Spagrud, L.J., 2007. Systematic review of observational (behavioural) measures for children and adolescents aged 3 to 18 years. Pain 127, 140–150.

Walker, L.S., Williams, S.E., Smith, C.A., Garber, J., Van Slyke, D.A., Lipani, T.A., 2006. Parent attention versus distraction: impact on symptom complaints by children with and without chronic functional abdominal pain. Pain 122, 43–52.

Wall, P.D., Melzack, R., 1989. Textbook of pain. Churchill Livingstone, Edinburgh.

Watson, K.D., Papageorgiou, A.C., Jones, G.T., et al., 2002. Low back pain in schoolchildren: occurrence and characteristics. Pain 97, 87–92.

Watt-Watson, J., Evernden, C., Lawson, C., 1999. Parents' perceptions of their child's acute pain experience. Journal of Pediatric Nursing 5 (5), 344-349.

Weisenberg, M., 2000. Cognitive aspects of pain. In: Wall, R.D., Melzack, R. (Eds.), Textbook of pain, 4th edn. Churchill Livingstone, Edinburgh, pp. 345–358.

Weydert, J.A., Shapiro, D.E., Acra, S.A., Monheim, C.J., Chambers, A.S., Ball, T.M., 2006. Evaluation of guided imagery as treatment for recurrent abdominal pain in children: a randomised control trial. BMC Pediatrics 6 (29), 1–10.

Wicksell, R., 2007. Values-based exposure and acceptance in the treatment of pediatric chronic pain: from symptom reduction to valued living. Pediatric Pain Letter 9, 13–20.

Wicksell, R., Dahl, J., Magnusson, B., Olsson, G., 2005. Using acceptance and commitment therapy in the rehabilitation of an adolescent female with chronic pain: a case example. Cognitive Behavioural Practitioner 12, 415–423.

Wicksell, R., Melin, L., Olsson, G., 2007. Exposure and acceptance in the rehabilitation of adolescents with idiopathic chronic pain – a pilot study. European Journal of Pain 11, 267–274.

Wilder, R.T., Berde, C.B., Wolohan, M., Vieyra, M.A., Masek, B.J., Micheli, L.J., 1992. Reflex sympathetic dystrophy in children. Clinical characteristics and follow-up of seventy patients. Journal of Bone Joint Surgery of America 74, 910–919.

Wilkins, K.L., McGrath, P.J., Finley, G.A., Katz, J., 1998. Phantom limb sensations and phantom limb pain in child and adolescent amputees. Pain 78, 7–12.

Wilson, G.A.M., Doyle, E., 1996. Validation of three paediatric pain scores for use by parents. Anaesthesia 51, 1005–1007.

Wolf, A.R., 1999. Pain. Nociception and the developing infant. Paediatric Anaesthesia 9, 7–17.

Woodgate, R., Kristjanson, L., 1996. A young child's pain: how parents and nurses 'take care'. International Journal of Nursing Studies 33 (3), 271–284.

World Health Organization, 1996. Cancer pain relief, 2nd edn. World Health Organization, Geneva.

World Health Organization, 1998. Cancer pain relief and palliative care in children. World Health Organization, Geneva.

Yaster, M., Karolinski, K., Maxwell, L., 1997. Opioid agonists and antagonists. In: Yaster, M., Krane, E.J., Kaplan, R.F., Cote, C.J., Lappe, D.G. (Eds.), Pediatric pain management and sedation handbook. Mosby, St. Louis, pp. 29–50.

Yura, H., Walsh, M.B., 1988. The nursing process: assessing, planning and implementation, 5th edn. Appleton Lange, Norwalk, CT.

Zeltzer, L., LeBaron, S., 1982. Hypnosis and nonhypnotic techniques for reduction of pain and anxiety during painful procedures in children and adolescents with cancer. Journal of Pediatrics 101 (6), 1032–1035.

Zeltzer, L., LeBaron, S., 1982. Hypnosis and nonhypnotic techniques for reduction of pain and anxiety during painful procedures in children and adolescents with cancer. Journal of Pediatrics 101 (6), 1032–1035.

Zeltzer, L.K., Tsao, J., C.I., Stelling, C., Powers, M., Levy, S., Waterhouse, M., 2002. A phase 1 study on the feasibility of an acupuncture/hypnotherapy intervention for chronic pediatric pain. Journal of Pain and Symptom Management 24, 437–446.

Children and surgery

18

Linda Shields Ann Tanner

ABSTRACT

The striking difference in nursing children, as opposed to adults, through a surgical experience is that they do not come alone but are an integral part of a family group, with parents and/or caregivers as advocates for their treatment, and often siblings and other relatives in their extended family (Alsop-Shields 2000, Smith & Dearmun 2006). As such, their care is more complicated and involved than it would be for a consenting adult patient. Parents of children admitted to hospital for surgery often have high levels of anxiety. If this anxiety is transmitted to the child, it can have a negative impact on the child's admission and surgery (Sadhasivam et al 2009). Increased availability of preoperative information, in the form of written information sheets, coupled with the exchange of information by nursing and medical staff is likely to reduce parental anxiety. Children undergoing surgery are often anxious. This anxiety may initiate a stress response, which can delay wound healing and suppress the immune system (Koinig 2002). Reduction of anxiety for the child and their parent is an important role for the perioperative nurse.

LEARNING OUTCOMES

- Gain an overview of the nature of paediatric surgery.
- Understand the role of parents and family-centred care in paediatric surgery.
- Gain an overview of common paediatric procedures of different age groups and developmental stages.
- Understand the importance of education for parents and children throughout any surgical experience.
- Understand the ethical and legal ramifications of surgery on children.
- Recognise and understand common paediatric emergencies.
- Understand the flow through the operating theatres: preparation, admission, induction, procedure/surgery/anaesthetic, recovery, discharge and education.

DOI: 10.1016/B978-0-7020-3183-0.10018-9

Why children need surgery

Paediatric surgery was not considered a specialised area separate to adult surgery until the first half of the 20th century (Mooney 1997). It encompasses a wide range of surgical procedures and differing ages, from premature infants weighing as little as 500–600 g to adolescents. There are many reasons why children need surgery. These can range from congenital malformations to accidental and non-accidental injuries, or a variety of disease processes (Shields & Werder 2002). A number of characteristic conditions and/or injuries for the varying age groups have been detailed in Table 18.1. These are representative of the general trends and are not indicative of all age groups or all types of surgery. Those highlighted have an accompanying photograph and a description of surgery.

Hernia repair

Hernias are one of the most common congenital abnormalities found in infants (Fig. 18.1). There are several different types of hernia affecting both male and female children. The most frequently occurring hernias are indirect and direct inguinal hernias and hydroceles. Hernias occur when the processus vaginalis (a peritoneal diverticulum that extends through the inguinal ring) remains as a patent conduit with the peritoneal cavity instead of closing off and disappearing. During fetal development, the processus vaginalis attaches itself to the testes and is pulled down into the scrotum as the testes descend. If the processus vaginalis remains patent it is a potential hernia. Twenty per cent of individuals have a patent processus but remain asymptomatic. If bowel or other contents from the abdomen enter the processus it becomes an actual hernia. If only peritoneal fluid enters the processus it becomes a communicating hydrocele (Weber & Tracy 2000). During male hernia

Table 18.1 A sample of paediatric surgical cases for different age groups

Age	Type of surgery	Figures
0–2	Hernia repair (most common-inguinal)	18.1
	Repair of tracheo-oesphageal fistula	
	Diaphragmatic hernia repair	
	Repair of gastroschisis and exomphalos	18.2, 18.3, 18.4
	Insertion of ventricular-peritoneal shunts for hydrocephalus	
	Circumcision (medical and cultural)	18.5
	Correction of congenital abnormalities (removal of extra digits, cleft palate repair, repair of imperforate anus)	
	Craniofacial surgery for congenital abnormalities such as fusion of cranial sutures	18.6
	Hypospadias repair	18.8
	Eye surgery such as probing of tear ducts and examination under anaesthetic for tumours	
2–5	Common ENT procedures such as:	
	• insertion of grommets	
	• adenoidectomy	18.9
	• tonsillectomy	18.10, 18.11
	Urological surgery such as cystoscopy and ureteric reimplantation	
	Lacerations, dog bites	
	Repair of fractured limbs	
	Dental restorations and extractions for multiple dental caries	
	Eye surgery for squint repair	
	Burns grafts for scald burns	
	Brain tumours	
5–10	ENT: adenoidectomy, tonsillectomy	18.10, 18.11
	Repair of fractured limbs	
	Accidental injuries	
	Appendicectomy	18.12
	Orthopaedic surgery for congenital skeletal deformities	
	Brain tumours	
10–15	Accidental injuries	
	Lacerations	
	Repair of fractured limbs	
	Torsion of testes	
	Laparoscopic appendicectomy	18.12
	Bone tumours	
	Burns, grafts for flame burns	

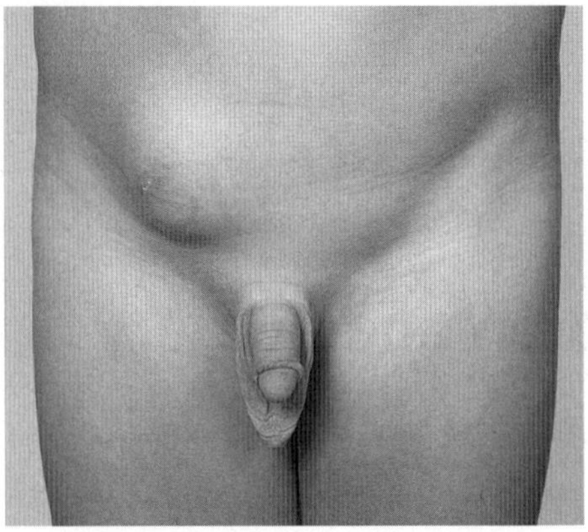

Fig. 18.1 • Inguinal hernia in a child.

repair, the hernial sac is dissected from the testicular structures; this dissection contains the risk of injury to the testicular blood flow (Palabiyik 2009).

Gastroschisis

Gastroschisis and omphalocele are two varieties of congenital abdominal wall defects resulting in a herniation of the abdominal contents in the developing fetus (Fig. 18.2). In gastroschisis the defect usually lies laterally to the umbilicus; the small and large bowel and often the stomach herniate through the defect and are not protected by a peritoneal membrane, but float freely within the amniotic fluid (Holcomb & Wallace 2000). The amniotic fluid acts as an irritant to the surface of the bowel, which forms a thick skin on the bowel surface. In an omphalocele, the umbilical ring is defective and can include a herniation of the entire small and large bowel, the stomach and the liver. Omphaloceles are protected by a layer of the peritoneal membrane. Atresia of the bowel can occur if the opening of the defect is narrow and the blood supply to the bowel has been compromised due to the subsequent stricture. For atresia, the affected bowel is resected. If the infant loses excess intestinal length – 'short gut syndrome', which impairs reabsorption of sufficient fluids and nutrients – the child may be dependent on total parenteral nutrition for life.

Treatment of gastroschisis depends on the size of the defect and the degree of herniation that has occurred. Elective caesarian of an infant with a known gastroschisis can limit the increased morbidity which may occur with prolonged labour and vaginal delivery (White 2009). Infants born with gastroschisis and omphalocele usually have surgery within the first day of life. Smaller defects may be manually reduced and the defect sutured as a primary closure. Larger defects may have a silo bag applied (Fig. 18.3), which contains all the abdominal contents. The bag hangs suspended above the infant and gravity and time aid in reducing the inflammation of the bowel, making it easier to manually reduce the hernia in a series of stages. If the abdominal wall defect is large, a prolene mesh graft may be used to assist in the closure of the defect. The defect can take years to close completely (Fig. 18.4).

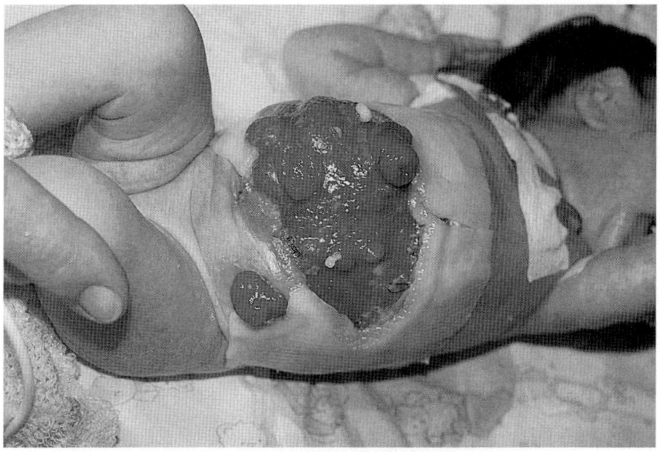

Fig. 18.2 • Gastroschisis.

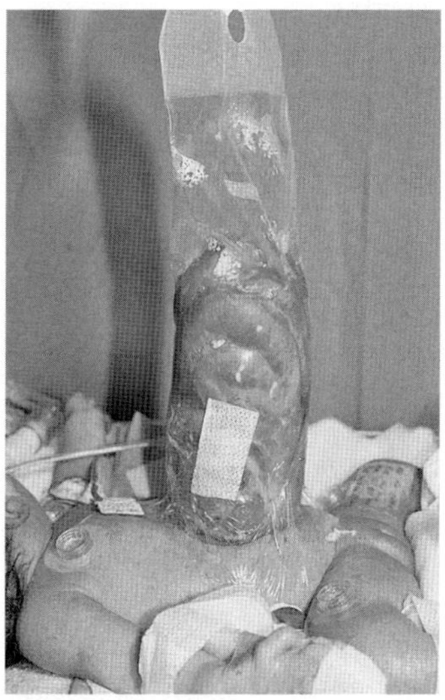

Fig. 18.3 • Repair of gastroschisis.

Circumcision

Circumcision was once routinely performed at birth in many countries, although this custom has now mostly disappeared. However, it remains a reasonably common procedure, although it is now performed for cultural/religious and medical reasons. There is some controversy surrounding male circumcision. In the UK about one-quarter of patients are circumcised for religious reasons (Mukherjee 2009). Medical circumcisions are required for two main conditions: phimosis, which is an inability to retract the foreskin, indicated by a ballooning of the foreskin on urination (Raynor 2000) and paraphimosis, which occurs when the foreskin which has retracted cannot be pulled back down, leaving it forming a stricture around the head of the penis.

Circumcision is usually performed under general anaesthetic and a penile nerve block. The surgeon makes a blunt dissection between the glans and the foreskin, the collar of the foreskin that has been isolated is then excised usually using diathermy, and the shaft skin is then sutured to the subcoronal skin using interrupted absorbable sutures (Fig. 18.5).

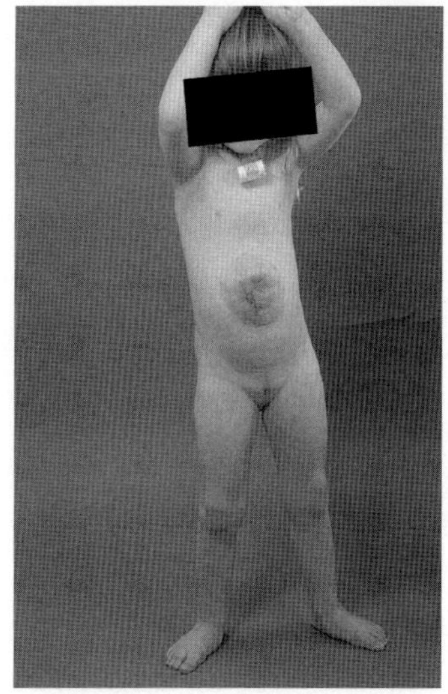

Fig. 18.4 • Child with healed gastroschisis at age 3.

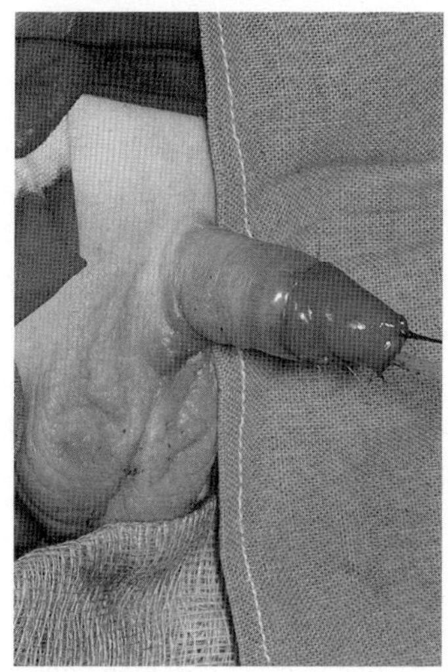

Fig. 18.5 • Circumcision.

Craniofacial surgery

One of the more frequent types of craniofacial surgery is cranial vault remodelling for the correction of fused cranial sutures (Herron et al 2002). These children require surgery at around 6 months of age. It is preferable to operate this young because the bones are relatively malleable and the fusion of cranial sutures has not yet caused any brain damage. The child is positioned either prone or supine, depending on the skull shape and the region of deformity.

Cranial vault remodelling involves a neurosurgeon and a plastic surgeon. A large hemicircular incision is made, within the hairline, from ear to ear. The scalp is retracted and periosteal elevators are used to scrape tissue off the periosteum (Fig. 18.6) in preparation for the craniotomy. The neurosurgeon performs the craniotomy (removal of the top half of the skull) and sutures any parts of the dura mater that might have been damaged during the removal. The plastic surgeon refashions the removed skull using bone cutters to make vertical cuts

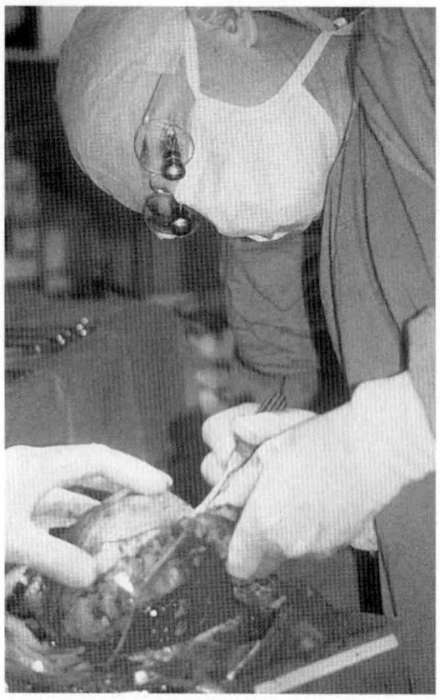

Fig. 18.6 • Craniofacial surgery.

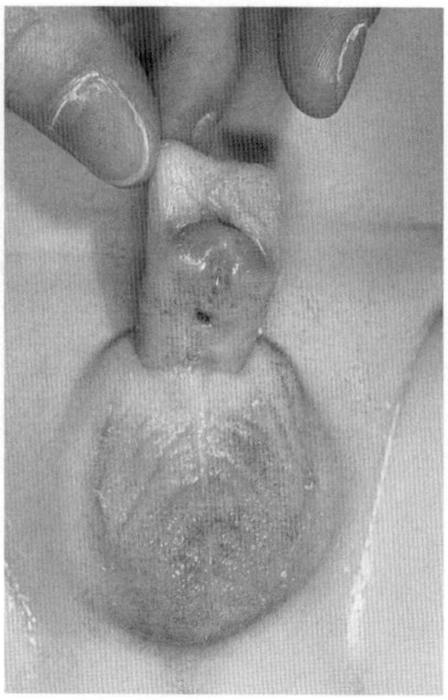

Fig. 18.7 • Hypospadias.

3–5 cm in length into the skull around its circumference to widen and enlarge the skull. The refashioned skull is either wired or plated back onto the child's head, and the scalp sutured back into place. In the instance of craniofacial deformities such as traumatic injury, biomaterials such as cement pastes, osteoactive biomaterials and prefabricated polymers are increasingly used. There is not the risk of donor site morbidity and they are not affected by the long-term re-absorption which can occur with autogenous bone grafts (Chim & Gossain 2009). A head bundle dressing is applied and drains are occasionally required to prevent a build up of old blood and subsequent wound infection and break down.

Hypospadias and repair

Hypospadias is one of the most common congenital anomalies. It occurs in 1:200 to 1:300 live births. The aetiology of hypospadias has been linked to environmental influences. There has been an increase over the past 30 years of male reproductive abnormalities occurring alongside the increased production and use of synthetic chemicals. Concerns have been raised that such environmental factors may play a role in the aetiology of hypospadias, undescended testes and lowered sperm count (Baskin & Ebbers 2006). Hypospadias (Fig. 18.7) is a developmental abnormality in which the urethra opens onto the ventral surface of the penis. The opening can occur anywhere from glans to the scrotum (Murphy 2000) (Fig. 18.8). Surgical repair of hypospadias is often two-staged. The repair involves the formation of a flap using the meatus to create a neourethra that opens at the tip of the glans. An indwelling catheter is left in situ for 7–10 days postoperatively, or until the dressing is removed.

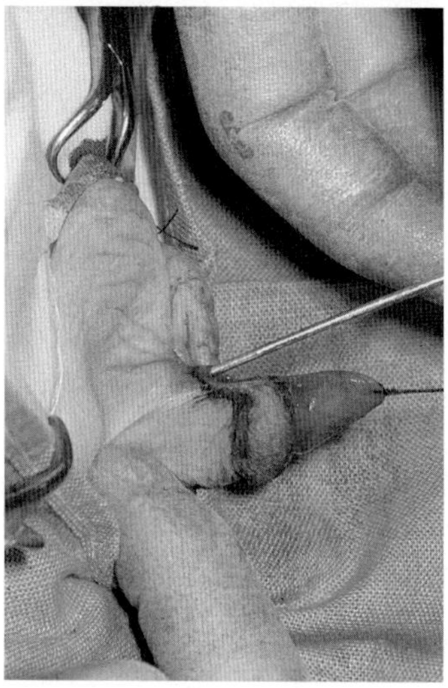

Fig. 18.8 • Hypospadias repair.

Adenoidectomy

Adenoidectomy is a common ENT procedure on children, particularly 2–5-year-olds. Some children in that age bracket have tonsils and adenoids so enlarged that they obstruct their breathing, particularly during sleep. Snoring is often an indicator. Paediatric sleep disorders such as obstructive sleep disorder are often associated with behavioural problems, poor school performance and decreased quality of life. Adenotonsillectomy resolves sleep disorder behaviours in 80% of children, and improves quality of life and behaviours (Mitchell 2008). General anaesthetic is given and the child lies supine, with a gel roll under the shoulders to tilt the head back (Herron et al 2002). The surgeon inserts a mouth gag, which both depresses the tongue and holds the jaw open. Two rods are used to support the gag in place and to keep the head in position (Fig. 18.9). An adenotome is used to scrape the adenoidal tissue from the adenoidal bed. Diathermy is not routinely used for adenoidectomy, rather haemostasis is obtained by firmly packing a swab into the adenoidal bed. This is removed after about 5 minutes and may be replaced with a fresh swab if bleeding persists. Adenoidal bleeding usually occurs if the adenoidal tissue has not been sufficiently scraped away, in this instance the surgeon may re-curette the tissue with the adenotome. Occasionally, suction diathermy is needed to cauterise any vessels

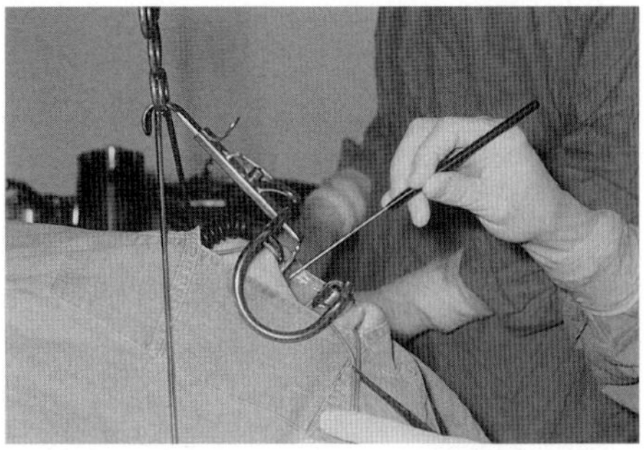

Fig. 18.9 • Adenoidectomy.

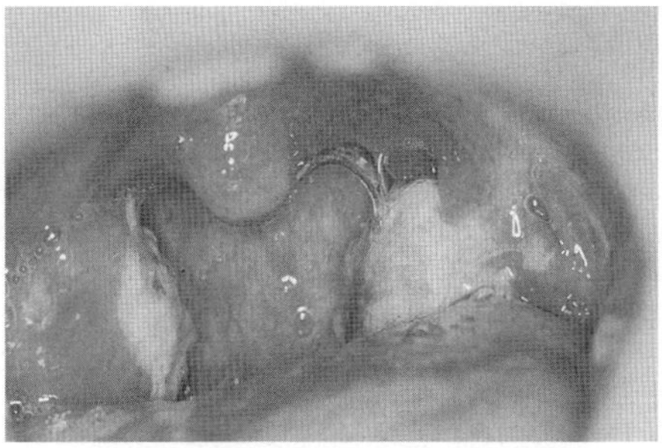

Fig. 18.10 • Tonsillitis.

that continue to bleed. Because Raytec® swabs are routinely packed into the adenoidal space for haemostasis, the scrub nurse's count is very important, as a bloody Raytec® is difficult to see and may cause a serious airway obstruction if left undetected.

Tonsillitis

Tonsillitis is a common illness of childhood, an infection which produces a purulent discharge which covers the inflamed tonsils (Fig. 18.10) and is accompanied by fever and often extreme discomfort. There is some controversy over the need for tonsillectomy (Fig. 18.11) and adenoidectomy and there is some suggestion that the operations are performed unnecessarily in some instances (Montgomery 1996). In children, adenotonsillectomy or adenoidectomy are performed to treat recurrent tonsillitis, obstruction of the nasopharynx and obstructive sleep apnoea (Nieminen et al 2000). Traditionally, there have been two methods for tonsillectomy – using a tonsil snare (guillotine) which loops over the tonsil and cuts it off at its base (Homer et al 2000), and more recently, by sharp or blunt dissection (Meeker & Rothrock 1999). Despite newer technologies, tonsillectomy is still associated with a relatively high risk of postoperative morbidity such as pain and bleeding (Sergi & Younis 2007).

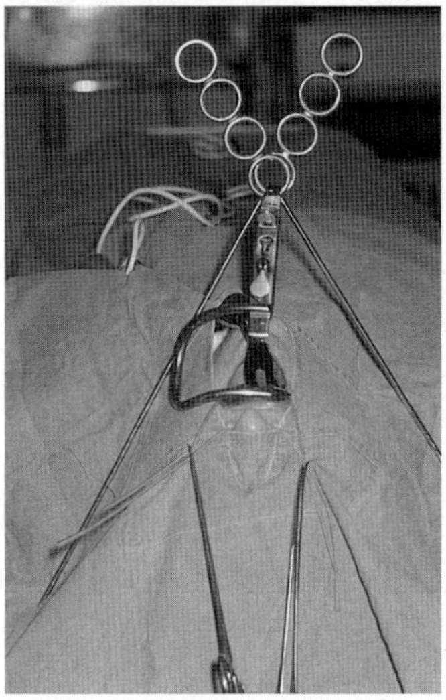

Fig. 18.11 • Patient prepared for tonsillectomy.

Laparoscopic appendicectomy

Children presenting with acute appendicitis usually have a number of tell-tale signs and symptoms. The onset of acute appendicitis is usually over a period of 6–36 hours. The child complains of abdominal pain, which commences around the umbilical area but moves to the right upper quadrant of the abdomen. If the appendix is inflamed the child may be febrile. In appendicitis, vomiting usually begins after the onset of pain; if the child begins vomiting before the onset of pain then the prognosis is more likely to be gastritis (Ein 2000). Diarrhoea does not usually commence unless the appendix has perforated, in which the case the sigmoid colon becomes involved and peritonitis may ensue.

Ultrasound is often performed to confirm a suspected appendicitis. Laparoscopic appendicectomy (Fig. 18.12) offers faster recovery times and a reduced rate of wound infection compared with open appendicectomy (Paterson 2008), and is now the preferred method. It involves the insertion of a large port or trocar for the camera at the umbilicus, and one to two other ports (usually 5 mm wide) for the grasping instruments. The appendix is ligated away from the appendiceal mesentery using diathermy. Once freed, the appendix is tied off, dissected from the bowel and removed via a 10-mm port (which is inserted to replace one of the 5-mm ports) and routinely sent for pathology.

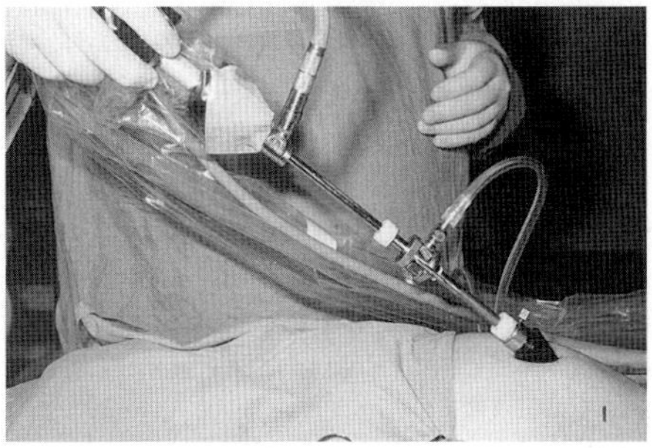

Fig. 18.12 • Laparoscopic appendicectomy.

Activity

Search the Cochrane Library for a copy of the protocol for the review about the use of topical anaesthetics for needle insertion in children (Kleiber et al 2002).

WWW

Visit the Association for the Wellbeing of Children in Healthcare website to order their publications about parents in the operating theatre: Parental involvement in their child's anaesthetic (video) and Policy relating to the provision of care for children undergoing anaesthesia:

- http://www.awch.org.au/policies.htm

WWW

Visit the Action for Sick Children website and see what information can be given to parents and children about going to the operating theatre:

- http://actionforsickchildren.org/index.asp?ID=206

The role of the family

In times past, parents (the child's natural parent, step-parent, legal guardian or carer) were excluded from the hospital during a child's admission (Glasper & Charles-Edwards 2002, Jolley & Shields 2008). Such attitudes are now not widespread and parents are encouraged, and often expected, to stay for the duration of the child's admission. However, parental presence in the operating room is a more contentious issue.

Forty years ago, admission to hospital was portrayed as a positive, growth-promoting experience for children (Jessner et al 1952, Oremland & Oremland 1973) and the experience of overcoming the emotional trauma associated with surgery was extolled as character-forming (Blom 1958); as late as 1992, Lansdown suggested that children could gain psychologically from a hospital admission. However, studies of the psychological trauma encountered by children and their parents before admission have highlighted the importance of adequate preparation of children for hospital admission and surgery (Strachan 1993).

Children have needs different to adults (Price 1994). The most important factor differentiating the needs of children from those of adults is their level of physical and psychological development.

A child's eye view of the operating room

Children are smaller and less developed physically and emotionally than adults, so have different visual and psychological perspectives to adults. Consequently, the environment of the operating room looks different to a child (Figs 18.13 and 18.14). Also, children lack the rationalisation skills that would allow them to integrate the environment perceptually, and so may become frightened.

The paediatric operating room environment must be planned with this in mind and should be as 'child-friendly' as possible, with pictures and cartoons on the walls, bright curtains and hangings, and colourful mobiles. Children are small, so pictures on walls need to be at relevant heights, for example, the bottom of walls for children who walk into the operating room, and higher

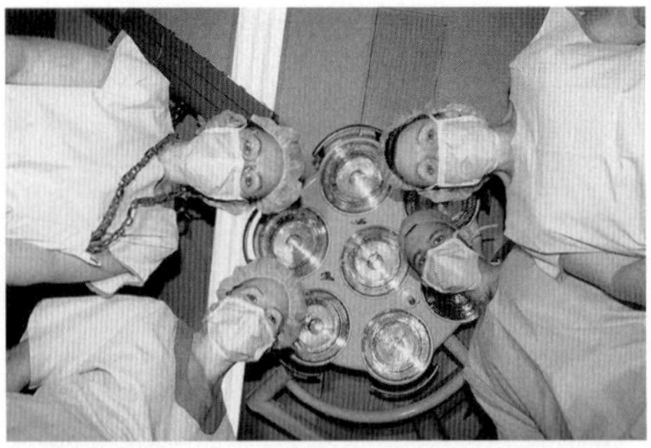

Fig. 18.13 • A child's view from the operating table.

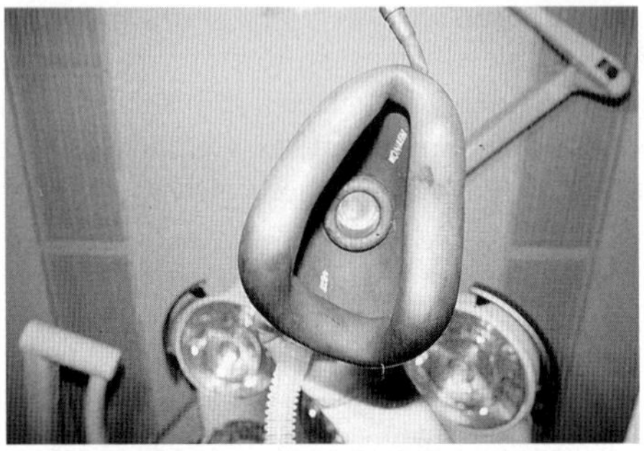

Fig. 18.14 • A child's view of an anaesthetic mask.

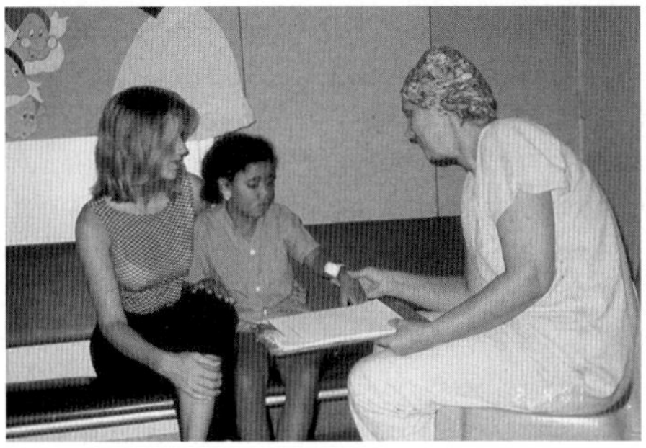

Fig. 18.15 • A child coming into the operating room in their own pyjamas.

for children who arrive on a trolley. Toys, books, television and videotapes are needed, as the children often are not premedicated and play until taken into the theatre. If possible, and if the parent is adequately prepared, parents should stay with the child until the child is anaesthetised, either in an induction room or in the operating theatre itself. Toy cars are fun for children to ride in from the ward to the operating room, or trolleys dressed up as boats or other 'fun' vehicles. Operating room dress is often redundant for children and they can be admitted to the operating room in their own pyjamas or clothes (Fig. 18.15).

Ethics and the law in paediatric perioperative settings

Informed consent

Most hospitals have rigid, mandatory policies for obtaining consent for operation from a parent before their child's surgery. It is imperative that the parents are fully informed as to the reason for the operation, what is going to happen to their child, and the risks involved (Steven et al 2008). By law in many countries, it is the duty of the surgeon to explain the procedure and accompanying risks (Perera 2008), and the anaesthetist has responsibility for explaining the anaesthetic and its implications to the patient before the operation (Australia, New Zealand College of Anaesthetists 2005). It is the nurses' responsibility to ensure that the child (if able), and the parents have been told and that they understand what has been said (Daly 2009). This confirmation is done preoperatively by nurses on the ward, and by the nurse who receives the patient in the operating suite. In some hospitals, it is the admitting nurse in the operating suite who must check that the consent form has been signed; in others, the child cannot leave the ward for the operating room until the consent form is signed. Except in the most extreme emergency situations, no operation can begin without a signed consent form.

In some hospitals, older children have the right to sign their own consent forms, although usually, by law, it must be countersigned by the parent. The child must understand what he or she is signing, must understand what the operative procedure is and what it is for, and must be informed of the risks involved. Any communication with a child has to be age appropriate; tools such as puppets and calico dolls are useful explanation tools.

Parents and children need to know what to expect. Even for the most informed, intelligent and knowledgeable person of any age, operating theatres and procedures are frightening, anxiety-causing events. The role of the paediatric perioperative nurse is to alleviate as much anxiety as possible for both children and parents (Shields & Waterman 2002).

Privacy

Children's privacy can be greatly compromised within the operating theatre. Some children are far more 'body-aware' and modest than many adults and to expose them unnecessarily is to affront their personal dignity, more so if they are anaesthetised. The anaesthetised child has no control over what is happening, his or her body may be exposed for the operation and there are numbers of people within the operating theatre at any one time. Theatre suites often have little provision for private conversations and procedure boards with patients' names and details are often on view to anyone who enters the suite. Perioperative nurses must ensure that children's privacy is respected at all times. Keep the patient covered as much as possible, restrict visitors to the operating theatres, and conduct conversations about private information away from heavy traffic areas. If a surgeon briefs the family on completion of a procedure, this should be done in a separate room away from other people (Fallatt et al 2007).

Patients' rights

Every child, regardless of sex, race, religion or class, has the right to be cared for with dignity and respect. This is as true in the perioperative area as in any other part of a healthcare facility (Perera 2008). Extraordinary procedures, an alien environment, odd smells and sounds, people in bizarre clothes and strange surroundings make up the milieu of the operating room suite. Many children and parents' perceptions of an operating theatre are gained from the media, and often these are unrealistic. Some are terrified at the thought of entering such a foreign place, and anyone who comes to the operating room area requires support. Nurses have the communication skills to make children and their families less frightened by touch, reassurance, talking and explaining what is happening.

Parents and children have the right to know that their safety and spiritual, emotional and physical well-being are assured while in the care of perioperative nurses (Ireland 2006). Children often have operations for life-threatening illnesses, possibly for palliative care or to improve quality of life. Parents often accept the risks of a new procedure in the hope that their life will be improved. Nurses are most often those who recognise the fear and foreboding felt by the children and parents and are most able to support them effectively.

Children and parents from a culture different to the prevailing culture of the hospital have a right to have their religious and spiritual needs met. For example, Muslim parents will feel much more comfortable about their child having an operation for removal of a body part if they know they have the choice to decide if that body part will be given to them to dispose of according to their religious laws (Ebrahim 1995). Nurses are best situated to find out the wishes of people and to afford them the opportunity of having their wishes respected.

Children and parents always have choice and it is an important part of operating room procedure to ensure these choices are open to the patient. If, at the last minute, a patient decides that he or she cannot go through with a procedure, then those wishes must be respected. Nurses require good counselling skills to talk with the family, help address any queries and issues, and allow them to discuss the issues with the appropriate person, be it the surgeon, the anaesthetist or both. The nurse assumes the role of patient advocate and coordinates communication for the child and family so their best interests are assured.

Preadmission programmes

Many paediatric hospitals use preadmission programmes as a means of educating the children and their caregivers about what to expect for their admission into theatre (The Hospital for Sick Children 2009). Because this occurs before admission, it is generally in a more relaxed environment, which in turn is more conducive for child and parent education. The child may have a visit to the theatre admission area and, if possible, the recovery room, and receive an explanation as to what to expect during his or her own admission to theatre. Preadmission clinics save time on the day of surgery, particularly for day-surgery procedures, and are a means of obtaining an informed surgical consent in advance, gaining a familiarity in the theatre environment and allaying anxieties. Information sheets, particularly for day-surgery, can be given to children and parents at this stage, or posted to those unable to attend the clinic.

Flow through the operating rooms

1. Admission: theatre reception

The first port of call in the operating rooms is the theatre reception area. Sometimes termed the 'holding bay', it is the public face of theatre. Unlike adults having surgery, the children, who are not usually premedicated, often walk in with their parents. They may ride in on a toy vehicle, or babies may be carried in by their parents. If the child is experiencing heightened anxiety, the anaesthetist may have ordered a pre-medication. Clonidine has become one of the drugs of choice as a pre-medication to alleviate anxiety (Bergendahl et al 2006). The role of the nurse in this area is to check the incoming child to ensure the name band is labelled correctly with the correct spelling, date of birth, weight and possible allergies. The child's identification band must be checked with the accompanying notes and X-rays, scans or pathology results to ensure they match the patient. The consent is confirmed by checking both written and verbal consent and confirming the type and location of surgery that the child and family believe they are about to undergo.

A preoperative checklist is completed to ensure that fasting times have been adhered to, that the presence of allergies and their reactions are documented, and that child and parent understand the procedure. During this admission, the nurse can ask the child and parent if they need to speak to the surgeon or anaesthetist once again before surgery. To alleviate anxieties, a relaxed, friendly, professional demeanour works best. This is the last stage for the child and their family before undergoing their anaesthetic, and can be a time of heightened emotions for both parties. Distraction works well at this time. Children's television and children's videos are often used as a distraction tool. Some operating rooms make use of volunteers, who help in play activities. Toys, books and ride-on cars and bikes can be effective. Some operating room staff encourage smaller children to ride a toy motor bike or car directly into the induction room, which keeps them distracted right up to anaesthetic induction. Of course, a quick assessment of the child's compliance needs to be done to ensure they can be coaxed off the bike or out of the car when it is time to do so. The aim is to minimise any preoperative anxiety as it is associated with adverse postoperative outcomes such as emergence delirium and increased pain (Zeev & Kain 2007).

2. Induction

Paediatric anaesthetic induction is the process where an anaesthetist administers an anaesthetic agent either as a gas via a mask or intravenously. The child is usually cannulated to provide intravenous access essential for the anaesthetic and for the administration of emergency drugs should the child suffer laryngospasm and require emergency intubation to maintain an airway. Both processes (gas or intravenous or a combination of the two) anaesthetise the child, who is then ventilated by means of an endotracheal tube, a laryngeal mask airway or a Guedel's airway with a ventilator bag and mask. Physiological signs are monitored. Electrocardiograph adhesive pads are placed on either side of the chest and one on the left flank. An oxygen saturation monitor is placed on the finger or toe so that the child can be safely monitored during surgery, and a blood pressure cuff is applied for further monitoring. The type of intubation and cannulation required depends on the type of surgery being performed. Once cannulated and intubated, the child is ready to be transferred onto the operating table and positioned appropriately for surgery.

The use of an induction room for paediatric anaesthesia is increasing. It provides a number of functions. First, based around the principles of family-centred care, it allows a parent or caregiver to accompany the child until he or she is anaesthetised, which in turn reduces the separation anxiety that may be felt by the child and parent. The presence of parents during the induction process arises from assessment of the child's developmental needs and the separation anxiety he or she might experience during traumatic events such as going to theatre. Unfamiliar faces and an unfamiliar environment impair the coping strategies in young children, and can cause feelings of vulnerability (LaRosa Nash & Murphy 1997). Adequate numbers of anaesthetic and paediatric nursing staff present facilitate case turnover, which vastly improves the turnaround time for longer lists. It also means that the instrument nurse can set up for the case in the theatre separate to the induction room. The anaesthetist is ultimately the one who decides if and when the parents can accompany their child during induction. Generally, for emergency anaesthetics when the standard fasting time is not possible, a rapid sequence induction is required and it is not common routine to have parents present.

Parental education is an effective means of reducing parental anxiety. The provision of information during the preoperative admission process may reduce anxiety and improve understanding of the anaesthetic and surgical process (Bellew et al 2002). Preparation of the parent and child improves outcomes. Preoperative anxiety is reduced and subsequently postoperative outcomes are improved. The reduction in anxiety has been linked to lower incidence of emergence delirium in the recovery unit, and the children require significantly less analgesia in the recovery unit (Zeev & Kain 2007). It is important that the accompanying adult is forewarned as to what to expect when the child is anaesthetised because, once induced, the child does not look to be merely asleep but looks lifeless. This can be extremely distressing for the parents and some will become upset and have to be escorted from the induction room. Obviously this is not the positive scenario sought during parent-present inductions.

Studies have found that it can be counterproductive to bring an anxious parent into the operating room without adequate preparation (Chan & Molassiotis 2002). Given sufficient education and reassurance before the day, and escorted immediately from the induction room once the child has received the anaesthetic agent, the process should successfully alleviate anxieties of the child by having the parent present until he or she is unconscious, and the parent is comforted by remaining with their child instead of leaving him or her among strangers (Fig. 18.16).

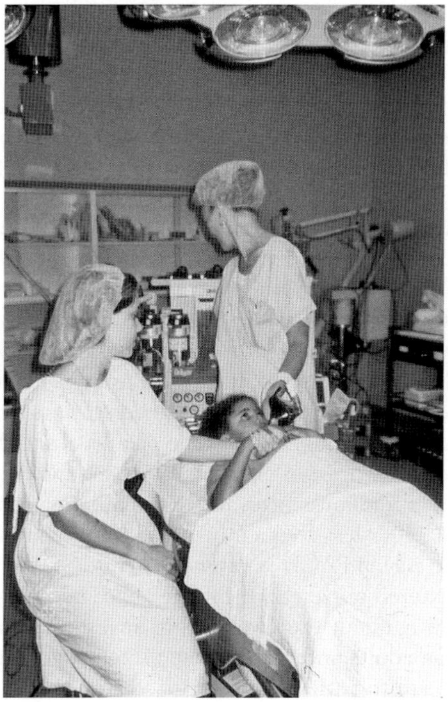

Fig. 18.16 • A parent present for induction of anaesthetic.

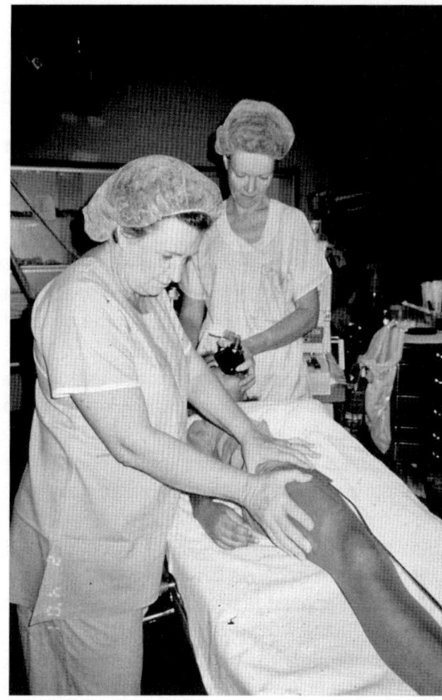

Fig. 18.17 • Positioning an anaesthetised child and applying the diathermy plate.

BOX 18.1

Factors which have a negative effect on a child's emotional experience of hospital admission:

- Age of child
- Child's personality traits
- Admission for longer than 2 weeks
- Painful and/or traumatic illnesses or injuries
- Inadequate preparation for routine admissions
- Previous experience of admission to hospital
- Parents not with child
- Staff with no specialist paediatric training
- Highly anxious parents
- Punitive parental style.

3. The operation

Once anaesthetised, the child is transferred from the induction room onto the operating table and is positioned as required. For example, the child may lie supine (which is the case for the majority of procedures) but could be placed prone or in a lateral position. Patient monitoring systems, such as oxygen saturation and an exhaled carbon dioxide monitor, are connected. These two non-invasive monitors provide the most valuable information to the anaesthetist regarding the child's condition during surgery (Binda & Mestad 2000). Blood pressure is monitored at regular intervals. If the surgery is major, arterial lines and central venous lines are inserted and taped securely so as not to dislodge once the child is positioned, prepared and draped. Most importantly, the airway is taped and secured and the child is not repositioned until the anaesthetist has control over the airway.

It is the instrument nurse's responsibility to check the patient's identification band with the chart, and to check the consent form. Usually, the scout nurse shows these to the instrument nurse, who is already 'scrubbed' and has set up for the case. The instrument nurse checks patient positioning and placement of the diathermy plate (Fig 18.17). The presence of allergies is rechecked. The child is then 'prepped' (using an antiseptic skin preparation such as aqueous betadine or chlorhexidine) and draped. Mayo tables and instrument trolleys are moved into position, suction and diathermy are connected before the surgeon puts knife to skin. The surgeon generally checks with the instrument nurse and the anaesthetist if they are ready to begin.

WWW

Examine pain management information on the internet:

- http://www.us.elsevierhealth.com/WOW/PainAssessmentInfantsChildren.ppt
- http://www.oucher.org/the_scales.html

The instrument nurse's legal responsibility is to maintain a correct count of any instruments or swabs that have been placed in or around the wound, and to ensure that all are removed from the wound before it is closed. There are a standard three counts completed by the instrument nurse and the scout nurse together: the first before the commencement of surgery, and after all accountable items have been taken onto the sterile field. The second is completed at the initial stages of wound closure and the third when the surgeon commences

BOX 18.2

Information for parents about anaesthetic induction

Educating parents before they accompany their child for an anaesthetic

1. Tell the parents what is going to happen once the child arrives in the OR reception room.
2. Explain that the child will be checked for name, operation, surgeon, side of operation if relevant, allergies, any loose teeth, when the child last ate and drank, and that the consent form has been legally signed.
3. Explain that while the parent does not have to, they are allowed to accompany their child into the induction room or theatre itself until the child is fully asleep.
4. Tell the parent and child that the parent will have to don an overgown, theatre cap and overshoes before going into the theatre.
5. Explain that if the anaesthetic induction is going to be intravenous it will not hurt because the child will have had topical anaesthetic cream applied ready for the needle insertion, or it may be by use of a mask held over the child's face.
6. Allow the child and parent to hold an anaesthetic mask, to smell it and to feel what it is like on the face. Explain how the gases flow through it and that it smells 'funny'.
7. Describe the process of anaesthetic induction:
   - They will be taken into the room, the child may be placed on the operating table itself.
   - Large lights will be overhead.
   - People in the room will all have theatre gowns, hats and masks on.
   - There will be a lot of activity going on around them.
   - The anaesthetist and nurse will stay with the child and parent all the time.
   - The anaesthetist will insert the needle into the child's hand, or will place the mask over his/her face and tell them to breathe deeply, when the child is ready.
   - Describe to the parent the quick action of the induction – the child will be awake one minute and within 5 seconds will have gone to sleep and be limp and may appear to be not breathing. Explain that this is completely normal and everything is under complete control. ***This is most important***, as parents may become frightened to see their child go limp so rapidly.
   - Tell the parent that they will be escorted out of the theatre by a nurse and that any questions they may have will be answered.
8. Ask the child and parent if they understand what you have told them, ask them questions so you can gauge that they have understood and answer any queries they may have.

Links to Websites

Read about parent-present induction as described to parents at the Children's Hospital Boston:

- http://web1.tch.harvard.edu/visiting/preparing/poparent.html

closing the skin. Dressings are applied, drapes and diathermy removed and, when the anaesthetist is satisfied that the child's condition is stable, the child is extubated (unless transferring directly to intensive care intubated) and transferred to the postanaesthetic care unit (PACU).

4. Postanaesthetic care unit

When the child arrives in the PACU the immediate tasks of the registered nurse are to secure the intravenous line, check that the child is breathing, ensure the airway is clear, reposition the airway (e.g. by supporting the jaw) if necessary, apply the oxygen saturation monitor, and place an oxygen mask on or next to the child's face, depending on the level of alertness and tolerance of the mask. Airway obstructions can occur in paediatric patients, particularly in those arriving deeply anaesthetised without mechanical airway support such as jaw support or a Guedel airway (Holm-Knudsen & Rasmussen 2009). Once these tasks have been done, the registered nurse checks the wound site for bleeding, assesses the pain level and documents vital signs. This process of checking, assessing and documenting is repeated at 5-minute intervals for the duration of the child's stay in PACU, or less frequently if the child's condition is stable and the stay in PACU is extended. This is at the discretion of the registered nurse caring for the child. Because children's metabolism is rapid, they wake from anaesthetic much more rapidly than adults and can become quite active. For this reason, the nurse to patient ratio for paediatric recovery units is routinely 1:1.

The child remains in the PACU until he or she is awake and responsive to stimuli (such as calling his or her name), maintaining his or her own airway, oxygen saturation is satisfactory on room air, pain is fully controlled and the wound dressing remains dry and intact. If any bleeding has occurred, the wound is reinforced and if significant, reassessed by the surgeon in case the child needs to return to theatre.

Pain management

Approximately 75% of children will say that they have considerable pain on the first day after surgery (Binda & Mestad 2000). Neonates are at risk of respiratory depression following the use of narcotics. For this reason, neonates require close monitoring if narcotics are required, preferably in an intensive care unit, and may need to remain intubated for their initial postoperative recovery. There is a greater risk of respiratory depression in any paediatric patient than in adults following narcotic use (Lundeberg & Lonnqvist 2004). An emergency scenario in the PACU is more likely to involve a respiratory arrest than a cardiac arrest. Close monitoring by experienced paediatric anaesthetic nursing staff is required.

When the child has undergone a major or significantly painful procedure, narcotic analgesia is administered by means of a metered dose system, which releases the prescribed amount (Lundeberg & Lonnqvist 2004). This can be patient-controlled analgesia (PCA) if the child is able to understand and use the device, or parent- or nurse-controlled analgesia (NCA) if the child is too young or not capable of administering a dose. Initially, these infusions may have a continuous background infusion and the parent, nurse or child can administer a bolus dose as prescribed according to a milligram per kilogram ratio. The pump is set with limits as to the number of bolus doses per hour. The child's level of pain and vital signs are closely monitored.

The role of the registered nurse in pain management is primarily one of acute assessment of the degree and severity of pain, and liaison with the anaesthetist to administer analgesics to bring the child's pain under control (Jonas & Worsley-Cox 2000). Experienced paediatric nurses are essential for this assessment because children may withdraw from those around them in response to their pain. In inexperienced hands this could be interpreted as an absence of pain. An increased understanding of the effectiveness of analgesia given as a premedication has markedly reduced the initial postoperative pain experienced by many children, particularly in the case of day-procedure surgery. In fact, pain is one of the factors inhibiting discharge following surgery and can significantly add to the health costs of day-case admissions if the child requires overnight stay for pain management.

5. Discharge from the postanaesthetic care unit

Once the child has satisfied the PACU discharge requirements, including maintaining his or her own airway, satisfactory oxygen saturation on room air, controlled pain and a dry and intact wound dressing, he or she is ready to be transferred back to the wards. As with the admission of parents into the induction room, it is now becoming standard practice in many PACUs to admit the parents once their child is stable and awake. However, the same principles apply in terms of educating and preparing the parent prior to their admission to PACU and reassuring them when they see their child (Smith & Dearmun 2006). If the parent is ill informed and not prepared for their visit to PACU they may become overcome with emotion. The role of the registered nurse is to support and explain procedural details and to outline the pain relief provided, and the location and type of dressings their child may have. Reassurance is the key word, and remaining calm, professional and friendly helps to comfort both the parent and child. The ward staff can be contacted to collect the child at the same time as the parents are invited into PACU. In this manner the parents and staff can benefit from the handover of the child's care.

Parents in the anaesthetic room and postoperative recovery

To ameliorate anxiety of both parent and child (Kain et al 2006), many hospitals and anaesthetists encourage parental presence during anaesthetic induction (PPI). Empirical evidence confirms benefits to both child and parent (Kain et al 2007, 2009), though some disagree (Sadhasivam et al 2009). It is important that parents are well prepared with thorough explanations of how their child will look as he or she becomes unconscious, that they are informed of everything that may occur, and that they are escorted from the theatre with positive assurances (Smith & Dearmun 2006) (Fig. 18.18). Although research about PPI has been extensive, little research exists about the presence of parents in the PACU, but it can be assumed that similar benefits to the family accrue. Anaesthetic induction can be very rapid so parents need to know what to expect, and how quickly their child can become unconscious.

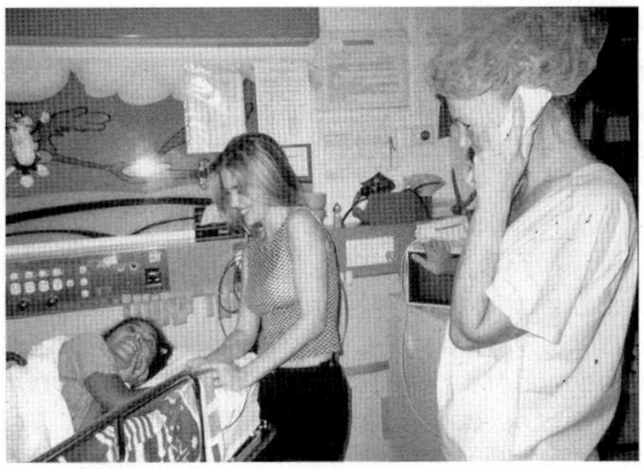

Fig. 18.18 • A parent present in PACU.

PowerPoint

Access the companion PowerPoint presentation: Ben's admission to PACU.

Standing orders

Standing orders (Shields & Waterman 2002), i.e. orders written by a team within a unit (usually, in this case, comprised of the head anaesthetist, nurse in charge of the PACU and, if different, the nurse in charge of the operating room) are often used in situations such as PACU where the nurses work autonomously. They save time while providing safe practice guidelines for care while a child is in the unit. A sample of standing orders for the postoperative recovery of children who have had adenotonsillectomy are shown in Box 18.3 at the end of this chapter.

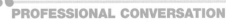

www

Examine the discharge planning in the parent information section of the website of the Morgan Stanley Children's Hospital in New York:

- http://childrensnyp.org/mschony/patients/discharge-planning.html

PowerPoint

Access the companion PowerPoint presentation to find out what happened to Ellie during her tonsillectomy.

PROFESSIONAL CONVERSATION

Rebecca is a registered children's nurse working in the recovery unit of a busy paediatric surgical suite.

Issues affecting discharge planning and parental anxiety during the child's discharge from the PACU/recovery unit

I like to invite the parents into the PACU once I have established that their child's condition is stable, that the child can maintain its own airway, and that any pain has been assessed and the child has been given appropriate analgesics.

One of the most important ways for me to alleviate parental anxiety is to welcome the parents into the unit and let them know that their help in settling or comforting their child is appreciated. I like to immediately reassure them that their child is fine. I give the parents an informal handover of care, any details of the surgery will be explained to them by the surgeons, but many parents like to hear how their child was in their absence. If the child has any intravenous lines, or indwelling catheters or other drainage tubes, I point these out to the parents and, if needs be, explain what they are for. This is also the time to explain any patient-controlled analgesia, and to educate the parents as to how long the child will require the intravenous access. For example, day-surgery patients will usually return to the ward with an intravenous bung only, which the ward staff will remove before discharge.

I show the parents the dressings covering the wound site. There is often a small amount of blood or serous ooze on a freshly applied dressing after surgery, particularly if the local analgesia was given after the wound was sutured, and this initial inspection for the parents' benefit provides a timely education session as well, which includes the dos and don'ts of care of the dressing, what signs to look for (i.e. bleeding or wound infection) and the number of days they need to keep the dressing dry and intact before their follow-up surgical review. It has been my experience that the better informed about the care of their child the parents are, the less anxious they tend to be.

The PACU provides the first point of contact for the parents as to what to expect after their child's surgery and provides the initial education of care and discharge planning advice. This education needs to be reiterated by the ward staff, and the child's condition reassessed before discharge.

Discuss the paediatric nurses' role when children return to hospital for complications following surgery.

Discharge

Children of various ages require different strategies for discharge planning but an important factor is to ensure the parents are comfortable about taking the child home and that they are fully prepared to do so. Similarly, the child, if he or she is old enough, must feel secure about going home. Children of appropriate ages should be involved in all stages of planning for their care, as should their parents.

In practical terms, discharge can be routine: when the child is awake, there is no bleeding from the wound site, the child has eaten and drunk and there is no vomiting or fever. The parents must be educated about:

- the child's care
- potential later complications
- when to call the hospital if something is wrong
- what the ward and A&E telephone numbers are
- what drugs to give and when and how
- when the child can return to a normal diet
- when the child can return to school, preschool, kindergarten or childcare
- how to identify infection
- when it is safe for the child to resume normal activity
- dressing and wound care
- potential changes in the child's behaviour relating to the hospital admission, how to recognise them and what to do about them
- appointment for the follow-up visit to the doctor or clinic.

However, with the best care in the world, things can sometimes go wrong.

BOX 18.3

Sample of standing orders for child with tonsillectomy and adenoidectomy and obstructive sleep apnoea

A sample of 'standing orders' used in PACU for children post-tonsillectomy (reproduced with the permission of Ms Lee-Anne Waterman and Greenwich Medical Media).

In the postoperative phase, a child with obstructive sleep apnoea (OSA) that has also had an ENT procedure is at risk due to post-op swelling and oedema. They should be closely monitored for signs of respiratory failure in addition to routine post-op observation.

Post-op oxygen standing orders

If a child's oxygen saturations drop below 90%:

1. Rouse the child.
2. Give oxygen if required.
3. If the child is unrousable commence resuscitation as per code procedure.
4. Call the consultant or registrar concerned.
5. 'Special' the child until review by medical staff.

   N.B. The child must not be left unattended with oxygen in situ while awaiting medical review.

Post-op pain relief orders for 'not for narcotic' children

It may be necessary for a child to be ordered narcotic pain relief and very close observation must then be undertaken for a minimum of 2 hours post administration. The child should be on pulse oximetry, and visual obs should include rousability and respiratory rate.

If a 'not for narcotic' child is in pain and requires stronger pain relief than ordered:

1. Call the ENT consultant or registrar concerned for a review of respiratory status and pain relief order.
2. Give pain relief as ordered.
3. Monitor oxygen saturations, respiratory rate and depth and rousability:
   - 5-minutely for 15 minutes.
   - 15-minutely for 2 hours.
4. If oxygen saturations drop below 90%:
   - Rouse the child.
   - Give oxygen as required.
   - If unrousable commence resuscitation as per code procedure.
   - Call ENT registrar or consultant concerned.
   - 'Special' the child until medical review.

References

Alsop-Shields, L., 2000. Peri-operative care of children in a transcultural context. AORN Journal 71, 1004–1020.

Australia, New Zealand College of Anaesthetists, 2005. P26 Guidelines for consent for anaesthesia or sedation. Australia, New Zealand College of Anaesthetists, Melbourne. Online. Available at: http://www.anzca.edu.au/resources/professional-documents/professional-standards/ps26.html.

Baskin, L., Ebbers, M., 2006. Hypospadius: anatomy, aetiology and technique. Journal of Paediatric Surgery 41, 463–472.

Bellew, M., Atkinson, K.R., Dixon, G., Yates, A., 2002. The introduction of a paediatric anaesthesia information leaflet: an audit of its impact on parental anxiety and satisfaction. Paediatric Anaesthesia 12 (2), 124–130.

Bergendahl, H., Lönnqvist, P.A., Eksborg, S., 2006. Clonidine in paediatric anaesthesia: review of the literature and comparison with benzodiazepines for pre-medication. Anaesthesiologica Scandinavia 50, 135–143.

Binda, R., Mestad, P., 2000. Anaesthetic considerations. In: Ashcraft, K.W., Murphy, J.P., Sharp, R.J. (Eds.), Pediatric surgery, 3rd edn. WB Saunders, Philadelphia, pp. 38–46.

Blom, G.E., 1958. The reactions of hospitalized children to illness. Pediatrics 22, 590–600.

Chan, C., Molassiotis, A., 2002. The effects of an educational programme on the anxiety and satisfaction levels of parents having parent present induction and visitation in a post anaesthesia care unit. Paediatric Anaesthesia 12, 131–139.

Chim, H., Gosain, A., 2009. Biomaterials in craniofacial surgery: experimental studies and clinical application. Journal of Craniofacial Surgery 20 (1), 29–33.

Daly, B., 2009. Patient consent, the anaesthetic nurse and the perioperative environment: Irish law and informed consent. British Journal of Anaesthetic & Recovery Nursing 10 (1), 3–10.

Ebrahim, A.F., 1995. Organ transplantation: contemporary Sunni Muslim legal and ethical perspectives. Bioethics 9, 291–302.

Ein, S., 2000. Appendicectomy. In: Ashcraft, K.W., Murphy, J.P., Sharp, R.J. (Eds.), Pediatric surgery, 3rd edn. WB Saunders, Philadelphia.

Fallat ME, Caniano DA, Fecteau AH and American Pediatric Surgical Association Ethics and Advocacy Committee 2007 Ethics and the pediatric surgeon. Journal of Pediatric Surgery 42(1),129–136.

Glasper, E.A., Charles-Edwards, I., 2002. The child first and always: the registered children's nurse over 150 years. Part one. Paediatric Nursing 14, 38–42.

Herron, A., Shields, L., Tanner, A., Waterman, L.A., 2002. In: Shields, L., Werder, H. (Eds.), Perioperative nursing. Greenwich Medical Media, London.

Holcomb, G., Wallace, N., 2000. Gastroschisis and omphalocele. In: Ashcraft, K.W., Murphy, J.P., Sharp, R.J. (Eds.), Pediatric surgery, 3rd edn. WB Saunders, Philadelphia.

Holm-Knudsen, R.J., Rasmussen, L.S., 2009. Paediatric airway management: basic aspects. Acta Anaesthesiologica 53 (1), 1–9.

Homer, J.J., Williams, B.T., Semple, P., et al., 2000. Tonsillectomy by guillotine is less painful than by dissection. International Journal of Pediatric Otorhinolaryngology 52, 25–29.

Ireland, D., 2006. Unique concerns of the pediatric surgical patient: pre-, intra-, and postoperatively. Nursing Clinics of North America 41 (2), 265–298.

Jessner, L., Blom, G.E., Waldfogel, S., 1952. Emotional implications of tonsillectomy and adenoidectomy on children. Psychoanalytical Study of Children 7, 126–169.

Jolley, J., Shields, L., 2008. The evolution of family centered care. Journal of Pediatric Nursing, October 2008 (on-line) DOI: 10.1016/j.pedn.2008.03.010

Jonas, D., Worsley-Cox, K., 2000. Information giving can be painless. Journal of Child Health Care 4, 55–58.

Kain, Z.N., Caldwell-Andrews, A.A., Mayes, L.C., et al., 2007. Family-centered preparation for surgery improves perioperative outcomes in children: a randomized controlled trial. Anesthesiology 106 (1), 65–74.

Kain, Z.N., Maclaren, J., Weinberg, M., Huszti, H., Anderson, C., Mayes, L., 2009. How many parents should we let into the operating room? Paediatric Anaesthesia 19 (3), 244–249.

Kain, Z.N., Mayes, L.C., Caldwell-Andrews, A.A., Saadat, H., McClain, B., Wang, S.M., 2006. Predicting which children benefit most from parental presence during induction of anesthesia. Paediatric Anaesthesia 16 (6), 627–634.

Kleiber, C., Sorenson, M., Whiteside, K., Gronstal, A., Tannous, R., 2002. Topical anesthetics for intravenous insertion in children: a randomized equivalency study. Pediatrics 110 (4), 758–761.

Koinig, H., 2002. Preparing parents for their child's surgery: preoperative parental information and education. Paediatric Anaesthesia 12, 107–109.

Lansdown, R., 1992. The psychological health status of children in hospital. Journal of the Royal Society of Medicine 85, 125–126.

LaRosa Nash, P., Murphy, J., 1997. An approach to paediatric perioperative care; parent-present induction. Nursing Clinics of North America 32, 183–198.

Lundeberg, S., Lonnqvist, P.A., 2004. Update on systemic postoperative analgesia in children. Paediatric Anaesthesia 14, 394–397.

Meeker, R.H., Rothrock, J.C., 1999. Alexander's care of the patient in surgery, 11 edn. Mosby, St Louis.

Mitchell, R., 2008. Sleep disordered breathing in children. Missouri Medicine 105 (3), 267–269.

Montgomery, W.W., 1996. Surgery of the nasopharynx. Surgery of the upper respiratory system, 3rd edn. Williams and Wilkins, Baltimore.

Mooney, K., 1997. Perioperative management of the pediatric patient. Plastic Surgical Nursing 17, 69–73.

Mukherjee, S., Joshi, A., Carroll, D., Chandran, H., Parashar, K., McCarthy, L., 2009. What is the effect of circumcision on risk of urinary tract infection in boys with posterior urethral valves? Journal of Paediatric Surgery 44 (2), 417–421.

Murphy, J., 2000. Hypospadius. In: Ashcraft, K.W., Murphy, J.P., Sharp, R.J. (Eds.), Pediatric surgery, 3rd edn. WB Saunders, Philadelphia.

Nieminen, P., Tolonen, U., Copponen, H., 2000. Snoring and obstructive sleep apnea in children: a 6-month follow-up study. Archives of Otolaryngological Head and Neck Surgery 126, 481–486.

Oremland, E.K., Oremland, J.D., 1973. The effects of hospitalization on children: models for their care. Charles C. Thomas, Springfield, MA.

Palabiyik, F., Cimilli, T., Kayhan, A., Toksoy, N., 2009. Do the manipulations in paediatric inguinal hernia operations affect the vascularisation of the testes? Journal of Paediatric Surgery 48, 788–790.

Paterson, H., Qadan, M., de Luca, S.M., Nixon, S.J., Paterson-Brown, S., 2008. Changing trends in surgery for acute appendicitis. British Journal of Surgery 95 (3), 363–368.

Perera, A., 2008. Can I decide please? The state of children's consent in the UK. European Journal of Health Law 15 (4), 411–420.

Price, S., 1994. The special needs of children. Journal of Advanced Nursing 20, 227–232.

Raynor, S., 2000. Circumcision. In: Ashcraft, K.W., Murphy, J.P., Sharp, R.J. (Eds.), Pediatric surgery, 3rd edn. WB Saunders, Philadelphia.

Sadhasivam, S., Cohen, L.L., Szabova, A., et al., 2009. Real-time assessment of perioperative behaviors and prediction of perioperative outcomes. Anesthesia and Analgesia 108 (3), 822–826.

Sergi, Z., Younis, R., 2007. Tonsillectomy and adenoidectomy techniques: past, present and future. Journal for Oto-Rhino-Laryngoscopy and its related specialties 69 (6), 331–335.

Shields, L., Waterman, L.A., 2002. Psychosocial care of children in the perioperative area. In: Shields, L., Werder, H. (Eds.), Perioperative nursing. Greenwich Medical Media, London.

Shields, L., Werder, H., 2002. Perioperative nursing. Greenwich Medical Media, London.

Smith, J., Dearmun, A., 2006. Improving care for children requiring surgery and their families. Paediatric Nursing 18 (9), 30–33.

Strachan, R.G., 1993. Emotional responses to paediatric hospitalization. Nursing Times 89 (46), 45–49.

Steven, M., Broadis, E., Carachi, R., Brindley, N., 2008. Sign on the dotted line: parental consent. Pediatric Surgery International 24 (7), 847–849.

The Hospital for Sick Children 2009 SickKids: pre-admission program. Available at http://www.sickkids.ca/ProgramsandServices/Pre-Admission-Program/index.html

Weber, T., Tracy, T., 2000. Groin hernias and hydroceles. In: Ashcraft, K.W., Murphy, J.P., Sharp, R.J., et al. (Eds.), Pediatric surgery, 3rd edn. WB Saunders, Philadelphia, pp. 654–662.

White, J., 2009. Gastroschisis: effect of mode of delivery. Journal of Paediatric Surgery 44, 657–660.

Zeev, N., Kain, M., 2007. Family centred preparedness for surgery improves perioperative outcomes in children. Anaesthesiology 106, 65–74.

Safeguarding children: the role of the children's nurse

19

Lorraine Ireland Catherine Powell

ABSTRACT

This chapter explores the role of the children's nurse in safeguarding children from maltreatment. The chapter aims to equip students of children's nursing with the knowledge and understanding that will enable them to identify, and respond appropriately to children who may be at risk of, or are actually suffering from, harm.

The chapter opens with an overview of child maltreatment that includes a definition of key terms, a discussion of the scale of the problem and a brief review of some of the theories and perspectives that seek to explain why some children and families are especially vulnerable to abuse. The chapter considers contemporary and emergent United Kingdom policy and guidance, and the way in which this impacts on nursing practice and professional responsibilities. However, since the 1990s, policy for children in the UK has been devolved to the governments and offices of the four countries of which it comprises – Wales, Scotland, Northern Ireland and England. This means that safeguarding children in each of these countries is informed by different legislation and guidance. This chapter does largely refer to the legislation and guidance within the English system, where it seems appropriate reference has been made to policy and research derived from the other countries. Practitioners looking for their key overarching policy guidance are directed as follows:

England: HM Government 2006 Working Together to Safeguard Children: A Guide to Interagency Working to Safeguard and Promote the Welfare of Children. Department for Education and Skills, London

Wales: Welsh Assembly Government 2006 Safeguarding Children: Working Together Under the Children Act 2004

Scotland: The Scottish Government 2004 Protecting Children and Young People: Framework for Standards Edinburgh, Scottish Government

Northern Ireland: Department of Health, Social Services and Public Safety (DoH SSPS) 2003 Cooperating to Safeguard Children. DoH SSPS. Belfast, Northern Ireland

In taking a children's rights perspective, particular emphasis is given to the nurse's role in the prevention of maltreatment and the promotion of positive parenting skills. Safeguarding children is a difficult and sensitive topic that touches the lives of many individuals and their families. Suggestions for accessing help and support are provided.

LEARNING OUTCOMES

- Define the major concepts associated with safeguarding children.
- Understand the challenges of measuring the problem of child maltreatment.
- Critically review the theories that seek to explain child maltreatment.
- Assume professional responsibility in the prevention, identification and reporting of child maltreatment.
- Identify how to access sources of help and support for safeguarding children.

Introduction

> The way in which a society treats its children is perhaps the best measure of its humanity
>
> (Lord Laming 2003)

Child maltreatment is a major health and social problem that has recently been suggested to be the single biggest cause of morbidity in children (Hobbs 2003). For many abused children, the adverse effects on health and well-being will be life long. Furthermore, each week in the UK at least one child will die as a result of cruelty (National Society for the Prevention of Cruelty to Children (NSPCC) 2007). There is little doubt that caring for a child who has been maltreated is one of the most difficult challenges that those working with children and families will face. It is work that is fraught with uncertainties and complexities, yet it can also be rewarding (Hall 2003).

DOI: 10.1016/B978-0-7020-3183-0.10019-0

Safeguarding is an 'umbrella' term encompassing actions to promote and maintain the well-being of children and young people (Powell 2007). Child protection falls within this remit and refers specifically to actions that may be undertaken to protect children who are at risk of, or who are suffering, significant harm. The findings of a statutory inquiry conducted by Lord Laming into the untimely death of Victoria Climbié in 2000 (Laming 2003) have been pivotal in shaping safeguarding policy. The inquiry highlighted how 'poor communication between agencies, a lack of attention paid to a child in her own right and failure to follow-up concerns can lead to disastrous consequences' Corby (2006 p 70).

Contemporary safeguarding policy aims to address these deficits, to promote the right of all children and young people to attain their potential and to recognise their particular vulnerability to different forms of abuse and neglect. The current framework for safeguarding children is based on 'The Every Child Matters' programme (DfES 2004) which has identified five key outcomes for all children and promotes the shared commitment of agencies in order to achieve them. The National Service Framework for Children, Young People and Maternity Services (DoH & DFES 2004) is an integral part of this programme and has promoted greater recognition of the need to protect children within the NHS. The Children Act (2004) introduced a statutory responsibility and formal structures within which a wide range of public services can work together to safeguard children. Statutory guidance for inter-agency working, including revised guidance for child protection procedures is detailed within the Government document 'Working Together to Safeguard Children' (HM Government 2006a).

The 3rd Chief Inspectors report (Ofsted 2008) identifies the many positive changes that have been made since the Laming inquiry and offers an invaluable review of safeguarding arrangements for Children's Nurses. However, the reports recommendations identify areas in need of improvement, including consistency in applying thresholds for concern, recognition of the needs of vulnerable and 'looked after' children, and the need for all agencies to make lines of responsibility and accountability explicit. At the time of writing this chapter the death of 'Baby P' provides further focus on some of these concerns (Department for Children, Schools and Families (DCSF) 2008a).

This chapter aims to equip students of children's nursing with the knowledge and understanding that will enable them to identify, and respond appropriately to, children who may be at risk of, or who are suffering from, harm. The chapter's underpinning philosophy reflects the words of the UK's best-known voluntary child welfare organisation, the NSPCC. This organisation acknowledges that the problem of child abuse and neglect will only be overcome when children's rights to physical and emotional integrity are respected (NSPCC 1996). We share this sentiment and hope that our readers will join with us in promoting and securing the best interests of children at individual, community and societal levels.

Definition of key concepts

Working at all levels to safeguard children requires a critical understanding of the notion of some key concepts; childhood, children's rights, child maltreatment and of child protection. This section considers these key concepts and encourages students of children's nursing to challenge some mainstream ideas as to how children should be treated.

Childhood

Safeguarding children is based on a tacit belief that children are a distinct group of vulnerable individuals who have not yet reached a certain chronological age. However, the notion of childhood (and therefore child maltreatment) is largely socially constructed and influenced by historical, social and cultural change. Although Qvortrup (1994 p 3) simply states that childhood is 'the life-space which our culture limits it to be', an analysis of contemporary childhood is an important precursor to an understanding of child maltreatment.

Activity

Discuss the nature and meaning of contemporary childhood in the UK. It may help to consider the following trigger questions:

- When does childhood start and end?
- Is childhood the 'golden age' it is often said to be?
- Are public places such as shops, pubs and restaurants 'child friendly'?
- Are school days really the 'best days of your life'?

Safeguarding policy in the UK rests on the legal definition of childhood that is reflected in the various Children Acts: The Children Act 1989, The Children Act 2004 (England and Wales), The Children (Scotland) Act 1995, The Children (Northern Ireland) Order 1995. Although this definition states that childhood lasts from birth to 18 years, recognition is given to the fact that action may need to be taken where there are concerns about an unborn child. Furthermore, in certain circumstances (i.e. for people with learning difficulties) children's services may incorporate provision for those aged up to 25 years (Children Act 2004).

Although attainment of a chronological age is a useful parameter for defining childhood, there is clearly much more to consider. Perhaps one of the most important aspects of contemporary childhood is that it is often circumscribed in negative terms (Archard 1993). A good illustration of this is the use of the term 'childish' in our society. The following quote, although being written more than 30 years ago, continues to reflect the subordinate and potentially damaging position of many children in the UK today:

> The fact of being a 'child', of being wholly subservient and dependent on being seen by older people as a mixture of expensive nuisance, slave and super-pet, does young people more harm than good
>
> (Holt 1975 p 15)

Children's rights

Children's rights theorists recognise the oppression of children as well as the lack of the constitutional rights that are accorded to others. Such oppression may be compared with the historical oppression of women, ethnic minorities and the proletariat. Franklin (1995) suggests that because children are politically disenfranchised they are frequently subjected to the sort of treatment that, if meted out to any other group in society, would be considered a moral outrage. The ongoing acceptance and use of corporal punishment in childhood, together with the readiness of the majority of adults to defend this practice, has been noted to be an 'obvious sign' of the low status of children (Newell 1995 p 215). In the UK children remain the only people who can in law be hit 'as reasonable punishment' (Children Act 2004, s 58).

Powell (2002) recognises that nurses' views on the issue of corporal punishment reflect prevailing social and cultural practices. However, she also argues that the loss of extended family, community networks and increasing social isolation of young families, mean that nurses should be actively seeking opportunities to offer support, information and guidance to promote positive parenting practices.

Furthermore, Alderson (2008) suggests that child maltreatment may be encouraged by beliefs about the inherent willingness of children and young people to inflict harm on others. This maligns children and young people and stigmatises those with 'problem behaviour' who are often the most vulnerable. Camila Batmanghelidgh's (2006) book 'Shattered Lives' bears witness to the lives of children who have experienced abuse and neglect and offers greater understanding for those confused by such hard-to-reach children.

Seminar discussion topic

At the current time, 'reasonable chastisement' remains legally acceptable in the UK. However, there is an increasing body of opinion among children's organisations that supports the view that hitting children is wrong. It is notable that all forms of physical punishment of children have been outlawed in Austria, Croatia, Cyprus, Denmark, Finland, Germany, Iceland, Israel, Latvia, Norway and Sweden. While recognising the effects of the prevailing social expectations, debate the case for a change in UK policy.

The children's rights movement is receiving support and global recognition following the inception of the United Nations (UN) Convention on the Rights of the Child, adopted by the General Assembly of the UN on 20 November 1989 (UN General Assembly 1989). The Convention, ratified by the UK in 1991, establishes a series of fundamental rights for children and young people and outlines the responsibilities of governments in ensuring that all services for children are offered in a child-centred, rights-based framework.

Article 19 of the Convention provides a clear message in relation to child protection activity:

> State parties shall take all appropriate legislative, administrative, social and educational measures to protect the child from all forms of physical or mental violence, injury or abuse, neglect or negligent treatment, maltreatment or exploitation, including sexual abuse, while in the care of parent(s), legal guardian(s) or any other person who has care of the child
>
> (UN General Assembly 1989)

Such protective measures should, as appropriate, include effective procedures for the establishment of social programmes to provide necessary support for the child and those who have care of the child, as well as for other forms of prevention and for identification, reporting, referral, investigation, treatment and follow-up of instances of child maltreatment. Progress towards the achievement of the UN articles is monitored periodically the most recent review identifies the attainments of the 4 countries which comprise the UK, continues to highlight the need to proactively seek out families experiencing difficulties and disadvantage (HM Government 2007).

Current policy developments that influence the provision of children's services (including child protection services) are increasingly seeking to address the needs of, and represent the views of, children and parents. 'Every Child Matters' (DfES 2004) outlined a cohesive framework of integrated services to help to support parents and carers and improve outcomes for all children and young people. Children were consulted in the process of development and wanted the provision of services and support that would help every child reach his or her potential, rather than a narrow set of services that intervened at times of crisis or failure. The key outcomes in childhood that are said to 'really matter' to children include: 'being healthy; staying safe; enjoying and achieving; making a positive contribution and economic well-being' (DfES 2004 p 9).

The National Service Framework (DoH & DFES 2004) sets out a 10-year programme for long-term and sustained improvement in children's health whilst The Children's Plan (DCSF 2007) identifies ways in which strengthened support may be provided for all families during the formative years of children's lives. 'The Staying Safe Action Plan' – produced following consultation with children, their parents, professional and members of the general public – makes explicit the scope of safeguarding practice and need for 'universal, targeted and responsive provision' (HM Government 2008b). Although 'coal-face' activity may sometimes seem far removed from the corridors of power, the safeguarding activities of children's nurses will be pivotal in transforming these policies into tangible and empowering action for children and their families. Having considered how an understanding of the nature of childhood, children's rights thinking and policy underpins child protection activity, the following section attempts to define child maltreatment.

Child maltreatment: defining the problem

Defining child maltreatment is challenging and rests on historical, cultural and social contexts and beliefs, as well as the interests and concerns of the definers. The consequence of this state of affairs is that differences of opinions are a key feature of child protection work. Differences of opinion can arise amongst health professionals, between health professionals and workers from other agencies (such as Children's Social Care Services or the Police) and, perhaps more importantly, they can arise between professionals and families and within families themselves.

PROFESSIONAL CONVERSATION

Katy White is a qualified children's nurse who has been working on an acute paediatric medical ward for a number of years.

Over the years that I have been staffing on this ward we have admitted a number of children who have raised concerns about possible child maltreatment. Sometimes the issues are difficult to disentangle. For instance, we had a baby in recently whose weight was a cause for concern. I think things had not been going well for a while.

The health visitor had had difficulty finding the family at home and they did not attend the Well Baby Clinic. I believe that grandma had called the clinic to say that she was worried that her daughter was not looking after the baby properly, but that she didn't want her daughter to know about the call. In the end the Health Visitor got the baby seen by the GP, who referred him to us.

The paediatrician wanted to run some tests to see if there was an underlying cause for the poor weight gain, but we could see that the baby was simply underfed. It turned out that the mother was spending a lot of time out with her friends and leaving her baby son with a variety of babysitters, which in my mind is neglect. He also had a terrible nappy rash, which proves that he wasn't being well cared for.

However, the younger staff on the ward felt sorry for the mother, who was their sort of age and had not wanted to be tied down by a child. She was also very reluctant to come into hospital with her son and I reckoned that she was grateful for some free babysitting. A number of us felt that a child protection referral should be made, but the Social Worker thought a family support route would be better. I think we'll see that baby again.

One of the ways of approaching the difficulties in definition is to spend some time reflecting on what child maltreatment is not. 'Good enough parenting' is a term that can be used to describe the provision of child care that will help to ensure that the health, safety and developmental needs of children are met. Good enough parenting can be discussed in terms of the provision of care and control. Care involves anticipating children's age-appropriate needs through prenatal care, adequate feeding, warmth and protection from harm. Control encompasses action to meet the child's safety requirements, as well as the setting of consistent limits to behaviour. Although the notion of 'control' might seem antithetical to the notion of children's rights, children must be treated as people in their own right and the parents able to put the child's needs above their own.

Reflect on your practice

- Is your interpretation of 'good enough parenting' congruent with that of your colleagues?
- Do you sometimes find yourself (or notice others) making negative judgements about parents' ability to parent their child?
- How can you ensure that the 'welfare of the child is paramount' when parents have a multiplicity of needs (e.g. they are trying to cope with financial difficulties, substance misuse, mental or physical health problems, domestic violence)?

Although it is helpful to consider the notion of 'good enough parenting' it is perhaps important to remember that, like child maltreatment, it is a concept that is heavily influenced by the prevailing social and cultural norms. Corby (2006 p 81) reminds us that professionals can become so accustomed to poor standards of parenting that they begin to accept them as normal, with potentially catastrophic consequences for children. Thus, although children's nurses clearly have a remit to provide culturally sensitive care and support to families, the focus on deciding whether or not a child has been maltreated should remain on the daily lived experience of the child.

The contextual nature of child maltreatment suggests that a broad sociological definition is a good starting point for determining what child maltreatment may be. The following definition, taken from a research report on prevention of maltreatment, remains one of our favourites:

> Child abuse consists of anything which individuals, institutions, or processes do or fail to do which indirectly harms children or damages their prospects of safe and healthy development into adulthood
>
> (National Commission of Inquiry into the Prevention of Child Abuse (NCIPCA) 1996 p 2)

Activity

- Try and think of examples of how individuals, institutions and processes may cause significant harm in children.
- Was it difficult to reach agreement on some of the examples you raised?

Section 31-10 of the Children Act 1989 similarly recognises the importance of children's health and development in ascribing a concept of 'significant harm' to denote the threshold that justifies compulsory intervention in family life (i.e. the initiation of statutory child protection procedures). Nevertheless, no detailed definition of what constitutes 'significant harm' is given. Indeed, it has recently been suggested that:

> Decisions about significant harm are complex and should be informed by a careful assessment of the child's circumstances, and discussion between the statutory agencies and with the child and family
>
> (HM Government 2006b p 8)

The NCIPCA (1996) definition of child maltreatment and the legal concept of significant harm offer excellent vehicles with which to challenge the infringements of children's rights to physical and emotional integrity. However, their scope may be too broad for everyday practice. A more practical definition of child maltreatment, which is broadly applicable throughout the UK, is provided by government guidance in the document 'Working Together to Safeguard Children (HM Government 2006a). Such guidance describes four 'categories' of maltreatment: physical abuse, emotional abuse, sexual abuse and neglect (note: there is significant comorbidity of the different types of abuse).The document 'What to do if you're worried a child is being abused' (HM Government 2006b) is a practitioner-friendly interpretation of the guidance providing the following definitions of each category:

> **Physical abuse** may involve hitting, shaking, throwing, poisoning, burning or scalding, drowning, suffocating, or otherwise causing physical harm to a child. Physical harm may also be caused when a parent or carer fabricates the symptoms of, or deliberately induces illness in a child.
>
> **Emotional abuse** is the persistent emotional ill-treatment of a child such as to cause severe and persistent adverse effects on the child's emotional development. It may involve conveying to children that they are worthless or unloved, inadequate, or valued only insofar as they meet the needs of another person, age or developmentally inappropriate expectations being imposed on children. These may include interactions that are beyond the child's developmental capability, as well as overprotection and limitation of exploration or learning or preventing the child participating in normal social interaction. It may involve hearing or seeing the abuse of another. It may involve serious bullying causing children to feel frequently frightened or in danger, or the exploitation or corruption of children. Some level of emotional abuse is present in all forms of maltreatment of a child although it may occur alone.
>
> **Sexual abuse** involves forcing or enticing a child or young person to take part in sexual activities, including prostitution whether or not the child is aware of what is happening. The activities may involve physical contact, including penetrative (e.g. rape or buggery or oral sex) or non-penetrative acts. They may include involving children in looking at, or in the production of on-line images, watching sexual activities or encouraging children to behave in sexually inappropriate ways.
>
> **Neglect** is the persistent failure to meet a child's basic physical and/or psychological needs, likely to result in the serious impairment of the child's health or development, such as failing to provide adequate food, shelter and clothing, or neglect of, or unresponsiveness to, a child's basic emotional needs. Neglect may occur during pregnancy as a result of maternal substance abuse. Once a child is born it may involve a parent failing to:
>
> – provide adequate food clothing and shelter (including exclusion from home or abandonment
>
> – protect a child from physical and emotional harm or danger
>
> – ensure adequate supervision (including the use of inadequate caregivers)
>
> – ensure access to appropriate medical care and treatment.
>
> It may also include neglect of or unresponsiveness to, a child's basic emotional needs.
>
> (HM Government 2006b pp. 8–9)

Children who are 'suffering from maltreatment' may present with overt signs of abuse that are immediately recognised (such as severe bruising in a non-mobile child) or abuse may be identified over a longer period of time (e.g. persistent failure to attend to health needs).

Identification of maltreatment will almost always depend on someone other than the child or parent recognising the problem. But this work is not easy, even for the most skilled and knowledgeable practitioner and it should never be undertaken in isolation. Thus we conclude this part of the chapter by returning to the work of Corby who notes that:

> The only safe definition of child abuse is that it is a judgement reached by a group of professionals on the examination of the circumstances of the child, normally (in Britain) at a child protection conference.
>
> (Corby 2006 p 84)

Activity

Are any of the following examples child maltreatment? Complete this activity alone and then discuss your responses with a partner.

	Yes	No	Not sure
A mother-to-be is using small amounts of heroin during her pregnancy			
An angry father lashes out at his child and causes minor bruising			
A teacher often tells a child that she is hopeless			
A 14-year-old girl is having sex with her 19-year-old boyfriend			
Parents with learning difficulties are feeding their small baby infrequently			
A 5-year-old frequently arrives at school without having had breakfast			
A 10-year-old is often left to care for her frail and demented grandmother			
A 14-month-old is found to have traces of cannabis resin in his urine			
A child with epilepsy has lower than expected levels of medication in his blood			
A stepfather insists on tucking his 10-year-old stepdaughter into bed – he says its their 'special time'			
A 3-year-old presents at the Emergency Department with a fractured femur – there is no clear history			
A 9-year-old with a squint has missed three appointments with an ophthalmologist			

The scale of the problem

There is no doubt that in the UK and elsewhere child maltreatment is a major health and social problem. However, as the above section indicates, accurate measurement of the scale of the problem is hindered by complex difficulties in defining and reporting maltreatment. A balanced perspective may be that whereas fatal or grievous abuse is extremely uncommon (but newsworthy), a very large number of children have their health and development compromised by less severe, but ongoing, abusive and neglectful situations. This section considers some of the statistical evidence.

Fatal maltreatment

Drawing on criminal statistics, the NSPCC reports that at least one child in the UK is killed every week as a result of maltreatment (NSPCC 2007). The risk of death from maltreatment is about three times greater for under-1s than for those aged between 1 and 4 years of age, with those aged 5 to 14 years facing half the risk of the 1 to 4 years age group (UNICEF 2003). With improvements to many areas of child health, deaths from maltreatment are becoming increasingly significant amongst the leading causes of death in childhood.

Some childhood deaths from maltreatment will be subject to a public inquiry, and thus become familiar to many of us through resultant press coverage e.g. Victoria Climbié and Baby P (Laming 2003, DCSF 2008a). However, most fatal abuse cases are not made public, although in all cases where a child dies or is very seriously injured, and maltreatment is thought to have contributed to the death, a Serious Case Review will be undertaken in line with government guidance (HM Government 2006a). Here, all agencies that cared for the child will be asked to review their records of contacts and services provided to the child and their family. Because of the universal nature of health services, this process will inevitably involve health professionals and underlines the importance of good record keeping at all times. The purpose of a Serious Case Review is to establish whether there are lessons to be learnt about the way in which local professionals and agencies work together to protect children, to outline action plans as to how any lessons will be responded to and to improve local inter-agency working in the future. Serious Case Reviews are not enquiries into how a child died, or who was responsible for their death; these processes are determined by the Coroner and Criminal Courts.

Many of those working in child protection are concerned that the fatal abuse statistics underestimate the true picture. Certainly, the use of criminal statistics may not accurately identify all deaths that result from maltreatment, particularly as neglect is the leading cause of childhood deaths from maltreatment (UNICEF 2003). From April 2008, new statutory child death review processes were introduced in England. The most important reason for reviewing child deaths is to improve the health and safety of children and to prevent other children from dying. The new processes put in place systems for collecting and analysing information about each childhood death (0–18 years) with a view to: identifying any case that gives rise to the need for a Serious Case Review; any matters of concern affecting the safety and welfare of children in the area; and any wider public health or safety concerns arising from a particular death or from a pattern of deaths.

Scenario

Jordan, aged 15 years, was being bullied at school for being overweight. Because of alcohol misuse and relationship difficulties, his parents were unable to provide adequate emotional support and guidance to their son. Deeply unhappy, Jordan took his own life.

How should this death be classified?

Non-fatal maltreatment

The NCIPCA (1996) report into the prevention of child maltreatment suggests a 'conservative estimate' of 1:10 of children in the UK experience abuse during the course of their childhood. Importantly (and at odds with a common misconception of 'stranger danger'), the NCIPCA report also recognises that most children who suffer maltreatment do so at the hands of someone that they know and trust. Although, the figure of 1:10 was put forward as an estimate, a research study into the prevalence of child maltreatment has provided some evidence to substantiate this figure (Cawson et al 2000). This important and influential study is outlined below.

Evidence-based practice

Cawson et al (2000) report on the results of computer-assisted interviews on childhood experiences carried out with a random probability sample of 2869 young people, aged between 18 and 24 years and drawn from the general population. The age group was selected to overcome the problems of interviewing children, yet include those individuals close enough to childhood to be able to recall experiences of growing up. The use of computers allowed the participants to enter sensitive data and protect their confidentiality.

Some of the findings are illustrated by the analogy of a double-decker bus taking children home from school. On the bus, at least seven children would be going home to families who were not perceived as loving or close, ten children would be going home to do housework and care for parents who were incapacitated by health or social problems (including substance misuse), two or three children would be going home to face domestic violence between their parents and two or three children would be returning to a threat of physical violence and/or emotional abuse. A number of the children on the bus would be returning to several or all of these conditions.

The authors note that the study may (in common with other retrospective prevalence studies) underestimate maltreatment because events in early childhood might not be remembered.

As well as raising concerns about the prevalence of abuse, the NCIPCA (1996) report also notes that in many cases maltreatment is neither reported nor identified. This failure to recognise and report maltreatment has been a recurring feature of studies that have interviewed adult 'survivors' of abuse. There still remains a substantial shortfall between the occurrence of maltreatment and reports to child protection agencies. Some 1.5–5% of children are reported to agencies annually in the UK, Canada, USA and Australia for all types of maltreatment (Gilbert et al 2008). However, according to survey data obtained from children, adolescents or parents the annual frequency of maltreatment is far greater (physical abuse 4–16%, psychological abuse 10%, neglect 1–15%, and exposure to intimate partner violence 10–20%; Gilbert et al 2008).

The prevalence of child maltreatment and the evidence of the 'hidden nature' of the problem provide a number of important challenges to those working in the field. The Professional Conversation box below gives insight into this work.

PROFESSIONAL CONVERSATION

Sarah Greene is a Child Protection Nurse Specialist at a Children's Trust.

Sarah has a background in health visiting and children's nursing and is the local 'Named Nurse' for child protection. Her role includes supporting and advising professionals who have child protection concerns, the development of local guidelines and policy, and the provision of training to a wide variety of healthcare staff. Sarah has been involved in three Serious Case Reviews.

The evidence base for child maltreatment is important in underpinning good practice. I try and encourage a broad awareness of the prevalence of the problem and ensure that practitioners explicitly 'rule out' possible abuse as part of their decision-making, particularly when children present with unusual or vague histories. I promote the value and importance of listening to children and advocate for the provision of opportunities for children to speak to us alone.

I am particularly conscious of the prevalence of maltreatment when I am facilitating a training session. Out of the 20 or so staff in attendance you have to remember the possibility that two people could have suffered an abusive or neglectful childhood – sometimes the sessions bring up issues that may have been hidden or never disclosed at the time. I always try and ensure that support is available for those who need it.

One of the difficulties for people who have experienced maltreatment is that such individuals may find themselves unwilling/unable to become involved in cases they might meet in the course of their work. If this is the case, it is an issue that other staff may need to recognise and respect. However, it is vitally important that no children who use our services fall through the safety net. Above all we encourage an open and supportive way of working that means that concerns can be identified and shared and measures put in place to safeguard the child.

Official statistics

A further source of statistics that may underpin our knowledge of child protection is the number of children who are subject to a child protection plan – this decision is made at child protection conference.

These figures are published each year as a point prevalence statistic (i.e. how many children have a child protection plan on a particular date). Although the figures may indicate some useful trends, we urge our readers to remember that this record is dynamic (with names being added and removed on a daily basis) and that the names held represent only those children who have identified, current and unresolved child protection concerns. Such concerns encompass children who are 'at risk' rather than suffering from 'actual harm'.

The DCSF website recorded a total of 29,200 children who were the subject of a child protection plan, as of 31 March 2008 (DCSF 2008c). This figure represents a rate of 27 children per 10,000 of the population and is for England only. If the figures are broken down by category of maltreatment (see the section on definitions above) these are as follows:

- Neglect: 45%
- Physical abuse: 15%
- Sexual abuse: 7%
- Emotional abuse: 25%
- Mixed categories: 8%.

Neglect is the most common category of abuse under which children became the subject of a child protection plan, 45% (which is one percentage point more than in 2007), whilst the percentage of children who became subject to a plan due to emotional abuse shows an increase from 23% in 2007. Children becoming subject to a plan due to physical abuse remains as in 2007 at 15%.

This section has attempted to portray the scale of the problem of child maltreatment. We have noted the impact of the difficulties of definition and the hidden nature of childhood abuse as fundamental to the challenge of portraying the scale of the problem with any great accuracy. However, we have seen that neglect (i.e. where there are acts of omission by parents and carers) features highly both in terms of its links with fatal maltreatment and as the leading reason for children to be subject to a Child Protection Plan.

Theories of maltreatment

Children's nurses pride themselves on being able to work openly and in partnership with children and their families. Clearly, when children require healthcare services and maltreatment (perpetrated by a parent or someone acting in that role) is suspected, the dynamics of this relationship will be compromised.

Two important points need stressing here: first, that the majority of children who suffer maltreatment will be returned to their families (albeit with the provision of services to monitor and safeguard their future well-being); second, that in many instances there will be a non-abusive parent who will be both witnessing the unnecessary suffering of their child and coming to terms with the fact that a much-loved spouse or partner may have perpetrated this event. An understanding of the aetiology of maltreatment may help the nurse to provide sensitive and supportive care to all the family.

Corby (2006) suggests that three main groups of theories seek to explain the causation of child abuse: psychological, social psychological and sociological. Within these groupings, a variety of ideas are proposed. These include such disparate theories as the survival instinct of the sociobiological school, the acceptance of intrafamilial violence of the social-cultural theorists and the institutionalisation of male power proposed by the radical feminists. However, as Corby recognises, there is an inherent danger to adopting single-cause explanations of the problem. What seems to be becoming more widely accepted is the notion of an integrated approach to understanding child maltreatment. Such an approach was postulated by Belsky (1993), whose ecological model recognises the dynamic and mutually dependent nature of individual characteristics, interactions within families, the social environment and the broader structural factors (such as societal attitudes to violence). Hence, the way in which these different levels interact with each other at specific moments in time will affect the likelihood of maltreatment (or not). An understanding of the ecological model of abuse may be useful in helping practitioners overcome prejudices and lessen the likelihood of the apportion of blame to the vulnerable and needy individuals who find themselves unwontedly harming their children.

Scenario

Jade, a preterm baby now aged 6 weeks, has been admitted to the Paediatric Intensive Care Unit after suffering a subdural bleed. Her condition is giving cause for concern and it is feared that she has suffered irreversible brain damage. Gemma, Jade's mother, has reported that Jade cried a great deal and that she was often anxious about upsetting the neighbours in the bed-sit where she has been living since being thrown out of her childhood home by her mother and step-father. Jade's father is a known drug user who has a number of other children. He is not allowed to visit the Children's Unit because he has been violent towards staff on another occasion. Gemma reports that she is depressed and lonely and that life with Jade has been a 'struggle'. She denies harming her. The health visitor has only managed to visit once because she is covering the caseload of a sick colleague.

Risk factors for child maltreatment

In an effort to apply theory to practice, a number of researchers have attempted to draw up checklists of risk factors (or vulnerability) for child maltreatment (e.g. see Browne et al 1988). However, as the researchers themselves acknowledge, this work is beset with difficulties that include high rates of false positives and the dangers of 'labelling' families. There is always a need to recognise that information gathering and assessment should balance the positive aspects of children's lived experiences against any possible concerns. However, some risk factors are worthy of special consideration here.

The particular vulnerability of children with disabilities to abuse and neglect is being increasingly recognised. A report by the National Working Group on Child Protection and Disability (2003) suggested that this vulnerability may be a result of a number of factors. These include societal attitudes and assumptions (e.g. disabled children are not abused), inadequacies in service provision (e.g. communication systems that lack the language necessary to disclose abuse) and factors associated with impairment (e.g. the need for intimate care that may increase the risk of exposure to abusive behaviour).

Reflect on your practice

- Children with disabilities are frequent users of community and hospital health services.
- How well are their special needs met?

Although children with disabilities represent an important group of vulnerable children, other groups have been identified. 'Working Together to Safeguard Children' (HM Government 2006a) outlines five key sources of stress for children and families that may negatively impact on the health and development of children, or impact on parental capacity to respond to the needs of their child:

- Social exclusion: caused by factors such as poverty, poor housing and racism.
- Domestic violence: including the threat to an unborn child where kicks and punches may be directed to the mother's abdomen.
- Mental illness in the parent or carer: including the effects of postnatal depression.
- Drug and alcohol misuse: including harm caused by maternal transmission of substances during pregnancy and the diminished parenting capacity of those under the influence of drugs and/or alcohol.
- Parental learning disability.

Children's nurses and others may be in a position to recognise these factors and offer early intervention and support to help to ensure the best outcomes for the child.

Research has tended to show a social class bias towards higher rates of child maltreatment in social classes D and E. However, it is important to remember that abuse and neglect feature across the social spectrum. Indeed, the authors of this chapter know of cases of overt child maltreatment, where there has been reluctance amongst health professionals to refer the case to Statutory Agencies simply because of the social standing of the parents. Likewise, although recognising that child maltreatment is more common amongst families on low incomes, Cawson et al (2000) suggest that the highest rates of undetected child maltreatment may rest in the professional classes.

In conclusion, this section has aimed to provide a brief overview of the factors that may cause a child to be maltreated. However, best practice rests on being open to a possibility of maltreatment in all contacts with children and, where age and developmental status allow it, listening to what the child has to say.

Professional responsibilities

This section considers the professional responsibilities of the nurse in safeguarding children and promoting their welfare. Before moving on to discuss the recognition and referral of child maltreatment, we will consider ways in which children's nurses may support vulnerable children and their parents and thus potentially help to prevent maltreatment.

Children in need

Children who are defined as 'children in need' under the Children Act 1989 (Section 17) are those who need extra support and services to help them reach or maintain a satisfactory level of health and development. Such children will include those with chronic health conditions, physical disabilities and learning differences, as well as those living in poor socioeconomic circumstances.

Changes in service provision have been made in response to the Children Act (2004) leading to the development of local partnerships 'Children's Trusts' whose aim is to safeguard children and to promote through integrated and local service provision the achievement of the 'Every Child Matters' outcomes (DFES 2004). To do this each Trust has to identify local challenges, resources and target their provision (HM Government 2008a).

Students of children's nursing will gain valuable experience of family life and the provision of health and social care services when undertaking their community placement. Exploration of your local Children's Trust and Children and Young People's Plan websites will inform your awareness of both the services available and the particular needs of children in your area. It is important that children's nurses seek and maintain links with health visitors, school nursing services and social workers, and know how to refer children and families in need of extra health, social or financial support. For children with complex needs, discharge planning should take into account the need to coordinate a range of services.

Activity

Find the details of any local Sure Start, Children's Fund and Connexions in your area. If possible, arrange to visit these projects and find out how children, young people and their families can access these services.

Support in the parenting role

For most children the central and most constant influence in their lives will be their parent(s) and children's nurses are in a position whereby they can help to advise and support parents on aspects of child care, thus reducing stress and possibly helping to reduce the likelihood of maltreatment. The rising birth-rate and increasing social isolation of young families, combined with geographical mobility, mean that many adults have extremely limited experience of child care before embarking upon parenthood. Children's nurses are well-placed to advise parents on normal development (e.g. when it is reasonable to expect a child to be clean and dry), positive parenting techniques (i.e. rewarding good behaviour and ignoring bad behaviour) and the benefits of play. Sometimes, however, it is just a sympathetic ear that is needed.

Proactive service delivery lies at the heart of safeguarding children and recognition of significant societal changes and public health concerns (such as childhood obesity, increased in emotional and behavioural problems in childhood, evidence of poor outcomes experienced by children in the most at-risk families). These factors must inform the development of local programmes, requiring an increased emphasis on parental support and a focus on the most vulnerable children and families.

In providing examples of how parents may be supported readers are directed to The Family Nurse Partnership Programme evaluation (Barnes et al 2008) which highlights the success of intensive home visiting by nurses or midwives and support for vulnerable first-time parents. The Child Health Promotion Programme (CHPP) (DoH, DFES 2008) provides further exemplars building upon the National Service Framework for Children, Young People and Maternity Services in demonstrating how preventative services can be tailored to meet the individual needs of children and their families.

For those who provide children's services, including children's nurses, the CHPP forms an invaluable guide to best practice and indicates how an evidence based and integrated approach can be used to support children and families. The programme begins in early pregnancy and ends in adulthood, informing those commissioning and providing a universal core programme (e.g. antenatal screening, immunisation and developmental reviews), plus programmes and services to meet different levels of need and risk (the principle of 'progressive universalism').

Recognition of child maltreatment

Children who have been maltreated may present for health care following a single traumatic event (such as a shake injury) or as a result of the compilation of a number of significant events, which may include neglect of healthcare needs. Child maltreatment may also be suspected during the course of a hospital admission or other encounters with health professionals for unrelated problems. Physical indicators of possible child maltreatment include bruising, bite marks, burns, scalds and fractures. Behavioural indicators include age-inappropriate behaviour, self-harm, wariness of certain individuals and 'frozen watchfulness'. A full review of physical and behavioural indicators of maltreatment is provided by Hobbs et al (1999).

Although there are no indicators that are 100% 'diagnostic' of maltreatment, it is important to carefully evaluate each child's history and presentation, taking into account their developmental needs and abilities.

Scenario

Scott, a 10-week-old baby, was seen in the Emergency Department with a cut above his left eye. He was accompanied by his mother, who explained that he had been out with his father that morning and managed to fall out of the buggy. On examination, bruising was noticed on Scott's abdomen.

Delays in presentation and inconsistencies in history giving are suspicious for maltreatment. Injuries of differing ages and repeated presentation to healthcare professionals are also of concern. Wherever possible, the child should be asked to give his or her own history. In some cases, children will spontaneously disclose abuse and, if this happens, it is vitally important that the child is allowed to talk freely, not openly questioned (this may affect criminal procedures), and that detailed, contemporaneous records are kept.

Fabricated or induced illness (FII) is a relatively rare, but important, form of child maltreatment that sometimes leads to the death of a child. Here, carers (usually the mother) repeatedly present the child to healthcare professionals with falsified accounts of various signs and symptoms. The child may then undergo multiple investigations (which in themselves may be harmful) without a firm diagnosis being reached. In more severe cases, symptoms are induced through the misuse of medication or other substances (e.g. table salt) or hospital equipment, such as infusion lines, might be tampered with. 'Safeguarding children in whom illness has been fabricated or induced' (HM Government 2008b) outlines what is known about this form of abuse, how difficult it may be to detect, and the importance of working within interagency child protection procedures. Health professionals who have unwittingly colluded with perpetrators of this type of harm will themselves need support through activities such as 'debriefing' (Terry 2004).

Recognition of maltreatment often relies on a professional's 'gut feeling' and a willingness to question 'puzzling' situations. In all cases it is important to check concerns with a senior colleague and to keep accurate records. Reviewing past records and history, including that of siblings, may also be helpful, as will informal discussions with other professionals who have contact with the child and family.

Responding and referral

Although it may well be a nurse who identifies possible indicators of child maltreatment, the decision to make a child protection referral to children's social care will normally be made by a senior paediatrician following careful evaluation of the child's presentation and history. Because nurses spend more time with patients there may be situations in which interprofessional disagreements arise. In these instances it is wise to seek the help of local child protection specialists (such as Named Professionals) to help to resolve differences in opinion and to ensure the child's welfare.

The process of referral described below is for England and, although parallels exist with the other countries of the UK, the reader is reminded of their responsibility to review their country-specific safeguarding policy guidance.

Following referral Children's Social Care will undertake an initial assessment and make a decision as to whether they believe that the child is at risk of, or suffering, actual significant harm. If this is the case they will call a Strategy Discussion, which will involve the Police and other relevant agencies. This process can take up to 7 working days but may be more immediate if there are urgent concerns about a child's welfare and a need for urgent protective measures. Should the Strategy Discussion lead to a decision that there are concerns about a child's safety then a full inquiry (under Section 47 of the Children Act 1989) will be undertaken. A social work manager will be responsible for convening a Child Protection Conference within 15 working days of the Strategy Discussion, if the enquiries substantiate the concerns. The purpose of a Child Protection Conference is to bring together and analyse information relating to the child and family, and decide whether the child is at continuing risk of harm and to identify future action to safeguard the welfare of the child.

If the child is at continuing risk of significant harm, then safeguarding the child will require interagency action and the implementation of an agreed 'child protection plan'. At the conference an outline of this plan will be formulated and a decision made and recorded, regarding which category of abuse or neglect the child is suffering, or is at risk of suffering. Alongside the child protection procedures, the police may undertake a criminal investigation. This may involve undertaking a joint interview with the child. Children who are not thought to be at risk of significant harm may nonetheless be identified by the conference participants (who normally include family members and the child if appropriate) as requiring services to promote their health and development. The conference will consider the child's needs and how best to support the family to meet them.

Child protection procedures involve detailed interagency working and rest on the principles of openness and partnership with children and their families. The document 'What to do if you're worried a child is being abused' (HM Government 2006b) provides more detailed guidance on procedures. To contribute to safeguarding children you may be required to share confidential information, without the consent of the patient or client. Although the Nursing and Midwifery Council's (NMC) Code of Professional Conduct (2008) requires nurses to protect confidential information, provision is made for nurses to act in the public interest and in accordance with national and local child protection policies (NMC 2008 Section 5.3 p 7–8). Readers are advised to consult guidance regarding when and how to share information professionally and legally (HM Government 2008c).

Summary

The chapter has aimed to equip students of children's nursing with the knowledge and understanding that will enable them to identify, and respond appropriately to, children who may be at risk of, or suffering from, harm. We hope that this work will give future children's nurses confidence in their abilities to be part of this important area of child health. The emphasis on the rights of the child has been deliberate – children's nurses will work with many vulnerable and needy families in the course of their practice. To lose the focus on the daily lived experience of the child is to court the possibility of another child maltreatment tragedy. We wish you well.

Child protection helplines and websites

Childline (24 hours): 0800 1111; http://www.childline.org.uk/

Contact-A-Family (9 a.m. to 5 p.m. Monday to Friday): support for parents of children with disabilities: 020 7222 2695; http://www.cafamily.org.uk/

Cry-sis (9 a.m. to 5 p.m. Monday to Friday): persistently crying and/or sleepless babies: 020 7404 5011; http://www.cry-sis.com/

Family Rights Group (1.30 p.m. to 3.30 p.m. Monday to Friday): support with child protection procedures: 020 7249 0008; http://www.frg.org.uk/index.asp

Kidscape (9.30 a.m. to 5 p.m. Monday and Wednesday): deals with bullying, stranger danger, threats of abuse: 020 7730 3300; http://www.kidscape.org.uk/

NCH Action for Children: 01772 25492; http://www.nchafc.org.uk/

NSPCC Child Protection Line (24 hours): acts in cases of neglect and abuse of children: 0808 800 500; help@nspcc.org.uk

National Association for People Abused in Childhood (NAPAC): for adult survivors of abuse: 0800 085 3330; http://www.napac.org.uk/

Respond: sexual abuse and people with learning disabilities: 0845 606 1503; http://www.respond.org.uk/

Survivors (Incest): 020 7833 3737; http://www.survivors.org.uk/

Women's Aid: emergency accommodation for abused women and children: 0117 963 3542; http://www.womensaid.org.uk/

References

Alderson, P., 2008. Young children's rights: exploring beliefs, principles and practice, 2nd ed. Jessica Kingsley Publishers, London.

Archard, D., 1993. Children: rights and childhood. Routledge, London.

Barnes, J., Ball, M., Meadows, P., et al., 2008. DCSF Research Report Nurse Family Partnership Programme: First Year Pilot Sites Implementation in England. Department for Children, Schools and Families. Department of Health, London.

Batmanghelidjh, C., 2006. Shattered lives: children who live with courage and dignity. Jessica Kingsley Publishers, London.

Belsky, J., 1993. Etiology of child maltreatment: a developmental-ecological analysis. Psychological Bulletin 114 (3), 413–434.

Browne, K., Davies, C., Stratton, P. (Eds.), 1988. Early prediction and prevention of child abuse. John Wiley, Chichester.

Cawson, P., Wattam, C., Brooker, S., Kelly, G., 2000. Child maltreatment in the United Kingdom: a study of the prevalence of child abuse and neglect. NSPCC, London.

Children Act, 1989. HMSO, London.

Children Act 2004 http://www.opsi.gov.uk/acts/acts2004/ukpga_20040031_en_1 (Accessed online February 13th 2009)

Children Act (Northern Ireland), 1995. Department of Health, Social Services and Public Safety (DHPSS) available on line at http://www.dhsspsni.gov.uk/childcare_guidance

Children Act (Scotland), 1995. HMSO, London. Available on line at http://www.opsi.gov.uk/ACTS/acts1995/ukpga_19950036_en_1

Corby, B., 2006. Child abuse: towards a knowledge base, 3rd edn. Open University Press, Maidenhead.

Department for Children, Schools and Families, 2007. The Childrens Plan. Building brighter futures. Available on line at http://publications.dcsf.gov.uk/eOrderingDownload/The_Childrens_Plan.pdf

Department for Children, Schools and Families (DCSF) 2008a Statement on Safeguarding of Children, Press Notice 2008/0271 available on line at http://www.dcsf.gov.uk (Accessed on line February 13th 2009)

Department for Children, Schools and Families (DCSF) 2008b Referrals and Assessments and Children and Young People who are subject to a child protection plan year ending 31st March 2008 available on line at http://www.dcsf.gov.uk/rsgateway/DB/SFR/s000811/index.shtml (Accessed online February 13th 2009)

Department for Children, Schools and Families, 2008c. Statistical release referrals assessments and children and young people who are subject to a child protection plan year ending March 2008. Available on line at http://www.dcsf.gov.uk/rsgateway/DB/SFR/s000811/sfr24_2008.pdf

Department for Education and Skills (DfES), 2004. Every child matters. The Stationery Office, London.

Department for Education and Skills (DfES), Department of Health (DoH), Home Office, 2003. Keeping children safe: the government's response to the Victoria Climbié inquiry report and joint chief inspectors' report safeguarding children. The Stationery Office, London.

Department of Health (DoH), 2002. Safeguarding children in whom illness is fabricated or induced. DoH, London.

Department of Health (DoH), Department for Education and Skills (DfES), 2004. National Service Framework for Children, Young People and Maternity Services: Care Standards. DoH, London.

Department of Health (DoH), Department for Education and Skills (DfES), 2008. The Child Health Promotion Programme. DoH, London.

Franklin, B. (Ed.), 1995. The handbook of children's rights, Routledge, London.

Gilbert R E, Spatz Wisdom C, Browne K 2008 Burden and consequences of child maltreatment in high income countries Lancet published on line Dec 3 DOI: 10.1016/SO140-6736(08) 61706-7 (Accessed online February 13th 2009)

Hall, D., 2003. Protecting children, supporting professionals. Archives of Disease in Childhood 88, 557–559.

Hobbs C 2003 In: Department for Education and Skills (DfES), Department of Health (DoH), Home Office (2003) Keeping children safe: the government's response to the Victoria Climbié inquiry report and joint chief inspectors' report safeguarding children. The Stationery Office, London.

Hobbs, C., Hanks, H., Wynne, J., 1999. Child abuse and neglect: a clinician's handbook, 2nd edn. Churchill Livingstone, London.

Holt, J., 1975. Escape from childhood: the needs and rights of children. Penguin, Harmondsworth.

HM Government, 2004. Every Child Matters Change for Children. Department for Education and Skills, London.

HM Government, 2006a. Working Together to Safeguard Children A Guide to Inter-agency Working to Safeguard and Promote the Welfare of Children. Department for Education and Skills, London.

HM Government, 2006b. What to do if you're worried a child is being abused. Department for Education and Skills, London.

HM Government, 2007. The Consolidated 3rd and 4th Periodic Report to the Committee on the Rights of Child. Department for Children, Schools and Families, London.

HM Government, 2008a Staying Safe Action Plan. Department for Children, School and Families, London.

HM Government, 2008b Safeguarding Children in whom illness has been fabricated or induced, supplementary guidance to Working Together to Safeguard Children. Department for Children, Schools and Families and Communities and Local Government, London.

HM Government, 2008c. Information sharing guidance for practitioners and managers. Department for Children, Schools and Families, London.

Lord Laming, 2003. The Victoria Climbié inquiry: report of an inquiry by Lord Laming. The Victoria Climbié Inquiry. Online. Available at: http://www.victoria-climbie-inquiry.org.uk/finreport/finreport.htm (Accessed online February 13th 2009).

National Commission of Inquiry into the Prevention of Child Abuse (NCIPCA), 1996. Childhood Matters. Stationery Office, London vol. I and II.

National Society for the Prevention of Cruelty to Children (NSPCC), 1996. A cry for children campaign: child protection agenda. NSPCC, London.

National Society for the Prevention of Cruelty to Children (NSPCC), 2007 Child Homicides: Key child protection statistics December 2007 Online. Available at: http://www.nspcc.org.uk/(accessed on line 2nd October 2008).

National Working Group on Child Protection and Disability, 2003. It doesn't happen to disabled children. Child protection and disabled children. NSPCC, London.

Newell, P., 1995. Respecting children's rights to physical integrity. In: Franklin, B. (Ed.), 1995 The handbook of children's rights, Routledge, London, pp. 215–226.

Nursing and Midwifery Council (NMC), 2008. Code of professional conduct. NMC, London.

Ofsted, 2008. Safeguarding Children: The third joint inspectors report on arrangements to safeguard children. Ofsted, London.

Powell, C., 2002. There is no such thing as a child receiving 'a good smack'. British Journal of Nursing 11 (22), 1425.

Powell, C., 2007. Safeguarding children and young people: a guide for nurses and midwives. Open University Press, Maidenhead.

Qvortrup, J., 1994. Introduction. In: Qvortrup, J., Bardy, M., Sgritta, G., Wintersberger, H. (Eds.), Childhood matters: social theory, practice and politics. Avebury, Aldershot, pp. 1–23.

Terry, L., 2004. Fabricated or induced illness of children. Paediatric Nursing 16 (1), 14–18.

United Nations Children's Fund (UNICEF) 2003 A league table of child maltreatment deaths in rich nations. Innocenti Report Card No. 5. UNICEF Innocenti Research Centre, Florence. Online. Available at: http://www.unicef-icdc.org (Accessed on line February 13th 2009).

United Nations General Assembly, 1989. Convention on the rights of the child. UNICEF, Geneva.

Web sites

The Victoria Climbié Inquiry Report can be read online at: http://www.victoria-climbie-inquiry.org.uk/finreport/finreport.htm (Accessed on line February 13th 2009)

Visit the United Nations Children's Fund (UNICEF) website to learn more about how this organisation advocates for children world-wide through facilitating the full implementation of the UN Convention of the Rights of the Child: http://www.unicef.org (Accessed on line February 13th 2009)

Keep up to date with developments in the UK National Service Framework on: http://www.doh.gov/nsf/children (Accessed on line February 13th 2009)

Every child matters and subsequent policy can be found on: http://www.dfes.gov.uk (Accessed online February 13th 2009)

Ethics in children's nursing

20

E Alan Glasper Jim Richardson

ABSTRACT

The primary aim of this chapter is to examine, within the context of recent developments in child health practice and research, some underlying ethical demands and dilemmas facing children's nurses. A description of the Nuremberg Code, the Helsinki Declaration, The UN Convention on the Rights of the Child and the Human Rights Act will form the backdrop to this chapter and a range of contemporary examples will be used to illuminate these issues. Within this arena, the four major principles that underpin healthcare ethics will be investigated and past examples of historical unethical practice and research acknowledged. The vulnerability of children and their families to potential coercion and the role of research ethics committees will be discussed.

LEARNING OUTCOMES

- Achieve an overview of the major ethical principles in child health care.
- Recognise how these principles can be applied in everyday child health nursing.
- Appreciate dimensions surrounding some ethical controversies in relation to research involving children.

Introduction

It might appear to the newly qualified children's nurse that the recent history of the profession is tarnished with examples of unethical healthcare practice and violation of basic human rights. With no less than four major official investigations related to ethical aspects of childcare published since the start of the 21st century (Department of Health (DoH) 2001a,b, National Assembly for Wales 2002, NHS Executive 2000) it can be appreciated that urgent action is necessary to restore public confidence in the NHS. However, before examining contemporary issues related to child health care it is worth remembering that it was the activities of German healthcare professionals during the years of the Second World War that finally galvanised an exhausted post-war world to do something about unethical healthcare practice and research. When the full scale of the dreadful experiments carried out on human beings, including children, against their will became fully known, perpetrators were prosecuted at the trials in Nuremberg, although not all were severely punished. In the wake of the Nuremberg trials, a code of practice was developed that became subsequently known as the Nuremberg Code (Eby 1995).

WWW

Read the Nuremberg Code online at:
- http://www.ohsr.od.nih.gov/nuremberg.php3

The Nuremberg Code particularly related to the ethical conduct of research. Although the elements that make up valid consent are the same in consent to research as in consent to treatment (information, capacity and freedom from coercion), research carries two extra dimensions that increase the potential vulnerability of research subjects to exploitation: (i) research may be risky and the potential benefit to the subject might be slight, unknown or absent; and (ii) the aims of the research may conflict with the therapeutic aims of treatment.

The Nuremberg code and past unethical practice

Ten key directives are highlighted, which pertain to the conduct of human experimentation. These include that:

- the voluntary consent of the human subject is absolutely essential
- the experiment should be designed to yield fruitful results for the benefit of society

DOI: 10.1016/B978-0-7020-3183-0.10020-7

- the experiment should avoid all unnecessary physical and mental suffering and injury
- no experiment should be conducted where there is reason to believe that death or disabling injury will occur, except perhaps where the experimenters themselves serve as subjects
- the degree of risk should never exceed the humanitarian importance of the problem to be solved through the research (adequate facilities should be provided to protect the experimental subject from injury, disability or death)
- experiments should be carried out only by appropriately qualified persons
- human subjects should be able to terminate the experiment whenever they wish
- during the experiment, the principal investigator must be prepared to terminate the experiment at any stage if there is reason to believe that continuation is likely to result in injury, disability or death of a subject

Despite the universal condemnation of the German atrocities committed in the name of scientific progress, unethical research on human beings has, unfortunately, continued. Perhaps the most flagrant abuse of human rights during a longitudinal government-sponsored medical investigation occurred in the USA between the years 1932 and 1972 during the Tuskegee syphilis study.

WWW

You can find out more about this infamous research at:

- http://www.med.virginia.edu/hs-library/historical/apology/index.html

In the study, 399 African–American men were denied treatment for syphilis; they were deceived by public health officials who were fully aware that effective treatment was available. Such has been the damage to the US government's reputation that it was necessary, in 1997, for the then President to issue a formal apology on behalf of the nation. Although the presidential words may have closed one chapter in the catalogue of human rights abuses, it would be naïve to believe that unethical research is currently not being conducted. A report in the Lancet (1997) revealed that the US Centre for Disease Control had supported unethical trials of new drugs for the treatment of human immunodeficiency virus (HIV), in which a placebo group of women were allowed to infect their children perinatally. These examples demonstrate the particular vulnerability of certain groups to exploitation. Children are a classic example of such a group.

The Helsinki declaration

Although the Nuremberg Code is explicit in its recommendations for healthcare researchers, the Tuskegee scandal demonstrated that harm was still being done in the name of good. The World Medical Association therefore adopted the recommendations contained in the document–Guiding physicians in biomedical research involving human subjects–at the 18th World Medical Assembly in Helsinki, Finland, in June 1964. This 'Helsinki Declaration' was subsequently amended several times, the last being at the World Medical Association General Assembly in Edinburgh in October 2000. Importantly, the Helsinki Declaration highlights the necessity of obtaining informed consent. Additionally, it advises caution if the research subject is in a dependent relationship with the researcher or if the individual might consent under duress. This is particularly pertinent for children's nurses, who purport to act as advocates for the family while also contributing to the research process.

The Declaration uses the term 'legal incompetence', whereby physical or mental incapacity makes it impossible to obtain informed consent or when the subject is a minor. In these cases the Helsinki protocol recommends the gaining of permission from a responsible relative. Although this is advocated, importantly the gaining of consent from the child is stressed in addition to that of the minor's legal guardian.

The UN Convention on the Rights of the Child and the Human Rights Act (1998)

The General Assembly of the United Nations adopted the convention on the Rights of the Child in November 1989; this came into force in the UK in January 1992.

WWW

You can access the UN Convention at:

- http://www.unhcr.ch/html/menu3/b/k2crc.htm

Activity

Read through the summary of the Convention on the Rights of the Child. Make notes against each article on its relevance to:

- research involving children
- clinical children's nursing practice.

When you have done this, consider to what extent the requirements of these two fields of practice differ from each other in their ethical requirements.

The UK's second report to The UN Committee on the Rights of the Child (DoH 1999) demonstrated that considerable effort was being made to meet the UN targets. However, UNICEF suggests that the government's 1999 report is 'little more than an uncritical review of aspects of government policy related to children' (UNICEF 2000).

The Human Rights Act of 1998, which came into effect on 2 October 2000, highlighted the potential of some areas of health and social care practice to affect the rights and freedoms promised under the Act. Power (2002) discusses Article 3, among others, of the Act, which relates to torture and degrading treatment or punishment and highlights the implications for child health nurses, especially when restraining children for healthcare interventions.

www

You can find the text of the Human Rights Act at:

- http://www.doh.gov.uk/humanrights/qa.htm

The implementation of these policies is beginning to impact on the way in which children are cared for in hospital and the Child Friendly Hospital Initiative spearheaded by UNICEF has been embraced by a number of children's hospitals in the UK such as The Royal Hospital For Sick Children Glasgow.

www

You can details of the Child Friendly Hospital initiative at:

- http://www.childfriendlyhealthcare.org

The four principles of healthcare ethics

Although the NMC Code of Professional Conduct (NMC 2002) provides explicit guidance on consent for all nurses, Section 3.9 discusses children in particular. Additionally the Royal College of Nursing (RCN) has issued guidelines for nurses involved with research (RCN 1977). These and other guidelines implicitly or explicitly use the four principles of healthcare ethics first proposed by Beauchamp & Childress in 1979.

1. Autonomy

The primary interpretation of this word is self-determination. The complexity of this concept is increased by its link with liberty. Personal liberty, although a common value of Western life, may have different value in other countries and other social groups, where decisions may be made by a group, such as a family, rather than espousing individual rights. Autonomy and childhood have in the past been perceived as mutually exclusive but there is now a growing awareness that children are able to make their own decisions if given information in an age-appropriate manner (Alderson 2000, British Medical Association (BMA) 2001).

When the term 'autonomy' is applied to contemporary healthcare practice and research the focus is on the right to informed consent (Behi 1995). Although every individual has this right, it must be appreciated that some, but especially children, may not be able to articulate this or may be prevented from doing so. The Gillick case (Gillick v West Norfolk and Wisbech AHA [1986]), in which a mother unsuccessfully challenged the legal right of doctors to withhold information about their advice and treatment of a minor from parents when it was thought to be in the young person's best interest, was a high-water mark in the enfranchisement of children (Alderson & Montgomery 1996). Since then, children who are deemed competent in line with 'Fraser guidelines' are, in the eyes of the law, able to make informed choices. When this conveniently matches the decision of the healthcare professional or guardian, this inclusion in decision making is seen as an example of good practice. When it does not, the rights of the child may be diluted on the basis that adults know best. Although this paternalistic approach within both treatment and research is in decline, competent children remain a group whose rights to consent or refuse consent are easy to overlook.

In the case of younger, pre-autonomous children, respect for autonomy is shown by ensuring that parents agree to give proxy consent to treatment and research. The cases detailed below demonstrate the loving commitment of parents to the well-being of their child and their deep sense of betrayal if their child is harmed by health professionals.

Scenario

14-year-old Sam has been suffering from lethargy, unusual tiredness and a tendency to bruise easily. Bloods drawn by his GP have yielded a very pathological result. Sam needs further investigation for a potentially serious illness. He absolutely refuses to tell his parents about this situation or to allow his parents to be told by a member of the care team.

Activity

Consider the factors to be taken into account in judging whether Sam is mature enough to make this decision alone. What are the ethical requirements of this situation, e.g. what are the rights and responsibilities of all the players in this scenario?

2. Beneficence

Beneficence means the duty to do good to others, to act in their best interests. However, if this principle was universal and we were required always to do good to everyone, the duty would be too onerous. Beneficence is a constituent part of a special duty of care such as that which exists between a nurse and patient or between a parent and child (Charles-Edwards 1995). Cases such as that of the GP Harold Shipman are particularly horrifying because of the breach of this duty of care.

One of the ambiguities at the heart of health care is the duty to act in the patient's best interests while avoiding the danger of following only the principle of beneficence and ignoring that of autonomy – 'the doctor knows best' phenomenon. The contemporary insistence that patient (and parent) must be given an informed choice attests to this and to the anachronism of paternalistic attitudes: 'Partnership between patient and healthcare professional is the way forward' (Kennedy 2001 p 13).

3. Non-maleficence

Florence Nightingale is reported to have said 'first do the patient no harm' and non-maleficence simply means to do no harm. However, this has to be tempered with the reality that inadvertent harm may befall a child during a caring intervention, which may not have been foreseen. Iatrogenic illness or illness precipitated by medical treatment is now a common cause of death and was first highlighted 25 years ago by Ivan Illich (1977). It is the duty of every nurse to avoid harming others, and this is reflected in the use of policies, procedures and protocols that are designed to minimise this. Some hospitals include this philosophy in their mission statements, e.g. The Great Ormond Street Hospital for Children has as its motto 'The child first and always'.

4. Justice

When applied to health care, justice is used in the context of an equitable use of healthcare resources. There is consequently a dichotomy between wanting to give the best for each patient (beneficence) and the recognition of competition for scarce resources among the whole of the client group. In the 1995 court case of Child B or Jaymee Bowen (R v Cambridge Health Authority, ex parte B [1995]) the principle of justice was at the heart of the controversy as portrayed by the media (Ham & Pickard 1998). Jaymee was aged 10 at the time and had suffered from acute lymphoblastic leukaemia, which she had developed at the age of 5 and for which she had a successful bone marrow transplant. She was admitted to hospital with acute myeloid leukaemia. Senior childhood cancer consultants advised against treatment believing it not to be in the child's best interests. Her father refused to accept this decision and sought other opinions. A London-based consultant offered to treat the child in the private sector at a cost of £75,000. The local health authority refused to underwrite the cost and the father started legal action, which was not successful. The case attracted much publicity and an anonymous benefactor eventually paid for the treatment. Sadly, the treatment did not have the lasting effects hoped for and Jaymee died just 17 months later. The case was cited as an example of healthcare rationing, now widely referred to as 'postcode health care', although the high-risk, low-benefit outcome of the proposed treatment was central to the medical decision that further treatment would be futile. The ethical dilemmas presented by participation in experimental treatment, such as that proposed in Jaymee's case, and not underpinned by peer-reviewed published evidence will always be problematical.

Activity

Consider the rights and responsibilities of each of the individuals/agencies involved in the above situation. Think about the ethical implications and consequences of the available courses of action, e.g. treating or not treating.

Advocacy

For the sake of completeness, it will be useful to consider the role advocacy might have in such ethically demanding situations. Advocacy is an idea that is widely discussed in nursing circles (Wheeler 2000). The concept is based on the fact that there will always be some who will need someone else to speak out on their behalf to protect their best interests. Although all of us are likely to require such assistance at some point in our lives, there are certain groups in society who have been identified as potentially in need of such help. Children who have not yet achieved the developmental skills for autonomous decision making are an obvious example of this (Mallik 1997).

Although advocacy is usually assumed to be benign in character and well-intentioned (Willard 1996), it must be recognised that the basis of advocacy is that the advocate has the power to speak with effect whereas the person advocated for does not. This power gradient must be recognised and acknowledged for what it is if advocacy is to be constructive. Checks and balances must be in place to ensure that paternalism, at best, and abuse, at worst, is avoided. With a realistic view of its potential advantages and disadvantages, advocacy can be a strong contributor to child well-being. Parents have long been advocates!

Contemporary examples of child healthcare practice and research where the rights of the child or family have been breached

Despite the existence of charters and declarations that purport to protect the public from the potential hazards of healthcare practice and research, pockets of questionable practice related to children and their families have undermined the otherwise good reputations of healthcare researchers.

Consent for organ retention at the Royal Liverpool Children's Hospital (Alder Hey)

As the news relating to the wholesale removal of organs from the bodies of dead children without parental consent at the Alder Hey Children's Hospital was breaking, it quickly became apparent that many other hospitals throughout the UK also had collections of children's organs. An audit conducted by the Chief Medical Officer Professor Liam Donaldson (DoH 2000) revealed that hospitals collectively had stored anywhere between 40,000 and 50,000 organs from deceased individuals. The scandal that emanated from the Alder Hey Children's Hospital covered the period 1988–1996, when organs were removed from the bodies of dead babies for research purposes without adequate consent.

The primary lesson of the Royal Liverpool Children's Inquiry (DoH 2001a; the Redfern Report, which represents the official report of events at the Alder Hey Children's Hospital) is that there was a gross mismatch between the understanding of the parents, who thought giving consent for tissue removal meant only small specimens, and the doctors, who believed such consent implied they could take what they wanted, including whole body systems.

It is perhaps timely to examine the origins of the Human Tissue Act, introduced in 1961. The law was originally introduced because of a shortage of eyes for corneal grafting. The Act made it lawful for doctors to authorise the removal of body parts for medical education and research purposes 'if having made such reasonable inquiry as may be practicable, he [sic] has no reasons to believe that any relative objects.' Hence a law introduced for medical expediency at a particular time in history opened the floodgates for abuse. It was the way in which some doctors interpreted and implemented this law that is the cause of this recent controversy (Glasper & Powell 2001).

Few people doubt the benefits to patients that are derived from human tissue research but the flagrant abuse of rudimentary consent procedures linked to the existing Human Tissue Act 1961 has resulted in a level of public scepticism that, if not rectified, will have a negative impact on future research and organ donation in particular. Indeed, in the days following the publication of the Redfern Report, world transplant pioneer Professor Magdi Yacoub was warning the public about a backlash against giving consent for organ donation and revealed an acute shortage of donors (2001).

The media reports also reveal the strength of public disquiet at the events at Alder Hey (Bentham 2001). A key finding of the report was the abundant evidence of failure on the part of clinicians to obtain appropriate consent. During the inquiry, doctors who gave evidence acknowledged that it was difficult to reconcile their traditional benign paternalistic attitudes, which made them seek to protect families from distressing events, to the wording of the Human Tissue Act in which the details of the procedure were supposed to be fully and frankly discussed. However, the inquiry concluded that, on the evidence, the medical profession did not properly consider the Act in the first place. This resulted in doctors believing they could have access to any part of a child's body that they wished. However, this only partially explains why the pathology department at Alder Hey systematically collected body organs from children in numbers that could not be reconciled with the research programmes being conducted at the hospital.

Nurses must acknowledge that existing consent procedures will have to be strengthened to avoid a repetition of the events at Alder Hey (Glasper & Powell 2000) and the other centres that retained organs. Although the DoH (2001c) has now produced a new reference guide to consent for examination and treatment, which includes a guide for children and young people, it must be acknowledged that families will continue to rely on nurses to be their advocates. This is particularly poignant in the light of the second scandal to encroach on the otherwise flawless reputation of Alder Hey. Only a year after the publication of The Redfern Report, the hospital was again accused of retaining the organs of children without parental consent, with managers being accused by the family solicitors of 'learning nothing' (Guardian, Editorial 2002).

Children's nurses are in a unique position to support the appropriate implementation of the enquiry's recommendations for consent. Alan Milburn, who was then the Secretary of State for Health, stated on the day of the report publication:

> For trust to thrive there has to be informed consent, not a tick-in-the-box regime – consent that is based on constructive dialogue and where consent is actually sought and positively given
>
> (Bosley 2001)

These recommendations emphasise that fully informed consent means that a person must have all the information required to make a final decision. Although many clinicians will find it difficult to provide the details recommended by the enquiry, e.g. about the post-mortem examination and what this entails, nevertheless it is now incumbent for this to become accepted and standard practice. The Chief Medical Officer (DoH 2000) stated:

> When a child dies that child is still the parent's child – not a specimen, not a cause, not an unfortunate casualty of a failed procedure, but someone's baby, someone's child. In life the parent is responsible for every aspect of a child's well-being. In death that responsibility should not be taken away.

To help parents fully understand the need to retain some organs for histological analysis, and that such examinations cannot take place for several weeks because of the scientific process, the information sharing that now must take place should also encompass parental wishes regarding the subsequent respectful disposal of the organ. Only if this process is strictly adhered to will relatives be able to begin, experience and complete the necessary process of human grieving.

Consent for major heart surgery at the Bristol Royal Infirmary

The situation of Bristol Royal Infirmary is linked to that of Alder Hey in that both concern children but also have ramifications for nursing as a whole. Alison Norman, the President of the UKCC said of the events 'it is a tragedy that it took the death of more than 30 children to act as a catalyst for cultural change within the NHS' (UKCC 2001). However, long before the 3-year public inquiry into children's heart surgery at the Bristol Royal Infirmary, chaired by Professor Ian Kennedy, was finally published, healthcare professionals were acknowledging that the old health service needed reform (Glasper 2001). The inquiry was initiated after it was revealed that mortality figures at Bristol for children undergoing heart surgery were higher than in comparable units in other parts of the country. The Bristol inquiry (DoH 2001b) showed that some healthcare professionals had not treated families with the proper respect due to them and had failed to obtain fully informed consent from parents before surgery. The lessons of Bristol emphasise the necessity for all children's nurses to accept the benefits of clinical governance, in which the family holds centre-stage in a continuous cycle of quality improvement. Furthermore, the recommendation that calls for children to be cared for only by professionals who have been specifically educated in the care of children reinforces the message of previous reports and has helped inform the ongoing development of the National Service Framework for Children.

The report had ramifications for the NHS in general, and in particular the need for openness in the giving of information. If information-giving is, indeed, the key to empowerment (Robertson 1995) then families must be given all the information they need to make critical decisions about their children. In the wake of Bristol a new regulatory body for NHS managers was being established whose maxim is a re-emphasis on patients first. The DoH's response to the public inquiry ratifies the findings and reaffirms the commitment of the government to transform the health service. Importantly, consent is highlighted as a continuous process, not a one-off event. This has important ramifications for children's nurses, as children, because of their developmental parameters, will require innovative methods of obtaining informed consent.

Conducting research and protecting the rights of children and their families

The BMA has been prompted to publish explicit guidelines for those who wish to conduct research with children (BMA 2001). Furthermore, the Royal College of Paediatrics and Child Health (RCPCH) have published guidelines on the involvement of children in research (RCPCH 2000 p 177) in which it states:

> Many children are vulnerable, easily bewildered and frightened, and unable to express their needs or defend their interests. Potentially with many decades ahead of them, they are likely to experience, in their development and education, the most lasting benefits or harms from research.

Activity

Obtain and read in detail the Royal College of Paediatrics and Child Health's useful set of guidelines (RCPCH 2000).

A number of questions related to research with children and young people have been raised and discussed by Alderson (1995):

- Are children likely to suffer any harm as a result of the research, in the form of emotional distress or intrusion?
- Do the benefits of the research clearly outweigh these possible risks?
- Who will benefit from the research – children or just the researchers?
- Are children given the proper information about the research?
- Are children offered the opportunity to refuse to participate or answer particular questions?

Despite the large volume of recommendations related to consent available to children's nurses from a variety of auspicious bodies, there is little evidence that children are actively involved with their own healthcare decision making in a meaningful way (Feasy 2001). Children are not used to being listened to and adults have difficulties about listening to children (O'Quigley 2000), and these inherent communication difficulties place children in a vulnerable position during healthcare interventions.

The role of local research ethics committees (LREC)

All NHS areas host research ethics committees, whose role it is to maintain high ethical standards in the conduct of all clinical research undertaken on patients and healthy volunteers and to safeguard the rights of human research subjects as defined by the Declaration of Helsinki, the reputation of the health professions and their institutions. It should be clarified that the LRECs are independent of the Trusts and are answerable to the National Health Service Executive outposts. The lines of accountability are changing with the introduction of a Research Governance Framework to ensure that any research carried out in health and social care has full ethical approval (for more information, see http://www.doh.gov.uk/research/rd3/nhsrandd/researchgovernance.htm):

- This includes all types of studies whether therapeutic or non-therapeutic on patients and normal subjects.
- The committees are accountable to a Health Authority and membership includes a lay chairperson and members in addition to doctors, nurses and other healthcare professionals. These committees meet monthly and consider all LREC applications.
- Applications can be approved fully, given conditional approval where amendments are necessary or approval can be withheld where there are concerns. It remains to be seen if newly organised LRECs will be able to safeguard children better than they did in the past.

Summary

The world of healthcare practice and research remains a moral minefield. Child health nurses, working within their philosophy of family care, are often at the forefront of activity and therefore open to criticism. It is incumbent upon all nurses to make themselves aware of the ethical dimensions of any research or clinical care they might be involved with no matter how peripherally. It will not be possible to protect the rights of the child unless they do so. If we do not learn the lessons of the past then we are destined to repeat them.

References

Alderson, A., 2000. exploring beliefs, principle and practice. Young children's rights. Jessica Kingsley, London.

Alderson, P., 1995. Listening to children; children, ethics and social research. Barnardos, Ilford

Alderson, P., Montgomery, J., 1996. Health care choices: making decisions with children. Institute of Public Policy Research, London.

Beauchamp, T., Childress, J., 1979. Principles of biomedical ethics. Oxford University Press, New York.

Behi, R., 1995. The individual's right to informed consent. Nurse Researcher 3 (1), 14–23.

Bentham, M., 2001. Report shows half of hospitals involved in body parts scandal. Headline News January 28 2001, p 26

British Medical Association (BMA), 2001. Consent, rights and choices in health care for children and young people. BMJ Books, London.

Bosley, S., 2001. Grotesque breach of trust at Alder Hey. The Guardian, January 29 2001, p 6

Charles-Edwards, I., 1995. Moral, ethical, and legal perspectives. In: Carter, B., Dearmun, A.K. (Eds.), Child health care nursing. Blackwell Scientific, London, pp. 61–74.

Department of Health (DoH), 1999. Convention on the Rights of the Child. DoH, London.

Department of Health (DoH), 2000. The removal, retention and use of human organs and tissue from post-mortem examination (Advice from the Chief Medical Officer). DoH, London.

Department of Health (DoH), 2001a. The Royal Liverpool children's inquiry: summary and recommendations. The Stationery Office, London.

Department of Health (DoH), 2001b. The report of the public inquiry into children's heart surgery at the Bristol Royal Infirmary 1984–1995. Learning from Bristol. DoH London.

Department of Health (DoH), 2001c. Reference guide to consent for examination or treatment. DoH, London.

Eby, M., 1995. Ethical issues in nursing research: the wider picture. Nurse Researcher 3 (1), 5–13.

Editorial, 2002. New organ retention row hits Alder Hey. The Guardian May 13.

Feasy, S., 2001. Children' participation in decision making (research and commentary). Paediatric Nursing 13 (10), 12.

Gillick v West Norfolk and Wisbech AHA [1986] AC 112, 1985 3WLR 830, 3 All ER 402 HL

Glasper, E.A., 2001. Nurses must enhance care in the wake of Bristol. British Journal of Nursing 10 (15), 966.

Glasper, E.A., Powell, C., 2000. Children need protecting in death as well as life. British Journal of Nursing 9 (1), 5.

Glasper, E.A., Powell, C., 2001. Lessons of Alder Hey; consent must be informed. British Journal of Nursing 10 (4), 213.

Ham, C., Pickard, S., 1998. Tragic choices in health care: the case of Child B. Kings Fund, London.

Illich, I., 1977. Limits to medicine; medical nemesis, the expropriation of health. Penguin, Harmondsworth.

Kennedy, I., 2001. Learning from Bristol: the report of the inquiry into children's heart surgery at Bristol Royal Infirmary 1984-1995. The Stationery Office, London.

Lancet, 1997. The ethics industry (editorial). Lancet 350, 297.

National Assembly for Wales, 2002. Too serious a thing/Peth rhy Ddifrif: the review of safeguards for children and young people treated and cared for by the NHS in Wales. National Assembly for Wales, Cardiff.

NHS Executive West Midlands Regional Office, 2000. Report of a review of the research framework in North Staffordshire Hospital NHS Trust (Griffiths Report). NHS Executive, Leeds.

Nursing and Midwifery Council (NMC), 2002. Code of professional conduct. NMC, London.

Mallik, M., 1997. Advocacy in nursing: a review of the literature. Journal of Advanced Nursing 25 (1), 130–138.

O'Quigley, A., 2000. Listening to children's views: the findings and recommendations of recent research. Joseph Rowntree Foundation, York.

Power, K., 2002. Implications of the Human Rights Act 1998. Paediatric Nursing 14 (4), 14–19.

R v Cambridge Health Authority, ex parte B [1995] 22 All ER 129(CA).

Robertson, R., 1995. The giving of information is the key to family empowerment. British Journal of Nursing 4 (12), 692.

Royal College of Nursing (RCN), 1977. Ethics related to research in nursing. RCN, London.

Royal College of Paediatrics and Child Health (RCPCH), 2000. Guidelines for the ethical conduct of medical research involving children. Archives of Diseases in Childhood 82, 177–182.

UKCC, 2001. UKCC response to Bristol public inquiry says that children should be nursed by properly-qualified children's nurses. Register Number 37, Autumn p 5.

UNICEF, 2000. The UN Convention on the Rights of the Child. UNICEF, London.

Wheeler, P., 2000. Is advocacy at the heart of professional practice? Nursing Standard 14 (36), 39–41.

Willard, C., 1996. The nurse's role as patient advocate: obligation or imposition. Journal of Advanced Nursing 24 (1), 60–66.

Yacoub, M., 2001. Heartless, mindless, living children should not pay the price for the dead (Editorial). The Times February 3.

21

Legal aspects of child health care

Louise M Terry Anne Campbell

ABSTRACT

This chapter summarises the judicial system and identifies the meaning of 'child' and 'parent' in law. It explores issues around consent to treatment. The concepts of 'duty of care' and 'negligence' are examined.

LEARNING OUTCOMES

- To appreciate significant aspects of child and family law and their impact on the well-being of children and their families.
- To understand and correctly apply key legal terms in a child health setting.
- To reflect on the relevance and impact of key cases on the present and future management of child health/illness situations.
- To understand consent issues.
- To appreciate what a 'duty of care' entails and to reflect on the impact and consequences of negligence.

The legal system

The legal system of England and Wales differs from that of Scotland and Northern Ireland. All share a common law tradition in which both judge-made law (case law) and parliament-made law (statutes) play a part. Judges interpret statutes (Acts of Parliament) and use previous case law (precedents) to guide their decisions. If no statute exists, judges rely on legal principles and precedent to reach a decision. The Civil courts are separate from the Criminal courts.

The Family Division of the High Court hears cases involving medical treatment decisions. Appeals against the decision can go to the Court of Appeal (Civil Division) and then to the House of Lords. In cases involving disputes over the treatment of children, the child will be represented by a guardian ad litem, usually from the Child and Family Court Advisory and Support Service (CAFCASS); the Official Solicitor may act as guardian ad litem. The guardian ad litem will try to ascertain the views of the child, if he or she is able to express them. Claims for compensation for negligently caused harm are heard in the Civil courts unless the negligence was criminally culpable. The Magistrates courts, which have a 'bench' of three lay Justices of the Peace, hear many criminal cases and some family cases, e.g. contact disputes.

Activity

Attend a session at your local Magistrates court to see justice in action.

Cases involving breaches of the 1950 European Convention for the Protection of Human Rights and Fundamental Freedoms can be heard in all British courts now since the Human Rights Act 1998 came into force in 2000. Appeals from the House of Lords can go to the European Court of Human Rights. However, although the UK has ratified the 1989 United Nations Convention on the Rights of the Child, this is not yet part of domestic law.

Activity

Visit the Houses of Parliament or listen to/watch a House of Lords debate on radio or television.

WWW

Look at the European Court of Human Rights website on:
- http://www.echr.coe.int

Who is a child?

The Family Law Reform Act 1969 confirms that a child or 'minor' is any person who has been born but is under the age of 18.

DOI: 10.1016/B978-0-7020-3183-0.10021-9

Seminar discussion topic

Should unborn children have rights? If so, what rights would you give them? Does the journey down the vaginal tract into the outside world change their moral status?

Who has parental responsibility?

1. The gestational mother (who may or may not be the biological mother).
2. The biological father if he:
   - was married to the gestational mother when the child was born
   - has since married the gestational mother
   - has, with the child's mother, jointly registered or re-registered the child's birth if the child was born after 1 December 2003, when relevant parts of the Adoption and Children Act 2002 came into force
   - has a residence order
   - has a court order that gives him parental responsibility
   - has a formal 'parental responsibility agreement' with the mother.
3. The husband of the gestational mother is presumed to be the legal father of the child but this can be rebutted by evidence, e.g. DNA samples. If the child was conceived using in vitro fertilisation treatment in a licensed clinic and the husband of the gestational mother consented to the use of another man's sperm, he will be the legal father.
4. A guardian of the child.
5. Someone who holds a custody or residence order in respect of the child.
6. A local authority that has a care order in respect of the child.
7. Someone who has an emergency protection order in respect of the child.
8. Any man or woman who has adopted the child.

There is a presumption by the courts that it is in the child's best interests to know his/her biological parentage: *Re H and A (paternity: blood tests)* [2002] 1 FLR 1145.

Seminar discussion topic

In the case of *The Leeds Teaching Hospitals NHS Trust v Mr and Mrs A and others* [2003] EWCA 259 (QB), Mrs A – the gestational mother – was found to be the biological mother of twins born using in vitro fertilisation but, because of a mix-up, Mr B's sperm was used instead of Mrs A's husband's. The presumption that Mr A was the legal father was rebutted and the court decided Mr B was the legal father. Mr and Mrs A may apply to adopt the twins to regain Mr A's legal status as father; Mr B can oppose the adoption order.

- Do you have concerns about this?
- What if the mix-up had occurred the other way around and Mr A was the biological father, Mrs A the gestational mother but Mrs B the biological mother?

Decision-making regarding children

The Children Act 1989 reflects the following principles:

1. The welfare of the child is paramount.
2. The child's views, in the light of his or her age and understanding, are to be taken into account.
3. There should be partnership with parents and other family members and support for the child within the family whenever possible.

Consent to treatment

Respect for autonomy is one of the principles underpinning the need to obtain consent before performing any healthcare intervention. Another is the right to bodily integrity. Lord Donaldson in *Re W (a minor) (medical treatment)* [1993] Fam 64 explains that consent has a clinical purpose of ensuring patient cooperation with treatment, and a legal purpose of providing a 'flak jacket' against criminal charges of assault or battery (e.g. Offences Against the Person Act 1869 s47 – liability for causing actual bodily harm), or civil claims for damages for trespass to the person. Failure to adequately inform or advise may give rise to negligence claims. In *Schloendorff v Society of New York Hospital* (1914), Cardozo said 'Every human being of adult years and sound mind has a right to determine what shall be done with his own body.' Increasingly, children's rights to determine what is done to them are being recognised in both law and ethics (Brazier & Bridge 1996, Hendrick 2000 pp 36–38, Terry & Campbell 2001).

Activity

Does your ward have information leaflets telling children what to expect from their stay? If not, why not design one? If you have got information leaflets, are they available in the languages your patients speak?

There are three forms of consent:

1. Orally, e.g. the patient says 'I need my dressing changed'.
2. Implied, e.g. the patient holds out his or her arm for a cannula to be inserted.
3. In writing, e.g. a signed consent form.

Each form is equally valid unless statute law expressly says otherwise, as in the Human Fertilisation and Embryology Act 1990, which requires written consent. The law also prohibits certain procedures regardless of patient or family wishes. For example, the Prohibition of Female Circumcision Act 1985 s1(1) makes it a criminal offence for any person (whether a healthcare professional or not) to 'excise, infibulate or otherwise mutilate the whole or any part of the labia majora or labia minora or clitoris of another person' or 'to aid, abet, counsel or procure' such mutilation. The Female Genital Mutilation Act 2003 made it a criminal offence to take a child abroad for such mutilation.

www

Look up 'female circumcision' on the internet to find information about this practice. Try:

- http://www.google.co.uk

  The following is one of the sites you might have found. How far should the law interfere with cultural norms?
- http://www. religioustolerance.org/fem_cirm.htm

Obtaining valid consent

Consent to medical or surgical treatment is usually obtained by a clinician but this duty can be delegated to a nurse who is suitably knowledgeable and competent to do this task. For consent to be valid, it must be:

- given by a competent person
- freely given
- informed.

Activity

Observe how different doctors inform patients and help children make decisions.

The giving of consent by a competent person

The competent person may be the child or someone with parental responsibility. The law treats the giving of consent to treatment differently depending on the age of the child. For instance, consent for very young children is very different from that for mature adolescents. Each situation will be considered in turn.

The infant or very young child

The obvious decisional incapacity of the child means that decisions will be made on its behalf usually by one or both parents. Usually, the consent of only one person with parental responsibility is required. Parental decisions should be made in the child's best interests and the welfare of the child is paramount. The ethical principles of beneficence (doing good) and non-maleficence (avoiding harm) underpin the decision (Beauchamp & Childress 2001). Doctors have dual obligations: to act in accordance with a responsible body of medical opinion when identifying treatment options and to act in the best interests of the incompetent patient (*Re S (Sterilisation: Patient's Best Interests)* [2000] 2 FLR 389).

Activity

Read the article by Bridgeman (2003). What can you learn for your practice?

When there is doubt or conflict over what constitutes a child's best interests, the court may be asked to decide. Education and communication are preferable to litigation, which can polarise views because of the adversarial nature of legal decision making in this country. The child might even be lost to medical scrutiny.

Reflect on your practice

How can you show respect for a person's religious or cultural beliefs while ensuring that you practice within legal and professional boundaries?

The school-age child

Normal childhood development leads to increasing ability to act autonomously (British Medical Association (BMA) 2001 pp 92–104). Alderson & Montgomery (1996) suggest that children as young as 5 years should be deemed as autonomous unless the evidence or the complexity of the decision suggests otherwise. Thus, a young child might be able to consent to a grazed knee being cleaned but not consent to X-rays and surgical resetting of a broken limb.

Nurses can help educate even very young children about medical treatment in a variety of ways. The child's views can be obtained, even though decisions will ultimately be taken in the child's best interests.

Scenario

Jake, a 6-year-old boy, is admitted for a tonsillectomy. His parents insist he is not told any details of his surgery, so he is not able to be fully informed and prepared by the health professionals.

- Identify the difficulties this could cause and evaluate possible interventions by healthcare professionals.

The mature minor under 16 years old

Maturity and insight into medical treatment has to be measured on an individual basis. A 10-year-old child who has undergone years of treatment for leukaemia might be sufficiently competent to make his or her own decisions regarding further chemotherapy. In *Gillick v West Norfolk and Wisbech AHA* [1986] AC112 at p114, the House of Lords held that a child under the age of 16 can consent to medical treatment if she had 'sufficient understanding and intelligence to enable her to understand fully what was proposed'. It is for the doctors to decide whether the child has a 'full understanding and appreciation of the consequences both of the treatment in terms of intended and possible side effects and equally important, the anticipated consequences of a failure to treat' (*Re R (a minor) (wardship: consent to treatment)* [1992] Fam 11 at p26 per Lord Donaldson MR). In this case, the girl who suffered from psychosis was deemed incompetent due to her fluctuating understanding.

'Gillick competent' children can consent to medical treatment even if their parents are opposed to it: 'parental right yields to the child's right to make his own decision' (per Lord Scarman), although their rights to refuse treatment are more limited. Their confidentiality should be upheld so their parents have no right to know that they have sought treatment. In *Re B (wardship: abortion)* [1991] 2 FLR 426, a 12-year-old girl was held to be 'Gillick competent' and could consent to a termination of pregnancy, although the court also said that had she not been competent the termination would be allowable in her best interests. Nurses should encourage children to involve their parents, particularly when surgery is proposed.

PROFESSIONAL CONVERSATION

Anne, a registered children's nurse on Part 15 of the professional Nursing and Midwifery Council (NMC) register works in Accident and Emergency.

Gillick competency, confidentiality and partnerships in care

I was on duty when a 13-year-old girl Muslim girl was brought in with abdominal pains. The doctor found she was 4 months pregnant and bleeding per vagina. She was very frightened and upset. Her parents were waiting outside asking what was wrong with her. I didn't know how to do my best for her. The doctor said she was Gillick competent but she seemed very immature to me so I wasn't sure. But I thought, 'If her parents are told what is wrong, what might happen to her?' All I could think of was reading in a newspaper about a Muslim girl who got pregnant and her family killed her for dishonouring it.

The 16–17-year-old child

The Family Law Reform Act 1969 s8(1) States that:

> The consent of a minor who has attained the age of sixteen years to any surgical, medical or dental treatment which, in the absence of consent, would constitute a trespass to his person, shall be as effective as it would be if he were of full age; and where a person has by virtue of this section given an effective consent to any treatment, it shall not be necessary to obtain any consent from his parent or guardian.

'Treatment' includes diagnosis, anaesthesia and ancillary procedures.

Activity

Compare and contrast examples of completed consent forms. Can you identify weaknesses?

The parent of questionable competency

Competency can be affected by learning disabilities, mental illness or other conditions. Where the parent is obviously incompetent, consent must be obtained from another person with parental responsibility or the court. In the case of adults and children over 16 years, competency requires being able to comprehend and retain the information given and weigh it in the balance to reach a decision: *Re C (adult: refusal of treatment)* [1994] 1 FLR 31 approved in *Re MB (medical treatment: consent)* [1997] 2 FLR 1097. Although Anglo-Welsh law does not fully recognise the concept of the emancipated minor, marriage or fighting for one's country have been deemed to free minors from parental control. Regardless of her age, the girl who becomes a mother has parental responsibility for her child. Her parents will not automatically have parental responsibility for the grandchild. In cases where the child-parent's ability to consent for her own child is doubtful, it may be necessary to apply to the court.

Freely given consent

Duress can invalidate consent, even if it has been applied in the best interests of the patient. Persuasion is acceptable, coercion is not and is likely to cause a breakdown in the relationship between the various parties. Even adults can be placed under duress to accept or reject treatment as in the case of *Re T (adult: refusal of treatment)* [1993] Fam 95, whose Jehovah's Witness mother persuaded her to reject blood transfusions. A court later allowed transfusion on the grounds that *T* was incompetent due to pain and pethidine at the time of her decision and was placed under duress. Children may be less able than adults to withstand emotional pressure. Regarding *Re E (a minor)(wardship: medical treatment)* [1993] 1 FLR 386, a 15-year-old Jehovah's Witness boy with leukaemia who was refusing blood transfusions, Brazier & Bridge (1996) question whether his refusal was 'free choice'.

Duress of circumstances is inadequately recognised within medicine. A 14-year-old may appear 'Gillick competent' but her fear of 'what my parents will say if they find out' might mean she does not fully consider the risks of abortion.

Scenario

A 15-year-old girl underwent a termination of pregnancy without her parents' knowledge. Complications arose and she underwent an emergency hysterectomy. On arrival in intensive care, a decision had to be made about notifying her parents but a senior manager was strongly opposed to this on confidentiality grounds. Discuss and justify your reasoning.

www

Look at the recommendations regarding the principles underpinning the use of patient information given to Caldicott guardians on:

- http://www.doh.gov.uk/confiden/cgmintro.htm

Informed consent

The World Medical Association's Declaration of Helsinki 1964 states:

> If it is at all possible, consistent with patient psychology, the doctor should obtain the patient's freely given consent after the patient has been given a full explanation.

Difficulties arise over provision of information. A balancing act is often performed, which can leave the patient or parent underinformed. The House of Lords decision in *Sidaway v Board of Governors of the Bethlem Royal Hospital and the Maudsley Hospital* [1985] AC 871 meant that for years the 'Bolam test' for negligence governed the provision of information about benefits, risks and side effects of treatment (*Bolam v Friern Hospital Management Committee* [1957] 1 WLR 582; see later). The standard was how much information would the 'reasonable' doctor disclose. In the Bristol Royal Infirmary inquiry, Professor Ian Kennedy was critical of the failure by surgeons to provide adequate information about the risks to children undergoing complex heart surgery (Kennedy 2001).

The Department of Health (DoH) now issues guidance and the standard of 'what would the reasonable patient want to know?' is appearing.

WWW

Read the DoH guidance on consent at:

- http://dh.gov.uk/(search for consent)

WWW

Read the recommendations made by Professor Ian Kennedy in the Bristol Inquiry report at:

- http://www.bristol-inquiry.org.uk

In *Chester v Afshar* [2005] 1 AC 134, the House of Lords held that patients are entitled to be given proper warnings about risks of surgery. They can recover damages for non-negligent complications if they can show they would not have had the operation at that particular time if warned, even if they might have had it later. Patients and parents are increasingly likely to actively seek medical information, particularly via the internet (Ham & Pickard 1998). The difficulty lies in understanding and interpreting it but patients, and families, are no longer silent partners in medicine.

Refusal of treatment

Refusal by parents

Decisions should be made in the best interests of the child. Cases may arise in which it is obvious that the parents' decision is coloured by personal preferences or beliefs and seems clearly contrary to the child's best interests. In the case of a life-threatening emergency, treatment can be given in the child's best interests to save 'life and limb' under the common law doctrine of necessity. In other cases, if doctors believe treatment is appropriate and persuasion has failed, they can refer the decision to the courts. A Specific Issue Order can be given under the Children Act 1989 or the court can exercise its inherent jurisdiction and make a declaration as to lawfulness of treatment.

Activity

When a child's treatment is the subject of dispute, a guardian ad litem will want to meet the child:

- What arrangements exist in your hospital regarding such meetings?
- How can you ensure that your professional responsibilities under the NMC Code of Professional Conduct, in particular, Clause 2, are fulfilled?

In *Re B (a minor) (wardship: medical treatment)* [1981] 1 WLR 1421, where the child had Down syndrome and needed life-saving emergency surgery but the parents refused consent, the Court of Appeal concluded 'it is not for this court to say that life of that description ought to be extinguished'. The lack of peer/judicial review contributes to the 'haphazard and often arbitrary nature of the practice' of interpreting best interests according to Robertson (1986). Caring for the disabled presents 'substantial burdens to parents, family, and even taxpayers', which not all are prepared to take on (Robertson 1986 p 217). The burdens on others are irrelevant under the Children Act 1989 according to Lord Justice Ward (*Re A (conjoined twins: medical treatment)* [2001] 1 FLR 1 at p52). In this case, the Catholic parents opposed the separation of conjoined twins, which would result in the inevitable death of the weaker twin. BMA (2001 p 4) advice that 'the implications for the family of treatment or non-treatment' should be considered when establishing a child's best interests now seems out-dated.

Activity

Next time the media discloses a contentious medical treatment case, read reports in different newspapers. Does your opinion change as you read the different versions?

Re J (a minor) (wardship: medical treatment) [1991] Fam 33 at p55, which involved a severely brain-damaged baby, held that 'the correct approach is for the court to judge the quality of life the child would have to endure if given the treatment'. *Re A (conjoined twins)* shows how difficult it is to determine 'best interests'. Sanctity of life, quality of life, the parents' views and the lawfulness of the operation were all considered. Lord Justices Ward and Brooke held the separation was not in Mary's best interests, although it was allowable. Lord Justice Walker was, according to Foster (2000), '... scarily clear [that] a short, terribly disabled and possibly painful life was a life not worth living' consequently, separation (and death) was in Mary's best interests. It was suggested that refusing to give one twin the chance of life could constitute abuse contrary to the Children and Young Persons Act 1933, which makes it a criminal offence to ill-treat, neglect or abandon a child under 16 years. In *Re S (a minor) (medical treatment)* [1993] 1 FLR 376, the court authorised blood transfusions for a 4-year-old child with T-cell leukaemia against her parents' religious objections.

Seminar discussion topic

In the case of *Re C (a child) (HIV testing)* [1999] 2 FLR 1004, the baby's mother was HIV positive and breast-feeding her infant against medical advice. She refused to allow the baby to be HIV tested or to be given prophylactic medication. The doctors obtained a court order for the child to be tested in his best interests but the mother went abroad with the baby before this could be done.

- Discuss the baby's rights versus the mother's.

In other cases, it is much less certain which viewpoint is the correct one. As Ham & Pickard (1998 p 22) point out, differences of opinion:

> ... reflect the individualistic values to which medicine has always subscribed, particularly in the case of clinicians who have reached the top of the hierarchy and feel they possess sufficient expertise to act on the basis of their own judgement.

In *Re ZM and OS (sterilisation: patient's best interests)* [2000] 1 FLR 523 at p533, a case involving incompetent adults, the judge held that expert opinion is not conclusive and should be 'weighed and judged by the court'. The seeking of independent medical advice by the Court of Appeal in *Re A (conjoined twins)* is new and to be encouraged but judges may struggle when critiquing medical information.

Only rarely is the refusal of treatment for minors allowed. In *Re T (wardship: medical treatment)* [1997] 1 FLR 502, involving a child in need of a liver transplant whose parents removed him from the UK, it was unclear that treatment was ethically appropriate and unlikely that the child would survive into adulthood even if the transplant went ahead. Freeman (2000 p 258) believes that the court was 'taken in' by the knowledge of the parents, who were healthcare professionals.

The emphasis placed on parental opinion in *Re T* cannot be seen as decisive following *Re MM (medical treatment)* [2000] 1 FLR 224. The child, *MM*, was a temporary resident in the UK while his Russian parents studied here. There was no definite diagnosis of his immunological condition and the parents seemed as knowledgeable as the doctors. The parents wanted to continue his existing treatment because, if started on immunoglobulins as English doctors wished, he would have to continue with them but they would be difficult to obtain in Russia. Using telephone conferencing, the judge was able to help the parents and doctors reach a compromise position.

Refusal by children

Young children lacking understanding may struggle and fight against those delivering necessary care. In such circumstances, when explanations or reassurances have failed to help, minimal restraint in the child's best interests is allowable. Guidance is available from the DoH (1993) and the Royal College of Nursing (1999).

Activity

Read the article by Jeffrey (2002).

Reflect on your practice

How would you give a 2-year-old child an intramuscular injection when she is fighting, crying and her mother can't stand injections either?

The Children Act 1989 (s38, 43, 44) gives the court powers to order medical or psychiatric examination and treatment but, if the child is of sufficient understanding to make an informed decision, the child has the right to refuse medical/psychiatric examination. If a competent child refuses examination, the doctor will be unable to make a diagnosis and recommend treatment. A competent child is unlikely to refuse examination because he or she will recognise the need for diagnosis. Consequently, a refusal of examination could be evidence of incompetence. The child's welfare is the paramount consideration, although the court should take into account the factors in s1(3) of the Children Act 1989. The child's wishes are only one factor to be considered.

Scenario

Jenny is 12 years old. She has achondroplasia. Her mother wishes her to have leg-lengthening operations but she refuses. Discuss.

The courts have held that a child's refusal of treatment can be overridden by anyone with parental responsibility or by the court. In *Re W (a minor) (medical treatment)* [1993] Fam 64, a 16-year-old girl with anorexia refused force feeding. As the Family Law Reform Act 1969 s8 does not use the word 'refuse' her powers to refuse treatment were not absolute – others could give permission. In *Re R (a minor) (wardship: consent to treatment)* [1992] Fam 11, the court held that even if the 15-year-old were 'Gillick competent', her refusal of antipsychotic medication could be overridden.

A Metropolitan Borough Council v DB [1997] 1 FLR 767 concerned a 16-year-old pregnant crack cocaine addict suffering from eclamptic fits who was admitted to hospital but discharged herself. Two days later she underwent a Caesarian section. The hospital wanted to monitor her so the local authority asked the court to place her in secure accommodation – the maternity ward. The court agreed she was incompetent to make her own decisions and granted the order.

The more sheltered an upbringing, the less likely a child is to be found competent, as in *Re L (medical treatment: Gillick competency)* [1998] 2 FLR 810. This involved a 14-year-old with epilepsy who had suffered serious scalding. She, and her parents, refused life-saving blood transfusions because of their Jehovah's Witness faith. Doctors preferred not to upset the child with details of how painful her death without treatment would be and asked the court for permission. Had she been told, she may have consented (Terry & Campbell 2001). The judge granted permission while acknowledging this could condemn her to 'life in the wings'. Judges, and doctors, must recognise that some patients may legitimately prefer death.

In *Re M (child: refusal of medical treatment)* [1999] 2 FLR 1097, a 15½-year-old girl refused consent to a heart transplant. Although her mother had consented, doctors wanted judicial backing and obtained it when the judge held *M* to be incompetent. Mason & Laurie (2005) suggest this represents 'the outermost reaches of acceptable paternalistic practices'. In a case involving an adult refusing consent to a life-saving Caesarian section (*R v St Georges NHS ex parte S* [1998] 2 FLR 728), the Court of Appeal held that even if the patient is not told of alternative procedures, the court should be if its permission is sought. In *Re M* (at p 1099) the court was told 'no other medical option was available', although life-saving alternatives such as mechanical hearts, which may have been medically better as well as more acceptable to the patient did, at the time, exist (Rogers 2000a). When treatment is refused, particularly if it involves physical maim, alternatives should be sought and considered before resorting to enforcement of the doctor's preference against the wishes of the mature minor.

A risk in *Re M* is non-compliance with antirejection medication once she reaches adulthood. The boy in *Re E* exercised his right to refuse further blood transfusions once he reached 18 and died. Bailey-Harris (2000 p 137) believes 'teenagers with deeply held convictions' should be regarded as mature and 'entitled to their full autonomy rights'. Douglas (1992) argues that the courts have rejected the right of a competent person to make mistakes and 'entrenched not welfare, but paternalism, as its guiding principle'. Bridgeman (1993) criticises the harsh treatment of *W*, who had already been dealt with harshly by fate. Huxtable (2000) questions the existence of the doctor's 'flak jacket' regarding mature minors.

The mentally ill child

If the child has mental illness, statutory powers under the Mental Health Act 1983 allow enforced treatment, although there is marked reluctance to use them because of the stigmatising nature of mental illness and being sectioned. Reluctance to use these powers left one child barricaded in her room, manipulating her family and not receiving the psychiatric help she needed before the court was eventually asked to exercise its jurisdiction (*South Glamorgan* CC *v W and B* [1993] 1 FLR 574). In *Re* C *(a minor) (detention for medical treatment)* [1997] 2 FLR 180, an order was made under s100 of the Children Act 1989 so that a 16-year-old with anorexia could be returned to a clinic for treatment. She had a history of absconding and was at risk of significant harm.

End-of-life issues

Lord Justice Hoffman, in *Airedale NHS Trust v Bland* [1993] AC 789 at p 834, felt that whether 'it would be lawful to provide or withhold the treatment or care is a matter for the law' not doctors. This reflects public opinion that doctors are accountable and patients have protectable rights. Imminent, unavoidable death constitutes well-established grounds for ending treatment (*Re* C *(a baby)* [1996] 2 FLR 43, concerning a baby left brain-damaged following meningitis). Establishing brainstem death is difficult in very young children but in *Re A* [1992] 3 Med LR 303, it was accepted that the 2-year-old was brainstem dead and that it was appropriate to disconnect the ventilator. In *Re* C *(a minor) (wardship: medical treatment)* [1989] 3 WLR 240, it was appropriate to withhold treatment enabling a baby with severe hydrocephalus to 'die peacefully with the greatest dignity and the least of pain, suffering and distress'. *Re J (a minor) (wardship: medical treatment)* [1991] Fam 33 (at p 53) held that 'it is settled law that the court's prime and paramount consideration must be the best interests of the child'. There is a 'strong presumption' in favour of preserving life except in 'exceptional circumstances', with Lord Justice Taylor stating 'it can not be too strongly emphasised that the court never sanctions steps to terminate life' (p 53). In *Re* C *(medical treatment)* [1998] 1 FLR 384, concerning a terminally ill child with spinal muscular atrophy type 1, the court held that 'whilst the sanctity of life is vitally important, it is not the paramount consideration. The paramount consideration here is the best interests of little C' (at p 393). The Orthodox Jewish parents wanted reventilation to remain an option because of their vitalist approach to sanctity of life.

Among other factors, the court will consider 'whether the life of this child is demonstrably going to be so awful that in effect the child must be condemned to die' (*Re B (a minor) (wardship: medical treatment)* 1981 1 WLR 1421, at p 1424). However, pain alone is no defence for ending life unlawfully, as Dr Cox found after he gave his patient potassium chloride to end her intolerable pain (*R v Cox* [1992] 12 BMLR 38).

In *A National Health Service Trust v D & Ors* [2000] FLR 677, the resuscitation status of a severely disabled child was considered. The court listed the four principles to be applied:

1. The paramount consideration is the best interests of the child.
2. The court has a clear duty to respect the sanctity of life, which imposes a strong presumption in favour of taking all steps to preserve it.
3. Actions to accelerate death or terminate life cannot be approved by the court.
4. The court cannot order a doctor to give treatment that the doctor is unwilling to give and which is contrary to the doctor's clinical judgement.

In *Re A (conjoined twins)*, Lord Justice Ward held that 'Mary may have a right to life, but she has little right to be alive' (p 54); in effect, Mary's twin, Jodie, had a stronger right to life than Mary. The impact of the Human Rights Act 1998, which came into force in October 2000 just after the conjoined twins case, has been considered in several end-of-life cases. In *NHS Trust A v Mrs M and NHS Trust B v Mrs H* [2000] it was held that Article 2 (the right to life), Article 3 (the right not to be subjected to degrading or inhuman treatment) and Article 8 (the right to respect for private life) did not bar the withdrawal of treatment that was not in the patient's best interests.

Conflict between parents and doctors

In *R v Cambridge District HA, ex parte B* [1995] 1 FLR 1055, the father of 'Child B' obtained a judicial review of the Health Authority's decision not to fund further treatment for his daughter, a 10-year-old suffering from leukaemia. His refusal to accept the doctor's non-treatment decision represented a 'direct challenge' to the doctors involved in her care (Ham & Pickard 1998). The court held that further treatment would not be in her best interests. If the court decides the doctor's stance is contrary to the patient's best interests, it can order the transfer of the patient to another doctor. This option was considered in *Re T* (the child needing a liver transplant). Doctors at Great Ormond Street Hospital requested the transfer of the conjoined twins in *Re A* on the grounds that they had the necessary expertise to do the separation, although they also said they might accede to the parental wishes not to operate (Rogers 2000b).

Parents may be concerned that their child is being used as a teaching tool and not receiving appropriate care, as in the case of a baby with Goldenhaar syndrome. When the parents sought to remove the child from the hospital, a child protection order banning this was obtained (Mahendra 2002).

Parents and doctors may conflict over when the child's condition should be considered terminal. In *Royal Wolverhampton Hospitals NHS Trust v B* [2000] 1 FLR 953, Bodley J concluded that the breakdown in trust between the parties required that the doctors were given permission to not treat the child dying from chronic lung disease due to prematurity if they thought fit, not just because this was in the patient's best interests but as 'a kindness to the parents' (p 957). The cases of babies Charlotte Wyatt ([2005] EWHC 693) and Luke Winston Jones ([2004] EWHC 2713) involved parents challenging medical decisions not to provide life-prolonging treatment and resuscitation.

Good care and communication seem vital to prevent conflicts

In the David Glass case, doctors gave David, a severely disabled boy with respiratory failure, the respiratory depressant diamorphine against his mother's clearly expressed objections (*R v Portsmouth NHS Trust ex parte Glass* [1999] 2 FLR 905). The family was outraged and, en masse, invaded the ward and resuscitated David amid scenes of violent disorder during which two doctors and the mother of another child were injured. Three of them were later jailed for assault (*R v (1) Davies (2) Wild (3) Hodgson* (2000) CA 28 July 2000 unreported). In March 2004, the European Court of Human Rights ruled that 'the decision to impose treatment on the first applicant (David) in defiance of the second applicant's (his mother's) objections gave rise to an interference with the first applicant's right to respect for his private life, and in particular his right to physical integrity' (*Glass v The United Kingdom* Application No 61827/00 ECHR 9 March 2004 paragraph 70). The Court concluded that the situation was not one of such urgency that treatment could proceed without the mother's consent because it was clear that the hospital had had sufficient time to secure a police presence on the ward and 'the doctors and officials used the limited time available to them in order to try to impose their views on [the mother]' (paragraph 81). In regard to the fact that the doctors' notes indicated the mother had consented at one point to the therapeutic use of diamorphine, even though a solicitor's letter the next day made her opposition clear, the Court held 'it cannot be stated with certainty that any consent given was free, express and informed' (paragraph 82).

The UK government was ordered to pay compensation to David and his mother jointly, because the Court recognised 'the stress and anxiety' she suffered in her own right as well as 'feelings of powerlessness and frustration in trying to defend her own perception of what was in the best interests of her child' (paragraph 87). David was discharged into the care of his GP a few hours after the violent incident and was still alive at the time of writing. The final word perhaps belongs to Judge Casadevall:

> In the particular circumstances of [this case] maternal instinct has had more weight than medical opinion.

WWW

Find the *Glass v United Kingdom* judgement on the European Court of Human Rights website:

- http://www.echr.coe.int/Eng/Judgments.htm

Conflict between parents

An exception to the rule that only one person with parental responsibility need consent arose in *Re J (child's religious upbringing and circumcision)* [2000] 1 FLR 571, when the non-practising Muslim father of a child wanted him to be circumcised against the non-practising Christian mother's wishes. The court ordered that circumcision required the consent of both parents or, when old enough to decide for himself, the child's consent.

In *Re C (welfare of child: immunisation)* [2003] EWHC 1376 (Fam), the fathers of two girls aged 4 and 10, both of whom lived with their mothers who were opposed to vaccination, asked the court to order that the children be vaccinated against tetanus, poliomyelitis and other diseases. The court held that immunisation was in the children's best interests. Article 8 of the European Convention on Human Rights did not mean that the right to privacy and family life meant the court could not protect the health of the child.

Consent to non-therapeutic, controversial or experimental treatment

Although the incompetent patient has a right not to be subjected to non-consensual touching, which is waived only if inhumane not to, children have been allowed to donate bone marrow to siblings or other relatives, with minimal, or no, interference by the courts. Child B's sister was the donor for the failed bone marrow transplant (*R v Cambridge District HA, ex parte B* [1995] 1 FLR 1055). In most such cases, providing the parents, doctors and child (if old enough to be involved) agree, the courts are not involved. In the Australian case of *Re GWW and CMW* (1997) 21 Fam LR 612, a 12-year-old boy was allowed to donate bone marrow to his aunt. It was clear that this was his own, voluntary decision. Although Month (1996) argues that preventing children from donating bone marrow may not be in their best interests, it is important for nurses to be alert for signs of duress or distress. In the American case of *Hart v Brown* (Super 1972) 29 Conn Supp 368, permission was given by the courts for a kidney donation from a healthy 7-year-old to his seriously ill, identical twin brother.

An example of controversial treatment is the use of plastic surgery to alter the facial features of Down syndrome children. One retired consultant paediatrician has called for such surgery to be outlawed like female circumcision (Jones 2000).

Where conventional medicine holds no hope, and death is certain, experimental treatment might be allowed. In *DS v (1) JS (2) An NHS Trust and PA v JA (2) An NHS Trust and Secretary of State for Health* [2002] EWHC 2734 (Fam) the court allowed two sufferers of variant Creutzfeld–Jakob disease (JS, an 18-year-old and JA, a 16-year-old, neither of whom had capacity any more to make their own decisions) to be given an untested treatment – pentosan polysulphate – directly into their brains, even though the procedure itself might kill them.

Reflect on your practice

What are the legal and professional responsibilities of the Named Nurse? Can conflict exist between the two?

Negligence

Healthcare interventions are not always successful. Where consent to risks has been sought and given, if those risks come about, the 'flak jacket' protects against being sued. When harm is caused through negligence, either by an omission to act appropriately or by errors in the actions performed, the injured child, or his or her family, might make a claim for compensation in the Civil Courts under the Tort of Negligence. To win compensation, the claimant must prove the following:

- The patient was owed a duty of care by the defendant.
- The defendant (doctor, nurse, hospital) breached the duty of care by failing to reach the standard required of them by law.
- The breach caused harm of a type that was foreseeable.

A request for patient records may indicate that a negligence action is being considered.

www

Read the DoH information on accessing patient information on:

- http://www.doh.gov.uk/ipu/confiden/faq.htm

Duty of care

A duty of care is owed once the hospital, doctor, surgeon, nurse or other person undertakes to perform certain tasks for the child. It is owed once the patient presents for treatment (*Barnett v Chelsea and Kensington HMC* [1968] 1 All ER 1068) and may continue after the patient has been transferred from one professional to another, has left the GP's surgery or hospital, or the nurse has left the patient's house.

Breach of the standard of care

Many nurses act in an extended role. The court will decide whether the healthcare professionals, or other carers, have met the standard that the law expects them to meet. The standard of care is found in *Bolam v Friern Hospital Management Committee* [1957] 1 WLR 582 (the 'Bolam test'):

> The test is the standard of the ordinary skilled man exercising and professing to have that special skill. A man need not possess the highest expert skill, ... It is a well-established law that it is sufficient if he exercises the ordinary skill of an ordinary competent man exercising that particular art.

The key words are 'exercising' and 'professing':

- Professing is what you say you are, e.g. children's nurse, doctor.
- Exercising is what you do: what task were you actually doing?

The court will hear expert witness evidence to determine what standard was acceptable. In *Bolitho v City and Hackney HA* [1998] AC 232, a child was left brain-damaged following a respiratory arrest. The ward sister had asked the doctor to attend with a view to preventively intubating him but the doctor failed to arrive. The House of Lords held that not only should a responsible body of opinion uphold the act or omission but there must be a logical basis to the opinion given. This reflects the trend for evidence-based health care.

Learners and their instructor must together meet the standard of the qualified person; inexperience is no excuse – the standard goes with the post. In *Wilsher v Essex AHA* [1986] 3 All ER 801, a junior doctor misplaced a catheter and miscalculated the oxygen for a premature baby who then suffered retrolental fibroplasia.

Written standards, guidelines, protocols, and Do Not Attempt Resuscitation (DNAR) policies are useful for providing consistent care. They need updating regularly and can be used as evidence in a court of law – failure to comply with standard guidance may be seen as proof of a failure to meet the relevant standard of care.

Activity

Attend a hearing of the NMC Professional Conduct Committee. Places are limited so book in advance.

Causation of foreseeable harm

Experts for the claimant will provide evidence to persuade the court 'on the balance of probabilities' that the breach of the standard of care caused the harm complained of. The defence will produce its own experts. The question the court asks is 'But for the negligent act or omission, would the harm complained of have occurred?' In *Barnett v Chelsea and Kensington* HMC [1968] 1 All ER 1068, a doctor who failed to examine three men who fell ill after night duty was found to have breached his duty of care. However, this breach did not cause the death of one of the men, which was held to be inevitable due to arsenic poisoning.

Where there are multiple possible causes of the harm, as in *Wilsher v Essex AHA* [1986] 3 All ER 801, unless the claimant can prove on the 'balance of probabilities' that one was the cause, the claim will fail. In *Wilsher*, the blindness could have been caused by several factors, not just the excess oxygen, so the child's claim failed. Likewise, in *Temple v South Manchester Health Authority* [2002] EWCA Civ 1406, negligent treatment of a 9-year-old's diabetic ketoacidosis had not, on the balance of probability, caused his irreversible brain damage. Where there are two equal acts of negligence, either of which could have resulted in the harm complained of, but science cannot provide the necessary proof, *Fairchild* [2002] 3 WLR 79 now holds that the court can decide that both were 'material causes'.

Compensation may sometimes be recovered for psychiatric damage. In *North Glamorgan NHS Trust v Walters* [2002] EWCA Civ 1792, a mother was compensated for suffering psychiatric injury caused by the shock of seeing the distressing final 36 hours of her son's life following a negligent failure to diagnose his acute hepatitis.

The doctrine of Res Ipsa Loquitur (the thing speaks for itself) simplifies the proof of negligence and causation. If forceps are left inside a patient after an operation, there was obvious negligence and the subsequent peritonitis will be attributed to this.

Unforeseeable harms cannot be protected or insured against so claimants will not be able to recover compensation for harms no one knew existed. If the professional should have known, liability can be established; continuing professional development is important.

www

Read the NHS Litigation Authority advice on how to reduce negligence in the NHS:

- http://www.nhsla.com

Accurate record keeping is vital. This is your defence when asked to justify your actions or inactions months or years later. In *Juliff v (1) Dr Hillard (2) Dr Trigg (3) Dr Lukaszewicz* (2001) QBD 24 June unreported, the medical notes were 'conscientiously, properly and accurately recorded' and demonstrated that the defendants had 'discharged their duties with conspicuous care and conscientiousness'. They were not to blame for the child's stroke, which followed a difficult-to-diagnose case of meningitis.

Reflect on your practice

Look at a nursing record you made a week ago. How clearly can you recall the patient's care? How well could you do this if asked in 8 years time when a solicitor's letter arrives?

www

Read the DoH (2001) guidance in 'The essence of care: patient-focused benchmarking for healthcare practitioners' on:

- http://www.publications.doh.gov.uk/essenceofcare/index.htm

Read the NMC's (2002) 'Guidelines for records and record keeping' on:

- http://www.nmc-uk.org

Activity

How can record keeping in your practice area be improved?

Vicarious liability

Under the doctrine of vicarious liability, the employer will be held liable for the employee's negligence providing the employee was working within the course and scope of his employment. In *Townsend v Worcester and District HA* [1995] 23 BMLR 31, the defendants were vicariously liable for brain damage caused by the excessive force applied to the baby's head during a forceps delivery.

Limitations for legal actions

In the case of negligent harm occurring during pregnancy, delivery or any time in childhood, the child retains a right to sue for 3 years after becoming an adult or becoming aware of the negligent act if no legal action has commenced before then.

Criminal liability

Gross negligence manslaughter

Where negligence causes death, criminal charges of gross negligence manslaughter might follow, as in *R v Adomako* [1993] 3 WLR 927 in which an anaesthetist's negligence led to his patient's death.

Activity

Visit your local Coroner's court, particularly if there is a paediatric case being heard.

Murder

Intentional neglect resulting in death may constitute murder or attempted murder. In *R v Arthur* [1981] 12 BMLR 1, Dr Arthur prescribed sedation and nursing care only for a Down syndrome baby rejected by his parents. Initial charges of murder were reduced to attempted murder when a post-mortem revealed the baby would have died anyhow because of his medical condition.

Deliberate harm by parents, carers or others

Child protection issues are covered in a separate chapter of this book. However, it is worth noting here that following Lord Laming's 2003 report into the death of Victoria Climbié, which identified failings on the part of health and other professionals in contact with Victoria, a new Children's Commissioner will be introduced, along with new duties of cooperation between all the different agencies in contact with children to minimise risk for all children as part of the Children Act 2004.

www

Look at the Children Act 2004 on:

- http://www.hmso.gov.uk/acts/acts2004/20040031.htm

and the explanatory notes on:

- http://www.parliament.the-stationery-office.co.uk/pa/ld200304/ldbills/035/en/04035x-.htm

Look at the Climbié report, in particular, the sections on the health services:

- http://www.victoria-climbie-inquiry.org.uk/finreport/finreport.htm

Summary

This chapter summarises legal issues relating to child health care as they stand at the time of writing. It is important for all health care professionals to remember that the law is not static. Changes to legislation and new cases testing out the boundaries of care occur regularly. It is your duty to keep yourself up to date to ensure that you continue to practice safely and within the law.

References

Adoption and Children Act. 2002. The Stationery Office, London.

Alderson, P., Montgomery, J., 1996. Health care choices: making decisions with children. Institute for Public Policy Research, London.

Bailey-Harris, R., 2000. Patient autonomy – a turn in the tide? In: Freeman, M., Lewis, A. (Eds.), Law and medicine: current legal issues, vol. 3. Oxford University Press, Oxford, pp 127–140.

Beauchamp, T.L., Childress, J.F., 2001. Principles of biomedical ethics, 5th edn. Oxford University Press, Oxford.

Brazier, M., Bridge, C., 1996. Coercion or caring: analysing adolescent autonomy. Legal Studies 16, 84–109.

Bridgeman, J., 2003. After Bristol: the healthcare of young children and the law. Legal Studies 23 (2), 229–250.

Bridgeman, J., 1993. Old enough to know best? Legal Studies 13, 69–80.

British Medical Association (BMA), 2001. Consent, rights and choices in health care for children and young people. BMA, London.

Children Act, 1989. HMSO, London.

Children Bill, 2004. The Stationery Office, London.

Department of Health (DoH), 1993. Guidance on permissible forms of control in children's residential care. HMSO, London.

Department of Health (DoH), 2001. Essence of care: patient-focused benchmarking for health care professionals. The Stationery Office, London.

Douglas, G., 1992. The retreat from Gillick. Modern Law Review 55, 569–576.

Family Law Reform Act, 1969. HMSO, London.

Foster, C., 2000. Rocks and hard places. Solicitors Journal 13 October, 922–923.

Freeman, M., 2000. Can we leave the best interests of very sick children to their parents? In: Freeman, M., Lewis, A. (Eds.), Law and medicine: current legal issues, vol. 3. Oxford University Press, Oxford, pp 257–268.

Ham, C., Pickard, S., 1998. Tragic choices in health care. the case of Child B. King's Fund, London.

Hendrick, J., 2000. Law and ethics in nursing and health care. Stanley Thornes, Cheltenham.

Human Rights Act, 1998. The Stationery Office, London.

Huxtable, R., 2000. Re M (medical treatment: consent) Time to remove the 'flak jacket'? Child and Family Law Quarterly 12 (1), 83–88.

Jeffrey, K., 2002. Therapeutic restraint of children. Paediatric Nursing 14 (9), 20–22.

Jones, R.B., 2000. Parental consent to cosmetic facial surgery in Down's syndrome. Journal of Medical Ethics 26, 101–102.

Kennedy I, (Chair) 2001 Learning From Bristol: the report of the public inquiry into children's heart surgery at Bristol Royal Infirmary Inquiry 1984-1995. Final Report. Cmd 5207. The Stationery Office, London. Online. Available on http://www.bristol-inquiry.org.uk.

Laming, Lord (Chair) 2003 The Victoria Climbié inquiry. The Stationery Office, London. Online. Available at: http://www.victoria-climbie-inquiry.org.uk/finreport/finreport.htm.

Mahendra, B., 2002. Facing up to a child's dilemma. New Law Journal 152 (7024), 426.

Mason, J.K., McCall Smith, R.A., Laurie, G.T., 1999. Law and medical ethics, 5th edn. Butterworths, London.

Mason, J.K., Laurie G.T., 2005. Personal autonomy and the right to treatment: a note on R (on the application of Burke) v. General Medical Council. Edinburgh Law Review 9, 123–132.

Mental Health Act, 1983. HMSO, London.

Month, S., 1996. Preventing children from donating may not be in their best interests. British Medical Journal 312, 241–242.

Nursing and Midwifery Council (NMC), 2002. Guidelines for records and record keeping. NMC, London.

Robertson, J.A., 1986. Legal aspects of withholding treatment from handicapped newborns: substantive issues. Journal of Health Politics. Policy and Law 11 (2), 215–230.

Rogers, L., 2000a, Mini heart pump to end transplants. The Times 9 April 2000.

Rogers, L., 2000b, Doctors may not operate on twins. The Sunday Times 1 October 2000.

Royal College of Nursing (RCN), 1999. Restraining, holding still and containing children: guide for good practice. RCN, London.

Terry, L.M., Campbell, A., 2001. Are we listening to children's views about their treatment? British Journal of Nursing 10 (6), 384–390.

The role of paediatric emergency assessment units

22

Penny Aitken E Alan Glasper Maureen Wiltshire

ABSTRACT

The primary aim of this chapter is to raise the understanding of the key issues surrounding the emergency assessment of the sick child and family. The specialist skills required by paediatric nurses and the importance of the environment in which the child is admitted and treated will be explored.

The introduction of NHS Direct, walk-in centres and the changing role of both the GP and community nurse require all nurses working within the NHS to explore new ways of working in line with recent government directives. These nurses work with the child and family to provide hospital acute care when appropriate and support for the child to be cared for at home whenever possible.

LEARNING OUTCOMES

- Recognise the nursing skills required in the assessment of the acutely ill child.
- Appreciate the development of nurse-led initiatives in the care of the child and family.
- Understand the importance of recent inquires and government policies in the development of evidence-based practice for emergency care.
- Recognise the importance of family-centred care in the emergency assessment setting.
- Appreciate that children should only be admitted as inpatients when other services are inappropriate.

Introduction

> Children should be admitted to hospital only if the care they require cannot be as well provided at home or on a short stay basis in hospital
>
> (DoH 1991)

The Royal College of Paediatrics and Child Health (RCPCH) supports this view and has highlighted the acute assessment unit as an example of best practice in the management of acute paediatric illness, which can prevent inappropriate admissions (RCPCH 1998). Such units are often sited adjacent to inpatient wards or within emergency departments and rely on skilled children's nurses. Meates (1997) has outlined the crucial role that they play in helping parents to provide self-care, thus reducing the need for overnight admission. Perhaps the most important objectives in establishing a Paediatric Emergency Assessment Unit (PEAU) are to place the child at the centre of care and to recognise the importance of the family in contributing to the care of their child (Department of Health (DoH) 2003).

Children admitted to hospital for assessment are often seen in inappropriate areas, such as Emergency Departments without designated paediatric areas or treatment areas on wards. Of great concern to nurses and paediatricians is the risk of premature discharge of children without the opportunity to evaluate treatment and monitor improvement at home for 24 hours. The key objectives in establishing a PEAU are to:

- assess all GP and other referrals and reduce unnecessary admission to hospital
- improve the quality of short-stay care and reduce family disruption
- adopt different ways of working to provide more effective use of resources
- provide the family with support to care for their sick child at home
- bridge any boundaries that may exist between primary and acute paediatric care.

This chapter and the companion PowerPoint presentation will follow an ill child from the initial consultation with the GP, admission to a PEAU, observation, discharge planning for care at home, follow-up next day telephone call and communication with other healthcare professionals.

DOI: 10.1016/B978-0-7020-3183-0.10022-0

Referral and admission to PEAU

Many PEAUs have been designed to enhance services to local GPs and a study by Aitken et al (2003) demonstrated that the majority of admissions were initiated from this source. The changing nature of initial contact between a family and the health service is ensuring that triage or the determination of urgency of healthcare intervention is taking place in a variety of geographical locations and mediums.

The use of the telephone by nurses has grown enormously in the UK since the inception of NHS Direct, and telephone nursing reflects the growth in the use of the telephone in contemporary British society (Glasper & Wilkins 1998). The safety and effectiveness of nurse telephone consultations was described by Lattimer et al (1998) who, in a seminal randomised controlled trial of equivalence between GPs and nurses, found that there were no adverse outcomes for patients.

WWW

Read summaries of the three chapters of the National Service Framework for Children's hospital services document and then look up the Chief Nursing Officer's ten key roles for nursing. In particular, explore the nurse's role in direct referrals:

- http://www.doh.gov.uk/NSF/children.htm
- http://www.doh.gov.uk/newrolesfornurses

Scenario

Ann-Marie is a 4-year-old girl who lives at home with her parents, her two sisters aged 12 and 10 years old and her 8-year-old brother. Ann-Marie attends a local playgroup and has no previous admissions to hospital. Ann-Marie was taken to her GP with a 3-day history of cough, a temperature and reluctance to eat and drink.

On arrival at the Paediatric Emergency Assessment Unit her respiratory rate = 40, pulse = 128, temperature = 38.2°C and oxygen saturations = 96% in air.

Activity

- What are the normal parameters for temperature, heart rate, respiratory rate, oxygen saturations and weight for a 4-year-old?
- What immediate nursing intervention would Ann-Marie require?
- In relation to the ten key roles of the nurse that you have previously explored, which patient group directives have been agreed in your clinical area?
- What training is required nationally to allow nurse prescribing?

WWW

Read the Paediatric Resuscitation guidelines online:

- http://www.resus.org.uk/pages/guide.htm

Explore a clinical decision support information system online:

- http://www.isabel.org.uk/

Birch et al (2005) reported a survey of GPs following a nurse-led initiative of accepting direct referrals. Following the introduction of a new nurse-led telephone referral service to a dedicated PEAU, they conducted a study to determine the views of GPs who used their service. The PEAU used to operate between 10am and 10pm on weekdays and between 10am and 6pm at weekends. The unit initially had four beds and treatment and stabilisation areas, plus associated services in a dedicated area of a regional child health unit. The study utilised a faxed questionnaire over a 1-month period to all consenting GPs using the PEAU with a postal questionnaire follow-up. Non-parametric Likert scores and qualitative data were used to determine levels of satisfaction with the service and the subsequent management of the referred children. Sixty-nine GPs referred 80 children to the PEAU via the service over a period of 1 month. All consented to participate and were sent a faxed questionnaire, which generated 39 (57%) responses. A follow-up questionnaire sent to the 39 respondents achieved a return of 25 (64%) responses. Thirty-four GPs agreed that referral via the dedicated nurse telephone service was easier than the previous senior house officer referral system.

This clearly demonstrated that GPs are happy to refer sick children to a PEAU via a dedicated telephone referral system. Although not all acute assessment units provide this service, the advantage of the GP speaking to the nurse ultimately receiving the child provides a clearer picture of the nature of the condition. This saves time for both the family and GP and therefore enhances a seamless service through the healthcare system.

Children's nurses working with ill children and their families are required to develop a wide range of advanced skills that meet the expectations of paediatric emergency assessment (Box 22.1). It is important that the nurse establishes a good professional relationship on meeting the child and family. This will enable the nurse to carry out a full nursing assessment to include a physical, developmental and social history and negotiate a plan of care. The very nature of childhood illnesses can result in some children presenting with a life-threatening condition and it is therefore essential that all staff undertake a recognised paediatric advanced life support course.

As the role of the children's nurse develops, the skills become more enhanced and the paediatric nurse practitioner will be first-line assessing and managing ill children. Although the majority of paediatric episodic illnesses are relatively benign and resolve completely, the implications of a missed diagnosis could become life threatening. Therefore, regardless of the type of illness, the basic information and skills required in the acute assessment of an ill child are for the most part the same in all children. Before the history-taking process begins it is essential that the nurse who is looking after the child and family introduces him- or herself, puts them at their ease and makes them feel welcome. A child-friendly environment should be encouraged, with age-appropriate toys and distraction. Privacy should be ensured throughout.

A well-taken and documented medical and social history of an ill child is crucial for the diagnosis and management of care for both the child and family. Open-ended questions should

Box 22.1

Types of conditions likely to be encountered in a PEAU

Although every assessment unit will offer slightly different services, the principles behind the units will be similar, in that they offer first-line emergency assessment of acute illness. Which specialties are seen within a unit will depend on the service requirements, however it is likely to include a vast variety of conditions and illness. Below are examples of the conditions that may be seen within a PEAU:

- abscesses
- appendicitis
- asthma
- bronchiolitis
- constipation
- convulsions
- croup
- diabetes mellitus/ketoacidosis
- failure to thrive
- gastroenteritis
- head injuries
- Henoch–Schönlein purpura
- hernias
- Hirschsprung's disease
- intussusceptions
- irritable hip
- jaundice
- Kawasaki disease
- meningitis
- pyrexia unknown origin
- rashes
- septic arthritis
- testicular problems
- urinary tract infection.

Child protection issues will also be encountered.

be used to ensure a full response from the child and family. At all times children should be encouraged to participate and tell their 'own story'. During the history-taking process it is helpful to maintain as much eye contact as possible with the child and family.

Even before the nurse lays a single hand on the child, a major element of the physical examination should have taken place. While undertaking the history from the child and family, the nurse will have been observing both child and family members to answer the questions:

- How do the parents relate to the child, and the child to its parents?
- Do the parents appear anxious, upset or distressed?
- Does the child happily separate from his or her parents?
- Does the child play age appropriately?
- Is the child unusually distressed?

Nurses working in an emergency assessment environment are frequently practising at a nurse practitioner level, which includes physical assessment, history taking, venesection, cannulation and prescribing (Box 22.2) (Dearmun & Gordon 1999, Rushforth 2002, Rushforth & Glasper 1999). Additionally, such nurses – using established protocols – admit children as inpatients and discharge them home with support of follow-up services (this will be discussed later in the chapter).

PROFESSIONAL CONVERSATION

Hayley Anderson is a second-year student nurse on clinical placement on a paediatric emergency assessment unit. Ellen Lancaster, her mentor, is a staff nurse within the unit.

Issues relating to physical and social history taking

While undertaking the assessment of Ann-Marie, Hayley asks her mentor to explain areas of the assessment and care that all children admitted to the unit are subjected to:

> *I've been on the ward for three shifts and I just don't understand why whenever a child presents we have to take such a detailed physical and social history – why do we need to know the surname of who lives in the home, if all the siblings have the same parents, and if they have a social worker or not? And why do we need to undress Ann-Marie, she's experiencing shortness of breath – she has a chest problem, she doesn't have abdominal pain, she hasn't experienced any lower limb trauma?*

Ellen explains to Hayley how every child requires a full social and medical history to ensure nothing is missed:

> *Bringing a child to hospital can be very stressful and therefore by ensuring we follow a structured assessment process we are reducing the risk of missing information that may be vital in the diagnoses and treatment of the child. By observing a child prior to a physical assessment, a relationship can be built and in taking this social and medical history, time is allowed for this.*

Reflect on your practice

Could you explain to a parent why there is a need for a full physical examination of all children presenting to an emergency assessment unit, as well as documenting a full social and medical history?

Activity

- Review the admission paperwork for children in your own practice area; do they meet the recommendations following the Victoria Climbié inquiry.
- Draw your own family tree. Could a colleague easily identify the age, sex and occupation of your parents and siblings? Could they identify who lives in the family home?

www

Read the Victoria Climbié report online:

- http://www.victoria-climbie-inquiry.org.uk/finreport/finreport.htm

Read the 'Safeguarding' Children document online:

- http://www.doh.gov.uk/safeguarding children/index.htm

Box 22.2

Types of skills likely to be developed when working on a PEAU

With the various learning opportunities offered within PEAU, both qualified and student nurses should have the opportunity to enhance their skills in many areas, not least in some of the examples below, whether by doing or assisting:

- cannulation
- collection of specimens
- distraction and play
- emergency procedures
- fluid management
- health promotion
- history taking
- inhaler techniques
- initial assessment of a sick child
- liaison with multidisciplinary team
- lumbar punctures
- managing pyrexia
- nasogastric tube management
- nebulisation
- negotiating with children
- negotiating with parents
- neurological observation
- ongoing assessment of a sick child
- pain management
- physical assessment
- pulse oximetry
- venesection.

Observation

The problems associated with short-stay admissions inappropriately admitted to acute children's wards are many but include time-consuming admission procedures and admissions to inappropriate wards where specialist nurses or equipment may not be at hand. Additionally, beds for elective admissions are effectively blocked. Consultant ward rounds are delays that impact on discharge and, importantly, an undermining of parental confidence in self-managing minor illnesses in the home. Furthermore, the economic costs in terms of bed occupancy and resource allocation should not be underestimated.

Although hospital inpatient care is undeniably expensive, in both fiscal and social domains, for the families of sick children and the admitting hospital, the reasons for admission to paediatric beds has only recently been investigated in the UK. Much of the literature is focused on the appropriateness of hospital admission and MacFaul (1997) has indicated that 50% of paediatric emergencies are discharged within 1 day and reports a significant reduction in overnight stays after the opening of a short-stay acute illness assessment facility.

Similarly, an Australian review of paediatric admissions (Numa & Oberklaid 1991) concluded that 65% of eligible admissions would have been fit for discharge within 12 hours had there been a short-stay unit available. A subsequent Australian study (Browne 2000) revealed considerable approval in terms of parental satisfaction with short-stay and cost savings when a 23-hour short-stay unit was attached to the emergency department.

The mean stay for children entering a PEAU in the study by Aitken et al (2003) was 2 hours 57 minutes. Although the NHS is inextricably focusing on waiting times, which are now linked to a wide range of Ministerial Directives, White Papers and Health Service Circulars (DoH 2000), the overall satisfaction of the family encounter with the healthcare facility must remain high. Accordingly, benchmark standards of care are a high priority for nurses and other healthcare professionals involved with service delivery. The publication of documents such as 'The essence of care' (DoH 2001) encourages all healthcare professionals to 'think out of the box' when reconciling innovation with improved levels of family satisfaction.

In the absence of such units, unnecessary delays often prolong the admission. Beattie & Moir (1993), in reporting the first annual audit of a 24-hour short-stay ward attached to an emergency department, studied 829 children of whom 25% stayed less than 12 hours. The most common cause of admission reported in this audit was head injury, with 479 cases documented.

Interestingly, the justification for a 24-hour PEAU service has been rejected in at least one large North American study (Bond & Weigand 1997), which concluded that a single observation bed would be inadequate 25% of the time and empty 37% of the time. In a retrospective study conducted by Rajaratnam (1991) of admission case notes of children, between 15% and 20% of the 620 randomly selected cases were considered by the assessors not to have required admission. Furthermore, between 3% and 9% of the admissions were judged to be for social and not medical reasons.

PROFESSIONAL CONVERSATION

Second-year student nurse Hayley Anderson is discussing Ann-Marie's case with staff nurse Ellen Lancaster, her mentor in the PEAU.

Nursing observation after medical treatment

Following a good response to paracetamol, when Ann-Marie's temperature has reduced and she appears much more happy and content in herself, student nurse Hayley Anderson asks her mentor Ellen (who is sharing Ann-Marie's care with her) when the family will be discharged home. Staff nurse Ellen explains the need for a period of observation to ensure that Ann-Marie's parents are happy with fever management at home, that she tolerates good volumes of oral fluids and that her condition remains stable.

Ellen goes on to explain to Hayley that this period of observation also gives the opportunity for the nurse to address any educational or health promotion needs of the child and family.

Medical and social factors associated with paediatric emergency admissions to hospital have been the subject of some scrutiny. Steward et al (1998) have linked self-referral by parents to an accident and emergency department as being associated with socioeconomic deprivation. It is the appropriateness of childhood emergency admissions that continues to be linked to the evolution of services such as a PEAU. Although Esmail et al (2000) cite evidence of rises in paediatric admissions to UK hospitals, with these possibly being linked to poor social circumstances, in a retrospective review of 3324 paediatric admissions from 13 district general hospitals only 8% were found to be inappropriate. This perhaps reflects the discriminatory prowess of the robust UK primary healthcare services and, importantly, in this study inappropriate admissions were not linked to GP referrals.

Of interest is a report of a study on 18,057 children by Raffles et al (1999), which compared admission rates to a child health unit before and after the creation of a dedicated six-bedded PEAU situated within a busy emergency department. The reduction in overnight admission rates was calculated at 19% in the first year of operation of the PEAU.

Reductions in overnight stays in a climate of increased emergency admissions of children generally to hospital are clearly linked to the development of PEAUs and a French report (Lamireau et al 2000) concludes that a short-stay unit can provide cost-effective, comprehensive care linked to a reduction of fears among clinicians of inappropriate discharge.

Discharge and follow-up care

Hospital admission involving an overnight stay is always disruptive to the families concerned and Rajaratnam (1991) highlights these and the potential opportunity costs in discussing the reconfiguration that some hospitals have made to their paediatric inpatient facilities in the light of changes in the management of emergency admissions.

A quadrennial review of data during 1 calendar month by Aitken et al (2003) related to emergency patient length of stay. It revealed a substantial rise in the number of children admitted for less than 1 day, therefore avoiding an overnight stay since the opening of the unit in 1998. The rise in overall numbers of short-stay children was also accompanied by a corresponding fall in the number of children staying overnight in hospital during the same time period. Lamireau et al (2000) and Beverly et al (1997) have reported similar magnitudes of raises in short-stay patients.

Activity

Discharge planning is a key part of the admission process. Review your local discharge process and paperwork in relation to Ann-Marie.

Reflect on your practice

What skills are needed to empower parents and children with both the knowledge and confidence to be cared for at home?

One of the increasing concerns expressed by some authors is that of inappropriate or premature discharge (MacFaul 1997). It is important to stress that during the study by Aitken et al (2003) only one child was readmitted to the PEAU within 24 hours of discharge; three children who had attended the PEAU within the previous week were readmitted, as were three who had been discharged within the previous month. A total of 20 children in the study had been inpatients within the previous month with 56 children attending the emergency department within the previous month.

In a study by Lal & Kibirige (1999), who investigated the relationship between paediatric assessment units, quality of care and unscheduled return visits, only 2% ($n = 65$) of children were identified. The primary identified reason stated for these returns was parental perceptions of the illness with only two re-referred by their family doctor. Such findings reinforce the crucial role of the PEAU nurse in the giving of discharge information, ensuring that in partnership parents are fully involved in the decision making process and that all concerns are fully addressed.

Proactively, the nursing staff in some PEAUs have introduced weekday 24-hour open access and an extended period to cover weekend and bank holiday readmission to PEAU for just such eventualities. The establishment of an open access process for children, without the necessity of re-consulting a GP is thought to be reassuring for parents who might have residual worries after discharge. Additionally, some PEAUs offer a routine, morning-after-discharge nurse-led telephone consultation to all parents. A survey of parental satisfaction with paediatric emergency care revealed that parents found both the open access arrangement and follow-up telephone call reassuring (Birch et al 2005).

PROFESSIONAL CONVERSATION

Hayley Anderson, a second-year student nurse on clinical placement on a PEAU, asks staff nurse Ellen Lancaster, her mentor, about follow-up procedures on the unit.

Follow-up after discharge from hospital

The morning after Ann-Marie's discharge, student nurse Hayley asks staff nurse Ellen why she is telephoning the family, as they have been discharged home and been given 24 hours open access if they are concerned. She expresses concerns about the amount of nursing time this takes up. She further discusses the view that NHS Direct gives advice over the telephone and that the NHS Direct nurses are supported by computerised decision support software. She asks 'Should nurses really be doing such telephone interaction without such tools?'

Ellen explains that although it is true that parents can contact the unit if they are concerned, the telephone follow-up allows nursing staff to reinforce any information given on discharge and provides an important link between the nursing staff and family. Parents/carers may well wish to clarify certain issues or concerns and feel reluctant to 'bother' busy health professionals. The follow-up telephone call allows parents to ask questions about the previous day's treatment and for nursing staff to address any concerns.

Activity

- Explore the cost of an overnight admission and the effect of an unnecessary admission to hospital on a child and their family.
- Examine the legalities of telephone advice and the introduction of NHS Direct.

Reflect on your practice

- Consider the importance of team working in the assessment and planning of individual care for the acutely sick child and the consequences of a breakdown of communication in the multidisciplinary team.
- Reflect on a recent example of a breakdown in communication within your own working environment.

Evidence-based practice

Aitkin et al (2007) conducted a study to assess the demand for a 24-hour service in one English regional health authority. The opinions of general practitioners (GPs) regarding the service were sought via a fax survey, and a retrospective analysis of out-of-hour admissions staying less than 24 hours, over two discrete 3-month periods. Differences in GP referral outcomes were also examined. GPs using the current PEAU (n = 431) were invited to participate. GP's responses and analysis of PEAU out-of-hours throughput and admission trajectories were obtained. Results indicate that 83.9% of respondent GPs strongly agreed or agreed that the unit should provide a 24-hour PEAU service. There was widespread approval by GPs to implement a 24-hour PEAU service and subsequent to this study many units have implemented a 24 hour service.

Summary

The study by Aitken et al (2003) reinforced the importance of service evaluation as part of a child health unit commitment to clinical governance. The development of the PEAU cited in this study was very much a nurse-led initiative and the success of the service is indicative of children's nurses' pledge to family-centred care. In avoiding an unnecessary hospital stay, potential emotional child and family upset may be avoided. In this way, seminal contemporary child health policy publications (DoH 1996) can be enacted and adhered to.

However, new opportunities for nurses to work in this expanding field of practice will require an appropriate educational preparation, which includes physical history taking and examination (Rushforth et al 1998).

Key points

- Emergency assessment short-stay units appear to be an effective way to manage some children not requiring overnight hospital stay.
- Although difficult to calculate, the economic benefits of short-stay units should not be underestimated.
- Fears of inappropriate premature discharge, although important, do not appear to be a cause for concern.

References

Aitken, P., Birch, S., Cogman, G., et al., 2003. Quadrennial review of a paediatric emergency assessment unit. British Journal of Nursing 12 (4), 234–241.

Aitkin, P., Glasper, E.A., Wiltshire, M., John, P., Abay, J., 2007. Ascertaining demand for a full time paediatric emergency assessment unit. Journal of Children's and Young People's Nursing 1 (2), 82–84.

Beattie, T.F., Moir, A., 1993. Paediatric accident and emergency short-stay; a 1 year audit. Archives of Emergency Medicine 10, 181–186.

Beverly, D.W., Ball, R.J., Smith, R.A., et al., 1997. Planning for the future; the experience of implementing a children's day assessment unit in a district general hospital. Archives of Disease in Childhood 77 (4), 287–292.

Bond, G.R., Wiegand, C.B., 1997. Estimated use of pediatric emergency department observation unit. Annal of Emergency Medicine 29, 739–742.

Browne, G.J., 2000. A short stay or 23 hour ward in a general and academic children's hospital; are they effective? Paediatric Emergency Care 16 (4), 223–229.

Birch, S., Glasper, E.A., Aitken, P., Wiltshire, M., Cogman, G., 2005. GP views of nurse-led telephone referral for paediatric assessment. British Journal of Nursing 14 (12), 667–673.

Dearmun, A., Gordon, K., 1999. The nurse practitioner in children's ambulatory care. Paediatric Nursing 11 (1), 18–21.

Department of Health (DoH), 1991. Welfare of children and young people in hospital. HMSO, London.

Department of Health (DoH), 1996. The patients charter. Services for children and young people. HMSO, London.

Department of Health (DoH), 2000. The NHS Plan. A plan for investment, a plan for reform. HMSO, London.

Department of Health (DoH) 2001 The essence of care. Patient-focused benchmarking for health care practitioners. Online. Available at: hhtp://www.doh.gov.uk/essenceofcare

Department of Health (DoH), 2003. The children's national service framework. DoH, London.

Esmail, A., Quayle, J.A., Roberts, C., 2000. Assessing the appropriateness of paediatric hospital admissions in the United Kingdom. Journal of Public Health Medicine 22 (92), 231–238.

Glasper, E.A., Wilkins V., 1998. Telenursing – the provision of information by telephone: the implication for paediatric nursing. In: Glasper, E.A., Lowson, S., (Eds.), Innovations in paediatric ambulatory care – a nursing perspective. Macmillan, Basingstoke, pp 31–47.

Lal, M.K., Kibirige, M.S., 1999. Unscheduled return visits within 72 hours to an assessment unit. Archives of Disease in Childhood 80 (5), 455–458.

Lamireau, T., Llanas, B., Fayon, M., 2000. A short stay observation unit improves care in the paediatric emergency care setting. Archives of Disease in Childhood 83 (4), 371.

Lattimer, V., George, S., Thompson, F., et al., 1998. Safety and effectiveness of nurse telephone consultation in out of hours primary care: randomised controlled trial. British Medical Journal 317, 1054–1059.

MacFaul, R., 1997. Commentary – planning for the future. The experience of implementing a children's day assessment unit in a district general hospital. Archives of Disease in Childhood 77 (4), 292–293.

Meates, M., 1997. Ambulatory paediatrics – making a difference. Archives of Disease in Childhood 76, 468–476.

Numa, A., Oberklaid, F., 1991. Can short hospital admissions be avoided? A review of admissions less than 24 hours duration in paediatric teaching hospital. Medical Journal of Australia 155 (6), 395–398.

Raffles, A., Foo, W.L., Chowdhurt, T., Dustagheer, L., 1999. Does a paediatric acute assessment unit influence paediatric admissions? Proceeding of the Royal College of Paediatrics and Child Health Spring Meeting. RCPCH, London Tuesday 13.

Rajaratnam, G., 1991. A study of admissions to paediatric beds. Postgraduate Medical Journal 67, 50–54.

Royal College of Paediatrics and Child Health (RCPCH), 1998. Ambulatory paediatric services in the UK. Report of a working party. RCPCH, London.

Rushforth, H., 2002. Study of the factors influencing decisions by acute care nurses to undertake expanded roles traditionally associated with medical practice. Final study report for the UKCC. UKCC, London.

Rushforth, H., Glasper, E.A., 1999. Implications of nursing role expansion for professional practice. British Journal of Nursing 8 (22), 1507–1513.

Rushforth, H., Warner, J., Burge, D., Glasper, E.A., 1998. Nursing physical assessment skills: implications for UK practice. British Journal of Nursing 7 (16), 965–970.

Steward, M., Werneke, U., MacFaul, R., et al., 1998. Medical and social factors associated with admissions and discharge of acutely ill children. Archives of Disease in Childhood 79, 219–224.

Emergency department management of children

23

Liz Gormley-Fleming Julie Flaherty E Alan Glasper

ABSTRACT

The primary aim of this chapter and its companion PowerPoint presentation is to review emergency care for children and the role of children's nurses in emergency departments. The role of the children's nurse in maintaining the integrity of the family unit during emergency interventions is highlighted. A case study scenario based around a child with epilepsy is utilised in this chapter.

LEARNING OUTCOMES

- Develop the specialist knowledge required to safely administer medicines to children.
- Understand how the triage process is operationalised in paediatric emergency departments.
- Explore how children presenting with fits are managed in emergency departments.
- Appreciate positive attributes of the environment of care in emergency departments in the overall care of children.
- Review pain management for children in emergency departments.
- Consider how the philosophy of family-centred care is promoted in emergency departments.
- Appreciate the role of paediatric emergency nurse practitioners.

The national picture

A 1997 report of national trends in the UK between 1979 and 1997 identified that in one year alone 459 children died as a result of accidents. Approximately 3.5 million children attend local A&E departments for their injuries each year and 10,000 children become permanently disabled every year. The cost to the NHS has been estimated at £100 million per annum; the personal cost is unquantifiable.

Since the inception of the NHS, medical care has been comprehensively provided for all. In the early 1960s the term 'casualty' became synonymous with that part of the NHS receiving and stabilising acutely ill and injured patients. The portal of entry into the hospital setting for the ill and injured was through the 'casualty' department. At the same time as the acutely ill and injured attended, those members of the public who felt their physical and mental health need required urgent medical attention took advantage of the casualty department's ever open door.

In 1961, the Standing Medical Advisory Committee of Central Health Services undertook an investigation into NHS acute hospital arrangements for receiving and stabilisation of acutely ill and injured patients. The subsequent report for the first time formally recognised the concept of 'casual attendees' within the casualty department. Within the report, acknowledgement was given to the very skilful and important work undertaken in casualty departments. In recognition that this work should continue to develop, the concepts of 'casualty' and 'casual attendees' needed to be refocused and the term Accident and Emergency (A&E) department was created.

Many subsequent reports, including the Court report 'Fit for the future' (Department of Health and Social Services (DHSS) 1976), 'Welfare of children and young people in hospital' (Department of Health (DoH) 1991), 'Children first. A study of hospital services' (Audit Commission 1993) and 'The patient's charter – services for children and young people' (DoH 1996), all advocated and determined recommendations and standards for health services, with specific reference to A&E services for children. Furthermore, there is now evidence that some of the recommendations of the many working groups are now taking shape, although slowly. Within the current climate of the modernising NHS (DoH 2000, 2004) there is now greater emphasis than ever on recognising and meeting the needs of families and children requiring A&E services.

DOI: 10.1016/B978-0-7020-3183-0.10023-2

There are currently many avenues to emergency services for children and young people. Importantly there are nine active children's A&E departments in the UK. Alternatively, there are 259 other A&E departments accommodating health needs of all ages either in teaching or district general hospitals. The general A&E departments vary tremendously from integrated child and family services, audiovisual separation of adults and children to co-location of child and adult services.

In an average year, 50% of children under 1 year of age will attend an emergency department, and 25% of older children. Additionally, one in 11 children will be referred to a hospital outpatient department (NHS Confederation 2003). Additionally, an important change has occurred in the utilisation of emergency departments in recent years, with increasing numbers of children seeking hospital assessment, largely via self-referrals, but not requiring hospital admission (Boyle et al 2000).

Given the high profile that children have within an emergency department and Watson (2000) indicates that this client group makes up 30% of all attendees to emergency departments every year, it is not surprising to note that the National Service Framework (NSF) for children, young people and maternity services (DoH 2003) includes specific recommendations for accident and emergency departments. These include physical separation between children and adult areas within emergency departments and environments that are accessible, safe and suitable for babies, children and families.

Partridge (2001) has highlighted that children attending emergency departments have not generally been either treated or seen in separate facilities by registered children's nurses. This situation will begin to change in light of the NSF recommendations, which will be audited by the Care Quality Commission. Furthermore, Partridge argues that nurses who work in emergency departments must recognise that the treatment of children and adults within the same space is fraught with difficulties. This sharing of facilities such as waiting rooms ensures that at least some children will be exposed unnecessarily to hostile sights and hostile sounds. It is, however, to be hoped that the token obligatory box of broken toys in a dark corner of the waiting room of some emergency departments, as described by Glasper (1995), is a thing of the past. However, nurse managers within emergency departments recognise these important aspects of care and are increasingly requiring registered nurses not holding a recognised children's nursing qualification to undertake shortened child branch courses at local universities.

Scenario

Sheila Putman is 4 years and 6 months. She had a grand-mal convulsion in the school playground and sustained a laceration to the scalp, which bled profusely. She is dazed and confused after the convulsion, crying and asking for her mother. The teacher calls an ambulance and travels with Sheila to the local emergency department. Sheila's mother is eventually located at her work address on the outskirts of the city. She arrives at the emergency department 30 minutes after Sheila's arrival.

Transportation to the emergency department

By far the best way for critically ill and injured children to travel to hospital is by ambulance. However, parents and carers are often unaware of the severity of illness and injury that children suffer. Often because of their size, children are 'scooped up' and brought by people unaware of the risks they are taking escorting children in critical conditions by private car, public transport or taxi. Only 6% of children attend emergency departments by ambulance.

Taking this figure into account, it is important that A&E staff are aware that seriously ill and injured children often arrive in the emergency department 'in arms', and should receive early triage for this very reason. Conveying to the public the message about appropriate use of ambulances in urgent and emergency situations has been ongoing for years. There are, however, numerous accounts of situations when an ambulance has been called inappropriately by someone who has misjudged the situation. The nationally available NHS Direct telephone advice service is available for parents and carers (tel: 0845 46 47). The nurses can provide emergency advice about a child's health status and mobilise an ambulance if necessary.

Ninety per cent of all children attending A&E do so between 8.00 a.m. and midnight; the remaining 10% attend between midnight and 8.00 a.m. The busiest period for children in A&E is between mid-day and 4.00 p.m., when over 55% children attend for unscheduled care; 80% of children with traumatic injury arrive between 4.00 p.m. and midnight.

MacFaul & Werneke (2001) conducted a study in which presenting problems were recorded in 842 admissions. Fifty-six per cent of children presented with one of three problems: breathing difficulty (25%), fit (16%), or feverish illness (15%). Feeding problems and diarrhoea together accounted for a further 21%. Seizures as a high cause of emergency admissions have come under considerable scrutiny by healthcare professionals working in such environments. The introduction of clinical guidelines (or care pathways) for the management of children presenting with fits in emergency departments is linked to improvements in the effectiveness of care delivery (Arnon et al 2004).

Activity

Critically review the Arnon et al (2004) paper. Access this online at: http://www.archdischild.com

Read the article by Watts et al (2003) and look at the Joanna Briggs Institute, Adelaide website. Access this at: http://www.joannabriggs.edu.au

What are fits, convulsions or seizures?

Many people in society suffer from fits, convulsions or seizures. One in 20 (5%) of all children will have a fit of some kind during childhood. About 1 in 200 (0.5%) children have epilepsy,

WWW

The following text is based on 'About seizures', a leaflet produced by the Royal Children's Hospital Melbourne. Access the original document at:

- http://www.rch.org.au/cep/epilepsy/

i.e. a neurological condition in which the child has a predisposition to recurrent, unprovoked fits.

Epileptic fits occur when there is a transient disarrangement of the electrical and chemical neurotransmitters in the brain, which results in brain cells discharging impulses in an abnormal fashion. This may create a temporary disturbance in the way the brain controls awareness and responsiveness, which commonly causes unusual sensations or abnormal movements and postures. What happens during a fit reflects what parts of the brain are involved.

There are many different types of fit. The following describes the classification of seizure types from the International League Against Epilepsy (ILAE). A major distinction that healthcare professionals try to make is between partial (focal) fits, where the abnormal activity arises in a localised part of the brain (usually on one side), and generalised fits, where epileptic activity begins all over the brain simultaneously.

Partial (focal) fits

Partial (focal) fits occur when the abnormal activity arises in a localised part of the brain, usually on one side, and consciousness may or may not be impaired. The manifestations of the seizure depend on the part of the brain involved with the abnormal electrical discharge. Partial fits are classified according to whether there is impairment of consciousness:

- **Simple partial fits**: arise in parts of the brain not responsible for maintaining consciousness, typically the movement or sensory areas. Consciousness is not impaired and the effects of the fit relate to the part of the brain involved. If the site of origin is the motor area of the brain, bodily movements may be abnormal (e.g. limp, stiff, jerking). If sensory areas of the brain are involved, the person may report experiences such as tingling or numbness, changes to what he or she sees, hears or smells, or very unusual feelings that may be hard to describe. Young children might have difficulty describing such sensations or may be frightened by these.
- **Complex partial seizures**: arise in parts of the brain responsible for maintaining awareness, responsiveness and memory – typically parts of the temporal and frontal lobes. Consciousness is lost and the person may appear dazed or unaware of his or her surroundings. Sometimes the person experiences a warning sensation, or aura, before losing awareness, essentially the simple partial phase of the fit. Behaviour during a complex partial fit relates to the site of origin and spread of the fit. Often, the person's actions are clumsy and the individual will not respond normally to questions and commands. Behaviour may be confused and the person might exhibit automatic movements and behaviours, e.g. picking at clothing, picking up objects, chewing and swallowing, trying to stand or run, appearing afraid and struggling with restraint. Colour change, wetting and vomiting can occur in complex partial fits. Following the fit, the person may remain confused for a prolonged period and may not be able to speak, see, or hear if these parts of the brain were involved. The person has no memory of what occurred during the complex partial phase of the fit and often needs to sleep.
- **Partial seizures becoming secondarily generalised**: fits that begin as simple or complex partial seizures may progress due to a spread of epileptic activity all over one or both sides of the brain, leading to a secondary generalised seizure. This part of the fit looks like a generalised tonic clonic seizure.

Generalised seizures

Generalised fits occur when epileptic activity begins all over the brain simultaneously and consciousness is always impaired in generalised seizures:

- **Tonic clonic fit**: sometimes called a 'grand mal' fit: produces a sudden loss of consciousness, with the person commonly falling to the ground followed by stiffening (tonic) and then rhythmic jerking (clonic) of the muscles. Shallow or jerky breathing, bluish tinge of the skin and lips, drooling of saliva and often loss of bladder or bowel control generally occur. The seizures usually last a couple of minutes and normal breathing and consciousness then returns. The person is tired following the seizure and may be confused. There is no aura prior to a tonic clonic seizure.
- **Absence fit**: sometimes called a 'petit mal' fit: produces a brief cessation of activity and loss of consciousness, usually lasting 5–30 seconds. Often, the momentary blank stare is accompanied by subtle eye blinking and mouthing or chewing movements. Awareness returns quickly and the person continues with the previous activity. Falling and jerking do not occur in typical absences.
- **Myoclonic fit**: sudden and brief muscle contractions that may occur singly, repeatedly or continuously. They may involve the whole body in a massive jerk or spasm, or may only involve individual limbs or muscle groups. If they involve the arms, the person might drop or spill what he or she was holding. If they involve the legs or body, the person may fall.
- **Tonic fit**: characterised by generalised muscle stiffening, lasting 1–10 seconds. Associated features include increased pulse, brief cessation of breathing, flushed face, bluish skin discoloration and drooling. If a tonic seizure

occurs suddenly while the person is awake, he or she may fall violently to the ground, causing injury. Tonic seizures often occur during sleep. Fortunately, tonic fits are rare and usually only occur in severe forms of epilepsy.
- **Atonic fit**: produces a sudden loss of muscle tone, which, if brief, may only involve the head dropping forward ('head nods'), but may cause sudden collapse and falling ('drop attacks').

From these descriptions, it can be appreciated that the exact type of fit may be difficult for a witness to determine. For example, a fit with stopping and staring could be a complex partial seizure or an absence seizure. A large, convulsive fit (grand mal) may be a generalised tonic clonic fit, a myoclonic fit, a tonic fit or a partial fit that became secondarily generalised. A sudden fall to the ground ('drop attack') can occur with a myoclonic, a tonic or an atonic fit or a partial fit involving the movement areas. Determination of the exact type of fit is important and is obtained from patient and observer descriptions, home video recordings, and EEG testing and sometimes video EEG monitoring.

It is also important to remember that many episodic behaviours and disorders in children can mimic epilepsy, including breath-holding spells, normal sleep jerks, daydreaming, fainting, migraine, heart and gastrointestinal problems, and psychological problems.

Managing acute seizures and status epilepticus

Activity

Think about the management of a brief seizure by putting yourself into the position of witnessing a child, known to have epilepsy, who is having a seizure in school:
- What would you do?
- What would you not do?

www

Advice relating to seizure management can be readily found on the following websites:
- Epilepsy Action (British Epilepsy Association) search for seizure-first aid: http://www.epilepsy.org.uk
- National Society for Epilepsy search for first aid for epilepsy: http://www.epilepsynse.org.uk

Rapid treatment has the potential to minimise the morbidity and mortality associated with acute seizures and convulsive status epilepticus (Scott et al 1998, Scott & Neville 1999). Although status epilepticus is described as a disorder in which epileptic activity, a seizure or series of seizures persists for 30 minutes or more, clinically, most seizures that do not stop spontaneously within 5 minutes progress for 30 minutes or more (Appleton et al 2000, Scott et al 1998, Tasker 1998). Seizure activity dramatically increases the brain's demands for oxygen and glucose. After 30 minutes compensatory mechanisms fail, resulting in cerebral oedema, metabolic acidosis and circulatory collapse and an increasing risk of cerebral damage (Shovron 2001). Causes of acute seizures in children include:

- acute cerebral dysfunction:
  - trauma
  - infection
  - tumours
  - metabolic disturbances
  - febrile seizures
- pre-existing epilepsy:
  - drug withdrawal
  - progression of underlying cause
  - acute illness
- pre-existing neurological abnormality, e.g. cerebral palsy.

The aim of management is to control the seizure before cerebral damage and life-threatening sequelae occur (Scott et al 1998, Tasker 1998). The neurological status should only be assessed after airway, breathing and circulation have been assessed and managed. Clear protocols with structured interventions are necessary to ensure prompt and consistent management of seizures and status epilepticus (Appleton et al 2000, Scott & Neville 1999, Shovron 2001, Tasker 1998) (Table 23.1).

Children who have repeated episodes of convulsive epilepticus may need an adapted acute protocol to reflect their individual response to treatments and interactions with regular anticonvulsants (Scott & Neville 1999, Tasker 1998). Individual protocols will require the inclusion of parental home treatment regimes.

Emergency care teams

Given that accidents are the foremost cause of death in children over 1 year of age, response to the care of the most seriously ill and injured children must be delivered speedily and following a professionally competent model backed up by the right facilities. A team approach allows critically ill and traumatised patients optimal chances for survival.

There has been a dramatic increase in the number of children attending hospital with head injuries in the last decade and this accounts for up to one-third of the incidence of accidental death in childhood. While there has been a marked improvement in the long-term outcome for children with traumatic brain injuries, there is an associated health impact for the child and their families (Parslow et al 2005). A systematic approach to the initial assessment and early management of head injuries is crucial to the long-term outcome (National Institute of Clinical Excellent (NICE) 2007).

The Royal College of Surgeons recommends that the emergency care team should include a team leader, usually the A&E consultant, a surgical consultant, a medical consultant, and an anaesthetic or intensivist consultant. Other team members will be registered nurses and allied health professionals (AHP); the numbers will vary but it has been

Table 23.1 Principles of managing acute seizures and status epilepticus (Appleton et al 2000, Scott & Neville 1999, Shovron 2001, Tasker 1998)

Stage	Action	Rationale
Immediate assessment and stabilisation	Rapid cardiopulmonary assessment If necessary maintain and secure airway Give oxygen Monitor vital signs and pulse oximetry Confirmation/history of seizure/child's past medical history	Recognise respiratory failure and shock Airway obstruction will compound hypoxia Ensure management is appropriate for the individual child
Immediate seizure control (5–10 minutes)	*Administer first-line anticonvulsant:* If IV access available, administer IV lorazepam If there is no venous access, administer either rectal diazepam or intramuscular midazolam or intramuscular paraldehyde Obtain IV or intraosseous access Obtain bloods for electrolytes and glucose Commence intravenous fluids. Repeat further IV dose of lorazepam if no response after 10 minutes Repeat cardiopulmonary assessment Prepare for intensive support	Lorazepam has longer duration of action compared with diazepam and lower risk of drug accumulation. It may be less effective in children taking regular benzodiazepine anticonvulsants Paraldehyde may result in abscess formation at injection site
Second-stage treatment (15 minutes onwards) Intensive care management	*If no response administer further anticonvulsants:* Phenytoin infusion Intubate and ventilate, transfer to intensive care Ventilate, monitor pulse/BP/temperature/urine output, EEG Phenobarbitone infusion If no response consider IV bolus of midazolam or thiopentone	Phenytoin is effective within 10–30 minutes and has a long duration of action and may prevent recurrent seizures Phenobarbitone is effective but may take time to reach therapeutic levels and may cause lowering of the blood pressure Midazolam is water soluble and easy to administer, less irritant to veins and appears to be effective in stopping seizures that have been unresponsive to other drugs

BP, blood pressure; EEG, electroencephalogram; IV, intravenous.

suggested that the trauma team should include four senior doctors, five nurses and a radiographer. It was clearly stated in the National Confidential Enquiry into Perioperative Deaths (1989 p 7) that:

> Consultants who take responsibility for the care of children … must be competent and must keep up to date in the management of children.

The Royal College of Paediatricians and Child Health stipulates that a nominated consultant anaesthetist, suitably trained in paediatric anaesthesia, should be responsible for children's services. It is important to train the right team members, with the right skills and abilities; successful results in a trauma situation are determined by the training and abilities of the trauma team.

A paediatrician should be included in the emergency care team for seriously traumatised children. After initial resuscitation and stabilisation, children should be transferred to the care of paediatric surgeons in a specialist facility with paediatric intensive care back-up. More recently, a joint report from the Royal College of Surgeons and the British Orthopaedic Association (RCS/BOA 2000) recommended that:

> Any hospital receiving and caring for the severely injured child must have on-site support from paediatricians and paediatric anaesthetists.

The Audit Commission (1993 p 48) highlights the fact that A&E departments do not always have or receive timely back-up from other specialists or allied health professionals to support diagnostic investigations. Further, the Audit Commission (1993 p 49) appraises a list of favourable specialists that should work synergistically with A&E services. Some specialty back-up seems obvious, such as anaesthesia, orthopaedics, general surgery and medicine. Support services that need to co-locate at A&E include critical care facilities, radiology, ultrasound, online CT scanner and 24-hour pathology services.

Disappointingly, the report 'Better care for the seriously injured' (RCS/BOA 2000) dedicates only one of 55 pages to the severely injured child. However, the report does acknowledge that there is a much higher frequency of serious head, chest and abdominal injuries in children than in adults. It berates less experienced doctors for their indecision and late intervention when managing a seriously injured child and is also the only report of all those mentioned above to relate and conclude that severely injured children present the greatest opportunity for organ salvage.

The Healthcare Commission 2009 identified that hospitals are still failing to provide adequate pain relief for children attending A&E Departments and that 74% of staff in emergency departments had not received basic training in resuscitation or in child protection. Staff working in emergency departments must be equipped with the appropriate skills and receive training to treat all children that attend the department.

Children's nurses in emergency departments

The development of A&E nursing has been at the forefront of role extension within the UK and the development of a faculty of emergency nursing within the Royal College of Nursing (RCN) has allowed nurses working within the domain to agree and establish levels of clinical competencies (Endacott et al 1999). Bentley (1996) has defined role categories for children's nurses who work in emergency departments, which include the development and use of protocols in the management of sick children. Despite this, Cleaver (2003) has highlighted the feelings of vulnerability experienced by children's nurses who work in emergency departments, who are perceived by their adult/general nurse colleagues as being experts in the care of sick children. Cleaver's study reveals that the children's nurses themselves, having acquired and mastered new roles, move from feeling vulnerable to feeling frustrated when they are not allowed to develop autonomous practice. However the Emergency Nurse Practitioner is now becoming an established role in many Children's A&E departments throughout the UK.

The environment in the A&E department

Often, the first point of contact or portal of entry to hospital is through the A&E department. The A&E department can be a distressing place, full of unfamiliar sights and sounds and little opportunity to prepare children for this experience (DoH 2003). Depending on their particular stage of cognitive development, children will interpret the situations into terms they can conceptualise. In turn, the child's perceptions and experiences in the A&E or emergency room will affect future attendances; the right staff and the right environment can have a dramatic impact (Audit Commission 1993, DoH 1991, 2003).

The provision of services for children should be appropriate to their cognitive and developmental needs. Children should be cared for in an environment that is audiovisually separate from the main A&E department and they should be attended to by staff who have been suitably trained and educated to care for children. The value of children's nurses in A&E is enormous; children's nurses possess skills in assessing children's development stage, communicating with child and family and developing care plans that meet the individual child's needs.

Triage in emergency departments

Triage is an integral part of the modern emergency department. The use of a recognised triage system has many advantages for the emergency department, including reference to a recognised decision-making structure and support in the form of a professionally accepted and validated system. Many units use the Manchester triage system, which is a method of identifying high-priority patients. The word 'triage' comes from the French 'to sort' and has its origins in the management of battlefield casualties. Although there are a number of definitions and Scoble (2004), for example, describes triage as a process of nurse assessment of a patient on arrival in an emergency department, all the definitions are consistent in that they describe triage as the categorising of sick or injured patients according to severity in order to coordinate care and ensure the most efficient and efficient use of emergency department staff and facilities (Box 23.1).

The Manchester triage system uses 52 flow charts, which allocate patients to one of the five national triage categories described above. Although the Manchester system is widely used and works well for prioritisation, Willis (2001) believes that it fails to encourage nurses using it to query in the case of a child the reason for the emergency attendance. In particular, the possibility of non-accidental injury as the cause of

Box 23.1

Triage categories

Triage category 1

- People who need to have treatment immediately (in practice, within 2 minutes) are called immediately life-threatening patients.
- People in this group are critically ill and require immediate attention. Most would have arrived at the emergency department by ambulance. They would probably be suffering from something like a critical injury or cardiac arrest.

Triage category 2

- People who need to have treatment within 10 minutes are called imminently life-threatening patients.
- People in this group would probably be suffering from something like a critical illness or very severe pain. People with serious chest pains, difficulty in breathing and severe fractures are included in this group.

Triage category 3

- People who need to have treatment within 30 minutes are called potentially life-threatening patients.
- People in this group would probably be suffering from something like severe illnesses, major bleeding from cuts, major fractures or dehydration.

Triage category 4

- People who need to have treatment within 1 hour are called potentially serious patients.
- People in this group would probably have less severe symptoms or injuries with something like a foreign body in the eye, sprained ankle, migraine or earache.

Triage category 5

- People who need to have treatment within 2 hours are called less urgent patients.
- People in this group probably have minor illnesses or symptoms that may have been present for more than a week, like rashes or minor aches and pains.

Triage categories 1 to 5 were previously described as resuscitation, emergency, urgent, semi-urgent and non-urgent.

admission has prompted Willis to describe an enhancement to the Manchester triage system known as CWILTED (Willis 2001):

- C = Condition: area of pain, problem, child protection.
- W = Witness: name, position and designation of person who actually saw the incident; if nobody saw the incident write 'none'.
- I = Incident: mechanism that caused the injury.
- L = location: home address, school, childminder (name and address), park or play area.
- T = Time: time accident occurred and date, time first aid given (including medication), time of last meal.
- E = Escort: it should not be automatically assumed that an accompanying adult is a parent. Does this person have parental responsibility? If he or she is not witness to the accident, how do they know what happened?
- D = Disability: initially this had been 'description' but this tended to repeat 'condition' and triage staff have modified this to be disability caused by the incident or diagnosis if known at the time. Willis (2001) notes that the staff of the emergency department at St Peters Hospital in Surrey reverted to 'description', i.e. to mean what the child looks like, is behaving like, etc., because 'disability' did not always appear appropriate when the child had a medical presentation.

www

CWILTED was cited by the Commission for Health Inspection (CHI) in a report of interagency working as being commendable practice. Read this report online at:

- http://www.chi.nhs.uk/eng/about/publications/safeguards/surry.pdf

Willis (2001) is critical of the Manchester triage system because important child protection issues might be missed and recommends that CWILTED is used as an adjunct to this method of identifying and prioritising patient problems. The Manchester system has also been criticised by Woolwich (1999), who laments the mechanistic approach of applying a computer algorithm to the identification of prioritised patient symptoms, believing that this empowers nurses conducting the triage by reducing their professional judgement, clinical expertise and intuitive acumen.

Triage using the National Triage Scale (Mackway-Jones 1997) has been widely adopted and is generally considered an efficient way of 'sorting' those very urgent needs from those with less urgent needs, and in managing emergency departments. Triage, however, can only be truly effective if the process takes place on arrival. Triage also needs to be a continual process, so that deterioration in children with initially lower priority can be recategorised (Mackway-Jones 1997 p 2). Immediate and continued triage requires nursing staff to be constantly available and assigned to triage duties. This is often difficult with a less than optimal nursing establishment. The emergency situation that can be visualised is more likely to take precedence than the potential one waiting for triage. One needs to be reminded of the 'duty care' to all patients and the emergency department shift coordinator holds the ultimate responsibility for deployment of nursing and medical colleagues.

Immediate triage is crucial for young children and babies. This can be a lengthy process because it can take some time taken to remove layers of clothing from small children. This will create a 'knock on' effect in delay for the next waiting child.

Less than 0.25% of all children attending emergency services require paediatric intensive care. However, it is widely known and accepted that half of this 0.25% will have been carried 'in arms' to the emergency department, with the consequent risks of further injury. Although only a small fraction of children attending emergency departments require paediatric intensive care services, level one dependency accounts for 61% of all PICU admissions.

Activity

Read the grey chapters in the Advanced Life Support Group (2003):
Chapter 1 Introduction
Chapter 2 Why treat children differently
Chapter 4 Basic life support
Chapter 5 Advanced support of the airway and ventilation
Chapter 6 Management of cardiac arrest
Chapter 8 The structured approach to the seriously ill child
Chapter 15 The structured approach to the seriously injured child

Scenario

What would really happen?

On arrival by ambulance, Sheila is taken into the paediatric emergency area, where the children nurse undertakes a quick visual assessment – Airway, Breathing, Circulation – to determine if there is any immediate life threat. Sheila is triaged and the nurse observes that she is in pain.

Sheila is known to suffer from epilepsy and has anticonvulsant therapy. She is alert and conscious and is able to express that she is feeling sore on her head. The nurse recognises that Sheila needs some analgesia. Paracetamol is the drug of choice.

The use of early warning scoring systems are now usurping many traditional systems of assessing the child in the emergency department.

The cause of Sheila's fit could range from meningitis or encephalitis, metabolic causes such as diabetic ketoacidosis, hypoglycaemia, electrolyte disturbances or from head injury, drug or poison ingestion or intracranial haemorrhage – all of which have the potential for respiratory, circulatory failure and shock. It should take less than a minute to identify any potential respiratory, circulatory or neurological failure, with resuscitation given immediately as necessary. Prompt recognition and treatment are essential if the extreme situation of cardiopulmonary arrest and a poor outcome is to be avoided. Respiratory failure is a clinical state characterised by inadequate ventilation or oxygenation and by circulatory failure. Because children have lower pulmonary reserves than adults they compensate quickly and are therefore susceptible to both cardiorespiratory failure and shock.

Recognition and assessment of pain

Integral to the process of triage, children have their pain assessed. Triage priority is often determined by severity of pain. This allows for the child's pain to be managed at the earliest opportunity. Once pain management is determined and the child made more comfortable, it may be possible to recategorise to a lower priority.

Pain assessment in the emergency department is often difficult, particularly with children. Having sustained an injury or illness causes the child anxiety. Children will be frightened of being in a strange environment and not knowing what is going to happen next, and often think that what happened is their fault and fear punishment. Children often imagine the worst outcome of their pain, or they will deny their pain entirely. Many healthcare professionals hold unfounded beliefs that because children are not crying they cannot be in pain. By the same rule it is often said, 'that children who make the loudest noise usually experience the least pain'.

Pain assessment tools used in conjunction with triage protocols, fall into three main types (Mackway-Jones 1997): verbal descriptor scales, visual analogue scales and pain behaviour tools. The ideal pain assessment tool in the emergency department should be age appropriate, user friendly and simple, quick to use and incorporate the three main types.

Verbal descriptor scales when working with children are extremely helpful. Depending on their cognitive stage of development, children often are unable to express the intensity of their pain. By understanding the mechanism of injury and the effect the injury has on the child, it is not unreasonable to anticipate the level of pain when a child is unable to express the intensity. An example of pain management would be the child who has amputated the end of a finger but is for many reasons unable to express how much pain he or she is experiencing. By using verbal descriptors weighted within a pain ruler (Mackway-Jones 1997 p 25) it would not be unreasonable to assess the pain between 6 and 7. Verbal descriptors for level 6 suggests pain is described as very bad/severe.

Pain relief for children in emergency departments

One of the elements of the Manchester triage scale is its insistence that a patient's pain must be assessed during the triage process. However, in reality, pain relief is often not managed to the patient's satisfaction. Maurice et al (2002) give a comprehensive review of emergency analgesia in childhood emergencies and counsel against using intramuscular injections because the rate of absorption of the drug is not predictable and, if the child is in shock, the drug will not be disseminated adequately around the body in the way that an intravenous injection would. Furthermore, the potential for the need for top-up injections coupled with the development of potential or actual needle phobia make this method of pain relief unacceptable. Maurice et al (2002) argue that the ideal analgesia in childhood emergencies is easily and painlessly administrated, has a rapid onset, and has predictable and effective pain reliving actions and importantly no unwarranted side effects (Box 23.2).

Activity

- What other methods of pain relief are available to emergency nurses?
- Discuss the role of distraction and complementary therapies.

Making medicine administration and drug calculations safer

After working through this section of the chapter you should be able to calculate drug doses accurately and safely. In the minds of most children, 'getting better' is associated with taking medicine. At a very early age children are introduced to paracetamol when they have a fever or feel unwell. At 3 months most children receive their first immunisation. If illness occurs then various drugs with a wide range of side effects will probably be required.

The treatment of an individual child or young person with medicine is a process that involves prescribing, dispensing, administering, receiving and recording. Thus treatment with medicines is a partnership between the doctor, the pharmacist, the nurse and the patient.

It is the trained nurses' responsibility to ensure safe and reliable medicine administration, to monitor the effects, to ensure patients understand their medication and to sign the prescription sheet. Familiarisation with the Nursing & Midwifery Councils (2008) Standards for Medicine Management is recommended. As a student nurse you should be able to assist the trained nurse to:

- identify the correct patient
- select the correct, in-date medicines
- calculate and measure the dose required
- administer the dose by the correct route.

Accuracy

When calculating drug doses for children, accuracy is of the utmost importance. Often, doses are very small, particularly for infants, and an overdose can have a catastrophic effect. In 1995 a junior doctor at Rotherham District General Hospital intended to give 150 micrograms of morphine to a premature

Box 23.2

Methods of relieving childhood pain in emergency departments (after Maurice et al 2002)

- Local anaesthesia infiltrated into the wound: simple and safe but potentially painful. This can be counteracted by using a small-bore needle or a warmed solution.
- Topical anaesthesia: ELA (not for infants under a year) or Ametop (not for infants under 1 month). Good for preparing for cannulation or venepuncture but not for use in open wounds or mucous membranes which makes them unsuitable for use in the cleaning or suturing of wounds.
- Field block: local anaesthesia is injected around the perimeter of a wound or abscess a centimetre away from the edge. Takes longer to work but prevents the reduction of the desired anaesthetic effect, which occurs when local is infiltrated into infected areas which have increased vascularity.
- Peripheral nerve block: this involves the injection of local into the area of a peripheral nerve to provide anaesthesia to the area of the body distal to the area being infiltrated. Commonly used to provide femoral (good for fractures of the shaft of femur before X-ray and application of traction) or digital nerve block (good for avulsed finger nails or draining of paronychia).
- Paracetamol: good for mild pain (can be given rectally).
- Non-steroidal anti-inflammatory drugs such as ibuprofen: not recommended for children younger than 1 year but useful for moderate pain, especially that caused by musculoskeletal trauma. Contraindicated in patients with a history of gastrointestinal bleeding or renal impairment. Can cause bronchospasm in asthmatic children.
- Nitrous oxide: in a mixture of 70% with 30% oxygen this gas is effective for venous cannulation. It is painless to administer and the children can control their own dispensation through a mouthpiece. In a 50:50 mixture, nitrous oxide has good analgesic effect.
- Opioids: codeine is a good drug for mild to moderate pain; its effect is enhanced when it is combined with paracetamol. Morphine is an excellent choice for severe pain such as that caused by burns or fractures; the intravenous route is preferred. Diamorphine administered intranasally has been shown to be effective in children with fractures of the long bones. Pethidine has shorter duration than morphine with less sedative effects. However, pethidine can cause nausea and sometimes convulsions. Fentanyl is a synthetic opioid that can be administered intravenously or intranasally. It has rapid onset and short duration but can cause respiratory depression. It should be used with caution in emergency departments. Ketamine has analgesic, anaesthetic and dissociative state properties but also has side effects such as increase in blood pressure, which makes it unsuitable for patients with raised intracranial pressure (RCPCH 2003). Paracetamol oral solution/suspension is available in 120 mg in 5 mL and 250 mg in 5mL. Calculate the dose of paracetamol for Sheila.
- 1% lidocaine is most commonly used for local anaesthetic infiltration prior to suturing children's wounds. This drug comes as 10 mg/mL and maximum dosages to achieve local anaesthesia are 3 mg/kg. Sheila weighs:

$$(\text{Age } 4\tfrac{1}{2} \text{ years} + 4) \times 2 = 17 \text{ kg}.$$

baby. She miscalculated the decimal point and gave 15 milligrams of morphine; the baby died. This is not meant to alarm you but to emphasise the importance of ensuring your ability to undertake calculations accurately. Please remember if you are unsure about a calculation stop and get help. Do not give medicines unless you are confident in your calculation. Practice calculations using the prescription charts on the wards and test your competence with your clinical assessor, clinical skills coordinator or academic tutor.

It is essential that you can undertake all medicine calculations without using a calculator. The reason for this is that it is too easy to press the wrong button and come out with an entirely wrong answer. Furthermore, you need to have a reasonable idea of the amount of drug you are expecting to give; in other words to understand what is a logical amount. If you work the dose out first by hand it is acceptable to then check it using a calculator.

Units used in medicine

Many different units are used in medicine for drug strength and dosages. You need to understand the units in which drugs can be prescribed and how to convert from one unit to another.

The first step is to check out your knowledge of these units, which are based on the International Systême of units (SI units) or metric system for weight, volume and amount of substances. Please ensure that you fully understand these units. If you have any difficulty you should consult one of the 'drug calculation for nurses' books (e.g. Lapham & Agar 2009).

You must be able to convert from one unit to another fluently, so practise until you can.

Activity

Complete the following:

- 1 kilogram (kg) = . . . grams (g)
- 1 gram (g) = . . . milligrams (mg)
- 1 milligram (mg) = . . . micrograms (mcg or μg)
- 1 microgram (mcg) = . . . nanograms (ng)
- 1 litre (L) = . . . millilitres (mL)
- 1 mole (mol) = . . . millimoles (mmol)
- 1 millimole (mmol) = . . . micromoles (mcmol or μmol)

Activity

Now try these unit conversions:

- 1 mol = . . . mcmol
- 1 kg = . . . mcg
- 1 mg = . . . mcg
- 1 g = . . . ng

Weight

Without doubt, the most rapid increase in height and weight occur in the first year of life. The average baby at birth weighs 3.2 kg and will treble its weight by its first birthday to 9.6 kg. By the second birthday the toddler will have quadrupled its birth weight to 12.8 kg.

In the emergency situation, it is important to ascertain the child's weight as a matter of urgency. Most drugs and therapies are given as the dose per kilogram. Given the impracticalities of weighing children in the emergency situation, a number of methods can be used to estimate a child's weight. The most widely known formula if age is known is:

$$\text{Weight}\,(\text{kg}) = 2 \times (\text{age in years} + 4)$$

Broselow tape may also be used.

Is the dose correct?

Before you give a medicine to the child you must be sure that the dose is correct. Drug dosages are commonly calculated on the child's weight. Every time you give medicines you must find out the child's weight and check in a paediatric formulary to find out the recommended dose per kilogram of body weight (the British National Formulary for children is a good reference source). If there is a discrepancy it must be checked with the prescriber.

Please remember that someone could have made a mistake when writing the child's weight on the drug chart. You must assess whether the weight shown makes sense in relation to the child's age. Until you are familiar with children's weights you should check using growth charts.

Activity

Check these calculations:

- Jennifer is 18 months old and weighs 14 kg. She has an abscess on her index finger and has been prescribed 200 mg of paracetamol 4–6-hourly for pain. The recommended dose is 15 mg/kg.
- Robert, aged 13, has had an accident. He chopped off the top of his finger with a skateboard. Following a course of intravenous antibiotics he has now changed to oral. He is prescribed oral cephalexin 500 mg at 06.00 hours and 18.00 hours. He weighs 43.3 kg. The Medicines for children formulary recommends 25 mg/kg daily in divided doses. What do you notice about this prescription?
- Paracetamol is the drug of choice for mild to moderate pain. A loading dose of paracetamol would be given at 20 mg/kg for children between 2 and 12 years of age (RCPCH 2003). Paracetamol oral solution/suspension is available in 120 mg in 5 mL and 250 mg in 5 mL. Calculate the dose of paracetamol for Sheila.
- 1% lidocaine is most commonly used for local anaesthetic infiltration prior to suturing children's wounds. This drug comes as 10 mg/mL and maximum dosages to achieve local anaesthesia are 3 mg/kg. Sheila weighs:

$$(\text{Age } 4.5 \text{ years} + 4) \times 2 = 17 \text{ kg}$$

Is the route correct?

Check in the formulary that the prescribed route is correct. Some drugs have different doses for different routes, so check correct dose for correct route. Also, check on the bottle or vial that you are using the correct formulation of the drug for the route you are using.

Side effects

It is also your responsibility to know the side effects and interactions of all the medicines that you give. Some of the side effects are pivotal to nursing care. For example, one of the side effects of morphine is respiratory depression. Thus it is vital that sedation level and respiratory function are rigorously monitored. Please ensure that you know and monitor the possible side effects for all the medicines commonly used in each of your clinical placements.

Activity

List ten medicines, with their side effects, which you have seen administered in your clinical placements. Include morphine whether you have seen it administered or not.

Calculations

If the prescribed dose is straightforward, calculation is simple. However, if the prescribed dose is a small fraction of the available medicine then this simple formula can be used:

$$(\text{Strength required [what you want]} \div \text{Strength available}$$
$$\text{[what you have got]} \times \text{stock solution)}$$
$$\text{(volume the drug is in)}$$

The 'what you want' and 'what you have got' should be in the same unit.

Activity

How many mL of paracetamol 120 mg in 5 mL will you give if the prescription is for:

- 50 mg?
- 75 mg?

How many mL of paracetamol 250 in 5mL will you give if the prescription is for?

- 100 mg?
- 150 mg?

www

Visit the Association of Chief Children's Nurses website and access the Paediatric Nursing Journal information on drug calculations

- http:\\www.accnuk.org

Box 23.3

Example

The prescription is for oral ampicillin 80 mg. The bottle contains 125 mg in 5 mL. How many millilitres should you give?

$$(80 \div 125) \times 5 = 3.2 \text{ mL}$$

There are various ways of denoting the concentration of drug in a liquid medicine. The most usual way is in mg of drug in mL of liquid, i.e. mg/mL. For example, paracetamol comes in oral suspensions of either 120 mg in 5 mL or 250 mg in 5 mL. Prescriptions must be:

- legible and not altered
- written in block capitals
- signed using a full name
- give the drug generic name, not the trade name.

Additionally, prescriptions for controlled drugs must:

- give maximum number of doses that may be administered
- give minimum dose interval
- have a separate prescription for each route of administration
- be administered and signed for by two people.

Any allergies must be recorded on the patient's prescription sheet. You must check for these.

Do not try to guess if you cannot read the prescription. A child was written up for 350 mg of an antibiotic. The prescription was illegible so the nurse guessed and gave 850 mg. The potential consequences of this guesswork are dangerous. There could be toxicity leading to permanent disability, severe reactions and litigation.

Activity

Try the following calculations:

Drug	Dose prescribed	Drug comes as:
Tegretol	70 mg	100 mg/5 mL
Paracetamol	60 mg, 240 mg	120 mg/5 mL
Erythromycin	100 mg	125 mg/5 mL
Flucloxacillin	62.5 mg	125 mg/5 mL
Atropine	150 micrograms	600 micrograms/1 mL
	240 micrograms	600 micrograms/1 mL
Digoxin	15 micrograms	50 micrograms/1 mL
	12 micrograms	0.05 mg/mL
Phenytoin	10 mg	30 mg/5 mL
Diazepam	3 mg	2 mg/5 mL
Morphine	3 mg	10 mg/1 mL

Answers can be found in the companion PowerPoint presentation.

Family-centred care in the emergency department

Traditionally, families have not been allowed to participate in or be present at certain invasive procedures involving children in emergency departments. There has been a growth in family-centred care in the UK and elsewhere, with writers such as Darbyshire (1994) and Smith et al (2002) articulating the role nurses can play in not only acting as family advocates but, importantly, in helping remove the barriers that impede the implementation of family-friendly protocols and procedures. The admission of parents/guardians to areas of the hospital that have traditionally excluded them has been slow and emergency departments have only recently acknowledged that the presence of parents during invasive procedures is actually helpful not only for the practising nurse but also for the child and family as a whole. Eppich & Arnold (2003) describe how family members can contribute to the overall care of the child during such procedures and, furthermore, can be present during cardiopulmonary resuscitation (CPR). A large body of evidence suggests that parental presence during hospital procedures is helpful to a child during a stressful procedure (Coyne 1995, Glasper & Powell 2000).

PROFESSIONAL CONVERSATION

Sue is a third-year child branch student who is undertaking a clinical placement in a mixed age continuum emergency department.

There are not always sufficient children's nurses on duty to ensure that all children are appropriately managed. Sue is working an early shift with her mentor Sally and they are reflecting on an event the previous day, when a mother was refused entry to the resuscitation room. The 18-month-old child was not successfully resuscitated and the mother later complained that she regretted not being present during this last period of her child's life.

Paediatric resuscitation

Although paediatric events that require resuscitation are rare, it is important that all nurses understand the principles of successful resuscitation. Castle (2002) suggests that most district general hospitals will have less than one paediatric cardiac arrest per week. It is the rarity of this event that makes it emotionally difficult for those in emergency departments. Seminal work by Ellison (1998) in Manchester showed that relatives want to be present during their child's resuscitation. It is, however, important to recognise that there are both positive and negative aspects of family presence during this stressful event. Although family presence during a resuscitation procedure is becoming more usual in emergency departments, many members of the interprofessional team still have concerns and doubts about it. Kidby (2003) believes that nurses should take into account the views of relatives, although resuscitation procedures should never be compromised by the presence of family members. Evidence suggests that it can improve the grieving process for families and be helpful to patients who survive (Rattrie 1999).

Paediatric intensive care

A study of trauma victims by the Royal College of Surgeons concluded that as many as one-third of those who died could have been saved. As discussed earlier, the starting point in caring for acutely ill and injured patients is an appropriate skilled workforce that is competent in assessment and management of such patients (Mackway-Jones 1997 p 35). The team approach allows critically ill or traumatised patients optimal chances for survival. The distribution of trauma deaths has been described as being 'trimodal'. Fifty percent of all trauma deaths occur before medical attention can be provided. The first peak in mortality occurs at the time of injury or shortly after. The second peak of the trimodal experience occurs within the first hours of injury. It is in this phase that the emergency care team response can make a difference in provision of care to prevent death as a result of 'airway, breathing and circulatory problems'. The term the 'golden hour' is often used to describe this second phase of the trimodal theory. Having survived the initial trauma, resuscitation and stabilisation patients who die in the third trimodal stage commonly die in intensive care from multisystem failure.

The paediatric intensive care report Framework for the future (NHS Executive 1997 p 7) describes three levels of care for the critically ill or injured child. Level one, often referred to as high-dependency care, is greater than that care provided on an acute paediatric ward or department. Children requiring level-one care require close observation, continuous heart monitoring, non-invasive blood pressure monitoring or single organ support not including respiratory support. Children who fall into level one may be experiencing severe breathing difficulties like croup, suspected intestinal obstruction or poisoning (NHS Executive 1997 p 9). Level two is defined as the level of care for children requiring assisted ventilation either due to respiratory absence or single system failure requiring respiratory support. Level three is defined as children with multisystem failure requiring advanced respiratory support.

Activity

Obtain the following references:

- Castle N 1999 Paediatric resuscitation. Emergency Nurse 7(1):31-39
- Castle N 2002 Paediatric resuscitation: advanced life support. Nursing Standard 17(11):47-52.
- Resuscitation Council (UK) guidelines: www.resus.org.uk

Discuss paediatric resuscitation in your clinical skills groups.

If you are a subscriber to any journal published by the RCN, you can obtain these papers from The Nursing Standard website searchable archive.

Child protection

Children's nurses must be able to recognise potential problems in relation to children and their interaction with their immediate family or carers. Child protection issues are often identified when observing the dynamics between the child and family. While undertaking assessment of any child it is important to identify non-verbal information as much as the verbal information gathered. The non-verbal clues might indicate lack of eye contact, withdrawn body posture, facial expression and tone of voice. These are all factors that can encourage or discourage the flow of information between the nurse and the parents.

Nurses who use verbal cues such as open-ended questions, active listening and empathy, can demonstrate to the parents that what they are saying is important and is helping in the care of their ill child. This is a continual process and should be two-way between the parent and nurse to facilitate the development of trust and confidence in the nursing and medical staff. This can begin the development in care of a partnership with the parents.

Social interaction manifest in numerous forms of non-verbal communication; children's nurses use non-verbal cues to eliminate, amplify or expand on what is expressed in words. The use of eye contact during conversations is a process by which each individual demonstrates attention and involvement in the conversation by regularly looking into the eyes of the other, staring intently can indicate evasiveness. Facial expressions, gestures and body posture can convey what is really meant even when nothing is actually said.

Parental involvement and partnership have been advocated since the publication of the Platt report (Ministry of Health 1959). Since this time, government policy has reaffirmed that the care of children should be provided in part by partnerships with parents and their families (DoH 1991). Most recently, 'Getting the right start: national service framework for children' (DoH 2003, 2004) advocates that children, young people and parents are partners in care and that partnership and parental involvement are recognised as important issues in services for children.

When children are unwell, parents often seek help because they do not have the knowledge or skills to care for their children at home; there is an implicit and explicit dependence on professional knowledge and expertise. However, this dependence is not one-sided. The professionals are dependent on the parents sharing information to enable appropriate care. This sharing of information can empower the family and reduce the vulnerability felt by the parents.

Partnership in care can have difficulties in the emergency situations as distress and anxiety can interfere with the parent's ability to formulate and rationalise decisions.

Scenario

In line with the NICE guidelines (available online at: http://www.NICE.org.uk) for head injuries, Sheila does not require a skull X-ray or computer tomography. However, her scalp wound does require closure. The wound to Sheila's head is no more than 3 cm in length and is deep dermal. The wound does not require to be sutured and can be closed by simple application of wound glue (of which there are many on the therapeutics market at the present time). Two of the most popular are Liquiband and Histoacryl.

Wound management in emergency departments

The wound on Sheila's head needs to be cleansed and closed. For a young child this is a very frightening procedure and Sheila will require a lot of psychological preparation for this to be accomplished. The hospital play therapist and Sheila's mother will try to distract her attention as much as possible. This may be by blowing bubbles or by playing a game or reading a storybook. Depending on the presentation of the wound there are different methods for closure. Sutures are still very common but will not be undertaken unless the child is able to understand what suturing entails. No child should ever be held down or wrapped in a blanket so that painful procedures can be undertaken. Children who have wounds and are non-compliant with therapies should either undergo conscious sedation or referral to surgeons. Often, wounds are 'steristripped' (previously known as butterfly stitches) and then kept dry for 5 days.

The role of play

The provision of therapeutic play facilities within emergency departments is of crucial importance in the management of children attending. The obligatory box of broken toys cited by Glasper (1995) is no longer acceptable and Smith (1998) believes that a play specialist in emergency departments can help reduce the fear and anxiety experienced by children attending. A good hospital play therapist will be aware of a child's developmental needs and can often determine the toys and therapeutics that each child needs for distraction from painful procedures.

Paediatric nurse practitioners

The expansion of roles within the emergency departments has been described by Jones & Smith (1998), who articulate the challenge of assessing and treating children in the emergency department for independent practitioners. To date, there is no national recognised course for the training and development of registered children's nurses to become ENPs. However, there has been an area of growth around clinical assessment of children, although again this has yet to gain national recognition.

Observations

Observation of all Sheila's vital signs remains stable throughout her treatment and stay in the emergency department. Her scalp wound has been cleansed and closed using wound glue. Sheila's immunisation status is checked and she is up to date with all her immunisation and does not require a tetanus booster. Having been given instructions and advice on how to care for Sheila at home, both Sheila and her mum are ready for discharge. Sheila is given an outpatient appointment for follow-up care for her epilepsy and her mum feels confident that she can manage Sheila's fits at home.

Summary

First contact emergency care for children and young people is a growing area of nursing. A number of national initiatives including the National Service Framework highlight the pivotal role of emergency departments in the care of sick children and their families. Children and young people nurses will continue to play a big role in ensuring that emergency care for their client group is commensurate with the age group continuum of growth and development.

References

Appleton, R., Choonara, I., Martland, T., et al., 2000. The treatment of convulsive status epilepticus in children. Archives of Disease in Childhood 83 (5), 415–419.

Arnon, K., MacFaul, R., Hemmingway, P., et al., 2004. The impact of presenting problem-based guidelines for children with medical problems in an accident and emergency department. Archives of Disease in Childhood 89, 159–164.

Audit Commission 1993. Children first: a study of hospital services. HMSO, London.

Bentley, J., 1996. Child-related services in general accident and emergency departments. Journal of Advanced Nursing 24, 1184–1193.

Boyle, R., Smith, C., McIntyre, J., 2000. The changing utilization of a children's emergency department. Ambulatory Child Health 6 (1), 39.

Castle, N., 2002. Paediatric resuscitation: advanced life support. Nursing Standard 17 (11), 47–52.

Cleaver, K., 2003. Developing expertise – the contribution of paediatric accident and emergency nurses to the care of children and the implications for their continuing professional development. Accident and Emergency Nursing 11, 96–102.

Coyne, I., 1995. Partnership in care: parents views of participation in their hospitalised child's care. Journal of Clinical Nursing 4, 71–79.

Darbyshire, P., 1994. Living with a sick child in hospital: the experiences of parents and nurses. Chapman and Hall, London.

Department of Health (DoH), 1991. Welfare of children and young people in hospital. HMSO, London.

Department of Health (DoH), 1996. The patient's charter – services for children and young people. HMSO, London.

Department of Health (DoH), 2000. The NHS plan: a plan for investment, a plan for reform. The Stationery Office, London.

Department of Health (DOH), 2003. Online. Available at: http://www.doh.gov.gov.uk/nsf/children/gettingtherightstart.htm

Department of Health (DoH), 2004. The national service framework for children, young people and maternity services. Online. Available at: http://www.dh.gov.uk

Department of Health and Social Security (DHSS), 1976. Fit for the future (the Court Report). The Report of the Committee on Child Health Services. HMSO, London.

Ellison, G., 1998. Witnessed resuscitation; the relatives' experience. Emergency Nurse 5 (8), 27–29.

Endacott, R., Edwards, B., Crouch, R., et al., 1999. Towards a faculty of emergency nursing. Emergency Nurse 7 (5), 10–15.

Eppich, W.J., Arnold, L., 2003. Family member presence in the paediatric emergency department. Current Opinion in Paediatrics 15 (3), 294–298.

Glasper, E.A., 1995. Paediatric ambulatory care: shop window or back door. British Journal of Nursing 4 (7), 384.

Glasper, E.A., Powell, C., 2000. First do no harm: parental exclusion from anaesthetic rooms. Paediatric Nursing 12 (4), 14–17.

Healthcare Commission, 2009. Improvement review – A Review of services for children in hospital. Healthcare Commission, London.

Jones, S.J., Smith, J.M., 1998. Expanding roles and practice within paediatric A and E departments – The children's nurse practitioner. In: Glasper, E.A., Lowson, S. (Eds.), Innovations in paediatric ambulatory care: a nursing perspective, Macmillan, Basingstoke.

Kidby, J., 2003. Family witnessed cardiopulmonary resuscitation. Nursing Standard 17 (51), 33–36.

Lapham, R., Agar, H., 2009. Drug calculations for nurses, a step by step approach, 3rd edn. Arnold, London.

MacFaul, R., Werneke, U., 2001. Recent trends in hospital use by children in England. Archive of Disease in Childhood 85, 203–207.

Mackway-Jones, K. (Ed.), 1997. Emergency triage. Manchester triage group, BMJ Publishing, London.

Maurice, S.C., O'Donnell, J.J., Beatie, T.F., 2002. Emergency analgesia in the paediatric population. Part II: pharmacological methods of pain relief. Emergency Medicine Journal 19, 101–105.

Ministry of Health, 1959. Committee of the Central Health Services Council. Report of the Committee on the Welfare of Children in Hospital. Ministry of Health, London.

National Institute of Clinical Excellence (NICE), 2007. Head injury, triage, assessment investigation and early management of head injuries in infants, children and adults, 2nd edn. NICE, London.

NHS Confederation 2003 Getting the right start: standard for hospital services. Briefing June 2003, N87.

NHS Executive, 1997. Paediatric intensive care: a framework for the future. Report of the National Co-ordinating Group on Intensive Care to the Chief Executive of the NHS Executive. NHSE, London.

Nursing and Midwifery, Council 2008. Standards for Medicines Management. NMC, London.

Partridge, T., 2001. Children in accident and emergency: seen but not heard? Journal of Child Health Care 5 (2), 49–53.

Parslow, R.C., Morris, K.P., Tasker, R.C., 2005. Epidemiology of traumatic brain injury in children receiving intensive care in the UK. Archives of Disease in Children 90, 1182–1187.

Rattrie, E., 1999. Witnessed resuscitation: good practice or not? Nursing Standard 14 (24), 32–35.

Royal College of Paediatrics and Child Health (RCPCH), 2003. Medicines for children. RCPCH, London.

Royal College of Surgeons (RCS) and the British Orthopaedic Association (BOA), 2000. Better care for the seriously injured. RCS, London.

Scoble, M., 2004. Implementing triage in a children's assessment unit. Nursing Standard 18 (34), 41–44.

Scott, R.C., Neville, B.R.G., 1999. Pharmacological management of convulsive status epilepticus in children. Developmental Medicine and Child Neurology 41, 207–210.

Scott, R.C., Surtees, R.A.H., Neville, B.R.G., 1998. Status epilepticus: patho-physiology, epidemiology, and outcomes. Archive of Diseases in Childhood 79 (1), 73–77.

Shovron, S., 2001. Management of status epilepticus in children. Journal of Neurology, Neurosurgery. Psychiatry 70 (suppl II), ii22–ii27.

Smith, F., 1998. Caring for children. Emergency Nurse 6 (6), 20–24.

Smith, L., Coleman, V., Bradshaw, M. (Eds.), 2002. Family centred care: concept, theory, and practice. Palgrave, Basingstoke.

Tasker, R.C., 1998. Emergency treatment of acute seizures and status epilepticus. Archives of Diseases in Childhood 79 (1), 78–83.

United Kingdom Central Council for Nursing, 2000. Midwifery and Health Visiting (UKCC). Guidelines for the administration of medicines. UKCC, London.

Watson, S., 2000. Children's nurses in accident and emergency department: literature review. Accident and Emergency Nursing 8, 92–97.

Watts, R., Robertson, J., Thomas, G., 2003. Nursing management of fever in children: a systematic review. International Journal of Nursing Practice 9, S1–S8.

Willis, M.A., 2001. CWILTED Emergency Nurse 8 (9), 18–22.

Woolwich, C., 1999. Putting the nurse back into triage. Emergency Nurse 7 (5), 8–9.

Website

The report of the National Enquiry into perioperative deaths www.ncepod.org.uk/pdf/1989/Full%20Report%201989.pdf

Advanced Life Support Group 2003 www.resuss.org.uk/pages/a/s.pdf

Section 2

Knowledge and skills for practice

Children with complex motor disability

24

Jackie Parkes Sonya Clarke

ABSTRACT

The aim of this chapter is to describe the needs and nursing care of children with complex motor disabilities, and to consider the support that the families of such children require. Complex motor disability has been defined as those conditions resulting in a significant motor impairment in association with other impairments affecting the senses, learning, communication and/or problems with active seizures. Particular reference is made to the condition cerebral palsy as an 'indicator' condition for complex motor disability.

This chapter is divided into two broad parts. The first part describes the wider context related to children with complex motor disability – the numbers of children with severe disability, sources of information, the impact of having a child with a complex disability, the aims of services and parents' expectations and need for those services. Reference is made to where the children's nurse 'fits in' to the wider service context. The second part of the chapter deals with a small number of care needs that are commonly present in children with complex motor disability, and includes a description of a nursing assessment and possible interventions related to these problems.

LEARNING OUTCOMES

- Appreciate the perspectives of individual level and population-based approaches to assessment and planning care for children with complex motor disability.
- Describe the leading causes of complex motor disability in childhood.
- Recognise the relative contribution to be made by the medical and social models of disability.
- Be able to locate and interpret information (routine and other) on children with complex motor disability in the UK.
- Recognise the central role of parents as experts in the management of children with complex disability.
- Understand the role of the children's nurse in identifying unmet need through competent nursing assessment of the child with complex motor disability and their family.
- Be able to critically apply proposed outlines for nursing assessment in the care of the child with complex motor disability and their families.

DOI: 10.1016/B978-0-7020-3183-0.10024-4

Introduction

The aim of this chapter is to focus on the care of the child with complex motor disability, and on the issues faced by their families, in the context of community and hospital. The chapter uses both an individual-level and a population-based perspective to explore both the needs of children with complex motor disability and the needs of their families. An individual level approach focuses on the needs and unique experiences of an individual – a child, his or her parents and siblings. This perspective is important in developing an individualised assessment of need and tailored plan of nursing care. It contrasts with a population-based approach, which considers the needs and experiences of groups of children and their families with similar conditions and usually living in the same geographic area (for example in a Health and Social Services Trust or one region of the UK). This perspective is important for prevention of disease, health promotion and planning and targeting services to those in greatest need. The children's nurse has a role to play at both levels of assessment and intervention in relation to child health and more specifically with regard to children with complex motor disability.

Definitions, numbers, needs and services

Definition of complex motor disability

The term 'complex motor disability' is interpreted here to mean children whose primary problem is a significant disorder of movement and whose condition is affected and complicated by the presence of other associated impairments such as sensory deficits, problems with learning, communication or active seizures. Cerebral palsy is a good example of such a condition and most children with cerebral palsy have at least one additional, associated impairment in conjunction with problems related to movement. Cerebral palsy can be severe: approximately one in three children are unable to walk and one in four have no useful arm or hand function (Parkes et al 2001a). The impact of disability experienced is further increased by the presence of other severe associated impairments: one in four children with cerebral palsy have severe learning disability (IQ < 50) and one in ten have no useful vision (Parkes et al 2001a).

In addition, some children with complex motor disability will depend on technology to sustain their lives, for example requiring assisted ventilation, artificial feeding or care associated with having a colostomy, ileostomy, urostomy or catheterisation (Glendinning et al 2001). It should be noted that the terms 'complex motor disability', 'complex healthcare needs' and 'technology-dependent children' are not interchangeable, although many of the same children are common to all three groups.

Leading causes of motor disability

The numbers of children with disabilities and conditions requiring medical intervention has increased in the last 30 years (Gordon et al 2000, Kirk 1999). Advances in medical care have helped to improve and prolong the life expectancy of some babies and children who would have previously died (Pharoah et al 1996). For example, neonatal intensive care has helped to improve the survival of extremely premature or low birthweight babies, who are at particularly high risk of developing problems like cerebral palsy (Johnson & King 1998, O'Shea et al 1998, Pharoah et al 1996). Also, interventions like chemotherapy and ventilation, now available in the community, have improved the life span of children with degenerative conditions.

Although it is important for the children's nurse to appreciate the underlying medical diagnoses and pathology of complex motor disabilities, medical diagnosis alone does not predict service needs (Gordon et al 2000, World Health Organization (WHO) 2001). For this reason, only a short overview of medical causes is presented here.

Activity

For a comprehensive overview of causes, complications and resulting conditions leading to complex physical disability, see McCarthy et al (1992) pp 18–21.

The leading causes of complex motor disability that may give rise to complex needs in children include cerebral palsy, spina bifida, Duchenne muscular dystrophy and other degenerative and neuromuscular conditions like spinal muscular atrophy. Cerebral palsy is the leading cause of physical disability in childhood (Parkes et al 2001a, Surveillance of Cerebral Palsy in Europe (SCPE) 2000) and has been defined as 'an umbrella term covering a group of non-progressive but often changing motor impairment syndromes secondary to lesions or anomalies of the brain arising in the early stages of its development' (Mutch et al 1992 p 549). A number of rare metabolic disorders (e.g. Lesch–Nyhan syndrome) and genetic syndromes (e.g. Turner syndrome) can also result in neuromotor impairments and disability. For some children, the underlying medical diagnoses remain uncertain.

Some of these conditions will invariably lead to premature death (e.g. Duchenne muscular dystrophy), whereas others are likely to mean the child and family will have a life-time of disability requiring specialist help and support (e.g. cerebral palsy). Although conditions like cerebral palsy and spina bifida are not fatal per se, premature death is associated with more severe forms (Crichton et al 1995, Hutton et al 1994). It has been estimated that of those with the most severe disabling cerebral palsy (unable to walk, no useful arm or hand function and with intellectual impairment) 70% will survive to age 10; 50% to age 20; and 40% to 30 years (Hutton & Pharoah 1998).

Medical and social models of disability

As children's nurses we need to be aware and appreciate the 'larger' issues around disability as a political, social and emerging academic discipline in its own right. Generally speaking, we are taught and tend to assume the 'medical model' in assessing and intervening in the care of children with disability and their families. The medical model supposes that disability is the result of pathology and impairment, resulting in deficit of function and rendering the person disabled and unable to participate fully in 'normal' life. Our interventions are aimed at the level of the individual and include pre- and postoperative surgical care, medication, rehabilitation and the provision of aids and appliances to help the individual adapt and 'fit into' mainstream society. Although it could be argued that this perspective is at least partially appropriate, the contrasting social model of disability has gained increasing validity and recognition.

The social model of disability conceives that impairments do not make a person disabled but rather that it is society who disables people by failing to accommodate their differences (Priestley 2003). The manifestation of this 'failure to accommodate' means that people with disabilities are excluded from mainstream life through segregated education, few and poorly paid employment opportunities, and difficulty gaining access to buildings and using public transport, among other things (Priestley 2003). In the social model of disability the level of intervention is aimed at changing societal attitudes and societal behaviour towards people with disability.

The distinction between these models is not merely an academic one because how we think about disability will influence our nursing practice. The children's nurse has a clear responsibility to provide nursing care and meet the immediate physical and psychological needs of the child and family. We also have a wider role to play.

Seminar discussion topic

Can children's nurses act as advocates at the societal level, raising awareness about inclusion for children with disability in 'mainstream' society and helping to change attitudes?

The World Health Organization and disability

In 1980, the World Health Organization (WHO) published the much cited International Classification of Impairments, Disabilities and Handicaps (ICIDH). This defined impairment as 'any loss or abnormality of psychological, physiological or anatomical structure or function'; disability as 'any restriction or lack (resulting from impairment) of ability to perform an activity in the manner within the range considered normal for a human being'; and handicap as 'a disadvantage for a given individual, resulting from an impairment or a disability, that limits or prevents fulfilment of a role that is normal'.

This framework has now been revised to form a more positive 'components of health' classification called the International Classification of Functioning, Disability and Health (or ICF; WHO 2002). Previously, the ICIDH was a 'consequences of disease' classification that focused on the impact of disease on the individual (WHO 1980). By contrast, the ICF focuses on health and measuring function regardless of the reason for the impairment (WHO 2002). The terms and concepts of 'disability' and 'handicap' have now been replaced by the terms 'activity limitations' and 'participation restrictions', respectively.

www

Read a beginner's guide to the ICF called 'Towards a common language for functioning, disability and health' online at:

- http://www3.who.int/icf/icftemplate.cfm?myurl=homepage.html&mytitle=Home%20Page

Click on 'Beginner's Guide'. In particular, see p 6 regarding ICF applications in service provision. Alternatively, for a more detailed account click on 'Introduction'.

The ICF provides a conceptual framework for the 'definition, measurement and policy formulations for health and disability' (WHO 2002 p 2) for use in health care and at the levels of individual, institution and population. Finally, one of the additional unique features of the ICF is recognition and classification of the environmental factors (such as social attitudes and social structures), which are derived from the social model of disability. Assessment of these features is necessary to complete the 'picture' of health and disability.

In the context of children's nursing it is important to appreciate the ICF because it is relevant and could be used in nursing practice in the following ways (adapted from WHO 2002):

- To provide standardised descriptions and a conceptual framework of health and health-related states for individual children and their families. For example, it could be used in relation to assessing and planning care for children with complex motor disability.
- Use of standardised language to promote interdisciplinary communication (with physiotherapists, occupational therapists, paediatricians for example) and make comparisons about health, health care and health outcomes in children with complex needs within geographic areas and between geographic areas.
- More generally, to provide reliable summary measures of population health for surveillance purposes and monitoring health outcomes.
- The ICF promotes assessment of the 'contextual factors' or barriers that limit the participation of individual children with complex motor disability or populations of children with complex motor disability and their families.
- It provides a systematic coding scheme for health care information systems.

Reflect on your practice

What would be the advantages and disadvantages of including the ICF as part of routine nursing assessment in the care of children with complex motor disability?

Sources of information on children with complex motor disability

Information about the numbers of children with complex motor disability or other forms of disability have been described as 'invisible' from the routine statistics published by government (Gordon et al 2000). Most regions within the UK have a formal, computer-based system for monitoring child health – a child health surveillance system. The sorts of information recorded on child health surveillance systems include birth notifications, immunisations, preschool health checks and the identification of any special needs. These systems tend to be orientated towards provision of services and have limited use as complete sources of information on specific conditions like cerebral palsy (Parkes et al 1998). Furthermore, these routine information systems could, but generally do not, publish information on children with complex needs as part of routine statistics.

Some of the gaps in the routine information about children with special and complex needs have been filled by ad hoc ('one-off') surveys carried out in Great Britain and Northern Ireland. In Great Britain, the Office of Population Censuses and Surveys conducted surveys of childhood disability in 1985 and 1988 (Bone & Meltzer 1989), which were subsequently reanalysed by Gordon et al (2000). Glendinning et al (1999, 2001) also reported on the numbers of technology-dependent children living in the UK; Beresford (1995) on the numbers of parents caring for a severely disabled child at home (in England) and Roberts & Lawton (2001) on severely disabled children whose families have accessed the Family Fund.

www

The Family Fund Trust is an independent organisation that provides financial support and information services to families caring for a severely disabled or ill child (under 16 years of age). The Family Fund Trust is government funded. Read more about the Family Fund at:

- http://www.familyfundtrust.org.uk

In Northern Ireland, sister OPCS surveys were conducted by the Policy, Planning and Research Unit in 1989 and 1990 (Duffy 1995, Smith et al 1992). A survey was undertaken in Scotland to identify the numbers and service needs of children with motor impairment and their families (Gough et al 1993). The results of these surveys are summarised in Table 24.1. Some caution must be used in the interpretation of Table 24.1 because

Table 24.1 Summary of surveys of childhood disability and technology-dependent children in the UK

Author and year	Geographical area	Definition used	Numbers and proportions of children with a disability (including children with severe/multiple problems where known)
OPCS Bone & Meltzer 1989	England, Wales, Scotland	'Disabled' as defined by the ICDIH (WHO); aged 0–15 years	360,000 disabled children (3.2% of the child population in the UK) 327,000 disabled children in England & Wales
OPCS Gordon et al 2000	As above	Re-analysed OPCS data and redefined disability and identified clusters of disability	45,000 children with the most severe and multiple disabilities
PPRU Smith et al 1992, Duffy et al 1995	Northern Ireland	'Disabled' as defined by the ICDIH (WHO); aged 0–15 years	14,600 disabled children (3.5% of the child population in NI) 2600 'severely disabled'
Gough et al 1993	Scotland	Motor impairment of central origin born 1985–86 and resident in Scotland 1991–92	244 children with a motor impairment of central origin (0.3% of child population in Scotland) Two-thirds had moderate–severe disability in relation to personal care; more than half had severe learning disability
Beresford 1995	UK (using the Family Fund database)	Been helped by the Family Fund and been in recent contact with the Family Fund; children < 16 years	Collected data on 1100 families caring for a severely disabled child Estimate 150,000 families are caring for a severely disabled child
Glendinning et al 2001	UK	Technology-dependent children	Estimates 6000 technology-dependent children in the UK (although some double counting may have occurred) 2800 children receiving artificial feeding (British Artificial Nutrition Survey cited by Glendinning et al)

Table 24.2 Studies of children and young people with cerebral palsy

Reference (alphabetical)	Geographical area	Method	Birth years	Number of children	Rate per 1000 live births
Colver & Mackie 1998	North East of England	Case register	1991–93	287	2.4
Edmond et al 1989	Great Britain	British Perinatal Mortality & Birth Survey	1958, 1970	40, 41	2.5
Ingram 1955	Edinburgh	Ad hoc survey	1938–52	208	1.9
Jarvis et al 1985	North East of England	Case register	1960–75	421	1.6
Johnson & King 1998	Oxford	Case register	1984–91	697	2.5
MacGillivray & Campbell 1995	Avon	Taken from a handicap register	1969–88	489	2.1
Parkes et al 2001b	Northern Ireland	Case register	1981–93	784	2.2
Pharoah et al 1990	Mersey	Case register	1980–84	309	1.9
Pharoah et al 1998	Mersey, Oxford & Scotland	Case registers	1984–89	1649	2.1
Williams et al 1996	North East Thames	Case register	1980–86	672	1.6

differences between surveys will be partly due to differences in the way 'disability' and 'severe disability' have been defined. It should be noted that the impact of disability may increase with age and studies of disability need to take this into account.

Some longitudinal studies of childhood motor disability do exist in the form of dedicated case registers of children with cerebral palsy. Currently, five such registers are actively recording cases in Northern Ireland, parts of England and Scotland. These registers fulfil an important function in providing unique information about the prevalence, severity and survival of children and young adults with cerebral palsy in the UK. The registers are also used to monitor trends over time and between areas and act as a sampling frame for research into causation and services. Table 24.2 summarises some of the literature on the numbers and prevalence of children with cerebral palsy in different parts of the UK, including information from the five registers referred to above.

www

The five registers of children with cerebral palsy in the UK are part of a working collaboration. Read about the UK Collaboration of Cerebral Palsy Registers online at:

- http://www.liv.ac.uk/PublicHealth/UKCP.htm

Although it could be argued that disability and complex motor disability remains relatively rare, the following extract written by a parent clearly highlights the impact on the child and family and their need for ongoing, intensive support to cope.

The impact of having a child with complex motor disability

The following 'real life scenario' written by a parent provides a unique and special insight into the parent's feelings and experiences of having a child with complex needs. It is strikingly similar to other accounts by parents who have reiterated many of the same messages (see Beresford 1994, Kingdom & Mayfield 2001).

In the account presented here, the parent does not elaborate on the precise 'medical equipment' she uses. However Beresford (1995) identified the following equipment being used by 1100 families for a severely disabled child at home: nasal feeding tubes (18%), suction equipment (16%), nebulisers and inhalers (10%), gastric feeding tubes (12%), a feeding pump (12%), catheters (7%), oxygen (9%), ventilators (7%), other things (14%). Clearly, parents have to develop advanced clinical skills to look after their child at home. The children's nurse has a clear role to play in teaching families these skills, sourcing and providing equipment, anticipating and preventing potential problems and supporting parents at home to provide the highest quality care.

Scenario

Real-life scenario by a parent of a child with complex motor disability

My son Daniel [a pseudonym] was born in 1998 and what should have been a wonderful event became a tragedy. Daniel has athetoid cerebral palsy. He is now 4½ years old and is a 24-hour job.

Apart from physical exhaustion looking after a handicapped child, the mental torment is nearly worse. Watching your child day to day and wondering if he will see another one or if the next illness will be the last and you have to say 'goodbye'.

The needs of the child are great and this can be where health services mainly focus. However, the needs of the parent often fall by the wayside. Practical help is required from the start in the form of advice, supplies and respite care. I 'fell' through the net and did not receive any real help until my son was 2½ years old. Daniel was then assigned a community nurse who realised our plight and set out to help. She organised all supplies, including nappies and medical equipment. Something as simple as this eased the load and was something less to worry about. She was excellent for advice on Disability Living Allowance and Motability transport. She also arranged hospice and respite care, which are wonderful, and tried to make life that little bit easier.

Too many parents are struggling on their own with limited information and resources as all too often one parent has to give up work to be the carer. This is what happened to me. There are few day-care facilities who can deal with a child with a nasogastric tube, a tracheostomy and epilepsy.

Emotional support is rare. It does not have to be an expensive organisation. Someone to talk to, have a coffee with and who does not mind if you have a good cry to get things off your chest, is often all that is required, but it is not out there. If it does exist, many parents are not told.

This might all sound like 'me, me, me', however to give Daniel a good life, I have to be strong mentally as well as physically. To put Daniel in care if I have a breakdown would cost approximately £700 per week. Me caring for my son is free.

I cannot describe the mental torture of knowing my son will die. Only a mother who walks a day in my shoes could possibly understand the constant struggle for help and advice. The situation has not improved a great deal in the last 20 years.

Aim of services

In 1991 the UK government ratified the United Nations Convention on the Rights of the Child (United Nations General Assembly 1989) and by doing so undertook to commit to the principles laid out by the Convention. Several articles within the Convention are relevant to children with disabilities (Articles 2, 3 and 12). More specifically, Article 23 states:

> … a mentally or physically disabled child should enjoy a full and decent life, in conditions which ensure dignity, promote self-reliance, and facilitate the child's active participation in the community.

Article 23 should form the basis for providing services and interventions to the child with complex motor disability and his or her family. The overall aim of services to children with complex motor disability must also include early detection (and prevention where possible), early intervention and family support. The ultimate aim for all children with health or special needs must be to help them achieve the maximum potential and the best quality of life possible:

> Children with profound and multiple disabilities and/or complex and continuing health care needs should enjoy the highest quality of life possible, receiving quality health, social and educational services which meet their needs and the needs of those who care for them, and respect their lifestyle and culture (Ward et al 2003)

Seminar discussion topic

Use the real-life scenario presented above and the account provided by Kingdom & Mayfield (2001):

- What issues or 'patient' problems can you identify? Distinguish between child-centred problems and parent-centred problems.
- To what extent do the parents' experiences and perceptions match the aims of services for children with disability specified above?
- Discuss the role of the children's nurse in addressing each of the issues or problems identified.
- What other professionals might the children's nurse interact with to help ensure the needs of this child and family are met?

Families' experiences of services

As we have already heard from parents, help and support is available from a wide range of services and professionals, some of whom focus directly on helping the child, whereas others concentrate on assisting the parents and family. Sloper & Turner (1992) found that parents of severely disabled children were in contact with a large number of professionals, as many as ten in any 1 year, with a range of 5–17. Similarly, in a study of children with moderate to severe cerebral palsy, Parkes et al (2002) also found that families were in contact with an average of seven service providers in a 6-month interval, range 1–13. Not surprisingly, parents of children with disability have reported problems related to coordination of services and fragmentation of care. Bamford et al (1997) described this as 'deficiencies in the total care concept'.

Sloper & Turner (1992) found that many parents reported that they had encountered problems in finding and coordinating services, particularly in the early days after diagnosis, as reported elsewhere (Bamford et al 1991, Haylock et al 1993, Watson et al 2002). In particular, parents have reported that professionals often duplicate work and seem unable to detect where the gaps in services are (Rees 1983). Haylock et al (1993) found school (i.e. special education) offered families a form of integration of care that they very much appreciated; again, this has been reported elsewhere (McConachie et al 1999).

The inadequacies of respite care for families with a child with special needs, both in terms of quantity and quality of services available, have been repeatedly identified in the literature (Beresford 1994, 1995, McConkey & Adams 2000, Stalker 1990). The children's nurse has a particular role to play here in terms of finding respite facilities, giving families good information and helping and preparing them psychologically to avail of services (Miller 2002, Ross & Parkes 2004). Families with a child with complex problems that require nursing care (e.g. problems with active seizures requiring medication) may find it more difficult to find respite from both the formal and informal sector because of their child's specialist requirements and the level of responsibility required of carers (Beale 2002, Parkes 1998). Families of children with severe and complex needs are at higher risk of stress and feelings of being unable to cope (Sloper & Turner 1993).

WWW

Read about a model of good practice in relation to providing holistic care for children with complex healthcare needs and their families. See the Children's Trust, Tadworth, Surrey, a charitable organisation providing specialist care, therapies and education for children with severe disabilities, at:

- http://www.thechildrenstrust.org.uk/

There are many examples of good practice in the care of children with complex motor disability both in the literature and in our local communities. Ross & Parkes (2004) outlined a model of good practice for the children's community nurse in relation to the care of a child with complex motor disability and the child's family. This paper highlights the unique role that the children's nurse can play in coordinating a multidisciplinary response that helps to 'cut down' excessive visits by numerous professionals while at the same time tailoring services to meet with the child and family's individual needs.

A number of 'care interfaces' and transitional phases may exist for the child with complex motor disability and their family, which the children's nurse must be aware of and anticipate. These interfaces exist where the child and family 'move' from one service arrangement to another, for example from community to hospital or from child to adult services, as a result of changing need or developmental stage. These interfaces and transitional phases are times when the child and family may need extra help and support to cope and where service providers are 'at risk' of failing due to inadequate planning, poor cooperation or coordination between multiagencies.

The children's nurse in collaboration with the child's paediatrician, the family and other members of the multidisciplinary team, can act as coordinator of health and social care services and ensure that adequate advance planning takes place before discharge from hospital or transfer to another setting. Children with complex needs often receive hospital services at a number of hospital locations (McConachie 1997) and this highlights the importance of children's nurses communicating with one another across institutional boundaries.

What families want from services

Based on research involving families with a disabled child, Baldwin & Carlisle (1994) identified the attributes of a quality service for children with disability. A number of their findings have been supported from research conducted by others. The results have implications for children's nursing practice and are summarised below.

Evidence-based practice

The following has been taken from Baldwin & Carlisle (1994), whose findings are supported by other research (the references of which are included here). Families with a disabled child want:

- an individual, comprehensive assessment of the needs of each child and family. Sloper & Turner (1992) also found that services that focus purely on the child's needs may put the family under more pressure
- regular review and assessment of need, particularly at times of transition. Hirose & Ueda (1990) identified the time of diagnosis, starting school, changing school and leaving school as times of stress for families with a child with disability
- an opportunity to make informed choices about services
- involvement in the design and delivery of a package of services
- a 'key worker' for each child and family, who maintains close contact, acts as a link person between the different agencies involved in their child's care, acts as an advocate and represents their views (Audit Commission 1994, Beresford 1994, Sloper 1999).

Research evidence additional to Baldwin & Carlisle's recommendations suggests that families need regular breaks that are tailored to their individual requirements (Beresford 1994, McConkey & Adams 2000).

For a more detailed account of the evidence regarding service models to support parents of disabled children, see Sloper (1999).

Setting standards: the children's national service framework

In 1998, the government launched a programme of National Service Frameworks (NSFs) for a number of key patient groups with the aim of 'driving the modernisation agenda' within the NHS. The aims of the NSFs are to set national standards for key interventions, develop strategies to support the implementation of interventions and to increase quality and decrease variation in service provision. An outline of the development of the Children's NSF is provided by Smith (2003). The Standards for Hospital Services is the first part of the Children's NSF and is available online.

WWW

Find the latest information on the development of the Children's National Service Framework, including a downloadable copy of the Standards for Hospital Services, at:

- http://www.doh.gov.uk/nsf/children/index.htm

There is also a Children's NSF Bulletin Getting the right start, which is available at the same website address.

An external working group on disabled children was set up to specifically address the unique and particular needs of children with disability and/or complex and life-limiting illness. This group comprises parents, professionals, voluntary workers and researchers. It also has a series of seven task groups set up to address specific issues related to early diagnosis task group, family support, equipment, therapy services, transition services, children's and family participation and children with severe disability and long-term conditions. Many of these priorities are reflected in the evidence-based work by Baldwin & Carlisle (1994) and from the accounts given by parents, including the real-life scenario described above. A number of key areas under consideration for the proposed standards and interventions for children with complex and continuing health needs have been specified in a draft 'work in progress' document.

WWW

Access the draft document at:

- http://www.doh.gov.uk/nsf/children/externalwgdisabled.htm

For earlier work on the development of a charter for children with disabilities and their families, see Milner et al (1996).

Nursing assessment and interventions

This section addresses a small number of activities of living that should be assessed by the children's nurse involved in the care of a child with complex motor disability – at home in the community, or on admission to hospital. Reasons for hospitalisation can include orthopaedic surgery, nutritional management including surgery, and other medical reasons such as management of a chest infection or pneumonia and respite care. The issues discussed here include mobility, eating and drinking and communication. These areas have been identified as the subject of specialist referrals in the literature (Cass et al 1999) and as relevant on the basis of our own clinical and research experience. Other problems not mentioned here, but addressed elsewhere in this book, include the management of the child with seizures, sensory impairments and pain management.

Many of the problems encountered by children with complex motor disability are interrelated and require complex analyses by the children's nurse to understand the relationship between patient problems and their underlying causes. Cass et al (1999) identified a useful hierarchy of assessment involving consideration of six levels. This model proposes that problem solving 'high'-level functions, like communication, depends on the resolution of lower-level functions affecting communication (e.g. head control). Sensory impairments can affect the ability to communicate; the presence of active seizures may impact on the child's general alertness and motivation and can affect eating and drinking. These examples underline the importance of taking a holistic approach to assessing and planning care for children with complex motor disability and listening carefully to parents and carers. They also highlight the importance of undertaking an assessment in a multidisciplinary environment where joint planning can be undertaken (Cass et al 1999).

In the context of children's nursing, the Roy adaptation model (1976) has much to offer the assessment of children with complex problems. This model focuses on the responses of the 'adaptive' person to a constantly changing environment (Fawcett 1995). Roy's nursing assessment comprises two stages:

1. Stage one: identification of 'adaptive' and 'maladaptive' behaviours in relation to four domains:
   - physiological mode
   - self-concept mode
   - role function mode
   - interdependence.
2. Stage two: identification of the stimuli that are thought to be responsible for the maladaptive behaviours. These stimuli are grouped into:
   - focal stimulus: the one most directly and immediately confronting the patient (as defined by nurse, child (where possible) and family)
   - contextual stimuli: all other stimuli present that influence the behaviour being observed
   - residual stimuli: the wider influences the patient may experience related to parent and family knowledge, beliefs, motivations, confidence and abilities.

The principles of competent nursing assessment include use of an appropriate model in which to frame: the assessment; the involvement of the parents and the child, where possible; use of positive language about what the child is able to do, as well as what he or she is unable to do; and regular review of the assessment undertaken. The emphasis within assessment will change according to the child's age and developmental stage and the family's needs (Cogher et al 1992). However, we propose core elements for consideration under the problems 'mobility', 'eating and drinking' and 'communication'.

Parents are increasingly being recognised for the experts that they are in the care and the management of their child with disability (Beresford 1994, 1995, de Geeter et al 2002, NSF 2003, Taanila et al 2002). It is vital that nursing assessment takes place in meaningful dialogue with the parent. Assessment will involve observation of the parent–child interaction and of the child alone and against developmental milestones, as well as through nursing interventions (e.g. taking vital signs).

The principles of competent nursing intervention with the child with complex motor disability include establishing a meaningful, working partnership with the child and family; meeting the child's prioritised needs for nursing care; identifying and meeting the child and family's information needs and promoting their adaptation to the environment in which they are being cared for. Communicating with and coordinating other service providers is vital to avoid duplication or the opposite – opening a new gap in the family's support network. In the case of hospitalisation, preparation for discharge should be begin on the day of admission.

www

Review Northern Ireland's 2007 Nursing response to children and young people with complex physical healthcare needs, online at:

- http://www.dhsspsni.gov.uk/complex_needs_report.pdf

Reflect on your practice

Read about an initiative to develop individualised, continuous documentation for children with special needs by Tippett (2001):

- What are the strengths of this approach?
- Are there any disadvantages to this approach?

Mobility

Complex motor impairment involves dysfunction of postural control, especially in children with cerebral palsy (Brogan et al 1998, Westcott et al 1997). Posture will be significantly affected in children with other conditions affecting truncal control and muscle strength (e.g. spina bifida, spinal muscular atrophy). Posture has been defined as the ability to maintain or control the centre of mass in relation to the base support (Westcott et al 1997). A sitting position is defined as a static balance, in comparison to a dynamic balance, which relates to walking. Attaining static balance is a prerequisite of dynamic balance.

In the long-term management of the child with complex motor disability, specialist physiotherapists and occupational therapists jointly oversee the assessment and planning of mobility (Fig. 24.1) and seating arrangements. This service is usually run in conjunction with the skill and expertise of specialist technicians in seating, aids and appliances. These professionals aim to optimise the child's posture and comfort, which will then enhance the child's respiration, eating, drinking, digestion, ability to communicate and help with moving and handling by the child's parents and carers. Physiotherapy services tend to be arranged, as might be expected, to provide the most intense levels of treatment to those most severely affected (Gough et al 1993, Haylock et al 1993, Parkes et al 2002). The aims of the physiotherapy for the child with complex motor disability are likely to be conservative and directed towards preventing further complications, as well as advising and supporting families to continue with 'good practice' at home.

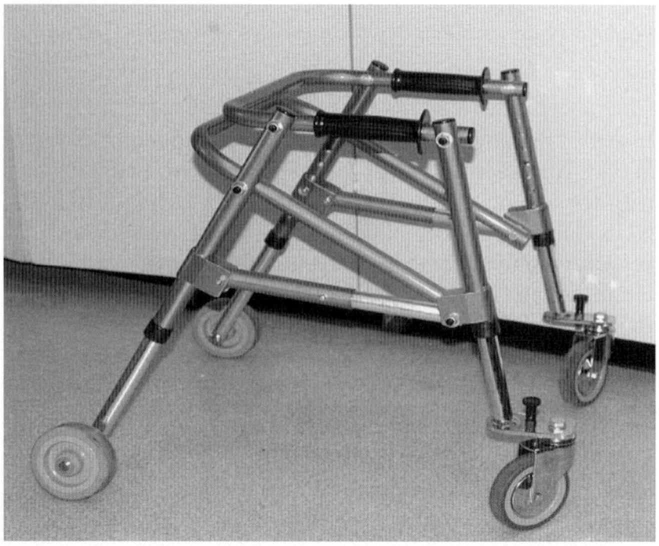

Fig. 24.1 • Postural control walker. This walker or rollator can be pushed or pulled (in reverse). It encourages the child to adopt a good posture, with the shoulders back, upright posture and leg extension.

The physiotherapist is the most common professional seen by the population of children with cerebral palsy (Parkes et al 2002), but is likely to be only one of the many key providers for children with complex problems. The children's nurse has a responsibility to liaise closely with the child's physiotherapist and occupational therapist to ensure good practice in relation to mobility, seating and positioning; and to adopt strategies aimed at preventing contractures or pressure areas and ensure these are incorporated in the plan of nursing care. Also any new developing problems, for example hip pain or dislocation, need to be identified and appropriate nursing interventions taken as early as possible. In the absence of independent walking, useful arm and hand function becomes particularly important to achieve independent mobility as a wheelchair user.

Bottos et al (2001) found that the introduction of powered wheelchairs (Fig. 24.2) for children with severe motor disability, including those with coexisting severe learning disability, enabled 21 of 27 children to move around independently and led to improved socialisation, but interestingly not to overall quality of life. The majority of parents in this study were not in favour of the introduction of powered wheelchairs at the beginning of the study but 23 of 25 expressed positive feelings at the end of the study.

There is evidence that the mobility of children with cerebral palsy is also affected by the environment or setting (Palisano et al 2003), which should be taken into consideration by the children's nurse when undertaking assessment of the child and family. Palisano et al (2003) found there was increased independence at school or in the community with wheelchair use, although few children self-propelled or used powered wheelchairs. However, this independence diminished at home for

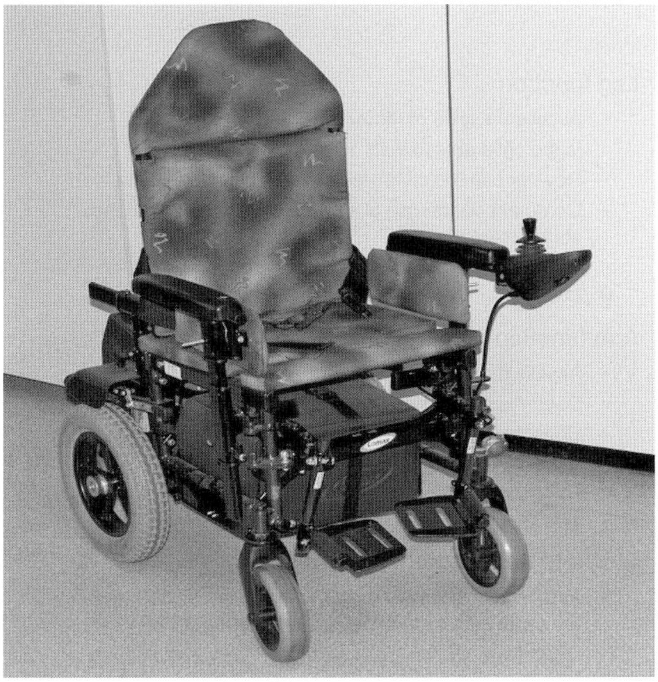

Fig. 24.2 • Powered wheelchair. This chair has a child-operated control panel to give the child more independence. This example is suitable for a child with head control, although a head rest can also be added, and should be for all children during transport. Note the seat belt and foot plates to ensure good positioning and safety. An electric battery sits under the seat and must be charged regularly.

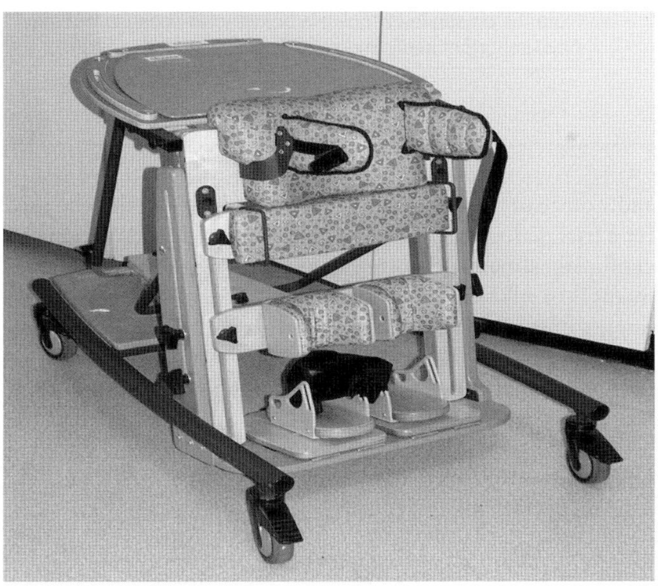

Fig. 24.3 • Prone stander. A prone stander offers an alternative position to help prevent deformities. It offers optimum hip symmetry and ensures a prolonged, passive stretch at the hips, knees and feet and ankles. This stander can also promote alertness and has an adjustable work surface to help prevent the child drooping forward.

the most severely affected children, 39% of whom were carried about by a parent. Capturing information about the child's functional abilities in different settings (Figs 24.3 and 24.4) is therefore very important and should include a description of abilities at home, in school and in the community.

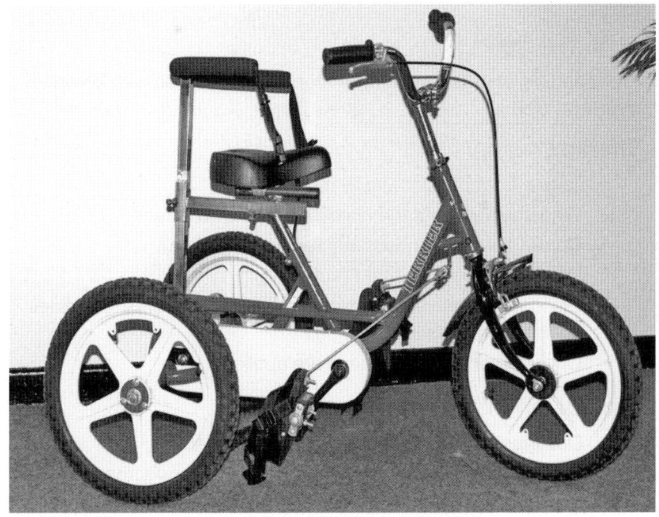

Fig. 24.4 • Adapted tricycle. This tricycle comes with a seat belt and foot plates with straps. Riding the tricycle encourages good positioning, postural control and muscle strength. It is suitable for children who are non-ambulant. It promotes reciprocal movement by breaking total body synergy associated with involuntary movements.

Orthopaedic surgery can lead to improvements in the day-to-day management of children in relation to personal hygiene, dressing and mobility. More specifically, the aims of orthopaedic surgery for the child with complex motor disability includes improving function, preventing pain, improving hygiene and appearance (Cogher et al 1992). Innovative treatments such as botulinum toxin also have a role in assisting management of limbs and joints affected by spasticity. Botulinum toxin is injected in minute amounts into targeted muscles and creates a temporary paralysis (see Korman et al (2003) for guidelines on the use of botulinum toxin injections for spasticity associated with cerebral palsy in children).

Nursing assessment of mobility

In relation to assessment of the child's mobility and seating, we suggest the criteria in Box 24.1 are considered as part of good practice to ensure a complete and accurate assessment of need is conducted. Some of these suggestions are derived from an assessment form developed by Evans et al (1989), aimed at standardising the description of children with motor impairment of central origin. We have adapted the content of the box to reflect an assessment form using the Roper, Logan, Tierney model for nursing practice (1990 p 56) and this template is used throughout.

Nursing interventions in mobility

The children's nurse, and particularly those with specialist orthopaedic training, has much to offer the child with complex motor disability and their family in terms of skill and knowledge in relation to mobility.

Adaptive seating can prevent or delay musculoskeletal deformities, enhanced postural control, upper limb control and oral motor control (Roxborough 1995). The treatment can also increase comfort, improve physiological function, enhance

Box 24.1

Proposed nursing assessment of mobility for children with complex motor problems

Therapy history

- Take a brief physiotherapy history.
- Who usually treats the child? Where? How often?
- Do the parents conduct any regimes at home?
- Describe usual parental practice.
- Discuss any preventive strategies with the parents, e.g. does the child wear splints at night?
- Check when and how these are applied.

Type of motor impairment

- Describe the nature of the motor impairment.
- Is there altered tone? If yes, is it increased or decreased?
- Are there abnormal or involuntary movements?

Extent of motor impairment

- Describe the distribution of the impairment.
- How many limbs are affected?
- Is one side of the body more affected than the other?
- Are the legs more affected than the arms?
- Are the arms more affected than the legs?

Head, neck and trunk control

- Describe the distribution of the impairment.
- Is the child able to hold his or her head up? For how long?
- If not, what is the most comfortable way to support the child's head?
- Can the child sit unsupported? For how long?
- If not, what is the best way to support the child in a sitting position?
- Is there any evidence of curvature of the spine?

Leg function

- Assess the level of motor independence.
- Is the child able to walk 15 steps unaided?
- How far can the child walk (give approximate distance)?
- Comment on the use of aids for walking (e.g. crutches, sticks, rollator).
- If the child uses a wheelchair, can he or she mobilise independently? How far?

Arm function

- Assess the level of motor independence.
- Does the child have any self-care or self-mobilising skills?
- Does the child require assistance with dressing? If yes, how much assistance?
- Does the child require any help with eating or drinking? If yes, how much?

Aids and appliances

- Assess and describe good handling and posture regimes for the child: include seating, standing and mobility.
- Describe any other appliances used, e.g. night splints.

Complications

- Assess if any complications exist.
- Describe any contractures that are present and describe position, severity and impact on child's ability. Check ankles, knees, hips, elbows and wrists.
- Describe the child's feet and footwear noting any abnormalities of posture (e.g. valgus) or problems related to comfort.
- Note the presence of scoliosis or kyphosis because this may have important implications for positioning and comfort.

function abilities and increase the child's social interaction. Cogher et al (1992 pp 152–166) provide a detailed description of the types of seating available. A wheelchair can offer not only independent mobility and transport, but also a position for eating and drinking, as well as a place to play with toys. Arranging suitable seating should include consideration of body posture, head control, and feet and limb positioning. Restraining straps, cushion requirements and material type are also vital in assuring the safe transport, tissue viability and hygiene needs of the child.

Providing equipment for mobility and positioning, especially if spinal curvature is present or has undergone correction, will often involve a dedicated orthotic team. Specialist technicians whose purpose is to maximise function, comfort and social acceptability will individually craft orthotic equipment (Fig. 24.5). Standard equipment will be adjusted to meet the needs of the individual. The parent will also require easy storage of equipment at home and during transportation, with ease of assembly and disassembly a high priority. If the equipment is static, consideration of space within the home is an important factor.

A main intervention in relation to seating and mobility is teaching parents about safe lifting and handling of the child, about continuing therapy routines at home and about safe use and storage of the equipment. The equipment can then be used for a trial period to review its effectiveness for both parent and child. Adjustments are often required, especially if the child's medical or physical status has changed. The developing child implies a limited life span for such equipment, for this reason, frequent check-ups and adjustments by technicians are essential for optimum use. Care must be taken not to 'overburden' the family with too high expectations about what they can manage at home, given that they may have other children or family commitments, and may also work.

Eating and drinking

An association between severe neurodevelopmental conditions like cerebral palsy and impaired oromotor function leading to eating problems has been identified (Gisel & Alphonce 1995). Samson-Fang et al (2003) cited that 27% of children with moderate to severe cerebral palsy included in a North American follow-up study were found to be malnourished (as measured by skin-fold thickness). Problems with eating and drinking vary from mild problems related to control of salvia or chewing ability to severe problems with disturbances of gut motility, reflux and vomiting.

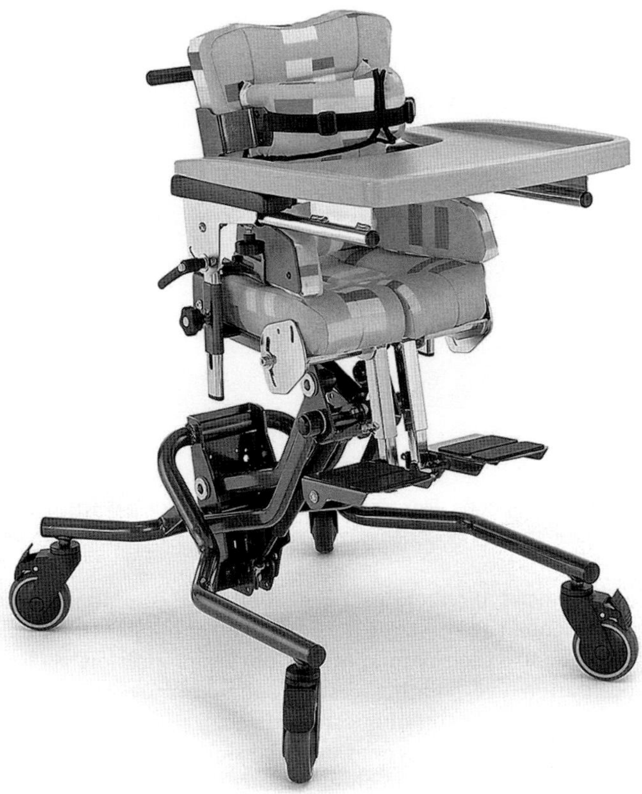

Fig. 24.5 • Adaptable chair. This chair can be raised or lowered, enabling the child to participate in different activities that take place at different heights – eating, playing or working at a desk. Note the knee blocks to help maintain hip position. The chair also has trunk and lateral supports with adjustable foot plates.

One of the most important assessment indicators of health in children is growth and a primary reason for intervening in eating and drinking is concern about the adequacy of nutrition as evidenced by poor growth. Children with severe oromotor impairment can take from 2–12 times longer to manipulate and swallow a standard amount of pureed food and 1–15 times longer to chew and swallow solid food (Gisel & Patrick 1988). These children are at higher risk of experiencing poor growth and weight gain, although artificial feeding techniques have been found to be effective in helping to establish weight gain. Furthermore, persistent feeding problems in young children with cerebral palsy have been identified as a marker for poor feeding, growth and developmental outcome later in childhood and could be used to identify those children with cerebral palsy who might benefit from gastrostomy feeding (Motion et al 2002). Given the complexity of the problems, a team approach to assessment is most effective and usually consists of parents, teacher, speech and language specialist, occupational therapist, physiotherapist, dietician, paediatrician and children's nurse.

Nursing assessment in eating and drinking

The severely affected child is assessed for his or her ability to coordinate sucking and breathing during feeds, with evidence of problems recognised during weaning. An inability to gain weight and the deterioration to low-weight-for-age-specific percentiles within the first year of life are characteristic. The assessment of eating and drinking impairment is based on measures of growth and eating skills: eating efficiency and oral motor skills (Gisel & Alphonce 1995). To make a detailed eating and drinking assessment, knowledge of what happens at meal times along with aspects of proposed change by the parent/carer is necessary. A profile of contributing factors is also required as part of the assessment and planning prior to professional intervention.

A second component that relates to the assessment and planning of eating and drinking is drooling. This problem is again often associated with cerebral palsy children with poor oromotor function. Intensive drooling leads to negative social interactions, schooling issues and physical effects: chapped and sore lips and chin, sodden clothes and often an unpleasant smell (Lloyd Faulconbridge et al 2001). The multidisciplinary team assesses such drooling along with individual planning and intervention.

In relation to assessment of the child's eating and drinking, the criteria in Box 24.2 are considered part of good practice to ensure that a complete and accurate assessment of need is conducted. Some of the suggestions in the box are derived from Evans et al (1989) and Cogher et al (1992).

Nursing interventions in eating and drinking

If it is apparent that adequate nutrition is being achieved, parents may just need reassurance, especially if eating is very messy. Simple alterations to posture and seating can prove very effective in enhancing dietary intake. Oral fluid intake may be altered through a thickening agent; a thicker consistency prevents reflux, choking and aspiration. This approach can also encourage a higher fluid intake and prevent dehydration. Food consistency may also be changed, for example from mashed to puréed textures. A change in equipment – spoons (Fig. 24.6) and cups (Fig 24.7) – often works in harmony with feeding techniques, which again reduce the risk of choking and aspiration. Cogher et al (1992) also suggest desensitising the child's face and mouth before eating by the use of touch if behaviour intolerance or an excess of involuntary movements are present.

Alternatively, a period of hospitalisation may be necessary often for the insertion and parental education of nasogastric tube feeding. Failure of such a system due to either non-compliance or tube insertion issues may lead to a long-term option, that of a gastrostomy feeding system. Gastrostomy is not without risk, although the benefits of adequate nutrition usually outweigh the risks of complications. Gastrostomy feeding has been associated with improved growth and quality of life in children with cerebral palsy (Smith et al 1999). This system, established by insertion of a tube through the abdominal wall into the stomach, is for long-term use. Regardless of the feeding method utilised, oral hygiene of the mouth is essential to reduce tooth decay and other related medical problems. Support and trouble-shooting for all feeding interventions can be sought within the community from a variety of healthcare professionals and at relevant hospital clinics.

Evidence-based practice

The American Academy for Cerebral Palsy and Developmental Medicine (AACPDM) undertook a systematic review of the outcomes of gastrostomy feeding in children with cerebral palsy (Samson-Fang et al 2003). The findings of the systematic review are summarised below:

- 10 studies met all the inclusion criteria and were included in the review. The 10 studies contain results on a total of 281 individuals.
- All the studies were described by Samson-Fang et al (2003) as comprising 'very low levels of evidence' when evaluated against the AACPDM quality rating scheme.
- Overall, however, there was consistency in the results, which favoured gastrostomy feeding.

This systematic review provides an excellent example of how to investigate the evidence base for practice in a rigorous way and could be used as 'gold standard' in assessing the evidence for children's nursing.

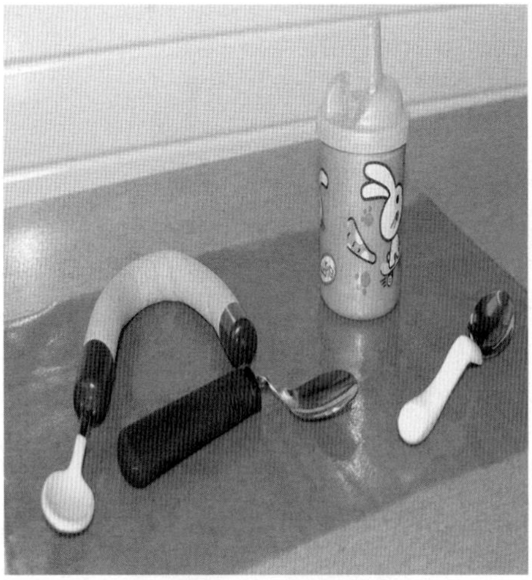

Fig. 24.6 • Spoons. Flexi-spoons are available to help children feed more easily and independently.

Feeding and language-related problems often go together in children with severe cerebral palsy, even though speech production does not inevitably correlate with earlier oral-motor patterns (Dormans & Pellegrino 1998). The next section considers the related area of communication.

Communication

Speech and language facilitate learning and regulate behaviour, they are also critical developmental tasks that form the basis for all social interactions. The ability to communicate is fundamental to expressing personal need or opinion. Children will often use their natural modes of communication, such as vocalisation, eye-pointing, gesture and body movements. Play can also enhance communication through motivation, imagination and the development of social skills. Several examples of good practice exist in the literature (Brodin 1999, Crawford & Raven 2002) and make useful suggestions to strengthen play opportunities for this group. Children restricted by physical and cognitive limitations who are not given adequate opportunities for free play are being further disadvantaged.

Box 24.2

Proposed nursing assessment of eating and drinking for children with complex motor problems.

Adequacy of nutrition

- Assess growth: height, weight.
- Assess rate of growth.
- Compare parent and professional assessment of growth and nutritional status.
- Take feeding history: length of time to complete a meal; assess daily intake and daily loss (vomiting).
- Describe amount and type of food intake.

History

- Find out about early feeding habits.
- Seek and include histories of dietetic and speech and language therapy input.
- Assess if any referrals might be necessary.

Oral skills

- Note dentition, any structural problems that might make eating or breathing while eating difficult.
- Observe and comment on ability to chew, swallow, clear palate, control saliva.
- Look for drooling.

Tolerance

- Assess if the child is prone to choking, coughing, spluttering, vomiting. Record frequency.
- Cogher et al (1992) emphasise the importance of assessing tolerance through behaviours – turning away, refusing to eat, crying, grimacing, gagging or vomiting.

Food preferences

- Describe the child's food preferences.
- Also describe the preferred texture (lumpy, solid, puréed); preferred feeding utensils.

Feeding technique

- Describe breathing pattern while eating and assess the risk of aspiration as far as possible.
- Describe the parents' technique.
- How do the parents position the child for eating and drinking?
- What special utensils do they have, or are preferred?

Digestion and elimination

- Is there any evidence of pain and discomfort on eating and drinking?
- Is there any history of constipation or other gastrointestinal problems: reflux, obstruction, rupture?

Parents' attitudes

- Find out about parents' feelings towards their child's nutrition and eating and drinking: are these associated with stress?

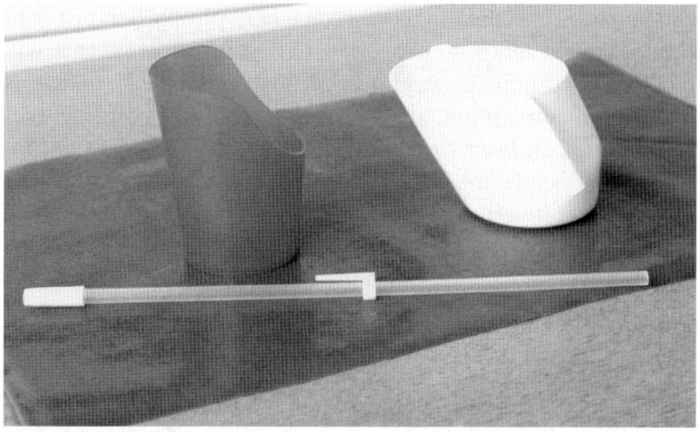

Fig. 24.7 • Cups and straws. A cup with an angled rim means that the child does not have to throw the head back if self-feeding. If being fed from these cups, the feeder has extra control in the amount of liquid the child receives. The straw has non-return valve that helps children with poor sucking ability. Note the non-slip mat to prevent spillages.

Children with significant neuromotor impairments may experience problems related to articulation of speech and language and/or problems related to intellectual ability and the ability to communicate and express themselves. Pennington & McConachie (1999) studied the interaction between non-verbal children with severe motor impairment and their carers. The findings indicated that the adults took control of conversations, instigated topics, asked questions and issued commands. The children provided the required responses, using a restricted range of communicative functions. This highlights the importance of children's nurses understanding how to communicate with non-verbal children. However, work conducted by Beail (1985) found that nurses had low-level and poor-quality interactions with children with multiple disabilities; it is to be hoped that awareness and practice have changed since then.

Nursing assessment in communication

In relation to the assessment of a child's communication abilities, the criteria in Box 24.3 are considered part of good practice to ensure a complete and accurate assessment of need is conducted. Some of the suggestions are derived from Evans et al (1989) and Cogher et al (1992).

Nursing interventions in communication

Effective assessment is imperative to optimise a child's communication and development potential. Impairments, including hearing, visual, cognitive (learning disability), attention deficits, respiratory problems, orthopaedic anomalies and other medical conditions (e.g. seizures, respiratory problems, gastroesophageal reflux), may all affect the child's ability to communicate (Cass et al 1999). The key interventions to facilitate communication in the child with complex motor problems, as described by Cogher et al (1992), should focus on good positioning – to maximise eye contact and minimise involuntary movements and facilitated expression through constructive play and augmented communication systems (Figs 24.8 and 24.9).

Box 24.3

Proposed nursing assessment of communication for children with complex motor problems

Oromotor abilities

- Are problems related to articulation of speech apparent (dysarthria)?
- Record history of speech and language therapy.

Social interaction

- What motivates the child to communicate: happy? sad? hunger? pain? Assess in conjunction with parents.
- Describe child's experiences and knowledge of play.
- Is the child able to participate in symbolic play?

Means of expression

- Describe means of expression: verbal or non-verbal.
- Alternative methods of communication: eye pointing? sounds?
- Formalised systems such as Makaton?
- Describe if any involuntary facial expressions are apparent – these can sometimes be misleading.

Non-verbal skills

- Describe non-verbal skills, especially if the child is unable to speak.
- Describe eye contact, vocalisation, body movements (head control, unwanted movements, facial grimacing).
- Describe if the child is able to 'take turns' in any interaction, assess attention span.

Comprehension

- Is there a reliable yes/no response: to nurse, to parents, to others?
- Ask parents level of understanding.
- Also record type of school attended; psychologist's reports.

Use of expressive language

- Describe use of expressive language: range and depth of vocabulary. Age appropriate?

Phonology

- Describe how the words sound: accurate?

Family communication

- Describe any child and family communication strategies that might exist, in particular the role of play, particular games.
- Describe how the parents and siblings communicate with the child.

To maximise the successful use of augmentative communication systems, the child should be introduced to the system as early as possible, professionals and parents need to be trained to facilitate the child and there needs to be planning and cooperation between the professional multi-agencies (Ko et al 1998). During a period of hospitalisation it is essential that the children's nurse supports the child to continue to use and develop his or her skills in augmentative communication systems as far as possible.

Ineffective communication can lead to frustration, which is sometimes interpreted as 'bad behaviour' in the child. Frustration can be expressed through non-compliance to care with

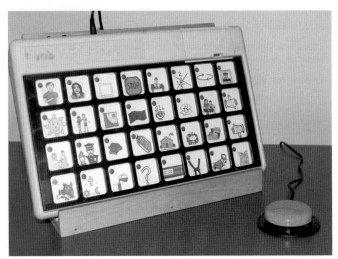

Fig. 24.8 • Symbols for communication. Picture symbols can be used to communicate. This communications board is activated by a switch. The child practises controlling the switch through work and play.

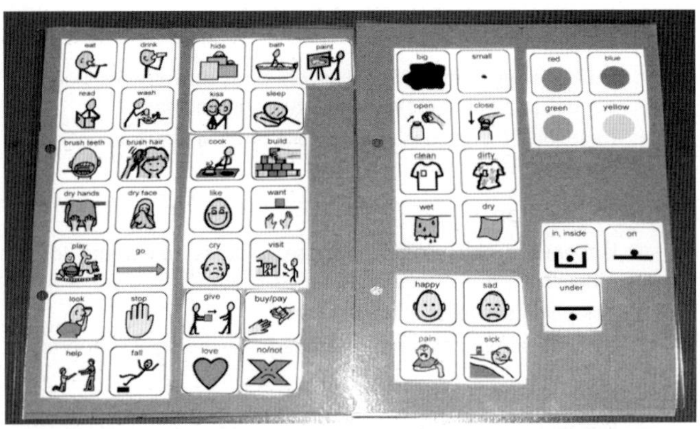

Fig. 24.9 • More symbols. This Makaton system is another example of symbols for communication. It is based on picture symbols. The child points at the words and, with practice, can build up relatively sophisticated communication. A booklet can be customised for each individual child.

rigid or thrashing torso and high vocalisation. The child may be expressing a need to change position or to resolve hunger, toiletry needs or pain. Free play can help alleviate such communication difficulties through development of the whole child. Behavioural cues may be misleading so parents and health professionals must be cautious in their assessment and planning. Facial impressions can be misunderstood due to low muscle tone and vocalisations can be misinterpretated due to increased laryngeal spasticity.

Promoting function requires the building of skills as well as developing compensatory mechanisms to help the child best function within the limits of his or her motor and cognitive abilities. Once a child's communication deficits and potential have been established, the specialist team of speech therapist and medical consultant must implement a phase of planning. Such planning will be shared within a larger team, to include paediatric nurse, health visitor, teacher, physiotherapist and occupational therapist. The aim is to develop all areas that will facilitate optimum communication for the child. If speech is not an available option, alternative skills such as pointing, picture boards, and non-verbal cues will be developed to ensure the child's needs are met. If the child is visually and hearing impaired, non-verbal responses such as body language along with the positive communication of a familiar parent/carer is vital for effective child communication.

Summary

This chapter has brought together a number of perspectives in the consideration of children with complex motor disability. Although complex motor disability is relatively rare, as are the conditions that give rise to it, the level of need and support required by children and their families is high and life long. Multiple agencies are involved in the provision of care and services to these children and care must be taken not to overburden families with too many professionals but at the same time ensure their needs are met. Parents caring for a child with complex motor disability are experts in their own right and a valued partner for the children's nurse. This chapter considered a small number of predominant problems experienced by children with complex needs. In particular, detailed consideration was given to what the children's nurse should assess and how they should intervene in the areas of mobility, eating and drinking and communication.

Acknowledgements

We would like to thank Daniel's Mum for her frank and honest account of her experiences caring for her son. We would also like to thank Mrs Sheila McNeill, Paediatric Physiotherapist, and Mrs Julia Maskery, Paediatric Occupational Therapist, for advice on the use of aids and adaptations as featured in the photographs and accompanying text; and Mrs Doris Corkin, Nurse Lecturer, for reading and commenting on an earlier draft.

References

Audit Commission, 1994. Seen but not heard: coordinating community child health and social services for children in need. HMSO, London.

Baldwin, S., Carlisle, J., 1994. Social support for disabled children and their families. A review of the literature. Social Work Services Inspectorate. HMSO, London.

Bamford, D., Griffith, H., Kernohan, G., 1991. I felt like running away: the social and emotional implications of cerebral palsy. Boys' and Girls' Welfare Society, London.

Bamford, D., Griffith, H., Kernohan, G., 1997. Analysis of consumer satisfaction with cerebral palsy care. British Journal of Social Work 27, 605–614.

Beail, N., 1985. The nature of interactions between nursing staff and profoundly multiply handicapped children. Child: Care, Health and Development 11, 113–129.

Beale, H., 2002. Respite care for technology-dependent children and their families. Paediatric Nursing 14, 18–19.

Beresford, B., 1994. Positively parents. Caring for a severely disabled child. Social Policy Research Unit. HMSO, London.

Beresford, B., 1995. Expert opinions. A national survey of families caring for a severely disabled child. Policy Press, Bristol.

Bone, M., Meltzer, H., 1989. The prevalence of disability among children. HMSO, London.

Bottos, M., Bolcati, C., Sciuto, L., et al., 2001. Powered wheelchairs and independence in young children with tetraplegia. Developmental Medicine and Child Neurology 43, 769–777.

Brodin, J., 1999. Play in children with severe multiple disabilities: play with toys – a review. International Journal of Disability. Development and Education 46, 25–34.

Brogan, E., Hadders-Algra, M., Forssberg, H., 1998. Postural control in sitting children with cerebral palsy. Neuroscience and Behavioural Reviews 22, 591–596.

Cass, H., Price, K., Reilly, S., et al., 1999. A model for the assessment and management of children with multiple disabilities. Child: Care,. Health and Development 25, 191–211.

Cogher, L., Savage, E., Smith, M.F., 1992. Cerebral palsy. The child and young person. Chapman & Hall Medical, London.

Colver AF, Mackie P 1998 North of England collaborative cerebral palsy survey. Annual Report.

Crawford, C., Raven, K., 2002. Play preparation for children with special needs. Paediatric Nursing 14, 27–29.

Critchton, J.U., MacKinnon, M., White, C.P., 1995. The life expectancy of person with cerebral palsy. Developmental Medicine and Child Neurology 37, 567–576.

de Geeter, K.I., Poppes, P., Vlaskamp, C., 2002. Parents as experts: the position of parents of children with profound multiple disabilities. Child: Care. Health and Development 28, 443–453.

Dormans, J.P., Pellegrino, L., 1998. Caring for children with cerebral palsy: a team approach. Brooks Publishing, London.

Duffy, B, 1995. PPRU surveys of disability report 5: disabled children in Northern Ireland: services, transport and education. Policy Planning and Research Unit, Belfast.

Edmond, A., Golding, J., Peckham, C., 1989. Cerebral palsy in two national cohort studies. Archives of Disease in Childhood 60, 1113–1121.

Evans, P.M., Evans, S.J.W., Alberman, E., 1989. A standard form for recording clinical findings in children with a motor deficit of central origin (letter). Developmental Medicine and Child Neurology 31, 121–127.

Fawcett, J., 1995. Analysis and evaluation of conceptual models of nursing, 3rd edn. FA Davis, Philadelphia.

Gisel, E.G., Alphonce, E., 1995. Classification of eating impairments based on eating efficiency in children with cerebral palsy. Dysphagia 10, 268–274.

Gisel, E.G., Patrick, J., 1988. Identification of children with cerebral palsy unable to maintain a normal nutritional state. Lancet 1, 283–286.

Glendinning, C., Kirk, S., Guiffridda, A., Lawton, D., 1999. The community based care of technology dependent children in the UK: definitions, numbers and costs. National Primary Care Research and Development Centre. University of Manchester, Manchester.

Glendinning, C., Kirk, S., Guiffridda, A., Lawton, D., 2001. Technology-dependent children in the community: definitions, numbers and costs. Child: Care. Health and Development 27, 321–334.

Gordon, D., Parker, R., Loughran, F., Heslop, P., 2000. Disabled children in Britain. A re-analysis of the OPCS disability survey. The Stationery Office, London.

Gough, D., Li, L., Wroblewska, A., 1993. Services for children with a motor impairment and their families in Scotland. Public Health Research Unit. University of Glasgow.

Haylock, C., Johnson, A.M., Harpin, V.A., 1993. Parents' views of community care for children with motor disabilities. Child: Care. Health and Development 19, 209–220.

Hirose, T., Ueda, R., 1990. Long-term follow up study of cerebral palsy children and coping behaviour of parents. Journal of Advanced Nursing 15, 762–770.

Hutton, J., Cook, T., Pharoah, P.O.D., 1994. Life expectancy in children with cerebral palsy. British Medical Journal 309, 431–435.

Hutton, J., Pharoah, P.O.D., 1998. Life expectancy in people with cerebral palsy. Abstract from an annual meeting. In: Colver A, Mackie P (Eds.), North of England collaborative cerebral palsy survey. Annual report, November: pp. 19–25 .

Ingram, T.T.S., 1955. A study of cerebral palsy in the childhood population of Edinburgh. Archives of Disease in Childhood 60, 1113–1121.

Jarvis SN, Holloway JS, Hey EN, 1985. Increase in cerebral palsy in normal birthweight babies. Archives of Disease in Childhood 60, 1113–1121.

Johnson A, King R 1998 Oxford register of early childhood impairments. Annual Report 1997. National Perinatal Epidemiology Unit, Oxford

Kingdom, S., Mayfield, C., 2001. Complex disabilities: parents preparing professionals. Paediatric Nursing 13: 34–38.

Kirk, S., 1999. Caring for children with specialised health care needs in the community. Health & Social Care in the Community 7, 350–357.

Ko, M.L.B., McConachie, H., Jolieff, N., 1998. Outcome of recommendations for augmentative communication in children. Child: Care. Health and Development 24, 195–205.

Korman, L.A., Paterson Smith, B., Ballrishnan, R., 2003. Spasticity associated with cerebral palsy in children. Pediatric Drugs 5, 11–23.

Lloyd Faulconbridge, R.V., Tranter, R.M., Moffat, V., Green, E., 2001. Review of management of drooling problems in neurologically impaired children: a review of methods and results over 6 years at Chailey Heritage Clinical Services. Clinical Otolaryngology 26, 76–81.

MacGillivray, I., Campbell, D., 1995. The changing pattern of cerebral palsy in Avon. Paediatric and Perinatal Epidemiology 9, 146–155.

McCarthy, G.T., Cork, M., Crane, S., et al., 1992. The baby and young child. In: McCarthy, G.T. (Ed.), Physical disability in childhood. An interdisciplinary approach to management. Churchill Livingstone, Edinburgh, pp. 13–52.

McConachie, H., 1997. Organization of child disability services. Guest editorial. Child: Care. Health and Development 23, 3–9.

McConachie, H., Salt, A., Chadury, Y., et al., 1999. How do child development teams work? Findings from a UK national survey. Child: Care. Health and Development 25, 157–168.

McConkey, R., Adams, L., 2000. Matching short break services for children with learning disabilities to family needs and preferences. Child: Care. Health and Development 26, 429–443.

Miller, S., 2002. Respite care for children who have complex healthcare needs. Paediatric Nursing 14, 33–37.

Milner, J., Bungay, C., Jellinek, D., Hall, D.M.B., 1996. Needs of disabled children and their families. Archives of Disease in Childhood 75, 399–404.

Motion, S., Northstone, K., Emond, A., et al., 2002. Early feeding problems in children with cerebral palsy: weight and neuro-developmental outcomes. Developmental Medicine and Child Neurology 44, 40–43.

Mutch, L., Alberman, E., Hagberg, G., et al., 1992. Cerebral palsy epidemiology: Where have we been and where are we going?. (Annotation) Developmental Medicine and Child Neurology 34, 547–551.

National Service Framework (NSF) 2003 Online. Available at: http://www.doh.gov.uk/nsf

O'Shea, T.M., Preisser, J.S., Klinepeter, K.L., Dillard, R.G., 1998. Trends in mortality and cerebral palsy in a geographically based cohort of very low birthweight neonates born between 1984 to 1994. Pediatrics 101, 642–647.

Palisano, R.J., Tieman, B.L., Walter, S.D., et al., 2003. Effect of environmental setting on mobility methods of children with cerebral palsy. Developmental Medicine and Child Neurology 45, 113–120.

Parkes, J., 1998. Children with cerebral palsy in Northern Ireland: needs and services. Unpublished PhD Thesis. Queen's University, Belfast.

Parkes, J., Dolk, H., Hill, A.E., 1998. Does the child health computing system adequately identify children with cerebral palsy? Journal of Public Health Medicine 20 (1), 102–104.

Parkes, J., Donnelly, M., Hill, N., 2001a. Focusing on cerebral palsy: reviewing and communicating needs for services. Scope, London.

Parkes, J., Dolk, H., Hill, N., Pattenden, S., 2001b. Epidemiology of cerebral palsy in Northern Ireland: 1981-1993. Paediatric and Perinatal Epidemiology 15, 278–286.

Parkes, J., Donnelly, M., Dolk, H., Hill, N., 2002. Use of physiotherapy and alternatives by children with cerebral palsy: a population study. Child: Care. Health and Development 28 (6), 469–477.

Pennington, L., McConachie, H., 1999. Mother–child interaction revisited: communication with non-speaking physically disabled children. International Journal of Language and Communication Disorders 345, 391–416.

Pharoah, P.O.D., Cooke, T., Cooke, R.W.I., Rosenbloom, L., 1990. Birthweight-specific trends in cerebral palsy. Archives of Disease in Childhood 65, 602–606.

Pharoah, P.O.D., Platt, M., Cooke, T., 1996. The changing epidemiology of cerebral palsy. Archives of Disease in Childhood 75, F169–F173.

Pharoah, P.O.D., Cooke, T., Johnson, A., et al., 1998. Epidemiology of cerebral palsy in England and Scotland 1984-1990. Archives of Disease in Childhood, F21–F25.

Priestley, M., 2003. Disability. A life course approach. Polity Press, Cambridge.

Rees, S.J., 1983. Families' perceptions of services for handicapped children. International Journal of Rehabilitation Research 6, 475–476.

Roberts, K., Lawton, D., 2001. Acknowledging the extra care parents give their disabled children. Child: Care. Health and Development 27, 307–319.

Roper, N., Logan, W.W., Tierney, A.J., 1990. The elements of nursing. Churchill Livingstone, Edinburgh.

Ross A, Parkes J 2004 Making doors open: the role of the children's community nurse in caring for a child with severe cerebral palsy. Paediatric Nursing.

Roxborough, L., 1995. Review of the efficacy and effectiveness of adaptive seating for children with cerebral palsy. Assistive Technology 7, 17–25.

Roy, C., 1976. Introduction to nursing: an adaptation model: Prentice-Hall, Englewood Cliffs, NJ.

Samson-Fang, L., Butler, C., O'Donnell, M., 2003. Effects of gastrostomy feeding in children with cerebral palsy: an AACPDM evidence report. Developmental Medicine & Child Neurology 45, 415–426.

Sloper, P., 1999. Models of service support for parents of disabled children. What do we know? What do we need to know? Child: Care. Health and Development 25, 85–99.

Sloper, P., Turner, S., 1992. Service needs of families of children with severe physical disability. Child: Care. Health and Development 18, 259–282.

Sloper, P., Turner, S., 1993. Risk and resistance factors in the adaptation of parents of children with severe physical disability. Journal of Child Psychology and Psychiatry 34, 167–188.

Smith, F., 2003. 'Getting the right start': the children's national service framework. Paediatric Nursing 15, 20–21.

Smith, M., Robinson, P., Duffy, P., 1992. PPRU surveys of disability report 2: the prevalence of disability among children in Northern Ireland. Policy. Planning and Research Unit, Belfast.

Smith, S.W., Camfield, C., Camfield, P., 1999. Living with cerebral palsy and tube feeding: a population-based follow-up study. Journal of Pediatrics 135, 307–310.

Stalker, K., 1990. Share the care: an evaluation of family-based respite care. Jessica Kingsley, London.

Surveillance of Cerebral Palsy in Europe (SCPE), 2000. Surveillance of cerebral palsy in Europe: a collaboration of cerebral palsy surveys and registers. Developmental Medicine and Child Neurology 42, 816–824.

Taanila, A., Syrjala, L., Kokkonen, J., Jarvelin, M.R., 2002. Coping of parents with physically and/or intellectually disabled children. Child: Care. Health and Development 28, 73–86.

Tippett, A., 2001. All about me: documentation for children with special needs. Paediatric Nursing 13, 34–35.

United Nations General Assembly, 1989. Convention on the Rights of the Child. UNICEF, Geneva.

Ward, T., Worswikc, J., Inglis, A. et al., 2003. Children with complex, continuing health needs and/or life-limiting conditions. Report of the task group. Children's national service framework: disabled children external working group. Online. Available at: http://www.doh.gov.uk/nsf/children

Watson, D., Townsley, R., Abbot, D., 2002. Exploring multi-agency working in services to disabled children with complex healthcare needs and their families. Journal of Clinical Nursing 11, 367–375.

Westcott, S.L., Lowes, L.P., Richardson, P.K., 1997. Evaluation of postural stability in children: current theories and assessment tools. Physical Therapy 77, 629–645.

Williams, K., Hennessey, E., Alberman, E., 1996. Cerebral palsy: effects of twinning birthweight and gestational age. Archives of Disease in Childhood 75, F178–182.

World Health Organization, 1980. International classification of impairments, disability and handicap (ICIDH). World Health Organization, Geneva.

World Health Organization, 2001. Beginner's guide. Towards a common language for functioning, disability and health (ICF). World Health Organization, Geneva.

World Health Organization, 2002. International classification of functioning, disability and health. World Health Organization, Geneva.

Caring for children and young people with body fluid and electrolyte imbalance

25

Agnes B Kanneh

ABSTRACT

Ensuring adequate hydration and electrolyte balance are essential aspects of care for children and young people in both health and disease. Balance in volume and solute composition of body fluids and electrolytes is ensured by the well-coordinated and integrated action of the homeostatic organs, carefully matching intake with output. Body fluids and electrolytes balance relates to equilibrium between intake and output, or between gain and loss in maintaining homeostasis. Imbalances occur when the body is deficient in, or has excess of the required amounts that ensure health and well-being. Recurrent imbalances in body fluids and electrolytes can have long-term adverse effects on the child's physical and cognitive growth and development (Petri et al 2008). This is because explanations offered on the structure and biological functions of water affirm the notion that water is the chemical of life, second only to oxygen (Eastwood 1997, Martini Nath, 2009).

The availability of and access to safe drinking water is a basic human right and, water has been suggested as a neglected nutrient in the young child (Bourne et al 2007).

In any human environment, safe water and electrolyte intake in the form of drinking is necessary to ensure a balance that maintains effective organ system function. Here, children – and especially the very young – are dependent on their parents and carers, including healthcare professionals, to meet this fundamental human need because of limited self-care ability. On an annual global scale, pneumonia and diarrhoea account for about 10 million deaths in children less than 5 years of age. Sadly, large numbers of children under 5 years of age worldwide present with acute gastroenteritis annually, causing nearly 2 million deaths. In the UK, 204 of every 1000 GP consultations and 7 of every 1000 hospital admissions of children under 5 years are due to gastroenteritis. Thus, acute diarrhoea is the leading cause of body fluid and electrolyte imbalance in children worldwide (Dalby-Payne & Elliott 2008).

DOI: 10.1016/B978-0-7020-3183-0.10025-6

LEARNING OUTCOMES

- Review key functions of water and electrolytes in children and young people.
- Identify and examine possible causes of body fluid and electrolyte imbalance in children and young people.
- Detail the regulatory systems that maintain body fluid and electrolyte balance.
- Specify common causes of body fluid and electrolyte imbalance in children and young people.
- Explain the clinical manifestations of dehydration and electrolyte imbalance in children and young people.
- Detail the principles of nursing care and evidence-based practice for the child who presents with body fluid and electrolyte imbalance caused by acute diarrhoea and vomiting.

Water composition of the body

Body fluids

The cell is the fundamental unit of life and metabolism and an adequate intake of water is essential to the survival and everyday activities of the metabolically active growing and developing child in both health and disease. Body fluids comprise total body water (TBW), with its dissolved chemical particles. Throughout life a large proportion of the body is water, changing as age progresses (Fig 25.1).

Water is vital to the existence of all living organisms and is the most abundant molecule of their cell mass (Campbell & Reece 2008). Two-thirds of the total body weight is water and it is the body's single most important constituent (Martini & Nath 2009). Table 25.1 shows the water composition of various tissues in the average individual. In the absence of water, chemical

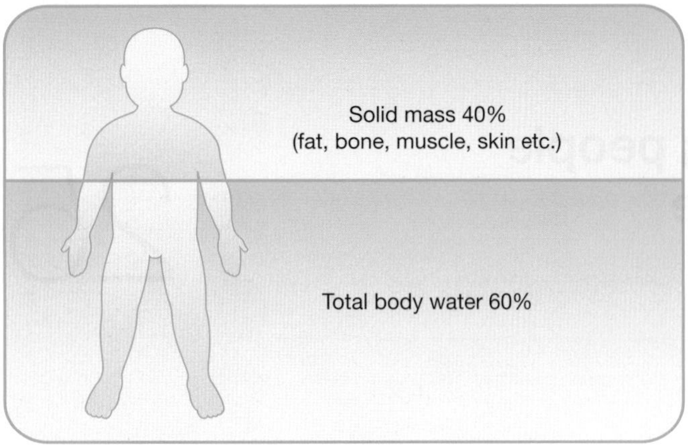

Fig. 25.1 • The percentage of total body water from age 1 year (Ichikawa 1990).

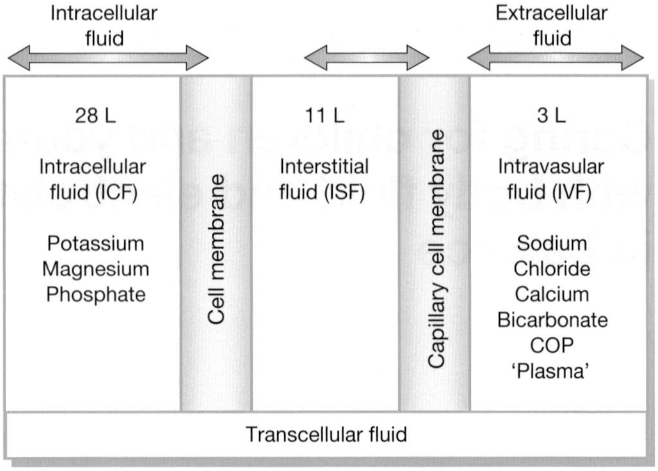

Fig. 25.2 • Distribution of total body water within compartments in the average adult; showing all the body fluid compartments and their corresponding constituents. The intravascular fluid (IVS) is the effective circulating blood volume (CBV), maintained largely with the help of the plasma proteins, with albumin maintaining 70–80% of the colloid oncotic pressure (COP). Colloid solutions with the same COP as plasma will stay in the IVS and thus are most efficient in restoring the CBV in hypovolaemia. Alternatively, crystalloid solutions administered intravenously are isotonic to plasma and thus distributed to the extracellular fluid (ECF), with the majority of it to the interstitial space (ISS). The sodium/potassium (Na/K) ATPase pump actively pumps sodium into the extracellular space (ECS) and potassium into the intracellular space (ICS), although glucose-containing fluids are evenly distributed in the ICS to rehydrate cells (Guyton & Hall 2005).

Table 25.1 Water composition of body tissues in the average 75-kg male

Tissue	Percentage of water	Litres of water	Percentage of total body water
Skin	72	9.72	22
Skeleton	22	2.47	5
Blood	83	3.11	7
Adipose	10	0.90	2
Muscle	76	24.51	55

reactions, metabolic processes and regulatory systems become severely compromised and eventually cease to function (Tortora & Derrickson 2009). A healthy adult can survive for around 10 days without water; a healthy child will survive only 3–4 days without water. For a thorough comprehension of the value of water to life, growth and development, and hence the deleterious effects of uncorrected body fluid and electrolyte imbalance, an understanding of the chemical and physical properties of water is essential (see Chapter 27 in Martini & Nath 2009). Daily fluid maintenance requirements take into consideration losses from the skin, airways, gastrointestinal tract and urine.

Body fluid compartments

TBW in multicellular human organisms is functionally divided into compartments. These are specific enclosures in which the fluid exists in relation to cell anatomy, with the cell membrane and capillary endothelum forming the interface between the compartments. Body fluid compartments differ in both their volume and solute composition. The solute composition, because of the osmotic movement of water, is in equilibrium between the extracellular fluid and intracellular space. Specific composition of each compartment establishes the optimal environment for the biochemical reactions that occur within them. The absolute and relative size and volume of each compartment varies with the age and sex of the individual. In relation to tissue cells, TBW exists in two main compartments and a third minor compartment:

- Intracellular fluid (ICF) compartment: comprises the fluid existing inside tissue cells.
- Extracellular fluid (ECF) compartment: comprises body fluid existing outside and between tissue cells.
- Transcellular fluid: an extra small compartment.

The body of the average adult contains approximately 42 L of water (Fig. 25.2), which is divided into the various body fluid compartments (Guyton & Hall 2005). Figure 25.2 and Table 25.2 illustrate the distribution of body water within the compartments and Figures 25.3 and 25.4 apply specifically in the various imbalances in the child, where fluid shifts can occur, thereby changing the osmolality of fluids within the three compartments.

Intracellular fluid

Intracellular fluid comprises the body water that exists inside the tissue cells that make up the child's body, and accounts for 35–40% of the total body water. The intracellular fluid is contained within a closed space (the cell) so it is not easy to estimate and there is a limit to which it can expand without causing stress to the cell membrane. For this reason, pure water (free water) is not administered intravenously because it is hypotonic relative to the intracellular solute composition.

Table 25.2 The body fluid composition during the lifespan (Ichikawa 1990)

Age	TBW (%)	ECF (%)	ICF (%)
Preterm neonate	80	45	35
Full-term neonate	75	40	35
1–12 months	65	30	35
1–12 years	60	20	40
Adult			
male	55	25	30
female	50	20	30

ECF, extracellular fluid; ICF, intracellular fluid; TBW, total body water.

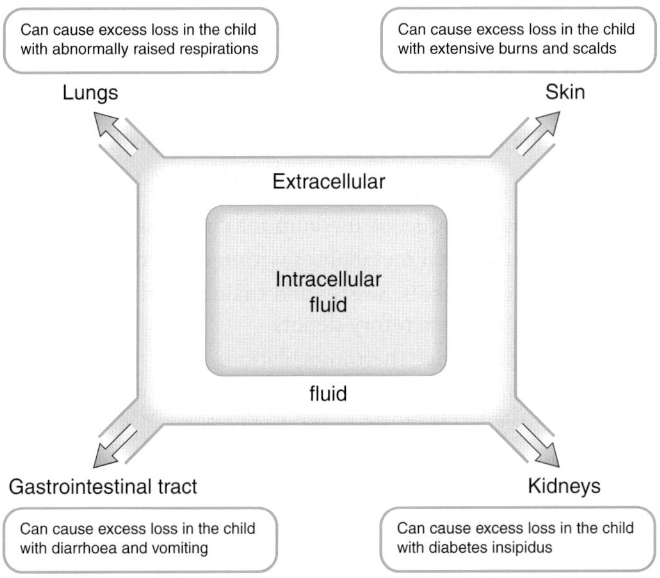

Fig. 25.3 • The relationship between intracellular fluid, extracellular fluid and exchange with the external environment within the body.

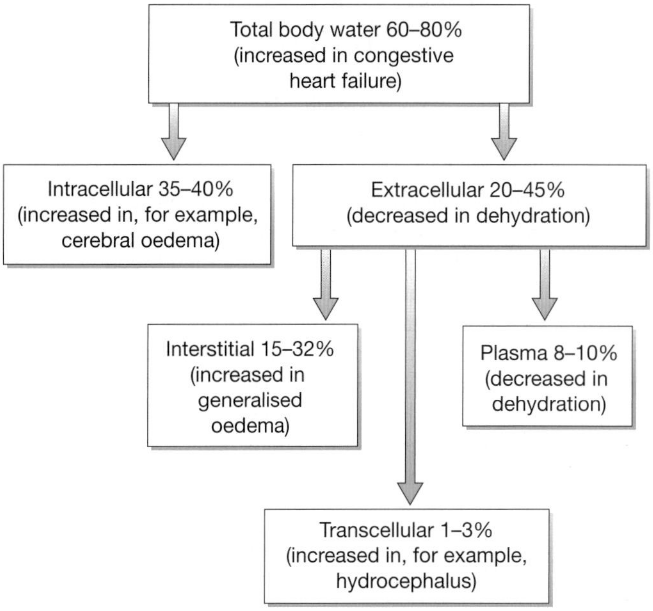

Fig. 25.4 • Total body water composition in children in health and disease.

Theoretical intravenous administration of pure water causes the cells (e.g. erythrocytes) to exist in a hypotonic environment relative to their intracellular space. Water will then move by the process of osmosis into the erythrocytes, causing them to swell until their cell membrane can no longer accommodate the increase in cell volume, causing them to burst (cell lysis). A similar situation will occur in water intoxication or overhydration with acute hyponatraemia. Here, the cells most vulnerable to osmotic fluid shift into their intracellular compartment are brain cells. Ultimately, cytotoxic cerebral oedema, with its attendant raised intracranial pressure (ICP), occurs. Cerebral function is altered, and this is reflected in an abnormal score on the Glasgow Coma Scale. Unrelieved, cerebral neuropathy resulting from the increased ICP can cause seizures, coma and death. There is increasing evidence to show that iatrogenic (treatment – induced) hyponatraemia is a real clinical threat to children especially in the postoperative period and the high-dependency setting. The only saving grace in preventing adverse outcomes in these circumstances is the careful monitoring of serum sodium levels in the children (Au et al 2008).

Extracellular fluid (Ichikawa 1990, Martini & Nath 2009)

Extracellular fluid exists (ECF) outside and between tissue cells, supporting and nourishing them as they bathe in it. ECF accounts for 20–45% of the total body weight in children and is further subdivided into two subcompartments:

- Intravascular fluid compartment – inside blood vessels
- Interstitial fluid – in between tissue cells.

Extracellular fluid is fundamental to the regulation and balance of body fluids and electrolytes because it is the changes in this compartment that act as a trigger for the activation of regulatory systems in the quest to maintain homeostasis.

Intravascular fluid compartment

The components in the intravascular fluid compartment enable the cardiovascular system to meet the metabolic needs of the body.

The cardiovascular system is a continuous, closed, blood-filled circuit equipped with a muscular and electrical pump (the heart) that maintains the pulmonary and systemic circulation. The cardiovascular system consists of:

- the heart: an electrical muscular pump that establishes the pressure gradient that ensures effective blood flow to tissue cells
- blood vessels: the channels or passageways through which blood flows within the body
- blood: the biological load and transport medium, which contains plasma, suspended blood cells and dissolved particles.

In plasma volume deficit, hypovolaemia occurs, increases blood viscosity and the packed cell volume, which can increase the propensity for thromboembolic episodes in a child with nephrotic syndrome, for example.

The intravascular fluid comprises plasma and makes up 8–10% of the total body water. It represents the entire amount of fluid inside the blood vessels, minus that inside the blood cells. The intravascular space is bounded by the capillary endothelial cell membrane. Plasma, the suspended blood cells and dissolved particles constitute the circulating blood volume (CBV). This is the actual fluid volume perfusing the tissue cells of the vital organs. It is in contact with and stimulates the volume receptors and baroreceptors in the vena cavae and aorta, respectively. Plasma, the fluid component of blood, contains salts, organic and inorganic compounds and hormones. Serum is plasma minus the clotting factors, in particular fibrinogen.

Interstitial fluid (Tortora & Derrickson 2009, Martini & Nath 2009)

The interstitial fluid (ISF) comprises the fluid interposed between the intravascular space and intracellular space. The interstitial fluid is the fluid between the cells, i.e. it bathes the cells. Nutrients and respiratory gases, plus enzymes, hormones and other substances, reach tissue cells via the arterial ends of the capillaries. Cells need to be cleared of their metabolic waste products and this is a function of the venous ends of capillaries; the process enables the waste products to reach their designated depots, such as the kidneys and lungs, for disposal.

ISF is tissue fluid and the interstitial space can be viewed as a 'biological bureau de change'. Effective distribution of fluid between the intravascular and interstitial compartments is determined by the difference between the hydrostatic pressure, which is generated by myocardial contractility and arteriolar vasoconstriction, and the opposing plasma oncotic pressure, generated by plasma proteins. This partially explains oedema in the child with nephrotic syndrome who becomes hypoproteinaemic.

Lymph, the fluid that circulates in the lymphatic vessels, is part of the interstitial fluid. It is an important fluid because it reclaims the small amounts of fluid that remains in the interstitial space back into the intravascular space, thus preventing fluid backlog leading to oedema. Although body fluids are compartmentalised, they are all in communication with one another with the help of their respective biophysical forces. Therefore fluid shifts occur in dehydration because fluid will tend to move into the compartment with the deficit.

Activity

Critical reflection on theory

With reference to the descriptions above, explain why a dehydrated child might manifest abnormal physical features of the skin and mucous membranes.

Transcellular fluid (Tortora & Derrickson 2009, Martini & Nath 2009)

Transcellular fluid is a minor part of the total body water, forming 1–3%. Its function is to lubricate and provide smooth movement between two closely related layers or membranes, e.g. the pleural membranes. In terms of the circulating blood volume, transcellular fluid is non-functional or vestigial. This is because it is not readily available to support the circulating blood volume in times of need, as in hypovolaemia for example. Transcellular fluid can, however, act as a third-space fluid in pathological conditions that cause accumulation of fluid in this space. Transcellular fluid comprises:

- cerebrospinal fluid (CSF) (excess = hydrocephalus)
- pericardial fluid (excess = pericardial effusion)
- pleural fluid (excess = pleural effusion)
- synovial fluid (excess = swollen joints)
- intraocular fluid (excess = glaucoma).

Biological functions of water

Essential functions of water in children and young people include:

- maintaining an adequate and effective CBV
- providing the aqueous medium for chemical reactions
- transporting vital metabolites within the body
- removing metabolic wastes and toxic materials from the body via their excretory depots
- ensuring effective thermoregulation
- maintaining balance in blood and other body fluids chemistry
- lubricating layers in close association and preventing friction on their movement
- supporting, cushioning and protecting body organs/structures.

These vital functions highlight the critical role adequate hydration plays in the effective functioning of the growing and developing child's body at any age, particularly infancy. Table 25.3 explains why children, especially the very young, are at increased risk of body fluid and electrolyte imbalance. Also, the organ systems that maintain water balance are immature in children, so young children in particular are at risk of body fluid and electrolyte imbalance. The well-hydrated child should therefore feel warm, have pink and moist mucous membranes, vital signs that are normal for their respective age band and pass a minimum of 1 mL of urine per kilogram of body weight per hour (Table 25.4).

The main electrolytes, their functions and regulatory systems

Electrolytes

Electrolytes/ions are inorganic molecules that, when dissolved in water, separate into their respective electrical charges: positive (cations) and negative (anions). It is essential that

Table 25.3 Why children need more water than adults

Concept	Rationale(s)
Higher ratio of extracellular fluid volume to that of intracellular fluid volume	Blood plasma forms part of the ECF and it is this body fluid that is in direct contact with the environment, e.g. perfusing the subcutaneous capillaries underneath the skin. The close encounter of ECF with the environment thus means a higher turnover rate of ECF in the child than the adult
Children have a large surface area-to-volume ratio meaning a higher insensible fluid loss from the skin and airways	The surface area-to-volume ratio of a small child is greater than that of an adult. This increases water loss from the child through the skin in heat loss by radiation to the environment. The concept thus adds to the child's increased biological need for water
Children have a higher metabolic rate	Children are highly metabolic individuals because of their ongoing growth and development, as well as their other life activities. Children therefore have a higher metabolic rate than adults, which in turn means that they proportionately require more water for both intercellular and intracellular synthesis and excretion of metabolic wastes
Children have a high rate of heat exchange	The high metabolic rate in the child means an increased energy expenditure, including thermal energy, thus a high rate of heat exchange. Water is required to facilitate this heat exchange, which increases the day-to-day water requirement for the child as compared with the adult
Children are not miniature adults	The homeostatic organs of children, especially infants, are immature and the control centre/brain (and their interconnecting pathways) require time to attain functional competence. Even the interaction between hormones and their target organ receptors takes time to mature in children. Therefore, the respective gains of control are less effective and at times exaggerated, as in the case of peripheral vasoconstriction in hypovolaemia. Children's homeostatic systems are thus not very well able to respond and make the necessary adjustments in sudden and extreme changes in set-points. Finally, the self-care abilities in particular in infants are limited resulting in a total dependence on parents/carers

ECF, extracellular fluid.

Table 25.4 Maintenance fluid requirement (Ryan & Molyneux 1996)

Weight (kg)	Fluid requirement
2.5–6 kg	150 mL/kg/24 hours
6–10 kg	120 mL/kg/24 hours
10–20 kg	100 mL/kg/24 hours
20 kg and over	75 mL/kg/24 hours

Table 25.5 Major metabolic cations and anions

Cations	Anions
Sodium (Na^+)	Chloride (Cl^-)
Potassium (K^+)	Bicarbonate (HCO_3^-)
Calcium (Ca^{++})	Phosphate (HPO_4^{2-})
Magnesium (Mg^{++})	'Proteins/amino acids' (A^-) Organic acids

the positively charged ions are in balance with the negatively charged ions. The physical and chemical properties of electrolytes and their existence in specific cellular compartments just as water enable them to carry out their respective biological roles in the body of the growing and developing child: maintaining total body water, acid–base balance, energy balance, effective enzyme function, the creation of muscle and nerve cell membrane potentials. Also, electrolytes composition of plasma is vital for effective functioning of tissue cells, in particular those of excitable form, i.e. neurons and myocytes. Key electrolytes in the body and their chemical symbols are shown in Table 25.5.

Most of the essential biological processes are dependent on electrolyte balance and affected by imbalance, which cannot be tolerated for a long time. Sodium and potassium are the chief positively charged ions. Sodium, potassium, chloride and bicarbonate are most likely to show in electrolyte imbalance. Sodium is the main extracellular cation and determines it's osmolality and CBV. Potassium is the main intracellular cation and determines intracellular fluid volume and cell membrance potential.

The high metabolic rate and the demands of growth and developmental of the child in health and disease make both electrolytes and water critical to their biological well-being. Table 25.6 shows the daily electrolyte requirements in children and Table 25.7 shows the normal reference values for electrolytes in children. These figures are biologically determined reference values but can vary in different clinical conditions on an individual basis (Ichikawa 1990, Somers & Harmon 1999, Tortora & Derrickson 2009).

Electrolytes are obtained from the child's diet in health (Martini & Nath 2009):

- Water is absorbed mostly by the process of osmosis, with sodium playing a major role.
- Sodium diffuses into the villi of the enteroctyes, then is actively pumped into the bloodstream by the Na^+/K^+ ATPase pump.

Table 25.6 Daily electrolyte requirements in children (Green 2004)

Electrolytes	
Sodium	1–3 mmol/kg/day
Potassium	1–3 mmol/kg/day
Chloride	2–3 mmol/kg/day
Calcium	0.7–1.5 mmol/kg/day
Phosphorus	0.9–1.5 mmol/kg/day

- Glucose is co-transported with sodium with the help of insulin, and used by the cells to make energy.
- Amino acids also use a co-transport system together with sodium.
- Calcium, phosphate and sulphate absorption require active transport, accelerated by calcitriol and parathyroid hormone.
- Magnesium absorption requires carrier proteins.
- Chloride and bicarbonate are absorbed by diffusion or carrier-mediated transport.
- Potassium absorption in the small intestine is mainly by passive diffusion, and cellular uptake is influenced by insulin in activating the Na+K+ APTase pump.

Urea

Urea is a waste product of protein catabolism and is removed from the blood via the kidneys. Neonatal and childhood plasma urea concentration levels are lower than in adulthood, reflecting the heightened amino acid utilisation for protein synthesis in childhood. Adult values are reached between 10 and 12 years of age.

Creatinine

Creatinine in the blood is the product of muscle energy metabolism and thus has a direct relationship with muscle mass. Plasma creatinine levels, therefore, vary with the age and sex of the individual. Creatinine is cleared/excreted from the blood via the kidneys (Linné & Ringrud 1999, Walmsley & White 1994).

Glucose

Glucose is the simple sugar that is the immediate energy source for cell metabolism. It is the preferred source of energy for brain cells, which rely on an adequate blood glucose because the brain has very limited glycogen stores. Together with oxygen, glucose is used by cells to synthesise adenosine triphosphate (ATP), that provides the chemical energy for continuous effective cellular function.

The anion gap

The anion gap is the calculation of the mathematical difference between the anions chloride (Cl^-) and bicarbonate (HCO_3^-) & the cations sodium (Na^+) and potassium (K^+):

- $[Cl^- + HCO_3^-] - [Na^+ + K^+]$ = Anion Gap
- Normal value in children is 5–12 mmol/L (Davies & Hassell 2007)
- Raised levels [>14 or more] suggest metabolic acidosis as in diabetic ketoacidosis.

Table 25.7 Plasma reference values for electrolytes in children and neonates (from Ichikawa 1990, Clayton & Round 1994)

Electrolyte	Childhood reference value	Neonatal reference value
Sodium	135–145 mmol/L	132–145 mmol/L
Chloride	100–106 mmol/L	90–110 mmol/L
Potassium	3.5–5.5 mmol/L	3.6–5.9 mmol/L
Calcium	2.2–2.6 mmol/L	1.9–2.85 mmol/L
Magnesium	0.75–1.0 mmol/L	0.71–1.1 mmol/L
Phosphorus	1.45–2.1 mmol/L	1.4–3.0 mmol/L
Bicarbonate	24–30 mmol/L	
Urea	3–7 mmol/L	1–5 mmol/L
Creatinine	18–70 micromol/L	<20–150 micromol/L
Glucose	3.9–6.9 mmol/L	
Osmolality	275–295 mOsm/kg H_2O	280–300 mOsmol/L
Anion gap	5–12 mmol/L	

Blood urea and electrolytes assay, although invasive and therefore unpleasant for the child and family, is a valuable biological and clinical assessment tool whenever the integrity of blood biochemistry is in question, as in dehydration for example. The test estimates essential elements and the chemical components in the blood and urine. Depending on the child's clinical state and technological facilities, the test result can be known within minutes, hours or days. Although reference values are offered here, individual units tend to operate on their laboratory-validated reference ranges that are calibrated to take into account the sources samples are obtained from and the machines used to carry out the assays. It is therefore the responsibility of all nurses to familiarise themselves with the accepted reference values in their own unit and to act promptly when results are outside these ranges.

Homeostasis (the regulation of body fluids and electrolytes) is a delicate, carefully orchestrated and balancing act between the hypothalamus and kidneys via a neurohormonal pathway regulates body fluids and electrolytes. The system works by a negative feedback in titrating intake and regulating output (see Tortora & Derrickson 2009).

The thirst mechanism

Thirst receptors present in the anterior hypothalamus are activated by low extracellular volume (hypothalamic thirst) and high EC solute concentration (osmotic thirst). The receptors detect changes in both volume and osmolality of their immediate extracellular environment to create the sensation of thirst in the individual thus, water/fluid ingestion (Stricker & Verbalis 1999). Interestingly, even though a time lapse of 10–20 minutes exist for the ingested water/fluid to be absorbed and restore homeostasis, we never drink (water) ourselves to death.

Here, in the phenomenon of oropharyngeal metering, the act of continuous swallowing (dipsogenic stimuli) forewarns the brain of the imminent restoration of CBV so the individual stops drinking before absorbing the ingested fluid/water (Figaro & Mack 1997). Figure 25.5 illustrates the behavioural response in body fluid and electrolyte homeostasis.

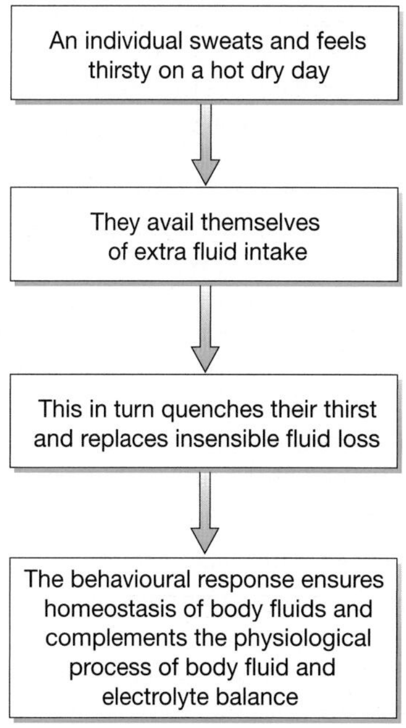

Fig. 25.5 • A behavioural response to increased insensible fluid loss on a hot day.

Antidiuretic hormone

Adaptive changes in TBW and Na^+ balance are regulated by the anterior hypothalamus. Hypothalamic cells in close contact with the osmoreceptors are activated by decrease in CBV or increase in plasma osmolality to produce antidiuretic hormone (ADH), transported to and secreted by the posterior pituitary into the bloodstream. ADH on reaching the renal distal tubules and collecting ducts causes the synthesis and positioning of water channels (aquaporins) on the luminal side, making them very permeable to water. This enables them to reabsorb water from the tubules back into the bloodstream to restore CBV. (Martini & Nath 2009, Porterfield 2001).

ADH Secretion = Concentrated Urine = Decreased Urine Output

thus explaining the term 'antidiuretic'.

Low plasma ADH levels = Dilute Urine = Increased Urine Output

Clinically, appropriate ADH secretion exists if it is in response to high plasma osmolality or hypovolaemia. Here the osmostat is reset at a lower level (Cheethan & Baylis 2002). Alcohol acts as a diuretic by inhibiting ADH secretion.

Aldosterone

Aldosterone, secreted by the adrenal cortex works on the principal cells of the renal distal tubules and collecting ducts. Stimuli for their release include low CBV, autonomic stimulation of renin release, and a rise in plasma potassium level. It promotes renal tubular sodium reabsorption by increasing the synthesis and activity of sodium channels, and the Na^+/K^+ ATPase pump. The increase in sodium reabsorption coincides with the excretion of potassium and hydrogen ions from the body in urine (Celsi & Aperia 1999). Caffeine acts as a diuretic by inhibiting the action of aldosterone on the renal tubules.

Conscientiousness and vigilance applies in managing fluid and electrolyte therapy in children, as these biological systems take time to acquire maturity (functional competence). Young children, especially infants, have impaired capacity to regulate body fluids and electrolytes due to the limited gain of control by the kidneys and a blunted response to the regulatory hormones (Guyton & Hall 2005, Holtbäck & Aperia 2003).

Dehydration in children

Children, especially infants, are at risk of body fluid and electrolyte imbalance. The reasons why children require a greater intake of water than adults are explained in Table 25.3. As the extracellular fluid is in direct contact with the outside world, and given that, the younger the child, the higher the proportion of extracellular fluid volume, any illness or situation in which fluid intake in the child is reduced or fluid is lost (e.g. acute diarrhoea and vomiting) creates potential for or actual imbalances (Elliot 2007, Endom et al 2008).

For example, a fever above 38°C requires an increase in the child's fluid intake of 10–12% because of the increased radiant heath, and thus water, loss. Tachypnoea similarly increases the child's fluid requirement two- to three-fold. Children undergoing surgery (because of the period of fasting involved and anaesthesia-related vasodilation), those on cancer chemotherapy, those who sustain moderate to severe burns and scalds, or present with vasco-occlusive sickle-cell painful crisis are all at risk of body fluid and electrolyte imbalance. Finally, any major systemic disease or trauma, and limited paediatric knowledge and expertise in both nursing and medical practice, can increase the risk of body fluid and electrolyte imbalance in children. Thus, it is important that when a child enters into a healthcare setting, the people caring for that child know and care about what they are doing, highlighting possible inadvertent care deficits and attendant risks in managing the child's fluid and electrolyte requirement.

Definition and causes of dehydration in children

Dehydration means an excessive loss of body water. Body fluid depletion occurs when EC loss exceeds fluid intake and retention. The phenomenon is usually accompanied by electrolyte imbalance, which causes fluid shifts to occur between all three compartments, with the child being in a negative fluid balance. Children, especially infants, have an increased propensity to dehydration because their total body water exceeds solid body mass.

Water forms a significant proportion of the child's body weight and therefore weight loss, except in circumstances such as malnutrition, is a reliable method of ascertaining body fluid deficit in children. Any recent weight loss in excess of 3% of previous weight is indicative of body fluid deficit. In circumstances where a previous or current weight cannot be ascertained, the physical appearance and cardiovascular parameters of the child are useful alternatives.

Acute diarrhoea and vomiting from gastroenteritis is the most common cause of dehydration in children caused by viruses, e.g. rotavirus or norovirus ~ 70%, bacteria, e.g. *Campylobacter jejuni* or *Salmonella* spp ~ 10–20% (Elliot 2007), (see the scenario later in this chapter). Dehydration in the child can occur for any of the reasons below:

Reduced fluid intake:

- frank neglect or water unavailability
- inadvertent fluid restriction that underestimates maintenance requirement
- poor swallowing as in severe cerebral palsy or undiagnosed oesophageal atresia
- uncompensated intake in excessive renal loss as the infant/toddler with diabetes insipidus
- anorexia due to psychiatric illness or adverse effects of drugs
- the unconscious child or one in a coma especially if they are alone/undiscovered.

- Increased body fluid loss:
  - excessive gastrointestinal loss
  - vomiting/emesis due to systemic disease or adverse effects of drugs, e.g. chemotherapy
  - acute or chronic diarrhoea, such as viral or bacterial infection of the gastrointestinal tract, or malabsorption syndromes causing osmotic diarrhoea
  - excessive loss from stomas or fistulae.
- Excessive renal loss:
  - adverse effects of osmotic or other forms of diuretics
  - adrenal insufficiency
  - salt-losing nephropathy
  - chronic renal failure
  - diabetes insipidus, especially in young children unable to compensate their renal loss by thirst satiety.
- From skin and respiratory tract:
  - hyperpyrexia
  - heat exposure
  - cystic fibrosis
  - severe burns.

Types of dehydration in children

Biochemical classification of childhood dehydration considers sodium as the principal extracellular cation and, as such, embodies the contextual classification. Symptoms usually appear in the child when the plasma sodium is less than 120 mmol/L or more than 150 mmol/L (Robertson et al 2007).

Isonatraemic dehydration

- plasma sodium 130–145 mmol/L
- plasma osmolality 275–295 mOsm/kg H_2O.

Isonatraemic dehydration is the most common form of dehydration, affecting approximately 70% of children who present with body fluid and electrolyte imbalance. Here, the solute loss equals water loss in the relatively healthy child with effective renal compensation. No change occurs in the tonicity or osmolality of fluids within the three compartments, thus there are no transmembrane fluid shifts. The extracellular compartment, being the most accessible to the external environment, bears the brunt of the fluid loss and contracts, reducing the CBV with the attendant hypovolaemia. Losses from the gastrointestinal tract, such as diarrhoea and vomiting, are the most common cause of isotonic dehydration in children (Dalby-Payne & Elliot 2008).

Hyponatraemic dehydration

- plasma sodium <130 mmol/L
- plasma osmolality <275 mOsm/kg H_2O.

Scenario

Nicola is a 12-week-old infant who presented with 10% (severe) dehydration caused by acute diarrhoea. She was born at term weighing 3.3 kg. She is admitted to the ward with her mother, and has a 2-day history of vomiting and passing frequent loose watery stools. She appears irritable, her cry is weak and she has poor muscle tone. Her recorded weight 1 week ago was 5 kg. Conclusion from investigations and clinical assessment indicates a state of 10% severe dehydration caused by her acute diarrhoea.

Nicola's clinical assessment and investigations

- Present body weight: 4.5 kg
- Blood urea: 8 mmol/L (normal range: 3–7)
- Axilla temperature: 38°C (normal range: 36–37°C)
- Plasma sodium: 146 mmol/L (normal range: 135–145)
- Plasma potassium: 5.4 mmol/L (normal range: 3.5–5.5)
- Plasma osmolality: 300 mOsm/kg/kg H_2O (normal range: 275–295)
- At rest:
  - heart rate per minute: 180 (normal range: 110–160)
  - packed cell volume: 48% (normal range: 28–42)
  - respiratory rate per minute: 52 (normal range: 30–40)
  - systolic blood pressure: 68 mmHg (normal range: 70–90)
- Extremities = cold and mottled
- Eyes contour = sunken
- Mucous membranes = dry lips and tongue
- Skin = hot, dry and lax
- Urine = small quantity; very concentrated
- Stools = loose and watery
- 10% dehydration from acute diarrhoea.

Hyponatraemic dehydration may be seen in about 10% of children. Causes include excessive solute loss in urine (as in diuretic therapy), severe burns, vomiting and acute/chronic diarrhoea. In this condition the net fluid loss contains more salt than water. Children may be managed inadvertently with hypotonic intravenous fluids (Robertson et al 2007) or encouraged to drink large volumes of sugary drinks to counterbalance the fluid loss. The cells will take up the glucose and leave the extra water in the extracellular compartment. As a result, a transmembrane fluid shift will occur from the extracellular to the intracellular compartment. So, the predominant water loss is once more from the extracellular compartment, resulting in reduced CBV and hypovolaemia. Here, the symptoms of dehydration can be more severe and should be considered in the child who presents with circulatory shock even in the absence of an apparent significant history of fluid loss.

Hyponatraemic dehydration should be distinguished from hyponatraemic water intoxication or hypervolaemia in the child with syndrome of inappropriate ADH (SIADH) where ADH is released in excessive amounts for a state of hydration.

Hypernatraemic dehydration

- Plasma sodium >145 mmol/L
- Plasma osmolality >295 mOsm/kg H_2O.

This form of dehydration affects about 20% of the children seen. Here, water loss occurs without the corresponding salt loss, i.e. a proportionally greater loss of water than salt. Examples include diabetes insipidus in the child with limited self-care, increased insensible loss in hyperyrexia and hyperventilation or inadvertent excessive administration of hypertonic intravenous fluid. As the extracellular fluid compartment is hypertonic, fluid moves across the membrane from the intracellular to the extracellular compartment to dilute the more concentrated plasma. It includes hyperglycaemia as in diabetes mellitus. In the end, both the intracellular and extracellular compartments are fluid depleted but the clinical manifestations may not be very obvious in the early stages. It can be difficult to predict the degree of dehydration in young children (Duggan et al 1996).

Principles of assessing and caring for the child presenting with dehydration

Nursing assessment is the first and principal step in the care of the child presenting with dehydration, as in the case of Nicola in the scenario. The assessment process should be holistic, comprehensive, child-focused and family-centred, regardless of the conceptual framework or nursing model around which it is based. Assessment is the systematic and continuous collection, organisation, validation and documentation of patient information, forming an integral part of the nursing process. It involves communicating accurate and reliable data about a child to relevant people in the healthcare team (Berman et al 2008, Smith et al 2004). To assist with Nicola's assessment, the following questions will be asked:

1. What evidence – from the most reliable clinical manifestations in Nicola's case – predicts the degree of dehydration?

This question is fundamental in the effective management of the child with suspected body fluid and electrolyte imbalance. Data derived during the assessment process must be reliable if effective decision making for the subsequent management of the child is to be achieved. There are differing opinions as to which clinical features suggest an accurate degree of dehydration. Categories such as 'mild', 'moderate' and 'severe' have been, and continue to be used in the clinical setting. Current evidence suggests that there is a fine divide between mild and moderate dehydration. Work by Duggan et al (1996) on the validity of the clinical signs of dehydration in young children identifies the following as the most reliable data source for estimating the degree of dehydration in infants aged 3–18 months with acute diarrhoea:

- Prolonged skinfold
- Altered neurological status
- Sunken eyes
- Dry oral mucous membranes.

Also, Steiner et al (2004) in work reviewing clinically useful signs for detecting 5% dehydration, concluded these to be:

- Abnormal capillary refill time
- Abnormal skin turgor
- Abnormal respiratory pattern.

Friedman et al (2004) in their study of 137 children averaging 18 months, diagnosed with gastroenteritis, proposed a four – item clinical scale of:

- General appearance
- Eyes
- Mucous membrances
- Tears.

Their scale, they explain, is intended to discriminate between and evaluate the responses to therapeutic strategies.

Weight loss is the 'gold standard' for estimating fluid deficit, and weight gain is used as the criterion from which to estimate progress or recovery from the state of dehydration. This is because recent weight loss in the otherwise well child usually means some loss of total body water, and not loss of mean mass. The evidence - based criteria hold individual merits in determining the degree of dehydration thus illness severity in the child and young person, provided the practitioner has insight into the biological and clinical relevance they hold in body fluid and electrolyte imbalance. Informed critical thinking is essential to safe, effective practice in the 21st century if best use is to be made of clinical data obtained on patient assessement (Berman et al 2008).

2a. What information is needed about Nicola?

- Medical examination and outcomes
- Blood investigations and results
- Urine investigations and results
- Her:
    - present and past illness history
    - physical appearance
    - physiological parameters
    - behaviour, activity, alertness.

Objective data are obtained by the nurse assessing the child; subjective data are information obtained from the child, as age permits, or their parent.

2b. Why is this information about Nicola required?

- Baseline observation of her vital signs provides a reference point for future care and management.
- Changes and/or trends in her baseline observations suggest improvement or further deterioration, and thus guide practice.
- It helps establish actual and potential problems to be used in planning, implementing and evaluating care.

3. How are data about Nicola ascertained?

- Prerequisite knowledge-base:
  - Common sense: assessment process
  - Intellectual sense: child development
- Age-related parameters
- Effects of hospitalisation on the child (Nicola) and family
- Effective communication skills: with Nicola, with her mother and with colleagues participating in her care
- Accurate measurement:
  - Technical skills and competence
  - Correct use of equipment
- Analysis and synthesis of data collected from which biological or clinical relevance should emerge
- Accurate documentation of data
- Clinical reasoning to guide timely appropriate and safe action in Nicola's care, e.g. nursing care, fluid and electrolytes therapy, communication/liaison with colleagues

4. What happens to the data after collection?

- Categorised and used to structure care
- Accurate, timely and complete documentation of care, i.e. not haphazard or on bits of paper
- Clinical analysis and reasoning
- What the data mean
- The significance of the data:
  - How ill she is?
  - Is she getting better?
  - Is she getting worse?
- Whether the findings from the data require immediate action
- Who to communicate with within the multiprofessional team
- Nursing care following observations in Nicola's best interest.
- Identification of Nicola's:
  - actual problems; potential problems
  - healthcare needs; parents' needs
- Planning Nicola's nursing care by setting child- and family-centred goals or suggesting child-focus expected outcomes of care
- Prioritising and implementing Nicola's care
- Evaluating her care
- Adapting/making changes in her care accordingly.

The above questions and their explanatory statements are expanded on in Chapter 11 of Berman et al (2008).

Nursing assessment and biochemical investigations

The scenario presents Nicola as very ill, with severe dehydration. As this is a life-threatening condition, her vital organs (brain, heart, lungs, kidneys) require effective physiological support. For this reason, the Roper–Logan–Tierney (1990) nursing model is applied for Nicola's care delivery and management. Data collection would start in the A & E department and be completed in the admission or ambulatory unit. It would include the following observations.

Breathing

This relates to Nicola's heart and lung function. Baseline observations will be made on admission onto ward:

- Readings at rest:
  - Respiratory rate per minute
  - Respiratory quality: effort, rhythm, depth
  - Heart rate per minute
  - Quality of heart rate: regularity; volume
  - Capillary refill less or over 2–3 seconds
  - Blood pressure: mean arterial pressure; systolic value.
- Colour and warmth of her limbs/extremities
- Comparison with age group as young infant.

The scenario indicates tachycardia and tachypnoea because the severe dehydration is compromising her heart and lung function.

Eating and drinking

Nicola's physical appearance, cardiopulmonary parameters and biochemical assays indicate that she is severely dehydrated, which is a life-threatening condition. The biological reasons for her clinical features are explained in Table 25.8. Her ongoing assessment should include:

- Body weight: degree of weight loss. A cloth or towel would be put on a clean scale, zeroed then used to record Nicola's weight without her nappies on.
- Whether she is formula or breast fed
- Amount of feeds for that day, if any
- Whether she is retaining or vomiting the feeds
- Consistency and amount of vomitus
- Onset and history of diarrhoea
- Volume, consistency and frequency of diarrhoea
- Integrity of Nicola's skin and mucous membranes
- Integrity and contour of her eyes.

Evidence suggests that the general appearance, skinfold integrity, dryness of mucous membranes, neurological, cardivascular

Table 25.8 Reasons for abnormal blood chemistry in diarrhoea

Nicola's blood chemistry	Possible reasons
Elevated plasma urea	Reduced CBV thus reduced GFR and excretory capacity of the kidneys as less water is delivered to them
Raised plasma sodium and potassium	Reduced ECF and ICF volume/water content means a higher solute concentration
Raised plasma osmolality	Reduced ECF means less water in blood vessels and thus a concentrated plasma
Raised packed cell volume	Reduced CBV means a reduction in the usual 55% plasma content of blood, thus a raised cellular component of the blood

CBV, circulating blood volume; ECF, extracellular fluid; GFR, glomerular filtration rate; ICF, intracellular fluid.

and respiratory status of the child who is dehydrated are the most reliable clinical data to show the degree of dehydration in children (Friedman et al 2008).

Personal cleansing and dressing

This aspect of assessment will focus on Nicola's general state, and will ascertain the following:

- Nicola's skin:
  - Cleanliness
  - Any rash
  - Redness
  - Integrity of her nappy area.
- Clothing: not necessarily new/expensive but clean
- How her mother usually meets her hygiene needs, i.e. baby soap/cream/lotion, as unit policy/guideline suggests
- General status of her scalp, eyes and face in general, e.g. cradle cap or sticky eyes
- Nicola's state of physical comfort
- The healthy state of her mouth, e.g. presence or absence of oral thrush/candida.

Microbiological studies to rule out any other forms of infection, e.g. urinary tract infection. Stool specimens may be requested to rule out any bacterial infection but, as the scenario shows, the conclusion is that she has acute diarrhoea of viral origin.

Maintaining a safe environment

Here, both the physical safety and psychological safety will be assessed:

- How restless or irritable Nicola is, in view of what is indicated in the scenario
- How settled she is between care or handling
- Whether she appears to be in pain or not
- Physical environment of her room and cot area:
  - Suction equipment, oxygen and emergency buzzer in working order
  - Equipment for basic life support
  - Safety of her cot in terms of contents/breaks
  - Safety of all other equipment required for her care, e.g. intravenous volumetric pumps, cardiac monitors, apnoea alarm
  - Equipment to facilitate effective infection control, e.g. hand washing utensils, disposable units, gloves and aprons.
- Nurse call alarm in her room in working order
- Necessary documents, e.g. fluid balance charts, observation charts, treatment chart, intravenous prescription chart
- Awareness of the nurse about their areas of accountability and responsibility
- Ensuring that Nicola's mother knows and understands the safety aspects of her care, in particular infection prevention and control
- How anxious Nicola's mother is
- Ascertaining main areas of anxiety for Nicola's mother, e.g. contact with her husband/partner about Nicola's admission
- Contacting Nicola's father – by her mother or ward if appropriate.

Eliminating

This will build on what was presented in the scenario, covering Nicola's:

- urine output:
  - volume
  - specific gravity (may not be a valid method to determine the degree of dehydration in children presenting with gastroenteritis (Steiner et al 2007)
  - frequency
- stools:
  - characteristics
  - consistency
  - amount
  - colour
  - frequency
  - odour
- changes in urine output and bowel habit as noted by her mother
- presence of tears when she cries
- vomitus:
  - amount
  - frequency
  - colour
  - consistency
- estimated production of 10 mL/kg/stool or vomitus.

A urine bag or pad may be applied on Nicola to obtain and carry out a clinitest on her urine. A concentrated urine with a raised specific gravity and osmolality that shows nothing else abnormal is indicative of dehydration.

Nicola's nappies may be weighed to assess urine output. The dry nappies are weighed before being applied on Nicola. The wet nappies are then weighed after removal and the gram-by-gram difference assumed as the amount of urine passed as 1 g dry weight is equivalent to 1 mL water.

Communicating

Communication with Nicola will be three-fold, i.e. that with Nicola even as an infant; with her parents, in particular her mother, on admission; and interprofessional and multidisciplinary communication:

- with Nicola: communication involves mainly obtaining data from her physical, behavioural, biochemical and physiological assessment:
  - making use of observation skills
  - concrete data
  - elusive/indirect subtle data
  - individual hunches
- with Nicola's parents:
  - history of the onset and progress of Nicola's diarrhoea and vomiting
  - changes observed in their child
  - their main worries and anxieties
  - specific information they wanted to know about Nicola, her care/treatment
- with colleagues:
  - accurate documentation
  - who the key members of the team are
  - their key areas of responsibility
  - nursing areas of accountability and responsibility: who is to be informed about her admission and assessment data

Mobilising

As well as the presentation in the scenario, the following areas will be assessed:

- Nicola's:
  - general activity
  - muscle tone: twitching; excessive tone
  - crying pattern
  - restful state or irritability
  - muscle weakness, abdominal distension: potassium deficit
  - sleep state/alert state
  - quality of chest wall movement on respiration.
- Nicola's physical care: how often she will be cared for physically.

- Anticipatory information on future care:
  - Home environment
  - Health education/health promotion.
  - Discharge home: any socio-economic issues to be addressed, e.g. home environment and parenting skills.

Working and playing

As Nicola is acutely ill at present, this relates mainly to her environment and the interaction with the following:

- How humanising or distressing her room/cot area is.
- What type of toys are safe and appropriate in the area.

Controlling body temperature

This area of assessment will similarly build on what was presented in the scenario.

- Ambient temperature: room temperature noted: too hot/too cold
- Nicola's body temperature:
  - Safest route of measurement per axilla or abdominal
  - Whether the pyrexia is resolving
  - How hot her skin/cheeks appear and feel
  - How warm her extremities feel.

Expressing sexuality

Nicola's assessment in this area will relate mainly to the manner in which her parents present the following:

- Clothes she wears
- Any preferred favourite clothing by her mother
- Which safe toys to be displayed in her cot.

Dying

Nicola's parents will be very anxious because their daughter is acutely ill. Many questions will be going through their minds about their daughter's illness, prognosis and future. Assessment thus includes:

- their main areas of worry
- their understanding of her illness
- their understanding about her treatment
- their conception of the reasons and use of machinery in her room
- areas they would like to discuss with medical staff
- specific close family members they would like to be informed and have present for support during their daughter's hospitalisation.

From the assessment and scenario content, the actual and potential problems are identified, care prioritised, planned, implemented and evaluated.

Biochemical investigations

Medical investigations of the child with body fluids and electrolytes imbalance include physical examination to establish the degree of dehydration. There is no evidence to support routine analysis of urea, electrolytes and creatinine. Children presenting with severe/moderate dehydration should have urea, electrolytes and creatinine estimated, e.g. Nicola in the scenario. Here, a combination of measures rather than a single one can improve diagnosis (Wilkinson et al 2008). Serum electrolyte measurements are essential before and after starting intravenous hydration or in suspected hypernatraemia (Elliot 2007). Biochemical assays should include plasma or serum electrolytes, osmolality, urea, pH, bicarbonate, glucose, calcium and also urine osmolality. Deviations from the norm or reference values shown in Table 25.7 usually mean that the child's body is unable to maintain normal control or balance either by excretion or conservation of body water or electrolytes (Linné & Ringrud 1999). Because an accurate chemical analysis of body fluids depends on their appropriate collection, handling and care, each specimen should be obtained, stored and transported to the laboratory in the correct manner. Hyperkalaemia can be misdiagnosed in the child who has had a traumatic specimen collection or a blood specimen stored or transported wrongly to cause haemolysis and thus release intracellular potassium from the red blood cells. Newer, quicker differential diagnostic stool tests include fahecal lactoferrin and real-time PCR (Gadewar & Fasano 2005)

Poor knowledge in nurses can contribute to problems in professional practice (Copnell 2008). Thus, it is essential that nurses know the age-related reference 'normal' values and understand the clinical significance of any changes in them. This way, practitioners can become aware of what the change means for the child's biological function (see Table 25.8) and take timely and appropriate nursing action, e.g. alerting or summoning medical staff to prescribe the necessary adjustment in the child's fluid and electrolyte therapy.

Personal experience shows that failure to take a timely and appropriate action on receiving a child's blood results may end with a gravely ill and prostrated/collapsed child by the end of a shift, so knowing the normal reference values and being aware of what they mean for the child are fundamental aspects of care in the child with body fluid and electrolyte imbalance. Work by Skinner (2007) supports these assertions.

There is evidence to suggest that simple urine tests for specific gravity and ketonuria are appropriate in assessing the child with a moderate (some) degree of dehydration (Nager & Wang 2002). Clincial manifestations are usually evident when the child has lost at least 5% of their body weight (Elliot 2007). High risk groups include infants up to 6 months, those that have more than eight diarrhoeal stools or more than four significant episocles of vomiting in 24 hours, and commorbity such as short gut syndrome or metabolic disease (Wilkinson et al 2008).

Therapeutic strategies in caring for the child with body fluid and electrolyte imbalance

The hydration state of the child including a recently documented weight loss will influence the child's immediate management strategies.

Severe dehydration and electrolyte imbalance such as that depicted in Nicola is a life-threatening situation. Indeed, body fluid loss (e.g. blood loss or acute diarrhoea) or fluid maldistribution (e.g. oedema in heart failure or nephrotic syndrome) are major causes of cardiac arrest in children. As such, the ABCD principles of paediatric resuscitation apply (BMJ 1999). The scenario shows that Nicola's respiratory status, although overworking to compensate for her dehydration state, is not in any immediate danger. However, her cardiovascular status is very compromised because of the 10% dehydration state. The ultimate goal of any therapeutic strategy is to restore her circulating blood volume and improve her tissue cell perfusion, especially her vital organs such as her brain, heart and kidneys. A rational fluid and electrolyte regime must therefore be commenced with the following therapeutic goals (Arfors & Buckley 1997, Armon et al 2001, Johnson & Sullivan 2003):

- Carry out a comprehensive and holistic assessment to accurately estimate Nicola's degree of dehydration and fluid deficit.
- Restore her circulating blood volume or intravascular fluid volume to establish an effective cardiac output, colloidal osmotic pressure and tissue perfusion.
- Maintain Nicola's interstitial and intracellular fluid and electrolytes by administering the most appropriate colloidal plasma substitute or physiologically balanced crystalloid solution.
- Establish and treat the cause of her dehydration through the most appropriate differential diagnosis.
- Prioritise and carry out her nursing care safely, effectively and humanely.
- Evaluate care and adapt management accordingly.
- Prepare Nicola's parents for a safe and smooth discharge home to prevent or minimise recurrence of her diarrhoea.

Evidence-based principles of care in dehydration and electrolyte imbalance caused by acute diarrhoea

Calculation of percentage dehydration

$$\text{Nicola's pre-illness weight} = 5\,\text{kg}$$

$$\text{Nicola's present weight} = 4.5\,\text{kg}\,[1\,\text{kg} = 1000\,\text{g}]$$

WWW

- http://www.archdischild.com
- http://www.WHO.org
- http://www.ESPGAN.org

Nicola's fluid deficit

$$\text{Pre-illness weight (kg)} - \text{present weight (kg)}$$

$$5000\text{ g} - 4500\text{ g} = 500\text{ g} = 500\text{ mL fluid deficit}: 1\text{ g} = 1\text{ mL}$$

Calculating Nicola's fluid requirement will determine her fluid deficit plus her maintenance requirement.

Prevention

- Is always better and more cost-effective than cure.
- Presently, several pathogens are targeted in developing new/improved vaccines, e.g: rotavirus and campylobacter (Gadewar & Fasano 2005).
- Breastfeeding, especially if exclusive and longer is protective against infectious gastroenteritis.
- Improved hygiene, safe water supply and infection prevention and control are the corner stone of care.

Nursing, as any other practice-based discipline, requires a body of professional knowledge, which is critical to effective clinical reasoning and decision making (Higgs & Tichen 2000). On this note, research evidence continues to highlight deficits in knowledge and practices of caregivers (Bachrach & Gardner 2002) and parents, (Datta et al 2001) and the conflicts between the beliefs and knowledge of doctors about the nutritional management of children with acute diarrhoea (Carral-Terrazas et al 2002). Such evidence has implications for the management and health promotion/education role of health professionals. Here, logical thinking and common sense should prevail, as this promotes safe use of knowledge that guides the clinical judgement, clinical reasoning and the decision-making process. Vandenplas et al (2007) suggest that treatment of these children should focus on the key pathology, i.e. body fluid and electrolyte loss and gut ecosystem disturbance.

Oral rehydration therapy (ORT) (Elliot 2007):

- Children with no or some dehydration can be managed at home if conditions permit.
- Oral rehydration solution (ORS) should be the standard treatment in moderate dehydration, preferable to other clear fluids.
- A fine bore nasogastric tube can be used to rehydrate children not well enough to feed orally.
- Cola, apple juice, fruit juice, cordials and sports drinks are hyperosmolar and low in sodium thus, may exacerbate diarrhoea and should be avoided. It can also compound the child's dehydration by causing osmotic fluid shift from blood vessels into the gut lumen.

Intravenous infusion therapy

- The circulating blood volume is restored in children with hypovolaemia prior to rehydration.
- Children with severe dehydration, like Nicola in the scenario, are admitted for intravenous infusion (IVI) therapy.

Hartling et al (2008) in a Cochrane review comparing ORT to IVI found no important clinical difference between ORT and IVI, and recommend that children with mild–moderate dehydration secondary to gastroenteritis should initially be treated with ORT. This review found that rehydration in 25 children treated with ORT failed and they required IV therapy.

In managing the child's fluid and electrolyte therapy, healthcare professionals should exercise diligence, conscientiousness and vigilance. Iatrogenic (treatment-related) hyponatraemia is a real health threat, attributed to the adminstration of hypotonia IV fluids, over hydration – in some cases > 120% maintenance fluid – and inadequate monitoring of the children's urea and electrolytes (Armon et al 2008, Hoorn et al 2006). Safe effective care includes cannula site care, 24-hour accurate fluid balance chart and careful documentation:

- NPSA Alert 22 – Use of hypotonic IV fluids see http://www.npsa.nhs.uk
- Coulthard (2008) puts an impressive argument forward for the use of the currently recommended IV fluid in childhood dehydration.

Diet

(See Elliot 2007, Gadewar & Fasano 2005, Harris et al 2008, Vandenplas 2007):

- The gastrointestinal tract continues to reabsorb nutrients.
- Breastfed infants should continue to be fed on demand.
- Over 80% of infants with diarrhoea and vomiting absorb their milk formula.
- Formula fed: infants should resume their full strength milk feeds as soon as rehydration is reestablished: amounts offered should be sufficient to satisfy energy and nutrients needs.
- Zinc supplements have considerable beneficial effects on the clinical course of acute diarrhoea and reduce associated complications and mortality.
- Probiotics are a useful adjunct to ORS, reduce diarrhoea duration and hospital stay. Selective strains of probiotics result in satistically significant and clinically moderate benefit. Their use is cost-effective.
- Children should resume normal diet once appetite returns.
- Early introduction of age-appropriate complementary (weaning) diets can include complex carbohydrates, lean meat, yogurt and vegetables.
- Foods high in fats and sugars should be avoided.
- Lactose intolerance is now rare, and considered if diarrhoea persists more than 7 days. Children should continue breastfeeding unless they have very sore buttocks: lactose-free formula can be given for 3–4 weeks, then the infant reintroduced to their usual milk formula.

Antidiarrhoeal agents

(See Gadewar & Fasano 2005, Su-Ting et al 2007, Tormo et al 2008)

- Motility-altering drugs can worsen colonisation.
- They can prolong microorganism excretion time through intestinal stasis.
- Opioids and anticholinergics are not recommended.
- Racecadotril is presently proposed as the new 'wonder drug' in acute diarrhoea, even though adverse drug reaction studies have not yet been carried out.
- Serious side effects were demonstrated in the use of loperamide in children younger than 3 years of age namely ileus, lethargy and death.
- Unit guidelines development groups recommend that no antidiarrhoeal agents should be used.
- Loperamide is not recommended in children for the treatment of acute gastroenteritis.

Thus, the risks of antidiarrhoeal agents outweigh the benefits in less than 3-year-olds, malnourished children, moderate–severely dehydrated children, and those presenting with bloody diarrhoea or systemic illness.

Antiemetics

(See Harris et al 2008, Szajewska et al 2007):

- Most studies in the area have focused on ondansetron.
- Position papers, scientific studies and expert groups recommend ondansetron use to be avoided in children with diarrhoea and vomiting.
- Metoclopramide does not reduce emesis and appears to increase illness duration and severity, thus it is not recommended for children with diarrhoea and vomiting.
- There is insufficient evidence to recommend the use of ondansetron during acute gastroenteritis in children.
- Alhashimi et al (2008) in a Cochrane review conclude that there is some, albeit weak and unreliable, evidence to favour the use of ondansetron and metaclopramide over placebo to reduce the number of episodes of vomiting in gastroenteritis.

Antibacterial agents

(See Gadewar & Fasano 2005):

- Viruses are the predominent causal agents in childhood acute infectious diarrhoea.
- Most cases are self-limiting.
- Disease duration is not shortened by antimicrobials.
- Antibiotics can increase cost, prolong illness and prolong carrier state especially in *Salmonella* infection.
- Available guidelines recommend specific anitbacterials for specific infections.
- The conclusion is that routine use of antibacterial agents is not recommended, especially in immunocompromised children.

Helmstadler (1998) contends that applied clinical knowledge, on which assessment skills and professional judgement depends, has always been the defining characteristic of an effective nurse. Ask any parent what they wish most for regarding their child's imminent hospitalisation and the answer will probably be that their child comes home intact in mind and body. This natural aspiration is unlikely to be realised if the healthcare professionals managing that child's care do not have an adequate and appropriate knowledge to inform their practice. This chapter has presented the applied biological sciences and evidence-based practice that promotes healing and uneventful recovery in the child or young person who presents in the healthcare setting with body fluid and electrolyte imbalance.

References

Alhashimi, D., Alhashimi, H., Fedorowicz, Z., 2008. Antiemetics for reducing vomiting related to acute gastroenteritis in children and adolescents (Review). The Cochrane Library Issue 2 John Wiley, Chichester.

Arfors, E.K., Buckley, P.B., 1997. Pharmacological characterists of colloids. Ballières Clinical Anaesthesiology 11 (1), 15–41.

Armon, K., Riordan, A., Playfor, et al., 2008. Hyponatraemia and hypokalaemia during intravenous fluid administration. Archives of Disease in Childhood 93, 285–287.

Armon, K., Stephenson, T., MacFaul, R., et al., 2001. An evidence and consensus based guideline for acute diarrhoea management. Archives of Diseases in Childhood 85, 132–142.

Au, A.K., Ray, P.E., McBryde, K.D., 2008. Incidence of postoperative hyponatraemia and complications in critically ill children treated with Au and normotenic solution. Journal of Pediatrics 152, 33–38.

Bachrach, L.R., Gardner, J.M., 2002. Caregiver knowledge, attitudes and practices regarding childhood diarrhoea and dehydration in Kingston, Jamaica. Revista Panamericana de Salud Publica 12 (1), 37–44.

Berman, A., Snyder, S.J., Kozier, B., et al., 2008. Kozier and Erb's Fundamentals of nursing. 8th edn. Prentice Hall, Upper Saddler River.

Bourne, L.J., Harmse, B., Temple, N., 2007. Water: a neglected nutrient in the young child? A South African perspective. Maternal and Child Nutrition 3, 303–311.

British Medical Journal (BMJ), 1999. Pre-hospital paediatric life support. BMJ books, London.

Campbell, N.A., Reece, J.B., 2008. Biology, 8th edn. Pearson Benjamin Cummings, San Francisco.

Carral-Terrazas, M., Martinez, H., Flores-Huerta, S., et al., 2002. Beliefs and knowledge of a group of doctors about the nutritional management of the child with acute diarrhoea. Salud Publica de México 44 (4), 303–314.

Celsi, G., Aperia, A., 1999. Endocrine control. In: Barratt, T.M., Avner, E.D., Harmon, W.F. (Eds.), Pediatric nephrology, 4th edn. Lippincott Williams, Baltimore.

Cheethan, T., Baylis, P.H., 2002. Diabetes insipidus in children: pathophysiology, diagnosis and management. Pediatric Drugs 4 (12), 785–796.

Clayton, B.E., Round, J.M., 1994. Clinical biochemistry and the sick child. Blackwell Scientific, Oxford.

Copnell, B., 2008. The knowledgeable practice of critical care nurses: a poststructural inquiry. International Journal of Nursing Studies 4, 588–598.

Coulthard, M.G., 2008. Will changing maintenance intravenous fluid from 0.18% to 0.45% saline do more harm that good? Archives of Diseases in Childhood 93, 335–340.

Dalby-Payne, J., Elliot, E., 2008. Grastroenteritis in children. Clinical evidence concise. American Family Physician 27 (3), February.

Datta, V., John, R., Singh, V.P., et al., 2001. Maternal knowledge, attitude and practices towards diarrhoea and oral rehydration therapy in rural Maharashtra. Indian Journal of Pediatrics 68 (11), 1035–1037.

Davies, J.H., Hassell, L.L., 2007. Children in intensive care: a survival guide. Churchill Livingstone Elsevier, Edinburgh.

Duggan, C., Refat, M., Hashem, M., et al., 1996. How valid are clinical signs of dehydration in children? Journal of Pediatric Gastoenterology and Nutrition 22, 56–61.

Eastwood, M., 1997. The principles of nutrition. Chapman and Hall, London.

Elliot, E.J., 2007. Acute gastroenteritis in children. BMJ 334, 35–40.

Endom, E.E., Somers, M.J., 2008. Treatment of hypervolemia (dehydration) in childen. Last Literature Review Version 16, 1 January.

Figaro, M.K., Mack, G.W., 1997. Control of fluid intake in dehydrated humans: role of oropharyngeal stimulation. American Journal of Physiology 272, R1740–R1746.

Friedman, J.N., Goldman, R.D., Srivastava, R., 2004. Development of a clinical dehydration scale for use in children between 1 and 36 months of age. Journal of Pediatries 145, 201–207.

Gadewar, S., Fasano, A., 2005. Current concepts in the evaluation, diagnosis and management of acute infections in diarrhoea. Current Opinion in Pharmacology 5, 559–565.

Green, M., 2004. Nutrition. In: O'Callaghan, C., Stephenson, T. (Eds.), Pocket paediatrics, 2nd edn. Churchill Livingstone, Edinburgh.

Guyton, A.C., Hall, J.E., 2005. Textbook of medical physiology, 11th edn. Elsevier, Edinburgh.

Hartling, L., Bellemeres, Wiebe, N., 2008. Oral versus intravenous rehydration for treating dehydration due to gastroenteritis in children (Review.) The Cochrane Library Issue 2 John Wiley, Chichester.

Holtbäck, U., Aperia, A.C., 2003. Molecular determinants of sodium and water balance during early human development. Seminars in Neonatolgy 8, 291–299.

Helmstadler, C., 1998. RCN annual conference paper. RCN, London.

Higgs, J., Tichen, A., 2000. Knowledge and clinical reasoning. In: Higgs, J., Jones, M. (Eds.), Clinical reasoning in the health professions. Butterworth-Heinemann, Oxford.

Hoorn, E.J., Lindemans, J., Ziete, R., 2006. Development of a severe hyponatraemia in hospitatized patients: treatment-related risk factors and inadequate management. Nephnelogy Dialysis Transplantation 21, 70–76.

Ichikawa, I. (Ed.), 1990. Pediatric textbook of fluids and electrolytes. Williams and Wilkins, Baltimore.

Johnson, J.E., Sullivan, P.B., 2003. The management of acute diarrhoea. Current Paediatics 13, 95–100.

Linné, J.J., Ringrud, K.M., 1999. Clinical laboratory science the basics and routine techniques, 4th edn. Mosby, St Louis.

Martini, FH., Nath, JL., 2009. Fundamentals of anatomy and physiology 8th edn. Pearson Benjamin Cummings, San Franciso.

Nager, A.L., Wang, V.J., 2002. Comparison of nasogastric and intravenous methods of rehydration in pediatric patients with acute dehydration. Pediatrics 109, 566–572.

Petri, W.A., Miller, M., Binder, H.J., et al., 2008. Enteric infections, diarrhoea and their impact on function and development. The Journal of Clinical Investigations 118 (4), 1277–1290.

Robertson, G., Carrihill, M., Heatherhill, M., et al., 2007. Relationship between fluid management, changes in serum sodium and outcome in hypernatraemia associated with gastroenteritis. Journal of Paediatrics and Child Health 43, 300–305.

Roper, N., Logan, W.W., Tierney, A.J., 1990. The elements of nursing. Churchill Livingstone, Edinburgh.

Ryan, S., Molyneux, E., 1996. Acute paediatrics. Blackwell Science, Oxford.

Skinner, S., 2007. Clinical investigations. In: Walsh, M., Crumbie, A. (Eds.), Watson's clinical nursing and related sciences, 7th edn. Balliere Tindall Elsevier, Edinburgh.

Smith, S.F., Duell, D.J., Martin, B.C., 2004. Clinical nursing skills: basic to advanced skills. Pearson Prentice Hall, Upper Saddle River, USA.

Steiner, M.J., Nager, A.L., Wang, V.J., 2007. Urine specific gravity and other indices: inaccurate tests per dehydration. Pediatric Emergency Care 23 (5), 298–303.

Stricker, E.M., Verbalis, J.G., 1999. Water intake and body fluids. In: Zigmond, M.J., et al., (Eds.), Fundamental neuroscience, Academic Press, San Diego.

Su-Ting, T., Crossman, D.C., Cummings, P., 2007. Loperamide therapy for acute diarrhoea in children: systematic review and meta-analysis. PLoS Medicine 4 (3), e98.

Szajewska, H., Grieruzzczak-Bialek, D., Dylag, 2007. Meta-analysis: for vomiting in acute gastroeteritis in children. Alimentary Pharmacology and Therapeutics 25, 393–400.

Tormo, R., Palanco, I., Salarzar-Lindo, E., et al., 2008. Acute infectious diarrhoea in children: new insights in antesecretary treatment with racecadotril. Acta Paediatrica 97 (8), 1008–1015.

Tortora, G.J., Derrickson, B.H., 2009. Principles of anotomy and physiology. 12th edn. John Wiley, Chichester.

Vandenplas, Y., Salvatore, S., Viera, M., et al., 2007. Probictics in infectious diarrhoea in children: are they indicated? European Journal of Pediatrics 166, 1211–1218.

Walmsley, R.N., White, G.H., 1994. A guide to diagnosis in clinical chemistry, 3rd edn. Blackwell Science, Oxford.

Wilkinson, H.C., Mazza, F., Turner, T., 2008. Evidence-based guideline for the management of diarrhoea with or without vomiting in children. Australian Family Physician 27 (6), 22–29.

Caring for children with genitourinary problems

26

Kevin McFarlane

ABSTRACT

The kidneys play a major role in maintaining homeostasis. They eliminate waste and maintain the balance of water, pH and electrolytes in the body. Disorders of the genitourinary system may impact on kidney function and present a severe threat to health. The aim of this chapter and the companion PowerPoint presentation is to provide the reader with an insight into common genitourinary tract problems. The chapter focuses on urinary tract infection, nephrotic syndrome, poststreptococcal glomerulonephritis, vesico-ureteric reflux, Wilms' tumour, hypospadias, cryptorchidism, circumcision, acute renal failure and chronic renal failure.

LEARNING OUTCOMES

- Discuss common genitourinary tract conditions with reference to:
  - pathology
  - presenting symptoms
  - diagnosis
  - nursing management
  - medical management
  - potential complications
  - education and prevention.

Introduction

Urinary tract infections (UTI) occur in 1% of boys and 3% of girls before they are 11 years old (Stull & Lipuma 1991). Overall, urinary tract infection is more common in girls but in the first 3 months after birth it is more common in boys. The term 'urinary tract infection' refers to an infection anywhere in the renal tract. It is convenient to categorise urinary tract infections into two groups:

- Lower urinary tract infection: involves the bladder and urethra and tends not to be associated with long-term sequelae.
- Upper urinary tract: involves the ureters and kidneys. Acute pyelonephritis (APN) is the most serious upper urinary tract infection. It is associated with arterial hypertension and chronic renal failure (Jodal 1987).

Escherichia coli

The most common causative organism associated with urinary tract infection is *Escherichia coli* (*E. coli*). This organism is responsible for 80% of infections. *E. coli* is normally found in the large bowel, where it is involved in vitamin K production. The bacteria enter the urethra via the perineum. The cell membrane of the *E. coli* bacterium contains protein structures called adhesions, which facilitate bacterial adhesion to the surface of urogenital cells. This adhesion prevents the bacteria from being washed away during micturition. The infection ascends the urethra and enters the bladder, where the bacteria adhere to the cells that line the internal surface.

Susceptibility to urinary tract infection

Some children are more susceptible than others to urinary tract infection. Uncircumcised boys under 1 year old are more prone than circumcised boys; the short female urethra increases susceptibility in girls. Constipation is linked to repeated urinary tract infection. Constipation impairs voiding by compressing the urethra or the bladder neck. It leads to a high urine residual. This creates the conditions in which bacteria can flourish. Treatment of constipation may result in the resolution of urinary tract infection (Loening-Baucke 1997). Finally, congenital abnormalities of the renal tract place the child at risk. Vesicoureteric reflux is the most common congenital abnormality of the genitourinary tract. Obstructive uropathies are also significant causes of urinary tract infection (Roth et al 2002b).

DOI: 10.1016/B978-0-7020-3183-0.10026-8

PowerPoint

Access the companion PowerPoint presentation, where you will find information on the common obstructive uropathies.

Diagnostic problems

Urinary tract infection in children is problematic because it is not always obvious. In addition, when it is identified it may be difficult to distinguish between a lower and upper urinary tract infection. The younger the child, the more likely these problems are to occur.

Diagnosis in an older child tends to be a little more obvious. An older child with a lower urinary tract infection may present with specific symptoms such as frequency, urgency, dysuria and secondary enuresis. If the infection is in the upper urinary tract, e.g. pyelonephritis, the child may present with fever, flank pain and is obviously ill.

Babies and infants are more difficult to diagnose. This is because presenting symptoms are often non-specific and may not particularly point to genitourinary origins. Possible non-specific symptoms are irritability, vomiting, diarrhoea, poor feeding and failure to thrive. These signs do not generally allow medical staff to predict whether the infection is in the upper or lower genitourinary tract. Fever is the only factor that may point to an upper urinary tract infection but its absence does not negate the possibility.

Collecting urine

In children older than 3 years, a midstream specimen of urine is the method of choice. The logic underpinning the collection of a midstream specimen is that the initial passage of urine flushes bacteria from the urethral orifice and thus reduces the likelihood of contamination. For those younger than 3 years who cannot or are unable to cooperate, an alternative approach is to obtain a clean-catch specimen. The procedure can be time consuming so it is helpful if a parent can be the person collecting the urine. The baby or infant is positioned over a sterile container until voiding takes place.

The use of U-bags is controversial. Collections made by this method are notorious for becoming contaminated; as many as one-third of specimens taken in this way yield false-positive results (Li et al 2002). Uncircumcised boys are particularly at risk. U-bags are commonly used for non-toilet trained children but should not be used in high-risk cases (Al-Orifi 2000).

Urine can also be gathered from absorbent collection pads placed inside nappies. The pads are checked every 10 minutes until the child is found wet. A syringe is then used to aspirate urine from the pad. Although pad specimens are still prone to contamination, there is some evidence that they are more effective than bag specimens (Feasey 1999). There is also evidence that parents prefer to use the pad method when home collection is required (Liaw et al 2000).

The most effective means of attaining an uncontaminated specimen of urine from a child is by suprapubic stab or by catheterisation. Because of pain and the invasive nature of these procedures, they are reserved for high-risk cases. Febrile babies less than 3 months old should have specimens taken by these means. Older non-toilet trained children with features of upper urinary tract infection or a history of urinary tract infection or with known abnormalities should be catheterised to obtain a specimen.

Irrespective of the method of obtaining urine for culture, the specimen should be transferred to a specimen bottle within 30 minutes of collection. It can then be stored in a fridge at 4°C until processing.

Reflect on your practice

- What methods of urine collection are you familiar with?
- Are you totally familiar with the manufacturer's recommendations concerning applying a U-bag?
- Are there times when you use U-bags when a more effective method could be used?

Urine testing

Urine should be screened at ward level. The nurse should be alert to the amount of urine that is produced; it may be diminished in urinary tract infection. The colour is also significant. Healthy urine will lie somewhere between clear and straw coloured. Infected urine is commonly cloudy. The smell of urine is traditionally thought to be a significant factor but it appears not to be a reliable indication of urinary tract infection in children (Struthers et al 2003).

Dipstick testing may prove positive for blood and/or protein. These substances are not particularly predictive of a urinary tract infection; they may be present but equally they may not. Much more predictive is the presence of nitrite and leucocyte esterase. Nitrate is a substance that is normally found in urine. Most bacteria convert nitrate to nitrite; it takes them around 4 hours to do this. This is why morning testing for nitrite is a good idea. A dipstick can also be used to detect the presence of leucocyte esterase. This is an enzyme produced by white blood cells; its presence indicates infection. A urine sample that is positive for leucocyte esterase and nitrites strongly suggests urinary tract infection. Definitive diagnosis is on urine culture.

Antibiotic therapy

Neonates (0–2 months) have immature immune systems. There is a likelihood that an infection could spread beyond the urinary tract. These babies are managed as if they have systemic sepsis and are prescribed parenteral antibiotics that are given for 2–3 weeks.

Children between 2 months and 2 years may also be hospitalised to receive intravenous antibiotics. A child who is unwell, with features such as fever, rigors, vomiting or dehydration, should be admitted. Rapid treatment is required because delay increases the risk of renal damage (Smellie et al 1994).

Parenteral antibiotics are administered for a period of 24–48 hours. This should be followed by a 7–10-day course of oral antibiotics.

Children who are considered to have a lower urinary tract infection and do not appear ill can be managed at home. They are prescribed oral antibiotics. There is a debate about how long the course should be. Some physicians prefer to prescribe a 7–10-day course whereas others prescribe a short course of 2–4 days. There is conflicting evidence in the literature (Keren & Chan 2002, Michael et al 2003) and the debate remains unresolved. Amoxicillin, trimethoprim-sulfamethoxazole and cephalosporin are the drugs of choice (Riccabona 2003).

Nursing considerations

Assessment must include pain, hydration stasis and temperature. The type of pain and the location varies. Pain may occur only on micturition. Bladder spasms may occur. Loin pain may be present. Non-pharmacological methods such as distraction and heat pads should be considered. Analgesia should be prescribed and administered as required. The child may be dehydrated because of reduced intake and increased insensible loss. It is necessary to observe for signs of dehydration and record input and output. The child's weight should also be recorded. Older children can be encouraged to consume adequate fluids but younger children might require intravenous support. Temperature control may be necessary. Children with lower urinary tract infections may have a mild temperature rise. Those with upper urinary tract infections may have more substantial temperature rises. Cooling measures should be implemented and antipyretics administered.

Investigations

Imaging is used during the acute illness and later to identify any damage to the kidneys and any predisposing causes of urinary tract infection. Babies and infants are most likely to be in danger of renal damage associated with genitourinary abnormalities (American Academy of Pediatrics (AAP) 1999). This age group is more likely to be investigated intensively. The diagnostic imaging methods that are usually considered include ultrasonography, dimercaptosuccinic acid scanning and voiding cystourethrogram.

Ultrasonography is a non-invasive test that provides information about the structure of the renal tract and dilation of the collecting system. It can identify dilated or duplicated ureters, ureteroceles and horseshoe kidneys. The test is limited because it cannot identify acute pyelonephritis or subsequent renal scarring. It may also fail to detect hydronephrosis.

Dimercaptosuccinic acid (DMSA) scanning is used during an acute urinary tract infection when an upper urinary tract infection is suspected. It can detect inflammation of the kidney substance and confirms the diagnosis of acute pyelonephritis. Later DMSA scanning can be used to determine the presence of any scarring. It is estimated that between 60 and 65% of children will have a renal scar following an initial insult of acute pyelonephritis (Jakobsson et al 1992).

Micturating cystourethrogram (MCU) provides information about the bladder and flow of urine. It identifies the presence of vesicoureteric reflux and the grade of reflux. An MCU can be carried out before or after the child has completed their initial antibiotic course (Mahant et al 2001). The procedure involves catheterisation and instillation of contrast media. Preparing the child and family before investigation can reduce the distress associated with the procedure. Story-telling and play have both been found to be effective (Phillips et al 1998).

Education and prevention

Children who have had one urinary tract infection are at risk of further infections. There are means of limiting the likelihood of a second infection. Detailed discussion concerning these means must take place. Information given to parents (and children) should be verbal and reinforced on paper.

Reflect on your practice

- Do you provide parents with information sheets on prevention of urinary tract infection?
- Are you satisfied with the clarity of these documents?
- Is the information comprehensive and accurate?

Parents and children should be taught the gross anatomy of the urinary tract and the nature of ascending infection. From this point they can then appreciate the recommended hygiene habits that must be practised. If a child is in nappies, these should be changed as soon as possible after soiling. Perineal hygiene is important in girls, stroking away from the urethra is recommended. Cotton underwear is advisable because synthetic materials may increase heat and sweating and encourage bacterial growth. Bubble baths should not be added to bath water and perfumed soaps are inadvisable. Using bubble baths and perfumed soaps may disturb the urethral flora and encourage bacteria to ascend.

Stasis of urine should be avoided so the child should drink frequently and also be given the opportunity to void every hour or two. Cranberry juice has been recommended as a suitable fluid because of its ability to acidify the urine, this is said to prevent binding of *E. coli*. Some authors find in its favour (Kontiokari et al 2001) whereas others debate its efficacy (Schlager 1999).

It is also necessary to teach parents to look for the features of a urinary tract infection. They may also have to learn how to obtain specimens and test them for nitrite and leucocyte esterase. Finally, the importance of complying with antibiotic therapy should be discussed and the necessity to attend follow-up clinic appointments and investigations should be stressed.

The nephrotic syndrome

The most common form of the nephrotic syndrome (NS) is idiopathic, which accounts for over 85% of presentations (International Study of Kidney Disease in Children 1978) and is the subject of this section. However, there are other causes: in a small number of cases the disorder is congenital, the most common congenital presentation being Finnish-type, an autosomal recessively inherited disease (Holmberg et al 1996). The nephrotic syndrome may also be a consequence of another disease; glomerulonephritis is most commonly implicated.

Pathology

Substances filter from the glomerulus into the nephron through a selective barrier called the basement membrane. Substances move through the barrier on the basis of size and electrical charge. In the nephrotic syndrome the selectivity of this membrane is impaired and the glomerulus allows albumin to escape from the blood into the filtrate. Urine therefore tests positive for protein; the amount of protein lost is often described as massive. The loss of albumin interferes with the body's ability to balance fluids between the various body compartments. Normally, albumin levels provide oncotic pressure that counterbalances the effect of hydrostatic pressure at capillary level. In effect, normal levels of albumin are necessary to maintain fluid within the vascular space. When albumin is lost in the filtrate, hypoalbuminaemia occurs and oncotic pressure falls. The effect is that hydrostatic pressure acts with minimum opposition, fluid shifts into the interstitial space and oedema results.

Sodium levels also play a role in oedema formation. Sodium retention occurs. Traditionally, it was thought that fluid shifts cause hypovolaemia, which triggers the renin-angiotensin mechanism, which, in turn, promotes sodium retention. An alternative view is that nephrotic syndrome causes a primary defect at the tubular level, and that this causes sodium retention (Orth & Ritz 1998).

PowerPoint

Access the companion PowerPoint presentation for a full explanation of fluid movement at the tissue level.

Hypoalbuminaemia is one consequence of the nephrotic syndrome; hyperlipidaemia is another. The levels of cholesterol and triglycerides in the blood rise as a result of increased synthesis by the liver and decreased clearance by the kidneys. Although the exact mechanisms for this are unknown, the potential consequences are a cause for concern. High cholesterol levels have a known association with atherosclerosis and high triglyceride levels may also have atherogenic properties and can cause further renal injury (O'Donnell 2001).

Diagnosis

Nephrotic syndrome should be suspected when a child presents with oedema and proteinuria. In the paediatric age group, urinary protein loss of 50 mg/kg per 24 hours or greater is a firm diagnostic criterion (Roth et al 2002a); other markers are hypoalbuminaemia and hyperlipidaemia. Diagnosis is usually made without resorting to biopsy during the initial illness. This approach is taken because the majority of children have idiopathic nephrotic syndrome and their biopsies reveal the same results: they demonstrate damage to the glomerular epithelial foot processes. This is called minimal change nephrotic syndrome. A biopsy is reserved for children who do not respond to treatment. Although biopsy in these cases is still likely to reveal minimal change nephrotic syndrome (International Study of Kidney Disease in Children 1978), a few will identify other microscopic changes that might signify a different approach to treatment and different long-term outlook.

Medical treatment

Corticosteroids are used to treat nephrotic syndrome, prednisolone being the drug of choice. The standard course is 8 weeks. A typical protocol might be 2 mg/kg daily for 4 weeks, then 1.5 mg/kg on alternate days for 4 weeks. Some children will relapse and require long-term maintenance. The earliest predictor that suggests a relapsing course is the time it takes the child to enter remission after prednisolone treatment is initiated (Constantinescu et al 2000). The child on long-term maintenance may receive prednisolone daily or every second day. There is evidence that alternate day regimes may be more beneficial and produce fewer side effects (Hiraoka et al 2003). If the child is commenced on long-term maintenance then the parents must be aware of possible side effects, such as increased appetite, weight gain and cushingoid symptoms. Parents also have to know about possible psychological side effects. Anxiety, depression and difficult behaviour are all possibilities (Soliday et al 1999).

Some children may be resistant to steroid therapy and others may suffer unacceptable side effects because of prolonged use. These children are likely to be prescribed immunosuppressive or immunomodulator drugs such as cyclosporine A, cyclophosphamide or levamisole. All these agents are associated with significant potential adverse effects and there is no consensus as to which is the most appropriate (Durkan et al 2001).

Diuretics are reserved for treating substantial oedema. Furosemide (Lasix) a loop diuretic is commonly prescribed. It is used judiciously because it may result in hypovolaemia, which in turn might increase the likelihood of thrombosis. Albumin may be used in conjunction with furosemide if severe oedema and complications such as pleural effusion or ascites are present.

Complications

Distribution of hydrostatic and oncotic pressure across the pleural and peritoneal membranes is altered. Fluid may shift into the pleural space and cause a pleural effusion. It may also shift into the peritoneal space and cause ascites. Both conditions impair lung expansion and respiratory distress may result. Treatment involves administration of diuretics and albumin.

Children with the nephrotic syndrome are prone to infection; chickenpox is a particular threat. Chickenpox is caused by the varicella-zoster virus and can have devastating effects on an immune-suppressed child. The child's immune status should be checked and, if not immune to varicella-zoster and exposed to chickenpox, then varicella-zoster immune globulin should be administered. Acyclovir prophylaxis may also be administered as an adjunctive (Goldstein et al 2000).

Peritonitis is also a potential threat. Any abdominal pain must be carefully assessed with this complication in mind. The causative organism is usually a pneumococcus and pneumococcal immunisation is recommended for all children. Penicillin prophylaxis may be given to some subgroups (McIntyre & Craig 1998).

The final complication is thromboembolism. Children are prone to both arterial and venous thrombosis. Disturbances in clotting and fibrinolytic systems occur; antithrombin III levels may be depleted and fibrinogen levels raised. High cholesterol and triglyceride levels and low levels of albumin are other risk factors. The presence of dehydration and the use of diuretic also increase susceptibility. Nurses should be cognisant of the features of deep venous thrombosis and pulmonary embolism. With regard to the latter, the development of tachypnoea should raise concern because this might be a sign of pulmonary embolism (van Ommen et al 1998). Thromboembolism requires immediate anticoagulant treatment.

Nursing management

Activity

A 10-year-old boy is admitted with significant oedema. His face, abdomen, legs and feet are particularly swollen. He reveals that his scrotum is also oedematous:

- What nursing interventions would you consider appropriate?

Check your answer with the companion PowerPoint presentation.

As the activity above suggests, caring for a child with oedema is a major focus when caring for a child with nephrotic syndrome. Fluid balance is also important. Fluid intake is normally controlled, the child's previous day's input and output being two of the factors that influence the amount prescribed. Diets high in protein (to increase albumin) or low in protein (to rest the kidneys) have been used in the treatment of this condition but they tend to be ineffective. The current approach is to determine the child's normal dietary protein requirements and ensure that these are met. Carbohydrate intake has to be sufficient to ensure that protein intake can be utilised appropriately and not used for energy purposes. Hyperlipidaemia is not generally a cause for concern during the initial illness. If the child does not respond to treatment and hyperlipidaemia becomes a chronic state, dietary measures such as reduced saturated fat and cholesterol intake are advisable. Medications to reduce cholesterol and triglycerides may also be recommended. Finally, because sodium levels may be elevated in the nephrotic syndrome, dietary sodium has to be controlled. Foods high in sodium should not be consumed and salt should not be added to foods during cooking or at meal times.

Measures must be taken to protect the child from infection and identify it if it occurs. To this end, visitors should be infection free and the number of visitors must be controlled. The child should also be observed for signs of infection such as cough, runny nose and sore ears. Temperature, pulse and respiration should also be recorded regularly.

Prognosis

Deaths due to the nephrotic syndrome are rare but do occur. These deaths are normally attributed to peritonitis and thrombus. Most children with idiopathic nephrotic syndrome respond within 10–14 days of treatment; of these, two-thirds will relapse. The parents need to know about this possibility and be in the position to recognise it. They should monitor the child's weight and test urine for protein. These children will require repeated courses of steroids, often for a prolonged period of time. Most will return to normal, although it may take many years.

WWW

Obtain a fact sheet on the nephrotic syndrome at the Great Ormond Street Hospital website:

- http://www.ich.ucl.ac.uk/factsheets/diseases_conditions/congenital_nephrotic_syndrome/

Poststreptococcal glomerulonephritis

Glomerulonephritis is an inflammation of the glomeruli of the kidneys. Poststreptococcal glomerulonephritis (PSGN) is the most common cause of acute glomerulonephritis in children and, as its name suggests, develops after a streptococcal infection. The site of infection is usually the pharynx or the skin. There is a latent period between the original infection and the presentation of poststreptococcal glomerulonephritis. If the source of infection is the pharynx the period is 1–2 weeks, whereas if the source is the skin it is 2–4 weeks. The condition is most often seen in boys and the age of onset is between 3 and 15 years (Simckes & Spitzer 1995).

Pathophysiology

The pathogenesis of poststreptococcal glomerulonephritis is not fully elucidated. There is evidence that a streptococcal component becomes lodged in the glomerular basement membrane (Cu et al 1998); this is the 'planted antigen' theory. Antibodies then fix to the component/antigen, forming an immune complex. The immune complex triggers a second phase, which involves activation of complement. Complement triggers a cascade of events that result in glomerular inflammation. Glomerular capillaries become blocked and impairment of glomerular filtering function occurs. Protein and blood are lost in the urine. The glomerular filtration rate (GFR) falls and urine output diminishes. In some patients, the reduction in the glomerular filtration rate may be significant and the child may develop acute renal failure. The fall in the glomerular filtration rate results in sodium and water retention and the expansion of the blood volume. Body fluid is redistributed and oedema results. Hypertension also occurs. This is partially due to sodium and water retention but other factors are thought to be involved.

PowerPoint

Access the companion PowerPoint presentation for a full explanation of glomerular filtration rate.

Signs and symptoms

The clinical severity of poststreptococcal glomerulonephritis is variable, with some children having mild disease and being asymptomatic (Tasic & Polenakovic 2003). When children have symptoms the onset is usually abrupt. The child suffers from haematuria, mild to moderate proteinuria and oedema. The degree of oedema varies. Mild periorbital oedema may occur or it may be more extensive. In some cases it may be severe with accompanying ascites or pleural effusion. Urine assumes a dark colour because of the presence of blood and protein. Urine output is diminished, some children are oliguric and, as mentioned above, may present with acute renal failure. Hypertension is common; this might be mild but can be severe. If severe, associated symptoms such as headache and visual disturbance occur. The child is usually fatigued. Anaemia, uraemia and hypervolaemia contribute to feelings of tiredness.

Diagnosis

Diagnosis is made on history, examination and a number of investigations. Urinalysis reveals blood, protein and high specific gravity. Throat swabs (or skin swabs) may be positive for streptococcal infection. Blood samples are taken and examined for antibody to streptococci and their extracellular products (Lang & Towers 2001). Antistreptolysin O (ASO) is one example. The normal ASO is < 166 Todd units, in poststreptococcal glomerulonephritis this is raised. Blood is also examined for evidence of complement activity. A reduction in complement elements C3 and C4 are suggestive of poststreptococcal glomerulonephritis.

Management

Antibiotics are administered to eliminate any persistent streptococcal infection; penicillin is the drug of choice. Hospitalisation is not always required but when hypervolaemia, oedema or hypertension are concerns the child is admitted.

Hypervolaemia and the resultant oedema make fluid balance an important focus. All input and output should be accurately documented. The child's weight should also be recorded. Hypervolaemia and oedema can be addressed by restricting fluids and sodium intake. The child's diet should not contain salty foods and salt should not be added. Dietary manipulation alone may be insufficient to deal with more severe problems and diuretics may be required. Loop diuretics such as furosemide act quickly and effectively.

Hypertension may be mild, moderate or severe. The frequency of recording will differ depending on the circumstance. The dietary measures and administration of diuretics taken to relieve oedema and hypervolaemia may be all that is required to reduce the blood pressure. If hypertension is not alleviated by these means then antihypertensive agents are employed. Severe rises in blood pressure require intravenous antihypertensive agents.

Prognosis

The prognosis of poststreptococcal glomerulonephritis is excellent (Kasahara et al 2001). Most children who develop the condition will recover, with blood pressure and renal function returning to normal. However, a small number of children do not recover and go on and develop renal failure (Baldwin et al 1974).

Vesicoureteric reflux

Vesicoureteric reflux (VUR) is the abnormal back flow of urine from the bladder into the ureter or into the ureter and kidneys. The condition may be unilateral or bilateral. VUR is usually a primary disorder caused by an anatomical defect at the junction between the ureter and the bladder. There is solid evidence that VUR has a familial basis (Noe et al 1992). Primary VUR is thought to be an autosomal dominant disorder with incomplete penetrance and variable expression.

Pathology

The ureters enter the bladder at an oblique angle on the posterior right and left lateral surface. The oblique course is continued through the bladder wall. Each ureter terminates in a ureteral orifice found at both sides of the upper level of the trigone. When the intravesical pressure is increased during micturition the detrusor muscle contracts and the intravesical section of the ureters are passively compressed. This valvular mechanism normally prevents reflux. The effectiveness of this mechanism is dependent on an adequate length of intravesical ureter (Belman 1997).

Reflux, urinary tract infection and scarring

VUR predisposes to urinary tract infection because urine that is refluxed into the ureter(s) trickles back into the bladder, producing an increased urine residual, which provides the conditions for an infection to take place. Reflux then provides a route by which the infection can reach the kidney. Urinary tract infection with VUR is associated with renal scarring and is an important cause of hypertension and chronic renal failure in later life.

Investigations

Children with urinary tract infection must be investigated promptly to determine VUR. Young children are particularly at risk and are usually prescribed prophylactic antibiotics until imaging is complete. One of the mainstays in the diagnosis of VUR is micturating cystourography (MSU). This is an invasive procedure involving the trauma of catheterisation, the potential for infection and exposure to radioactivity. There is controversy concerning when it should be used and protocols vary. Because children under 3 years are more prone to VUR, they tend to routinely undergo the procedure. Abdominal X-ray and ultrasound are also usually carried out. Older children, who are not as at risk, may be spared MCU, although this is not always the case. Primary investigation of these children may include abdominal X-ray, ultrasound and DMSA scanning. If these tests suggest reflux then MCU may be required. A positive MCU allows reflux to be graded. Grading influences management.

PowerPoint

Access the companion PowerPoint presentation for further information about grading.

Management

The objective of medical management is to keep the urine infection-free while waiting for spontaneous resolution. This is an effective treatment and can work in all grades of reflux, but the higher the grade the less likely spontaneous resolution is. Medical management involves the prescription of continuous low-dose antibacterial prophylaxis. The drugs are usually given in a single nightly dose.

Prophylaxis is usually discontinued when reflux disappears. This can be expected between 6 and 10 years (Huang & Tsai 1995). Management also emphasises the importance of measures designed to minimise the likelihood of urinary tract infection. The parent/child is taught the importance of adequate fluid intake, appropriate wiping action, regular toileting, double voiding to expel refluxed urine, and avoidance of constipation.

Surgery is considered for patients with grade IV and V reflux. It is considered as an option because spontaneous resolution is less likely. Surgery is also considered when prophylaxis fails to prevent urinary tract infection or further renal damage. Open surgery involves re-implantation of the offending ureter or ureters. The aim of re-implantation is to create an adequate intravesical tunnel, to allow compression of the ureter against the detrusor muscle. The success rate of reimplanation is 95% (Birmingham Reflux Study Group 1984).

An alternative surgical technique avoids open surgery. Endoscopic injection therapy involves using a standard operating cystoscope to visualise the ureteric orifice. A substance is then injected below the epithelial layer, just inside the edge of the orifice. This narrows the lumen. The technique takes about 15 minutes and can be done on a day-patient basis. Teflon was the original injected substance but concerns arose concerning particle migration to lymph, liver and lungs. Bovine collagen was then used but was also considered unsatisfactory because it was reabsorbed. Other products are on the market but it seems that the ideal material has yet to be developed (Leonard 2002). The operation is available in some centres but it is not as successful as open surgery and reoccurrence is a problem.

Follow-up

Children who are being treated prophylactically have to attend clinics on a regular basis, usually 3-monthly. They have their urine checked for infection, and undergo blood pressure and growth monitoring. Clinic appointments also provide the opportunity to reinforce the importance of compliance with medication. Further radiological studies are always necessary to ensure that reflux has not worsened or, more hopefully, that it has actually resolved. If the child has been treated surgically, follow-up continues to be important but the nature of the surveillance changes with fewer specimens required and fewer radiological studies.

Wilms' tumour (nephroblastoma)

Wilms' tumour is the most common abdominal tumour in childhood, affecting 1 in 10,000 children (Birch & Breslow 1995). It most commonly presents between the ages of 1 and 3 years and is seen equally in boys and girls. The condition may be bilateral or unilateral and it may occur as an isolated problem or may be associated with other syndromes or abnormalities.

Wilms' tumour is a malignancy associated with the embryonic cells that form the kidney. Renal stem cells differentiate and are responsible for forming the nephrons and connective tissue. In Wilms' tumour, some of these stem cells are thought to persist and are referred to as 'nephrogenic rests'. These are present at birth and retain their embryonic differentiation potential; they are the precursors of Wilms' tumour. The cells that constitute the rests begin to multiply and differentiate. Wilms' tumours are found to contain normal kidney tissue but they may also contain squamous epithelium, skeletal muscle and cartilage tissue (Coppes et al 1999); sometimes the tumours do not contain any of these recognisable cell types. Anaplasia is the presence of uncharacteristic cell types. These tumours tend to be more aggressive and difficult to treat. Wilms' tumour invades local structures and spreads via the lymphatic system. The most common sites of metastasis are the lungs, liver and brain.

Genetic alterations

The genetic mechanism responsible for Wilms' tumour is complex. Approximately 1% of presentations occur in families in which susceptibility appears to be inherited. The pattern of inheritance is autosomal dominant with incomplete penetrance.

There is strong evidence that the gene that predisposes to this is to be found on chromosome 17 (Rahman et al 1996). A similar percentage of presentations occur as part of recognised syndromes such as aniridia and Beckwith–Weidemann. The majority of cases of Wilms' tumour present sporadically. A number of genes that are implicated in sporadic cases have been identified. One such gene is found on chromosome 11 (11p13). It is known as the Wilms' tumour suppressor gene. Only 5–10% of sporadic Wilms' tumour cases are characterised by this defect. Circumstantial evidence suggests that other genes are involved but the location and identification of these genes are unknown. The involvement of different genes helps to explain why different areas of the kidney are affected and different cell changes take place. It may also explain why the condition is unilateral or bilateral. It is possible that increasing knowledge about the genetic origins of the disorder may lead to earlier diagnosis or even prevention of the condition.

Presentation and diagnosis

The most common initial indication of an isolated Wilms' tumour is an abdominal mass (McLorie 2001). These, often massive, tumours may be identified by a parent or by the GP. Alternative presenting features are malaise, hypertension, abdominal pain and haematuria. Following identification of the mass, an ultrasound is carried out. The ultrasound can detect the solid nature of the tumour and distinguish it from other conditions such as hydronephrosis. Abdominal computerised tomography is then performed, followed by magnetic resonance imaging.

Grading and staging

Therapy involves chemotherapy and surgery for all patients. Radiotherapy is not usually used but may be required when metastasis is present or following surgery when remnants of the tumour are still present. The International Society of Paediatric Oncology (SIOP) has developed protocols that determine management. Staging and grading determine the duration of chemotherapy, and the specific chemotheraputic agents. Staging involves determining the position and extent of the tumour. Staging is determined by visualising techniques such as computerised tomography and magnetic resonance imaging. Grading is concerned with histology; it involves determining the nature of the tumour cells. A needle biopsy of the renal mass prior to initiation of chemotherapy is recommended (Vujanic et al 2003). The histology is described as 'favourable' or 'unfavourable'. A favourable histology demonstrates a tumour composed of recognisable cell types; an unfavourable histology demonstrates anaplasia.

Chemotherapy and surgery

When grading and staging are complete, the child commences on prenephrectomy therapy. The grading and staging determine the protocol the child embarks on. Cytotoxic therapy involves using at least two chemotheraputic agents. The first-line chemotherapy agents used to treat Wilms' tumour include vincristine, actinomycin D and doxorubicin. Pre-nephrectomy chemotherapy induces a dramatic reduction in the size of the tumour (McLorie 2001). Following chemotherapy surgery is conducted. In the case of a unilateral tumour surgery is aimed at complete removal of the affected kidney. Bilateral tumours require a different approach. Surgery is carried out to remove the tumour while conserving functional kidney tissue.

Nursing considerations

The child may present with an abdominal mass but might not feel ill. The focus of care at this point will be on the parents, who will be devastated when the diagnosis is made. One concern in terms of the child is related to the possibility of metastasis. Unnecessary palpitation of the abdomen should be avoided. The child should be handled carefully. There is a danger that malignant cells could be liberated from the tumour if these measures are not taken. Later nursing interventions will focus on problems associated with chemotherapy. Following chemotherapy, interventions are concerned with the preoperative and postoperative care of the child with a nephrectomy.

Prognosis

There is an overall survival rate of 80% (Wilms' tumour: status report 1990). As SIOP continues to fine-tune drug therapy protocols and new drugs become available, even better results may be achieved. There is a low risk of developing secondary cancers related to treatment. Renal malignant neoplasms are more common in children who have been treated for Wilms' tumour than the general population (Cherullo et al 2001).

WWW

For information about cancers see the Cancer UK Research website. Information on Wilms' tumour can be found at:

- http://www.cancerhelp.org.uk/help/default.asp?page=6521

Hypospadias

Hypospadias is a congenital anomaly of the male genitalia in which the urethral meatus is abnormally located on the ventral side of the penis anywhere from the glans to the perineum. In Europe, hypospadias has an estimated prevalence of 4.1 per 1000 male births (Calzolari et al 1986). Hypospadias may be proximal or distal; most are distal. In these situations the meatus is positioned in the glans.

The proximal form of hypospadias is more serious. Hypospadias here may be penoscrotal, scrotal or perineal. The condition may also be associated with other congenital malformations, such as undescended testes, inguinal hernias, upper urinary tract anomalies, and cardiac and gastrointestinal malformations (Albers et al 1997). Chordee may accompany both types of hypospadias; this term refers to curvature of the penis. It occurs in 15% of distal and at least 85% of proximal hypospadias (Snodgrass 1999).

Causes

There are a number of known causes of hypospadias. It is a feature of several chromosomal abnormalities. It is seen in XX male syndrome, Wolf–Hirschhorn syndrome and Drash syndrome. It is also a feature of a number of endocrine anomalies. Urethral development takes place between 8 and 20 weeks' gestation. Before 8 weeks, male and female external genitalia appear identical. The action of androgens (e.g. testosterone, androsterone) triggers the development of the male genitalia. Partial androgen receptor insensitivity is a recognised cause of hypospadias. Another related cause is 5-alpha-reductase deficiency. Testosterone has to be transformed by 5-alpha-reductase so that it can activate androgen receptors. A deficiency of 5-alpha-reductase impairs testosterone action; hypospadias is one of a number of possible consequences.

Surgery

Surgery is carried out between 6 and 18 months. Most hypospadias require a one-stage repair (because most are distal). A one-stage repair may also be sufficient to reverse proximal hypospadias but a two-stage repair may be necessary. Irrespective of the number of stages required, the objective is the same: to bring the urethral meatus to the tip of the penis, correct any chordee, and create a cosmetically acceptable glans and penile shaft. Numerous procedures have been developed to achieve this. Commonly documented examples are the Thiersch-Duplay, Mathieu, Mustardé, meatal advancement and glanuloplasty and tubularised incised plate (TIP) urethroplasty.

Postoperative care

Pain is one of the major problems in the immediate postoperative period. Penile block, caudal or epidural analgesia are employed to minimise this. Postoperative pain assessment and regular analgesia are required. Following surgery, a dressing is wrapped round the penis to provide support and protection and to minimise discomfort. Because different techniques are used, there are variations in the use of catheters and stents; some techniques employ them and others do not (Bernie & Alagiri 2003). Irrespective of whether these adjuncts are used, assessment of adequate urinary output is essential. The nurse should attempt to ensure that the child does not tamper with the dressing, stents or catheters. Doing so is associated with negative postoperative outcomes such as fistula development (Grobbelaar et al 1996). The dressing stays on for 4–7 days.

Removal of the dressing is a source of anxiety for parents and is painful and upsetting for the child. Before removal of the dressing, the child is given analgesia. It is common practice to then place the child in a bath to soften the dressing material. Despite this, the dressing is often still difficult to remove without upsetting the child. Distraction techniques can be employed and parent participation encouraged as a means of reducing distress. This procedure is a focus of attention in the literature. Sanders (2003) suggests that a barrier film can be applied before a dressing is attached to ease removal. Alternative modes of dressings that promote ease of removal have been suggested. Other authors question the efficacy of using dressings, as there is evidence to suggest that dressings might not be necessary in routine hypospadias repair (McLorie et al 2001, van Savage et al 2000).

Immediate postoperative concerns

Postoperative complications include infection, retention and fistula formation. Antibiotics are prescribed to minimise the likelihood of infection. The nurse must still be alert for signs of infection such as elevated temperature, discharge from the wound and foul-smelling urine. Retention may be anatomical or drug induced. All children, irrespective of the surgical technique employed, should be observed for this complication. A fistula may occur in the week following surgery. Urine leaks may appear from a point along the reconstructed tract. Spontaneous closure is rare and a second operation is required in this case.

Outcome and long-term problems

Studies have identified a high level of satisfaction with the outcome of hypospadias surgery. Long-term problems concern micturition difficulties and problems with sexual function. Micturition difficulties are generally caused by stricture. Urethral dilation may be necessary and in some cases open urothroplasty may be required. Sexual function problems, such as erection and ejaculation difficulties, have been reported following repair of severe hypospadias.

WWW

For further information see the links on the Hypospadias and Epispadias Association (HEA) web page:

- http://www.hypospadias.net/

Cryptorchidism

Cryptorchidism (undescended testis) is categorised as congenital or acquired. The incidence of congenital cryptorchidism in full-term males at birth is 2–4% (Barthold & González 2003). In early fetal development the testes are located within the abdominal cavity. Mediated by hormonal and mechanical factors, the testes descend into the scrotum. Migration begins at 17 weeks' gestation and is usually complete by 33 weeks (Malas et al 1999). Sometimes one or both testes fail to descend; the former is more common. If one or both fail to descend they may still fall within the first year; this is particularly true in the case of premature babies. If by 1 year testes are still undescended then orchidopexy is normally required. Cryptorchidism may also be acquired. In this situation the testes are in a normal scrotal position initially but one or both become undescended later. The pathogenesis of acquired cryptorchidism is unknown, although possible causal factors such as failure of the spermatic cord to elongate have been proposed. Because cryptorchidism can be diagnosed during infancy (congenital) and later childhood (acquired) boys undergo the operation at different ages.

Undesirable consequences

Children with cryptorchidism are at risk from a number of undesirable consequences. Compared with other males they have a greater risk of testicular torsion. This occurs when the testicle twists on the spermatic cord and results in disturbance of blood flow, ischaemia and infarction of the testicle. Emergency surgery is required to save the testicle.

Infertility

The condition is also associated with infertility. If bilateral cryptorchidism remains untreated the adult male will be infertile. However, surgery does not ensure fertility. The treated male may be fertile, subfertile (Coughlin et al 1997) or infertile. A successful outcome appears to be related to the position of the testes before operation, the age at operation and an adequate blood supply to the testes following surgery.

Testicular cancer

Cryptorchidism is an established risk factor for testicular cancer. It is possible that hormonal conditions cause both cryptorchidism and testicular cancer. Another possibility is that the higher temperature, to which the undescended testicle is exposed, promotes tumour formation. There appears to be a relationship between the age at which the male undergoes orchidopexy and the likelihood of testicular cancer (Herrinton et al 2003). Early orchidopexy appears to be associated with a more positive outcome.

Surgery

Trends in orchidopexy have fallen in recent years. This may be due to better diagnosis or a simple decrease in frequency (Mireille et al 2003). The operation is often carried out as a day-case procedure and involves mobilising the testes, spermatic cord and blood supply. The testes or testicle is then brought down into the scrotum and secured by suture.

On return from theatre a dry dressing may be in place. It is removed prior to, or during, a shower the following day. The stitches dissolve a week later. Initially there is considerable swelling and bruising of the scrotum. This will cause discomfort and moderate pain relief will be required. Quiet play should be encouraged. Energetic play/exercise should be avoided for 10–14 days. There are complications associated with the procedure. There may be damage to the blood supply or spermatic cord during the operation, testicular function may be lost, wound infection may occur but is rare.

The risk of testicular cancer is still present even though orchidopexy has been carried out. All males should carry out testicular examination at regular periods. Those who have had cryptorchidism have added reason to do so.

WWW

For information about self-examination for testicular cancer, see:

- http://tcrc.acor.org/tcexam.html

Circumcision

Circumcision refers to excision of the prepuce, the outer portion of the foreskin covering the penis. The prepuce normally covers the glans. In infancy the inner surface of the prepuce, the mucosa, adheres to the glans and over the next 2 years retraction normally becomes possible. The foreskin protects the glans and keeps it soft and moist. Circumcision may be carried out for religious reasons, prophylactic reasons or for phimosis.

Religious reasons

The most common reason for circumcision is religious. Circumcision is a sacred ritual for Muslims and Jews. The timing differs for each religion. Jewish babies are circumcised on the eighth day of life. Muslim children are circumcised between the seventh day following birth and up to puberty.

Prophylaxis

Arguments in favour of routine circumcision for prophylactic reasons focus on a number of conditions. Urinary tract infection is one. The literature suggests that there is an increased risk of urinary tract infection in the uncircumcised child in the first year of life (Schoen et al 2000). Human papillomavirus (HPV) is another condition in which circumcision may be beneficial. HPV is a sexually transmitted disease and strains of the virus are linked to cancer of the cervix. Castellsague et al (2002) present evidence that male circumcision is associated with reduced risks of penile HPV infection and cervical cancer in female partners. Circumcision may also have a positive impact on the transmission of human immunodeficiency virus (HIV). Szabo & Short (2000) explain that the inner lining of the foreskin, the mucosal layer, contains Langerhans' cells. These cells are targets for HIV. The authors suggest that during heterosexual intercourse the foreskin is pulled back leaving the vagina exposed to an area rich in virus. Circumcision, it is thus argued, would reduce the likelihood of HIV transmission. In sub-Saharan Africa, where HIV is rampant, circumcision as a means of prevention of HIV is being advocated as an additional HIV prevention strategy (Rain-Taljaard et al 2003). This position is not without its critics. Others argue that it is not acceptable citing medical, ethical and legal reasons (Hill & Denniston 2003).

Phimosis

Phimosis refers to a non-retractable foreskin. It is the most common medical indication for circumcision (Rickwood 1999). Balanitis xerotica obliterans is an inflammatory disorder that affects the prepuce and glans; it is rare before 5 years and it peaks before puberty. Features include phimosis (requiring circumcision), which may be accompanied by bleeding, dysuria and acute retention. Phimosis can also be diagnosed in the absence of balanitis xerotica obliterans and circumcision is carried out in these cases too. Circumcision in these situations is contentious. It is argued that it may not be necessary because the foreskin will retract in time without surgical intervention (Farshi & Atkinson 2000).

Management

No matter what the reason for circumcision, there are risks attached. Bleeding, infection and retention are all possible complications. On return from theatre the wound may be exposed or a dressing such as Vaseline gauze may be in place. The penis will look swollen and child and parents should be prepared for this. The wound can be cleaned with moistened cotton balls. It should be observed for infection and bleeding. If bleeding does occur it is usually minor and self-limiting, severe bleeding is uncommon. A white/yellowish exudate forms after 48 hours; this should not be confused with pus. It is granulation tissue and part of the healing process. Pus has a thicker consistency and smells malodorous. Infection is a rare occurrence but if it does occur the wound is cleansed regularly and antibiotic therapy commenced.

www

For further information read the circumcision information and resource pages at:

- http://www.cirp.org/

Acute renal failure

Acute renal failure (ARF) is the sudden loss of renal function. Failure occurs over a period of hours or days. The kidneys play a major role in maintaining homeostasis. They maintain the body's water, electrolyte and acid–base balance, as well as eliminating waste from the body. In acute renal failure this homeostatic balance is lost and waste is not eliminated effectively. The causes of acute renal failure are traditionally divided into three categories: pre-renal, post-renal and intrinsic.

Activity

- Make a list of the functions of the kidneys.
- Compose a brief statement explaining each of the functions.
- Access the companion PowerPoint presentation and compare your answers.

Pre-renal causes of acute renal failure are associated with impaired renal blood flow. The kidneys are structurally normal. All types of shock possess the capability to cause acute renal failure. Shock results in inadequate perfusion pressure and reduction in glomerular filtration rate. Oliguria occurs and the kidneys can no longer maintain their homeostatic functions. If the initiating condition is reversed promptly, kidney damage is prevented. If the initiating condition is not reversed, sympathetic and hormonal activity cause intense renal vasoconstriction and ischaemic renal injury and cell death occurs.

Intrinsic renal failure is concerned with pathology within the kidney. Glomerulonephritis and nephrotic syndrome are both possible causes but the most common cause, across all age groups, is haemolytic uraemic syndrome (Moghal et al 1998). This condition is caused by verotoxin-producing *E. coli*, a strain that is carried by cattle. It is thought that meat becomes contaminated during the slaughter process. The organism is destroyed if food is cooked properly but when a child consumes infected meat, colitis occurs. The verotoxin is then absorbed from the intestinal tract and enters the circulation, where it fixes to receptor sites on renal epithelium. Damage to the glomeruli result in a significant reduction in glomerular filtration thus impairing the kidneys' regulatory functions.

Post-renal causes of acute renal failure are associated with obstruction. Common conditions that cause obstruction are posterior urethral valves, ureteropelvic obstruction and neurogenic bladder. These conditions impair the flow of urine and back pressure results. The pressure in the renal tubules rises. As filtration depends on the pressure in the glomerulus being higher than that in the tubules, the gradient diminishes and the glomerular filtration rate falls. The kidneys fail.

Diagnosis

The predisposing causes of acute renal failure will alert those caring for the child to the possibility of the development of acute renal failure. The signs and symptoms are varied and may include oliguria (less than 0.5 mL/kg/h in children) or anuria, oedema, nausea, vomiting, hypertension, confusion or seizures. Blood chemistry reveals increasing blood urea nitrogen (BUN) and creatinine. Abnormalities in electrolyte and acid balance are also evident. Imaging studies such as ultrasound may be ordered to determine whether obstruction is a cause. Renal biopsy is not routine but may be carried out if diagnosis is unexplained (Kersnik et al 2001).

Nursing management

This is a life-threatening condition and enormous sensitivity is required when dealing with the parents. They should be encouraged to verbalise their feelings. Issues should be discussed with honesty and information provided should be accurate. The parents should be encouraged to participate in care but only to the degree that they are comfortable with.

Physical management is aimed at eliminating the underlying cause, balancing fluid and electrolytes, controlling acidosis, sustaining nutrition and protecting the child from infection. There may be fluid depletion or overload, thus fluid may have to be replaced or removed. This makes accurate recording of the child's input and output critical. The child's weight is also significant and should be documented twice daily. If fluid has to be replaced, the choice is between crystalloid, colloids and blood. The cause of the renal failure influences the choice of fluid. In the case of fluid retention dietary measure can be taken. Sodium and fluid intake can be restricted. Diuretics such as mannitol and furosemide may be prescribed; dopamine is an alternative.

Electrolyte balance focuses on sodium and potassium. High sodium levels may occur and are associated with fluid retention and oedema formation and are thus undesirable. In the event of hypernatraemia, sodium restriction is necessary. High potassium levels are also cause for concern. They may approach dangerous levels due to increased production and decreased elimination.

Hyperkalaemia is life threatening because it disturbs the conductive mechanism of the heart. This may result in dysrhythmia. Cardiac monitoring may be ordered in anticipation of such an event. Initial management involves restricting potassium intake, administration of potassium binding agents, control of acidosis and diuretic therapy aimed at increasing urinary output. Glucose metabolism causes potassium to move into cells. Glucose and insulin may be administered to induce these events (Kemper et al 1996). Severe hyperkalaemia is one of the reasons for commencing renal replacement therapy.

Acidosis is undesirable for a number of reasons. Prominent among these is its impact on potassium levels. It promotes the movement of potassium from the intercellular fluid into the extracellular compartment, and thus promotes hyperkalaemia. Acidosis also impacts on cerebral function. Neurological observations are implemented if there is any evidence of confusion or mental impairment. Acidosis may be treated with sodium bicarbonate.

Acute renal failure is highly catabolic. Parenteral nutrition or enteral feeding may be ordered to meet the child's nutritional requirements. The nutritional components are tailored to the child's needs. The amount of energy provided is usually high so that the body does not metabolise body tissues. If body tissue is metabolised for energy, potassium is liberated into an environment where hyperkalaemia may already exist.

The child has to be protected from infection because the immune system is compromised when homeostasis is impaired. Sepsis is a frequent cause of death. Great care has to be taken to protect the child from nosocomial infections. Hand-washing and implementation protocols designed to eliminate the possibility of cross-infection should be strictly applied. The child should be observed for signs of infection and antibiotic therapy should be implemented promptly if infection is discovered.

The interventions described above, plus treatment of predisposing causes, may produce the desired response. In the event of continued fluid overload, hyperkalaemia, acidosis or severe uraemia renal replacement therapy will be required until renal function returns. Common modalities include peritoneal dialysis, intermittent haemodialysis and continuous haemofiltration or haemodiafiltration (Flynn 2002). The choice of modality depends on the child's age, clinical condition and local experience with the particular modalities.

Prognosis

Prognosis depends on the underlying cause. The outcome for those suffering from haemolytic-uraemic syndrome is excellent. The mortality rate for other illnesses that cause acute renal failure is much higher. Wong et al (1996) recorded a mortality rate of 27%.

Chronic renal failure

There are numerous causes of chronic renal failure in children. The most common cause is VUR. Other significant causes are the obstructive uropathies such as posterior urethral valves, ureterocele and ureteropelvic junction obstruction (Roth et al 2002b). Medical conditions that may result in chronic renal failure are nephrotic syndrome and glomerulonephritis.

Chronic renal failure is categorised according to changes in glomerular filtration rate. This is the amount of filtrate that flows into all nephrons in 1 minute. The normal rate in a child is 110–120 mL/min.

Creatinine is a waste product of protein metabolism. Serum levels of creatinine can be measured. Creatinine is eliminated from the body by the kidneys. A 24-hour collection of urine is obtained to determine the amount cleared. By comparing serum creatinine to levels cleared in the 24-hour collection, the glomerular filtration rate can be calculated.

Chronic renal failure is regarded as mild, moderate or severe. The criteria are as follows:

- Mild: glomerular filtration rate 50–75 mL/min
- Moderate: glomerular filtration rate 25 mL–50 mL/min
- Severe: glomerular filtration rate less than 25 mL/min.

Clinical features

The kidneys are multifunctional. Impairment of these functions produces a variety of clinical features. Common features are poor appetite, stunted growth, anaemia (with associated features), increased or decreased urine output, oedema, hypertension, skin discoloration and pruritus.

Diagnosis

Chronic renal failure diagnosis is based on history, clinical examination, altered laboratory values, various scanning techniques and biopsy. Laboratory values reveal elevated blood urea nitrogen, elevated creatinine, altered calcium:phosphorus ratio, acidosis and electrolyte imbalance. The diagnosis is confirmed by kidney biopsy.

Management

There are a number of causes of chronic renal failure and these affect the management. There are also different stages of severity and variable progression. Thus the management described here is generalised.

The child's dietary protein intake should be based on the recommended dietary allowances (RDA) for his or her chronological age. Additional increments may be desirable to ensure growth. Increasing dietary protein intake above the RDA has to be balanced against the kidneys' ability to rid the body of waste products of protein metabolism. The energy portion of the diet has to be high; it is given in the form of fat and carbohydrates. If energy intake is insufficient then protein will be utilised for energy purposes. This will impair the child's growth. Maintaining strict records of intake and output are necessary. Height and weight are also documented.

High sodium levels encourage fluid retention, oedema and also contribute to hypertension. In chronic renal failure, sodium and fluids are usually restricted. Sodium should not be added to cooked food and foods high in salt should be avoided. These measures may not suffice and sodium intake may have to be restricted to a specific amount. Elevated potassium levels due to decreased excretion are associated with arrhythmias and cardiac arrest. Foods high in potassium should thus be avoided.

Attempts to curb the onset of anaemia are initially made by encouraging the anorexic child to eat. The diet should be attractive and small portions offered. It should be rich in iron, folic and vitamin B12. These substances may also be given in supplement form. Anaemia is inevitable in chronic renal failure because of loss of erythropoietin production. As the degree of kidney failure progresses, erythropoietin production fails and anaemia breaks through. Treatment involves administration of erythropoietin. Elimination of anaemia with erythropoietin is very effective; it is known to enhance cardiac, muscular and immune functions (Vijayan et al 2000) and generally improve quality of life.

Hypertension has been linked to the progression of chronic renal failure. There are a number of mechanisms that may be responsible for hypertension in chronic renal failure. Sodium and fluid retention is one factor. Controlling sodium and fluid intake is therefore employed to control blood pressure. Another mechanism involves the triggering of the renin-angiotensin system (RAS). The mechanism is activated by a falling glomerular filtration rate. Angiotensin II (produced when the renin-angiotensin system is triggered) promotes sodium and water retention and causes widespread vasoconstriction. It also promotes inflammation, fibrosis and scarring of the kidneys (Soergel & Schaefer 2002). Diuretics and acetylcholinesterase inhibitors are used to counteract the activities of the renin–angiotensin system.

Activity

- Describe the renin-angiotensin system.

Compare your recall of the mechanism with the companion PowerPoint presentation.

A precursor of active vitamin D is manufactured in the skin. Another precursor is consumed in the diet and is absorbed from the bowel. Both liver and kidneys modify these precursors and produce biologically active forms. Active vitamin D stimulates the absorption of dietary calcium from the bowel. By doing so, it helps to maintain serum calcium levels. In chronic renal failure the damaged kidneys do not activate the precursors of vitamin D. The result is that calcium absorption from the bowel is impaired and hypocalcaemia results. The problem is compounded by abnormalities in serum phosphorous levels.

Serum phosphorous levels tend to be elevated in chronic renal failure. This is partly due to the damaged kidneys, which fail to eliminate the substance. High serum phosphate is undesirable. It binds to calcium and lowers blood levels and also impairs vitamin D action, which also adversely affects calcium levels. Hypocalcaemia stimulates the production of parathyroid hormone that promotes movement of calcium out of bones. Bone demineralisation takes place and the child develops osteodystrophy.

Efforts are made to maintain calcium levels. Because the damaged kidneys do not activate precursors of vitamin D, an active form has to be prescribed. Calcium supplementation may also be provided. Attempts are also made to control serum phosphorous levels. Food high in phosphorous should be avoided and binding agents, such as aluminium hydroxide or calcium carbonate, which prevent phosphorous absorption, are prescribed. These measures have a positive impact but as failure progresses bone demineralisation becomes inevitable.

Acidosis adversely affects protein metabolism and is strongly implicated in growth delay (Boirie et al 2000). As kidney disease progresses there is a failure to synthesis ammonia (a process necessary to ride the body of hydrogen ions). There is also a failure to effectively reabsorb bicarbonate. These two factors combine to cause acidosis. When serum bicarbonate falls to levels below 22 mmol/L it should be corrected (National Kidney Foundation 2000). Sodium citrate or sodium bicarbonate may be administered orally. When a child is on dialysis, the problem can be met by adapting the dialysate solution to include high sodium bicarbonate concentrations.

Dialysis

Continuous ambulatory peritoneal dialysis is the preferred form of dialysis. Its main advantage is that the child can pursue his or her normal activities. A catheter is inserted into the child's abdomen. Gravity is utilised to allow dialysate to flow into the abdominal cavity. It lies on one side of the peritoneal membrane. An exchange between dialysate fluid and body fluid on the opposite side of the membrane takes place. The process takes about 2 hours and then the now altered dialysate is removed by allowing it to drain into a bag attached to the catheter and placed below the abdomen. Peritonitis is a complication of peritoneal dialysis. If this occurs it may be necessary for the child to convert to haemodialysis. This is more efficient than peritoneal dialysis but is much more restrictive. The child has to attend a specialist unit for 3 or 4 hours two or three times a week.

WWW

For information about dialysis, refer to the National Kidney Federation website:

- http://www.kidney.org.uk/Medical-Info/pd.html

Transplant

The child is tissue-typed to ensure compatibility. The outcome has improved in recent years thanks to pharmacological innovations designed to prevent rejection. These pharmaceuticals suppress the child's immune system. T cell induction therapy, steroid therapy and chemotherapy are all utilised.

Summary

Paediatric nurses are required to care for children with congenital and acquired anomalies of the genitourinary tract. This chapter has attempted to offer an insight into some of the more common anomalies. Nurses caring for children must have a well-developed knowledge of urinary tract infection (UTI) because it is very common and because of its association with impaired renal function, hypertension and end-stage renal disease. VUR was given prominence in this chapter because it is intrinsically linked to UTI and is the most common congenital abnormality of the renal tract. The nephrotic syndrome and poststreptococcal glomerulonephritis warranted attention because they are the commonest disorders associated with glomerular pathology. Children are commonly subject to surgical procedures involving the genitourinary tract. To this end, circumcision, hypospadias, cryptorchidism and Wilms' tumour were included. Finally, acute and chronic renal failure were given prominence because they are complications associated with most of the previously mentioned anomalies.

References

Albers, N., Ulrichs, C., Gluer, S., et al., 1997. Etiologic classification of severe hypospadias: implications for prognosis and management. Journal of Pediatrics 131 (3), 386–392.

Al-Orifi, F., McGillivray, D., Tange, S., et al., 2000. Urine culture from bag specimens in young children: are the risks too high? Canada Journal of Pediatrics 137, 221–226.

American Academy of Pediatrics (AAP), 1999. Practice parameter: the diagnosis, treatment, and evaluation of the initial urinary tract infection in febrile infants and young children. Pediatrics 103, 843–852.

Baldwin, D.S., Gluck, M.C., Schacht, R.G., Gallo, G.R., 1974. The long-term course of poststreptococcal glomerulonephritis. Annals of Internal Medicine 80, 342–358.

Barthold, J., González, R., 2003. The epidemiology of congenital cryptorchidism, testicular ascent and orchiopexy. Journal of Urology 170 (6), 2396–2401 Pt 1.

Belman, A.B., 1997. Vesicoureteral reflux. Pediatric Clinics of North America 44 (5), 1171–1190.

Bernie, J., Alagiri, M., 2003. Tubeless barcat: a patient-friendly hypospadias procedure. Urology 61 (6), 1230–1232.

Birch, J., Breslow, N., 1995. Epidemiological features of Wilms' tumor. Hematology/Oncology Clinics of North America 9, 1157–1178.

Birmingham Reflux Study Group, 1984. A prospective trial of operative versus non-operative treatment of severe vesico-ureteric reflux: 2 years' observation in 96 children. Contributions to Nephrology 39, 169–185.

Boirie, Y., Broyer, M., Gagnadoux, M.F., et al., 2000. Alterations of protein metabolism by metabolic acidosis in children with chronic renal failure. Kidney International 58 (1), 236–241.

Calzolari, E., Contiero, M.R., Roncarati, E., et al., 1986. Aetiological factors in hypospadias. Journal of Medical Genetics 23 (4), 333–337.

Castellsague, X., Bosch, F., Munoz, N., et al., 2002. Male circumcision, penile human papillomavirus infection, and cervical cancer in female partners. New England Journal of Medicine 346, 1105–1112.

Cherullo, E.E., Ross, J.H., Kay, R., et al., 2001. Renal neoplasms in adult survivors of childhood Wilms' tumor. Journal of Urology 165 (6), 2013–2016 Pt 1.

Constantinescu, A.R., Shah, H.B., Foote, E.F., et al., 2000. Predicting first-year relapses in children with nephrotic syndrome. Pediatrics 105 (3), 492–495 Pt 1.

Coppes, M.J., Wolff, J.E., Ritchey, M.L., 1999. Wilms' tumour: diagnosis and treatment. Paediatric Drugs 1 (4), 251–262.

Coughlin, M., O'Leary, L., Songer, N., et al., 1997. Time to conception after orchidopexy: evidence for subfertility? Fertility and Sterility 67 (4), 742–746.

Cu, G.A., Mezzano, S., Bannan, J.D., et al., 1998. Immunohistochemical and serological evidence for the role of streptococcal proteinase in acute post-streptococcal glomerulonephritis. Kidney International 54 (3), 819–826.

Denton, M.D., Chertow, G.M., Brady, H.R., 1996. 'Renal-dose' dopamine for the treatment of acute renal failure: scientific rationale, experimental studies and clinical trials. Kidney International 50 (1), 4–14.

Durkan, A., Hodson, E., Willis, N., et al., 2001. Non-corticosteroid treatment for nephrotic syndrome in children. Cochrane database of systematic reviews (4) CD002290.

Farshi, Z., Atkinson, K., 2000. A study of clinical opinion and practice regarding circumcision. Archives of Disease in Childhood 83 (5), 393–396.

Feasey, S., 1999. Are Newcastle urine collection pads suitable as a means of collecting specimens from infants? Paediatric Nurse 11 (9), 17–21.

Flynn, J.T., 2002. Choice of dialysis modality for management of pediatric acute renal failure. Pediatric Nephrology 17 (1), 61–69.

Goldstein, S.L., Somers, M.J., Lande, M.B., et al., 2000. Acyclovir prophylaxis of varicella in children with renal disease receiving steroids. Pediatric Nephrology 14 (4), 305–308.

Grobbelaar, A., Laing, J., Harrison, D., et al., 1996. Hypospadias repair: the influence of postoperative care and a patient factor on surgical morbidity. Annals of Plastic Surgery 37 (6), 612–617.

Herrinton, L., Zhao, W., Husson, G., 2003. Management of cryptorchidism and risk of testicular cancer. American Journal of Epidemiology 157 (7), 602–605.

Hill, G., Denniston, G., 2003. HIV and circumcision: new factors to consider. Sexually Transmitted Infections 79 (6), 495–496.

Hiraoka, M., Tsukahara, H., Matsubara, K., et al., 2003. A randomized study of two long-course prednisolone regimens for nephrotic syndrome in children. American Journal of Kidney Diseases 41 (6), 1155–1162.

Holmberg, C., Laine, J., Rönnholm, K., et al., 1996. Congenital nephrotic syndrome. Kidney International Supplement 53, S51–S56.

Huang, F.Y., Tsai, T.C., 1995. Resolution of vesicoureteral reflux during medical management in children. Pediatric Nephrology 9 (6), 715–717.

International Study of Kidney Disease in Children, 1978. Nephrotic syndrome in children: prediction of histology from clinical and laboratory characteristics. Kidney International 13, 159–165.

Jakobsson, B., Soderlundh, S., Berg, U., 1992. Diagnostic significance of 99mTc-dimercaptosuccinic acid (DMSA) scintigraphy in urinary tract infection. Archives of Disease in Childhood 67, 1338–1342.

Jodal, U., 1987. The natural history of bacteriuria in childhood. Infectious Disease Clinics of North America 1, 713–729.

Kasahara, T., Hayakawa, H., Okubo, S., et al., 2001. Prognosis of acute poststreptococcal glomerulonephritis (APSGN) is excellent in children, when adequately diagnosed. Pediatrics International 43 (4), 364–367.

Kemper, M.J., Harps, E., Müller-Wiefel, D.E., 1996. Hyperkalemia: therapeutic options in acute and chronic renal failure. Clinical Nephrology 46 (1), 67–69.

Keren, R., Chan, E., 2002. A meta-analysis of randomized, controlled trials comparing short- and long-course antibiotic therapy for urinary tract infections in children. Pediatrics 109 (5) E70–0.

Kersnik Levart, T., Kenig, A., Buturovic Ponikvar, J., 2001. Real-time ultrasound-guided renal biopsy with a biopsy gun in children: safety and efficacy. Acta Paediatrica 90 (12), 1394–1397.

Kontiokari, T., Sundqvist, K., Nuutinen, M., et al., 2001. Randomised trial of cranberry-lingonberry juice and Lactobacillus GG drink for the prevention of urinary tract infections in women. British Medical Journal (Clinical research edition) 322 (7302), 1571.

Lang, M.M., Towers, C., 2001. Identifying poststreptococcal glomerulonephritis. Nurse Practitioner: American Journal of Primary Health Care 26 (8), 34–42.

Leonard, M., 2002. Endoscopic injection therapy for treatment of vesicoureteric reflux: a 20-year perspective. Paediatrics and Child Health 7 (8), 545–550.

Li, P.S., Ma, L.C., Wong, S.N., 2002. Is bag urine culture useful in monitoring urinary tract infection in infants? Journal of Paediatric and Child Health 38 (4), 377–381.

Liaw, L.C., Nayar, D.M., Pedler, S.J., 2000. Home collection of urine for culture from infants by three methods: survey of parents' preferences and bacterial contamination rates. British Medical Journal 320 (7245), 1312–1313.

Loening-Baucke, V., 1997. Urinary incontinence and urinary tract infection and their resolution with treatment of chronic constipation of childhood. Pediatrics 100, 228–232.

Mahant, S., To, T., Friedman, J., 2001. Timing of voiding cystourethrogram in the investigation of urinary tract infections in children. Journal of Pediatrics 139 (4), 568–571.

Malas, M., Sulak, O., Oztürk, A., 1999. The growth of the testes during the fetal period. British Journal of Urology 84 (6), 689–692.

McIntyre, P., Craig, J.C., 1998. Prevention of serious bacterial infection in children with nephrotic syndrome. Journal of Paediatrics and Child Health 34 (4), 314–317.

McLorie, G., 2001. Wilms' tumor (nephroblastoma). Current Opinion in Urology 11 (6), 567–570.

McLorie, G., Joyner, B., Herz, D., et al., 2001. A prospective randomized clinical trial to evaluate methods of postoperative care of hypospadias. Journal of Urology 165 (5), 1669–1672.

Michael, M., Hodson, E.M., Craig, J.C., et al., 2003. Short versus standard duration oral antibiotic therapy for acute urinary tract infection in children. Cochrane database of systematic reviews 1 CD003966.

Mireille, B., Toledano, L., Anna, L., et al., 2003. Temporal trends in orchidopexy, Great Britain, 1992–1998. Environmental Health Perspectives 111, 129–132.

Moghal, N.E., Brocklebank, J.T., Meadow, S.R., 1998. A review of acute renal failure in children: incidence, etiology and outcome. Clinical Nephrology 49 (2), 91–95.

National Kidney Foundation, 2000. Clinical practice guidelines for nutrition in chronic renal failure. American Journal of Kidney Disease 35 (6 Suppl 2), S1–S140.

Noe, H.N., Wyatt, R.J., Peeden Jr., J.N., et al., 1992. The transmission of vesicoureteral reflux from parent to child. Journal of Urology 148 (6), 1869–1871.

O'Donnell, M., 2001. Mechanisms and clinical importance of hypertriglyceridemia in the nephrotic syndrome. Kidney International 59 (1), 380–382.

Orth, S.R., Ritz, E., 1998. Medical progress: the nephrotic syndrome. New England Journal of Medicine 338 (17), 1202–1211.

Phillips, D.A., Watson, A.R., MacKinlay, D., 1998. Distress and the micturating cystourethrogram: does preparation help? Acta Paediatrica 87 (2), 175–179.

Rahman, N., Arbour, L., Tonin, P., et al., 1996. Evidence for a familial Wilms' tumour gene (FWT1) on chromosome 17q12-q21. Nature Genetics 13 (4), 461–463.

Rain-Taljaard, R., Lagarde, E., Taljaard, D., et al., 2003. Potential for an intervention based on male circumcision in a South African town with high levels of HIV infection. AIDS Care 15 (3), 315–327.

Riccabona, M., 2003. Urinary tract infections in children. Current Opinion in Urology 13 (1), 59–62.

Rickwood, A., 1999. Medical indications for circumcision. British Journal of Urology 83 (Supplement 1), 45–51.

Roth, K., Amaker, B.H., Chan, J.C.M., 2002a. Nephrotic syndrome: pathogenesis and management. Pediatrics in Review 23(7):237–248

Roth, K., Koo H.P., Spottswood, S.E., et al., 2002b. Obstructive uropathy: an important cause of chronic renal failure in children. Clinical Pediatrics 41(5):309–314

Sanders, C., 2003. Comparison of dressing removal following hypospadias repair. British Journal of Nursing 12 (15), S21–S28 Supplement.

Schlager, T.A., Anderson, S., Trudell, J., et al., 1999. Effect of cranberry juice on bacteriuria in children with neurogenic bladder receiving intermittent catheterization. Journal of Pediatrics 135 (6), 698–702.

Schoen, E., Colby, C., Ray, G., 2000. Newborn circumcision decreases incidence and costs of urinary tract infections during the first year of life. Pediatrics 105, 789–793.

Simckes, A.M., Spitzer, A., 1995. Poststreptococcal acute glomerulonephritis. Pediatrics in Review/American Academy of Pediatrics 16 (7), 278–279.

Smellie, J.M., Poulton, A., Prescod, N.P., 1994. Retrospective study of children with renal scarring associated with reflux and urinary infection. British Medical Journal 308, 1193–1196.

Snodgrass, W., 1999. Changing concepts in hypospadias repair. Current Opinion in Urology 9 (6), 513–516.

Soergel, M., Schaefer, F., 2002. Effect of hypertension on the progression of chronic renal failure in children. American Journal of Hypertension 15 (2), 53S–56S Pt 2.

Soliday, E., Grey, S., Lande, M.B., 1999. Behavioral effects of corticosteroids in steroid-sensitive nephrotic syndrome. Pediatrics 104 (4), e51.

Struthers, S., Scanlon, J., Parker, K., et al., 2003. Parental reporting of smelly urine and urinary tract infection. Archives of Disease in Childhood 88 (3), 250–252.

Stull, T.L., Lipuma, J.J., 1991. Epidemiology and natural history of urinary tract infections in children. Medical Clinics of North America 75, 287–297.

Szabo, R., Short, R.V., 2000. How does male circumcision protect against HIV infection? British Medical Journal 320, 1592–1594.

Tasic, V., Polenakovic, M., 2003. Occurrence of subclinical post-streptococcal glomerulonephritis in family contacts. Journal of Paediatrics and Child Health 39 (3), 177–179.

van Ommen, C.H., Heyboer, H., Groothoff, J.W., et al., 1998. Persistent tachypnea in children: keep pulmonary embolism in mind. Journal of Pediatric Hematology and Oncology 20 (6), 570–573.

van Savage, J., Palanca, L., Slaughenhoupt, B., 2000. A prospective randomized trial of dressings versus no dressings for hypospadias repair. Journal of Urology 164 (3), 981–983 Pt 2.

Vijayan, A., Behrend, T., Miller, S.B., 2000. Clinical use of growth factors in chronic renal failure. Current Opinion in Nephrology and Hypertension 9 (1), 5–10.

Vujanic, G.M., Kelsey, A., Mitchell, C., et al., 2003. The role of biopsy in the diagnosis of renal tumors of childhood: Results of the UKCCSG Wilms' tumor study 3. Medical and Pediatric Oncology 40 (1), 18–22.

Wilms' tumour: status report, 1990. National Wilms' tumour study committee. Journal of Clinical Oncology 9, 877–887.

Wong, W., McCall, E., Anderson, B., 1996. Acute renal failure in the paediatric intensive care unit. The New Zealand Medical Journal 109 (1035), 459–461.

Respiratory illness in children

27

Janet Kelsey Gill McEwing

ABSTRACT

The primary aim of this chapter is to give the reader a theoretical grounding from which to care for children and young people with respiratory illnesses. The anatomy of the respiratory tract and the mechanism of external respiration are described. The effects of incomplete development of the respiratory system in children, and its impact on nursing care, are discussed. A detailed account of respiratory assessment is given, outlining some of the skills and specialised equipment required. The common respiratory infections encountered in children are discussed with their nursing management.

LEARNING OUTCOMES

- Demonstrate an understanding of the anatomy and physiology of the respiratory tract.
- Gain an overview of the nature of respiratory illness in children.
- Appreciate the role of the nurse in caring for children with respiratory illness.
- Identify the signs of respiratory distress.
- Use relevant literature and research to inform the nursing care of children with respiratory illness.

Introduction

The most common illnesses in infants and children in the UK are disorders of the respiratory system. Respiratory tract infections in children, although common, are not usually serious. Frequent infections occur in children because the immune system has not been exposed to common pathogens and therefore infections tend to develop with each new exposure. The risk of infection is also increased in children because the respiratory tract is relatively short. Most of these infections do not cause a serious problem to the child; however children are particularly vulnerable to respiratory problems because of their relatively high oxygen requirements and the immaturity of their respiratory system (Carter 1995). Respiratory disease in early childhood can interfere with the development of the lungs and cause permanent lung damage. Acute respiratory failure can result from any airway, pulmonary or neuromuscular disease that impairs oxygen exchange or elimination of carbon dioxide.

Some respiratory problems are more common at specific ages. The same organism can cause different illnesses at different ages. For example, the respiratory syncytial virus (RSV) frequently causes bronchiolitis in infants but causes only a sore throat and cold symptoms in older children (Meadow & Newell 2002).

The majority of infections (80%) are restricted to the upper respiratory tract and approximately 20% of these will become severe and require medical intervention. These include conditions such as bronchiolitis, laryngotracheobronchitis, epiglottitus, pneumonia and acute asthma (Morton & Phillips 1992, Thompson 1990). These are major causes of morbidity in children and a common reason for admission to hospital (Meadow & Newell 2002).

Respiratory illness accounts for 30–40% of acute medical admissions to hospital of children and over 450 deaths in England and Wales each year. The Child Health Committee (1997) reported that the principal cause for admission to hospital (30.9%) of children aged 0–4 years in England between 1993 and 1994 was a respiratory problem.

Anatomy and physiology of the respiratory tract

The human body requires a constant supply of oxygen. Children have a higher metabolic rate than adults, and thus an increased need for oxygen, which demands that their respiratory system functions effectively. The respiratory system consists of the lungs, the airways, the chest wall and the pulmonary

DOI: 10.1016/B978-0-7020-3183-0.10027-X

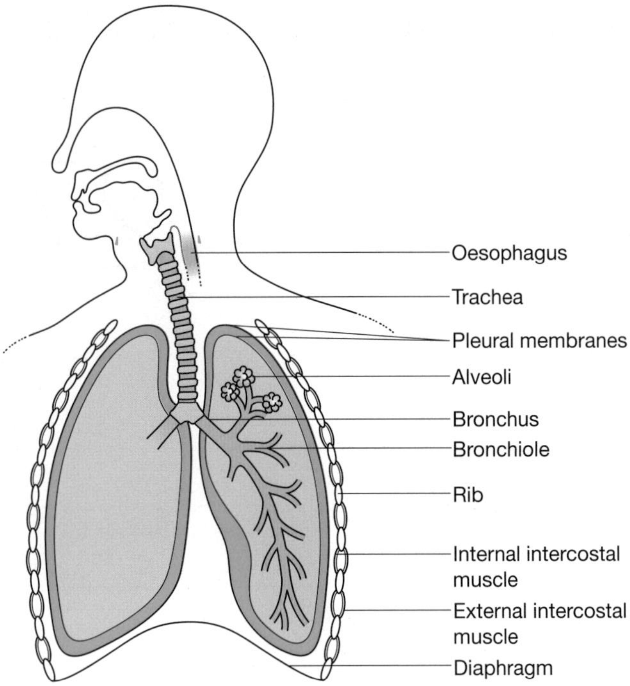

Fig. 27.1 • Basic structure of the lungs.

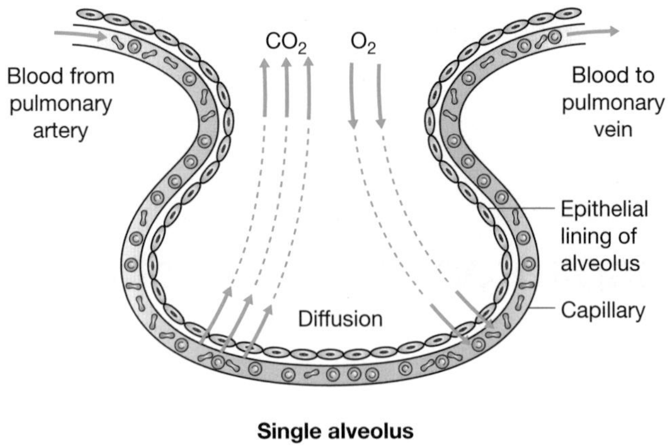

Fig. 27.2 • A single alveolus.

circulation. The lungs (Fig. 27.1) are situated in the thorax, the sides of the thorax are bounded by the rib cage; linking the ribs are the intercostal muscles. At the base of the thorax is a flexible sheet of muscle known as the diaphragm.

The primary function of the respiratory system is the exchange of gases between the environmental air and the blood. There are three steps in this process: the movement of air in and out of the lungs, the movement of gases between air spaces in the lungs and the blood, and the movement of blood from the capillaries surrounding the lungs to the body's organs and tissues. The first two processes are functions of the respiratory system, the third is performed by the cardiovascular system (McChance & Heuther 2002).

The respiratory system can be divided into the upper and lower airways. The upper airways consist of the nasopharynx and the oropharynx. These structures are lined with highly vascular, ciliated epithelium. This warms and moistens the inspired air and removes foreign particles from it as it passes into the lungs. During quiet respiration, air passes through the nose, nasopharynx and oropharynx to the lower airways. During exercise or when the nose is obstructed the mouth and oropharynx are used for ventilation, however by this route the air is not filtered or humidified as efficiently as via the nasopharynx. The larynx connects the upper and lower airways; it is a cartilaginous structure that prevents collapse of the airways during inspiration. Air then flows into the trachea, which is supported by U-shaped cartilage. The trachea divides into the two main bronchi, which in turn divide into bronchioles; there are 16 divisions in total, ending in the terminal bronchioles. This multiple subdivision causes a decrease in the velocity of the air flow into the lungs, which allows for maximum gaseous exchange to take place. The bronchioles have cartilage within their walls until the tenth division. The terminal bronchioles continue to divide into smaller respiratory bronchioles, and then into the alveolar ducts. These lead to the alveolar sacs, which are made up of numerous alveoli. The alveoli (Fig. 27.2) are the primary gas-exchange units of the lungs; it is here that oxygen enters the blood and carbon dioxide is removed (McChance & Heuther 2002).

PowerPoint

Access the companion PowerPoint presentation.

There are 20 million alveoli at birth, increasing to 300 million alveoli in the fully formed lungs of the adult (Meadow & Newell 2002). This means that infants and young children have a relatively small alveolar surface area for gaseous exchange. Each alveolus has a network of capillaries wrapped around it. The walls of the alveoli and the capillaries are only one cell thick. A thin layer of liquid covers their surface, which aids gaseous exchange between the inhaled air and the circulating blood.

Inhalation involves the diaphragm contracting and flattening and the external intercostal muscles contracting, pulling the ribcage upwards and outwards. This increases the volume inside the thorax, decreases the pressure inside the lungs, and air is sucked in. When the diaphragm relaxes it domes up into the thorax and, as the external intercostal muscles relax, the rib cage drops down and moves inwards. This increases the pressure inside the lungs and forces air out. The internal intercostal muscles contract during strenuous breathing to pull the rib cage down to produce a forced expiration. There are two main considerations in infants and children. First, in the newborn, the diaphragm is not able to contract as effectively as in an older infant or child because it is attached higher at the front and is therefore longer. Second, infants and children have a relatively round thoracic cavity due to the horizontal position of the ribs, this places increased dependence on the diaphragm and abdomen as the primary means of ventilation.

PowerPoint

Access the companion PowerPoint presentation.

www

See respiratory movements online at:

- http://mywebpages.comcast.net/wnor/respiratory movements.htm

Lung volumes

The total capacity of a child's lungs increases from 1.4 L in the 5-year-old child to 4.5 L at the time of puberty (MacGregor 2000):

- At the end of quiet respiration, the air that remains in the lungs is termed the **functional residual capacity**.
- Following forced expiration, between 0.5 and 1.5 L (depending on age) of air remains trapped in the alveoli; this minimal volume is called the **residual volume**.
- The additional volume of air forced out of the lungs during a forced expiration of between 0.5 and 1.5 L is known as the **expiratory reserve volume**.
- During quiet respiration, the amount of air in the lungs increases from 0.7 L at 5 years (or 2.25 L at puberty) at the end of expiration to 0.8 L at 5 years (or 2.55 L at puberty) at the end of inspiration; this 0.1 L (0.3 L at puberty) of air moving in and out of the lungs is called the **tidal volume**.
- The **vital capacity** of the lungs is the amount of air moving when the patient is performing forced inspiration and forced expiration, which will be the sum of the inspiratory reserve volume, the expiratory reserve volume and the tidal volume. This volume is related to the size of the patient; at age 5 years it is approximately 1 L and this increases to 3 L at puberty (MacGregor 2000). The vital capacity can be increased if the patient stands up because the volume of blood in the lungs is reduced.
- The **peak flow** is the maximum velocity of air flow produced in a forced respiration. When this value is low it suggests that expiratory respiratory muscle activity is weak or that there is an obstruction to expiratory air flow due to some form of bronchoconstriction such as asthma.

Nervous control of breathing

The respiratory centre is situated at the base of the brain and is made up of the medulla oblongata and the pons. The control of breathing has both automatic and voluntary components. Voluntary control allows for breathing to be integrated with voluntary actions such as blowing, singing and speaking. Automatic control involves input from two types of receptors; those that monitor the pH, carbon dioxide and oxygen levels in the blood, and those that monitor breathing patterns and lung function.

Chemoreceptors assess the level of carbon dioxide and oxygen in the blood, messages are transmitted to the respiratory centre and ventilation is adjusted to maintain arterial blood gases within a normal range (Table 27.1). How much oxygen is in the blood depends on the:

- haemoglobin concentration in the blood (Hb g/dL)
- oxygen saturation of the haemoglobin (SaO_2)
- partial pressure of oxygen (PaO_2).

Table 27.1 Normal arterial blood gas values in children neonate at birth child

pH	7.32–7.42	7.35–7.45
$PaCO_2$	30–40 mm Hg	35–45 mmHg
HCO_3	20–26 mEq/L	22–28 mEq/L
PaO_2	60–80 mmHg	80–100 mmHg

The central chemoreceptors located in the medulla oblongata monitor the carbon dioxide level in the blood by assessing the number of free hydrogen ions in the cerebrospinal fluid circulating around the medulla. This is important because the carbon dioxide level in the blood affects the pH level of the extracellular fluid of the brain. These receptors are extremely sensitive in the short term but long-term elevation of carbon dioxide levels, such as can occur in chronic respiratory disease, causes desensitisation of these receptors.

The carotid and aortic bodies are chemoreceptors that are sensitive to oxygen levels in the carotid artery and aorta, respectively. They are less responsive than the central chemoreceptors and are activated only when the oxygen level falls below 60 mmHg. Therefore hypoxia is the main stimulus for ventilation in persons with chronic hypercarbia (Porth 1994).

Reflect on your practice

How would you explain to a junior nurse the importance of the correct level of oxygen administration when assisting a child with a chronic respiratory condition experiencing an acute respiratory illness?

PowerPoint

Access the companion PowerPoint presentation.

The anatomy and physiology of the respiratory and cardiovascular systems of children differs from that of adults. This influences the care given to children and hence must be considered when assessing and managing children with respiratory problems.

It is important to remember that anatomical differences influence the degree to which children respond to respiratory

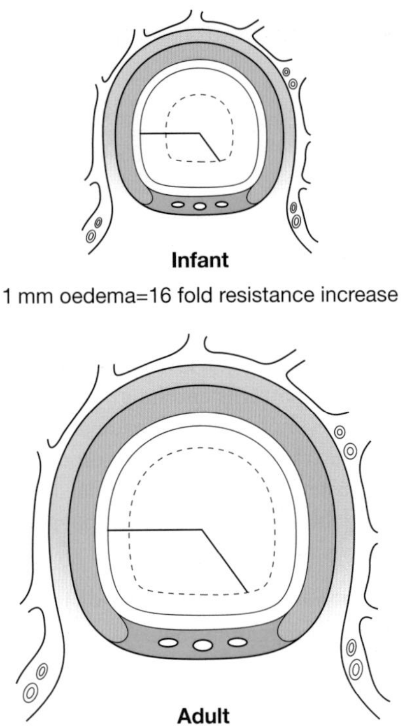

Fig. 27.3 • Anatomical differences between the airways of an infant and of an adult.

illness because of the smaller diameter of the airways (Fig. 27.3 and Table 27.2). Poiseuille's law states that:

$$\text{Resistance } \alpha = 1/\text{Radius}^4$$

That is, resistance to airflow is inversely proportional to the fourth power of the radius. In other words, a small amount of mucous or oedema in the airways will significantly increase resistance to airflow and therefore increase the work of breathing.

Respiratory assessment and examination of the chest

A calm manner should always be adopted when assessing any child with respiratory problems. The 'hands-off approach' can generate a lot of useful information gained through careful observation and this is particularly useful in very young children, who may resist physical examination. It is always important to leave the child with his or her carer in an upright position. Although observations focus on the respiratory status of the child, it is important to note the child's general appearance, level of engagement with carer, colour, hydration status and temperature. In addition, the ability of infants to feed should be noted. If at any time you feel the child needs immediate intervention, for example they are having difficulties breathing, then the assessment should be stopped and emergency care given to stabilise the child.

Assessment follows the ABC criteria for assessment in conjunction with neurological observations and provides a framework for rapid and effective nursing assessment of the child with respiratory problems. The survey should therefore include assessment of the following:

A. Airway

Patency of the airway is assessed, observing for spontaneous ventilation, and look, listen and feel. Note any presence of inspiratory noises. If the child is able to speak or is crying this indicates that the airway is patent. If there is no evidence of air movement then chin-lift or jaw-thrust should be carried out and the basic life support algorithm commenced.

B. Breathing

To assess the adequacy of breathing the chest should be examined and the following assessed:

- The effort of breathing including respiratory rate, recession, grunting, use of accessory muscles and nasal flaring.
- The efficacy of breathing including breath sounds and chest expansion/abdominal excursion.
- The effects of inadequate respiration including heart rate, oxygen saturation, skin colour and mental status.

Assessment of breathing therefore involves examination of the chest for the following:

- Respiratory movements
- Number rhythm, depth and quality of respirations
- Character of breath sounds utilising the skills of palpation, auscultation and percussion.

Chest wall movement should be symmetric bilaterally and coordinated with breathing.

On inspiration, the chest rises and expands (Fig. 27.4A); on expiration, the chest descends and decreases in size (Fig. 27.4B). In children less than 6–7 years of age, respiratory movement will be mainly abdominal or diaphragmatic; in older children respirations are mainly thoracic.

To observe for chest expansion, stand at the child's head or feet and, looking down the midline, note any asymmetry of movement. Decreased movement on one side may be the result of foreign body obstruction, pneumonia, pneumothorax or atelectasis.

Respiratory movements can be felt by placing each hand flat against the chest or back with thumbs in the midline along the lower costal margin (Fig. 27.5). The hands move with the chest wall during respiration. The amount of respiratory excursion is evaluated and asymmetry is noted.

PowerPoint

Access the companion PowerPoint presentation.

Palpation is carried out for voice conduction (vocal fremitus). Place the palmar surface of the hand on the child's chest and feel for vibrations as the child speaks. At the same time, move the hand symmetrically on either side of the sternum and

Table 27.2 The differences in the anatomy and physiology of the respiratory and cardiovascular systems of children (Cosby 1998 cited by Dolan & Holt 2000)

Factor	Nursing considerations
Airway	
Large head, short neck, inability to support head	Assistance required to maintain position of comfort
Large tongue	Airway is easily obstructed by tongue; proper positioning is often all that is necessary to open the airway
The floor of the mouth is easily compressible	Care is required when positioning of the fingers when holding the jaw
Infants less than 6 months old are obligate nose breathers	Obstruction of the nasal passages by mucus can compromise the infant's airway
Smaller diameter of all airways in a 1-year-old child. Tracheal diameter is less than the child's little finger	Small amounts of mucous or swelling easily obstruct the airways; child normally has increased airway resistance
The epiglottis is horseshoe shaped and projects posteriorly at 45%. The larynx is high and anterior	Tracheal intubation can be more difficult. A straight blade laryngoscope is used, cricoid pressure may be necessary to facilitate intubation
The trachea is short and soft. The cricoid cartilage is the narrowest portion of neck	Airway of infant can be compressed if neck is flexed or hyperextended. Tube displacement is more likely. Provides a natural seal for endotracheal tube
The cricoid ring is lined by pseudostratifed ciliated epithelium loosely bound to areolar tissue	Particularly susceptible to oedema. Uncuffed tubes are preferred in pre-pubertal children
Breathing	
Infants rely mainly on diaphragmatic breathing. The ribs lie more horizontally in infants and contribute less to chest expansion. Their muscles are more likely to fatigue compared with adults	Children are more prone to respiratory failure. Anything that impedes diaphragm contraction or movement, e.g. abdominal distension can contribute to the development of respiratory failure
Sternum and ribs are cartilaginous; chest wall is soft; intercostal muscles are poorly developed	Infant's chest wall may move inwards instead of outwards during inspiration (retractions) when lung compliance is decreased; greater intrathoracic pressure is generated during inspiration. The compliant chest wall may allow serious parenchymal injuries to occur without rib fracture
Increased metabolic rate (about twice that of an adult); increased respiratory demand for oxygen consumption and carbon dioxide elimination	Respiratory distress increases oxygen demand, as does any condition that increases metabolic rate, e.g. fever
Lung compliance and high chest wall compliance in the neonate	Respiratory function inefficient during episodes of respiratory distress
Smaller amount of elastic and collagen tissue in the paediatric lung	May contribute to the increased incidence of pulmonary oedema, pneumomediastinum and pneumothorax in infants
Circulation	
Child's circulating blood volume is larger per unit of body weight (70–80 mL/kg) but absolute volume is relatively small; 70–80% of newborn's body weight is water, compared with 50–60% of an adult body weight; about half of this volume is extracellular Stroke volume is small and relatively fixed in infants. Cardiac output is directly related to heart rate	Blood loss considered minor in an adult may lead to shock in a child; decreased fluid intake or increased fluid loss quickly leads to dehydration Acute blood loss produces symptoms when 20–25% of circulating volume has been lost Dehydration will compromise peripheral perfusion when 7–10% of the infant or child's body weight and 5–7% of the adolescent or adult body weight is lost Stroke volume cannot increase to improve cardiac output. Response to volume therapy is therefore blunted
By the age of 2 years the myocardial function and response to fluid is similar to that of an adult	Tachycardia is the child's most efficient method of increasing cardiac output. However ventricular rates of > 180–220 beats/min compromise diastolic filling time and coronary artery perfusion
Systemic vascular resistance rises after birth and continues to do so until adulthood	Children's normal values for blood pressure increase with age

vertebral column. Vocal fremitus is usually most prominent at the apex and least prominent at the base of the lungs. Absent or diminished vocal fremitus in the upper airway may indicate asthma or foreign body obstruction. Increased vocal fremitus may indicate pneumonia or atelectasis.

During palpation other abnormal vibrations that indicate pathological conditions are noted. These include pleural rub, which is felt as a grating sensation and is synchronous with respiration and crepitation, which can be felt as a coarse crackly sensation and is the result of air escaping from the lungs to the

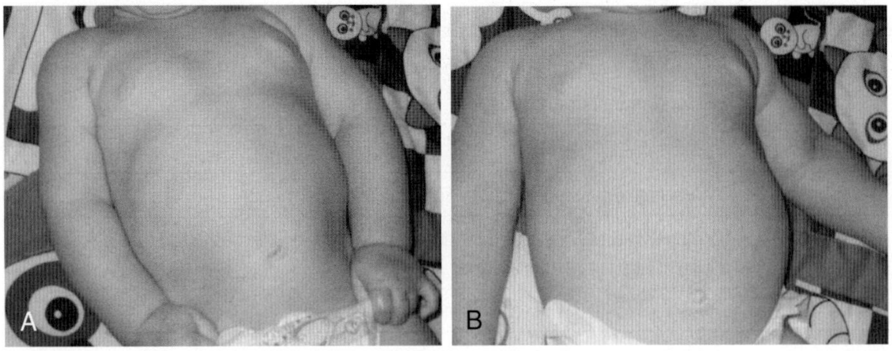

Fig. 27.4 • Chest expansion.

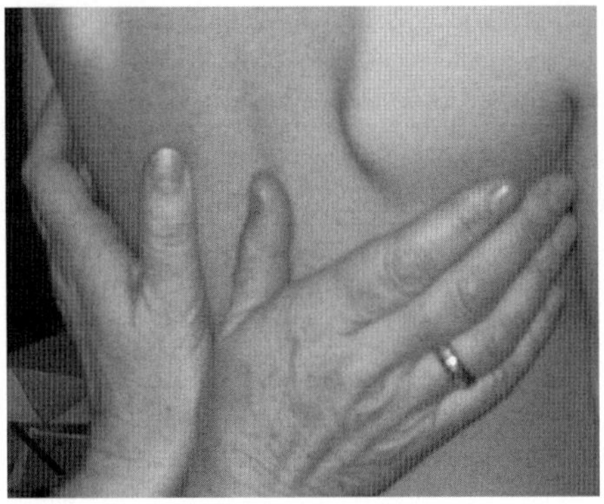

Fig. 27.5 • Respiratory movements.

subcutaneous tissue. This may be caused by injury or surgical intervention. Both crepitation and pleural rub can often be heard as well as felt.

The sinking-in of soft tissues relative to the cartilaginous and bony thorax may be noted in some respiratory disorders. This is recession, it is described as intercostal, subcostal, substernal, clavicular and suprasternal and it demonstrates increased work of breathing:

- Intercostal, subcostal or sternal recession show increased work of breathing.
- Recession is more easily seen in younger children whose chest wall is more compliant.
- In children over 6 or 7 years, recession suggests severe respiratory problems.
- The degree of recession gives an indication of the severity of the breathing difficulty.

Nasal flaring is also an indication of increased work of breathing. The enlargement of the nostrils helps to reduce nasal resistance and maintain airway patency; it is usually described as either minimal or marked. Head bobbing in the infant is a sign of dyspnoea.

Respiratory rates should be measured over a full minute (Table 27.3). It should be remembered that young children breathe diaphragmatically and therefore are observed by watching abdominal movement rather than the movement of the chest. A decreasing rate or rhythm may indicate deterioration rather than improvement in the child's condition (Mackway-Jones et al 1997). A resting rate of >60 breaths/minute is a sign of respiratory distress in a child irrespective of age (Cosby 1998 cited by Dolan & Holt 2000). Tachypnoea at rest indicates a need for increased ventilation.

Respiratory rate

Further information about the severity of the child's illness may be gained by measurement of oxygen saturation (SaO_2) levels with a pulse oximeter (Fig. 27.6). A saturation of less than 92% while breathing air, or less than 95% when breathing oxygen, is low. Rajesh et al (2000) evaluated respiratory rate as an indicator of hypoxia in infants <2 months of age and concluded that a respiratory rate of >60/minute is a good predictor of hypoxia and that the infants should be treated with oxygen should the facility to measure SaO_2 not be available. It should be remembered that pulse oximetry is less accurate when the SaO_2 is less than 70%, when shock is present, and in the presence of carboxyhaemoglobin. If there is evidence of respiratory or circulatory failure then arterial blood gases are needed.

WWW

Learn about the oxyhaemoglobin dissociation curve at:

- http://www.ebme.co.uk

The effectiveness of breathing is also assessed by observing breath sounds. Auscultation allows assessment of breath sounds for pitch, intensity, quality, location and duration. Breath sounds are best heard if the child inspires deeply. Normal breath sounds are vesicular, soft and low pitched on inspiration followed by shorter sound on expiration; bronchial or tubular are similar to the sounds heard upon auscultation over the larynx during respiration; and bronchovesicular is a

Table 27.3 Normal respiratory rates (Mackway-Jones et al 1997)

Age (years)	Breaths/min
<1	30–40
2–5	20–30
5–12	15–20
>12	12–16

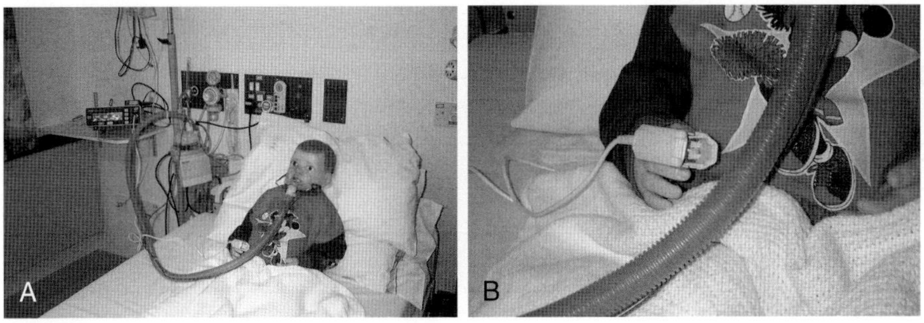

Fig. 27.6 • Measurement of oxygen saturation levels.

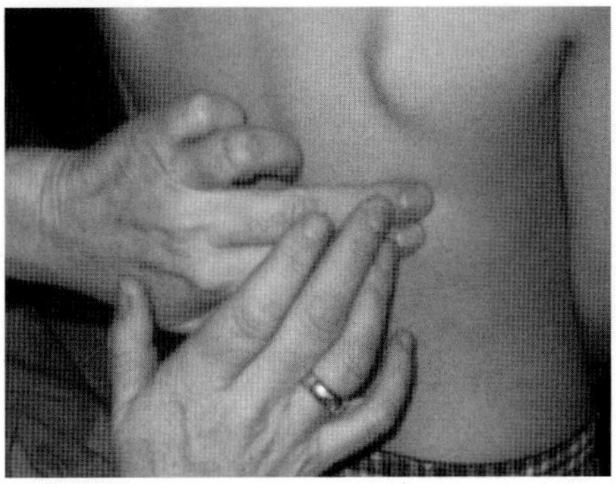

Fig. 27.7 • Percussion

mixture of bronchial and vesicular sounds. Vesicular are heard over most of the chest, except over the larynx and trachea, and, in infants, over the upper chest. Infants' breath sounds are bronchovesicular in the upper chest because of increased transmission (Thompson 1990). Fluid, air or solid masses in the pleural space all interfere with the conduction of breath sounds.

Consolidation or solidification of a portion of the lung caused by, for example, pneumonia will result in tubular or bronchial breathing being heard over the posterior chest due to increased transmission between the trachea and the periphery of the chest (Thompson 1990).

Alert, diminished or absent breath sounds are always abnormal.

Percussion or tapping of the lungs (Fig. 27.7) is carried out to determine the presence and location of air, liquid and solid material in the lung and to evaluate the densities, position and landmarks of the underlying organs. Normally, the percussion note in a lung full of air is resonant. When there is fluid in the chest, e.g. pleural effusion, the note becomes flat. With pneumonia where there is an increased amount of fluid but not in the chest the note becomes dull. With excess air, e.g. asthma, the note is hyper-resonant. It is normal to find dullness over the liver and heart.

Activity

To help discriminate between hollow and flat sounds
Try tapping various parts of an internal wall, see if you can distinguish between the hollow sound of the unsupported plaster board and the flat sound of the solid wood or concrete support.

Voice sounds are also part of auscultation of the lung. Normally, vocal resonance or voice sounds are heard but the sounds are muffled and indistinct. Hearing clear distinct sounds is an abnormal finding and is caused by the same conditions causing abnormal vocal fremitus.

Various respiratory illnesses produce adventitious sounds that are not normally heard over the chest; these are not alterations in normal breath sounds but are additional abnormal sounds.

The effects of inadequate respiration can be seen by examining heart rate, skin colour and mental status. These are linked to the examination of circulation and disability.

C. Circulation

Adequacy of circulation is assessed by examining the cardiovascular status and looking for the effects of circulatory inadequacy on other organs.

Vital signs

The child's vital signs should be appropriate for the child's age and clinical condition. A child normally has a faster heart rate (Table 27.4) and respiratory rate and a lower arterial pressure than an adult. The child's heart rate and pulse volume should be assessed by palpating both central and peripheral pulses. It is important to note that normal vital signs are not always appropriate when a child is seriously ill, indeed a normal heart rate and respiratory rate may indicate cardiopulmonary arrest is imminent. Hypoxia produces tachycardia and is to be expected; bradycardia is a sign of respiratory failure and a preterminal sign. Absent peripheral and weak central pulses are signs of advanced shock and hypotension in children.

An accurate pulse should be measured for a full minute and be consistent with the apex beat. If measuring the heart rate

Table 27.4 Normal heart rates

Age (years)	Beats/min
<1	110–160
2–5	95–140
5–12	80–120
<12	60–100

Table 27.5 Systolic blood pressure by age

Age (years)	Systolic blood pressure
<1	70–90
2–5	80–100
5–12	90–110
>12	100–120

Table 27.6 Normal variations in temperature related to age

Age (years)	Temperature (°C)
<1	37.5–37.7
2–5	37.0–37.2
5–12	36.7–36.8
>12	36.6

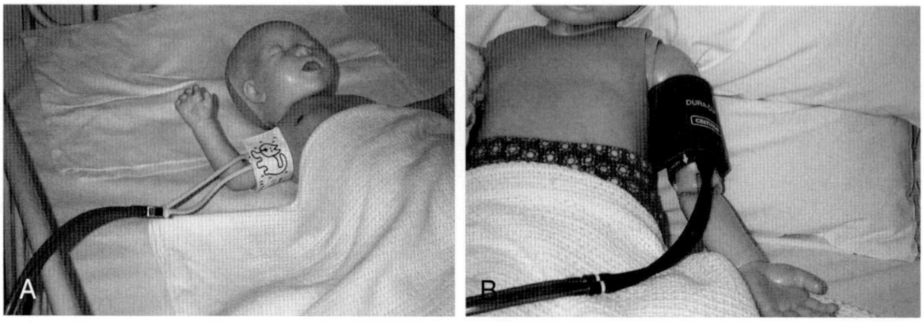

Fig. 27.8 • Observation of a child's blood pressure.

of children less than 2 years of age, a stethoscope should be placed over the apex of the heart and the beats counted for a full minute. Sinus tachycardia is common in the unwell anxious child and further assessment should be carried out to identify the cause.

Blood pressure (Table 27.5)

Expected systolic blood pressure (BP) = 80 + (age in years × 2)

The size of the child's limb must be taken into consideration when taking blood pressure. Make sure the width of the blood pressure (BP) cuff is about two-thirds the length of the child's upper arm (Fig. 27.8). A cuff that is too large may produce a reading that is too low; a cuff that is too small may give a false high reading (Brown 2007).

Children in early shock may have a normal blood pressure reading initially, hypotension is often a late sign and preterminal sign of circulatory failure. Small quantitative changes in the child's blood pressure may indicate significant qualitative changes in the child's clinical condition. It is therefore imperative that accurate and current observations are taken into account when assessing the child's circulatory status.

Skin perfusion and body temperature

The skin colour and temperature should be consistent over the trunk and limbs. Clinical signs of poor perfusion include peripherally cool skin, pallor, mottling, peripheral cyanosis and capillary refill >2 seconds. By the time central cyanosis is visible in acute respiratory distress respiratory arrest is very close. Capillary refill is a quick and easy method for determining the efficacy of respiratory function. A raised digit is pressed for 5 seconds and the time taken for blood to return to the area is estimated in seconds. A capillary refill time of greater than 2 seconds in a child and 3 seconds in a neonate is a sign of poor oxygenation. Ambient temperature should always be considered in the interpretation of capillary refill.

The normal circadian range of infant's temperatures over the 24-hour period has been described as ranging from 36°C at night to 37.8°C during active periods in the day (Table 27.6). In addition, there is now recognised to be a variable fluctuation between individuals of 0.5°C (Mackowiak et al 1992). Therefore we should accept individual variations in normal body temperature, recognising that time of day and age of child may affect expected normal values.

D. Disability

Parents are usually the first to recognise any changes in their child's level of consciousness and it is therefore important to listen to what they say. A hypoxic child may be irritable or agitated early on but increasingly lethargic later. He or she might fail to recognise or interact, e.g. maintain eye contact, with the parents or might not respond to stimuli, e.g. unfamiliar nurses. A progressive drop in level of consciousness is a late sign of hypoxia and may be an indication of impending respiratory distress. Other factors that may lead to a decreasing level of consciousness are shock, sepsis, ingestion of depressants, metabolic abnormalities, hypothermia and head injuries. The level of consciousness should be assessed using the AVPU scale:

A = alert
V = responds to voice
P = responds to pain
U = unresponsive.

Any problem with ABC must be addressed before assuming that a decrease in conscious level is due to a primary neurological problem.

The final but integral part of the child's assessment is their medical history. Factors to be taken into consideration include the following symptoms:

- Is the child breathless:
  - When? At rest, walking, talking, sleeping, feeding?
- Does the child have a cough?
  - What type?
  - How long has the child had this?
- When do the symptoms occur – daytime, night-time?
- Are the symptoms improving or worsening?
- Are there any aggravating or precipitating factors? Does anything relieve the symptoms?
- Are the symptoms associated with anything, e.g. feeding? Is the child able to take feeds?
- How long has the child been unwell, has this happened suddenly, did it occur over time?
- Does the child have a sore throat?
- Is there any nasal discharge, has the child a cough, is the cough productive, what colour is the sputum, how long have these been present?
- Has the child's sleep been affected?
- Is the child's breathing noisy, in what way? Ask the parents to describe any noises they have heard.
- What has the child's activity level been like?

Less specific symptoms to observe for include:

- pyrexia
- urinary output
- anorexia
- vomiting
- diarrhoea
- abdominal pain
- meningism.

In addition, the family will be asked about the child's previous medical history, family and social history, environmental factors and developmental history including immunisation status. It is of interest to note that Elphick et al (2001) found 'wheeze' to be a commonly chosen word used by parents to describe their child's noisy breathing. However, there was wide variation in what parents meant by this term, with many using the word inappropriately. The authors conclude that:

> This highlights the need for accurate history taking, as parents' initial response may be to use words that they perceive as being a medical term. The responsibility lies with the doctor to ensure that interpretation of the language used by parents reflects accurately the noise they mean to describe (Elphick et al 2001) (Table 27.7)

Summary

The diagnosis of acute respiratory disease in childhood is largely a clinical one. It rests on history and examination with the aid of chest radiograph when necessary. The clinical signs of respiratory failure include those demonstrating evidence of a significant increase in the work of breathing, e.g. severe retractions or grunting, inadequate ventilation rate, apnoea or gasping, reduced or absent inspiratory breath sounds and alterations in level of consciousness and evidence of compromise in systemic perfusion, e.g. significant tachycardia, bradycardia and extended capillary refill. Central cyanosis is a late sign of severe hypoxia and requires urgent treatment (Morton & Phillips 1992).

Table 27.7 Terminology used to describe different patterns of respiration

Term	Description
Tachypnoea	Increased rate
Bradypnoea	Decreased rate
Dyspnoea	Difficulty in breathing
Apnoea	Cessation or inability to breathe
Hypoventilation	Decreased and irregular depth of respirations
Hyperventilation	Increased rate and depth
Hypercapnia	Increased levels of carbon dioxide
Hypoxia	Low level of oxygenation
See-saw	Chest falls on inspiration and rises on expiration
Cheyne–Stokes	Altered rate and depth of respirations with periods of apnoea

Management of respiratory illness in children

The aims of the management of respiratory disease are applicable to all respiratory illnesses in addition to the disease-specific treatments. These aims of management are to:

- monitor the child's vital signs, effort and efficacy of breathing and effect of inadequate respiration, i.e. oxygen saturations, colour and mental status
- facilitate respiratory effort and maximise oxygen delivery to maintain O_2 saturations above 92%:
  - position the child for maximum comfort and to facilitate respiratory movements
  - decrease oxygen demand by reducing stress, minimal handling and fever
  - provide humidified and monitored supplemental oxygen by age-appropriate means, i.e. head box for infants, mask for older children
- minimise intrusive examinations and treatments
- prevent complications such as hypoxia
- promote hydration and prevent dehydration by utilising nasogastric or intravenous fluids to maintain adequate fluid intake
- evaluate the effect of pyrexia on the child and administer antipyretics as appropriate
- provide nutrition

- instigate appropriate pharmacological interventions
- communicate effectively with the child and family
- provide psychological support for the child and family
- provide opportunistic health education
- prevent spread of infection
- provide clear and explicit discharge advice.

Respiratory infection

Infections of the respiratory tract are described in a number of ways depending on the area of involvement (Fig. 27.9). However, the infections tend to spread from one area to another because of the continuous nature of the mucous membrane that lines the respiratory tract and the shorter distance between the anatomical structures in children. In addition, the short, open Eustachian tube allows easy access to the middle ear. Infections of the respiratory tract may therefore involve more than one structure.

The largest percentage of infections accounting for acute illness in children is caused by viruses. Infants under 3 months of age have a lower infection rate, which then rises between the ages of 3 and 6 months and remains high through the toddler years. However, by the age of 5 years viral infections are less frequent, although the incidence of *Mycoplasma pneumoniae* and group B streptococcal infections rises.

Upper respiratory tract infection

The average child has between four and twelve upper respiratory tract infections a year and 90% of these are viral, requiring symptomatic management only. Of the remaining 10%, group B

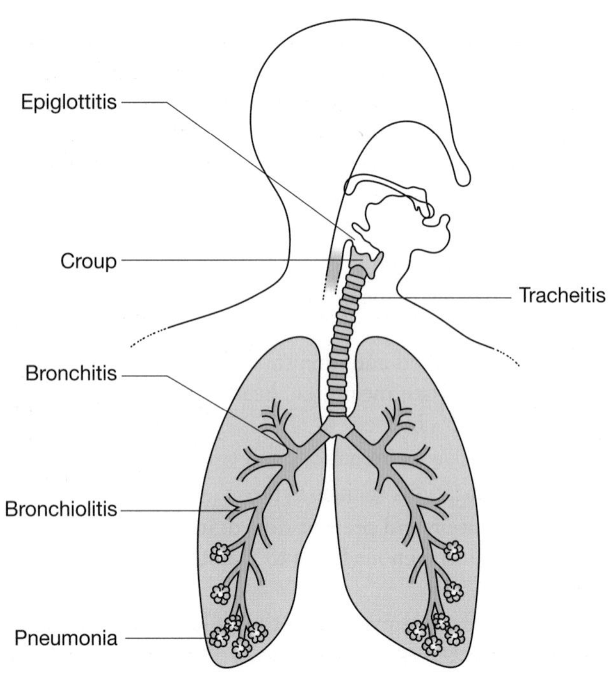

Fig. 27.9 • Anatomic location of respiratory infections.

haemolytic streptococcus is common and requires treatment with penicillin. However, we should always remain vigilant for the possibility that a child with a mild upper respiratory tract infection may have an accompanying illness such as meningitis.

Whooping cough

Pertussis or whooping cough is an acute respiratory infection caused by *Bordetella pertussis*. It occurs mainly in non-immunised children and a single attack confers lifetime immunity.

Characteristics of whooping cough

Begins with the symptoms of an upper respiratory tract infection:

- Coryza
- Sneezing
- Low-grade temperature
- Cough, which continues for some weeks and becomes more severe and paroxysmal. May consist of short rapid coughs followed by an inspiratory 'whoop' sound during which the child's face becomes flushed. This can continue until mucus is vomited.

Specific treatment

The management of whooping cough includes administration of antimicrobial therapy, e.g. erythromycin, as this may reduce the period of infectivity. However, it does not alter the course of the illness. Household and other close contacts should also be treated.

Croup syndromes

Croup is a general term that applies to any condition producing inspiratory stridor. Stridor is a harsh vibratory sound caused by partial obstruction of the upper airway. Croup syndromes include laryngotracheobronchitis (LTB), spasmodic croup, bacterial tracheitis and epiglottitis. LTB and croup are often used synonymously.

LTB is common cause of upper airway obstruction in children and is usually mild but sometimes can be serious (Knutson & Aring 2004). It is an acute inflammation of the upper and lower respiratory tract. The symptoms are initially in the larynx causing stridor and then in the trachea and bronchi leading to a cough and wheeze that occurs in children aged 6 months to 2 years, usually occurring in the winter months. The peak incidence is during the second year of life with boys more affected than girls.

Characteristics of croup

Croup is usually preceded by an upper respiratory tract infection:

- Rhinorrhea
- Coryza
- Low-grade fever
- Sudden onset – often at night.

It presents with:

- inspiratory stridor
- barking cough
- harsh cry/hoarseness.

If obstruction is severe there is:

- tachypnoea
- stridor
- intercostal, supraclavicular, substernal and suprasternal inspiratory retractions.

As the condition worsens there is:

- cyanosis
- increased respiratory effort
- restlessness
- reduced stridulous sound (Rudolf & Levene 2006).

These symptoms are a result of oedema of the larynx and trachea. They are usually triggered by recent infection with the parainfluenza virus (Ausejo et al 1999), although other pathogens can be involved (respiratory syncytial virus, adenovirus, enterovirus and rhinovirus). The incidence of croup is 1.5–6% of children less than 6 years of age, of these 1.5–31% are admitted to hospital (Marx et al 1997, cited in Ausejo et al 1999).

Specific treatment

- Maintain airway, less than 5% require intubation and this is usually due to gradual deterioration rather than acute obstruction.
- Nebulised and/or oral glucocorticoids (Russell et al 2003) usually nebulised budesonide and oral dexamethasone (Rudolf & Levene 2003).
- Inhaled steroids reduce upper airway oedema (Rudolf & Levene 2006), which has a rapid and sustained effect (D'Amore & Campbell Hewson 2002).
- Nebulised adrenaline has been shown to provide temporary relief to patients with croup but is not thought to have long-term benefits (Mathew et al 2005).

Activity

Review Poiseuille's law and consider the effect of a distressed child with a more turbulent airflow.

Evidence-based practice

Cold humidified air (mist therapy) is not effective in improving clinical symptoms in children with moderate croup. Discuss.

www

Childhood immunisation: familiarise yourself with the guidance notes for professionals:

- http://www.doh.gov.uk/greenbook/greenbbookpdf/chapter-16-layout.pdf

Epiglottitis

This is mainly seen in children aged 2–5 years. The infection is usually caused by *Haemophilus influenzae* B and the condition is becoming rare as a result of the introduction of the HIB immunisation of infants (Tanner et al 2002).

Characteristics of epiglottitis

- Short history
- Fever
- Stridor
- Dyspnoea
- Systemically unwell: pale, toxic, lethargic
- May drool and be unable to swallow but have minimal cough (Tanner et al 2002)
- Child often adopts the characteristic posture of sitting upright, mouth open and their chin thrust forward (Rudolf & Levene 2006)
- Extreme anxiety.

The infection causes inflammatory oedema of the supraglottic area, which includes the epiglottis and the pharyngeal structures. If the condition is suspected, examination of the mouth must be avoided because acute or total airway obstruction could result. The child should be examined only with an experienced anaesthetist ready to intubate if required (Rudolf & Levene 2006). Do not lie the child down because this forces the epiglottis to fall backwards, leading to complete airway obstruction. Radiography of the neck is justified only if diagnosis is in doubt and should take place only if the child is stable; radiography in lateral position may also precipitate respiratory arrest due to complete airway obstruction (Tanner et al 2002). It is also not advisable to perform any procedure that may increase the child's anxiety (e.g. taking a blood specimen) as this could precipitate airway spasm and cause death (Rudolf & Levene 2006).

Specific treatment

If epiglottitis is suspected then emergency intubation should be performed to protect the airway (Tanner et al 2002). Intravenous antibiotics are required immediately following intubation, usually chloramphenicol or ampicillin (Rudolf & Levene 2006). Recovery is usually rapid once the airway is established and antibiotic therapy given.

Apnoea

Temporary cessation of breathing can be the result of central respiratory depression or from mechanical obstruction. It can occur in the first 2 days of infections, particularly respiratory syncytial virus and pertussis (Meadow & Newell 2002). When apnoea is associated with cyanosis or unconsciousness then possible causes that need to be considered are seizures, congenital heart disease or airway obstruction.

Aspirated foreign body

Usually occurs in toddlers who are mobile and put small objects in their mouths. Small beads, coins and foodstuffs are the most common objects aspirated. Peanuts are the most dangerous because they swell in the airway, becoming firmly embedded and difficult to remove because they fragment (Rudolf & Levene 2006). Initially, the child may suffer from acute choking but the aspiration of a foreign body may not be recognised. Obstruction may be complete or incomplete. Incomplete obstruction usually allows the passage of air either in both directions or one only. Complete obstruction prevents either inspiration or expiration.

Characteristics of aspirated foreign body

- Acute onset
- Respiratory distress
- Wheeze often unilateral
- Persistent cough
- Asymmetry of chest
- Mediastinal shift
- Dull percussion if collapse has occurred (Rudolf & Levene 2006).

Specific treatment

A bronchoscopy under general anaesthetic to remove the foreign body is required. It is important that this is performed as soon as possible to prevent coughing moving the object back up into the trachea, which may lead to more severe obstruction of the airway (Mackway-Jones et al 2005).

Activity

Look at your local health education literature to find the advice given to parents regarding suitable toys for toddlers and first aid in the event of aspiration of a foreign body.

www

Read the advice from the Child Accident Prevention Trust:

- http://www.capt.org.uk

Bronchiolitis

This condition is the most common cause of severe respiratory infection in infancy, usually occurring in the winter months. It is a viral infection with 75% of cases due to respiratory syncytial virus; other pathogens implicated include adenovirus, parainfluenza and rhinovirus. By the age of 2 years 90% of children are immune to respiratory syncytial virus (Meadow & Newell 2002). It usually occurs in children under the age of 18 months; the most serious cases are infants under 6 months old. The mortality rate is 1 in 5000–20,000.

The infection causes inflammatory obstruction of the small airways and necrosis of the cells lining the lower airways. The ciliary damage impairs the clearance of secretions and this combined with increased mucosal secretion, submucosal oedema and desquamation of cells results in obstruction at the bronchiolar level with atelectasis and hyperinflation. The child is often able to inhale but has difficulty exhaling. Air becomes trapped below the obstruction and interferes with gaseous exchange. Hypoxia and in severe cases hypercapnia may occur (Porth 1994).

Characteristics of bronchiolitis (Meadow & Newell 2002)

- Initial coryza
- Fever
- Tachycardia
- Tachypnoea
- Irregular breathing, recurrent apnoea
- Cough
- Subcostal and intercostal recession
- Irritability
- Poor feeding
- Widespread wheeze and crepitations
- Hyperventilated chest
- Cyanosis/pallor.

The typical appearance of a baby with acute bronchiolitis is therefore one of:

- marked breathlessness
- rapid respirations
- distressing cough
- retraction of lower ribs and sternum
- wheezing depending on degree of airway obstruction.

Many infants with bronchiolitis can be managed at home, however careful assessment is required in deciding which infants need hospitalisation. The NHS Executive guidelines for the management of acute respiratory failure in normal infants and children recognise that a respiratory rate of > 50/minute, a heart of > 140/minute and O_2 saturation of < 92% in air, with the use of accessory muscles defines a moderately severe episode and requires hospitalisation (Table 27.8).

Respiratory failure may be preceded by cyanosis, pallor, listlessness and reduction or absence of breath sounds (Porth 1994) and hypoxia requires urgent interventions.

Specific treatment

- Because of the risk of apnoea, small infants should be nursed using apnoea monitors or O_2 saturation monitors.
- Antibiotics, bronchodilators and steroids have no positive effect on this condition.
- Some infants (2%) suffer recurrent apnoea attacks, exhaustion or hypercapnia and hypoxia, and require mechanical ventilation.

Reflect on your practice

What advice have you witnessed being given to children's families regarding the spread of RSV?

Activity

Review the effect of a raised temperature on an infant's metabolic rate and oxygen requirements.

- Why is this important in infants with bronchiolitis?

Table 27.8 Assessment of Illness severity

Clinical parameter	Severity	
	Mild	**Moderate to severe**
Activity level	Alert	Reduced level of consciousness, exhausted or fatigued
Heart rate	<140/minute	>140/minute
Respiratory rate	<50/minute	>50/minute
Oxygen saturation	>92%	<92%
Temperature	<380	>380
Recession	Mild	Marked
Nasal flaring	None	Some
Feeding	Taking three-quarters or more than half of normal feeds	Taking less than half of normal feeds
Colour	Pink	Pallor, mottling, cyanosed or grey
Level of hydration	Normal	Evidence of dehydration
Apnoea	None	History of
Capillary refill	<2 seconds	>2 seconds

PowerPoint

Emma's scenario is repeated on the companion PowerPoint presentation. Work through it here or on the PowerPoint. Answers are provided at the end of the chapter or on the presentation.

Scenario

Emma is 3 months old, she is admitted to the assessment ward accompanied by her anxious parents. The GP visited her at home and organised for an emergency admission.

Emma has had a runny nose for 2 days and is off her feeds. She has felt hot since yesterday evening and over the past few hours she has become quite pale. However, her mother reports that Emma is not as irritable as last night and has at last stopped crying:

- What framework would you utilise to assess Emma's physiological status?
- What observations do you need to carry out?
- What would you expect these observations to be?
- Would you categorise Emma's present condition as mild, moderate or severe?
- Is there any information in the history given that would cause concern?
- What care would you expect to be initiated?
- What ongoing care would Emma require?

Lower respiratory tract infection

Pneumonia

Pneumonia is an infection of the lower respiratory tract most commonly due to bacterial or viral pathogens. Pneumonia can be classified according to its anatomical distribution:

- Lobar pneumonia occurs when there is involvement of a large portion of or an entire lobe of a lung.
- In bronchopneumonia there is patchy consolidation involving several lobes of the lungs.
- Interstitial pneumonia involves the walls surrounding the alveoli and bronchioles; this type of pneumonia is usually caused by viral or mycoplasmal infections (Porth 1994).

Pneumonia is also classified by the infective pathogen, e.g. streptococcus or mycoplasma. The incidence of bacterial pneumonia is highest amongst children < 2 years of age, with boys affected more than girls (2:1 ratio). Viral infections with RSV are also common in this age group; this is the most common cause of viral pneumonia. Death rates from pneumonia in England and Wales for children under 1 year are 111 per million population; children aged 1–4 years 14 per million population; and children 5–14 years 3 per million population (Office of National Statistics 2003). Children who are chronically sick or have congenital abnormalities are at greater risk. Predisposing factors should always be considered in children who present with pneumonia, such as congenital abnormality of the bronchi or inhaled foreign body (Rudolf & Levene 1999).

Bronchopneumonia

This condition occurs in young children and older children with chronic conditions that affect their respiratory function (Meadow & Newell 2002). A large number of different organisms can be responsible. Bronchopneumonia usually follows another respiratory illness such as bronchiolitis, whooping cough or viral infection.

Characteristics of bronchopneumonia (Meadow & Newell 2002)

- Tachypnoea
- Dry cough initially then productive with purulent sputum
- Fever
- Fretfulness
- Intercostal/subcostal recession
- Grunting in infants
- Nasal flaring
- Generalised crepitations
- Cyanosis in severe cases.

Lobar pneumonia

Around 90% of cases of lobar pneumonia are caused by *Streptococcus pneumoniae*.

Characteristics of lobar pneumonia (Meadow & Newell 2002)

- Sudden illness
- High fever
- Flushed
- Tachypnoea
- Cyanosis in severe cases
- Respiratory distress
- Intercostal/subcostal recession
- Grunting in infants
- Nasal flaring
- Pleuritic pain – child leans forward towards affected side
- May have referred pain in abdomen or shoulder tip.

Specific treatment

Broad-spectrum antibiotics are usually administered, with one choice of an antibiotic being based on the most likely pathogen dictated by the child's age and clinical presentation. Physiotherapy is no longer considered beneficial in children with pneumonia.

WWW

Read more about this condition online:

- http://kidshealth.org/parent/infections/index.html

Seminar discussion topic

There is an increased risk of pneumonia in the first year of life if parents smoke:

- What other potential health risks are there to children in a smoking household?
- Should smoking be banned completely?

Tuberculosis

After years of decline in the incidence of this disease, the global incidence is now increasing. The World Health Organization (WHO) estimates that one-third of the world's population is infected with *Mycobacterium tuberculosis*. Global infection rates are 1.86 billion people and are highest in south-east Asia (Dye 1999). Watson & Moss (2001) report that, in the year 2000 in England and Wales, 235 schoolchildren aged 5–14 were notified as having tuberculosis (TB). Most of these will not have been infectious but some will have been smear positive and therefore potential sources of infection. Most children are infected by someone close to them but outbreaks also occur in other meeting places, e.g. schools. In 2001, the biggest ever school outbreak of TB recorded in the UK occurred in Leicester.

Common presenting symptoms

- Cough and respiratory symptoms
- Mild dyspnoea
- Weight loss and anorexia
- Fever may occur.

These are gradual in onset and increase in severity as the disease progresses. Investigations include chest radiography, tuberculin test, gastric aspiration and sputum testing. Treatment is by antituberculosis drugs for between 3 and 6 months under the care of a clinician with experience in tuberculosis care.

Asthma

The changes in prevalence of asthma in children are difficult to determine because of changes in diagnostic practice (Magnus & Jaakkola et al 1997) but, however defined, asthma and wheezing in children has increased dramatically over the past few decades (Kaur et al 1998). Asthma is thought to affect approximately 10% of children and the incidence and severity of the disease appears to be increasing (Cross 1999). This increase is thought to be due to environmental factors (Caldwell 1998). It is difficult to diagnose asthma in the very young because it is hard to distinguish between asthma and other causes of wheezing. Epidemiological studies suggest that up to 30% of all children under the age of 3 years have had an acute episode of wheezing (Barnes 2003). This makes asthma the most common medical condition of childhood (Asthma UK 2004). There are approximately 2000 deaths (adult and children) each year in the UK due to asthma; 80% of these are thought to be preventable.

Asthma is a chronic inflammatory condition of the airways, the cause of which is still not completely understood (Kieckfeler & Ratcliffe 2004). Asthma is described as, 'airway obstruction that is reversible, airway inflammation, and increased airway responsiveness to a variety of stimuli'.

The aetiology of asthma is multifactorial (Barnes 2003). There is often a family history of atopy, asthma or allergies and, in addition to this, there are precipitating factors such as infection, allergic triggers, tobacco smoke or physical or emotional stress. Some of the possible reasons for an exacerbation of an asthma attack are:

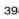

- predisposing factors such as:
  - a strong genetic factor (Frew & Holgate 2005)
  - maternal smoking
  - not breast-fed for the first 4 months of life (Oddy et al 1999)
  - family atopy (Frew & Holgate 2005)
- indoor triggers such as:
  - allergy to house-dust mite (Frew & Holgate 2005)
  - allergy to animal dander (Caldwell 1998)
  - tobacco smoke (Simon et al 2005)
  - moulds and fungal spores from *Aspergillus fumigatus* (Frew & Holgate 2005, Zureik 2002)
- outdoor triggers:
  - allergy to pollen
  - cold weather (Caldwell 1998)
  - air pollutants
  - industrial chemicals

- other possible triggers:
  - viral infection (Cates & Fitzgerald 2001)
  - exercise (de Bisschop et al 1999)
  - food allergies (Simpson 2007)
  - stress, emotion and laughing (Meadow & Newell 2002).

Weekly or daily use of paracetamol has been linked with increasing the severity of asthma in some individuals (Shaheen 2000).

Asthma is a hyper-responsiveness of the airways induced by a trigger (Barnes 2003). It commonly presents as a lower airway obstruction; the wheezing is generated by turbulent airflow causing oscillation of the bronchial wall. Three factors are involved in the asthmatic response:

1. Bronchospasm:
  - narrowing of the bronchial walls due to contraction of the smooth muscle
  - more severe in the smaller bronchi and bronchioles, where there is no cartilage in the walls.

2. Inflammation:
  - causes the airways to become hyper-responsive and narrow easily in reaction to a wide range of stimuli
  - further narrowing of the airways by the invasion of the mucosa, submucosa and muscle tissue by inflammatory cells.

3. Inflammatory cells:
  - mainly eosinophils but also contain neutrophils macrophages and mast cells
  - contain chemical mediators, including histamine, prostaglandins and leukotrienes, which cause vasodilation and increased capillary permeability
  - result in mucus production and oedema.

The lumen of the airways is therefore narrowed by contraction of the smooth muscle, mucosal oedema and the hypersecretion of mucus (Fig. 27.10) (Hockenberry et al 2003).

Scenario

It is 6pm and Jason, a 12-year-old boy, is to be admitted to the children's ward. His mother is with him. Jason is a known asthmatic and he is prescribed regular medication. He was sent home from school earlier in the day with an acute exacerbation of his asthma. He is breathless and unable to carry out a conversation:

- What additional equipment would you get ready prior to Jason's arrival on the ward?
- When they arrive, what questions would you ask Jason and his mother?
- What observations would you carry out?
- What are the normal ranges for these observations for a child this age?
- What medications should have been administered during the day?
- What treatment should be given?
- What advice should be given to Jason and his mother before discharge from hospital?

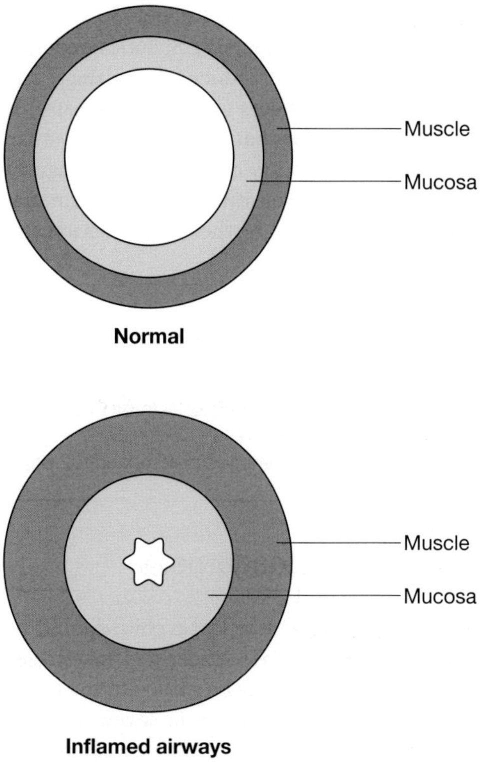

Fig. 27.10 • The asthma response.

Characteristics of severe asthma

- Too breathless to talk
- Chest recession/use of accessory muscles
- Respiratory rate >50 breaths/minute (children under 5 years) or respiratory rate >30 breaths/minute (children 5 years and over)
- Heart rate >130 beats/minute (children under 5 years) or >120 beats/minute (children 5 years and over)
- Peak flow reduced to <50% of expected
- Wheezing may or may not be a prominent feature
- Use of accessory muscles of respiration.

(Barnes 2003).

Characteristics of life-threatening asthma

- Conscious level depression
- Agitation
- Exhaustion
- Poor respiratory effort
- Cyanosis
- Oxygen saturation levels < 85% in air
- Silent chest
- Peak expiratory flow rate (PEF) < 30%.

(Barnes 2003).

There are two phases of the asthmatic response (Kieckfeler & Ratcliffe 2004). The first phase occurs within minutes of the exposure to the stimuli, reaches a peak in about 30 minutes and subsides after approximately 2 hours. It includes oedema, mucus secretion and bronchospasm-induced wheezing. The second phase occurs about 4–12 hours after the exposure; it reaches a peak after about 4–8 hours but can last for more than 24 hours. This inflammatory reaction can lead to damage of lung tissue. The airways are hypersensitive to allergic stimulation in this phase, which can result in further inflammation and bronchoconstriction.

WWW

Read the most recent audits on the prevalence of asthma in the UK:

- http://www.asthma.org.uk/about/images/childrenaudit02.pdf

Principles of asthma management

In the event of an acute asthmatic attack the child should be given 2–4 puffs of a beta 2 agonist, via spacer and face-mask; repeated every 20–30 minutes. This may be sufficient for a mild asthma attack; up to 10 puffs can be given in severe asthma. If the child has not improved after 10 puffs they should be taken to hospital immediately (British Thoracic Society/Scottish Intercollegiate Guidelines Network 2008 – BTS/SIGN). When waiting for transfer to hospital the child can continue to have puffs of beta 2 agonist as necessary, during the transfer by ambulance the child should be given oxygen and nebulised beta 2 agonists.

A bolus of intravenous salbutamol can be effective in cases of severe asthma.

The early use of steroids is recommended, therefore oral soluble prednisolone should be given early in the attack as it can prevent the relapse of symptoms and reduce the need for hospital admission (BTS/SIGN 2008).

Intravenous hydrocortisone can be given every 4 hours in children with severe asthma who are unable to take oral medication.

Ipratropium bromide used in addition to beta 2 agonists used in the first 2 hours of an acute attack has been shown to be safe and effective particularly in severe cases (Vondra et al 2002). In children who respond poorly to beta 2 agonists repeated doses of ipratropium bromide should be given early in the treatment.

Intravenous drugs may be necessary because inhaled drugs are not effective during severe asthmatic attacks because the airways are completely obstructed by inflammation and mucus (Jordan & White 2001). ECG monitoring should be used if frequent doses of nebulised salbutamol or intravenous salbutamol are given.

In cases of severe or life-threatening asthma which is not responding to beta 2 agonists and steroids then aminophylline can be given in a high dependency setting (Goodman et al 1996).

The use of intravenous magnesium sulphate by slow infusion has not been confirmed but is a safe treatment for acute asthma management (Ciarallo et al 2000).

Children may require intravenous fluids to avoid dehydration if severe asthma is prolonged and they are not tolerating oral fluids.

Humidified oxygen may be required to maintain the child's oxygen saturation. The method of oxygen administration chosen depends on the child's age and condition. Transcutaneous measurement of oxygen saturation is used for continuous oxygen assessment if the child is hypoxic, so that oxygen therapy can be titrated against the oxygen saturation levels. Arterial blood gas monitoring may be necessary if the child shows signs of severe respiratory distress; this will help determine if the child is in respiratory failure and needs respiratory support. If necessary, assisted ventilation using endotracheal intubation may be used for a short period of time, usually 8–12 hours.

PowerPoint

Access the companion PowerPoint presentation.

The decision to admit the child to hospital or to discharge the child home is often difficult. Clear guidelines are available from (BTS/SIGN 2008).). These are available on the Society's website (http://www.brit-thoracic.org.uk).

The step approach to drug management is advised by both national and international guidelines for the management of asthma in children (www.sign.ac.uk – BTS/SIGN 2008). The National Institute of Clinical Excellence (NICE 2000) has also published a guide to the management of asthma and a useful review of the use of inhaler systems/devices in children.

WWW

Read the guide produced by NICE at:

- http://www.nice.org.uk

Look up the Kids Club for 7–14-year-olds to help gain their compliance:

- http://www.asthmabusters.org

Discussion of the scenarios

Bronchiolitis scenario: Emma

What framework would you utilise to assess Emma's physiological status?

Assessment follows the ABC criteria for assessment in conjunction with neurological observations and provides a framework for rapid and effective nursing assessment of the child with respiratory problems. The survey should therefore include assessment of:

- airway
- breathing
- circulation
- disability.

What observations do you need to carry out?

- Vital signs: temperature, pulse and respiration. Remember that normal vital signs are not always appropriate when a child is seriously ill, indeed a normal heart rate and respiratory rate may indicate cardiopulmonary arrest is imminent.
- Respiratory rates: should be measured over a full minute.
- Assessment of breathing: involves examination of the chest including observation of respiratory movements, number, rhythm, depth and quality of respirations, and character of breath sounds utilising the skills of palpation, auscultation and percussion.
- Remember that the degree of recession gives an indication of the severity of the breathing difficulty and nasal flaring is a further sign of increased work of breathing. A resting rate of > 60 breaths/minute is a sign of respiratory distress in a child irrespective of age and an oxygen saturation of less than 92% while breathing air is low.
- The child's heart rate and pulse volume should be assessed by palpating both central and peripheral pulses for 1 minute. The skin colour and temperature should be consistent over the trunk and limbs. Clinical signs of poor perfusion include peripherally cool skin, pallor, mottling, peripheral cyanosis and capillary refill > 2 seconds. Remember that by the time central cyanosis is visible in acute respiratory distress respiratory arrest is very close.

What would you expect these observations to be?

- Mum reports Emma as struggling to get her breath and you count her respirations as 52 breaths/minute.
- Her peripheral temperature is 38°C.
- Her pulse is 155 beats/minute on an apex recording.
- Her oxygen saturations are 90% in air.
- She has marked recession and nasal flaring.
- She is pale and her capillary refill time is 3 seconds.

Would you categorise Emma's present condition as mild, moderate or severe?

Most likely she would be classed as severe because her pulse rate is above 140/minute, her oxygen saturations are below 92% in air, she has marked recession and nasal flaring. She has also become pale and stopped crying, which may be an indication of fatigue.

Is there any information in the history given that would cause concern?

Emma has not been eating for 2 days. You need to ask exactly how much feed she has taken. You also need to ask when she last had a wet nappy and assess if her anterior fontanelle is sunken. You are assessing her state of hydration. She has had a reduced fluid intake, a raised temperature and fewer wet nappies, therefore you would expect her to be dehydrated. If you cannot remember how to classify dehydration, please review this now.

Emma has stopped crying, which may indicate that she is becoming fatigued and that her decreased oxygen saturation is altering her mental status. You would need to assess her against the AVPU scale.

What care would you expect to be initiated?

- Regular observations of vital signs and capillary refill, continuous monitoring of oxygen saturations.
- Humidified and monitored oxygen therapy in a head box to maintain oxygen saturation > 92% (Fig. 27.11).
- Obtain a specimen of nasopharyngeal aspirate to determine cause of bronchiolitis.
- Nursing assessment of state of hydration to include amount of feed taken, urine output, temperature of peripheries, peripheral pulses, skin turgor, temperature gap, capillary refill time, state of mucous membranes and specific gravity of urine.
- Assessment of ability to feed orally and care planned accordingly to progress to either orogastric/nasogastric or intravenous fluids as condition determines.
- If oral feeding continues then reduce feed volume and increase frequency offered as condition determines returning to normal feeds and frequency as condition improves.
- If oral feeding discontinues then commence mouth care.
- If intravenous fluids are initiated then commence care of intravenous infusion and intravenous cannula site.
- Monitor urine output. Minimum required for an infant is 2 mL/kg/h. Weigh nappies before and after use; 1 g = 1 mL.
- Manage fever as appropriate. Remember that an increase in temperature raises basic metabolic rate and increases oxygen demand.
- Prevent spread of infection.

What ongoing care would Emma require?

Continuation of all above care and in addition:

- minimal handling
- care of family to include all aspects of family-centred care

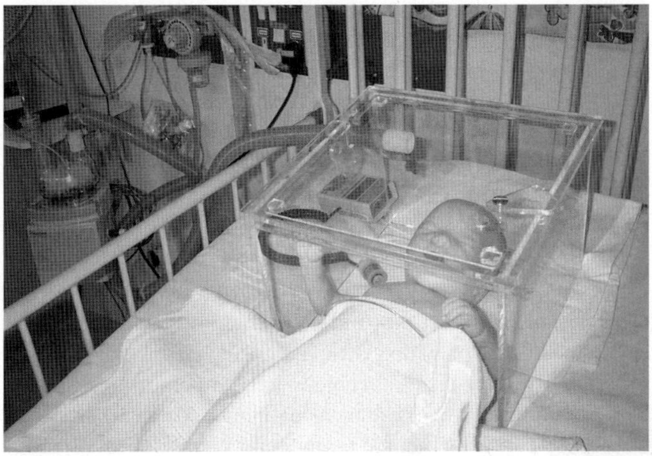

Fig. 27.11 • Oxygen therapy.

- education of family regarding ongoing care needs at home
- discharge planning including outpatient appointment, health visitor liaison and referral to community team as appropriate, discharge summary, completion of health visitor red book, medication and provision of written information/advice.

Asthma scenario: Jason

What additional equipment would you get ready prior to Jason's arrival on the ward?

- Oxygen
- Nebuliser
- Oxygen saturation monitor
- Equipment for intravenous therapy
- Extra pillows.

When they arrive, what questions would you ask Jason and his mother?

- What is his normal medication?
- What medication has he taken today, how frequently and when was it last given?
- What may have triggered this attack?
- Is his condition worsening or improving?
- How long has been breathless?
- Has he been in hospital recently for asthma?
- Response to treatment previously?
- How much has he had to drink today?

What observations would you carry out?

- Vital signs: temperature, pulse and respirations. Remember that normal vital signs are not always appropriate when a child is seriously ill, indeed a normal heart rate and respiratory rate may indicate cardiopulmonary arrest is imminent.
- Respiratory rates: should be measured over a full minute.
- Assessment of breathing involves examination of the chest including observation of respiratory movements, number, rhythm, depth and quality of respirations, and character of breath sounds. The child's inability to speak is a relevant factor when assessing their respiratory distress.
- Remember that the degree of recession gives an indication of the severity of the breathing difficulty and nasal flaring is a further sign of increased work of breathing. A resting rate of >60 breaths/minute is a sign of respiratory distress in a child irrespective of age and an oxygen saturation of less than 92% while breathing air is low.
- The child's heart rate and pulse volume should be assessed by palpating both central and peripheral pulses for 1 minute. The skin colour and temperature should be consistent over the trunk and limbs. Clinical signs of poor perfusion include peripherally cool skin, pallor, mottling, peripheral cyanosis and capillary refill >2 seconds. Remember by the time central cyanosis is visible in acute respiratory distress respiratory arrest is very close.
- The child's level of consciousness should be noted. Is the child agitated or becoming lethargic?

What are the normal ranges for these observations for a child this age?

- Normal respiratory rate 15–20 breaths per minute
- Normal heart rate 80–120 beats per minute
- Temperature 36.6–36.8°C
- Oxygen saturation level 95–98%
- Capillary refill < 2 seconds.

What medications should have been administered during the day?

The following answers are based on British Thoracic Society/Scottish Intercollegiate Guidelines Network (2008):

- Normal medications prior to acute exacerbation probably beta 2 agonist
- When exacerbation occurred 2–4 puffs beta 2 agonist via spacer
- Beta 2-agonist increased to 2–4 puffs every 20–30 minutes up to total 10 puffs according to response
- Soluble oral prednisolone 30–40 mg may have been given under the direction of the GP
- If seen in A&E department then nebulised beta 2 agonist driven by oxygen may have been administered.

What treatment should be given?

- Depending on severity, continue treatment as above administering nebulised beta 2 agonist driven by oxygen until the attack is under control
- Continue oxygen via face-mask or nasal prongs
- If required give intravenous hydrocortisone 100 mg
- Monitor Jason's vital signs
- Position Jason for maximum comfort
- Prepare for intravenous cannulation and infusion.
- Provide psychological support for Jason and his mother.

What advice should be given to Jason and his mother before discharge from hospital?

The following answers are based on British Thoracic Society/Scottish Intercollegiate Guidelines Network (2008):

- Continue with beta 2 agonist as prescribed
- Continue with oral prednisolone for up to 3 days
- Contact GP if asthma not controlled on prescribed treatment
- Provided written asthma action plan
- Check inhaler technique
- Arrange GP follow-up.

References

Asthma, U.K., 2004. Where do we stand? Asthma in the UK today. Asthma UK Publications.

Ausejo, M., Saenz, A., Pham, B., et al., 1999. The effectiveness of glucocorticoids in treating croup: meta-analysis. British Medical Journal 319, 595–600.

Barnes, K., 2003. Paediatrics – a clinical guide for nurse practitioners. Butterworth Heinemann, London.

British Thoracic Society, 2002. British Thoracic Society guidelines for the management of community acquired pneumonia in childhood. Thorax 57 (suppl I), i1–24.

British Thoracic Society/Scottish Intercollegiate Guidelines Network 2008 British Guideline on the Management of Asthma. A national clinical guideline. Revised May 2008. www.sign.ac.uk.

Brown, A., 2007. Assessing a child's blood pressure. In: Glasper, A., McEwing, G., Richardson, J. (Eds.), Oxford handbook of children's and young people's nursing. Oxford University Press, Oxford.

Caldwell, C., 1998. Management of acute asthma in children. Nursing Standard 12 (29), 8–14 49–54.

Carter, B., 1995. Nursing support and care: meeting the needs of the child and family with altered respiratory function. In: Carter, B., Dearman, A.K. (Eds.), Child health care nursing. Blackwell, London, pp. 275–305.

Cates, C., Fitzgerald, M., 2001. Asthma. Clinical Evidence 5, 1011–1027.

Child Health Committee, 1997. The specific health needs of children and young people, 2nd report. Child Health Committee, London.

Christopher, A., Crowley, S., 2003. The burden of respiratory disease in childhood. Lung & Asthma information agency Factsheet 2003/2.

Ciarallo, L., Brousseau, D., Reinert, S., 2000. Higher-dose intravenous magnesium therapy for children with moderate to severe acute asthma. Archives of Pediatric and Adolescent Medicine 154 (10), 979–983.

Cross, S., 1999. Better care for people with asthma. Nursing Standard 13 (46), 4–10 51–54.

D'Amore, A., Campbell Hewson, G., 2002. The management of acute upper airway abstruction in children. Current Paediatrics 12, 17–21.

de Bisschop, C., Guenard, H., Desnot, P., Vergeret, J., 1999. Reduction of exercise-induced asthma in children by short, repeated warm ups. British Journal of Sports Medicine 33 (2), 100–104.

Dolan, B., Holt, L., 2000. Accident and emergency theory into practice. Ballière Tindall, London.

Dye, C., Scheele, S., Dolin, P., Pathania, V., Ravigalione, M.C., 1999. Aug 18. 1999 Consensus statement. Global burden of tuberculosis: estimated incidence, prevalence, and mortality by country. WHO Global Surveillance and Monitoring Project. Journal of the American medical association 282 (7), 677–686.

Elphick, H.E., Sherlock, P., Foxall, G., et al., 2001. Survey of respiratory sounds in infants. Archives of Disease in Childhood 84, 34–39.

Frew, A.J., Holgate, S.T., 2005. Respiratory medicine. In Kumar, P., Clark, M. (Eds.), Clinical medicine, 6th edn. Elsevier, London.

Goodman, D.C., Littenberg, B., O'Connor, G.T., Brooks, J.G., 1996. Theophylline in acute childhood asthma: a meta-analysis of its efficacy. Pediatric Pulmonology 21 (4), 211–218.

Hall, C.B., 1998. Respiratory syncytial virus. In: Feigin, R.D., Cherry, J.D. (Eds.), Textbook of pediatric infectious diseases. WB Saunders, Philadelphia, pp. 2084–2111.

Johnson H 2007 Croup. British Medical Journal Clinical Evidence. http://clinicalevidence.bmj.com (Accessed 7 November 08).

Joint Committee on Vaccination and Immunisation (2007) BCG statement Executive summary. http://www.advisorybodies.doh.gov.uk/jcvi/statements.htm (Accessed 11 November 2008).

Jordan, S., White, J., 2001. Bronchodilators: implications for nursing practice. Nursing Standard 15 (27), 45–55.

Kaur, B., Anderson, H.R., Austin, J., et al., 1998. Prevalence of asthma symptoms, diagnosis, and treatment in 12–14-year-old children across Great Britain (International Study of Asthma and Allergies in Childhood; ISAAC UK). British Medical Journal 316, 118–124.

Kieckfeler, G., Ratcliffe, M., 2004. Asthma. In: Allen, P., Vessey, J. (Eds.), Primary care of the child with a chronic condition, 4th edn. Mosby, Missouri.

Knutson, D., Airing, A., 2004. Viral croup: a current perspective: differential diagnosis http://www.medscape.com/viewarticle/493855_4.

MacGregor, J., 2000. Introduction to the anatomy and physiology of children. Routledge, London.

Mackowiak, P., Wasserman, S.S., Levine, M.M., 1992. A critical appraisal of 98.6°F the upper limit of the normal body temperature and other legacies of Carl Reinhold August Wunderlich. Journal of the American Medical Association 268, 1578–1580.

Mackway-Jones, K., Molyneux, E., Phillips, B., Wieteska, S., 2005. Advanced paediatric life support, 4th edn. Blackwell Publishing, Oxford.

Magnus, P., Jaakkola, J., 1997. Secular trend in the occurrence of asthma among children and young adults: critical appraisal of repeated cross sectional surveys. British Medical Journal 314, 1795–1803.

McChance, K., Heuther, S., 2002. Pathophysiology – the biologic basis for disease in adults & children. Mosby, London.

Meadow, R., Newell, S., 2002. Lecture notes in paediatrics, 7th edn. Blackwell Science, Oxford.

Morton, R.J., Phillips, B.M., 1992. Accidents and emergencies in children. Oxford University Press, Oxford.

The National Institute of Clinical Excellence (NICE), 2000. Online. Available at: http://www.nice.org.uk.

Oddy, W.H., Holt, P.G., Sly, P., et al., 1999. Association between breastfeeding and asthma in six year old children: findings of a prospective birth cohort study. British Medical Journal 319, 815–819.

Office of National Statistics 2003 Online. Available at: http://www.statistics.gov.uk.

Porth, C.M., 1994. Pathophysiology – concepts of altered health states, 4th edn. Lippincott, London.

Rajesh, V.T., Singh, S., Kataria, S., 2000. Tachypnoea is a good predictor of hypoxia in acutely ill infants under 2 months. Archives of Disease in Childhood 82, 46–49.

Russell, K., Wiebe, N., Saenz, A., Ausejo Segura, M., Johnson, D., Hartling, L., Klassen, T.P., 2003. Glucocorticoids for croup. Cochrane Database of Systematic Reviews Issue 4, Art. No: CD001955. DOI: 10.1002/14651858.CD001955.pub2.

Rudolf, M., Levene, M., 1999. Paediatric and child health. Blackwell Science, Oxford.

Scottish Intercollegiate Guidelines Network (SIGN), 2006. Bronchiolitis in children. NHS Quality Improvement Scotland.

Shaheen, S., Sterne, J., Songhurst, C., Burney, P., 2000. Frequent paracetamol use and asthma in adults Thorax 55, 266–270.

Simon, C., Everitt, H., Kendrick, T., 2005. Oxford handbook of General Practice, 2nd edn. Oxford University Press, Oxford.

Simpson, A.B., 2009. Food allergy and asthma morbiditity in children. Paediatric Pulmonology 42 (6), 489–495.

Tanner, K., Fitzsimmons, G., Carrol, D., et al., 2002. Haemophilus influenzae type b epiglottitis as a cause of acute upper airways obstruction in children. British Medical Journal 325, 1099–1100.

Thomas, D.O., 1996. Assessing children – it's different. RN 59 (4), 33–44 (quiz 45).

Thompson, S.W., 1990. Emergency care of children. Jones & Bartlett, Boston.

Watson, J.M., Moss, F.M., 2001. TB in Leicester: out of control, or just one of those things? British Medical Journal 322, 1133–1134.

Westley, C.R., Cotton, E.K., Brooks, J.G., 1978. Nebulized racemic epinephrine by IPPB for the treatment of croup: a double-blind study. American Journal of Diseases of Childhood 132 (5), 484–487.

Vondra, V., Sladek, K., Kotasova, J., Terl, M., Rossetti, A., Cantini, L., 2002. A new HFA-134a propellant in the administration of inhaled BDP via the Jet spacer: controlled clinical trial vs the conventional CFC. Respiratory Medicine 96 (10), 784–789.

World Health Organization (WHO), 1995. The management of acute respiratory infections in children. In: Practical guidelines for outpatient care. WHO, Geneva.

Zureik, M., Neukirch, C., Leynaert, B., et al., 2002. Sensitization to airborne moulds and severity of asthma: cross sectional study from European Community respiratory health survey. British Medical Journal 325, 411–418.

Caring for children with gastrointestinal problems

28

Julia M Winter

ABSTRACT

The aim of this chapter is to review the types, causes and management of both acute and chronic gastrointestinal disorders in infants and children. The chapter content will focus primarily on the most common causes of gastrointestinal disturbance, likely to be encountered by the children's nurse. Management will be considered both with reference to best evidence and also within the context of a family-centred approach to care. Additional information relevant to this chapter will be available on the Evolve website, with PowerPoint presentations on the chapter content.

LEARNING OUTCOMES

- Identify the causes and management of vomiting in infants and children.
- Identify the causes of acute and chronic diarrhoea in infants and children.
- Recognise and distinguish between presentation of acute and chronic disorders.
- Identify the causes of sudden acute gastrointestinal problems requiring surgery.
- Consider the management of both acute and chronic gastrointestinal disorders, adopting a family-centred approach to care.
- Review the changes in incidence in chronic gastrointestinal disorders, considering causes and implications for healthcare practice.

Glossary

Anal stenosis: Narrowing or stricture of the anal canal and sphincter.

Atresia: Absence or closure or a natural passage or channel, imperforation.

Bulimia: An eating disorder, which is characterised by self-induced vomiting after eating.

Cell hyperplasia: The abnormal multiplication or increase in the number of cells in normal arrangement in a tissue.

Cirrhosis: Liver disease characterised pathologically by loss of the normal microscopic structure.

Fundoplication: Mobilisation of the lower end of the oesophagus and wrapping (plication) of the fundus of the stomach around it. Done as a treatment for reflux.

Haemolytic uraemic syndrome: A pathological condition with involves the rupture (haemolysis) of red blood cells, subsequent anaemia, low platelet count and kidney failure.

Hirschsprung's disease: Congenital aganglionosis of colon leading to loss of gut motility.

Imperforate anus: A congenital obstruction of the anal opening.

Intussusception: Telescoping of one portion of the intestine into another.

Jejunal biopsy: Tissue sampling of the jejunum.

Malrotation: Failure during normal embryonic development of normal rotation of all or part of an organ.

Meconium ileus: Obstructed bowel due to impacted, tenacious meconium.

Myopathies: Disease of muscles.

Neurofibromatosis: Growth of neurofibromas (smooth soft or firm tumours) anywhere in the myelinated nervous system (autosomal inheritance).

Organic causes: A disease that occurs as a result of anatomical or physiological abnormality.

Pyloric stenosis: A congenital disorder in which the pylorus is thickened causing obstruction of the gastric outlet.

Scleroderma: Hardening of skin.

Steatosis: Fatty degeneration.

Systemic lupus erythematosus: A chronic autoimmune disease.

Villous atrophy: Wasting or flattening of the villi.

WWW

Use this site, or similar, to look up terms you are not sure of:

- http://www.nlm.nih.gov/medlineplus/mplusdictionary.html

DOI: 10.1016/B978-0-7020-3183-0.10028-1

Vomiting

Vomiting in infants and children is a common problem and therefore likely to be experienced by the majority of families and all children's nurses. Causes of vomiting are diverse and are summarised in Table 28.1. This table shows that causes of vomiting differ between infants and older children. Some are associated with anatomical dysfunction requiring surgery. Other causes of vomiting can be medically managed. One common problem, which lends itself in most cases to medical management, is gastro-oesophageal reflux.

Activity

Choose one of the problems requiring surgery:

- Using a systematic approach, plan the care the child would require before and after surgery.
- How could you make sure you adopted a family-centred approach?

You can check principles of pre- and postoperative care on the companion PowerPoint presentation.

www

Go to:

- http://www.surgical-tutor.org.uk

and using the search facility identify:

- incidence
- pathophysiology
- diagnosis
- management

of pyloric stenosis, intussusception and Hirschsprung's disease.

You can find images of most of the conditions mentioned at:

- http://images.google.co.uk

Table 28.1 Causes of vomiting

Infant	Older child/adolescent
Overfeeding (> 200 mL/kg/day)	Gastroenteritis
Gastrointestinal obstruction	
Pyloric stenosis	
Duodenal or ileal atresia	
Congenital malrotation	
Hirschsprung's disease	
Meconium ileus (in cystic fibrosis)	
Intussusception	
Gastro-oesophageal reflux	Systemic infection
Whooping cough	Raised intracranial pressure
Systemic infection (e.g. urinary tract)	Migraine Bulimia Poisoning Pregnancy

Gastro-oesophageal reflux

Gastro-oesophageal reflux (refluxing of stomach contents into the oesophagus) is frequently seen, to varying degrees, in infants.

Aetiology

The most common cause is functional immaturity of the gastro-oesophageal sphincter. It is more frequently seen in children with a neurological condition, such as cerebral palsy, and also in children with Down syndrome. Whereas mild reflux (possetting) is generally harmless (although it increases the amount of laundry!) it becomes problematic when associated with failure to thrive or complications develop. These include oesophageal scarring, due to refluxing of gastric acid, which can lead to strictures. There is also the risk of aspiration and potentially apnoea. Diagnostic investigations aim to assess any aspiration risk, degree of severity and structural abnormality such as hiatus hernia.

www

Look at the diagram showing relevant anatomy and position of affected sphincter at:

- http://www.empowereddoctor.com/library/photo/gerd.jpg

Diagnosis

Diagnostic investigations include:

- contrast studies: show degree of reflux, strictures, altered anatomy of oesophageal junction
- 24-hour pH probe studies: detect presence of gastric acid in oesophagus
- ultrasound of gastro-oesophageal junction: can demonstrate reflux but no other anatomical defects
- radionuclide scan: aspiration.

Management

Management centres mainly on thickening feeds with products such as Carobel® and nursing the infant in a more upright position. In more severe cases, drugs to increase gut motility and speed stomach emptying have been used. However, the condition is viewed by some as a normal physiological variant (Bourke & Drumm 2002) and only those infants whose condition is complicated, for example, by aspiration, need further medical of surgical intervention.

www

Look at the information for parents offered online by Great Ormond Street Hospital:

- http://www.ich.ucl.ac.uk/

It is important that an accurate medical and nursing assessment is made of infants and children presenting with vomiting to identify and treat quickly any significant underlying medical problems. Key points to consider are (Miall et al 2003):

- the overall state of the child, including level of consciousness, circulatory and respiratory function. Does the child need urgent resuscitation?
- feeding history: the child who is being overfed and vomiting the excess will seem happy and thriving, as will a child with some minor regurgitation. However, other more serious causes of vomiting will lead to weight loss, failure to thrive and, in more severe cases, potentially dehydration and death
- pattern of vomiting, e.g. projectile vomiting presenting from 3 to 6 weeks may indicate pyloric stenosis. Bile-stained vomiting is suggestive of obstruction and needs further investigation as a matter of urgency
- vomiting following paroxysms of coughing is suggestive of whooping cough: check immunisation status
- access to poisons such as medication, alcohol and other chemicals
- febrile: infection both within and outside of the gastrointestinal systems can cause vomiting. If diarrhoea is present, gastroenteritis is likely. If not it is useful to consider urinary tract infection, meningitis and middle ear infection.

Key investigations are summarised in Table 28.2.

Diarrhoea: acute and chronic

As with vomiting, diarrhoea is also a common childhood problem and may be experienced in conjunction with vomiting or on its own. Causes of diarrhoea can be broadly categorised as infectious, inflammatory/allergy mediated or due to malabsorption.

Table 28.2 Key investigations for vomiting (Miall et al 2003, Smart & Nolan 2000)

Investigation	Significance
Urea and electrolytes	Imbalance in gastroenteritis and pyloric stenosis
Chloride	Depleted in pyloric stenosis
pH and bicarbonate	Metabolic alkalosis common in pyloric stenosis
Toxicology	If poisoning suspected or to exclude
pH monitoring and barium swallow	To show gastro-oesophageal reflux
Presence of gastric peristalsis during feeding and presence of pyloric tumour on palpation	Indicate pyloric stenosis
Bile-stained vomit	Intestinal obstruction
Urine for culture	Presence of infection

Acute infectious diarrhoea

Acute infectious diarrhoea is a common medical problem of childhood accounting for significant numbers of hospital admissions. Although most cases are an unpleasant and debilitating experience, poor management – particularly in the vulnerable young child or in severe cases – can lead to life-threatening dehydration. It is a major cause of morbidity and mortality in developing countries.

Causative organisms

These can be both viral and bacterial, with trends in seasonal causes seen and a correlation between age group and vulnerability to type of organisms. A summary is shown in Table 28.3.

Activity

Other less common bacterial causes of diarrhoea include *Yersinia enterocolitica, Vibrio cholerae,* staphylococci and *Clostridium* spp:

- What can you find out about these organisms?

As most acute episodes of gastroenteritis are self-limiting, management focuses primarily on assessment of the degree of dehydration and replacing fluid loss. This is successfully achieved in most cases with the use of oral rehydration solution (ORS). Other factors to consider from a nursing perspective include enabling family management of the child with an acute attack at home and education to minimise the risk of further episodes that might be caused, for example, by poor food handling and preparation techniques. If the child is admitted, minimising the risk of infection to other patients is also of considerable importance.

Although acute gastroenteritis is the most common cause of diarrhoea, particularly in the preschool child, other causes of diarrhoea could be considered.

Reflect on your practice

- What nursing interventions can you implement to reduce the risk of infection to others in the ward environment?
- How can you ensure that resident family is not posing an infection threat?
- Using Paediatric Early Warning Scoring Systems (Haines et al 2005), what signs would alert you to a deteriorating child?

You will find additional guidance in the Royal College of Nursing (RCN) publication 'Good practice in infection control' (RCN 2004).

Malabsorption and food allergies

Cystic fibrosis

Aetiology

Cystic fibrosis (CF) is an autosomal recessive inherited disorder. It is more common in the Caucasian population, and currently affects 1:2500 live births in the UK. The gene responsible is located on the long arm of chromosome 7, with

Table 28.3 Summary of the causative organisms of diarrhoea (McVerry 1999, Wong 1999)

Organism	Epidemiology/pathology	Symptoms
Rotavirus	Most common causative organism in UK, Particularly affecting the under 2s More common in cooler times of year Damages mucosa with severe inflammatory changes Incubation 1–3 days Transmission: faecal/oral	Fever >38°C for approx. 48 hours Vomiting, profuse watery diarrhoea, may last up to a week
Adenovirus	Second most common viral cause, most common in younger age groups More common in cooler months Mucosal damage (check if Norwalk group) Incubation within 24 hours Transmission: faecal/oral, person to person or droplet	May have associated respiratory infection Diarrhoea not usually vomiting
Giardia (protozoan)	Most common cause of non-bacterial diarrhoea in North America Favours cool moist conditions More common in children May be asymptomatic carriers Pathophysiology not proven – suspect either produces toxin or causes mechanical obstruction of the absorptive surface of intestine Incubation up to 1 week Transmission: contaminated food, water sources, person to person	Diarrhoea average 1 week May be longer and may be transient or persistent disaccharide intolerance
Escherichia coli	Common in newborns More common in summer Produces toxins, which bind to mucosal villi and cause profuse secretion of water and electrolytes. Can also invade and destroy epithelium Incubation variable Transmission: contaminated and undercooked food, person to person	Fever, green watery and explosive diarrhoea, abdominal distension Usually settles 3–10 days *Note: E. coli* 157 also causes abdominal cramps, haemorrhagic colitis and haemolytic uraemic syndrome
Salmonella spp	More common in toddler age groups More common in summer Invades connective tissue of small bowel and colon – local inflammation and secretion of fluids. Local oedema Incubation period 6–72 hours Transmission: carried in poultry, eggs and other food sources; also by pets	Variable degrees of symptoms, including fever and chills, vomiting cramps and diarrhoea (may be bloody) Can have infection at other sites causing local symptoms or septicaemia *Note: S. typhi* causes fever, fatigue, cough, diarrhoea and weight loss
Shigella	More common in toddler age groups More common in late summer Causes enterotoxin production – see above Incubation 1–7 days Transmission: person to person or fomites	Sudden high fever Abdominal cramps Watery diarrhoea with mucus and blood May also have headache, neck stiffness and potential for convulsions with fever
Campylobacter jejuni	More common in toddler age groups and young adults More common in late summer Enterotoxin production and loss of absorptive surface from villi Incubation 1–7 days Transmission: birds are most common host. Carried on foods and milk	Fever, watery or sticky diarrhoea may be blood and leucocytes Vomiting Usually self-limiting rarely leads to complications such as haemolytic uraemic syndrome, septicaemia Infectivity can be limited with erythromycin

<F508 being the most common mutation, although 900 other variations were found between 1989 and 2001 (Cystic Fibrosis Trust 2001); 1 in 20 individuals is likely to be a carrier.

The disease primarily affects the exocrine glands. Sufferers do not have normal life expectancy, although this is improving with treatment advances.

Activity

Check your understanding of autosomal recessive inheritance. Draw a diagram to illustrate this and check if you are correct by checking on the companion PowerPoint presentation.

Exocrine glands regulate production of sweat and mucous. Affected individuals may present with varying symptoms, dependent on the degree of severity. Symptoms commonly include digestive and respiratory problems but overall can include:

- shortness of breath
- persistent cough
- hyperhydrosis (excessive sweating)
- limited lung capacity
- 'salty' skin
- wheezing
- abdominal pain
- pneumonia
- excessive appetite but little weight gain
- large, foul-smelling stools
- diarrhoea
- impaired fertility
- reduced bone mass.

Children affected by cystic fibrosis, regardless of symptom severity, have increased sodium and chloride levels in saliva and sweat. Children with cystic fibrosis are unable to effectively reabsorb sodium and chloride leading to increased losses, particularly in warmer conditions. This creates an increased risk of dehydration, hypochloraemia and hyponatraemia.

Symptoms are caused by production of viscous mucous, which accumulates, obstructing the mucous-secreting glands in affected organs. There is also obstruction of small passages, namely the bronchioles of the lungs, pancreatic and biliary ducts.

Respiratory function

Failure to expectorate bronchial secretions by normal ciliary movement results in accumulation of secretions, which then create a medium for infection. Lung damage is progressive over time as continued obstruction causes atelectasis and emphysema. Colonisation with *Pseudomonas aeruginosa* is specific to cystic fibrosis sufferers. Eventually, there is destruction of bronchial epithelium and progressive fibrosis with impaired pulmonary function. Long-term treatment options include lung transplant.

Gastrointestinal function

Gastrointestinal problems are due to occlusion of the pancreatic ducts with mucous concretions. Outflow of pancreatic enzymes is obstructed, resulting in impaired digestion and absorption of nutrients, particularly fats and proteins. Over time, fibrosing of the pancreas occurs, which may account for the increased incidence of insulin-dependent diabetes in cystic fibrosis sufferers.

Diagnosis

Early diagnosis is now possible as, since 2007, all parents are offered neonatal screening using a heelprick blood test (UK Newborn Screening Programme Centre 2009). Later diagnosis is supported by presence of the symptoms described above but is confirmed by a 'sweat test'. This is achieved by collection of a minimum of 100 mg of sweat and measuring the quantity of sodium chloride contained within. Many parents of infants with cystic fibrosis will remark that their child 'tastes salty'. Normal sodium chloride levels are <40 mmol/L; sodium levels of >50 mmol/L and chloride levels of >60 mmol/L are abnormal (Smart & Nolan 2000).

Other diagnostic tests include (Cystic Fibrosis Trust 2001):

- prenatal chorionic villous sampling
- meconium ileus in neonatal period
- genotyping
- pancreatic function
- stool elastase.

Management

Gastrointestinal symptoms

The aim of gastrointestinal management is to ensure the child achieves adequate nutrition for optimal growth with minimum gastrointestinal symptoms. The mainstay of treatment is pancreatic enzyme replacement (pancreatin), which contains the enzymes protease, lipase and amylase, which assist in the digestion of protein, fats and starch, respectively. Supplements are given orally. Pancreatin is inactivated by gastric acid and heat; therefore supplements are most effective in an enteric-coated form and given immediately prior to or with meals and snacks. If mixed with food and drink, care should be taken that it is not too hot. Pancreatin can cause perioral and buccal mucosa irritation, so children should be taught to swallow quickly and not retain it in the mouth. Large doses may cause perianal irritation. Pancreatin is currently available in both capsule and granular form. It is usually porcine in origin so this factor should be considered in relation to the child and family's religious beliefs. The dosage required is variable, influenced by the severity of the child's disease and the individual child's response to medication. However, it should be noted there is also an identified association between high-dosage pancreatin and fibrosing colonopathy, a condition that can lead to pain and intestinal obstruction (Dodge 2000).

Dietary management

As absorption of nutrients from the small intestine is reduced in children with cystic fibrosis, their carbohydrate, fat and protein calorie requirements are in excess of the norms for their age, if optimal height and weight is to be maintained. It is recommended that their overall calorie requirements are between 120 and 140% of the RDA, with 40% of intake provided by fats. However, studies have found that within both preschool and school-age groups, a minimum of one-third of children did not meet the recommended calorie and fat intakes, demonstrated more mealtime negative behaviours and had lower measures of weight and height than children in the control groups (Powers et al 2002, Stark et al 1997).

Survival in cystic fibrosis is mostly mediated by the rate of deterioration in lung function, as the disease progresses (Steinkamp & Widermann 2002). Deterioration in lung function is associated with worsening nutritional status. Although it is yet to be confirmed which of these factors is a precursor for the other, there is evidence that poor nutrition in childhood has a negative effect on lung growth, which may result in more rapid progression of lung disease. De Vizia et al (2003) found that omega-3 fatty acid supplements resulted in a decrease in inflammatory responses and antibiotic use in cystic fibrosis patients, so this may be a useful form of nutritional supplement. Optimal calorie intake may be supported by enteral and parenteral feeding in the community. However, the burden of responsibility and the resource implications for the child's family are significant and an assessment of benefits to the child and family and ongoing support is required (Puntis 2001).

Achieving optimal nutritional management in a family-managed setting requires focused education in relation to the disease and nutritional needs. Although there is sometimes the belief among health professionals that the child and family with a chronic illness become 'experts', it has been shown that some children and caregivers are not fully aware of how to meet nutritional needs. Families showed a better understanding of the management of pancreatic enzyme supplements than of nutritional requirements overall (Stapleton et al 2000). Arguably, a key nursing management focus should be supporting optimal nutrition in the infant and growing child. Given the impact of chronic disease on the child and family as an integrated unit, adopting a family-focused approach is good practice. The best outcomes are likely to be achieved by working with the multidisciplinary team members, including dieticians and community nurse specialists, where available. Clear communication and agreed care strategies should be developed between the acute and ambulatory care settings. Consideration should be given to the financial support the child and family might need.

As with all chronic health deficits, there is potential for emotional stress. There are indicators that children with cystic fibrosis have an altered perception of body image, which although negative, differs from the distortions shown by healthy children in control groups. It was shown that self-esteem in relation to body image was similar between groups of 7–12-year-olds with cystic fibrosis and a control group who were cystic fibrosis free. However, children with cystic fibrosis were significantly more likely to report their ideal body size as larger, differing from the control group, who were more likely to identify their ideal body size as smaller and thinner (Truby & Paxton 2001). This would seem to indicate the significance of the efforts children with cystic fibrosis must make to maintain their weight.

Coeliac disease

Aetiology

Coeliac disease (gluten-sensitive enteropathy), although characterised by problems with absorption, is in origin a food allergy. Gastrointestinal food allergies include a range of disorders, which result from adverse responses to dietary antigens (Sicherer 2003). These are listed below:

- Immediate gastrointestinal hypersensitivity (anaphylaxis)
- Oral allergy syndrome
- Allergic eosinophilic oesophagitis
- Gastritis
- Gastroenterocolitis
- Dietary protein enterocolitis
- Proctitis
- Enteropathy
- Coeliac disease.

Attributed, but not proven, are colic, gastro-oesophageal reflux and constipation.

Coeliac disease is still thought as of a relatively rare condition, known to affect 1 in 1000 individuals in the UK. However, it is thought that this figure could be higher – up to 1 in 300 (Sullivan 1999). It has historically been thought of as a disease predominantly affecting the Caucasian population, with the classic phenotype described as blonde and blue eyed. However, there is an increasing incidence amongst Afro-Caribbean races, and suggestion that it may be a major cause of chronic diarrhoea in North Africa, India and the Middle East (Catassi 2002). Those affected have a permanent intolerance to the α-gliadin protein that is found in wheat, barley and rye, and in hybrids of these. The mechanisms and origins of the abnormal allergic response to gluten are not fully understood, although some individuals have a genetic predisposition, which is dependent on specific alleles of the HLA system, the DQ2 and, less frequently, the DQ8.

On ingestion of gluten-containing cereals, first of all wheat and, secondly, barley and rye, traces of gluten-derived peptides come in contact with the antigen-presenting cells (APC) located in the lamina propria of the intestinal mucosa. This activates, in DQ2- or DQ8-positive subjects, an abnormal immune response leading to the typical coeliac enteropathy – intestinal villous atrophy with crypt hyperplasia (Catassi 2002). Essentially, there is an abnormal immune response, which is thought to be triggered by unknown factors such as an acute viral illness. As with many immune-mediated illnesses, the disease has familial tendencies and an increased risk of developing it if a close relative is affected.

The villous atrophy decreases the absorptive surface of the gut wall and the amount of enzymes usually available on the villous surface. The result is passage of partly undigested food through the intestinal tract. This leads to diarrhoea or, because of the large amounts of undigested fat, bulky, foul-smelling stools, which are pale in colour. These fatty stools are termed 'steatorrhoea'. As the disease pathology progresses, the ability to absorb proteins, carbohydrates, calcium, folic acid, iron and some vitamins also decreases and the child presents with diarrhoea/steatorrhoea and weight loss, including both fat and muscle. Symptoms may be noted from infancy as weaning introduces gluten-containing foods, but progresses until symptoms become noticeable, usually in early toddler years (Hockenberry 2003). The classic 'coeliac toddler' presents with thin arms and legs, flat wasted buttocks, bloated abdomen, and with a miserable and lethargic appearance. Commonly, they are anaemic and may have rickets; slowing of bone growth may show on X-ray examination. However, it should be noted that coeliac disease is increasingly being identified in asymptomatic patients or with atypical presentation (Davison 2002). This is particularly relevant in children who have related or associated disorders, as discussed later.

Diagnosis

Diagnosis is made on history and presentation, although Walters (2007) identifies that the majority of diagnoses are now made in patients over the age of 50. Classic early childhood presentation of abdominal distension, fatty stools and signs of malabsorption are no longer the most common presentation, rather more children present with anaemia. Familial trend is also a characteristic of coeliac disease. Initial blood tests for tissue transglutaminase with findings confirmed by the presence of α-gliadin antibodies (present in response to gluten) and anti-reticulin and anti-endomysial antibodies (which are present when the gut mucosa is damaged) may be made. Definitive diagnosis is made by duodenal biopsy and microscopic examination of the structure of the villi. Additionally, children with coeliac disease will demonstrate clinical remission of signs when given a gluten-free diet.

Management

The management is quite simple in that there is complete remission of gut changes if a gluten-free diet is followed. The diet is a permanent lifetime requirement. Oats are also usually excluded from the diet, as they are often contaminated with wheat (Sullivan 1999).

Managing the diet effectively and consistently can pose challenges for the child and family. Obvious gluten-containing foods such as bread, biscuits and cakes can be replaced but many of the products are less palatable, especially breads. In addition, gluten appears under many guises within foods. Examples include thickeners for commercially prepared meals and desserts, and flavourings in snack foods, such as crisps. Generally, food labelling is improving and many products now state whether they are gluten free, or use the symbol of two crossed heads of grain to show that the product is coeliac friendly. Support groups such as the Coeliac Society and the Coeliac Resource Centre offer advice on gluten-free commercial products, recipes and special dietary products. Major supermarket chains are steadily increasing their range of specialist dietary products. Staple foods such as bread and flour are available on prescription. Referral to a paediatric dietician is useful.

Activity

Think of an average menu for a birthday tea party for a 4-year-old. How much of it is likely to contain gluten?

How could you advise a parent to manage the normal social activity of party invitations?

Useful addresses:

- The Coeliac Society, PO Box 220 High Wycombe, Buckinghamshire. Website: http://www.coeliac.co.uk
- Coeliac Disease Resource Centre (Part of Nutricia Dietary Care), Newmarket Avenue, White Horse Business Park, Trowbridge, Wiltshire BA14 0XQ. Website: http://www.glutafin.co.uk

Complications/related problems

It is known that coeliac disease coexists in children with other conditions; they may be asymptomatic. As the potential complications of untreated coeliac disease include reduced fertility, reduced bone density and gastrointestinal malignancy, routine screening for coeliac disease may be considered for children with

- Down syndrome (prevalence of coeliac disease = 4–17%)
- insulin-dependant diabetes (prevalence of coeliac disease = 1–17%)
- ulcerative colitis and Crohn's disease (Gale et al 1997, Holmes 2001).

The common factor with some of the above seems to be the existence of autoimmune problems. Coeliac disease is also associated with other complications or disorders, including:

- arthritis: an association between coeliac disease and arthritis is suggested, with remission of arthritis symptoms with successful dietary treatment of coeliac symptoms
- dental problems such as defects in dental enamel: these are prevalent in children with coeliac disease. Children with enamel defects and a history of non-specific diarrhoea should be considered for further gastroenterology investigations
- infertility: has been shown to be a presenting factor in women with undiagnosed coeliac disease. Fertility improved with introduction of a coeliac diet
- liver dysfunction: is a noted complication in coeliac patients (Davison 2002) and the recognition of the autoimmune component to coeliac disease has led to the recognition of its association with other autoimmune disorders, including liver disease. Three types of liver disease are described:
  - Mild liver dysfunction: characterised by raised liver enzymes and some changes in histology, including Kupffer cell hyperplasia, mononuclear cell infiltration, mild fibrosis and steatosis. In most cases, liver enzymes revert to norm within 12 months of establishing a gluten-free diet.
  - Chronic liver disease: characterised by severe cirrhosis, fibrosis and hepatitis with associated biochemical changes. Despite the underlying damage, gluten free diets are shown to result in significant improvement.
  - Autoimmune liver disease: encompasses autoimmune hepatitis, primary and autoimmune sclerosing cholangitis. Some links with coeliac disease for these conditions has been established (Davison 2002).

It is not known if the types of liver disease described above are separate entities or if they fall on a pathological spectrum.

Cow's milk allergy

Cow's milk allergy is primarily a disease of childhood and affects an inexactly determined number of the population, but it has been suggested that the figure can be estimated as 1–3% of the general population and 3–5% of bottle-fed infants. There is an increased prevalence in infants in whom there is history of prematurity, atopy or other gastrointestinal disorders (Bahna 2002). Cow's milk protein comprises of two major fractions – casein and whey – in a proportion of approximately 80:20. Casein and the β-lactoglobulin component of whey are the most allergenic, with varying degrees of sensitivity shown in affected individuals. Sensitivities are manifest in specific gastrointestinal symptoms or severe systemic and life-threatening reactions. The most hypersensitive individuals can react not only to ingested proteins but also if there is skin contact.

Aetiology

Hypersensitivity to cow's milk can be mediated by one of four immunologic reactions (Bahna 2002):

- Type I (anaphylactic or intermediate): most common, mediated by IgE antibodies.
- Type II (cytotoxic): least common, IgM, IgG or IgA antibodies activate complexes.
- Type III (arthus type): second most common, formation of immune complexes that comprise antigen, involves IgA, IgG, IgM and occasionally IgE.
- Type IV (delayed): mediated by sensitised T lymphocytes.

Diagnosis

Whereas type 1 reactions are relatively easy to clinically evaluate, the other three types are more difficult. Assessment particularly addresses the relationship between the ingestion of cow's milk protein and manifest symptoms. However, all possible symptoms are shared with other disorders. Specific diagnosis therefore rests most conclusively with measuring serum IgE antibodies for specific foods.

Management

Ideally, management should be considered from the proactive and preventative viewpoint. There is evidence that food allergies may be related to early exposure to food allergens. In some cases, exposure may be via maternal breast milk. In terms of general protection against a range of food allergies there is evidence that breast-feeding contributes to prevention, but this protection may be lessened where there is high maternal fat intake (Hanson et al 2003). There is also evidence that early gut colonisation with Gram-negative organisms lessens the incidence of food allergy developing. Current hygiene practices (enthusiastically rigorous) in early infant care detract from this early colonisation process. The practice of supporting early neonatal feeding with cow's milk formula, before establishing breast-feeding, may contribute to cow's milk allergy developing in early childhood. Studies so far do not suggest that restricting maternal diet in pregnancy mediates against cow's milk allergy (Fiocchi et al 2003).

Once the problem exists effective management requires introduction of alternatives to cow's milk protein. Soya food products and soy formulas are usually well tolerated, but other options are hydrolysed cow's milk protein formula, e.g. Pregestemil.

Lactose intolerance

The terms 'cow's milk allergy' and 'cow's milk intolerance' are often used interchangeably and it is important to note that they are two distinct entities.

Whereas cow's milk allergy is an immunologically mediated reaction to cow's milk proteins, characterised by local and systemic reactions that can be fatal, cow's milk intolerance refers to problems with the digestion, absorption or metabolism of components of cow's milk, which are non-immunological. Cow's milk allergy primarily affects infants and young children and the majority of those affected will experience spontaneous resolution, whereas cow's milk intolerance tends to have its onset in later childhood or young adulthood, and persists (Bahna 2002). The exception to this is when it develops secondary to acute gastroenteritis in infancy or early childhood, when it is usually a transient problem. Lactase (β-galactosidase) is required to hydrolyse lactose (carbohydrate component of mammalian milk) into the monosaccharides glucose and galactose. If insufficient lactase is produced to complete this process, lactose with water passes on to the colon where it undergoes a fermentation process, producing hydrogen, carbon dioxide and lactic acid. This causes the symptoms of bloating, flatulence, abdominal pain and watery diarrhoea. Severity of symptoms is variable dependent on individual degrees of insufficiency. The problem has racial prevalence, with the highest incidence in races with darker skins and the least affected being the very fair skinned. Primary lactose intolerance is rare in infants and may be an inherited autosomal trait (Bahna 2002, Fiocchi et al 2003).

Diagnosis

Various tests support diagnosis, including blood glucose monitoring post-ingestion of a measured 'dose' of lactose. The simplest test is to measure hydrogen levels in exhaled breath, as the hydrogen produced in the colon is excreted via the lungs. Definitively, individuals whose symptoms resolve on introduction of a lactose-reduced diet can have diagnosis confirmed.

Management

Dietary exclusion of lactose, as the primary 'milk' source will be effective in controlling symptoms. Other than in infants with primary intolerance, most individuals can tolerate some lactose, particularly in live yoghurts and non-pasteurised cheeses where the lactose-digesting enzymes produced by the *Lactobacillus* aid its digestion. Infants can be swapped to a soybean formula (Bahna 2002). Of interest is the finding of Fiocchi et al (2003), whose small study found that even children with hypersensitive reactions of cow's milk proteins were not intolerant of lactose.

Inflammatory bowel disease

Crohn's disease and ulcerative colitis are distinct forms of inflammatory bowel disease (IBD). Although their histology differs, they share many symptoms and have a similar impact on the child and family's life. Studies suggest that their incidence has increased since the 1980s, although it is not clear whether this is a true increase or due to better diagnosis (Jenkins 2001). The incidence of newly diagnosed cases seems now to have settled, which would lend support to the increase being due, at least in part, to increasing skills in diagnosis.

Currently, the British Paediatric Surveillance Unit (BPSU) identifies incidence as 5.3 cases per 100,000 children under the age of 16. This equated to 700 new cases per annum in the UK. Average age at diagnosis is 11–12, with 13% of cases occurring in children under 10.

Aetiology

Research to date is unable to offer any definitive causes for IBD. There appears to be a genetic predisposition with 'susceptibility' genes being located. This is more likely in individuals affected by Crohn's disease. However, findings are not consistent across different groups, suggesting the need for further studies. Environmental factors, which are likely to include specific infectious pathogens, dietary elements and common childhood infections, are also thought to trigger the disease. Limited exposure to gut pathogens in early childhood may also increase the likelihood of developing inflammatory bowel disorders. The suggestion that the measles vaccine or virus is a predisposing factor has yet to be supported, and several studies have concluded that the there is no statistical support to link measles vaccine with either IBD or autism (Black et al 2002, Davis et al 2001). In affected individuals, immunologically mediated inflammatory responses in the intestinal mucosa are exaggerated.

Evidence-based practice

We have seen much published on the safety or otherwise of the MMR vaccination and its links with both gut disorders and autism. The initial research (Wakefield 1998), which suggested the association between MMR and autism, has been discredited. The popularising of Wakefield's initial theories was largely via the non-professional press. Consider how you can ensure that children and their families can be helped to make decisions about their care and treatment, based on accurate interpretation of the evidence available.

Table 28.4 Differences between Crohn's disease and ulcerative colitis (Jenkins 2001, Metcalf 2002, Walker-Smith 2000)

Feature	Crohn's disease	Ulcerative colitis
Location	Can affect whole of GI tract but mouth, stomach and oesophagus rare	Ulceration confined to the colon
Diarrhoea	Type varies dependent on area of gut involved	Loose stools, blood
Pain	Present	Usually dull ache
Bleeding	Present	Present
Linear growth delay	May be most obvious feature prior to diagnosis	Less common, however diagnosis made earlier due to acute onset of gastro symptoms
Gut mucosal inflammation and ulceration	Present – patchy, plus may develop strictures	Present, diffuse
Mucous	Present in stool in Crohn's colitis	Depletion
Extra intestinal signs		
Anaemia		
Raised ESR and platelets	Present	Present
Increase in inflammatory mediators (cytokines, leukotrienes, prostaglandins)	Erythema nodosum	
Skin manifestations		

ESR, erythrocyte sedimentation rate; GI, gastrointestinal.

Diagnosis

Some symptoms are shared between Crohn's and ulcerative colitis but there are differences, which are summarised in Table 28.4. Whereas diagnosis of IBD may be suspected on symptom history and initial blood testing, visual examination of the gut using endoscopy, radiological tests and gut biopsy is needed to confirm and differentiate diagnosis. Magnetic resonance imaging (MRI) has been found to be an accurate diagnostic procedure (Laghi et al 2003).

Management

Physiological management approaches differ, to some extent, between ulcerative colitis and Crohn's disease, although the aims are shared, including the need to induce and maintain remission, secure a reduction in symptoms and promote normal physical, social and emotional growth and development.

Currently 5-aminosalicylates (5-ASAs) are used to support remission induction in mild to moderate ulcerative colitis and in mild Crohn's disease. Corticosteroids are used for more moderately severe disease, but their long-term use as a maintenance therapy is contraindicated due to side effects. Other therapies used in more severe or unresponsive disease include immunomodulators and monoclonal antibodies. Surgery is an option, but is more successful where disease is localised, as found in ulcerative colitis.

Activity

Using either web-based resources or pharmacology texts:

- Identify the different actions of each of the groups of drugs listed in the above text.
- How would you explain their actions to an 11-year-old child?

www

Useful web address:

- http://www.livingwithcrohnsdisease.com/livingwithcrohnsdisease

Use this website to look at living with inflammatory bowel disease from the patient's perspective.

Some children may develop perianal lesions or proctitis, both of which are difficult to treat. Rectal water-soluble steroids or 5-ASA drugs may be used successfully for management of proctitis.

Emergency care is required for the child who develops severe colitis, including administration of intravenous fluids, electrolytes, antibiotics and steroids. Perforation is a risk and surgery may be required.

Arguably, physical care and management is clearly described, with specific protocols to follow. However, the potential impact of inflammatory bowel disease on the child and family, both socially and mentally, is worthy of consideration within nursing strategies. Some studies suggest that young adults who developed IBD as children have problems with self-esteem. The average age at diagnosis coincides with onset of puberty and adolescence.

Reflect on your practice

How might the adolescent child with inflammatory bowel disease be supported, using a multidisciplinary approach, to minimise the threat to self-esteem? You may find it useful to read: Vitulano-Lawrence (2003).

Constipation

Constipation, which can be defined as delay or difficulty in defecation, is a common paediatric problem. Normal frequency of bowel movements varies from child to child, ranging from more than once per day to none for several days, and infrequency alone is not necessarily a problem. Causes of constipation are broadly differentiated into organic and non-organic. Organic causes are shown in Table 28.5.

Table 28.5 Organic causes of constipation (Baker et al 1999)

Cause	Examples
Anatomic malformations	Imperforate anus Anal stenosis Pelvic mass
Metabolic and gastrointestinal	Cystic fibrosis Diabetes mellitus Coeliac disease Hypothyroidism
Neuropathic	Spinal cord problem Neurofibromatosis
Intestinal nerve or muscle disorders	Hirschsprung's disease Visceral myopathies and neuropathies
Abnormalities of abdominal muscles	Prune belly syndrome Gastroschisis Down syndrome
Connective tissue disorders	Systemic lupus erythematosus Scleroderma
Drugs	Opiates Phenobarbitone Antihypertensives Antidepressants
Miscellaneous	Lead poisoning Vitamin D overdose

However, for the majority of children presenting with constipation problems, the cause is non-organic. Non-organic causes include poor dietary management, including insufficient fibre, and dehydration, developmental problems that complicate toilet training, emotional abuse, depression and also inappropriate/punitive toilet training practices in the younger child. There are also those who have a familial tendency and sedentary lifestyle. In early years the most common cause of constipation is functional – meaning it exists in the absence of obvious cause. It is thought to commonly develop in response to the child experiencing unpleasant emotional experiences or pain associated with defecation. This results in the child deliberately holding faeces and actively working against the impulse to defecate. Ignoring the urge to defecate results in retention of faeces in the colon, fluid is reabsorbed and the faecal mass becomes, large dry and hard, termed 'impacted'. As a consequence, liquid faeces leak around the impacted mass, causing involuntary soiling (encopresis). The problem is progressive as the child becomes frightened, anticipating that the experience of defecation will be painful and difficult, and resisting the urge to defecate. Soiling is unpleasant and may create tension in the home, nursery or school, which can lead to social isolation and feelings of poor self-worth.

Soiling is usually involuntary but it may be a behaviour learnt after toilet training has been achieved. This is often indicative of stress or emotional upset; 80–95% of encopresis is associated with functional constipation.

Diagnosis

Functional non-organic constipation is diagnosed on the basis of medical and psychosocial history taking and physical examination. Initially, organic causes need to be excluded. Indicators of organic causes would include general malaise or other systemic signs such as weight loss, nausea/vomiting, and blood in the stools or abdominal distension. Rectal examination allows size of the rectum to be assessed and also amount and type of stool. The perineum and perianal area can be examined at the same time to assess for signs of trauma. If there is nothing of note and there is a history of toileting difficulties and stool-withholding behaviour, it is likely that the cause is functional. If it is inappropriate to conduct a rectal examination, for example if the child refuses or abuse is suspected, abdominal X-ray can be used to determine whether impacted faeces are present.

Reflect on your practice

Consider the kind of questions that might be asked to establish the state of a child's bowel function (colour, shape, frequency, size, associated with pain…):

- How might some children and families find this interview?
- How can it be facilitated to be more comfortable?

Management

Baker et al (1999), based on a review of evidence and practice, suggested a staged approach to management. This is described as follows:

1. Determine if there are impacted faeces
2. Remove/resolve impaction
3. Maintenance: using education, support, diet and medications
4. Follow up.

Successful and complete disimpaction is arguably a precursor to successful ongoing management. Removal of impacted faeces can be achieved using oral or rectal medication or a combination of the two. Choice should centre on child and family preference. Oral medication may be perceived as less invasive.

Oral medications include electrolyte solutions, either alone or in combination with high-dose laxatives, for example lactulose or senna. Ideally, stool softeners, such as lactulose, should be used before stimulants to minimise the pain of passing a large, hard stool. Rectal preparations can also be used, including saline and phosphate enemas, and some success has been achieved using glycerol suppositories. Mineral oils, which act as stool lubricants, are also favoured in the US and Australia, and feature in practice guidelines developed by the North American Society for Paediatric Gastroenterology and Nutrition (NASPGN). Their use in the UK is not widely accepted because of concerns about aspiration pneumonias, gut changes and altered vitamin absorption. However, the evidence to support these concerns is insubstantial (Sharif et al 2001).

Having removed the impacted faeces, management moves to maintenance using a 'whole child' approach. Therapy includes dietary management, maintaining laxative therapy and also behaviour modification, focusing on making toileting and bowel evacuation into a non-stressful experience.

Dietary changes aim to increase fluids and include fruit, fibre and non-absorbable carbohydrates. Laxatives can include osmotic laxative, such as lactulose, docusate sodium and polyethylene glycol (Movicol). The latter has a limited licence for use with children, with restrictions on period of use. Softeners are combined with bowel stimulants, which include senna and sodium picosulphate. Rectal medication may be used, but with caution, given the associated unpleasant experiences it may engender. Medication programmes require use of dosage adequate to establish bowel function, which is regular and characterised by absence of straining, soiling or discomfort. Careful weaning from medication can then begin. Behaviour modification makes use of diary keeping, unhurried regular toileting, ideally shortly after meals to capitalise on the effect of the gastrocolic reflex, and also reward systems for successful evacuations (ERIC 2001).

A Cochrane review found that combining behavioural and/or cognitive interventions with drug therapies resulted in better outcomes at 6- and 12-month follow-ups (Brazelli & Griffiths 2004). During the treatment and management phases, close family support and education is required. Families need to understand the origins of the problem and where additional problems such as soiling have developed, make clear that this is likely to be non-intentional. Families may need support to set realistic objectives, in terms of outcomes over time, and to develop the ability to manage behaviour reinforcement using positive learning approaches. Education and encouragement to change the family diet to one that is more balanced may also be required.

WWW

The following websites offer further reading and management guidelines. You could consider to what extent guidelines are consistent between organisations and care teams:

- http://www.eric.org.uk

Summary

This chapter has offered an overview of some of the major gastrointestinal problems likely to be encountered by children's nurses. Additional information can also be found on the Evolve website. Generally, acute problems can be managed effectively, with positive outcomes expected in most cases. However, there is an increase in the incidence of chronic illnesses in child health, some of which have been explored in this chapter. This is creating a need to focus on long-term family-centred care and to continue to develop strong links between ambulatory and acute care settings. Continuing to strengthen multiprofessional cooperation in care commissioning and delivery remains a child health professional responsibility. It is envisaged that this will continue to be a key challenge in child health care for the foreseeable future.

References

Baker, S., Liptak, G., Colletti, R., et al., 1999. Constipation in infants and children: evaluation and treatment. Journal of Paediatric Gastroenterology and Nutrition 29, 612–626.

Bahna, S., 2002. Cow's milk allergy versus cow's milk intolerance. Annals of Allergy Asthma and Immunology 89 (6), 56–60.

Black, C., Kaye, J., Jick, H., 2002. Relation of childhood gastrointestinal diseases to autism: nested case control study using data from UK General Practice Research Database. British Medical Journal 325 (7361), 419–421.

Bourke, B., Drumm, D., 2002. Cochrane's epitaph for cisapride in childhood gastro-oesophageal reflux. Archives of Disease in Childhood 86 (2), 71–72.

Brazelli, M., Griffiths, P., 2004. Behavioural and cognitive interventions with or without other treatments for defecation disorders in children (Cochrane Review). The Cochrane Library, issue 1. John Wiley, Chichester.

Catassi, C., 2002. Coeliac disease, an emerging problem in developing countries. Celiachia News Inglese. Online. Available at: http://www.celiachia.it.news/page33.html [accessed 3 November 2003].

Cystic Fibrosis Trust, 2001. National consensus standards for the nursing management of cystic fibrosis. Cystic Fibrosis Trust. Bromley, Kent.

Davis, R., Karmarz, P., Bohlke, K., et al., 2001. Measles-mumps-rubella and other measles-containing vaccines do not increase the risk for inflammatory bowel disease: a case-control study from the vaccine safety datalink project. Archives of Pediatrics and Adolescent Medicine 155 (3), 354–359.

Davison, S., 2002. Coeliac disease and liver dysfunction. Archives of Disease in Childhood 87 (4), 293–296.

De Vizia, B., Raia, V., Spana, C., Pavlisis, C., 2003. Effect of an 8-month treatment with omega-3 fatty acids (eicosapentaenoic and docosahexaenoic) in patients with cystic fibrosis. Journal of Parenteral and Enteral Nutrition 27 (1), 52–57.

Dodge, J., 2000. Fibrosing colonopathy. Gut 46 (2), 152–153.

ERIC, 2001. Childhood soiling, minimum standards of practice for treatment and service delivery: benchmarking guidelines. ERIC, Bristol.

Fiocchi, A., Martelli, A., de Chiara, A., et al., 2003. Primary dietary prevention of food allergy. Annals of Asthma. Allergy and Immunology 91 (1), 3–13.

Gale, L., Wimalaratna, H., Brotodiharjo, A., Duggan, J.M., 1997. Down's syndrome is strongly associated with coeliac disease. Gut 40 (4), 492–496.

Haines, C., Perrot, M., Weir, P., 2005. Promoting care for the acutely ill child. Development and evaluation of a Paediatric Early Warning Tool. Intensive and Critical Care Nursing 22 (2), 73–81.

Hanson, L., Korotova, M., Telemo, E., 2003. Breast feeding, infant formulas and the immune system. Annals of Allergy. Asthma and Immunology 90 (6), 59–63.

Hockenberry, M., Wilson, D., Winkelstrin, M., Kline, N., 2003. Wong's Nursing care of infants and children. Mosby, St Louis.

Holmes, G., 2001. Coeliac disease and type 1 diabetes mellitus-the case for screening. Diabetic Medicine 18, 169–177.

Jenkins, H., 2001. Inflammatory bowel disease. Archives of Disease in Childhood 85 (5), 435–437.

Laghi, A., Borrelli, O., Paoloantonio, P., Dito, L., 2003. Contrast enhanced magnetic resonance imaging of the terminal ileum in children with Crohn's disease. Gut 52 (3), 393–397.

Metcalf, C., 2002. Crohn's disease: an overview. Nursing Standard 16 (31), 45–52.

Miall, L., Rudolf, M., Levene, M., 2003. Paediatrics at a glance. Blackwell Science, Oxford.

McVerry, M., 1999. Managing the child with gastroenteritis. Nursing Standard 13 (37), 49–52.

Powers, S., Patton, S., Byars, K., Mitchell, M., 2002. Caloric intake and eating behavior in infants and toddlers with cystic fibrosis. Pediatrics 109 (95), 75–79.

Puntis, J., 2001. Nutritional support at home or in the community. Archives of Disease in Childhood 84 (4), 295–301.

Royal College of Nursing (RCN), 2004. Good practice in infection control – guidance for nursing staff. RCN, London. Online. Available to RCN members at: http://www.rcn.org.uk.

Sharif, F., Crushell, E., O'Driscoll, K., Bourke, B., 2001. Liquid paraffin: a reappraisal of its role in the treatment of constipation. Archives of Disease in Childhood 85 (2), 121–124.

Silbermintz, A., Markowitz, J., 2006. Inflammatory bowel disease. Paediatric Annals 35 (4), 269–274.

Sicherer, S., 2003. Clinical aspects of gastrointestinal food allergy in childhood. Pediatrics 111 (6), 1609–1619.

Smart, J., Nolan, T., 2000. Paediatric handbook, 6th edn. Blackwell Science, Australia.

Stapleton, D., Gurrin, L., Zubrick, S., Silburn, R., 2000. What do children with cystic fibrosis and their parents know about nutrition and pancreatic enzymes? Journal of the American Dietetic Association 1000 (12), 1494–1500.

Stark, L., Mulvihill, M., Jelalian, E., Bowen, M., 1997. Descriptive analysis of eating behavior in school age children with cystic fibrosis and healthy control children. Pediatrics 99 (5), 665–670.

Steinkamp, G., Wiedemann, B., 2002. Relationship between nutritional status and lung function cystic fibrosis: cross sectional and longitudinal analyses from the German CF quality assurance project. Thorax 57 (7), 596–611.

Sullivan, A., 1999. Coeliac disease. Nursing Standard 14 (11), 48–52.

Truby, H., Paxton, A., 2001. Body image and dieting behavior in cystic fibrosis. Pediatrics 107 (6), E92.

UK Newborn Screening Committee, 2009. A laboratory guide to Newborn Screening in the UK for Cystic Fibrosis. UK National Screening Committee, Great Ormond Street, London.

Vitulano-Lawrence, A., 2003. Psychosocial issues for children and adolescents with chronic illness: self-esteem, school functioning and sports participation. Child and Adolescent Psychiatric Clinics of North America 12 (3), 585–592.

Wakefield, A., 1998. Ileal-lymphoid-nodular hyperplasia, non-specific colitis, and pervasive developmental disorder in children. Lancet 351, 637–641.

Walker-Smith, J., 2000. Chronic inflammatory bowel disease in children: a complex problem in management. Postgraduate Medical Journal 76 (898), 469–473.

Walters, J., 2007. Gastroenterology: coeliac disease often goes undiagnosed. Practitioner Oct 25, 43 Accessed via Proquest Nov 2009 ID1372341131.

Caring for children with cardiovascular problems

29

Barbara V Novak

ABSTRACT

The purpose of this chapter and its companion PowerPoint presentation is to explore advances in understanding of cardiovascular problems that occur in infants and children and address issues regarding the delivery of evidence-based care. The ranges of cardiovascular problems that occur in children, the expanse of knowledge concerning these problems and the variations in clinical management do not permit a full and comprehensive exploration of all the relevant factors. Nevertheless, this chapter will explore a range of biological, developmental and therapeutic principles fundamental to knowledgeable and competent, child-centred practice.

LEARNING OUTCOMES

- Critically review the embryonic and fetal development of the cardiovascular system.
- Demonstrate understanding of the specific anatomical and physiological features of the cardiovascular system.
- Detail the nomenclature of congenital cardiovascular disease in childhood.
- Outline the nature of acquired cardiovascular problems in childhood.
- Outline the assessment of a child with suspected cardiovascular problem.
- Detail the strategy for evidence-based nursing care of a child with cardiovascular problems.

Introduction

Some of the most complex childhood health problems are related to cardiovascular defects and anomalies. The cause of these defects and anomalies are not always known, although a range of contributing factors such as folate deficiencies, intrauterine infection and chromosomal abnormalities may play decisive roles. In general, congenital cardiovascular defects and anomalies occur in 8–10% of children born alive (Hoffman 2003, Sommer et al 2008). Given the complexities involved in the development of the embryonic cardiovascular system it is not surprising that they occur this frequently. Many of the congenital cardiovascular defects and anomalies can be diagnosed in utero before birth. Other problems may be detected within the first few months of birth, usually due to the child manifesting persistent central and peripheral cyanosis often accompanied by respiratory difficulties. A small number of defects and anomalies may not be detected until later in childhood or during adult life. Irrespective of when the symptoms appear in most instances the clinical management of congenital cardiovascular problems will require specialist medical, surgical and nursing interventions.

Improved health care and better infection control are known to have reduced the incidence of acquired cardiovascular disease such as bacterial endocarditis in childhood. Nevertheless, viral myocarditis, cardiomyopathies and secondary cardiovascular disease caused by metabolic problems can arise in children and will require specific, at times life saving, evidence-based therapeutic interventions.

The normal cardiovascular system

The normal circulatory system can be divided into two functional compartments: the systemic circulation, which is supported by the left ventricle; and the pulmonary circulation, which is supported by the right ventricle. The right and the left ventricles work in relative harmony. This ensures that the systemic circulation transports oxygenated blood and nutrients from the left ventricle through the aorta to the systemic arteries and capillaries. The pulmonary circulation receives its deoxygenated blood from the right ventricle. This blood is then pumped through the pulmonary artery to lungs. Here a complex capillary bed surrounds the alveoli and facilitates gaseous exchange across the capillary-alveolar membranes. This mechanism ensures that oxygenated blood is transported to the left atrium by way of pulmonary venules, which anastomose giving rise to four pulmonary

DOI: 10.1016/B978-0-7020-3183-0.10029-3

veins which commonly attach to the posterior wall of the left atrium. The oxygenated blood flows from the left atrium to the left ventricle which ejects it into the aorta ensuring that the metabolic needs of all organs and tissue are met.

The development of the cardiovascular system

The developed cardiovascular system is an adaptive but relatively efficient transport network supported by a rhythmically pulsatile four-chambered heart. Its role is to transport blood within the closed circuit of semi-compliant vessels, delivering nutrients and metabolic substrates from the placenta to the embryo/fetus and removing fetus metabolic waste products back to the placenta. The anatomical developments and corresponding functional adaptations are dependent on the existence of a vast range of factors including the appropriate expressions of the human genome which masterminds the embryonic development and contributes to the establishment of the primitive cardiovascular system.

Scenario

Christopher, a third-year child branch student nurse, reported to his seminar colleagues that a number of children had been admitted to his ward with a history of respiratory difficulties and cyanosis. The evidence drawn from the physical assessments suggests that these children are suffering from congenital cyanotic cardiac anomalies. The severity of the respiratory difficulties and cyanosis means that these children require specialist hospitalised care. Christopher asked that the seminar should focus on the normal embryonic development of the heart and then critically examine the anatomy and physiology of the cardiovascular system in children.

The origins and development of the embryonic and fetal heart

The heart and its corresponding blood vessels develop from the splanchnopleuric mesoderm (embryonic tissue adjacent to the endoderm) in the cardiogenic region. The underlying endoderm contributes to this development by signalling to the primitive angioblastic cords to converge and form a pair of lateral endocardial tubes, which are then gradually fused and reshaped as the embryo grows and folds. This gradual, but carefully orchestrated, fusion of these tubes shapes the single primitive heart tube, which is then remodelled by a sequential process of septation and folding that transforms the single lumen into the four chambers of the definitive heart. The initial chambers are primitive, and require considerable development.

Activity

Read Chapter 7 (Development of the heart, pp 151–188) and Chapter 8 (Development of the vasculature, pp 189–223) in: Larsen W 2008 Human embryology. Churchill Livingstone, Edinburgh.

Activity

Critically reflect on the embryonic developments of the heart and the blood vessels and consider how such developments contribute to the shaping of the fetal circulation.

The shaping of the embryonic cardiovascular system

The primitive heart tube consists of endothelium which is shaped by a series of definitive expansions, shallow ridges and crevices (sulci). By the 22nd day a thick mass of splanchnopleuric mesoderm surrounds this heart tube, differentiating into the loosely organised myocardium and cardiac jelly, a layer of thick acellular matrix synthesised by the developing myocardium (Larsen 2008). The visceral pericardium lies externally to the myocardium. It evolves from mesothelial cells, which are derived independently from the splanchnopleuric mesoderm. These cells are believed to migrate onto the surface of the developing heart from the regions of the septum transversum or the sinus venosus.

Approximately, from the 23rd day, the single heart tube begins to elongate, simultaneously loop and fold. This displaces the bulbus cordis to the right and adjusts the position of the primitive ventricle to the left, allowing the primitive atrium to move in an upward direction. The complex cardiac folding is believed to be completed by the 28th day of embryonic life. According to Larsen (2008), this highly organised looping of the primitive heart tube may be intrinsically motivated and possibly influenced by the state of hydration of the cardiac jelly, active migration and development of the primitive myocytes (cardiac muscle cells), and local haemodynamic forces initiated by the embryo's circulating blood. This early cardiac morphogenesis includes the formation of the coronary vascular plexus, which later forms the coronary vessels.

The mesoderm, mesodermal growth factors and other factors expressed in the developing myocardium influence tissue differentiation and regulate the course of atrial and ventricular development. The cardiac neural crest contributes to the formation of the primitive ventricular outflow tracts. The internal septation of the heart, and the formation of the heart valves, are attributed to the development of the mesenchymal tissue at the atrioventricular and proximal outflow regions of the heart. The structural developments in the heart and blood vessels may play a role in regulating the functions of the cardiovascular system. For instance, marginal increases in blood pressure may contribute to the development of the embryonic myocardium and the smooth muscle of the blood vessels.

The primitive heart begins to contract on approximately the 22nd day (Larsen 2008) and blood begins to circulate through the primitive vessels within the next 2 days. The first blood cells found in the embryo's circulation are formed in the yolk sac, although embryonic and later fetal haematopoiesis occurs in the liver, spleen, thymus and, of course, eventually the bone marrow. The sustained rhythmic myocardial contractility may, in part, be dependent on myocardial hypertrophy, which is a basic adaptive response of the cardiac myocytes to an increasing workload. Polin & Fox (2004) suggest that myotropin (which may play an important part in the pathogenesis of myocardial hypertrophy) could act as an important primary modulator responsible for enhancing myocyte protein synthesis and myocyte growth and differentiation.

The developing atria

The right atrium is remodelled during the 4th and 5th weeks of gestation. This initiates the gradual incorporation of the enlarged right sinus horn and the development of the venae cavae. A single pulmonary vein sprouts from the posterior wall of the left atrium and then divides to form the right and left pulmonary veins, which grow in the direction of the primitive lungs, where they join the smaller pulmonary veins which develop around the primitive bronchial tissue. The right and left pulmonary veins are eventually reconstructed forming, in most instances, four pulmonary veins.

The anatomical divisions between the atria and the common atrioventricular canal separate the systemic from the pulmonary circulation. This separation also depends on the gradual fusion of the septum primum and the septum secundum. The septum primum establishes a firm interatrial muscle and the septum secundum contributes to the development of the foramen ovale, or oval window. Throughout the embryonic and early fetal life, all septal structures form large openings that allow blood to flow in a specific direction. The foramen ovale is one of the most important of these openings because it permits shunting of blood from the right atrium to the left atrium. This mechanism allows the blood to bypass the right ventricle, the pulmonary artery and its tributaries. The foramen ovale normally closes soon after birth, partly because of the abrupt cessation of fetal circulation at birth, with the first breath and the eventual dilatation of the pulmonary vessels. These mechanisms reverse the pressure difference between the atria and push the flexible membranous part of the septum against the less conforming muscular septum thus closing the foramen ovale and blocking any shunting of blood from the right to the left atrium.

Division and shaping of the common atrioventricular canal by the septum intermedium (the middle segment of the intraventricular septum) into the right and left atrioventricular canals ensures that the right atrioventricular canal aligns the right atrium with the right ventricle and the left atrioventricular canal aligns the left atrium with the left ventricle. The division and reshaping of the common atrioventricular canal initiates the development of the primitive left ventricle, which establishes a firm contact with the proximal portion of the truncus arteriosus, a major vessel, which ultimately divides to form the future aorta and the main pulmonary artery. The four main cardiac valves begin to form in the 5th week of gestation, almost immediately following the division of the atrioventricular canal, and the septation of the truncus arteriosus, and is initially supported by growth and shaping of ventricular muscle from below. However, proliferating cells, which surround these orifices eventually, form the distinctive mitral and tricuspid valves.

The developing ventricles

The right and the left ventricles are composite structures. According to Larsen (2008) the right ventricle is derived predominantly from the inferior aspects of the bulbus cordis and the right aspect of the conus cordis. The left ventricle develops mainly from the primitive ventricle and the left wall of the conus cordis. Corresponding outflow tracts, namely, the main pulmonary artery and the aorta, complete the morphogenesis of the heart and its major vessels. The intraventricular septum is formed by the developing right and left ventricular walls opposing one another (Collins 2008). The growth of the muscular part of the septum halts just before its superior edge meets the inferior membranous surface of the septum intermedium in the middle segment of the intraventricular septum. This temporary arrest in growth is associated with a number of developmental benefits including ventricular enlargement and formation of the ventricular trabeculae (ridges in the myocardium), which shape the ventricular chambers and their respective outflow tracts so that the heart can function as a competent mechanical pump.

The truncus arteriosus, which serves as the main cardiac outflow pathway, is divided by a septum which shapes the distal aspects of the right and left outflow tracts for the right and left ventricles respectively. As the aorta separates from the main pulmonary artery three distinctive swellings (tubercules) evolve initiating the development of the semilunar valves, also known as the aortic and the pulmonary artery valves which direct the intracardiac blood flow (Larsen 2008).

The final stage in the intracardiac development involves the growth of the membranous interventricular septum, which is originally derived from the inferior endocardial cushion. As the membranous septum fuses with the muscular interventricular septum at about 8 weeks of gestation blood flow between the right and the left ventricles ceases. The aorta and the pulmonary artery ensures that both ventricles can now function autonomously with respect to their own outflow tracts. In instances where fusion between the membranous and muscular parts of the septum fails a septal or intra-ventricular septal defect (VSD) will persist. This is the most common type of congenital cardiac anomaly that occurs in children.

The development of the valves

The atrioventricular valves begin their development in the 5th week of gestation with the formation of cusps within the atrioventricular canals. Generally, the left atrioventricular valve has only two cusps, which form the bicuspid valve, also known as the mitral valve. In contrast, the right atrioventricular valve usually, but not always, develops three cusps, which shape the tricuspid valve. The free edges of these cusps attach to the sinew-like chordae tendineae, which insert into the ventricular papillary muscles. The design of these valves ensures that during diastole the cusps fold back allowing the blood to flow uninhibited from the atria to the ventricles. Significantly, during systole, the tight closure of these cusps prevents a backflow of blood from the atria into the ventricles.

Chamber and vessel concordance

Primitive blood vessels begin to appear in the splanchnopleuric mesoderm of the yolk sac on the 17th day. A similar aggregation of cells, also known as blood islands, appears in the embryonic disc on the 18th day. These cells initiate the formation of the embryo's blood vessels which, according to Colins (2008), are initially surrounded by a fibronectin rich matrix which is later incorporated into the endothelial lamina. The early development and subsequent reshaping of the endocardial tubes allows a pair of dorsal aortas to attach to their cranial axis and then form the first pair of aortic arches. Four additional aortic arches develop during the 4th and 5th weeks, connecting the rudimentary aortic sac (also known as the truncus arteriosus) to the dorsal aortas, which fuse later to form the median dorsal aorta. This complex network of the aortic arches is eventually remodeled to establish arteries within the upper thorax, neck and head. The dorsal aorta gives rise to three distinctive sets of arterial vessels (Collins 2008, Larsen 2008):

- The ventral arteries, which supply the gut
- The lateral arteries, which supply the retroperitoneal organs such as the kidneys and the gonads
- The intersegmental arteries, which supply, in part, the head, the neck and body walls.

The arteries supplying the gastrointestinal tract are derived from remnants of vitelline arteries and the vitelline duct, which anastomose with the paired dorsal aortae. The dorsal aortae in turn connect to the umbilical arteries, which carry blood from the embryo, and later the fetus, to the placenta.

The primitive venous system consists of three major components:

- The cardinal veins, which drain the head, neck, body walls and limbs
- The vitelline veins, which initially drain the yolk sac
- The umbilical veins, which carry oxygenated blood from the placenta to the embryo/fetus.

All three sets of veins initially drain into the right and left sinus horns but their extensive modification shapes the distinctive systemic venous connection with the right atrium. The left sinus horn is eventually transformed into the coronary sinus and the oblique vein of the left atrium. The coronary sinus receives most of the venous blood returning from the coronary vascular bed. The vitelline venous system gives rise to the liver sinusoids and the portal system that transports venous blood from the intestinal tract to the liver. The vitelline system further subdivides within the liver establishing the ductus venosus, a small vessel that directs the embryonic/fetal blood from the umbilical vein directly into the inferior vena cava.

The complex arrangement of the heart is attained by the 55th day of gestation (Larsen 2008). The remaining period of gestation facilitates growth and relative maturation of the cardiovascular structures and corresponding haemodynamic adaptation. Myocardial cells proliferate in conjunction with the rapid accumulation of contractile proteins and metabolic substrates.

Activity

Read

- Chapter 22 (The circulatory system) in Hoffman (2003 pp 1745–1904).
- Chapter 21 (Blood vessels and circulation) in Martini and Nath (2009 pp 719–775).
- Critically review the anatomical and physiological characteristics of the fetal circulation.
- Give a reasoned account of the adaptations, which need to occur in the fetal circulation shortly after the birth of a child.
- Give a rationale for the differences between the fetal circulation and the assumed normal circulation of a 7-year-old child.

Developmental changes in the cardiovascular system

The normal position and shape of the heart in children

In children, the heart is a small, rounded, three-dimensional pyramid that lies in the mediastinal cavity more horizontally than in adults. The apex of the heart is normally higher and located in the fourth left intercostal space, extending only to the fifth intercostal space by 7 or 8 years of age. The base of the heart lies in an oblique position behind the sternum. It consists of the atria and their respective auricles (small appendages of each atrium). The two ventricles form the inferior aspect of the cardiac silhouette coming together to form the apex.

A mature heart weighs between 230 and 340 g, and this weight generally reflects the person's body size. However, according to Gatzoulis (2008), this weight is achieved only between 17 and 20 years of age. In children, the normal heart is relatively small, the size varying with age and body surface area. The heart is suspended in a pericardial sac by its attachments to the aorta and the pulmonary artery. This leaves the apex relatively free and allows the ventricles to move the apex forward to strike against the left side of the chest wall during contraction (systole). This characteristic thrust is best heard as the apex beat on auscultation and is frequently referred to as the point of maximal intensity.

Activity

- Name the three anatomically distinctive layers of the heart.
- Give a reasoned account of the functions of these distinctive layers.

The pericardium

The fibrous pericardium encloses, and to some extent protects, the heart. It forms a continuum with the adventitia of the major veins and arteries that communicate with the heart. The serous pericardium is a double-layered membrane that consists of flat secretory epithelium, connective tissue and some adipose tissue, which is present in insignificant quantities in children. The two layers of the serous pericardium form a pericardial cavity, which holds a very small volume of serous fluid that acts as a lubricant preventing the occurrence of friction as the two membranes glide over each other during systole.

The myocardium

The myocardium, the contractile muscle of the heart, is composed of highly specialised small myocytes rich in specialised contractile proteins, mitochondria and sarcoplasmic reticulum. During embryonic and fetal life the myocardium develops as a result of a gradual increase in myocyte numbers and the intrinsically sustainable contractility. The relatively slow development of myofibrils (contractile elements) within the myocytes throughout fetal life, during infancy and childhood appears to contribute to a characteristic myocyte hypertrophy (i.e. an increase in the size of the myocytes). After birth, in children of all ages, the capacity for myocyte hyperplasia may be limited but myocyte hypertrophy will continue, under normal physiological conditions, up to 20 years of age.

Sources of chemical energy for the myocardium

The chemical energy for the contraction of heart muscle is derived from the metabolism of carbohydrates and fatty acids. However, because the amount of oxygen required for fatty acid metabolism is 11% more than that required for carbohydrate metabolism, to produce an equivalent quantity of adenosine triphosphate, fatty acids are not as efficient as glucose in terms of providing metabolic fuel or energy. Nevertheless, the adult myocardium has a strong preference for fatty acids. This contrasts with the preferences of the fetal and neonatal myocardium for carbohydrates or glucose. This may be clinically significant in circumstances of hypoglycaemia, which could compromise myocardial contractility and so cardiovascular function in neonates and possibly young children (Gluckman & Heymann 1996). Booker (1998) reported significant postnatal increases in myocardial contractility possibly attributable to increases in contractile protein, the delivery of Ca^{2+} to the myofilaments, enhanced sensitivity of troponin to Ca^{2+} and reduced sensitivity to acidosis. The timing of the transition from the use of glucose to fatty acids as the dominant metabolic fuel is not known, although it is possible that this transition is a gradual process influenced by the child's diet and maturation of the myocardium.

The endocardium

The endocardium is composed of a specialised endothelium and a layer of fibroelastic connective tissue that lines the inner surfaces of the heart including the four cardiac valves. Characteristically, the endocardium is thicker in the atria than the ventricles and this may have a functional significance yet to be determined.

Electrophysiology: functional features of the heart

The coordinated contraction of myocardium provides the mechanical energy for the transportation of blood throughout the entire vasculature. Both the electrodynamic controls of the heart and the force of myocardial contractility are the consequence of the sophisticated cellular mechanisms that bring about the rhythmic excitation–contraction coupling phenomena. In the fetus, the right ventricle ejects approximately 60% of blood while the left ventricle ejects only 40% of the total cardiac output (Hoffman 2003). As both ventricles pump blood against a similar vascular resistance, there is little difference in the thickness of the myocardium as the two ventricles develop. However, in some instances the right ventricular wall is slightly thicker than the left ventricular wall, and this persists for a considerable time after birth. Electrocardiographic (ECG) recordings reflect this phenomenon as a relative right ventricular dominance (Hoffman 2003 pp 1757–1762). The right ventricular hypertrophy is generally attributed to the workload of the right ventricle and associated physical development of the myocardium during fetal life. A clear distinction must, however, be made between the physiological right ventricular hypertrophy and a hypertrophy initiated by some form of pathophysiological change that may affect the competence of the entire cardiovascular and pulmonary systems in neonates and children.

Activity

- Give a reasoned explanation for the significant differences in the normal ranges in children's heart beats identified in Table 29.1.
- Define bradycardia in the context of each of the age groups in Table 29.1.
- Define tachycardia in the context of each of the different age groups.
- In your view, is bradycardia or tachycardia more clinically significant in children; and why is this the case?

Table 29.1 Normal range of heart rates in children at rest

Age of the child	Normal range (beats per minute)	Average (beats per minute)
Newborn–6 months of age	90–160	120
6–12 months of age	80–140	110
1–3 years	80–120	100
3–6 years	75–115	90
6–9 years	70–110	90
9–11 years	70–105	85
11–14 years	65–100	80

The faster heart rate in neonates and infants is largely attributed to the smaller size of the ventricular chambers, which are capable of ejecting only a small amount of blood, commonly referred to as the stroke volume, on each ventricular contraction. However, as the child's metabolic demands are high, and these have to be met by an effective cardiac output (the quantity of blood pumped by the left ventricle per minute), the potential deficits created by the small stroke volume are corrected by the higher heart rate. As children grow older, their hearts – and especially the ventricular chambers – evolve, the stroke volume increases, and this contributes to the significant reduction of the heart rate. It is important, however, to appreciate that the normal heart rate and stroke volume in all children fluctuate with activity and crying.

The cardiac cycle

The cardiac cycle is defined as the time from the beginning of one heart beat to the beginning of the next. Each cardiac cycle is initiated and governed by an action potential generated within the sinoatrial node and conveyed rapidly to both atria. The fractional delay in the transfer of the impulse from the atria to the ventricles ensures that the atria contract before the ventricles, as a result of which the blood is pumped by the atria into the ventricles, increasing the ventricular volume, which in turn raises the stroke volume. The four phases of the cardiac cycle are commonly known as:

- contraction (phase I)
- ejection or systole (phase II)
- relaxation (phase III)
- filling or diastole (phase IV).

Although the rhythmic contraction of the heart is intrinsic (a mechanism frequently referred to as myogenic), the harmonising of the cardiac cycle, in terms of rate, force of contractility and volume output, is accomplished by the autonomic nervous system (Priebe & Skarvan 2000). The autonomic nervous system has a direct effect on the nodal tissue, the coronary vessels, atrial and ventricular myocardium and so, to some extent, augments and supports the adapting cardiac function. Physical activities or crying will also increase the child's heart rates significantly by, among other factors, increasing oxygen demand.

At the onset of ventricular contraction, the atrial and ventricular pressure are fairly equal. However, as the ventricular blood volume increases, the ventricular pressure rises, initiating the closure of the atrioventricular valves. This gives rise to the first heart sound (called 'lub'). Because the pulmonary artery and aortic valves remain closed, the ventricles are said to be in isovolumetric contraction. This raises the ventricular pressure further and causes a bulging of both the semilunar and the atrioventricular valves. The semilunar valves open when the left ventricular pressure exceeds the aortic pressure and the right ventricular pressure exceeds the pulmonary artery pressure. The rapid expulsion of blood during the early phase of systole raises the ventricular pressures further establishing a maximum ejection point. This is followed by the last systole phase, which influences the gradual decline in the ventricular and aortic pressures, and the onset of ventricular diastole or early isovolumetric relaxation which culminates in the closure of the semilunar valves and the initiation of second heart sound ('dub').

The volume of blood ejected on each ventricular contraction is defined as the stroke volume. The cardiac output is defined as the amount of blood ejected by the heart during each minute (cardiac output = stroke volume × heart rate/min). The cardiac index takes into consideration the child's body surface area and is therefore a measure of the cardiac output per square metre of body surface area. In children, cardiac index values continue to rise to above 4.0 L/min/m^2 up to 10 years of age, and then declines, falling to a new lower normal value of about 2.4 L/min/m^2 (Guyton & Hall 2006). This phenomenon may be attributed to the normally high metabolic rate in younger children. Exercise and crying will also influence the child's stroke volume, cardiac output and cardiac index, but this is usually transitory in contrast to the factors that have a more definitive effect on cardiac output such as the child's age, size, metabolism and body surface area.

Although the function of the heart shows some degree of adaptability, four constant factors are critical to effective cardiac output and corresponding tissue perfusion. These are the:

- heart rate
- myocardial contractility
- preload (the volume of blood that returns to and stretches the ventricles prior to contraction)
- afterload (the resistance to the ejection of blood from the ventricle into the great vessels), and total peripheral resistance.

Although the heart rate and myocardial contractility are of cardiac origin both can be augmented by neural and humoral mechanisms. By contrast, the preload and afterload are dependent on blood volume, the size of the heart and the dimension of the blood vessels. There is, however, a cyclical nature to this, in that both preload and afterload are important determinants of cardiac output, which is influenced by the heart rate and myocardial contractility.

Scenario

Christopher's knowledge of the developmental anatomy and physiology of the cardiovascular system now leads him to focus on the nature of cardiovascular problems that can occur in infancy and childhood.

Determining the origins and extent of cardiovascular problems in childhood

Children of all ages can present with signs and symptoms that suggest underlying cardiovascular or pulmonary problems that invariably require therapeutic interventions that are dependent on precise diagnosis of the problem and competent delivery of evidence-based care designed to meet the individual child's health needs. Knowledge of structural anomalies and functional problems is indispensable in the competent assessment of a child with suspected cardiovascular or respiratory problems as it serves as a basis for critical analysis of the evidence collected during various clinical assessments, and more invasive investigations, which such children require.

Evidence-based practice

The professional context

Children's nurses need to be fit for practice. This includes being knowledgeable about the:

- normal anatomical features of the child's heart
- normal functional scope of the child's cardiovascular system
- possible deviations from such norms and how these might affect a child.

It requires the nurse to be competent in:

- assessing such children for evidence of a cardiovascular problem
- monitoring the physical, physiological and behavioural changes that may appear as a consequence of an underlying cardiovascular problem
- communicating the findings to other practitioners in a professional manner
- using the empirical evidence in the formulation of diagnosis, therapeutic interventions and appropriate care
- communicating with the child and the parents in an informed and professional manner.

Cardiovascular problems, which present in childhood, are commonly classified according to their congenital or acquired origins. The purpose of the systematic observation, assessment and rigorous investigation is to establish the structure and functions of the cardiovascular and respiratory system, and identify the precise nature of the problem. In general, children with acquired heart disease, such as myocarditis, commonly present with symptoms that suggests generalised ill health. In contrast, some children with congenital heart disease can be asymptomatic, whereas others present with signs and symptoms that are confined to the cardiovascular and sometimes the respiratory system at a very early stage. The most common features are cyanosis, failure to grow, a cardiac murmur, dysrhythmia and symptoms of congestive cardiac failure.

Activity

- Access the companion PowerPoint presentation and define congenital cardiovascular disease that occurs in children.
- Distinguish between the common features of acyanotic and cyanotic congenital cardiovascular lesions that occur in children.
- Distinguish between congenital cardiovascular disease and acquired cardiovascular disease that may occur in children.

Congenital cardiovascular problems can be grouped into two distinctive classifications: the acyanotic cardiovascular lesions and the more profound cyanotic cardiovascular lesions. The acyanotic cardiovascular lesions generally include structural problems such as patent ductus arteriosus, atrial septal defects and some ventricular septal defects. In general, children with these defects are initially asymptomatic. The first indication of an underlying cardiovascular problem may be the child's history of recurrent respiratory infection, failure to grow or poor exercise tolerance.

Ventricular septal defects are the most common congenital cardiovascular defects occurring in isolation or in association with more complex cardiovascular anomalies. These defects are commonly classified according to their size and position in the interventricular septum. Defects are most common in the membranous part of the septum, although they do extend into the muscular part of the septum. A wide range of defects can also occur in the muscular part of the septum. The position, size and complexity of the defect (Hoffman 2003, Sommer et al 2008) determine the signs and symptoms with which the child presents. For instance, the size of the defect determines the magnitude of the shunting of blood from the left ventricle to the right ventricle. Larger defects tend to have a more profound effect on the right ventricle as a consequence of which infants present early with respiratory difficulties and congestive cardiac failure. Both problems are caused by an increase in pulmonary blood flow caused by the amount of oxygenated blood being shunted from the left ventricle across the defect into the right ventricle. This additional volume of blood is then directed to the lungs. This leads to pulmonary plethora as a consequence of which normal pulmonary ventilation and gas exchange may be compromised. In time, the haemodynamic disturbances caused by the abnormal inter-ventricular shunting of blood causes right ventricular hypertrophy and left atrial and ventricular dilatation (Hoffman 2003, Sommer et al 2008). This augments the normal shape of the heart, a feature that is observed on the child's chest X-ray.

Congenital cardiovascular lesions that cause the baby to be cyanotic from birth account for less than 25% of all congenital cardiac defects. Many of these defects are life threatening, such as, for instance, tricuspid atresia, and early diagnosis and therapeutic intervention is essential. The severity of the cyanosis is invariably determined by the restrictions to pulmonary blood flow, which has a compromising effect on pulmonary gas exchange. Transposition of the great arteries is one of the most common forms of cyanotic congenital cardiac defects that presents in neonates. It occurs more commonly in males than females with a ratio of 3:1 (Flanagan et al 1999, Hoffman 2003).

The abnormality is confined to the ventricular-arterial connections in which the aorta is attached to the right ventricle and the pulmonary artery is attached to the left ventricle. This means that the pulmonary and systemic circulation run in parallel to each other, a process that interferes with the normal oxygenation of blood in the lungs, as a consequence of which the blood in the systemic circulation is oxygen poor and the baby suffers from severe cyanosis. In this instance, the baby's survival depends on the presence of other defects, such as a patent ductus arteriosus or atrial or ventricular septal defects, which permit mixing of blood between the pulmonary and systemic circulation. The presence of these associated defects and the degree of mixing between the two bloodstreams also determine the haemodynamic findings.

Most commonly, such babies present with only a small patent foramen ovale, which does not facilitate adequate mixing between the pulmonary and the systemic blood, and thus contributes to severe cyanosis shortly after birth. As a consequence, such babies experience low PaO_2, which leads to metabolic acidosis and depression of myocardial function. The normal fall in pulmonary vascular resistance and the corresponding increase in pulmonary blood flow that occurs soon after birth leads to left atrial and left ventricular volume overload. The combination of metabolic acidosis with depression of myocardial contractility and volume overload may be contributing to heart failure and rapid deterioration in the infant's haemodynamic status.

Acquired cardiovascular disease is relatively uncommon in children in the developed world. Nevertheless, awareness of the existence of such problems is important if children are to receive the most appropriate treatment that their condition warrants. The acquired cardiovascular diseases can be grouped into those that are caused by:

- infection, as in endocarditis, myocarditis and pericarditis
- systemic metabolic problems, as in myocardial disease
- unknown factors, as in cardiomyopathy and cardiac tumours.

Depending on the primary cause, each of these conditions may affect the child in a very different ways, for instance, the nature and virulence of the pathogen, the magnitude of the metabolic problem or the severity of the abnormal morphological change to the heart. It is therefore important to recognise that children affected by any of these problems can present acutely ill with severe haemodynamic instability and signs of low cardiac output. Alternatively, some children may experience more subtle forms of ill health and present with failure to grow, reduced exercise tolerance and occasionally cardiac dysrhythmias (Bristow 2003, p 1860) that if untreated may result in sudden death.

The common denominator in the acute and the more long-standing acquired form of heart disease is congestive cardiac failure, which must be treated in conjunction with any treatment for the underlying cause of the primary disease. However, supportive therapeutic interventions culminating in a successful eradication of the primary disease is not always possible. Surviving children with myocardial disease may, in some circumstances, require cardiac transplantation as a means to enhancing their quality of life.

Reflect on your practice

A 6-week-old baby is admitted to the cardiac unit with a short history of breathlessness, difficulties with feeding and increasing cyanosis, especially during crying. Following a thorough physical assessment and ultrasonic scan of the baby's heart and greater blood vessels, a diagnosis of ventricular septal defect is made. On arrival to the cardiac unit the baby is found to be in congestive cardiac failure and, therefore, will require swift therapeutic intervention and competent nursing care:

- How should this baby's care be managed to maximise the best therapeutic outcome?
- Give a systematic account of the nursing care that this baby will require.
- Give a reasoned account of the medical treatment that this baby will require.

Congestive cardiac failure

The differences between the various kinds of congenital and acquired heart disease in childhood are determined, to a large extent, by the impact of the primary problem on the function of the cardiovascular and respiratory systems. Respiratory difficulties and hypoxia are common clinical features in children with altered pulmonary blood flow. Furthermore, as children's myocardium is more oxygen dependent (Hoffman, 2003) hypoxia is likely to have a compromising effect on cardiovascular and other major organ function and eventually contribute to the development of heart failure.

Congestive cardiac failure occurs when the heart is unable to pump sufficient amounts of blood to the systemic (and pulmonary) circulation required to meet the metabolic demands of the body. Congestive cardiac failure is invariably the result of some structural or morphological defects in the cardiovascular system, which in time, give rise to characteristic haemodynamic changes that lead to the following:

- **Volume overload**: commonly caused by left-to-right intracardiac shunts that give rise to right ventricular hypertrophy and increased pulmonary blood flow.
- **Pressure overload**: commonly caused by obstructive lesions such as coarctation of the aorta and valve stenosis.
- **Impaired contractility**: caused by factors that affect myocardial contractility, such as cardiomyopathy, myocarditis, hypoglycaemia and low serum potassium, calcium or magnesium.
- **High cardiac output demands**: caused by such problems as septicaemia, in which peripheral vasodilatation allows an abnormal redistribution of the child's circulating blood volume away from the vital organs.

The pathophysiology of congestive cardiac failure can be viewed in terms of right ventricular failure and left ventricular failure. Right ventricular failure is characterised by suboptimal ventricular function. This leads to an abnormal rise in end-diastolic pressure, which in turn raises the central venous pressure and causes systemic venous engorgement. The ensuing systemic venous hypertension causes hepatomegaly and, in some instances, dependent tissue oedema. In contrast, left ventricular failure is characterised by abnormal increases in the left ventricular end-diastolic pressure, resulting in haemodynamic changes in the left atrium and the pulmonary veins. As a consequence, the lungs become congested with blood that then raises the pulmonary pressures and contributes to pulmonary oedema. However, because both sides of the heart depend on an adequate function of the other side, failure of one ventricular chamber invariably also causes reciprocal changes in the opposite chamber. This is particularly so in children whose hearts are small and functionally immature. Nevertheless, the cardiovascular system is capable of initiating compensatory mechanisms that result in a sustainable increase in cardiac output in keeping with the metabolic needs of the body. These compensatory mechanisms include activation of the sympathetic nervous system, increased heart rate, ventricular hypertrophy and dilatation. The failing heart and the compensatory mechanisms are responsible for the clinical features with which the child presents. The four most distinctive features that must be recognised in children are:

- impaired myocardial contractility
- pulmonary congestion
- systemic venous congestion
- fluid retention.

Each of these features must be critically and methodically evaluated. The intention being to ensure that the:

- severity of congestive cardiac failure is recognised
- primary cause is identified
- best therapeutic and caring interventions are utilised.

Diagnostic assessment and evaluation of the child

The child's health and appearance frequently reflects the competence of the cardiovascular system, although this cannot always be assumed without careful physical assessment and evaluation. Therefore, a typical physical assessment should consist of inspection, palpation and auscultation. These will be followed by a range of more invasive assessments, such as evaluation of blood gases, echocardiography and cardiac catheterisation, which will provide more definitive evidence regarding the specific nature of the cardiovascular problem. The collected evidence must be documented and critically evaluated as part of the process of establishing the diagnosis.

Inspection

Inspection of the child's general appearance must include the body size, proportions, skin colour, visible pulsations and exaggerated shapes to the thorax. Assessment of the respiratory rate and pattern will also contribute to a better evaluation of the cardiovascular function. The child's response to stimuli and the surrounding environment will give an indication of the developmental milestones that have been reached. In health, a child's core body temperature is relatively constant at 36.0–37.5°C and the peripheral temperature is no lower than 34–35°C. However, if the peripheral skin temperature is found to be consistently lower it is important to distinguish between the possible contributing factors, such as low environmental temperatures or the child's compromised peripheral perfusion.

Palpation

This involves tactile skills that contribute to the evaluation of the child's haemodynamic status. The pulse can be palpated in superficial arteries such as the brachial, radial, femoral artery and dorsalis pedis. The qualities of the pulse can be describes in terms of:

- frequency
- rhythm
- amplitude.

However, it must be appreciated that pulses may be difficult to feel in neonates and infants because of the relatively low arterial resistance to blood flow generated by the comparative thinness of the tunica media within the walls of the arteries and arterioles. For this reason, in children under 1 year of age, the heart rate should be recorded over the apex of the heart, using a stethoscope rather than by means of palpation of the radial pulse as it may not be possible to reliably feel the radial pulse. However, as the child grows older, the muscle fibres of the tunica media enlarge, augmenting the internal diameter of the arteries and raising the resistance to arterial blood flow, which in turn influences the magnitude of the pulse wave.

The intensity of a pulse can be rated on a scale of 0 to 4 as follows:

- An absent pulse is graded as 0.
- A palpable but weak and easily obliterated pulse is graded 1.
- A normal easily palpable pulse is graded as 2.
- A full pulse is graded as 3.
- A bounding pulse that is easily visible is graded as 4.

Blood pressure

This term generally applies to the arterial pressure in the systemic circulation. Blood pressure fluctuates with each heart beat, between a maximum value (systolic pressure) achieved during cardiac systole and a minimum value (diastolic pressure) that reflects the diastolic phase. The blood pressure can be measured by invasive methods, which involve inserting a needle, attached to a monitoring device, into a peripheral artery. More commonly, however, blood pressure is measured externally, or is estimated by using an inflatable cuff on the upper arm or sometimes on the leg (below the knee). The accuracy of the measurement is dependent on the size of the cuff and this must be proportional to the length and diameter of the limb (two-thirds of the limb must be covered, e.g. on the upper arm this is two-thirds of the distance between the shoulder and the elbow). Alternatively, a Doppler percutaneous flow probe can be used to measure the systolic and a diastolic pressure. This device detects cessation of blood flow very accurately. The difference between the systolic and the diastolic pressure values is known as the pulse pressure. The major physiological factors that affect the pulse pressure are the stroke volume, the force of ventricular ejection and the compliance of the arterial vascular network. The greater the stroke volume, the greater is the amount of blood that must be accommodated in the arterial network. This produces a rise in the systolic pressure and a fall in the diastolic pressure, which will culminate in a wider pulse pressure.

Wide ranges of factors influence the child's blood pressure such as maturation of the autonomic nervous system, developments and maturation in the cardiovascular system and corresponding reflex mechanisms. Furthermore, there is some evidence to suggest that the intrauterine environment which influences low birth weight may also contribute to the development of hypertension in adulthood (Barker et al 1993). In health, children's blood pressure parameters vary with age and under normal physiological conditions there should be a gradual increase in the systolic and diastolic pressures according to age (Table 29.2).

The physiological adaptation and maintenance of normal blood pressure is attributed principally to baroreceptors, which are present in the carotid and aortic bodies. These receptors are thought to augment and sustain the normal systemic blood pressure by reflex. However, in children with hypoxia, fluid retention and congestive cardiac failure the function of these baroreceptors could be compromised and so contributing to the changes in blood pressure that is sometimes observed in these children.

Auscultation

This involves listening to the specific sounds generated by the heart as a consequence of the:

- systematic opening and closing of atrioventricular valves
- systematic opening and closing of the semilunar pulmonary artery and aortic valves
- vibration of blood against the walls of the heart and major blood vessels.

It is not uncommon for neonates and young children to present with a range of heart sounds and murmurs that are not always indicative of an underlying cardiovascular problem. Nevertheless, the presence of cardiac murmurs must be taken into consideration in the overall assessment of the child's cardiovascular system. The two distinguished heart sounds that must be heard are known as S_I and S_{II}. Under normal circumstances, S_I is louder at the apex of the heart in the mitral and tricuspid valve area. Conversely, S_{II} is best heard near the base of the heart in the pulmonary artery and the aortic valve area. Two further heart sounds may be audible and these are known as S_{III} and S_{IV}. S_{III} is thought to be produced by vibrations caused during ventricular filling and may be heard in some children and young adults. By contrast, S_{IV} is generally attributed to the reduction in vibration initially caused by atrial contraction at the end of diastole. This sound is seldom heard and, when audible, further cardiovascular assessments should be considered. Cardiac murmurs are important sounds in neonates and young children, and must not be ignored, as they can suggest underlying cardiac or major blood vessel anomalies that will require further systematic screening and critical evaluation.

Table 29.2 Blood pressure in childhood. Readings are the 50th centile for boys (taken from Second Task Force on Blood Pressure Control in Children 1987)

Age	Systolic blood pressure (mmHg)	Diastolic blood pressure (mmHg)
Newborn	73	55
6 months	90	53
1 years	90	56
3 years	92	55
6 years	96	57
9 years	100	61
12 years	107	64
15 years	114	65

Chest radiography

This can determine the position of the heart, its size and shape, chamber and major vessel enlargement or hypoplasia. It depicts the anatomical size and shape of the trachea, the bronchi, and the lungs in relation to the heart. It provides considerable evidence regarding air entry and pulmonary ventilation and demarcates the extent of the pulmonary blood flow and pulmonary venous return. In children with cardiac problems such as congestive cardiac failure, chest radiography will help to establish the extent of the primary anatomical anomalies as well as the severity of path physiological problems such as cardiomegaly, pulmonary plethora and pulmonary congestion. In isolation, such evidence may be inconclusive; however, when considered in conjunction with other factors it can contribute to a definitive diagnosis.

Electrocardiography

This records the changes in the electrical potentials during cardiac activity (Table 29.3). Such data also provide information about the anatomical orientation of the heart; the relative size of the chambers of the heart; heart rate, rhythm and origin of excitation; and the spread of the impulse. Disturbances in the normal conduction process can be suggestive of a primary cardiovascular problem.

Electrocardiography in children will also reflect some age-related changes, which must be taken into consideration in the

Table 29.3 Electrocardiograph recording of the function of the heart as a pump

Electrocardiographic event	Corresponding physiological event in the heart
P wave	Depolarisation (excitation) of the atria prior to their contraction. The action potential (impulse) is initiated in the sinoatrial node. It spreads through the atrial muscle reaching the atrioventricular node
P-R segment	Atrial depolarisation and conduction of impulses through the atrioventricular node
QRS complex	Depolarisation (excitation) of the ventricles, the repolarisation (relaxation) of the atria is masked by the ventricular depolarisation
S-T segment	End of ventricular depolarisation and the beginning of the ventricular repolarisation
T wave	Repolarisation (relaxation) of the ventricles

overall evaluation of the child's cardiovascular system. A summary of the age-related significant points may be detailed as follows:

- At birth, the thickness in the right ventricular muscle exceeds the thickness of the left ventricular muscle. This is a physiological phenomenon reflecting the right ventricular workload during fetal life. However, the significant increase in the left ventricular workload, after birth, gradually augments this. Thus, the right ventricular dominance normally seen in neonates and young infants is gradually replaced by left ventricular dominance in later childhood. The ratio of left to right ventricular muscle mass in young adults is believed to average at 2.5:1 (Gatzoulis 2008, Houston 1998, Park & Guntheroth 1987) and the electrocardiography recording reflects this ratio.
- The gradual increase in the chambers of the heart, in conjunction with the ongoing maturation of the myocardium, allows the heart to handle greater quantities of blood volume. In the healthy child this results in increasing stroke volume and cardiac output as a consequence of which the heart rate decreases.
- In conjunction with the decreasing heart rate all lengths and intervals (PR interval, QRS duration, QT interval) of the cardiac cycle increase (Houston 1998).

Existing cardiovascular problems can, however, interfere with the electrophysiological conduction throughout the atrial and ventricular myocardium, and these are then reflected in the electrocardiographic recordings.

Echocardiography

This technique uses high-frequency sound waves to document detailed images, from which the atria, ventricles, the septal tissue, the atrioventricular and semilunar valves, and the great vessels can be identified and their dimensions measured. Most congenital cardiovascular defects and major myocardial changes may be identified using this technique. However, the correct diagnosis and therapeutic intervention is dependent on the precise measurement and critical evaluation of the size and complexity of the cardiovascular problem.

Cardiac catheterisation

This is the most invasive procedure that a child with a suspected cardiovascular problem may have to undergo. It involves inserting a radio-opaque catheter through a peripheral blood vessel into the respective chambers of the heart. This procedure is usually combined with angiocardiography in which a radio-opaque die is injected through the catheter into the circulation. Combined, these procedures facilitate the collection of evidence regarding:

- oxygen saturation of the blood within the four chambers of the heart and the greater blood vessels
- haemodynamic pressure values within the four chambers and the greater blood vessels
- stroke volume and cardiac output values
- the position, size and complexity of the cardiovascular defects and anomalies.

Nursing care considerations

Children born with cardiovascular anomalies, and those that acquire cardiovascular disease, will require extensive diagnostic, therapeutic and nursing interventions. The specific range and sequence of interventions will be dictated by the severity of the cardiovascular problems with which the child presents. For instance, cardiovascular anatomical problems are likely to require surgical and supporting pharmacological interventions. In contrast, functional problems within the cardiovascular system, such as congestive cardiac failure, may be resolved by appropriate pharmacological interventions. In both instances, however, these children will require nursing care and their families will require support and education.

Evidence-based practice

The nursing care of a child with a suspected cardiovascular problem can be challenging because such children do not consistently display symptoms until the child's energy expenditure exceeds the ability of the heart to meet the metabolic needs of the body. With the exception of children born with cyanotic cardiovascular disease, the onset of signs and symptoms, in many children, is gradual and at times inconsistent requiring the nursing and medical staff to be vigilant in obtaining the appropriate clinically and socially significant evidence.

Methodical assessments of the child will enable the nurse to identify several nursing diagnoses that will require attention. All assessments must take into consideration the history of the child's physical growth, intellectual and psychosocial development, nutritional preferences and exercise tolerance. This information forms a critical part of the evidence about the child's general state of health and gives an indication about the kind of supportive nursing care and therapeutic interventions that the child may require.

In all circumstances, nursing interventions must be driven by the evidence collected during methodical assessments, or derived by critical evaluation of the child's:

- general physical appearance
- responsiveness
- behaviour
- restfulness and sleep
- vital signs: body temperature, heart rate/rhythm, respiratory rate/effort, blood pressure
- presence of hypoxia
- state of hydration
- elimination: extent of perspiration, urine output, emesis, faeces.

Activity

- Give a reasoned account as to why the above assessments are required.
- Critically evaluate the available evidence and demonstrate how this evidence can be used in the overall management of this child.

Children with established cardiovascular disease, especially congestive cardiac failure, must be cared for in a manner that will ensure comfort, maximise rest and support cardiac, respiratory, digestive and renal function. Nursing and therapeutic interventions must be coordinated so as to ensure the child's energy expenditure is minimised. Positioning the child in a manner that promotes comfort, facilitates lung expansion and minimises distress and cardiac workload is an important aspect of nursing. Allowing for frequent rest and sleeping periods will also reduce the workload of the heart, promote the child's scope for healing and restoration of health where this is possible.

Invasive diagnostic procedures such as thoracic surgery are painful and frightening. These children will, therefore, require emotional and psychological support from their parents, siblings and the practitioners caring for them. It must also be recognised that the child's parents, siblings and significant others will find such situations justifiably stressful. Every effort must be made to support them by involving them in the decision-making process. They should be given explanations about the evolving symptoms and how these can impact on the child's well-being. Similarly, explanations must be offered about care and treatment options if the parents are to make informed decisions.

Children are not always able to communicate verbally their pain, discomfort or distress and every effort must be taken to monitor their emotional, physical and physiological state to ascertain that comforting interventions and appropriate analgesia are administered proactively. For instance, children who have undergone surgery may require continuous intravenous infusion of opioids such as morphine sulfate or fentanyl for a period of 24–48 hours. Providing the dosages are calculated carefully in relation to the child's body surface area, these drugs are considered as safe and effective in relieving severe forms of pain. However, milder forms of oral analgesia, such as paracetamol, may be given at regular intervals or when required to control less severe forms of pain. Providing the child is haemodynamically stable, provision must be made to encourage active play and mobilisation. Children who are comfortable, pain free and happy are likely to make a quicker recovery in health.

Activity

Most infants with congenital or acquired cardiovascular problems develop, at some stage, congestive cardiac failure, which contributes to difficulties with feeding due to breathlessness caused by other factors such as ventilation–perfusion mismatch. Give a reasoned account of the nutritional needs of such children and how these needs can be best met without causing distress to the individual child.

Small, nutritious and appetising meals should be offered to these children. Infants should be offered small but frequent bottle feeds and, where this is not possible, nasogastric tube feeding may have to be considered, especially if the infant manifests respiratory distress or cyanosis. Managing the child's hydration is an important aspect of care and all fluid intake must therefore be monitored carefully to ensure that episodes of overhydration or dehydration are avoided.

Children with congestive cardiac failure frequently experience problems of systemic fluid retention and hepatomegaly. This may further aggravate the child's respiratory distress and cardiac workforce, and compromise cardiac output and organ perfusion. Digestion and absorption of nutrients and elimination of metabolic by-products may be adversely affected.

Activity

- Critically review the impact of systemic fluid retention and hepatomegaly on the child's ability to feed and absorb nutrients.
- Establish as to why hepatomegaly could have a compromising effect on the function of the diaphragm and the gastrointestinal tract.
- Explain why these children may be failing to grow.

The limited availability of nutrients combined with the child's greater respiratory effort can have a devastating effect on the child's metabolism and might ultimately lead to metabolic acidosis, hypoglycemia, inappropriate activation of the renin-angiotensin-aldosterone system, electrolyte imbalance and concomitant fluid retention.

Activity

- Give a reasoned account how each of these problems can be recognised.
- Explain why each of these problems could have a detrimental effect on the child.
- How can the above problems be avoided?

Congestive cardiac failure compromises myocardial contractility and reduces cardiac output. This invariably leads to reduced renal perfusion and activation of renin-angiotensin-aldosterone system which causes retention of sodium and water. The persistent, unchecked, retention of sodium and water not only reduces urinary output but also contributes to the development of pulmonary and systemic oedema. The retention of fluid contributes to weight gain despite the child's reduced nutritional intake and occasional vomiting. It is worth noting that significant fluid retention causes weight gain and tends to mask the child's cachexic state.

Activity

- Outline the measures that can be taken to monitor the child's fluid intake and elimination.
- Give a reasoned account as to why the child's blood electrolyte values should be monitored.

Therapeutic intervention

Even in the most difficult situation, the primary cause of congestive cardiac failure needs to be determined and managed proactively. Correctable problems must be resolved expediently. One of the most successful interventions of congestive cardiac failure is likely to consist of the use of medication such as furosemide (a loop diuretic), lanoxin (a cardiac glycoside) or spironolactone (a potassium-sparing diuretic). In some circumstances, children who need such medication may also be given potassium supplements to maintain physiologically desirable plasma potassium values.

Cardiac rhythm disturbances may occur in children. Some of these disturbances resolve spontaneously, although more persistent disturbances will require definitive therapeutic interventions. For instance, a child with persistent bradycardia caused by conduction problems will require a permanent pacemaker to sustain acceptable cardiac rhythm. In contrast, children with recurrent episodes of profound supraventricular tachycardia may require suitable antiarrhythmic drugs. The primary rationale for both therapeutic interventions is to normalise cardiac rhythm in order to sustain good cardiac output.

Activity

Read:

- Chapter 18 (The heart) and Chapter 19 (The vascular system) in Rang et al (2007 pp 277–2297 and pp 298–320).

Reflect on your practice

- How would this medication affect the child's congestive cardiac failure?
- Give a reasoned account of the improvements in the child's health as a consequence of the appropriate therapeutic intervention.
- Consider the kind of preparation the child and family will require in instances where surgical intervention is required in order to safeguard the child's quality of life and long-term survival.

Key points

Following a methodical assessment of the child and a critical review of the clinically significant evidence, every effort must be made to assist the child in a manner that will reduce the cardiac workload. Such therapeutic and nursing interventions must also make every effort to reduce the child's respiratory distress, improve cardiac output and assist in elimination of undesirable quantities of retained body fluids. Care must be taken to ensure that the child's hydration and nutritional intake meets the metabolic demands and that the child is showing signs of growth and development.

Major anatomical defects that present at time of birth in the form of cyanotic congenital heart defects will require palliative or corrective surgical intervention at the most clinically appropriate time. The central aim here is to reconstruct the heart and, where necessary, the blood vessels in a manner that will restore normal cardiovascular haemodynamics and avoid the long-term complications that are commonly associated with congenital heart disease. Functional problems, such as myocarditis, congestive cardiac failure and low cardiac output must also be dealt with as they arise. In these instances, swift diagnostic and therapeutic interventions consisting of finely balanced hydration, nutrition, notropic agents and antifailure drugs, among others, are essential.

Activity

Critical reflection on theory and practice:

- Review the therapeutic intervention that should be considered for a child with a known cyanotic congenital cardiovascular anomaly and evidence of congestive cardiac failure.
- Critically review the nursing diagnoses that will have to be considered in the planning of nursing care for a child with congestive cardiac failure.
- Critically examine the merits of evidence-based practice in your consideration of holistic nursing care for a child with congestive cardiac failure.

Evidence-based nursing interventions are fundamental in the overall management of the child and family. These interventions begin with a methodical assessment of the child, documenting the available evidence. A critical exploration of this evidence will inevitably lead to informed decisions regarding the specific care that a child with a cardiovascular problem may require. Proactive holistic care must take into consideration the child's need for comfort, rest, sleep and nutrition. The more technical aspects of care, such as monitoring the child's haemodynamic values and evaluating the child's response to planned therapeutic and nursing interventions, must also form an important part of competent nursing practice.

Summary

It is not possible to consider here the full extent of the complex nature of cardiovascular problems that are known to encroach on children's lives. Nevertheless, attempts have been made to draw attention to the embryonic and fetal developments of the cardiovascular system with a view to establishing a basis for understanding the normal cardiovascular function in children. This approach has in turn prepared the background for understanding some of the common congenital and acquired cardiovascular problems that some children present with. The therapeutic interventions must be decided according to the specific problems with which such children present. This suggests that the ethos of best practice requires children's nurses to collect and critically consider the evidence that will significantly influence the therapeutic and nursing management in a manner that will result in a more restful child with improved cardiac function.

References

Barker, D.J.P., Osmond, C., Golding, J., et al., 1993. Growth in utero, blood pressure in childhood and adult life, and mortality from cardiovascular disease. In: Baker, D.J.P. (Ed.), Fetal and infant origins of adult disease. British Medical Association Publishing, London.

Booker, P., 1998. Myocardial stunning in neonates. British Journal of Anaesthesia 80, 371–383.

Bristow, J., 2003. Acquired cardiovascular disease. In: Rudolph, C., Rudolph, A., Hostetter, M., et al (Eds.) Rudolph's paediatrics, 21st edn. McGraw Hill, New York, pp. 1860–1865.

Collins, P., 2008. Embryogenesis. In: Standring, S. (Ed.), Gray's anatomy – the anatomical basis of clinical practice. Churchill Livingstone, New York.

Flanagan, M., Yeager, S., Weindling, S., 1999. Cardiac disease. In: Avery, G. et al (Ed.), Neonatal pathophysiology and management of the newborn. Lippincott Williams and Wilkins, New York.

Gatzoulis, M., 2008. Thorax. In: Standring, S. (Ed.), Gray's anatomy – the anatomical basis of clinical practice. Churchill Livingstone, New York.

Gluckman, P., Heymann, M., 1996. Paediatrics and perinatology: the scientific basis. Edward Arnold, London.

Guyton, A., Hall, J., 2006. Textbook of medical physiology. WB Saunders, Philadelphia.

Hoffman, J., 2003. The circulatory system. In: Rudolph, C., Rudolph, A., Hostetter, M. et al (Eds.), Rudolph's paediatrics, 21st edn. McGraw Hill, New York, pp. 1745–1905.

Houston A, 1998. Cardiovascular Disease. In: Campbell A, McIntosh N (Eds) Forfar and Arneil's Textbook of paediatrics. Churchill Livingstone, Edinburgh.

Larsen, W., 2008. Human embryology. Churchill Livingstone, London.

Martini, F., Nash, J., 2009. Fundamentals of Anatomy and Physiology. Pearson International Editions, London.

Park, M., Guntheroth, W., 1987. How to read paediatric ECGs. Mosby Year Book, Baltimore.

Polin, R., Fox, W., 2004. Fetal and neonatal physiology. WB Saunders, Philadelphia.

Priebe, H.J., Skarvan, K., 2000. Cardiovascular physiology. BMJ Books, London.

Rang, H., Dale, M., Ritter, J., Moore, P., 2007. Pharmacology. Churchill Livingstone, Edinburgh.

Second Task Force on Blood Pressure Control in Children, 1987. Normal blood pressure readings for boys. National Heart. Lung and Blood Institute, Bethesda, MD.

Sommer, R., Hijazi, Z., Rodes, J., 2008. Pathophysiology of congenital heart disease: shunt lesions. Circulation 117, 1090–1099.

Wong, D., Hockenberry-Eaton, M., Wilson, D., et al., 2008. The child with cardiovascular dysfunction. In: Wong, D. et al (Ed.), Nursing care of infants and children, 6th edn. Mosby, St Louis, pp. 1464–1529.

Suggestions for Further Reading

Chien, K., 2000. Genomic circuits and the integrative biology of cardiac diseases. Nature 407, 227–232
This article explores some of the complex interactions between possible genetic and environmental factors and how these could act as modifiers of human health, particularly cardiovascular disease. Considerable attention is given to the distinctions between the pathogenesis of congenital and that of acquired cardiovascular problem.

Doyle, R., Goldberg, K., Harold, C., Poeggel, J., 2000. Handbook of paediatric drug therapy. Springhouse Corporation, Pennsylvania
This book offers a succinct résumé of drugs that may be used as part of a treatment regimen for infants and children with congestive cardiac failure.

Kitchiner, D., 2004. Antenatal detection of congenital heart disease. Current Paediatrics 14 (1), 39–44
This article offers an informative account of the methods used to detect structural and functional cardiac anomalies that present in fetuses during the antenatal period.

Nolan, G., 1998. Transcription and the broken heart. Nature 392, 129–130
This article offers an invaluable insight into some of the factors that may influence the development of the embryo's heart.

Seale, A., Shinebourne, E., 2004. Cardiac problems in Down syndrome. Current Paediatrics 14 (1), 33–38
This article provides an excellent account of the spectrum of heart defects, therapeutic interventions and anticipated outcomes in children with Down syndrome.

Srivastava, D., Olson, E., 2000. A genetic blueprint for cardiac development. Nature 407, 221–226
This article offers an invaluable insight into some of the genetic factors that may influence the development of the embryo's heart.

Walsh, K., 2004. Interventional cardiology. Current Paediatrics 14 (1), 45–50
This article gives an excellent account of the current ranges of therapeutic interventions, which should be considered when managing the care of a child with congenital cardiovascular problems.

Yaffe, S., Avanda, J., 1992. Paediatric pharmacology: therapeutic principles in practice. WB Saunders, Philadelphia
This book provides an excellent account of a range of pharmacological principles that need to be taken into consideration when caring for a child with compromised cardiovascular function.

Caring for children: the role of the immune system in protecting against disease

30

Maureen R Harrison

ABSTRACT

The aim of this chapter is to provide an overview of immunology, in particular barrier defence, and therefore to increase the children's nurses' understanding of how this knowledge can relate to the prevention and process of infection in infants and children.

LEARNING OUTCOMES

- Be able to understand the different phases of the immune response.
- To identify how innate immunity provides the first line of defence in protecting against infections.
- Be aware of the physiological barriers that prevent infection occurring.
- To understand other factors of first-line defence, such as cell-mediated and humoral immunity, which enable most infants and children to respond to microbial attack.
- To apply knowledge of innate immunology to principles of nursing practice, in particular infection control.
- To outline the assessment of a child with acute infection.

Introduction

The efficiency of the immune system in protecting against infection is often taken for granted in countries such as the UK. Even the World Health Organization (WHO) has demonstrated that, in developed countries like the UK, death from respiratory infections is not as significant as other causes of death, being only fourth in ranking from the ten leading causes of death in high income countries (WHO 2008). However, in low income countries, six of the top ten causes of death have infectious and perinatal causes. Figure 30.1 demonstrates causes of death among children under the age of 5 worldwide. It is important to note that 54% of deaths are also associated with malnutrition.

A limited number of viral and bacterial pathogens are responsible for infectious disease among neonates and infants. The most pathogenic bacteria are encapsulated bacteria, such as *Streptococcus pneumoniae*, *Streptococcus pyogenes*, *Staphylococcus aureus*, *Escherichia coli*, *Neisseria meningitidis*, and *Haemophilus influenza* (Klouwenberg & Bont 2008) and immunity against these organisms protects an infant from disease. An understanding of the nature of the battle between humans and microorganisms, and the role of the immune system in protecting children from infectious diseases, is important. This knowledge then needs to be linked to how the children's nurse can promote and optimise health.

Many infectious agents (bacteria, viruses, fungi and protozoa) would use any opportunity to utilise the human body as a means for growth and proliferation. However, the human body has developed a series of very effective defence mechanisms to establish immunity against infection (Roitt et al 2006). The word 'immunity' comes from the Latin word immunitas, meaning 'freedom from'. In most instances, the human body is very efficient at avoiding attack but at certain times the infectious agents win, the result being the development of an infection (Roitt et al 2006).

There are many interindividual variations in how the immune system functions such as genetics, age, gender, diet, history of infections and vaccination (Clader & Kew 2002), and Figure 30.1 demonstrates the importance of nutrition; however, this chapter is concerned predominantly with the main process of immunity. The immune system has three phases in the overall response to attack:

- Phase 1: immediate response – innate immunity
- Phase 2: the inflammatory response
- Phase 3: the adaptive immune response.

Each of these phases has its own unique strategies of warfare. However, only the first and second phases will be discussed with particular application to the developing immunity in a child. This will then be linked to the relevance of certain aspects of care for children.

DOI: 10.1016/B978-0-7020-3183-0.10030-X

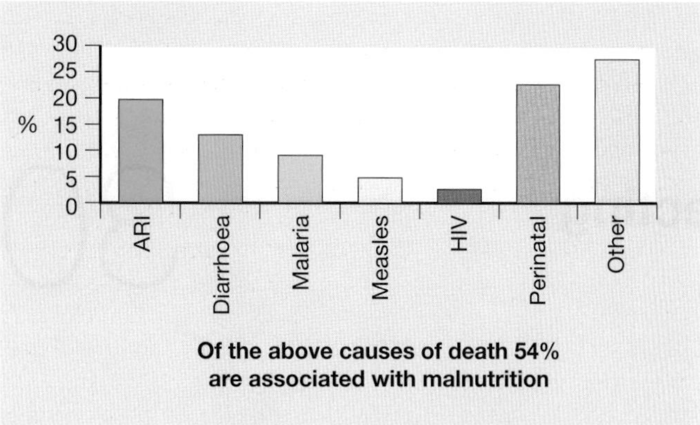

Fig. 30.1 • Proportional mortality among under fives worldwide, 2001. Of the causes of death shown, 54% of deaths are associated with malnutrition (reproduced with permission from WHO 2003).

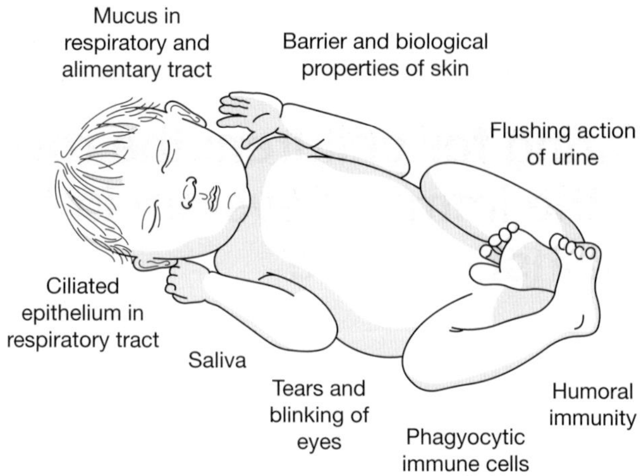

Fig. 30.2 • The key features of innate immunity.

Phase 1. The immediate response to infection: innate immunity

At birth, most infants have the capacity to develop a very efficient immune system, as is demonstrated by the majority of infants who survive their first year of life without suffering from major life-threatening infections. Indeed, from as early as 20–26 gestational weeks, the fetus has been observed to be capable of mounting a sophisticated immune response, as evidenced by those fetuses who were infected with rubella during pregnancy (Warner 2004) and were shown to have antibodies against the rubella in their blood. However, the immune system is not fully developed at birth, and certain 'units' need to undergo learning programmes that will eventually enable them to recognise and destroy the huge dimension of immunogens (agents that are harmful to the human host) (Stiehm 1996). That part of the immune system involved in learning is referred to as the 'adaptive immune response' and includes the development of specific immune cells, lymphocytes and the production of antibodies (immunoglobulins) against all harmful microorganisms. This arm of the immune system will be not be discussed in any depth in this chapter, although aspects of it will be referred to.

The first means of defence against microorganisms that would cause harm to the body is called 'innate immunity' or 'non-specific immunity' and previous exposure to these organisms is not needed to provide protection against infection. In other words, this part of the immune system does not need to learn how to destroy or render inactive these organisms because the ability to know how to fight against them is inherent, and from birth most babies have these fundamental immunological capabilities. The three main mechanisms of innate immunity are (Fig. 30.2):

- barrier mechanisms
- cell-mediated mechanisms
- humoral mechanisms.

These non-specific resistance mechanisms are responsible for the major part (> 95%) of host defence, the 'host' being the human body; they will therefore be studied in detail in this chapter (Zinkernagel 2003).

Barrier mechanisms

Many of the essential components of the immune system develop very early in fetal life and most healthy newborn babies are prepared to deal with antigen challenges (Janeway et al 2004, Newell & McIntyre 2000). An antigen is any molecule that can stimulate an immune response, in particular a response that mobilises the adaptive immune system. The first lines of defence against infection are the external systems, which are commonly described as the barrier mechanisms. These are so called because they protect individuals by stopping harmful microorganisms from entering the body, and inhibit colonisation of the same.

Skin

The skin is the largest organ in the young baby and it provides an intact, dry surface that is resistant to the penetration of microorganisms. Not all microorganisms are harmful and the skin of children and adults is normally host to a number of bacteria, such as harmless diphtheriods, Gram-positive cocci and yeasts, which are called commensal microorganisms (Greenwood et al 2002). They are called 'commensal' because they have been 'permitted' to live on the skin and they provide some protection by taking up space and competing for nutrients that cannot then be used by more harmful disease-causing bacteria. They also produce by-products that inhibit the growth of other organisms (Greenwood et al 2002).

At birth, the skin is sterile because it has been contained within amniotic fluid. A biological advantage of an infant being nursed in close skin-to-skin contact with the mother immediately after birth is to encourage the rapid colonisation of the infants previously sterile skin, with the mothers harmless commensal bacteria and fungi (Inglis 2003).

Nurses must remember that they also carry commensal bacteria on their skin. In most instances the bacteria on their skin will remain harmless if transferred to children by contact. However, stringent infection control measures are paramount to reduce transfer of potentially harmful pathogens through skin contact (RCN 2009).

Activity

Review the following online course on infection prevention, in particular with relation to hand washing:

- http://www.engenderhealth.org/ip/

Also go through the publication 'The management and control of hospital acquired infections in acute NHS Trusts in England' (DoH 2003, DoH 2006):

- http://www.nao.org.uk/publications/nao_reports/9900230.pdf

Analyse the implications for your own practice.

The Health Protection Agency (2008) has identified that the very young are particularly vulnerable to hospital acquired infections (HAI) and that most infections were associated with hospital strains of MRSA (methicillin-resistant *Staphyloccoccus aureus*). Hand-washing has proven to be one of the most effective preventative measures against HAIs (Bissett 2003, NICE 2003, Parker 1999, Ward 2000).

Scenario

Khaleda has been admitted with infected atopic dermatitis and microbiology reports indicate that her skin is infected with MRSA:

- From your understanding of the barrier properties of innate immunity, identify why she is more prone to developing an infection in her skin.
- Discuss how you will manage her care. To inform your discussion these are topics you must address:
  - infection control procedures
  - risk factors for developing MRSA
  - the rationale behind presenting symptoms
  - treatment strategies
  - the evidence base for treatment.

Non-compliance with hand-washing policies is a well-known problem and Ng et al (2004) found that a technique of hand rub with alcohol preparations and the wearing of non-sterile gloves led to a considerable reduction in infection episodes. Although this procedure can be monitored more overtly than straightforward hand-washing, it cannot fully replace the need to adequately wash the hands before any procedure involving an infant and child.

Serious bacterial infections in infants are not solely attributable to hand-washing and the mode for infection spread can also include nasopharyngeal colonisation and through penetration of microorganisms into the blood (Brook 2003). These organisms can gain access to the blood through microscopic tears in the skin, such as those caused by intravenous access devices (Inglis 2003). Other organisms cited as responsible for early onset neonatal sepsis are the group B streptococcus, *Escherichia coli* and *Staphylococcus epidermidis*, all of which are both commensal and nosocomial organisms, and most of which can be eliminated by meticulous hand-washing (Ballot 2000, Nenstiel et al 1997).

The skin controls the numbers of commensal bacteria through various secretions such as sweat and sebum. There are two types of sweat gland, one of which – the eccrine glands – are functional at birth. Apocrine sweat glands, which are found mainly in the axillae, groin, face and scalp are stimulated by the sex hormones and therefore do not become fully functional until puberty (McCance & Huether 2005). Sweat contains mostly water, salts, traces of metabolic wastes and some immunoglobulin A (IgA). Immunoglobulins are produced by B lymphocytes, very specialised immune cells and part of the adaptive immune system, which are produced from the lymphoid lineage in the bone marrow (Parham 2005). In the newborn infant, IgA antibodies in sweat are quite limited, but fortunately the concentration of salt and a fairly acidic pH 4–6 is inhibitory or lethal to the survival of many microorganisms (Rennie & Roberton 1999, Whaley & Wong 1995).

The sebaceous glands, which also produce sebum, are stimulated by maternal androgens and become very active in the last trimester and early infancy. In utero, these produce vernix caseosa, a white, waxy substance that gives an additional layer of protection in terms of its antimicrobial and mechanical properties (Greenwood et al 2002, Marchini et al 2002). Following the birth of the baby, the mother is advised not to wipe away vernix caseosa because not only does it protect the skin against microorganism attack, it is one of nature's most efficient emollients. Many mothers worry about the white spots on their babies faces and they need to be assured that these are not acne but the final remnants of vernix in the skin pores.

The skin is also protected by mechanical means, which is the thickness of the skin and the hardness of keratinised cells, however the delicate neonate's skin lacks the hard extra layers of the skin of an older child. In the very low birthweight infant the stratum corneum is absent or deficient (Bautista et al 2000, Marchini et al 2002), therefore awareness of these infants' lack of the immunological barrier properties of the skin is crucial.

In fully developed skin, cells divide rapidly, the top layers constantly being renewed and dead cells sloughing away. An example of how proliferate the sloughing action is can be seen in the dust that relentlessly collects on furniture, most of which is dead skin cells. This sloughing action provides protection, because any harmful bacteria that are starting to colonise the skin will be sloughed away (Janeway et al 2004). Regular cleansing of an infant and child's skin not only facilitates the sloughing action but the massaging action stimulates the blood supply to the skin, which protects the skin immunologically and encourages growth of new cells.

Activity

Basic hygiene care

Prepare written guidelines for new parents on the hygiene needs and principles of care for their baby. Identify actions required in a step-by-step approach and provide a simple rationale for each action taken.

Activity

Reflecting on practice

Review the guidelines in caring for the skin of premature and low birthweight infants in Storm & Lund Jensen (1999):

1. Due to the immaturity of the skin of the preterm infant, it is particularly susceptible to damage.
2. Adhesives for attaching probes, etc., should be used as little as possible and should be removed with great care.
3. Bathing is not recommended for very low birthweight babies for at least 7 days after birth.

Are there variations in the way these recommendations have been implemented in your experience of neonatal care?

Box 30.1

Summary of protective properties of skin

- Intact skin resistant to microorganisms
- Presence of commensal organisms
- Skin secretions such as sweat and sebum
- Thickness of skin
- Sloughing off of old skin cells and rapid replacement of new skin cells
- Presence of immune cells within the dermis of skin
- Presence of immune proteins such as antibodies and complement

Cleansing is of particular importance in the nappy area, because the combination of microorganisms and urine together in a damp environment will encourage the growth of certain organisms, and in turn, their by-products will contribute to skin breakdown.

The final means of the skin providing protection is through Langerhans cells (immature dendritic cells) and macrophages, which are found in the dermis. These cells arise from the myeloid lineage of cells produced in the bone marrow (Parham 2005), all of the cells from this line providing innate protection. The role of dendritic cells, Langerhans cells and macrophages is to recognise, ingest and destroy antigens, presenting them later to T and B lymphocytes, for future recognition. Most of the cells from the myeloid lineage release lysozymes and cytokines from granules within their cytoplasm. Lysozymes are enzymes that damage and cause the death of bacteria by splitting the sugars found in their cell walls, thus destroying the bacterial cell wall. Cytokines will be discussed later but they are protein messengers that affect the behaviour of other cells (Parham 2005).

Like all soldiers, Langerhans cells need to be fully equipped for killing and to have the ability to recognise the enemy before they can attack. Mature Langerhans cells, which are ready for attack, can be found from the 5th month of gestation, but some of their action is limited until well after birth, owing to their lack of opportunity to have previously met and therefore recognised antigens in utero (Ballot 2000, Rennie & Roberton 1999). This final means of control is vital, especially when the top epidermal layer of the skin is broken by small cuts or erosions, and it is another reason why nurses must be aware that skin damage in a very young baby, even through a tiny venepuncture site, will render the infant more prone to attack, invasion from microorganisms and the development of infection (Janeway et al 2004).

A summary of the protective properties of skin is shown in Box 30.1.

Respiratory tract

Mucous lines the surface of many areas in the body, such as the respiratory tract. To some extent, these areas are more prone to infection than skin, because their moist and sticky surface provides a good breeding environment to bacteria (Janeway et al 2004). In the respiratory tract, microorganisms and unwanted dust particles that have been inhaled are trapped in the mucus, which is constantly being driven upwards, by the action of cilia, towards the pharynx. The mucus, with all its debris, is then either coughed out or swallowed. Cough and swallow reflexes have been demonstrated as early as 12 weeks' gestation (McIntosh et al 2003), and are therefore well developed in a full-term healthy neonate. These reflexes are both efficient means of expelling unwanted invaders to the body.

However, the ability of the entire respiratory tract to produce mucus is reduced in infancy (McIntosh et al 2003) and breach of this fine layer of mucus through a number of factors (Rona 2000, Schwartz 2004, von Mutius 2000) will cause a breach in the protective properties and render the infant very prone to colonisation by airborne microorganisms or antigens (Janeway et al 2004). Viruses in particular are very quick to take advantage of this reduced protection in the young baby, hence the relatively frequent occurrence of symptoms of 'snuffles', caused in response to viral attack.

The antibody immunoglobulin A (IgA) is secreted into the mucous linings. Two of the roles of IgA are to inhibit the adherence and proliferation of any antigens, such as bacteria, on epithelial surfaces. In the infant, IgA is one of the last immunoglobins to reach competent levels, therefore the neonate has relatively less protection against infection from those parts of the body where microorganisms can gain such easy entry, such as the respiratory tract (Newell & McIntyre 2000). However, IgA protection can be provided from the mother as discussed later.

It has been found that those children who have enhanced responsiveness to allergens (produce more immunoglobulins) in the neonatal period (Warner 2004) have been associated with a later risk of developing allergies such as asthma. These infants produce IgE instead of IgA. Subsequent exposure to the allergen that has resulted in the production of IgE, causes binding of the allergen to the IgE on the mast cell. This triggers the inflammatory response, which can vary in severity and, in some circumstances, produce life-threatening reactions such as severe asthma or anaphylaxis. Unfortunately, the damage caused by the allergic reaction is out of proportion to the threat posed by the allergen.

Eyes

The eyes are potentially an area where microorganisms can gain access into the body. Protection is provided by the conjunctiva, which is covered by a film of tears, and the constant blinking of the eyes flushes and cleanses the eye surface. Tears contain antibacterial products such as lysozyme but tear glands do not normally function until the child is 2–4 weeks old. Because of their narrow lumen, the tear glands are liable to blockage, which prevents the properties of tears from washing the eyes and renders the small baby prone to invasion by microorganisms that can cause conjunctivitis (Greenwood et al 2002, Kreir & Mortensen 1990). Parents should be shown how to clean their babies eyes by taking a damp piece of soft material from the area nearest the nose, the caruncle, and then across to the other side. This action helps to clear the tear ducts.

The gastrointestinal tract

The large surface area of the gastrointestinal tract is covered by a single layer of columnar epithelium and mucus, which allows for absorption of nutrients but also for entry of microbial pathogens (Garside & Mowat 1999). Within moments of birth, the gastrointestinal tract is challenged by myriads of bacterial and food antigens. There is evidence to suggest that even before birth the gastrointestinal tract is exposed to some antigen challenges as the fetus swallows amniotic fluid (Warner 2004). These swallowed antigens are met by antigen-presenting cells (APCs, e.g. macrophages and dendritic cells) in the fetus' gastrointestinal tract. For lymphocytes from the adaptive immune system to recognise antigens, they must first be presented by these antigen-presenting cells and the gastrointestinal tract is one of the only organs in the newborn infant with mature antigen-presenting cells.

The adaptive immune system, which allows for the formation of immune memory, is prominent at the mucosal site within the gastrointestinal tract. There are two subsets of memory T cells, natural and acquired. The natural memory T cells are self-specific, responding to self-antigens such as stressed and worn out epithelial cells. The acquired memory T cells gain their memory from antigens presented by antigen-presenting cells (Cheroutre & Madakamutil 2004). They then stimulate B cells to produce immunoglobulins specific to the antigens, such as IgA and IgG. In most cases, the presence of those immunoglobulins induces tolerance to those antigens within the gastrointestinal tract (Warner 2004) by neutralising the antigen and rendering it harmless. Unfortunately, there are instances when the antigen introduced to the gastrointestinal tract becomes immunogenic, meaning that it will cause a reaction including inflammation of the local tissues within the gastrointestinal tract. The result of this reaction is once again because of the production of IgE rather than IgA and IgG. Examples of this are those babies who develop intolerance to the proteins, carbohydrates or fats in manufactured baby milks, or the immune responses to gluten in patients with coeliac disease.

Seminar discussion topic

Read the article by Sicherer (2003). This article discusses a range of food allergies seen in infants and children:

- Discuss the common symptoms demonstrated by food allergies.
- Differentiate between what is an allergy and a hypersensitivity.

Many food intolerances do resolve in time but management of children's diets can be a problem for parents. Choose a couple of the more common disorders and identify what the problems might be and the advice you would give to parents regarding dietary management.

There is a huge network of immune tissue called gut-associated lymphoid tissue (GALT), which acts as a selective barrier to prevent the entry of these antigenic or infectious material into the body. The gastrointestinal tract is therefore considered the largest 'immune organ' in the body, with more than 70% of immune cells, both innate and adaptive, located there (Garside & Mowat 1999, Grönlund et al 2000).

Neonates have a limited amount of GALT but this develops rapidly over the first 2 years of life and certainly feeding is associated with the maturation of gut-associated lymphoid tissue (Flidel-Rimon et al 2004). Immunological protection is also provided by secretory IgA, which is quantitatively and functionally defective for a variable period after birth (Flidel-Rimon et al 2004). The number of IgA plasma cells (B lymphocytes) in the duodenal mucosa reaches that of adults by 2 years of age, whereas the level of mucosal secretory IgA antibodies reaches adult levels only at the age of 6–8 years (Grönlund et al 2000). Owing to the undeveloped mucosal immunological protection, there is higher vulnerability to infection and possibly more sensitisation to dietary antigens (MacDonald 1994, Warner 2004).

The saliva in the mouth has protective properties, which include IgA, lysozymes, mucopolysaccharides, which block some viruses, and glycolipids that compete with bacterial cell wall products for attachment to the mucous membranes (Greenwood et al 2002, Janeway et al 2004).

The newborn infant is unable to gain the full protective benefits of saliva because saliva production is limited in comparison to the amount produced later in life. However, this is compensated for as the different shape of the mouth and oral cavity facilitates efficient sucking and allows milk to be swallowed almost immediately. As milk does not stay in the mouth long, saliva is not needed for its protective action. Breastfeeding counteracts most of the immunological deficiencies because breast milk passively prevents infections getting into and crossing the intestinal barrier, and it also promotes the infant's immunity (Filteau 2000). For example the IgA concentrations found in breast milk are very high in the first few months of feeding (Weaver et al 1998). Other protective properties of breast milk include lysozyme and lactoferrin, which is an iron-binding protein that has a bactericidal effect on *E. coli*. Breast milk also contains macrophages and lymphocytes, which play a vital role in the immune response (Cushing et al 1998, Howie et al 1990, Oddy et al 2003, Wilson et al 1998, WHO 2002).

Early introduction of enteral feeding in preterm infants is recommended (Flidel-Rimon et al 2004, Okada et al 1998) owing to the reduced risk of nosocomial infection such as neonatal sepsis, maintenance of the intestinal barrier and development of competent mucosal immunity.

The production of saliva is only noticeably increased around 4 months. Around about this time, as the child starts weaning, the shape of the mouth changes, food is kept in it for longer periods and production of saliva is noticeably increased through the baby drooling (Weaver et al 1998). The salivary glands continue to increase in size while the child is undergoing the oral phase of development. In their attempts to understand the world better, children will put almost anything into their mouth to be sucked or chewed and the protection the saliva affords is very advantageous (Greenwood et al 2002).

Saliva can protect the mouth from many microorganisms but an organism that is particularly resistant to the effects of saliva is *Streptococcus mutans*, an organism that has been very closely linked to cause dental caries and has been found in the saliva of infants even as young as 1 year old (Radford et al 2000). Studies have suggested that mothers are the principal source of *S. mutans* to their infants (Li & Caufield 1995). Because of this, the practice of mothers sucking their infant's dummy (pacifier) to 'clean' it is not to be recommended! Saliva has the capabilities of easily protecting the infant from those organisms that would have attached to the dummy after rolling on the floor!

The pH of the stomach in older babies is between 1.5 and 3.5, which is not conducive to the survival of many microorganisms (McCance & Huether 2005). However, in the first week of life it has been found that the gastric pH is often higher than pH 4, and the acidity is not increased until the establishment of feeds at 2 week (Sonheimer et al 1985). Again, this is not a problem for breast-fed infants, but is a factor to be considered for those who are bottle fed.

The large intestine contains a substantial and diverse population of commensal bacteria that are important for health (Fingold et al 1983). These bacteria have a protective function in that they secrete bacteriocins, which are substances that inhibit the growth of other pathogens that cause disease, and they stimulate the maturation of the adaptive immune system and IgA-secreting cells (Grönlund et al 2000). It is very important that, soon after birth, bacteria that are beneficial rather than harmful to health colonise the colon. Beneficial genera include *Bifidobacterium* spp, *Bacteroides fragilis* and *Lactobacillus* spp. Breast milk contains 'bifidus factor', which promotes the growth of *Bifidobacterium*, which is a significant contribution that breast-feeding provides against gut infections. Only one feed of commercial milk can upset the very delicate balance of beneficial versus harmful bacteria in the first week of life (McKay & Perdue 1993).

As faeces move through the intestinal tract, the inner lining of the intestinal tract is cleared and any harmful pathogens, which may have adhered to the lining, are removed. As young infants have shorter colonic transit times, this clearance process occurs at faster rates. (Arhan et al 1981, Kreir & Mortensen 1990). A summary of the protective properties of the gastrointestinal tract is shown in Box 30.2.

Box 30.2

Summary of protective properties of gastrointestinal tract

- Presence of mucus
- Huge numbers of innate immune cells such as macrophages and dendritic cells
- Large quantities of IgA and IgG produced from B cells
- Gut-associated-lymphoid tissue (GALT)
- Saliva
- Protection from breast-feeding
- Hydrochloric acid in stomach
- Commensal bacteria
- Movement of faeces

Evidence-based practice

Evidence suggests that the most common enteric pathogens causing gastroenteritis are caused by self-limiting viral infections, notably rotavirus, adenovirus, adenovirus, astrovirus, Norwalk-like viruses and bacterial agents such as Salmonella and Campylobacter (McIver et al 2001).

Young children are vulnerable to dehydration owing to profuse diarrhoea and in most cases the treatment recommended is oral rehydration therapy to replace lost fluids, continuation of breast-feeding and early reintroduction of food when vomiting has stopped (Candy 1987).

Administration of the oral rehydration therapy via a nasogastric tube is a reliable and safe method of managing mild to moderate dehydration (Armon et al 2001, Callaghan et al 2003).

On recovery, recommended treatments include the introduction of live microbial food supplements (probiotics) such as foods containing Bifidobacteria and Lactobacteria to re-establish the intestine's natural defence barrier (Isolauri et al 2002).

Urogenital tract

The urinary tract is protected primarily against microorganisms by being flushed by sterile urine, and babies and toddlers who wear nappies certainly void more frequently than older children. Urinary stasis and bacterial virulence are risk factors for bacterial invasion, resulting in urinary tract infections. This problem is demonstrated in children with congenital, structural abnormalities that prevent complete emptying of urine from the genitourinary tract (Jakobsson et al 1999, Smellie et al 1998).

Cell-mediated mechanisms of innate immunity

If microbes succeed in breaching the external barrier defences, protecting the blood are a group of immune cells called monocytes, which eventually enter the tissues and become macrophages. From the same myeloid lineage there are also polymorphonuclear leucocytes (PMNs); the most numerous polymorphonuclear leucocyte is the neutrophil. Neutrophils, and a variety of antimicrobial substances found in the blood and body fluids, can be rapidly mobilised to enter any site of infection (Parham 2005).

From the lymphoid lineage comes a group of highly specialised innate cells called the natural killer (NK) cells. NK cells are very important in the defence against viral infections (Roitt et al 2006, Ward 2000). They are almost absent during fetal life and their numbers are seen to rise considerably 3 weeks after birth, reaching peak activity by 8 weeks of age, after which their activity slows down (Stiehm 1996).

Polymorphonuclear leucocytes have a variety of functions, one of which is phagocytosis – a feeding process whereby the phagocytic polymorphonuclear leucocytes engulf and digest particles recognised by them as foreign to the body. Many of these particles are antigens, which stick to the surface of the phagocyte and are then engulfed within the cell by a process in which parts (pseudopods) of the polymorphonuclear leucocyte surround the antigen. Once inside the polymorphonuclear leucocyte, the antigen is enclosed in a vacuole so that it

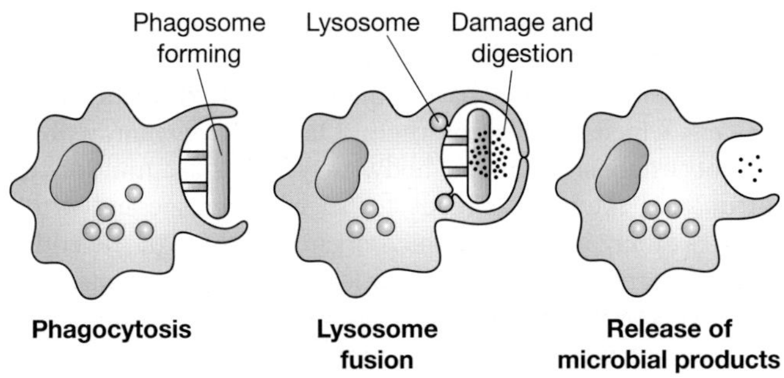

Fig. 30.3 • The action of polymorphonuclear lymphocytes.

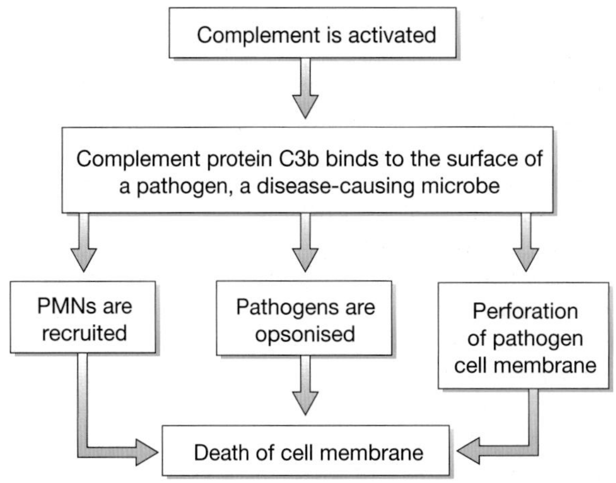

Fig. 30.4 • The role of complement.

cannot harm the cell, lysozyme then fuses with the vacuole and destroys the antigen (Fig. 30.3) (Roitt et al 2001).

Some microorganisms can be very 'slippery', making it difficult for phagocytic polymorphonuclear leucocytes to grab and keep hold of them. To overcome this problem, the polymorphonuclear leucocytes coat the microorganisms with antibodies (immunoglobulins) and with a group of proteins such as complement and C-reactive protein (CRP).

Phagocytosis in the neonate is often impaired because there is diminished attachment of the microorganism to the polymorphonuclear leucocytes (McIntosh et al 2003), and certain antigens on bacteria promote a thymus independent response which means that T helper cells do not stimulate B cells to produce antibodies. This in turn results in a reduced immunologic memory (Klouwenberg & Bont 2008). Also in the neonate, once engulfed by the polymorphonuclear leucocyte, killing of microorganisms can be depressed by the poor production of oxygen free radicals, which are essential in the destruction process. These functions are further depressed when the infant is stressed and otherwise compromised physiologically (McIntosh et al 2003).

Innate humoral defence mechanisms

A number of antimicrobial proteins are present in the tissue and body fluids. These are collectively known as humoral defence mechanisms, which are used predominantly to prevent attachment by microbes to cell and tissue surfaces. 'Complement' is a generic term encompassing a very complex group of about 20 serum proteins that have the ability to lyse (break down) red blood cells, and destroy Gram-negative bacteria. Complement proteins interact with each other, and with antibodies, together greatly assisting in the war against harmful microorganisms by inducing opsonisation (i.e. preparing the microorganisms to be 'eaten') and therefore aiding phagocytosis (Janeway et al 2004, Kreir & Mortensen 1990, Roitt et al 2006) (Fig. 30.4).

There are decreased complement levels in the neonate, however, the complement system matures more rapidly than any other innate immune systems, and, within weeks of birth, complement levels in a baby are comparable to adult levels (McIntosh et al 2003).

Other humoral factors include antibodies (immunoglobulins) from B lymphocytes and plasma cells. Antibodies produce precipitation, agglutination and neutralisation of many antigens, including bacteria and viruses, and they also enhance phagocytosis considerably (Roitt et al 2006). Immunoglobulin M (IgM) and IgG protect against antigens in blood and the lymphatic system, and IgA protects mucosal membranes, as already discussed. During gestation and after birth, the developing fetus and infant are relatively immunoincompetent and very dependent on maternal antibodies transferred transplacentally (IgG) and through breast milk (IgG and IgA). These maternal antibodies attenuate systematic infections when the infant's own antibodies are slowly being produced and eventually providing effective protection on their own by 3–6 months of age (Zinkernagel 2003).

Many tissues synthesise proteins that can be referred to as basic polypeptides, which help to destroy microorganisms by inhibiting cellular respiration, inhibiting the synthesis of DNA and RNA and increasing the permeability of bacterial cell membranes. The liver also produces CRP, which stimulates the complement cascade, enhances the release of cytokines, and activates phagocytic cells that bind to and disrupt the cell wall of certain microorganisms (Cermak et al 1993). CRP is synthesised within 6–8 hours of exposure to a pathogen and it can increase 1000-fold during the inflammatory response, hence it is a very useful diagnostic marker (from a blood sample) for the presence of infection. Unfortunately, the delay in the synthesis of CRP can mean the early detection of an infection using this CRP marker can be a problem (Da Silva et al 1995, Ng et al 1997).

Cytokines

Cytokines are glycoproteins that are rapidly synthesised by many immune cells, in response to any antigen. Cytokines are 'cellular messengers'. They have different names depending on where they originate. They not only have an effect on the cells of the immune system, they also generate a response with many other physiological systems. Each cytokine that has been identified has its own function(s). Collectively, their functions include the stimulus and activation of cells of the immune system. An example is interleukin-1, a cytokine known for its fever-producing properties and also its ability to stimulate white cell production in the bone marrow (Ballot 2000).

Cytokines are partially responsible for many of the symptoms that are recognised as a deviation from health

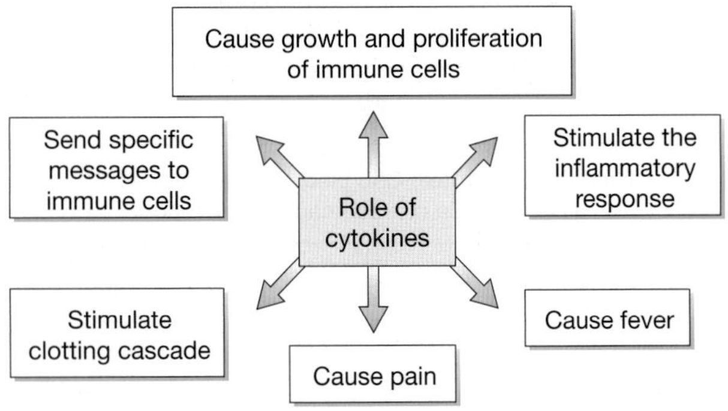

Fig. 30.5 • The role of cytokines.

(Duramad et al 2007) and their role is very important in the next stage of immune protection, the inflammatory response (Fig. 30.5).

Activity

Neonatal sepsis

The main bacterial causes for infections in children under 1 month are group B streptococcus, *Escherichia coli, Listeria monocytogenes, Streptococcus pneumoniae, Haemophilus influenzae, Staphylococcus aureus, Staphylococcus epidermidis, Neisseria meningitidis* and Salmonella spp (Brook 2003). Signs and symptoms of infection in the very young infant include (McIntosh et al 2003):

- lethargy
- poor feeding, vomiting, abdominal distension
- apnoea and respiratory distress
- pallor
- temperature instability
- seizures
- prolonged capillary refill time
- mottling of skin.

1. What procedures would you undertake to detect the source of infection?
2. What other factors (other than barrier functions) would predispose a newborn to infection.

Having identified many of the factors in innate immunity, this section has shown the diverse ways that foreign substances are dealt with so efficiently. If bacteria or viruses manage to avoid all the barriers and innate mechanisms of protection, the body is still able and ready to fight against the invading organisms by bringing into play another very sophisticated means of protecting itself, ensuring that infants and children do not succumb to every infection.

Phase 2. The inflammatory response: the response after microbial attack

In the first part of the chapter, various strategies used by the body to prevent infection occurring were discussed. In the above activity, you would have described symptoms that are caused by the inflammatory response.

Over the years, certain microorganisms have evolved very clever strategies to avoid the body's attempts to prevent their entrance and, once they have gained entrance, they then resist the cells which can destroy them. Once microorganisms have become established in the body, they will start multiplying. Fortunately, the body is ready for such subterfuge and within minutes of any invasion by microorganisms through the body's defence barriers, a highly sophisticated series of events takes place. This protective, healing response involves inflammation, and it is put into motion by a number of immune cells such as dendritic cells, macrophages, neutrophils, T and B lymphocytes and mast cells, through the cytokines that they release.

The classic signs of this stage – the inflammatory response – are heat, swelling, redness, pain and loss of function (McCance & Huether 2005). To briefly summarise, this response is as follows. After microorganisms have gained entrance into tissues, heat in the area is caused by localised vasodilatation, which is an opening up of arteries or capillaries that allows increased amounts of blood to flow into the area. In the innate response it was identified that blood contains many components that are vital to the war against microorganisms. Heat is also caused by the increased amount of cellular and metabolic activity in the area. The local blood capillaries become permeable, which means leakier than normal, allowing plasma proteins, phagocytic cells and leucocytes to exude out from the blood into the extracellular spaces where the microbes have become established. The end result of the extra flow of blood and blood products to the area causes swelling and redness to tissues.

During the inflammatory response the pain is caused by pressure on the nerve endings in the swollen tissue and the effects of prostaglandins released from locally damaged cells.

The whole of the inflammatory response however is far more complex, and this detail will be discussed in the context of an infection, under the following headings (Kreir & Mortensen 1990):

- Microorganisms that are successful in breaking the defence barriers
- The changes in blood circulation in the inflamed area
- The effects of inflammatory mediators
- The effect of inflammation on the whole body: the febrile response.

Microorganisms that are successful in breaking the defence barriers

Many microorganisms, such as bacteria, have evolved mechanisms aimed at avoiding some of the innate defences of the human body and some pathogens even have genes devoted to this purpose (Parham 2005). The whole immune response to any pathogen involves complex molecular and cellular reactions whereby immune cells recognise the bacteria through the proteins, some of which are antigens, on the bacterial cell wall. Many of these antigens are complex carbohydrate and protein structures. If the structure of these antigens becomes slightly changed through evolution, the body's immune system will not recognise the antigen as quickly as it previously did and action taken against the bacteria is delayed. Another common method of pathogenic bacteria avoiding is the synthesis of an outer capsule, which is very hard for phagocytic cells to attach to (Roitt et al 2006). An example of the effects of evolution on *Staphyloccocus aureus* is the development of methicillin-resistant *S. aureus* (MRSA).

Viruses are good examples of the ability to genetically mutate. The common cold and influenza virus passed from person to person through coughs and sneezes is destroyed by antibodies that bind to its outer envelop. It takes 1–2 weeks for the immune system to produce these antibodies and, once produced, the virus is soon cleared and symptoms subside. However, in the meantime the virus might have spread to a large number of individuals. Over a period of time new viral strains are produced that have slightly different molecules on the viral envelope. These are therefore not immediately recognised by the immune system and there are not specific antibodies within the system against these new strains. Therefore, if these new strains manage to evade defence systems, once again an individual will have cold and influenza symptoms (Parham 2005).

Having avoided phagocytosis, once in the tissues, microorganisms will rapidly reproduce and increase their numbers. Despite the genetic mutations to avoid detection, once in the tissues these agents will soon be met by dendritic cells and macrophages. Molecules on the outer surface of microorganisms are characteristic of pathogens but absent from human cells. Examples of these are lipopolysaccharide (LPS), peptidoglycan, lipoteichoic acid and flagellin (Bochud & Calandra 2003). Complement binds with these molecules, allowing opsonisation and phagocytosis. Macrophages also have sensors (Toll-like receptors, TLR) on their surface for pathogenic components and, when macrophages come into contact with these components, they secrete cytokines (Bochud & Calandra 2003, Parham 2005). The cytokines then recruit other immune cells, in particular neutrophils into the infected area, initiating and continuing the inflammatory response until all the microorganisms have been destroyed.

The degree of inflammation is usually associated with the success with which the organism has established itself; the greater the numbers of bacteria or virus, the greater the inflammation. Until the inflammatory response has been fully initiated, there will be very few symptoms to affect and warn the child of the presence of the bacteria.

Changes in blood circulation in the inflamed area caused by cytokines

Cytokines produced by activated macrophages include interleukins (IL) such as IL-1, IL-6, IL-8 (also known as CXCL8), IL-12 and tumour necrosis factor alpha (TNF-α) (Fig. 30.6). Other molecules are released by macrophages and mast cells include histamine, bradykinin, prostaglandins, oxygen radicals, nitric oxide, leukotrienes and platelet activating factor (PAF). Collectively, these substances are called inflammatory mediators because they all contribute to tissue damage and inflammation.

On their release, these substances cause the local blood capillaries to relax, dilate and become permeable 'leaky'. This increases the blood flow to the area, resulting in redness and plasma and immune proteins leaking from the vessels causes swelling of the tissues. The neutrophils can leave the circulation by adhering to blood vessel walls and then squeezing through the walls by a process called diapedesis. The process of attraction is called chemotaxis (Janeway et al 1999).

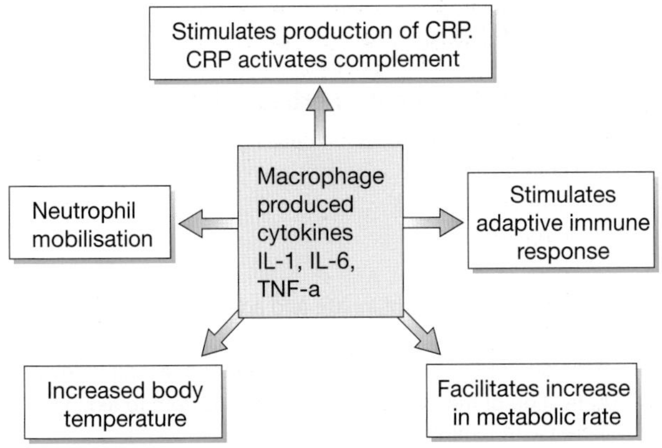

Fig. 30.6 • The role of cytokines released from macrophages.

Once at the site of infection and inflammation, neutrophils and tissue macrophages work very quickly to fight against the microbes through phagocytosis. The site of inflammation becomes a real battleground, where cells from both sides of the conflict die. The accumulation of white blood cells, dead tissue cells, fluids leaked from the circulation and microbes, all contribute to 'pus'.

Typical examples of the inflammatory response can be seen in the inflamed skin in dermatitis and in tonsillitis. If the tonsils were examined they would look more red and swollen than normal with spots of pus. The child with tonsillitis may have a difficulty in swallowing owing to increased pain. Eventually the body will get rid of the pus via the lymphatic system or by using tissue macrophages to remove it.

Tonsillitis is an example of 'local' inflammatory responses and in most instances the effects of cytokines are contained within tissues. However, if the infection is more widespread in the body (systemic) and is bacterial, the effects of the inflammatory response are seen throughout the body. Inflammatory reactions vary slightly dependent on the type of bacteria, whether they are Gram positive or Gram negative, but it has been clearly demonstrated that if TNF-α is released into the circulation, the effect of vascular dilatation and permeability can lead to severe shock (Dellinger et al 2008).

As the cytokines are produced at the start of the inflammatory response, their presence in blood samples can be indicative of an infection. Even though preterm and term infants have immature inflammatory responses, it has been demonstrated that they display a higher percentage of IL-6 and IL-8 (Ng 2004) and high plasma levels of IL-6, IL-10 and TNF-α often signify severe infection. IL-6 is an important cytokine because it coordinates the body's response to infection. For example, with IL-1, IL-6 is responsible for resetting the hypothalamic thermostat to raise body temperature. It also stimulates the liver to produce CRP and it mobilises neutrophils to enhance their phagocytic activity. Recently, IL-6 has been used as a marker with a sensitivity of up to 89% in detecting infection early in neonates (Ng 2004). Unfortunately, soon after the initial inflammatory response and if a child receives antibiotic

Box 30.3

Summary of protective properties of inflammation

- Changes in blood circulation causing:
  - heat
  - swelling
  - redness
  - pain
- Further mobilisation of innate and adaptive defence mechanisms
- Resetting of the thermoregulatory centre resulting in fever
- Activation of the sympathetic nervous system to aid in the increase in temperature
- Symptoms associated with sympathetic nervous system activation: nausea and vomiting
- Lethargy and malaise to promote rest

therapy, IL-6 levels fall and become almost undetectable after 24 hours (Ng 2004).

A summary of the protective properties of inflammation is shown in Box 30.3.

The effects of other inflammatory mediators

Histamine and serotonin are some of the cytokines released from granules within damaged mast cells. Other substances are manufactured from arachidonic acid, a molecule found within the cell walls of mast and local tissue cells. These substances are prostaglandins and leukotrienes. They are responsible for the pain that comes with inflammation. They cause pain by further increasing the vascular permeability, therefore increasing the swelling, which produces pressure on the nerve endings. Prostaglandins also intensify pain by sensitising nerve receptors.

Bacteria that enter into tissues will damage the lining of blood vessels exposing collagen. On contact with collagen, a plasma protein, factor XII (the Hageman factor), is activated and initiates the clotting cascade: platelets start adhering to each other, forming tiny clots within the local vessels and in the blood products at the site of inflammation. At the same time, the damaged endothelial cells release platelet-activating factor, a cytokine that encourages platelet aggregation. Clots help to immobilise microorganisms and prevent them entering the blood and lymph tissues, as well as preventing significant blood loss from the blood capillaries, which have been made permeable. During the clotting process, platelets release prostaglandins, which further promote inflammation and the start of tissue healing (Parham 2005).

The effect of inflammation on the whole body: the febrile response

Inflammation in any localised tissue can, and often does, result in a response by the whole body, such as fever, tiredness and general malaise.

Fever, as mentioned, results following the release of IL-1, IL-6 and TNF-α, endogenous pyrogens (fever-producing substances) released by macrophages and, through the release of prostaglandins, produced by tissue cells and neutrophils. These fever-producing substances have a direct action on the hypothalamus, causing the hypothalamus to reset the thermoregulatory set point, so instead of the normal body temperature of 36.0–37.2°C, the new set point will be at a higher rate. The new set point is determined by the number of endogenous pyrogens in the circulation, the more pyrogens, the higher the set point and the resulting body temperature (Klugger 1995).

To facilitate the rise in temperature, the hypothalamus stimulates the sympathetic nervous system, causing vasoconstriction, whereby the arteries in the body's peripheries become narrowed. This helps to conserve any body heat that might be lost through radiation from the skin surfaces. The sympathetic nervous system raises the metabolic rate and glycogen stores are mobilised to provide extra fuel for the energy and heat produced from increased metabolism. Oxygen demands are increased because it is also a fuel needed by cellular metabolism, therefore the child's respiratory rate will increase; the heart rate will also increase to deliver the oxygenated blood to the cells and remove the by-products of metabolism.

The additional heat created by the enhanced metabolic rate is retained by the body, causing an increase in body temperature.

While the body temperature is rising, the child will look pale and will often feel anorexic and tired, both effects of the sympathetic nervous system. The observant mother or a nurse would notice an increase in respiratory and pulse rate. The child's trunk might feel warmer than normal, but the peripheries will feel cool. The child might be shivering, an attempt of the body to create more heat through muscular activity. At this point the kindest treatment would be to tuck the child up in bed to let him or her sleep and allow the body to wage war against the bacteria. Once the raised hypothalamic temperature point has been reached, the body will commence its cooling-down process. Only in extremely rare conditions (associated with altered fluid and electrolyte balance) does the body temperature keep rising relentlessly. In most instances, once the raised hypothalamic set point has been reached the body will start cooling itself and the child will kick off the covers.

Fever is thought to have many beneficial effects for the host because it accelerates many of the innate and acquired or specific immune reactions. Fever causes a reduction of the iron and zinc levels in the blood, both of which are needed for bacterial growth. Fever increases the movement of neutrophils and lymphocytes into the war zone and, on its own, fever can kill or dramatically reduce the ability of bacteria to function and reproduce. Many bacteria cease to function at temperatures of 38°C and above. However, the negative aspects of fever are discomfort of the child and potential dehydration. Dehydration in the case of tonsillitis would result from the child not drinking, owing to the discomfort in the throat, and increased loss of insensible fluids as the temperature rises, and possibly vomiting.

When caring for a child all these factors must be considered, and it must be remembered that fever is a very important diagnostic sign and need therefore not be actively reduced (NICE 2007). It is generally considered that the benefits of fever far outweigh the disadvantages. If the child is well hydrated, antipyretics need not be given. However, if the resulting inflammatory response has caused many symptoms of malaise and the child is in a lot of discomfort, it is better to consider the administration of these medications for their analgesic rather than their antipyretic properties.

The NICE (2007) guidelines identify a traffic light warning symptom giving guidelines on managing children's fever. Children who are very unwell, unrousable, with very poor colour and evidence of any respiratory distress need to be seen by medical practitioners urgently as these symptoms often indicate that the child has contracted an overwhelming infection and the inflammatory response is significant and in part contributes to the child's deteriorating health. However, that is an entirely different subject involving the inflammatory and the adaptive immune response.

Summary

Having identified the events of the inflammatory process, it is easy to liken it to the body being at war against an unwelcome and unwanted invasion of enemies. If the body fails to meet the challenge, bacterial invasion would soon overwhelm the body and the prognosis of recovery would be poor. The fact that so many children survive infections is credit to their very efficient immune systems. The reaction of the body to the enemy results in some unpleasant side effects, such as fever, but they usually serve the important purpose to cause the individual to rest to allow the immune army and other body systems, such as the sympathetic nervous system, to win the battle.

References

Arhan, P., Devroede, G., Jehannin, B., et al., 1981. Segmental colonic transit time. Diseases of the Colon and Rectum 24 (8), 625–629.

Armon, K., Stephenson, T., MacFaul, R., et al., 2001. An evidence and consensus based guideline for acute diarrhea management. Archives of Diseases in Childhood 85, 132–145.

Ballot, D.E., Sepsis Neonatal, Newell, M.L., McIntyre, J., 2000. Congenital and perinatal infections. Cambridge University Press, Cambridge pp 321-336.

Bautista, M.I.B., Randall Wickett, R., Visscher, M.O., et al., 2000. Characterisation of vernix caseosa as a natural biofilm: comparison to standard oil based treatments. Pediatric Dermatology 17 (4), 253–260.

Bissett, L., 2003. Interpretation of terms used to describe handwashing activities. British Journal of Nursing 12 (9), 536–542.

Bochud, PY., Calandra, T., 2003. Pathogenesis of sepsis: new concepts and implications for future treatment. British Medical Journal 326, 262–266.

Brook, I., 2003. Unexplained fever in young children: how to manage severe bacterial infection. British Medical Journal 327, 1094–1097.

Callaghan, S., Hughan, J., Johnson, L., 2003. The use of a nasogastric tube for rehydration therapy in the dehydrated paediatric patient with gastroenteritis: a clinical audit of adverse events associated with its use. Neonatal and Paediatric Child Health Nursing 6 (1), 13–17.

Candy, C.E., 1987. Recent advances in the care of children with acute diarrhea: giving responsibility to the nurse and parents. Journal of Advanced Nursing 12 (1), 95–99.

Cermak, J., Key, N.S., Bach, R.R., et al., 1993. C-reactive protein induces human peripheral blood monocytes to synthesis tissue factor. Blood 82, 512–520.

Cheroutre, H., Madakamutil, L., 2004. Acquired and natural memory T cells join forces at the mucosal front line. Nature Reviews. Immunology 4 (4), 290–300.

Clader, P.C., Kew, S., 2002. The immune system: a target for functional foods? British Journal of Nutrition 88 (Suppl 2), S165–S177.

Cushing, A.H., Samet, J.M., Lambert, W.E., et al., 1998. Breastfeeding reduces risk of respiratory illness in infants. American Journal of Epidemiology 147, 863–870.

Da Silva, O., Ohlsson, A., Kenyan, C., 1995. Accuracy of leukocyte indices and C-reactive protein for diagnosis of neonatal sepsis: a critical review. Pediatric and Infectious Diseases 14, 362–366.

Dellinger, P.R., Levy, M.M., Carlet, J., et al., 2008. Surviving sepsis campaign: international guidelines for management of severe sepsis and septic shock. Intensive Care Medicine 34 (1), 17–60.

Department of Health (DoH), 2003. Winning ways, working together to reduce healthcare associated infection in England. Central Office of Information, London.

Department of Health (DoH), 2006. Essential steps to safe, clean care. Central Office of Information, London.

Department of Health (DoH), 2008. The Health and Social Care Act, 2008. Code of practice for the NHS on the prevention and control of healthcare associated infections and related guidance. Central Office of Information, London.

Duramad, P., Tager, I.B., Holland, N.T., 2007. Cytokines and other immunological biomarkers in children's environmental health studies. Toxicology letters 172, 1–2 48-59.

Fingold, S.M., Sutter, V.L., Mattisen, G.E., 1983. Normal indigenous intestinal flora. In: Hentges, D.J. (Ed.), Human intestinal microflora in health and disease. Academic Press, New York.

Filteau, S.M., 2000. Symposium on nutrition and immunity. Role of breast-feeding in managing malnutrition and infectious disease. Proceedings of the Nutrition Society 59 (4), 565–572.

Flidel-Rimon, O., Friedman, S., Lev, E., 2004. Early enteral feeding and nosocomial sepsis in very low birthweight infants. Archives of Diseases in Childhood. Fetal and Neonatal edition 89, F289.

Garside, P., Mowat, A.M., 1999. Oral tolerance in disease. Gut 44, 137–142.

Greenwood, D., Slack, R.C.B., Peutherer, J.F., 2002. Medical microbiology: a guide to microbial infections, 16th edn. Churchill Livingstone, Edinburgh.

Grönlund, MM., Arvilommi, H., Kero, P., 2000. Importance of intestinal colonization in the maturation of humoral immunity in early infancy: a prospective follow up study of healthy infants aged 0-6 months. Archives of Diseases in Childhood. Fetal and Neonatal Edition 83, F186–F192.

Health Protection Agency 2008, 2008. Surveillance of healthcare associated infections report. Health Protection Agency, London.

Howie, P.W., Forsyth, J.S., Ogston, S.A., et al., 1990. Protective effect of breast feeding against infection. British Medical Journal 300, 11–16.

Inglis, T.J.J., 2003. Congenital and neonatal infections. In: Inglis, T.J.J. (Ed.), Microbiology and infection: a clinical core text for integrated curricula with self assessment, 2nd edn. Churchill Livingstone, Edinburgh, pp. 159–169.

Isaacs, D., Fraser, S., Hogg, G., 2004. *Staphylococcus aureus* infections in Australasian neonatal nurseries. Archives of Diseases in Childhood. Fetal and Neonatal Edition 89, F331.

Isolauri E, Kirjavainen P.V., Salminen S., 2002. Probiotoics: a role in the treatment of intestinal infection and inflammation? Gut 50:iii54–iii59.

Jakobsson, B., Jacobson, S.H., Hjalmas, K., 1999. Vesico-ureteric reflux and other risk factors for renal damage: identification of high and low-risk children. Acta Paediatrica 431 (Suppl), 31–39.

Janeway, C.A., Travers, P., Walport, M., Capra, J.D., 2004. Immunobiology: the immune system in health and disease, 6th edn. Churchill Livingstone, London.

Klouwenburg, P.K., Bont, L., 2008. Neonatal and infantile immune responses to encapsulated bacteria and conjugate vaccines. Clinical and Developmental Immunology. Published online September 23, 2008.

Klugger, M.J., 1995. The mechanism of fever. In: David, T.J. (Ed.), Recent advances in paediatrics. Longman, Harlow p 13.

Kreir, J.P., Mortensen, R.F., 1990. Infection, resistance and immunity. Harper and Row, New York.

Li, Y., Caufield, P.W., 1995. The fidelity of initial acquisition of mutans streptococci by infants from their mothers. Journal of Dental Research 74 (2), 681–685.

MacDonald, T.T., 1994. Development of mucosal immune function in man: potential for GI disease states. Acta Paediatrica Japan 36, 532–536.

Marchini, G., Lindow, S., Brismar, H., et al., 2002. The newborn infant is protected by an innate antimicrobial barrier: peptide antibiotics are contained in the skin and vernix caseosa. British Journal of Dermatology 147, 1127–1134.

McCance, K.L., Huether, S.E., 2005. (eds) Pathophysiology: the biological basis for disease in adults and children, 5th edn. Mosby, St Louis.

McIntosh, N., Helms, P.J., Smyth, R.L., 2003. Forfar and Arneil's textbook of pediatrics, 6th edn. Churchill Livingstone, Edinburgh.

McIver, C.J., Hansman, G., White, P., et al., 2001. Diagnosis of enteric pathogens in children with gastroenteritis. Pathology 33, 353–358.

McKay, D.M., Perdue, M.H., 1993. Intestinal epithelial function: the case for immunophysiological regulation. Digestive Diseases and Sciences 38 (8), 1377–1387.

National Institute for Health and Clinical Excellence with National Collaborating Centre for Women and Children's Health, 2007. Fever illness in children assessment and initial management in children under 5 years. NICE & RCOG Press, London.

National Institute for Health Clinical Excellence, 2003. Infection control: prevention of infection in primary and community care CG2. NICE, London.

Nenstiel, R.O., White, G.L., Aikens, T., 1997. Handwashing a century of evidence ignored. Clinical Reviews 7 (55-58), 61–62.

Newell, M.L., McIntyre, J., 2000. Congenital and perinatal infections. Cambridge University Press, Cambridge.

Ng, P.C., 2004. Diagnostic markers of infection in neonates. Archives of Diseases in Childhood. Fetal and Neonatal Edition 89, F229–F244.

Ng, P.C., Cheng, S.H., Chui, K.M., et al., 1997. Diagnosis of late onset neonatal sepsis with cytokines, adhesion molecules, and C-reactive protein in preterm, very low birth weight infants. Archives of Diseases in Childhood. Fetal and Neonatal Edition, F221–F227.

Ng, P.C., Wong, H.L., Lyon, D.J., et al., 2004. Combined use of alcohol rub and gloves reduces the incidence of late onset infection in very low birthweight infants. Archives of Diseases in Childhood. Fetal and Neonatal Edition 89, F336.

Oddy, W.H., Sly, P.D., de Klerk, N.H., et al., 2003. Breast feeding and respiratory morbidity in infancy: a birth cohort study. Archives of Diseases in Childhood 88, 224–228.

Okada, Y., Klein, N., van Saene, H.K., et al., 1998. Small volumes of enteral feedings normalise immune function in infants receiving parenteral nutrition. Journal of Pediatric Surgery 33, 16–19.

Parham, P., 2005. The immune system, 2nd edn. Garland Science, Abingdon.

Parker, L.J., 1999. Importance of hand washing in the prevention of infection. British Journal of Nursing 8 (11), 716–720.

Radford, J.R., Ballantyne, H.M., Nugent, Z., et al., 2000. Caries associated microorganisms in infants from different socio-economic backgrounds in Scotland. Journal of Dentistry 28 (5), 307–312.

Rennie, J.M., Roberton, N.R.C., (Eds.), 1999. Textbook of neonatology, 3rd edn. Churchill Livingstone, Edinburgh

Roitt, I.M., Brostoff, J., Male, D.K., Roth, D.B., 2006. Immunology, 7th edn. Mosby Books, Edinburgh.

Royal College of Nursing (RCN), 2009. Infection prevention and control: minimum standards. RCN, London. Online. Available at http://www.rcn.org.uk/downloads/publications/public-pub/002725.pdf

Rona, R.J., 2000. Asthma and poverty. Thorax 55, 239–244.

Schwartz, J., 2004. Air pollution and children's health. Pediatrics 113 (4), 1037–1043.

Sicherer, S.H., 2003. Clinical aspects of gastrointestinal food allergy in childhood. Pediatrics 111 (6), 1609–1616.

Smellie, J.M., Prescod, N.P., Shaw, P.J., et al., 1998. Childhood reflux and urinary infection: a follow up of 10–41 years in 226 adults. Pediatric Nephrology 12, 727–736.

Sonheimer, J.M., Clark, D.A., Gervaise, E.P., 1985. Continuous gastric pH measurement in young and older healthy preterm infants receiving formula and clear liquid feeds. Journal of Pediatric Gastroenterology and Nutrition 4 (3), 352–355.

Stiehm, R.E., 1996. Immunologic disorders in infants and children, 4th edn. Harcourt Brace, New York.

Storm, K., Lund Jensen, T., 1999. Skin care of preterm infants: strategies to minimise potential damage. Journal of Neonatal Nursing 5 (2), 13–15.

von Mutius, E., 2000. The burden of childhood asthma. Archives of Diseases in Childhood 82 (Suppl II), ii2–ii5.

Ward, D., 2000. Hand washing facilities in the clinical area: a literature review. British Journal of Nursing 9 (2), 82–86.

Warner, J.O., 2004. The early life origins of asthma and related allergic disorders. Archives of Diseases in Childhood 89, 97–102.

Weaver, L.T., Arthur, H.M.L., Bunn, J.E.G., et al., 1998. Human milk IgA concentrations during first year of lactation. Archives of Diseases in Childhood 78, 235–239.

Whaley, L.F., Wong, D.L., 1995. Whaley and Wong's nursing care of infants and children, 5th edn. Mosby, St Louis.

Wilson, A.C., Stewart Forsyth, J., Greene, S.A., et al., 1998. Relation of infant diet to childhood health: seven year follow up of cohort of children in Dundee infant feeding study. British Medical Journal 316, 21–25.

World Health Organization, 2002. Infant and young child nutrition: global strategy on infant and young child feeding. 55th World Health Assembly, Geneva A55/15.

World Health Organization, 2003. Child and adolescent health development; overview. Online. Available at: http://www.who.int/child-adolescent-health

World Health Organization, 2008. Global Burden of Disease: The 10 leading causes of death by broad income group (2004), Fact sheet No 310 Online. Available at: http://www.who.int/mediacentre/factsheets/fs310/en/index.html

Zinkernagel, R.M., 2003. On natural and artificial vaccinations. Annual Review of Immunology 21 (1), 515–542.

Caring for children and adolescents with malignant disease

31

Beth Sepion

ABSTRACT

Cancer is a group of malignant diseases that are rare in childhood and adolescence. The aim of this chapter is to give an overview of the care of children/adolescents with a malignant disease. It will begin with a brief explanation of what cancer is and an overview of shared care. The main focus will be on the challenges, physical and psychological, facing children's nurses when caring for a child/adolescent and his or her family as they undergo treatment. The majority of children/adolescents with cancer experience care over a period of months or years, in regional centres, district general hospitals and the community. Few nurses, therefore, will experience caring for a child and their family from the time of diagnosis to the completion of treatment. The concept of the illness trajectory, identified by Corbin & Strauss (1991), has been used to offer an insight into the journey, physical and emotional, that these families travel and the variety of healthcare professionals they will encounter during their individual journeys. The companion PowerPoint presentation provides the background information about the common treatment modalities, side effects and management strategies.

LEARNING OUTCOMES

- Identify common childhood malignancies.
- Describe the different treatment modalities and common associated side effects.
- Discuss the impact of a cancer diagnosis on the patient and different members of the family.
- Discuss the role of the nurse caring for the child with a malignancy and his or her family throughout the illness trajectory.
- Identify the skills required to work with children/adolescents with cancer and their families.
- Discuss the strategies that different families develop to cope with cancer and its treatment throughout the illness trajectory.
- Discuss interdisciplinary and transdisciplinary care for the child with cancer and the family.

Introduction

Childhood malignancies are considered to be a chronic illness and, although rare, nurses may care for these children/adolescents in a variety of healthcare settings. It is important, therefore, to have an understanding of the disease, its treatment and the impact this can have for the children/adolescents and their family as they undergo intensive and complex treatment regimens. The NICE Guidance on Cancer Services 'Improving Outcomes in Children and Young People with Cancer' (2005) identified key recommendations concerning the delivery of care for this group of patients. Implementation of these recommendations is currently being carried out and evaluated.

Malignancy/cancer/tumour

The terms cancer, tumour and malignancy are often used synonymously. Cancer is a name given to a group of diseases that share common characteristics of uncontrolled cell growth following a genetic mutation. In childhood, in particular, there is invasion to local tissue with spread to distant sites via the lymphatic and blood system. The names of the specific cancers signify the tissue of origin, e.g. nephroblastoma, a malignant tumour of the kidney.

A tumour is a swelling; it can be benign or malignant. Benign refers to a swelling that does not invade its surrounding tissue, it causes damage by local pressure and/or obstruction.

Activity

- What is the more common name for a tumour of the kidney? What is the common age of children presenting with this condition, why is this?

DOI: 10.1016/B978-0-7020-3183-0.10031-1

Malignant tumours are invasive, they cause damage by invading surrounding tissue and they have the ability to establish new tumours at distant sites (metastases). Cancer (from the Greek work karkinos, meaning crab) was described by Hippocrates as growths that invaded other tissues.

Malignancies in childhood are rare. There are approximately only 1470 new cases each year in the UK (2004 data available at: http://www.statistics.gov.uk). However, despite the dramatic improvement in the cure rate over the past 25 years (60–70%), cancer remains one of the most feared diagnoses (Parry 2003). The improvement in success rate is due to a greater understanding of the nature of childhood malignancies, including refined diagnostic and prognostic investigations, knowledge of treatment modalities, supportive care and the establishment of regional centres where participation in multicentre trials is acknowledged as being essential (Children's Cancer and Leukaemia Group (CCLG) 2007).

PowerPoint

Access the companion PowerPoint presentation to learn more about the common childhood cancers:

- List the common presenting signs and symptoms for each of the diseases.

Shared care

Many of the children/adolescents diagnosed with cancer will participate in a system of care known as 'shared care'. Within this approach, the individual may receive care at the regional oncology centre, the district general hospital and at home from the primary healthcare team and, in some areas, paediatric oncology outreach nurses.

The concept of shared care is not unique to cancer but its adaptation within childhood cancer services has had to embrace the challenges of developing a countrywide transdisciplinary service for patients with rare diseases. In the 1970s, the UKCCSG recognised the need to treat children/adolescents in regional oncology centres to develop specialist knowledge and a multidisciplinary team with specific skills to care for this group of patients (UKCCSG 1997). Twenty-two regional centres within the UK were created. This meant that many patients had to travel significant distances, which in turn meant disruption for other family members, potential lack of family support for the patient and family at the hospital, and financial implications.

It also resulted in the deskilling of staff at the district general hospitals in relation to care of the patient with cancer (Patel et al 1997). However, as mortality and morbidity rates improved, it was decided to assess the feasibility of children/adolescents with acute lymphoblastic leukaemia receiving part of their treatment at their local district hospital. Muir et al (1992) demonstrated that 'sharing care' was safe practice and the service, for children/adolescents with other malignancies as well as acute lymphoblastic leukaemia, has continued to develop. However, it is not without its problems, especially the need to educate staff in the shared-care, community and regional centres, about caring for, and working with this group of patients (Patel et al 1997).

The Calman–Hine report (Department of Health (DoH) 1995) identified shared care as an important approach for the care of patients with cancer. Having been established within paediatric oncology since the early 1990s, the NHS Cancer Plan (DoH 2000) acknowledged the childhood cancer services success in developing such a service.

Activity

Read Sepion (2004) to discover how some parents felt about participating in shared care.

However, if families are to participate in shared care they require contact names, telephone numbers and information regarding the roles of the shared care centre, the regional centre and in some cases the paediatric oncology outreach nurses. Patient/parent-held records have been developed to facilitate resolution of some of the problems associated with all the information that the parents require. They provide resources for the parents when they get home and help with the communication between regional centres, shared care and the community (Hooker & Williams 1996).

The illness trajectory

Pre-diagnosis

The illness history for a child with a malignancy may be relatively short; parents may take their child to the GP with a history of a persistent infection, as with Jonathan in the following case scenario. GPs are usually the first professional encountered by the family. A common investigation for children/adolescents with a history of recurrent infection, abnormal bruising or bleeding, lethargy or abnormal lumps is a blood count for the assessment of their haemoglobin, platelets and white cell count including a differential.

Scenario

Jonathan, aged 6 years, was taken to his GP with a chest infection; he was treated with antibiotics for a week. As his chest infection did not improve after the course of antibiotics his mother returned to the GP with Jonathan. The GP requested a chest X-ray and a full blood count. That evening, Jonathan's parents were telephoned by the GP, who explained to them that as Jonathan's blood count was abnormal, they needed to take him to their local hospital immediately. On arrival at the hospital, Jonathan's parents were advised that his blood results were indicative of leukaemia and the next morning, following a blood transfusion overnight, he would be transferred to a regional cancer unit where he would undergo investigations for leukaemia.

His blood results were haemoglobin 6.8 g/dL, platelets 48×10^9, and total white cell count 25.4×10^9. The differential showed 95% blast cells.

Activity

- What are the normal ranges for a full blood count and differential?
- What do the terms anaemia, neutropenia, thrombocytopenia and pancytopenia mean?

GPs are likely to see only one or two cases of childhood malignancy in a 20-year practice but education regarding the signs and symptoms of these conditions and the need for prompt intervention has seen a significant improvement in GPs' responses to such symptoms over the last 30 years (Pinkerton et al 1994).

It is likely that the admission to the district general hospital will be for a short period of time, in some cases just an overnight stay while arrangements are made for transfer to the regional paediatric oncology centre where the diagnosis and prognosis will be confirmed and treatment commenced. Transfer to another centre will raise the patient's and parents' anxiety levels. They require written details and an explanation of how to get there, the name of the ward and staff that are expecting them. It is also useful to be able to advise them what to expect when they arrive at the centre. This can help the parents prepare themselves and their child to face a children's ward where they will see children/adolescents who are undergoing treatment and who have altered body images such as alopecia.

Information booklets about the regional cancer unit are useful for the patient and family to enable them to prepare for the transfer.

Activity

Discover the number and location of regional centres in the UK at:

- http://www.cclg.org

Many families may well have to travel a significant distance away from home to their nearest centre. Make a list of the advantages and disadvantages for the patient and family members when being transferred to a regional oncology centre.

Reaching a diagnosis

Due to a greater knowledge about childhood malignancies, the confirmation of the diagnosis is rarely a medical emergency. However, for the child/adolescent and parents it will be a time of great emotional distress and uncertainty (Kars et al 2008). It is vital, therefore, that the investigations are planned to cause the minimum amount of physical and psychological stress for the child and family. However, due to the neutropenia, children/adolescents can become acutely ill very quickly, therefore nurses need to be able to identify children/adolescents at risk of developing septic shock, recognising subtle changes in their condition, and be able to prioritise appropriate emergency care.

Activity

- What are the normal ranges of observations for Jonathan?
- List the signs and symptoms of septic shock?

Establishing venous access is often the first priority, both for assessment of blood values and to facilitate the administration of medications, hydration and the correction of haematological and electrolyte abnormalities prior to further investigations being carried out. The type and variety of investigations required will be decided upon depending on the suspected diagnosis. Bone marrow aspirates and trephines are carried out to confirm and determine the type of leukaemia (acute lymphoblastic leukaemia and acute myeloid leukaemia), lumbar punctures are required to identify the presence of leukaemia cells in the cerebrospinal fluid. Children/adolescents with solid tumours are likely to undergo a combination of:

- X-rays
- computerised tomography (CT) scans
- radioisotope scans, e.g. bone scans, renal function scans
- magnetic resonance imaging (MRI) scans.

Effective communication between the different departments involved in the investigative procedures is essential. It is also important to remember, however, that the patient may have to experience the investigations numerous times throughout treatment – the preparation for the procedures is, therefore, crucial.

Consideration for the use of pharmacological interventions, such as sedatives or anaesthesia, and non-pharmacological methods, such as distraction, play and hypnosis, for procedures that are invasive, painful or that require the patient to remain still should be given (Christensen & Fatchett 2002). Assessment and intervention by the play therapist is valuable as relationships are just beginning to be established. Carrying out many procedures under one anaesthetic or sedative requires expert planning and negotiation skills. If the investigation is deemed not to be invasive or painful, or the patient is considered to be able to comply with instructions, it will still be necessary to assess that the patient is free from physical and/or emotional pain/discomfort and establish appropriate therapeutic interventions where required (Pinkerton et al 1994).

This is an extremely difficult time for the patient, parents, other family members and the members of the healthcare team. Effective communication is vital to minimise additional stress and to establish trusting relationships that are essential to assist the child and family as they start this journey (Clarke et al 2005).

Parents see themselves as advocates for their child (Holm et al 2003), making medical decisions, limiting the actions of healthcare professionals and learning about their child's condition. Their education in order to participate, therefore, is paramount.

Activity

- List the different healthcare professionals that the patient and parents are likely to come into contact with or require the services of during the diagnostic phase of their illness.
- What are the advantages and difficulties for the parents and child meeting all these people?
- Having done this, now think about the role of the nurse, what skills will the nurse require to minimise the additional stress for the child and family?

Confirming the diagnosis

The confirmation of the diagnosis will bring many mixed reactions and emotions. The family whose child has had a short history of a mild illness may find it difficult to accept that their child has a life-threatening illness, whereas for the family who have encountered a delay or complications in the confirmation of diagnosis and whose child's condition has continued to deteriorate, it may come as a relief in that they can now begin treatment. Buckman (1992) advises that, although specific details of what was said will be forgotten, the way in which the news of the diagnosis is given to the family will be remembered. It is important, therefore, that the confirmation of the diagnosis is a planned event. Privacy, an appropriate environment, time and honesty are key issues. Parents will search for a cause for their child's illness and a meaning of the illness (Ruccione et al 1994). Parents feel responsible for their child, yet at this stage they lack knowledge, authority and power to participate in healthcare decisions. It is important that they receive the right amount of information and feel listened to (Clarke & Fletcher 2003). Interestingly, Clarke-Steffen (1993) identified that once parents felt they had been told the details of the worst things that could happen to their child, they felt more able to trust the professionals to be honest with them about subsequent information or news.

Activity

Read Dickinson (2008) and McNally & Eden (2004). What are the current issues concerning the causes of childhood cancer in the UK?

It is recommended that children/adolescents are informed of their diagnosis, treatment and prognosis (Eiser et al 1994). However, many factors need to be taken into consideration, such as the existing communication strategies within the family, cultural and religious beliefs, and the child's age and level of development (Price 2003).

Activity

Read 'The private worlds of dying children' by Myra Bluebond-Langner (1978), who was one of the first people to research the informational needs of children with a life-limiting illness. How have attitudes changed over the past 25 years?

It must be remembered that parents will react in different ways depending on their coping strategies, previous experiences, relationships and culture. The grief that the families experience when they hear the diagnosis has been likened to Kubler Ross's (1969) model of grief.

Activity

Describe why theories of grief and loss are applicable to the parents of children/adolescents following a diagnosis of cancer.

Although it is recognised that children/adolescents have a right and a need to know their diagnosis (Eiser et al 1994), negotiation with the parents will help to decide the best way this is carried out for their child. Parents may need time to come to terms with the diagnosis first, but delay in confirming the diagnosis with the child/adolescent might result in finding out via an alternative source, which can subsequently lead to difficulties in establishing trusting relationships. Telling the patient and family together may be valuable for some families, for others the parents may prefer to break the news themselves. Price (2003 p 38) identifies the following strategy to assist information giving to children:

C = consider age and cognitive development stage carefully
H = highlight and establish child's current level of understanding
I = include other members of the multidisciplinary team (MDT) as appropriate, e.g. play specialist
L = language that is simple and age appropriate should be used
D = discuss with and involve parents
R = restrict the time of the session: remember a child has limited attention
E = employ a range of strategies, e.g. play, stories, etc.
N = necessary to elicit feedback and evaluate effectiveness.

It is recognised that the confirmation will come as a shock and the ability to remember information will be reduced; it is vital, therefore, that the patient and parents feel reassured that they can ask staff to go over information as often as is required for them (Pinkerton at el 1994).

Activity

Do an internet search and discover how many different sources of information regarding childhood tumours are available. Think about how you might guide parents to use this source and variety of information.

Commencement of treatment

An outcome of the establishment of the UKCCSG in 1978 and the organisation of the 22 regional centres has been the increase in the number of children/adolescents that are entered into clinical trials, which evaluate current treatments, test new drugs or test existing drugs in different dosages, ways of administration or combinations.

PowerPoint

Access the companion PowerPoint presentation for the section on clinical trials.

WWW

Log onto the following website for information regarding current trials:

- http://www.ukccsg.org

Although recruitment of adults with cancer into trials is low (approximately 30%) the figures for children/adolescents is much higher; 90% of children/adolescents with a malignant disease are registered with the UKCCSG, 80% of these are eligible for entry onto trials and 70% actually participate in trials (more details are available at: http://www.cancerresearchuk.org). As previously mentioned, the rarity of childhood cancer makes this vital because the significance of findings would be difficult to evaluate if the numbers entered onto trials was low.

The aim of treatment is to remove or to kill the malignant cells and achieve a cure. The term 'cure' refers to the patient who can be expected to have the same life expectancy as any other child/adolescent who does not have a malignancy. Quality of life (QoL) for patients is an important consideration when deciding upon treatment approaches. QoL for cured patients is also very important and will be discussed in more depth in the cure/survivorship section. Cure usually refers to patients that have not been receiving treatment for 5 years and have no evidence of disease.

The main treatments for childhood malignancies are:

- chemotherapy
- radiotherapy
- surgery
- biotherapy/immunotherapy.

Chemotherapy

Chemotherapy is a systemic treatment and is widely used in childhood malignancies as the tumours have a high rate of proliferation and dissemination (metastatic spread). A helpful analogy for children/adolescents is that chemotherapy is like a spaceship that boldly goes where other treatments cannot go.

WWW

Log onto the following website and follow the links to patient information and the adventures of Captain Chemo:

- http://www.royalmarsden.org.uk

An interesting information guide for children/adolescents undergoing chemotherapy is an interactive cartoon character, called Captain Chemo (www.royalmarsdenhospital.org.uk), which was created by a patient.

Chemotherapy may be used in the following way:

- Definitive/primary: when it is used as the sole treatment
- Adjuvant: when it is administered following the removal of a primary tumour to destroy any remaining micrometastases
- Neoadjuvant: when it is used to shrink a tumour prior to surgery
- Salvage: when it is administered to a patient who has relapsed following treatment using a different modality
- Palliative: when it is administered to manage symptoms in patients with advanced/incurable disease.

Chemotherapy attacks rapidly reproducing/dividing cells. Three systems in particular are affected: the haemopoetic (bone marrow; BM), the gastrointestinal (GI) and the skin. These are often the most common and most well-known associated side effects. Key issues of these more common side effects will be explored following the outlines of the different treatments.

Activity

Using the three headings above, make a list of the potential side effects and symptoms that may occur when cells are destroyed or damaged. You could have up to seven side effects for the GI tract, three for the BM and up to four for the skin.

As previously mentioned, children/adolescents will face repeated courses of chemotherapy and it is important, therefore, to aim for the first one to be a positive experience in order to prevent anticipatory problems with subsequent courses (Gibson & Soanes 2008, Tomlinson & Kline 2008).

Radiotherapy

Radiotherapy is the use of ionising radiation. To begin to understand the principles of radiation, it is necessary to undertake some physics revision, in particular the atom, which can be found on the companion PowerPoint presentation. The different types of radiotherapy used in the treatment of childhood malignancies are also described. Like chemotherapy, radiation has different uses, it may be used for:

- the eradication of the disease, e.g. cure
- the control of symptoms: this may be as a planned treatment or as an emergency, e.g. for children/adolescents with raised intracranial pressure
- imaging
- treatment.

Another useful resource for staff, patients and their families is a video 'It's all in the zap' made by a group of teenagers who had received radiotherapy.

PowerPoint

View the extract from the video 'It's all in the zap' on the companion PowerPoint presentation.

WWW

A web page has also been created for information and communication. Log on and read the information provided by the teenagers for other patients:

- http://www.allinthezap.com

Members of the public and healthcare professionals are frightened of radiation because it is invisible and is highly technical. Parents and patients require up-to-date information and supportive advice to help them through this treatment. The majority of children/adolescents will receive radiotherapy as an outpatient, the treatment is usually daily, Monday to Friday, and can last for a period of 2–6 weeks. Families often feel isolated during this time, as the radiotherapy department may not be in the hospital where they are receiving the other treatment. It is useful, therefore, to ensure that the families have contact names and telephone numbers of appropriate personnel to enable them to seek help, reassurance and advice. They may also require financial help or other social support to manage the impact of daily outpatient trips to the radiotherapy department (Gibson & Soanes 2008, Tomlinson & Kline 2008).

Surgery

Surgery for childhood cancer was the only treatment until the 20th century, when radiotherapy and subsequently chemotherapy became available; cure rate at this time was very low. These have risen considerably since multimodality treatment approaches have been developed.

Activity

Explain why surgery in childhood/adolescent cancer is rarely used as a single treatment modality.

Surgical services for childhood malignancies have developed over the past 25 years and now include important roles such as:

- aiding a diagnosis, e.g. biopsy
- aiding treatment, e.g. central venous line, gastrostomy tube
- a treatment, e.g. complete resection, partial resection
- assessing response to treatment, e.g. bone marrow aspirates and trephines
- limb conservation surgery, e.g. endoprosthesis
- the management of metastasis.

It is almost inevitable that children/adolescents with a malignancy will undergo a surgical procedure in some form and, although it may appear to be the most straightforward of all the treatments, it may, as Hollis (1997) identifies, result in loss of function, a cosmetic insult or both, for example a teenager with an osteosarcoma who undergoes limb amputation as part of a treatment protocol.

Throughout their treatment, children/adolescents will encounter repeat investigations and procedures to assess the response of the treatment. For example, patients with leukaemia will undergo repeated bone marrow aspirates and trephines, and lumbar punctures. Assumptions may be made that because this is the 5th or 10th time, the patient will be used to it and the appropriate psychological care and support may not be offered. Models of nursing such as family-centred care, primary nursing or named nurse (Bishop 2000) offer the opportunity to establish therapeutic relationships that facilitate nurses' understanding of the coping strategies used by individual patients. This also applies to knowledge of how the parents cope as their child undergoes yet another general anaesthetic.

It is also worth remembering that major surgery, such as orthopaedic surgery, may be carried out in specialist units, possibly even in other centres. This again adds to the patient and families' need for appropriate advice and information. Once more, the patient and parents may be faced with meeting yet another group of healthcare professionals, establishing relationships and learning to trust them.

The nurse has a major role to play in ensuring that the patient is prepared, physically and emotionally, for the procedure.

Another important consideration is the outcome of the surgical procedure. This may determine the long-term outcome for the patient – is he or she cured or is yet more treatment required? In addition to being worried about surviving the procedure, and perhaps the potential of altered body image, parents and the patient will be anxious to know whether the tumour was completely removed, whether further treatment will be needed or if there is a viable next option (Gibson & Soanes 2008, Tomlinson & Kline 2008).

Biotherapy

Biotherapy refers to the manipulation of the immune system to treat diseases. Other terms used to describe this approach are biologic response modifiers and immunotherapy. The common biotherapy used in childhood/adolescent malignancy treatment is granulocyte colony stimulating factor (GCSF), which is used to support patients going through intensive chemotherapy regimens and peripheral stem cell transplants (Gibson & Soanes 2008, Tomlinson & Kline 2008).

Common side effects of treatment

Children/adolescents undergoing treatment for a malignancy are likely, therefore, to receive a combination of therapies, which may last for months or, in the case of leukaemia, years. Some patients will undergo long periods of hospitalisation, others will receive much of their treatment as outpatients, attending both the regional centre and the shared care hospital. The effective management of side effects, therefore, is vital.

Effective management incorporates the physical and psychological care for the patient and the psychological care of family members. Symptom management for a patient undergoing treatment for a malignant disease requires nurses to have knowledge of the:

- disease and its symptoms
- treatments and their side effects
- management of both of the above.

Nurses must be able to prioritise their care and show flexibility in the way that the care is delivered (Pinkerton et al 1994). Many of the skills that nurses demonstrate will be carried out by the parents once the patient is discharged and, therefore, negotiation and education are key aspects of care.

Activity

- List the body's normal defence mechanisms.
- Why is the patient with a malignant disease, who is receiving treatment, at risk from infection?

Neutropenia

The treatment of a malignant disease attacks the body's normal defence mechanisms directly and indirectly. The direct effects are on the white cells and the immune system. The indirect effects are through the methods of administration, e.g. via long lines that puncture the skin, other procedures such as venepunctures, bone marrow aspirates and lumbar punctures, which increase the risk of infection. In addition, poor nutritional intake due to nausea and/or vomiting has an effect, as does the use of antibiotics, which damages normal flora. For the children/adolescents who have received chemotherapy, the greatest risk is of developing septicaemia. However, they are also susceptible to haemorrhage, anaemia and anorexia leading to cachexia.

The prevention and early detection of infection is, therefore, a priority. Regular observations of temperature, pulse, respirations and blood pressure and an accurate fluid balance are essential for the patient who is neutropenic. The nurse also needs to be able to recognise subtle changes such as skin colour, position, the patients' interest in ward activities, even personality traits which may indicate the need to initiate repeat observations or other investigations. Recognition of the early signs of septicaemia is essential to prevent septic shock. Oral hygiene, skin integrity and nutritional intake must also be regularly evaluated.

Reflect on your practice

Nursing tip

The definition of neutropenia is the absence of neutrophils. Neutrophils are white cells and, therefore, when observing for the classic signs of infection, patients who are neutropenic will not produce pus!

Management of neutropenia regarding where the patient is nursed will vary depending upon local policy. In regional centres, neutropenic patients are unlikely to be isolated as there are insufficient facilities. However, in district general hospitals they may be routinely isolated because of other infections on the ward. The most important aspect for the prevention of infection is hand washing (Pinkerton et al 1994).

Nausea and vomiting

Nausea and vomiting are immediate side effects of chemotherapy but they can persist for several days following administration of the drug, especially nausea. Children have identified nausea as being worse than vomiting, and assessment, which includes the patient and family, is therefore essential. Various rating scales have been developed (Le Baron et al 1988) but as yet they have not been seen universally in practice. There are debates about young children's ability to accurately report their feelings. Zelter et al (1988) recommend that children as young as 5 years are able to use a rating scale, whereas Abu-Saad (1993) does not fully agree.

Knowledge of the emetogenic potential of the chemotherapy drugs and combinations of antiemetic drugs can be found on the companion PowerPoint presentation.

Hawthorne (1995) suggested that the best approach is prevention rather than control once it has occurred. Some patients experience anticipatory nausea and vomiting, this is a complex reaction that triggers memories, thoughts, images from previous experiences. It could be a particular smell, such as disinfectant, food or a nurse's perfume, a particular room, generally something that the patient associates with nausea and/or vomiting.

Pharmacological, non-pharmacological and complementary methods all have a role to play in establishing individualised approaches.

Scenario

Pete, aged 16 years, felt nauseous as soon as the car turned into the drive of the hospital. He was treated with Nabilone (a cannabinoid) taken the evening prior to admission. This helped him sleep better on the night before admission and prevented the experience of nausea as he arrived at the hospital.

Activity

Read Pearman (2002), who explores the management of nausea and vomiting from a health promotion base.

Stomatitis

There is conflicting evidence as to the number of children who experience oral complications (stomatitis) following chemotherapy (Aitkin 1992, Holmes 1991). However, as with nausea and vomiting, prevention is better than cure. The term 'stomatitis' refers to inflammation of the oral mucosa. It occurs as a direct effect of the chemotherapy and is indirectly complicated by the decreased myeloproliferation of the bone marrow. The clinical picture is one of ulceration, swelling, pain, dry, cracked bleeding lips and desquamation of the gums and palate (Hooker & Palmer 1999). This can have a direct effect on the patients' quality of life, affecting the ability to eat, drink, communicate and, in severe cases, even swallow saliva. Some patients require continuous morphine analgesia to control pain and facilitate oral care (Pinkerton et al 1994).

Although it is recognised that oral care is essential, there is again conflicting evidence as to oral care regimens. The principles are identified in Box 31.1. How this is achieved is strongly debated. Although there is no disagreement regarding assessment being the first vital step in planning effective care (Campbell et al 1995), the type of oral assessment guide for children is an issue where there is conflicting evidence (Holmes & Mountain 1993).

Activity

Read Gibson & Hayden (2004) for a description of the development of an oral assessment tool by Great Ormond Street Hospital for Children. This tool is based on Eilers et al's (1988) tool and the discussion includes an analysis of the predominantly adult-based evidence with regard to the applicability of the equipment and solutions for use with children.

Box 31.1

Aims of oral care

To maintain oral function and promote patient dignity, comfort and well-being by maintaining:

- a clean and healthy oral cavity
- moist mucosa
- mucosal integrity

and preventing:

- plaque
- infection
- dry cracked lips.

Constipation

As previously identified, many of the side effects that the patients experience are compounded by the combination of direct and indirect effects. Constipation is another example of this. Patients in hospital are often at an increased risk of developing constipation because of inactivity and a change in their diet and fluid intake, this may then be complicated by medications such as analgesics, especially opioids, and some of the chemotherapy drugs. For example, vincristine, a drug commonly used in the treatment of leukaemia, causes autonomic neuropathy. Educating the patient and family about the importance of appropriate nutrition and hydration and the monitoring of bowel actions is essential. Initiating, maintaining and evaluating accurate fluid, diet and bowel records is a responsibility of the nurse, even if parents decide to participate by carrying out the documentation.

Activity

- With reference to the side effects of chemotherapy, what are the potential risks for a patient who develops constipation?

Nursing tip: patients who are prescribed opioids for pain relief should always receive laxatives to prevent constipation

Anorexia/cachexia

The importance of adequate nutritional intake has been highlighted several times already but it is important to recognise the challenges for the patient and his or her family. Once again, there are compounding issues. The treatment is likely to result in the patient's nutritional intake being altered, through nausea (with or without vomiting), stomatitis, anorexia and taste alteration, or food restriction prior to procedures. Working with the dietitian, identifying at-risk patients, initiating flexible meal ordering, and facilities for parents to cook or to bring food in are ways of preventing or minimising severe problems (Pinkerton et al 1994).

Steroids, used as part of a treatment protocol or as an anti-emetic, can also affect the appetite of patients. Patients with tumours of the central nervous system who may be receiving steroids to reduce raised intracranial pressure often experience problems associated with weight increase. Children/adolescents with leukaemia receive pulses of steroids, which can alter their eating habits. Parents require advice and support to enable them to cope with the impact of having a child whose interest in food varies from waking in the night because they are hungry to one who has no interest in food at all.

Pain

Patients may experience pain as a result of their disease, the investigative procedures, facilitation of treatment, treatment and side effects. Effective assessment and management is essential because, as previously mentioned, many of the patients will experience some or all of the above repeatedly throughout their illness trajectory.

Effective pain strategies have been discussed elsewhere in this book, as has the use of pharmacological, non-pharmacological and complementary approaches, but it is important to remember spiritual pain. These patients will be exposed to other children/adolescents with malignant disease, they will observe them at different stages of their illness trajectory and may well see those suffering painful experiences (Pinkerton et al 1994). They may be aware of, or even witness, death – possibly the death of a close friend, a friendship that has developed through the camaraderie of sharing the same illness and, therefore, the same or similar experiences. It is vital, therefore, to acknowledge this and to work with the patient to develop coping strategies. Effective communication, which is an essential part of transdisciplinary working, becomes vital.

Fatigue

Cancer-related fatigue (CRF) has been recognised as a distressing and debilitating symptom in the adult cancer arena for over a decade but has only recently been explored in children/adolescents (Gibson et al 2004a). Fatigue has been identified in adolescents as being multidimensional and multifactorial (Edwards et al 2003, 2004). It can affect the patient's ability to cope with the disease and treatment, participate in normal activities of daily living and can have long-lasting impact. Coping strategies suggested by patients include medical interventions such as blood transfusions, nutrition, sleeps/naps and distraction.

Activity

Think about the ward environment and the activities that nurses carry out and identify factors that may contribute to the patients experiencing fatigue.

Altered skin integrity

This is particularly relevant to children/adolescents receiving external beam radiation. The reaction is likened to having sunburn. The first sign is redness, the skin then becomes dry and flaky (dry desquamation) and can proceed to being wet and flaky (moist desquamation). The key principles are to promote comfort, prevent infection and minimise trauma. Faithfull (2001) discusses evidence on the prevention and management of skin side effects – whilst it is adult-based it is applicable with adaptation for children and adolescents.

Altered body image

Children/adolescents are concerned about their appearance, and it is important to be able to look and dress like their peers. Treatment, as already identified, can result in undesirable physical changes that make them look and feel different (Thompson 2001). Although it is important to stress the temporary nature of side effects such as alopecia and weight gain/loss, patients, and other family members will require help from the multidisciplinary team to develop coping strategies to deal with these, especially for permanent side effects such as amputation or surgical scars.

Other body changes may not be visible, such as infertility, but can have a major impact for males as well as females. Again, psychological support to develop coping strategies is essential. Two cancer charities, the Teenage Cancer Trust and Teencancer, have developed web pages that give adolescents the opportunity to share experiences of coping with these and other problems.

Activity

Log onto the following websites. List the facilities that are available for teenagers. Identify the common questions asked by this group of patients:

- http://www.teencancer.org
- http://www.teenagecancer.org

Psychological care

In the 1980s, when improvements in the remission and cure rates were becoming evident, new problems for the psychological care of the patient and family were being identified. Koocher & O'Malley (1985) interviewed survivors and their families who described the problems of living with cancer. One of the key factors identified was the need for the preparation to be able to live with cancer. For the parents, it included advice and support to let their child live as 'normal a life' as possible and to be able to facilitate all members of the family to live with the impact of the disease and treatment.

More recent research by Clarke-Steffen (1997) explored how current families managed 'living' with childhood cancer. She identified the concept of 'reconstructing reality' (Box 31.2) and explains the stages that the parents, patient and family members go through to develop these strategies. She begins with the impact of the potential diagnosis and uses the analogy of being in 'limbo', when the patient, parents and family members are waiting to know the diagnosis, and are experiencing feelings of vulnerability and helplessness. When the diagnosis is confirmed, there is a new daily routine to adjust to and with this are feelings of uncertainty, and a change in the way that life is viewed. Reconstructing reality provides evidence of the challenges that the family faces and the importance of the role of the members of the professional healthcare team. An interesting finding from this qualitative study was that parents appreciated nurses 'being there'. Being there when families are in 'limbo' requires very special skills.

Box 31.2

Reconstructing reality (from Clarke-Steffen 1997 p 281):

- Managing the flow of information
- Reorganising roles
- Evaluating and shifting priorities
- Changing future orientation
- Assigning meaning to the illness
- Managing the therapeutic regimen.

Activity

Imagine how it would feel to be with the parents of Jonathan as they waited for the confirmation of his diagnosis. How would you feel, what would you say, and what would you do?

Sadly, nothing we can say will make it better but, as mentioned earlier, the way that we say things and the courage to stay with the family – just 'being there' – can make a memorable difference.

Quality of life

Quality of life (QoL) for children/adolescents with cancer has also been researched (Eiser & Morse 2001, Gibson et al 2004b, Hicks et al 2003) and the following issues explored:

- physical well-being and symptoms
- psychological well-being
- social well-being
- spiritual well-being.

Hicks et al (2003 p 192) identified the following five themes, which can have an effect on the psychosocial well-being of the patient and subsequently the ability to become well-adjusted survivors:

- fatigue
- effect on activities
- medication and treatment effects
- relationship changes
- hair loss.

The philosophy for treatment in the 1960s and 1970s, when cure was rare, was 'cure at whatever cost'. The philosophy is now 'cure with the least cost' (Pinkerton et al 1994).

As previously mentioned, children/adolescents will receive multimodal therapy and, therefore, may experience some or all of the side effects identified. Healthcare professionals, therefore, require knowledge of the compounding factors associated with the treatments and the appropriate skills to identify at-risk patients, initiate appropriate assessment strategies, implement effective management plans and evaluate all aspects of the care. Some patients will receive treatments during which intensive or high doses of chemotherapy and/or radiotherapy are used. These treatments will result in an increase in the severity of the side effects, both from the symptoms themselves and also the length of time they persist. As the risk of complications increases with the intensity of the treatment, the skill and role of the healthcare professional must also be extended and developed.

Scenario

Jonathan was in the regional centre for 10 days. On discharge his white cell count was 1.9×10^9 with 30% neutrophils, haemoglobin 10.9 and platelets 68×10^9. He had started his first course of chemotherapy, which was to be completed as an outpatient at his local hospital. He had a skin-tunnelled catheter in situ.

Going home

It has already been identified that once the diagnosis of a malignancy has been confirmed, the ability to remember details about the disease and treatment is reduced. When planning the discharge, providing the information is only a small part of the process. Nurses caring for these families need to be able to negotiate with them to provide information at an appropriate and convenient time, in a format that is acceptable and as frequently as is required by individual families (Cox 2000). The families will require information and advice regarding:

- identification of infection (including temperature monitoring)
- medication administration
- care of the central venous device
- nutrition
- oral hygiene
- contact names and numbers/who to call in an emergency
- how to recognise an emergency
- outpatient appointments
- details of shared care.

Several of these require the parents to be proficient in new skills, for example, caring for the central venous device and administering cytotoxic medication, as well as managing all the information and coping without having knowledgeable, supportive people, such as staff and other parents, around.

Although it is acknowledged that discharge planning begins on admission, the planning and timing of patient and parent education must be negotiated in a way that acknowledges and recognises the impact that the diagnosis may have had.

Activity

- Write a detailed plan of how you would structure the teaching for Jonathan and his parents.
- What factors will you take into consideration when planning the timing?
- What specific nursing skill is central to the success of your plan?

Remission

Remission is the term used to describe no evidence of disease. It is most commonly used in the leukaemias to describe the amount of blast cells in the bone marrow. A remission marrow will have less than 5% blast cells (blast means immature), it is normal for bone marrow to have up to 5% blast cells present, therefore a remission marrow is one that has less than 5% blast cells.

Once in remission, patients with acute lymphoblastic leukaemia will commence the treatment phase known as maintenance therapy. This is to maintain the remission and minimise the chance of relapse, i.e. the disease returning. Boys will undergo a 3-year maintenance protocol, whereas girls have 2 years of maintenance therapy.

Protocols for acute myeloid leukaemia and the solid tumours last for months rather than years. The chemotherapy is more intensive, requiring frequent and/or extended hospitalisation and inpatient supportive care.

Relapse/recurrence

Parents in Koocher & O'Malley's (1985) study likened the threat of relapse as the sword of Damocles. Even after being pronounced 'cured', the fear did not disappear. Relapse rates vary with individual diseases and depend on prognostic features and the stage of the disease at diagnosis. Relapse brings with it the need for information regarding confirmation and extent of the spread of recurrent disease and the possibility of further treatment. This may include the opportunity to gain second opinions.

Having experienced them once, it is important that the patients' feelings regarding QoL issues are taken into consideration when treatment opportunities are being discussed. This poses the potential for ethical debates regarding the use of experimental treatments.

WWW

Read Dyer (1995) and Entwistle et al (1996) on the case of child B, and the surrounding media coverage, at:

- http://www.bmj.com

Previous knowledge of how the patient has coped with treatment will be useful but it is essential that a trusting and supportive relationship be established at the time of relapse. As a decision is reached, the family needs to feel supported by all members of the healthcare team.

If further treatment is not an option, discussion about the provision of appropriate palliative care will be required. Parents will need support and advice regarding communicating the results and their implications to the patient. Harris & Curnick (2000) recommend that parents are given time to assimilate the information before they can begin to discuss it with the patient. Bluebond-Langner (1992) suggests that openness within a family is more likely if the parents feel supported. The skills and approaches used at the time of diagnosis will be required again, incorporating the knowledge gained through the previous treatment experience. At this time, however, parents may feel the need to protect their child from the pain of facing death.

Activity

In 'The private worlds of dying children', Bluebond-Langner (1978) identified the concept of 'mutual pretence':

- In the current climate where 'openness' is recommended, list the difficulties for nurses working with a family where mutual pretence may be utilised as a coping strategy.

PowerPoint

Access the companion PowerPoint presentation for information relating to the incidence of patients developing a second malignancy

End of life care and death

Although cure rates are improving, cancer is the highest cause of death due to illness in the UK (data available at: http://www.statistics.gov.uk). The majority of children/adolescents dying from cancer are cared for at home with the support of appropriately experienced nurses (Hunt 1996). A small number, however, will die in hospital. Some of these will be anticipated deaths, when the parents and/or patient have chosen to receive end of life care in hospital or when a decision is reached that further active treatment is no longer appropriate but the patient is too ill to be transferred home. Rarely, unexpected death due to oncological emergencies such as septic shock, an allergic reaction to medication, haemorrhage or tumour lysis syndrome, can occur.

PowerPoint

Access the companion PowerPoint presentation to learn more about oncological emergencies.

Sudden death prevents the establishment of effective palliative and end of life care, the opportunity to prepare for the death and the chance to say goodbye. Black (1991) advocates that managing and coping with sudden death requires specific skills, especially the ability to communicate effectively and offer appropriate support. Sudden death can impact on normal grieving and can exacerbate grief reactions.

Activity

Read Curnick & Harris (2000) for issues related to the child dying with cancer.

Long-term survivors

The introduction of multimodal treatment has seen an improvement in survival rates to almost 70% (data available at: http://www.statistics.gov.uk). This has posed new challenges for the healthcare team in the prevention, recognition and management of long-term side effects. The UKCCSG has developed guidelines for long-term follow-up care (UKCCSG 1995). Specialists in paediatric respiratory, endocrinology, cardiology, neurology and psychology are part of the long-term follow-up team.

Long-term side effects are related to the combination and dosage of drugs used – multimodal therapies can exacerbate any toxicity. The body systems where toxicities are anticipated include the:

- lungs
- heart
- renal system
- liver
- gonads: fertility
- endocrine: growth and puberty
- hearing
- central nervous system
- skin
- skeletal
- eyes.

Chesterfield (1999) advocates the nurse's responsibility of facilitating survivors' adaptation to the physical and/or psychological disabilities they may have. However, for some patients this may be a life-long challenge. For children/adolescents who have missed a significant amount of schooling and have received treatment such as cranial irradiation, which has detrimental effects on some aspects of intellect (Anderson et al 1994), the choice of further education/employment may be restricted.

The decision-making skills of adolescents who had received treatment for cancer were explored by Hollen & Hobbie (1996). They concluded that, for some, the ability to make decisions was affected by the combination of treatment and the impact of hospitalisation, which had resulted in them missing out on normal developmental interaction. This is particularly important when the role of the nurse as health promoter is considered. Giving advice about not smoking to a teenager who has received lung irradiation may not be enough for patients who have difficulty in making decisions. The context in which they may be tempted to smoke – being out with their peers when perhaps they are the only one not smoking – needs to be considered. Advice on strategies to prepare them to be able to say no are also required.

Health promotion regarding sexual health for adolescents may present challenges for some parents and healthcare professionals. Information regarding safe sex, for example the use of condoms, may prevent difficulties in families where the parents may be unaware that their son/daughter is sexually active. Adolescents who may have been told that their fertility has been impaired, may decide to experiment without the use of contraception and are therefore at risk of an unwanted pregnancy as well as of developing life-threatening infections. Support groups with other survivors and interactive internet networks (e.g. http://www.allinthezap.com, http://www.teencancer.org, and http://www.teenagecancer.org) have been developed by young people to help each other.

Adolescents and young adults

Adolescents and young adults have very specific needs in relation to achieving their unique developmental tasks (Taylor & Muller 1995) and adapting to their disease, its treatment and the restrictions that may result as a direct consequence

(Kelly & Gibson 2008). Their ability to comprehend the illness and its implications, the restrictions made by the treatment and the physical changes, can lead to lowered self-esteem and depression (Ritchie 1992) and increase their sense of personal vulnerability (Eiser 1996). To help them cope and maintain hope, Hooker (2004) identified the need for accurate, truthful information that enables them to participate in decision-making, assess the threat of the illness and gain a sense of control. There is debate as to the most appropriate place for this group to receive treatment (Whelan 2003). They have been described as being at the edge of no-man's land by Hollis & Morgan (2001) and in need of dedicated services. NICE (2005) recommended that a specific registry for the over-15-year-olds is developed as well as age-specific treatment services and environments. Morgan & Hubber (2004) describe the challenges of establishing such a service, identifying the problems associated with acting as the mediator between the patients, their families and the adult and paediatric healthcare professionals.

Activity

Read Thompson (2004).

Surviving cancer and cure

The treatment of cancer is often depicted as a battle, with patients either winning the battle or losing the fight. Survival could, therefore, be associated with winning the battle. Lozowski (1993) proposes that survival begins at the time of diagnosis, with the patients surviving the many components of cancer and its treatment, living with their cancer through periods of remission and relapse. However, as the definition of cure is that there is no evidence of disease 5 years after completion of treatment, there are children/adolescents who are survivors but who are not cured – they have won the battle but not necessarily the war.

Significantly, Van Eys (1991) suggests that as well as biological cure, psychological and social cure is also required and, therefore, biological cure alone could be viewed as only part success if the patient is left with psychological and/or social needs. Research by Eiser & Jenney (1996) has identified a correlation between duration and intensity of treatment and the prevalence of psychological late effects. Medical interventions such as venepuncture or side effects affecting body image, such as alopecia or altered weight, can affect the patient's psychological well-being, reiterating the importance of managing the procedure effectively.

Earlier in the chapter, Clarke-Steffan's (1997) model of family adjustment identified the important role that parents have in managing the flow of information regarding the treatment and the day-to-day care of the patient. Children/adolescents with cancer have to cope with being different, of living a different type of life to that of their healthy peers, and this can leave them with feelings of abandonment, loneliness and loss of control. Time away from school may leave them with different career choices, perhaps being dependent on their parents when their peers are experiencing and enjoying their growing independence.

Interestingly, a study of school-age children with acute lymphoblastic leukaemia by Dowling et al (2003) explored the relationship between childhood cancer stressors and the psychological adjustment to cancer and identified a direct correlation. Although the authors acknowledge limitations with the study and recommend further research, it does raise questions regarding personal factors that may help children/adolescents cope with the stressors of cancer and its treatment, and hypothesises whether personal traits such as humour, resilience, hardiness and optimism can be learnt and developed.

The role of parents, peers and schools in providing psychosocial support has also been explored by Suzuki & Kato (2003). A review of the literature identified a variety of resources available to facilitate the education and skill development of the parents, peers and schools to help the patient adjust and cope. The internet and video games were particularly useful for education and provided an opportunity to practice or rehearse communications with the patient.

Hicks & Lavender (2001) promote the development of psychosocial support interventions to facilitate improvement of QoL regardless of the eventual outcome of the illness. Acceptable QoL is linked to rehabilitation by Bradwell & Hawkins (2000), who advocate that rehabilitation begins at diagnosis. Although this is important, Selekman's (1991) suggestion of a revision of the concept of rehabilitation for children is compelling in that she advocates the philosophy of habilitation. This recognises the need to continue normal development to prevent developmental delay. She advocates supporting children to achieve levels of development as yet unknown to them. For patients facing months of hospitalisation, isolation from peers, school and social activities, this is an important aspect of care.

The child/adolescent with cancer, and the family, face many hurdles as they try to reconstruct reality (Clarke-Steffan 1997). The patient will miss school, peers and social activities, and might have to cope with altered body image and come to terms with uncertainty about the future, even as a survivor.

Siblings also have to adjust to the change in their life brought about by the reconstruction. The impact of this depends on their age and relationship with the ill sibling. Initially, it may be separation from the family (Foley et al 1993) followed by non-negotiated routine changes and altered family plans for holidays, etc., as a result of adaptation to the treatment and its restrictions. They experience the same fears and incomprehension as the parents but often they do not have someone to talk to or confide in (Faulkner et al 1995). Parents require guidance to meet the needs of all family members throughout the illness trajectory, but especially at times of crisis. They may feel that they are protecting their healthy children/adolescents but they may be adding to their burden by making them feel excluded, unable to participate in the care and decisions. Simms et al (2002) advocate involving them in the care of their sick sibling.

Summary

Childhood malignancy has been described as a chronic illness. It is essential, therefore, that children/adolescents receive comprehensive care that encompasses their physical, psychological and psychosocial well-being within a philosophy of family-centred care, preparing and supporting them as they live with cancer, its treatment and the side effects (Langton 2000). Working with this group of patients, whether in a regional centre, shared care or primary healthcare environment, can be very rewarding but is also stressful (Bulley 2000). Maintaining clear professional boundaries when working closely with families can be difficult, but it is essential because the patient and family need professional care and, to continue to provide this care, nurses are required to identify and develop their own coping strategies.

The concept of the illness trajectory (Fig. 31.1) (Corbin & Strauss 1991) has been used to identify the challenges that a child/adolescent with cancer, and his or her family, will face as treatment is undergone. The number of healthcare professionals and care environments they may encounter on this journey has also been highlighted. Many nurses will see the patient and family in the context of only one healthcare setting and it is important, therefore, to have an understanding of the challenges facing these families as they receive transdisciplinary care. The Cancer Plan (DoH 2000) identified a seamless approach to care, which is difficult when care is shared between different healthcare professionals and environments.

However, the last three decades have seen remarkable improvements, both in the approach to the care of the child/adolescent with a malignant disease and in the success of treatments. The enthusiasm and determination to deliver improved evidence-based care for the child/adolescent and their family continues.

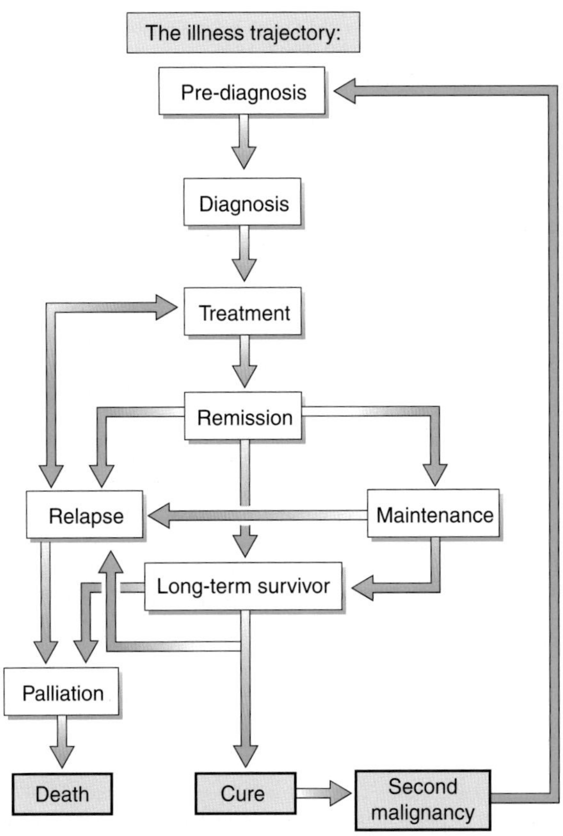

Figure 31.1 • The illness trajectory (reproduced with permission from Corbin & Strauss 1991).

References

Abu-Saad, H., 1993. Paper presented at Royal College of Nursing 1st International Conference in Paediatrics. Paediatric pain management. An intervention study. Cambridge, UK.

Aitkin, T.J., 1992. Gastrointestinal manifestations in the child with cancer. Journal of Pediatric Oncology Nursing 9 (3), 99–109.

Anderson, V., Smibert, E., Ekert, H., Godber, T., 1994. Intellectual, educational and behavioural sequelae after cranial irradiation and chemotherapy. Archives of Diseases in Childhood 70, 476–483.

Bishop, J., 2000. Partnership in care. In: Langton, H. (Ed.), The child with cancer: family centred care. Baillière Tindall, London.

Black, K., 1991. Sudden unexpected death: caring for the parents. Paediatric Nursing 17 (6), 571–574.

Bluebond-Langner, M., 1978. The private worlds of dying children. Princeton University Press, Princeton, NJ.

Bluebond-Langner, M., 1992. Children and death: directions for the 90s. Princeton University Press, Princeton, NJ.

Bradwell, M., Hawkins, J., 2000. Survivorship and rehabilitation. In: Langton, H. (Ed.), The child with cancer; family centred care in practice. Baillière Tindall, London.

Buckman, R., 1992. How to break bad news. A guide for health care professionals. Papermac, London.

Bulley, S., 2000. Impact of treatment on the nursing team. In: Langton, H. (Ed.), The child with cancer; family centred care in practice. Baillière Tindall, London.

Campbell, S.T., Evans, M.A., MacTavish, P., 1995. Guidelines for mouth care. The Paediatric Oncology Nurses Forum. Royal College of Nursing, London.

Chesterfield, P., 1999. Late effects of chemotherapy. In: Gibson, F., Evans, M. (Eds.), Paediatric oncology acute nursing care. Whurr, London.

Christensen, J., Fatchett, D., 2002. Promoting parental use of distraction and relaxation in pediatric oncology patients during invasive procedures. Journal of Pediatric Oncology Nursing 19 (4), 127–132.

Clarke, J.N., Fletcher, P., 2003. Communication issues faced by parents who have a child diagnosed with cancer. Journal of Pediatric Oncology Nursing.

Clarke, S.A., Davies, H., Jenny, M., Glaser, A., Eiser, C., 2005. Parental communication and children's behavior following diagnosis of childhood leukaemia. Psycho-Oncology 14 (4), 274–281.

Clarke-Steffen, L., 1993. Waiting and not knowing: the diagnosis of cancer in a child. Journal of Pediatric Oncology Nursing 10 (4), 146–153.

Clarke-Steffen, L., 1997. Reconstructing reality: family strategies for managing childhood cancer. Journal of Pediatric Nursing 12, 278–287.

Corbin, J.M., Strauss, A., 1991. A nursing model for chronic illness management based upon the trajectory framework. Scholarly Inquiry for Nursing Practice: An International Journal 5, 154–174.

Cox, A., 2000. Discharge – a planned event. In: Langton, H. (Ed.), The child with cancer; family centred care in practice. Baillière Tindall, London.

Curnick, S., Harris, A., 2000. The dying child. In: Langton, H. (Ed.), The child with cancer: family centred care in practice. Baillière Tindall, London.

Department of Health (DoH) 1995. A policy for commissioning cancer services. A report by the expert advisor on cancer of the Chief Medical Officers of England and Wales (the Calman–Hine report). HMSO, London.

Department of Health (DoH) 2000. The cancer plan. DoH, London.

Dickinson, H., 2008. The causes of childhood leukaemia. Editorial. British Medical Journal 330, 1279–1280.

Dowling, J.S., Hockenberry, M., Gregory, R.L., 2003. Sense of humor, childhood cancer stressors, and outcomes of psychosocial adjustment, immune function, and infection. Journal of Pediatric Oncology Nursing 20 (6), 271–292.

Edwards, J., Gibson, F., Richardson, A., et al., 2003. Fatigue in adolescents with and following a cancer diagnosis; developing an evidence base for practice. European Journal of Cancer 39 (18), 2671–2680.

Edwards, J., Gibson, F., Sepion, B., 2004. Cancer-related fatigue in teenagers: a journey of discovery. In: Gibson, F., Soanes, L., Sepion, B. (Eds.), Perspectives in paediatric oncology nursing. Whurr, London.

Eilers, J., Berger, A.M., Petersen, M.C., 1988. Development, testing and application of the oral assessment guide. Oncology Nursing Forum 15, 325–330.

Eiser, C., 1996. The impact of treatment: adolescents' views. In: Selby, P., Bailey, C. (Eds.), Cancer and the adolescent. BMJ Publishing, London.

Eiser, C., Jenney, M.E.M., 1996. Measuring symptomatic benefit and quality of life in paediatric oncology. British Journal of Cancer 73, 1313–1316.

Eiser, C., Morse, R., 2001. A review of measures of quality of life for children with chronic illness. Archives of Diseases in Childhood 84, 205–211.

Eiser, C., Parkyn, T., Havermans, T., McNinch, A., 1994. Parents' recall of the diagnosis of cancer in their child. Psycho-oncology 3, 197–203.

Faithfull, S., 2001. Radiotherapy. In: Corner, J., Bailey, C. (Eds.), Cancer nursing care in context. Blackwell Science, Oxford.

Faulkner, A., Peace, G., O'Keefe, C., 1995. When a child has cancer. Chapman & Hall, London.

Foley, G.V., Hochtrian, D., Hardin Mooney, K., 1993. Nursing care of the child with cancer. WB Saunders, Philadelphia.

Gibson, F., Hayden, S., 2004. Development of an oral care protocol. In: Gibson, F., Soanes, L., Sepion, B. (Eds.), Perspectives in paediatric oncology nursing. Whurr, London.

Gibson, F., Edwards, J., Sepion, B., 2004a. Cancer related fatigue in teenagers: a journey of discovery. In: Gibson, F., Soanes, L., Sepion, B. (Eds.), Perspectives in paediatric oncology nursing. Whurr, London.

Gibson, F., Soanes, L., 2008. Cancer in children and young people. Wiley, Chichester.

Gibson, F., Soanes, L., Sepion, B., 2004b. Perspectives in paediatric oncology nursing. Whurr, London.

Harris, A., Curnick, S., 2000. Care in the community. In: Langton, H. (Ed.), The child with cancer: family centred care in practice. Baillière Tindall, London.

Hawthorne, J., 1995. Understanding the management of nausea and vomiting. Blackwell Science, Oxford.

Hicks, M.D., Lavender, R., 2001. Psychosocial practice trends in pediatric oncology. Journal of Pediatric Oncology Nursing 18 (4), 143–153.

Hicks, J., Bartholomew, J., Ward-Smith, P., Hutto, C.J., 2003. Quality of life among childhood leukaemia patients. Journal of Pediatric Oncology Nursing 20 (4), 192–200.

Hockenberry-Eaton, M., Hinds, P.S., 2000. Fatigue in children and adolescents with cancer. Evolution of a programme of study. Seminars in Oncology Nursing 16, 261–272.

Hollen, P., Hobbie, W., 1996. Decision and risk behaviours of cancer surviving adolescents and their peers. Journal of Pediatric Oncology Nursing 13 (3), 121–134.

Hollis, R., 1997. Childhood cancer into the 21st century. Paediatric Nursing 9 (3), 12–15.

Hollis, R., Morgan, S., 2001. The adolescent with cancer – at the edge of no-man's land. Lancet Oncology 2 (1), 43–48.

Holm, K.E., Patterson, J.M., Gurney, J.G., 2003. Parental involvement and family centred care in the diagnostic and treatment phases of childhood cancer: results from a qualitative study. Journal of Pediatric Oncology Nursing 20 (6), 301–313.

Holmes, S., 1991. The oral complications of specific anticancer therapy. International Journal of Nursing Studies 28 (4), 343–360.

Holmes, S., Mountain, E., 1993. Assessment of oral status: evaluation of three oral assessment guides. Journal of Clinical Nursing 2 (1), 35–40.

Hooker, L., 2004. Teenagers' information needs. In: Gibson, F., Soanes, L., Sepion, B. (Eds.), Perspectives in paediatric oncology nursing. Whurr, London.

Hooker, L., Palmer, S., 1999. Administration of chemotherapy. In: Gibson, F., Evans, M. (Eds.), Paediatric oncology acute nursing care. Whurr, London.

Hooker, L., Williams, J., 1996. Parent-held shared care records: bridging the communication gaps. British Journal of Nursing 5 (12), 738–741.

Hunt, J., 1996. Paediatric oncology outreach nurse specialist: the impact of funding arrangements on their professional role. Paediatric Oncology Nurses Forum. Royal College of Nursing, London.

Ishibashi, A., 2001. The needs of children and adolescents with cancer for information and social support. Cancer Nursing 24 (1), 61–67.

Kars, M.C., Dunijnstee, M.S.H., Pool, A., Van Delden, J.J.M., Grypdonck, M.H.F., 2008. Being there: parenting the child with acute lymphoblastic leukaemia. Journal of Clinical Nursing 17 (12), 1553–1562.

Kelly, D., Gibson, F., 2008. Cancer care for adolescents and young adults. Wiley, Chichester.

Koocher, G.P., O'Malley, J.E., 1985. The Damocles syndrome. McGraw Hill, London.

Kubler Ross E, 1969. On death and dying. MacMillan, New York.

Langton, H., 2000. The child with cancer-family centred care in practice. Ballière Tindall, London.

Le Baron, S., Zeltzer, L.K., LeBaron, C., et al., 1988. Chemotherapy side effects in pediatric oncology patients; drugs, age, sex as risk factors. Medical and Pediatric Oncology 16 (4), 262–268.

Lozowski, S., 1993. Views of childhood cancer survivors. Selected perspectives. Cancer 71 (Suppl), 3354–3357.

McNally, R., Eden, T., 2004. An infectious aetiology for childhood leukaemia: a review of the evidence. British Journal of Haematology 27, 243–263.

Morgan, S., Hubber, D., 2004. Setting up an adolescent service. In: Gibson, F., Soanes, L., Sepion, B. (Eds.), Perspectives in paediatric oncology nursing. Whurr, London.

Muir, K.R., Parkes, S.E., Boon, R., et al., 1992. Shared care in paediatric oncology. Journal of Cancer Care 1, 15–17.

National Institute for Health and Clinical Excellence, 2005. Improving outcomes with children and young people with cancer. NICE, London.

Parry, C., 2003. Embracing uncertainty: an exploration of the experiences of childhood cancer survivors. Qualitative Health Research 13 (1), 227–246.

Patel, N., Sepion, B., Edwards, J., 1997. Development of a shared care programme for children with cancer. Journal of Cancer Nursing 1, 1–4.

Pearman, K., 2002. Chemotherapy-induced nausea and vomiting: a health promotion resource. Paediatric Nursing 14 (6), 30–32.

Pinkerton, C.R., Cushing, P., Sepion, B., 1994. Childhood cancer management: a practical handbook. Chapman & Hall, London.

Price, J., 2003. Information needs of the child with cancer and their family. Cancer Nursing Practice 2 (7), 35–38.

Ritchie, M.A., 1992. Psychosocial functioning of adolescents with cancer. Oncology Nursing Forum 19, 1947–1501.

Ruccione, K., Waskerwitz, M., Buckley, J., et al., 1994. What caused my child's cancer? Parents' responses to an epidemiology study of childhood cancer. Journal of Pediatric Oncology Nursing 11 (2), 71–84.

Selekman, J., 1991. Pediatric rehabilitation from concepts to practice. Pediatric Nursing 17 (1), 26–27.

Sepion, B., 2004. Shared care. In: Gibson, F., Soanes, L., Sepion, B. (Eds.), Perspectives in paediatric oncology nursing. Whurr, London.

Simms, S., Hewitt, N., Vevers, J., 2002. Sibling support in childhood cancer. Paediatric Nursing 14 (7), 20–22.

Suzuki, L.K., Kato, P.M., 2003. Psychosocial support for patients in pediatric oncology: the influences of parents, schools, peers and technology. Journal of Pediatric Oncology Nursing 20 (4), 159–174.

Taylor, J., Muller, D., 1995. Nursing adolescents: research and psychological perspectives. Blackwell Science, London.

Tomlinson, D., Kline, N., 2008. Pediatric oncology nursing: advanced clinical handbook. Springer, New York.

Thompson, J., 2001. The needs of children and adolescents. In: Corner, J., Bailey, C. (Eds.), Cancer nursing in context. Blackwell Science, London.

Thompson, J., 2004. Preface. Personal reflections on the development of paediatric oncology nursing as a speciality. In: Gibson, F., Soanes, L., Sepion, B. (Eds.), Perspectives in paediatric oncology nursing. Whurr, London.

United Kingdom Children Cancer Study Group (UKCCSG), 1987. Report on cancer services for children. UKCCSG, London.

United Kingdom Children's Cancer Study Group (UKCCSG), Late Effects Group, 1995. Long term follow up therapy-based guidelines. UKCCSG, Leicester.

United Kingdom Children Cancer Study Group (UKCCSG), 1997. The resources and requirements of a UKCCSG treatment centre. UKCCSG, London.

Van Eys, J., 1991. The truly cured child. Pediatrician 18, 90–95.

Whelan, J., 2003. Where should teenagers with cancer be treated? European Journal of Cancer 39 (18), 2573–2578.

Zelter, L.K., LeBaron, S., Richie, M., et al., 1988. Can children understand and use a rating scale to quantify somatic symptoms? Journal of Consulting and Clinical Psychology 56 (4), 567–572.

Useful Websites

http://www.bmj.com
http://www.cancerresearchuk.org
http://www.childbereavement.org.uk
http://www.royalmarsden.org
http://www.statistics.gov.uk
http://www.teenagecancer.org
http://www.teencancer.org
http://www.cclg.org
http://www.winstonswish.org.uk

Non-malignant haematological disorders of childhood

32

Kate Khair

ABSTRACT

The aim of this chapter is to discuss the anatomy and physiology of blood and its production and the impact that abnormalities of these systems, which lead to a variety of non-malignant haematological disorders, have on children The most common of these disorders, which are often chronic conditions that may have a genetic inheritance pattern, are described. The nursing care of children with these diseases will be discussed.

LEARNING OUTCOMES

- Demonstrate an understanding of the anatomy and physiology of the haematological system.
- Gain an overview of the common haematological disorders of childhood.
- Understand the role of nurses for caring for children with non-malignant haematological disorders.
- Use relevant contemporary literature to inform the nursing care of children with non-malignant haematological disorders.

Introduction

There are two aspects of haematology which form part of the normal haematological system. The first is haematopoiesis (from the Greek, haem = blood and poiesis = to make) which involves the general aspects of blood cell formation in the bone marrow, the second is haemostasis (also from Greek haem = blood and stasis = stagnation) which is the process of blood clotting. Abnormalities within either of these two systems lead to disorders which cause significant clinical symptoms of bruising, bleeding, anaemia or infection. Some of these conditions can be acute, e.g. ITP, although the majority, e.g. sickle cell disease or haemophilia, are chronic conditions, which used to be fatal in childhood but with contemporary management can also now be seen as chronic diseases of adolescence and adulthood. Children with these conditions receive nursing care at home, given by their parents (Burnes et al 2008, Vidler 1999) and themselves, as well as by community nurses, in local general hospitals, and also in tertiary care centres which may be either paediatric or haematological, or both. There are regional haemoglobinopathy centres and haemophilia comprehensive care centres which provide 24-hour access and advice about treatment of children with these complex conditions.

Anatomy and physiology of the haematological system

Haemopoiesis

Haemopoiesis occurs from the first few weeks of embryo development predominantly in the liver and spleen. In later fetal life (at about 6–7 months of gestation) the bone marrow takes over and during childhood and adulthood becomes the source of blood cell production (Hoffbrand et al 2001). In children the bone marrow in all bones is active in cell production; in adolescence as bone growth ceases cell production occurs only in the sternum, vertebrae, pelvis and ribs. The sternum and pelvis are the sites most commonly used for bone marrow aspiration to establish diagnosis of bone marrow disease/dysfunction.

Haemopoiesis begins with a stem cell which gives rise to separate lineages and develops into a variety of cells which in turn become erythrocytes (red blood cells (RBC)) leucocytes (white blood cells (WBC)) and thrombocytes (platelets) (Fig. 32.1). The normal ranges for these cells are dependant upon age and sex (Table 32.1). The specific actions of these cells are discussed below.

Erythrocytes

Erythrocytes are bi-concave discs which have a lifespan of approximately 120 days. They transport haemoglobin which carries oxygen around the body. As the RBC grows old it becomes fragile, the cell ruptures and the haemoglobin is broken down into haemosiderin and bile pigments which are excreted by the liver.

DOI: 10.1016/B978-0-7020-3183-0.10032-3

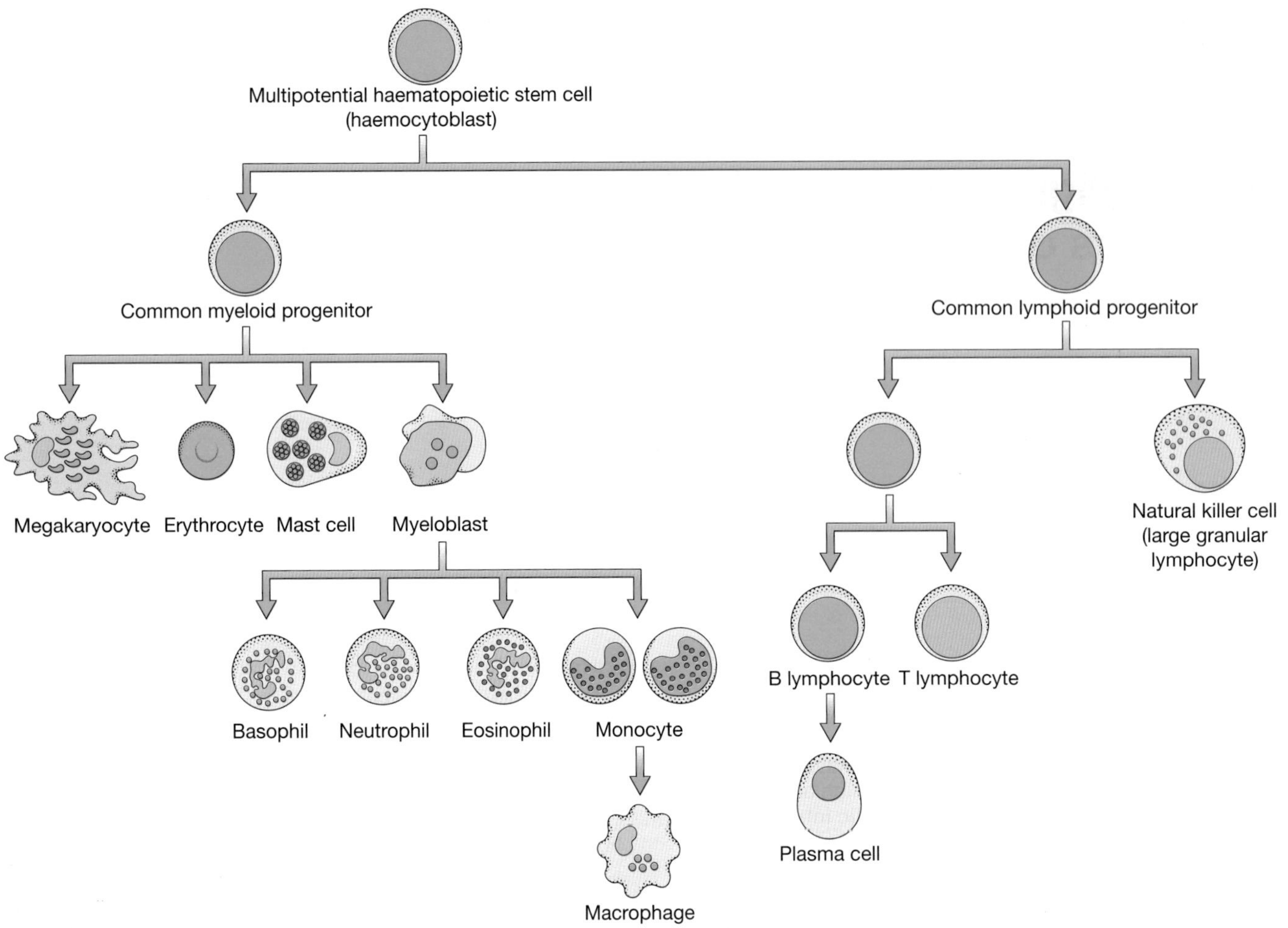

Fig. 32.1 • Haemopoiesis

Table 32.1 Normal FBC ranges

Age	Hb (g/dL)	MCV (fL)	Neutrophils (10^9/L)	Lymphocytes (10^9/L)	Platelets (10^9/L)
Birth	14.9–23.7	100–125	2.7–14.4	2–7.3	150–450
2 weeks	13.4–19.8	88–110	1.5–5.4	2.8–9.1	170–500
2 months	9.4–13.0	84–98	0.7–4.8	3.3–10.3	210–650
6 months	10.0–13.0	73–84	1.0–6.0	3.1–11.5	210–560
1 year	10.1–13.0	70–82	1.0–8.0	3.4–10.5	200–550
2–6 years	11.5–13.8	72–87	1.5–8.5	1.8–8.4	210–490
6–12 years	11.1–14.7	76–90	1.5–8.0	1.5–5.0	170–450
Adult ♀	12.2–15.1	77–94	1.5–6.0	1.5–4.5	180–430
Adult ♂	12.1–16.6	77–92	1.5–6.0	1.5–4.5	180–430

Reproduced, with permission, from Oxford Handbook of Clinical Haematology, 3rd edn.

Leucocytes

There are five types of white cells (leucocytes): lymphocytes, monocytes, neutrophils, eosinophils and basophils. Each of the subgroups of WBC plays a different role in immune processes and are involved in inflammation, phagocytosis, allergy and healing. All of these cells have a nucleus but have a much shorter lifespan than the RBC, being measurable in the blood for a matter of hours; however WBC leave the blood and move into tissues where they act as a reservoir to fight infection where they die after a matter of a few days (Campbell et al 1995 p 610)

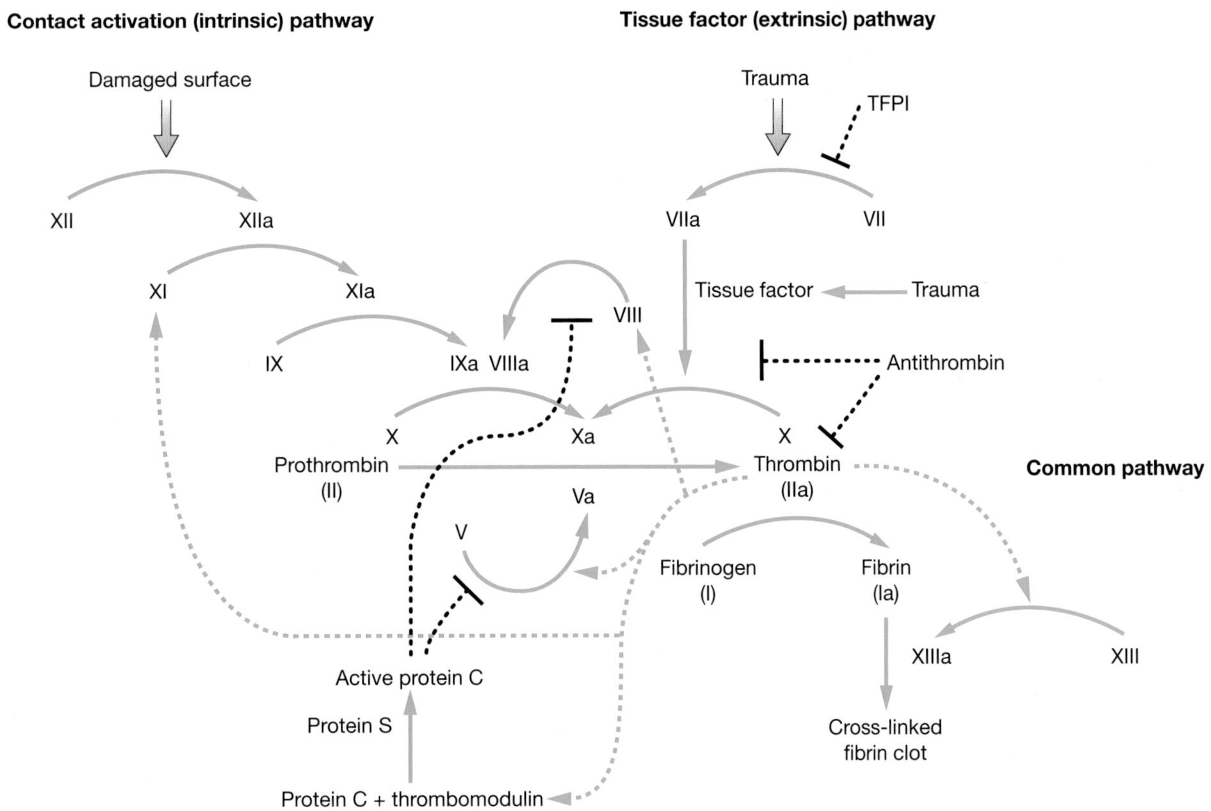

Fig. 32.2 • Coagulation cascade

Thrombocytes

Thrombocytes (platelets) are the smallest cells, originating from megakaryocytes in the bone marrow, and have a lifespan of 8–10 days. They are round discs, which are able to change shape due to their structure, they adhere to each other as well as coagulation factors to cause a platelet plug at the site of damage to the blood vessel. The surface of the platelet is coated with glycoproteins which are particularly important for adhesion and aggregation and which are fundamental for the formation of the platelet plug. Platelets are instrumental in protection from and treatment of bleeding disorders

Coagulation

Coagulation is a complex cascade of actions, involving a variety of mechanisms from blood vessel wall constriction and platelet adhesion to activation of coagulation factors which adhere to the platelets to form a clot to stop bleeding. If this mechanism was left 'unchecked' thrombosis would occur; to prevent this, coagulation factor inhibitors 'switch off' the coagulation cascade once bleeding has ceased. The coagulation cascade is defined as three interdependent parts: the intrinsic, the extrinsic and the common pathways. The intrinsic pathway begins with 'contact activation' with factor XII becoming activated, this converts factors XI, IX, and VIII into their active parts which work with factor X to initiate clot formation. At the same time the extrinsic pathway generates a 'thrombin burst' when tissue factor is released at the site of injury: activated factor VII circulates in high levels, in turn further activating factors VIII, and factors V and X, within the common pathway where finally thrombin acts to convert fibrinogen to fibrin and a haemostatic plug is formed.

With the exception of von Willebrand factor (which is produced in the endothelium) coagulation factors are produced or synthesised by the liver, therefore liver disease can present with and be complicated by coagulation disorders (Fig. 32.2).

Interpretation of blood results

Full blood count

The full blood count (FBC) is a broad screening test looking at bone marrow cell production which screens for red cell, white cell and platelet abnormalities. FBC is a relatively easy test to perform, but normal ranges will vary from hospital to hospital. FBC results should be interpreted with knowledge of the normal range of the hospital as well as the child's age, sex and ethnicity as these will affect the results, e.g. the haemoglobin varies between the sexes and with age.

Bone marrow aspiration

Bone marrow aspiration (where the cells of the bone marrow are aspirated in a liquid form into a syringe) and bone marrow trephine (where a core of bone marrow is removed through a large bore needle) are tests to examine the cellular content (aspirate) and the structure (trephine) of the bone marrow. In children these are most commonly performed under general anaesthesia from the posterior iliac crest (Sepion 1990) as a diagnostic test when bone marrow failure, leukaemia, metabolic or immunological conditions are suspected. The bone marrow aspirate is spread onto a slide and is easily examined using a microscope; diseases affecting the marrow can be easily diagnosed.

Clotting screen

The clotting screen is a screen of the three aspects of coagulation described above. The activated partial prothrombin test (APTT) is a test of the intrinsic pathway; the prothrombin time (PT) is a test of the extrinsic pathway, whilst the thrombin time (TT) tests the conversion of fibrinogen to fibrin in the common pathway. If the clotting screen suggest that a coagulation disorder may be the cause of bruising/bleeding further investigations are required. Interpretation of an abnormality in the initial coagulation screen and further tests required are detailed in Table 32.2. Not all haematology laboratories will be able to perform all of these tests; referral to a regional paediatric haemophilia centre should be considered if an inherited coagulation disorder is suspected.

Non-malignant haematological conditions

Non-malignant haematological conditions lead to a variety of disorders, which present throughout childhood. The majority of these conditions are inherited, e.g. sickle cell anaemia and haemophilia, and usually present in infancy and early childhood. Acquired diseases, which may present in later childhood and adolescence are often severe and may be life threatening causing problems of infection and bleeding. The commonest non-malignant disorders seen in childhood are discussed below; further information on these disorders can be obtained from the paediatric haematology reference books listed in the bibliography.

Bone marrow failure syndromes

Bone marrow failure can be either congenital or acquired. Although extremely rare the commonest form of congenital bone marrow failure is Fanconi anaemia (FA), which is inherited in an autosomal manner and is associated with growth retardation, defects of the skeleton, kidneys or skin, with occasional mental retardation (Hoffbrand et al 2001 p 91). Children with FA usually present at around 5–10 years of age

Table 32.2 Interpretation and further investigation of coagulation screen results

PT	APTT	TT	Possible abnormality	Further investigation required
↑	N	N	Factor VII deficiency (extrinsic pathway) Liver disease Vitamin K deficiency	Measurement of PT based factors
N	↑	N	Deficiency of factor VIII (haemophilia or vWD) factor IX, XI, XII or contact factors (intrinsic pathway) Lupus anticoagulant or other coagulation factor inhibitor	Measurement of APTT based factors vWD screen DRVVT, Exner
N	N	↑	Hypofibrinogenaemia Dysfibrinogenaemia	Reptilase time and other thrombin time corrections
↑	↑	N	Deficiency of factor II, V, X (common pathway) Vitamin K deficiency Liver disease Massive transfusion Oral anticoagulants	PT and APTT based factors, INR
N	↑	↑	Heparin	Reptilase time and other thrombin time corrections
↑	↑	↑	Disseminated intravascular coagulation Large amounts heparin Severe hypofibrinogenaemia	D-dimers, reptilase time and other thrombin time corrections
N	N	N	All tests normal but history of bleeding – consider: • Factor XIII deficiency • Mild platelet disorders	vWD screen Factor XIII screen/activity Platelet function tests

PT = prothrombin time; APTT = activated partial thromboplastin time; TT = thrombin time; N = within normal range; ↑ = prolonged; vWD = von Willebrand's disease; DRVVT = dilute Russell Viper venom time; INR = international ratio.

Adapted, with permission, from Khair et al 2003.

Table 32.3 Haemoglobin gene variants

	Haemoglobin variant	Clinical features
Fetal haemoglobin (HbF)	Normal feature of infancy Switch to adult Hb (HbA) at 6 months of age	Hereditary persistence of HbF caused by genetic abnormalities – leads to anaemia.
Haemoglobin A (HbA)	Normal adult haemoglobin	None
Haemoglobin C (HbC)	Most frequently seen in children of west African decent	Mild haemolytic anaemia with splenomegaly
Haemoglobin D (HbD)		No haematological abnormality to mild haemolytic anaemia
Haemoglobin E (HbE)	Most frequently seen in children of south east Asian decent	Mild hypochromic anaemia
Haemoglobin S (HbS)	Sickle haemoglobin	Sickle cell trait (HbAS) – not usually clinically significant Additional care with anaesthesia Sickle cell disease (HbSS) – severe haemolytic anaemia with sickle cell crises including stroke in young children
Haemoglobin SC (HbSC)		Particular risk of thrombosis and pulmonary embolism
α thalassaemia	Most commonly seen in children from Mediterranean/Asian/ Oriental descent	Can be mild causing moderately severe hypochromic anaemia but in severe cases is incompatible with life, can cause hydrops fetalis and intra uterine death
β thalassaemia	Most commonly seen in children from Mediterranean/Asian/ Oriental decent	Severe anaemia from 6 months of age requiring transfusion Hepatosplenomegaly Infections Osteoporosis

with increasing signs of bone marrow failure that may include pancytopenia (reduction in blood count of red and white blood cells and platelets) or leukaemia.

Aplastic anaemia (AA) also presents with pancytopenia which may be either congenital or acquired. Causes of acquired AA include infection, drugs (especially chemotherapy) and exposure to radiation or pesticides. Kostmann syndrome is rare, also known as severe congenital neutropenia (SCN), and usually detected soon after birth when severe and/or life-threatening infection occurs (Ancliff 2003).

Osteopetrosis (literally 'stone bone') is a rare inherited disorder where bones harden becoming brittle. Mild osteopetrosis is usually asymptomatic but severe forms result in stunted growth, deformity, anaemia from bone marrow failure, blindness and deafness due to increased pressure on nerves from bone overgrowth (Hamdan et al 2006).

Haemoglobinopathy – in infancy children have a variant of haemoglobin known as fetal haemoglobin or HbF. After about 6 months of age they begin to express adult haemoglobin (HbA). Children inherit two sets of haemoglobin genes, one set from each parent. In haemoglobinopathies there is an abnormality in one or both sets of the haemoglobin genes giving rise to an abnormal haemoglobin molecule, which leads to diseases known collectively as haemoglobinopathies.

One of the most significant genetic abnormalities in haemoglobin causes sickle cell anaemia, which is the most common genetic defect in England, affecting 1:2000 births (Dick 2007) this is most commonly seen in people of Afro-Caribbean decent. The abnormal haemoglobin (HbS) is fragile and unable to carry oxygen effectively, the red cells 'sickle' and breakdown causing symptoms such as pain, anaemia and stroke. Children with only one copy of this gene are said to have sickle cell trait (HbAS). Sickle cell disease occurs when two copies of the HbS gene are inherited (HbSS) – one from each parent. See Table 32.3 for a list of haemoglobin gene variants.

Thalassaemia is a group of disorders of the globin genes where one or more of the genes is either missing or is inactive, this is most commonly seen in children of Mediterranean and Asian decent (Modell et al 2001). There are two subtypes of thalassaemia: α (alpha) and β (beta) thalassaemia. The α subtype causes moderately severe anaemia and splenomegaly unless two copies of the abnormal α-thalassaemia haemoglobin are inherited which results in incompatibility with life often resulting in inter uterine death with hydrops fetalis (Yang & Li 2009). The β subtype is a much more clinically severe disease presenting in infancy with anaemia, hepatosplenomegaly, bone marrow hyperplasia, infection and osteoporosis (Clarke & Higgins 2000).

There is now an national newborn haemoglobinopathy screening programme, with all neonates in the UK undergoing haemoglobin analysis as part of the neonatal screening programme (previously known as the Guthrie test) (NHS 2006). This has resulted in 'at risk' children being diagnosed at an average of 6 weeks before they become symptomatic (Bain 2009).

Bleeding disorders

The disorders which result in bleeding can be mild to severe, inherited or acquired, as a result of bone marrow abnormalities in platelet production or function or in a reduction or absence of any of the coagulation factors. The commonest causes of bleeding are discussed below as either disorders of platelets or coagulation.

Platelet disorders

Thrombocytopenia

The full blood count will show if there is thrombocytopenia; this should be repeated to confirm this finding. The commonest cause of thrombocytopenia in children is immune thrombocytopenic purpura (ITP), which is often occurs following viral infections (Vora & Makrish 2001). Whilst bruising is common severe bleeding is rare if the platelet count is above 20×10^9/L. If there is persistent thrombocytopenia, referral to a paediatric haematology centre should be considered, aiming to exclude a congenital platelet disorder, leukaemia or a bone marrow failure syndrome. Congenital thrombocytopenias are rare but may present with symptoms of bruising or bleeding soon after birth. Thrombocytopenia with absent radii ('TAR syndrome') is an autosomal recessive disorder characterised by bilateral absence of the radii, which is clinically obvious at birth (Al-Jefri et al 2000). Wiskott–Aldrich syndrome is an X-linked immune deficiency disorder associated with bacterial infections and/or eczema (Mullen et al 1993). Bernard–Soulier syndrome is an autosomal recessive disorder most commonly seen in consanguineous families which causes mild to severe bleeding in both boys and girls (George et al 1981).

Functional

These are platelet disorders with normal platelet numbers but abnormal function and can be minor causing bleeding following surgery, through to life threatening such as Glanzmann's thrombasthenia. Transient abnormalities in platelet function causing easy bruising are common and are often associated with the use of anti-platelet drugs such as non-steroidal anti-inflammatory drugs or aspirin. Other drugs that are known to affect platelet function are listed in Table 32.4.

Table 32.4 Drugs which may affect platelet function

Cytotoxic therapy
Ethanol
Chloramphenicol
Arsenic
Benzene
Non-steroidal anti-inflammatory drugs
Aspirin
Rifampicin
Penicillin
Sulphonamides
Trimethoprim
Diazepam
Sodium valproate
Carbamazepine
Frusemide
Tolbutamide
Digoxin
Heparin
Warfarin
Methyldopa
Oxyprenolol
Quinine

Inherited platelet function defects are very rare, the most severe of these is Glanzmann's thrombasthenia – an autosomal recessive disorder which results in severe often spontaneous bleeding usually from the mucous membranes, which can be life threatening (Hardisty 2000). Platelet storage pool disorders, where there is a deficiency in the nucleotide content of the platelet, and platelet release defects, where the nucleotides cannot be released properly, both result in mild to moderate bruising and bleeding following trauma or surgery.

Coagulation disorders

Von Willebrand disease (vWD) is the commonest inherited bleeding disorder with an incidence of 1:100 to 1:1000. The inheritance varies according to the subtype and affects boys and girls equally. There are three major subtypes of vWD; bleeding in type 1 and 2 is usually mild but in type 3, which is inherited in an autosomal recessive manner, there is usually severe bleeding often from mucous membranes from early childhood resulting in mouth and nose bleeds (Mannucci 2001).

Haemophilia is an X-linked condition in which boys experience bruising and bleeding which can be severe (Khair et al 2003). Haemophilia A (classical haemophilia, a deficiency of factor VIII) affects about 1:10,000 boys, whilst haemophilia B (Christmas disease or factor IX deficiency) affects about 1:50,000 boys. The bruising/bleeding is dependent upon the level of factor in the plasma, with the severest bleeding occurring in those with the lowest factor levels. Although considered an inherited disorder, approximately 1 in 3 boys with haemophilia have no previous family history with there being a new genetic mutation in their FVIII or FIX gene. Girls who are haemophilia carriers may also suffer bruising/bleeding and mennorhagia when in adolescence as they may also have low factor levels.

Scenario 1

Jennifer is a 4-year-old girl who has sickle cell disease. She has been admitted to the ward from the A&E department with acute chest syndrome and is accompanied by her mum. Jennifer has been 'off colour' for the last 4 days with fever and cough, her brother has similar symptoms though not sickle cell disease.

- What framework would you use to assess Jennifer?
- What observations do you need to do?
- What do you expect these observations to be?
- Is Jennifer's condition mild, moderate or severe?
- Is there anything in the history that would give concern?
- What care would you expect to be initiated?
- What ongoing care does Jennifer need?

The other coagulation disorders are very rare compared with haemophilia and vWD; however they can cause life-threatening bleeding. Deficiency of factor II, V, VII or X can cause significant bleeding when autosomal recessive inheritance has occurred, however carriers of these disorders can also experience mild bleeding/bruising (Bolton-Maggs et al 1995). Factor XI deficiency is most commonly seen in children of Ashkenazi Jewish decent; the bleeding tendency is usually mild (Collins et al 1995). Factor XII deficiency is commonly seen but rarely if ever predisposes to bruising/bleeding. Factor XIII deficiency is an autosomal recessive condition which presents in the neonatal period with umbilical cord bleeding, delayed cord separation or intracranial haemorrhage (Anwar & Miloszeski 1999). Disorders of fibrinogen can be both in quantity and/or quality, often presenting in early childhood with bruising and bleeding whilst dysfibrinogenaemia may also cause thrombosis (Lak et al 1999).

Acquired coagulation disorders are commonly seen in children who are unwell. Vitamin K deficiency is the most common acquired bleeding disorder of childhood being seen in liver disease, gastrointestinal disorders and cystic fibrosis. Neonates who have not received vitamin K prophylaxis at birth can develop haemorrhagic disease of the newborn which usually presents in the first few days of life (Sutor et al 1999) and is preventable with the administration of IM vitamin K at birth. Children with severe liver disease may have abnormal coagulation due to impaired synthesis of coagulation factors. Disseminated intravascular coagulation is uncontrolled activation of coagulation, causing coagulation factor and platelet consumption and usually occurs in children who are critically ill. It is most commonly seen in children in intensive care units.

In summary, the diagnosis of haematological diseases of childhood is predominantly a clinical laboratory test based on sound knowledge of the haematological system and the symptoms produced when this fails. Nursing and medical care is often supportive for what are often life-long and potentially life-threatening diseases.

Management of children with haematological disorders

The aims of management of any malignant haematological disease are applicable to all the conditions discussed in this chapter, although there are some disease specific considerations that need to be taken into account. Management aims are:

- to monitor the child's vital signs and overall condition
- to minimise invasive investigations and treatments
- to deliver treatments, many of which are intravenous, safely
- to minimise the risk of side effects and complications of treatment
- to evaluate the effectiveness of treatment
- to communicate effectively with the child and family
- to provide clear discharge advice
- to provide on going, home/community-based care.

The haematological conditions discussed in this chapter are likely to be life-long, potentially life-threatening disorders which may be inherited and have genetic implications for the child, their current family and their future family. Children with these conditions are likely to be treated with blood or its constituents, the rationale for this best practice in administration and monitoring are described in Table 32.5. Specific requirements for some children/conditions are addressed later in the chapter.

Table 32.5 Transfusion of blood products including coagulation factors

Procedure	Process	Rationale
Preparation of child and family	Inform child and family that transfusion is necessary, the reason for the transfusion and what this entails Document consent Ensure venous access is secured	To gain understanding and to document consent To enable transfusion to commence
Prescription	Blood products *must not* be administered unless prescribed by a doctor The prescription should include the infusion rate, volume and infusion time of < 4 hours If antihistamine pre-medication is prescribed administer prior to transfusion	Recommendation of British Committee for Haematology Standards in Blood Transfusion Task Force Reduced risk of fluid overload and infection Reduce allergic reactions
Transfusion preparation	Arrange for collection of blood products from blood bank or pharmacy On receipt of blood products onto the ward the collection slip and/or other documentation should be signed Check that the child's details are the same on the blood product, the prescription and the child's wristband	To ensure product on ward in timely manner to be administered to the child To provide audit trail of safe transfusion practice To ensure the correct product is being administered to the correct child
Infusion	Observe the child closely for the first 30 minutes of blood product infusion (not necessary for coagulation factors) Record date and time of start of infusion Monitor vital signs – temperature, pulse, blood pressure as per local (hospital/unit) policy (not necessary in coagulation factors) Monitor infusion site if infusion is being given peripherally	This is when transfusion reactions are most likely to occur To monitor complications such as allergic reactions To monitor for extravasation and phlebitis
Complete transfusion	Remove blood product administration set Dispose of giving set and bag	To reduce risk of infection To ensure safe disposal

Adapted, with permission, from Great Ormond Street Hospital for Children NHS Trust, Clinical Practice Guidelines for Coagulation factors, Cryoprecipitate; Platelet and Red Cell Products transfusion. Available at www.ich.ucl.ac.uk

Table 32.6 Bone marrow failure syndromes seen in children

Aplastic anaemia
Fanconi anaemia
Myelodysplasia syndromes
Schwachman's
Diamond–Blackfan anaemia
Kostmann's syndrome
Osteopetrosis
Dyskeratosis congenita

Bone marrow failure

Although rare, the commonest bone marrow (BM) failures syndromes seen in children are listed in Table 32.6. Depending upon the degree of BM failure children will present with a variety of signs and symptoms which may include anaemia, bleeding and infection. Anaemia in BM failure is caused by low haemoglobin production. Bleeding is due to a thrombocytopenia and/or over production of immature platelets, which do not work effectively, and infection is due to leucopoenia. A combination of low levels of haemoglobin, platelets and white cells is known as pancytopenia.

Characteristics of anaemia

- Pallor
- Hypoxia
- Lack of energy/lethargy
- Shortness of breath – particularly on exercise.

Characteristics of thrombocytopenia

- Petechiae/bruising
- Wet petechiae
- Mouth/nose bleeding.

Characteristics of leucopoenia

- Recurrent infection which may be viral in origin
- Sepsis
- Overwhelming bacterial infection
- Fungal infection.

Specific treatment

The initial management of BM failure is supportive care: including blood product support when red cell and platelet transfusions are given. The care of children receiving blood products is detailed in Table 32.5. These should be used to relieve symptoms rather than to treat the FBC – children with BM failure may have a platelet count which runs in single figures, if there is no bleeding this should be monitored and only treated if they become symptomatic or are to undergo surgery.

Appropriate anti-infective therapy should be used; infection control measures should be strictly adhered to including avoidance of large groups of other children who may be carrying viral infections such as chickenpox. Bone marrow transplantation may be used as a cure for these children (see below).

Haemoglobinopathy

Sickle cell disease

Children with sickle cell disease (SCD) present with a variety of symptoms ranging from painful episodes of 'sickle cell crisis' due to occlusion of blood vessels following sickling of red cells; acute chest syndrome, which may be caused by infection (Vichinsky et al 2000); liver disease due to gallstones (Bond et al 1987); leg ulcers; stroke, which most commonly presents between the ages of 2 and 5 years of age (Ohene-Frempong et al 1998); priapism in adolescent boys and, in unvaccinated undiagnosed children, rapid death from pneumococcal sepsis.

Treatment of children with SCD will be individualised and based on their symptoms. All children in the UK are now vaccinated against pneumococcal infection, but it remains of even greater importance that children with SCD are vaccinated against this as well as all routine childhood vaccinations as this will protect them from infections and reduce the risk of fever and acute chest syndrome. Additionally in those children who are (blood) transfusion dependant, vaccination against hepatitis B should also be offered. Reduced function of the spleen (splenic hypofunction) caused by infarction within the spleen by sickled red cells also leads to increased susceptibility to infection, therefore children with SCD are offered penicillin prophylaxis in an attempt to reduce mortality from sepsis (Gaston et al 1986).

Children with SCD suffer recurrent painful episodes (crises) which are caused by vaso-occlusion; these can vary from mild occlusion with mild to moderate pain which can be managed at home with mild analgesia such as paracetamol or ibuprofen, through to severe crises which requires hospitalisation and codeine, pethidine or morphine administration. A child-focused pain score such as the faces pain rating scale (Wong & Baker 1998) should be used to assess pain and monitor analgesia response. Intravenous fluids should be given if there is dehydration as this will further exacerbate the crisis.

Acute chest syndrome is a potentially fatal complication of SCD which may present with acute respiratory failure which may require intensive care and ventilation. On admission to the ward the child should have a full respiratory assessment (see Chapter 27) including oxygen saturation testing. Sleep studies should be undertaken to observe for obstructive sleep apnoea, an echocardiogram should be undertaken to look for pulmonary hypertension which is part of chronic sickle lung conditions. If present, a transfusion programme may be initiated. Hydroxyurea, a chemotherapy agent, has been shown to be effective in reducing the recurrence of acute chest syndrome and is used effectively in many children with SCD (Mueller 2008).

Stroke, which is caused by cerebral ischaemic damage, occurs most often in children aged 2–5 years with as many as

11% of children with SCD suffering clinically evident stroke (Ohene-Frempong et al 1998). Stroke in SCD is thought to be caused by stenotic lesions in the cerebral arteries, which can be detected as high blood flow abnormalities on transcranial Doppler (TCD) scanning. All children with SCD should undergo annual TCD scanning as there is evidence that exchange transfusion programmes in children with high blood flow abnormalities can prevent stroke. It is now UK practice for children aged over 3 to have at least annual TCD scanning. Additional risk factors in children with SCD who have had a stroke include low haemoglobin levels and obstructive sleep apnoea, both of which lead to hypoxia. Children who have had strokes are most commonly managed on a transfusion programme throughout childhood and adolescence, this can lead to iron overload which will itself need management (see Thalassaemia below). Children with SCD who have suffered a stroke should be assessed in a specialist sickle centre where they can be seen by a paediatric neurologist for initial care, they will require intensive rehabilitation from a multidisciplinary team including nursing, physiotherapy, psychology and occupational therapy.

Priapism is a prolonged (lasting more than 3 hours), painful, unwanted erection, commonly seen in adolescent and young adult males that can be a surgical emergency. Minor attacks can be treated with analgesia, emptying the bladder and taking a warm bath. In severe attacks an urgent urological opinion should be sought. Irrigation of the penis with epinephrine is often an effective treatment but if this fails emergency venous shunting surgery is necessary. Liver disease is most commonly caused by gallstones and obstructive jaundice; appropriate surgical intervention should be offered if this becomes problematical.

Characteristics of sickle cell crisis

- Pain
- Respiratory distress ± fever in chest syndrome
- Acute anaemia
- Priapism
- Stroke.

Specific treatment

- Analgesia
- Keep warm
- Keep well hydrated – including IV fluid administration if necessary
- Full respiratory assessment for children with chest syndrome (see Chapter 27) including:
  - oxygen saturation monitoring and therapy
  - ventilation if indicated
  - overnight sleep studies in non-acute phase of illness
  - pulmonary function testing
- Full neurological assessment for children with stroke
- Transfusion programmes for children with stroke and frequent sickle crises
- Annual transcranial Doppler scanning in all children aged > 3 years
- Bone marrow transplantation.

Scenario 2

John is a 7-year-old boy who has severe haemophilia A. He is accompanied to the ward by his father following a football injury causing an acute knee bleed which had occurred on the previous day. John usually has prophylaxis every other day and before sport given by his mum who is currently in hospital following the birth of a baby. Dad reports that he had three attempts to treat John after the injury, he only managed to give about half the dose as the needle 'tissued'.

- What framework would you use to assess John's joint?
- What observations do you need to do?
- What do you expect these observations to be?
- Is John's condition mild, moderate or severe?
- Is there anything in the history that would give concern?
- What care would you expect to be initiated?
- What ongoing care does John need?

Thalassaemia

Children with thalassaemia are now surviving into adulthood with good health and are able to lead essentially normal lives (Weatherall & Clegg 2001). However, thalassaemia remains a severe disease that requires life-long management and care and, even with the best care, complications such as growth failure can occur. Standard treatment of regular blood transfusions given every 2–3 weeks to correct anaemia enables normal growth and development, limits splenomegaly and the bone marrow expansion which causes the typical facial bone features of thalassaemia and prevents cardiac failure (Standards for the clinical care of children and adults with thalassaemia in the UK 2008).

Treatment of children with thalassaemia will be individualised and based on symptom management. The majority of children are transfusion dependent by the age of 3. This means that they are anaemic, usually with a haemoglobin of <7 g/dl without transfusion. This leads to fatigue, poor appetite, developmental delay, failure to thrive and cardiac failure. A transfusion programme that keeps the haemoglobin >10 g/dl is usually successful in alleviating most of these symptoms, although this requires frequent hospital attendances for cross matching and transfusing. A small number of children may be transfused at home following parental training (Madgwick & Yardumian 1999).

Repeated transfusions lead to iron overload which can be fatal. Unbound iron that is in the plasma is toxic to cardiac and liver tissue, which can result in cardiomyopathy, cardiac arrhythmia and failure. There can be liver fibrosis leading to cirrhosis, liver failure and liver cancer. There is good evidence that these side effects of transfusion can be overcome through the use of iron chelation therapy where free iron in the plasma is bound to the chelating agent and is excreted via the urine or faeces. The commonest of these chelating therapies is desferoxamine, which is given as an 8–12-hour subcutaneous infusion 5–6 times per week. This has been shown to be effective in reducing the toxic effects of iron, reducing liver and cardiac toxicity (Brittenham et al 1994). However, this places a significant burden upon the child and family with time taken to site needles and infuse products being cited as reasons for poor continued adherence to treatment (Telfer et al 2005). Recent enhancements to improve adherence include 'balloon pumps' which automatically infuse and oral chelation agents, two of which have been licensed for use in children in the UK.

Specific treatment

Blood transfusion

- Pre-arranged transfusions should be given following guidelines in Table 32.6.
- Peripheral cannulation should be undertaken only by experienced staff.
- Central venous access devices may be implanted.

Chelation

- Subcutaneous overnight infusions 5–6 nights per week:
  - subcutaneous infusion needles
  - mechanical pump/infusor
  - monitor treatment success by measuring serum ferritin levels
- Bone marrow transplantation.

Bleeding disorders

Although in itself rare, the commonest significant bleeding disorder is haemophilia which causes bleeding mainly in the weight bearing (ankle and knee) joints. Children with haemophilia will present with acutely hot, painful joint swelling (haemarthrosis) usually preceded by trauma. The joint will be flexed (as this reduces pressure within the joint and is less painful) with a limited range of movement. These are treated initially in three ways: by replacement of the missing coagulation factor, by administration of analgesia (avoiding non-steroidal anti-inflammatory drugs as these affect platelet function and worsen bleeding) and implementing physiotherapy guidelines of PRICE (see Table 32.7). Recurrent haemarthrosis leads to significant arthritic joint damage, therefore children with severe haemophilia, who are most likely to have bleeding are treated with prophylactic factor replacement therapy. This is given as an individualised, tailored dosing/frequency regimen enabling children to participate in sporting activity with reduced risk of bleeding (Khair & Geraghty 2007).

Nose and mouth bleeds are common in children with coagulation disorders following trauma and occur spontaneously in children with platelet abnormalities. Usual first aid measures for managing nose bleeds (compression of the nose, application of ice packs, sitting with head forward) should be instituted. Mouth bleeds are more difficult as they often fail to respond to first aid measures, however giving an ice lolly may help as this reduces the blood flow to the mouth due to vasoconstriction secondary to cold therapy! In many children this proves ineffective and administration of intra-nasal or intravenous desmopressin (Khair et al 2007), tranexamic acid (an anti-fibrinolytic drug which slows down clot breakdown), clotting factors or platelet transfusions may be necessary. In children with severe platelet disorders activated factor VII may be a useful adjunctive therapy and may avoid exposure to blood products (Almeida et al 2003).

Table 32.7 Management of soft tissue injury/joint bleeds with PRICE

Protection	Use of splints, slings, crutches as applicable. Splints should be individually made, reflecting the degree of swelling and position of the affected joint. Children should be instructed in the use of crutches by an appropriately trained health care professional.
Rest	Use of 'relative rest' or 'controlled activity'. Bed rest is virtually impossible in children with painful, swollen joints, 'sofa rest' whilst watching television should be encouraged. Controlled activity should be introduced once the joint has settled and normal mobility has been regained.
Ice	Use of cold therapy, either through cold wraps (gel filled refrigerated bandages) or cold compresses where crushed ice can be applied to the affected area for short, timed, periods. The skin should be protected from contact with the ice by use of a towel or pillowcase.
Compression	Use of supportive elastic wraps or bandage, applied loosely so as not to constrict the limb causing more oedema, swelling and pain.
Elevation	Supported elevation (sofa rest for legs, pillows supporting arms) for up to 72 hours following injury. Compression should not be used at same time as elevation.

Characteristics of bleeding disorders

Joint bleeds

- Pain
- Swollen, hot joint
- Decreased range of movement
- Unable to weight bear.

Nose/mouth bleeds

- Last > 20 minutes
- Shown no signs of clotting
- Child becoming hypovolaemic:
  - tachycardia
  - hypotensive
  - pale
  - sweaty.

Specific treatment

Joint bleeds

- Use PRICE therapy
- Nurse in position most comfortable to child

- Administer appropriate analgesia
- Administer coagulation factors as prescription
- Monitor range of movement and joint size to ensure bleed has ceased.

Mouth bleeds

- Use local first aid measures including cold therapy if possible
- Monitor airway – clots in throat may obstruct airway
- Administer coagulation factors/platelets as prescription
- Continue tranexamic acid for 5 days post bleed
- Give dietary advice – soft diet until bleeding fully ceased, avoid crisps!

Blood-borne viruses

Pathogens which can be transmitted through blood and/or blood products are hepatitis (A, B and C), cytomegalovirus (CMV), human T-cell leukaemia viruses (HTLV) human immunodeficiency virus (HIV) and variant Creutzfeldt–Jakob disease (vCJD). In all cases except vCJD tests have been developed to screen donors who are excluded from blood donation if they test positive, therefore the risk of being infected with these viruses from UK donated blood components is now extremely low. However, blood components should still be considered to be potentially infectious and their administration should be avoided unless there is no other option.

Viral inactivation processes, such as heat treatment and/or solvent detergent treatment of plasma and its products (coagulation factors, immunoglobulins), make these products theoretically safer than cellular blood products. Due to transfusion of vCJD in the UK all children born since January 1 1996 are treated with plasma products imported from the USA. It is good practice to regularly screen children who receive repeated blood transfusions for known blood-borne pathogens and to vaccinate them against hepatitis A and B.

Bone marrow transplantation

Recently bone marrow transplantation (BMT) has been used as a therapeutic option in children with aplastic anaemia (Myers & Davies 2009), Fanconi anaemia (Wagner et al 2007), Glanzmann's thrombasthenia (Connor et al 2008), Bernard–Soulier syndrome (Reiger et al 2006), thalassaemia (Rajasekar et al 2009) and sickle cell anaemia (Krishnamurti 2007). Unlike children having BMT for leukaemia, children with the diseases discussed above are unlikely to have experienced prolonged hospitalisation and intensive chemotherapy. Specific attention should be paid to their psychological preparation pretransplant (Bennett-Rees et al 2008 p 107). BMT is undertaken in specialist regional paediatric BMT centres and further information on nursing care of children undergoing BMT can be obtained by contacting your local centre.

Discussion of the scenarios

Haemophilia scenario: John

What framework would you use to assess John's joint? Assessment follows the PRICE criteria for assessment and treatment of haemarthrosis – this provides a uniform and rapid assessment tool that can readily be used by nurses. The assessment should therefore include:

- Protection
- Rest
- Ice
- Compression
- Elevation.

What observations do you need to do?

- Pain assessment: asking John and his dad if analgesia has already been given
- The position that the knee is held in
- Can John walk?

What do you expect these observations to be?

- Dad reports that he gave John paracetamol when the injury occurred
- The knee is held in a flexed position even at rest
- John is unable to walk, even standing is painful

Is John's condition mild, moderate or severe?

- John's knee bleed will most likely be assessed as severe as he has had little response to factor VIII given at home by his Dad, he is still unable to weight bear and is still in pain.

Is there anything in the history that would give concern?

- John had substandard treatment of his bleed as his dad couldn't give the factor
- The factor should have been given before sport and not after the bleed occurred
- Mum is in hospital with a new baby.

What care would you expect to be initiated?

- Analgesia
- Factor VIII
- PRICE ± physiotherapy assessment
- Crutches to avoid weight bearing.

What ongoing care does John need?

- Daily doses of factor VIII until bleed has settled
- Analgesia until knee no longer painful
- Physiotherapy to achieve pre bleed range of movement on the knee.

Sickle scenario: Jennifer

What framework would you use to assess Jennifer?

- Airway
- Breathing
- Circulation.

What observations do you need to do?

- Vital signs
- Recession?
- Cough
- O_2
- Pain
- Colour.

What do you expect these observations to be?

- Back pain
- Fever
- Pallor.

Is Jennifer's condition mild, moderate or severe?

- Severe because of acute chest syndrome.

Is there anything in the history that would give concern?

- Brother – who is looking after him?
- Delay in Rx.

What care would you expect to be initiated?

- Analgesia
- O_2
- IV fluids
- Bronchodilators
- Physio
- Blood?

What ongoing care does Jennifer need?

- Hydroxyurea
- Referral to respiratory paediatrician
- Pulmonary function
- Parent.

References

Al-Jefri, A., Bussel, J., Freedman, M., 2000. Thrombocytopenia with absent radii: frequency of marrow megakaryoctye progenitors, proliferative characteristics, and megakaryoctye growth and development factor responsiveness. Pediatric Hematology & Oncology 17, 299–306.

Almeida, A.M., Khair, K., Hann, I., et al., 2003. Use of recombinant factor VIIa in children with inherited platelet function disorders. British Journal of Haematology 3, 477–481.

Ancliff, P., 2003. Congenital neutropenia. Blood Reviews 4, 209–216.

Anwar, R., Miloszeski, K.J.A., 1999. Factor XIII deficiency. British Journal of Haematology 107, 468–484.

Bain, B.J., 2009. Neonatal/newborn haemoglobinopathy screening in Europe and Africa. Journal of Clinical Pathology 1, 53–56.

Bennett-Rees, N., Hopkins, S., Stone, J., 2008. Preparation for bone marrow transplant. In: Gibson, F., Soanes, L. (Eds.), Cancer in children and young people. Wiley, London.

Bolton-Maggs, P.H.B., Hill, F.G.H., 1995. The rarer inherited coagulation disorders: a review. Blood Reviews 9, 65–76.

Bond, L.R., Hatty, S.R., Horn, M.E., et al., 1987. Gall stones in sickle cell disease in the United Kingdom. British Medical Journal (Clinical Research Edition) 295, 234–236.

Brittenham, G.M., Griffith, P.M., Nienhuis, A.W., et al., 1994. Efficacy of desferrioxamine in preventing complications of iron overload in patients with thalassaemia major. New England Journal of Medicine 331 (9), 567–573.

Burnes, D.P., Antle, B.J., Williams, C.C., et al., 2008. Mothers raising children with sickle cell disease at the intersection of race, gender, and illness stigma. Health and Social Work 3, 211–220.

Campbell, S., Glasper, A.E. (Eds.), 1995. Whaley and Wong's Children's Nursing UK edition. Times Mirror, London.

Clarke, G.M., Higgins, T.N., 2000. Laboratory investigation of hemoglobinopathies and thalassemias: review and update. Clinical Chemistry 46, 1284–1290.

Collins, P.W., Goldman, E., Lilley, P., et al., 1995. Clinical experience of factor XI deficiency: the role of fresh frozen plasma and factor XI concentrate. Haemophilia 1, 227–231.

Connor, P., Khair, K., Liesner, R., et al., 2008. Stem cell transplantation for children with Glanzmann thrombasthenia. British Journal of Haematology 140, 568–571.

Dick M 2007 Sickle cell disease in childhood. Standards and guidelines for clinical care. Detailed guidance 2007. Online: www.nhs.uk/sicklandthal (accessed April 2009)

Gaston, M.H., Verter, J.I., Woods, G., et al., 1986. Prophylaxis with oral penicillin in children with sickle cell anaemia. New England Journal of Med 314, 1593–9.

George, J.N., Reiman, T.A., Moake, J.L., et al., 1981. Soulier disease: a study of four patients and their parents. British Journal of Haematology 48(3), 456–467.

Guideline for the physiotherapy management of soft tissue injury with PRICE during the first 72 hours (ACSPM). June 1988. Available from National Library for Health: www.library.nhs.uk (accessed May 2209)

Hamdan, A.L., Nabulsi, M.M., Farhat, F.T., et al., 2006. When bone becomes marble: Head and neck manifestations of osteopetrosis. Paediatric Child Health 1, 37–40.

Hardisty, R.M., 2000. Platelet function disorders. In: Lilleyman, J., Hann, I., Blanchette, V. (Eds.), Paediatric hematology. Churchill Livingstone, Edinburgh.

Khair, K., Baker, K., Mathias, M, et al., 2007. Intranasal desmopressin (Octim): a safe and efficacious treatment option for children with bleeding disorders. Haemophilia 5,548–51

Khair, K., Geraghty, S.J., 2007. Haemophilia A; meeting the needs of individual patients. British Journal of Nursing 16, 987–993.

Khair, K., Hann, I.M., Liesner, R., 2003. The investigation of easy bruising. In: David, T. (Ed.), Recent advances in paediatrics. The Royal Society of Medicine Press, London.

Krishnamurti, L., 2007. Haematopoetic cell transplantation: a curative option for sickle cell disease. Pediatric Hematology and Oncology, 8569–8575.

Lak, M., Keihani, M., Elahi, F., et al., 1999. Bleeding and thrombosis in 55 patients with inherited afibrinogenaemia. British Journal of Haematology 107, 204–206.

Madgwick, K.V., Yardumian, A., 1999. A home blood transfusion programme for beta thalassaemia patients. Transfusion Medicine 9 (2), 135–138.

Mannucci, P.M., 2001. Treatment of von Willebrand disease. Thrombosis and Haemostasis 86, 149–153.

Modell, B., Khan, M., Darlison, M., et al., 2001. A national register for surveillance of inherited disorders: beta thalassaemia in the United Kingdom. Bulletin of the WHO 79 (11), 1006–1012.

Mueller, B.U., 2008. When should hydroxyurea be used for children with sickle cell disease? Pediatrics 122, 1365–1366.

Mullen, C., Anderson, K., Blaese, R., 1993. Splenectomy and/or bone marrow transplantation in the management of the Wiskott-Aldrich Syndrome: Long term follow-up of 62 cases. Blood 10, 2961–2966.

Myers, K.C., Davies, S.M., 2009. Haematopoietic stem cell transplantation for bone marrow failure syndromes in children. Biology of Blood Marrow Transplantation 15, 279–292.

NHS sickle cell and thalassaemia screening programme. London, 2006. www.screening.nhs.uk/sickleandthal (accessed April 20 2009)

Ohene-Frempong, K., Weiner, S.J., Sleeper, L.A., et al., 1998. Cerebrovascular accidents in sickle cell disease: rates and risk factors. Blood 91, 288–294.

Rajesekar, R., Mathews, V., Lakshmi, K.M., et al., 2009. Cellular immune reconstitution and its impact on clinical outcome in children with beta thalassemia undergoing a matched related myeloablative allogeneic bone marrow transplant. Biology of Blood Marrow Transplantation 15, 597–609.

Rieger, C., Rank, A., Fiegl, et al., 2006. Allogeneic stem cell transplantation as a new treatment option for patients with Bernard-Soulier syndrome. Thrombosis and Haemostasis 95, 190–191.

Sepion, B., 2000. Investigations, staging & diagnosis: implications for nurses. In: Thompson, J. (Ed.), The child with cancer – nursing care. Scutari Press, London.

Standards for the clinical care of children and adults with thalassaemia in the UK. www.ukts.org/pdfs/awareness/ukts (accessed June 7 2009)

Sutor, A.H., von Kries, R., Cornelissen, E.A., McNinch, A.W., Andrew, M., 1999. Vitamin K deficiency bleeding (VKDB) in infancy. Thrombosis and Haemostasis 81, 456–461.

Telfer, P., Constantinidou, G., Andreou, P., et al., 2005. Quality of life in thalassaemia. Annals of the New York Academy Sciences 1054, 273–282.

Vichinsky, E., Neumayr, L.D., Earles, A.N., et al., 2000. Causes and outcomes of acute chest syndrome in sickle cell disease. National Acute Chest Syndrome Study Group. New England Journal of Medicine 342, 1855–1865.

Vora, A.J., Makris, M., 2001. An approach to investigation of easy bruising. Archives of Diseases of Childhood 84, 488–491.

Vidler, V., 1999. Teaching parents advanced clinical skills. Haemophilia 5, 349–353.

Wagner, J.E., Eapen, M., MacMillan, M.L., et al., 2007. Unrelated donor bone marrow transplantation for the treatment of Fanconi anemia. British Journal of Haematology 5, 2256–2262.

Weatherall, D.J., Clegg, J.B., 2001. The thalassaemia syndromes, 4th edn. Blackwell Sciences, Oxford.

Wong, D., Baker, C., 1998. Pain in children: comparison of assessment scales. Pediatric Nursing 1, 9.

Yang, Y., Li, D.Z., 2009. A survey of pregnancies with Hb Bart's disease in Mainland China. Haemoglobin 2, 132–136.

Further reading

Hoffbrand, A.V., Pettit, J.E., Moss, P.A.H. (Eds.), 2001. Essential Haematology, 4th ed. Blackwell Science, London.

Gibson, F., Soanes, L. (Eds.), 2008. Cancer in children and young people. Wiley & Sons, London.

Provan, D., Singer, C., Baglin, T., Dokal, I., (Eds.), 2009. Oxford handbook of clinical haematology, 3rd edn.

Lilleyman, J., Hann, I., Blanchette, V., (Eds.), 2000. Paediatric haematology. Churchill Livingstone, Edinburgh.

Websites

Aplastic anaemia: *www.theaat.org.uk*

Fanconi anaemia: *www.fanconi.org*

Haemophilia: *www.haemophilia.org.uk*

Thalassaemia: *www.ukts.org*

Sickle Cell Disease *www.sicklecellsociety.org*

Caring for a child with a neurological disorder

33

Joanna Smith Catherine Martin

ABSTRACT

The aim of this chapter and companion PowerPoint presentation is to provide an overview of neurological problems in childhood. This will be achieved by introducing the nervous system and the principles of caring for a child with a neurological disorder, and outlining common childhood neurological disorders.

LEARNING OUTCOMES

At the end of reading this chapter you will be able to:

- Outline the overall structure and function of the nervous system.
- Understand the general principles of caring for a child and family, where the child has a neurological disorder.
- Appreciate the range of neurological disorders in childhood and the potential impact on the child and family.
- Describe the common neurological disorders of childhood.

Introduction

Disorders of the nervous system are an important group of childhood conditions; central nervous system malformations account for approximately 75% of fetal deaths and 40% of deaths within the first year of life (Padgett 2006). Approximately 15–20% of hospitalised children have a neurological problem either as the sole or associated complaint. Diseases of the neurological system have a profound effect on the lives of the child and family and are probably the most disruptive of all ailments. Caring for the child with a nervous system disorder and their families is challenging because the outcome is often uncertain, many disorders are rare and the family will have expert knowledge of the child's needs, which can lead to frustration for parents and feelings of inadequacy for healthcare professionals. Traditional models of care focusing on the disease process (illness, dependence and treatment) are inappropriate. Although key principles can be applied, care must be individually designed, have a developmental focus and be influenced by encouraging the child to reach their full potential.

The role, structure and function of the nervous system

The nervous and endocrine systems are the main regulatory systems of the body. The nervous system is the most rapid means of maintaining homeostasis, which is achieved by reacting and responding to internal and external stimuli. The nervous system is descriptively divided into the central nervous system (CNS) and the peripheral nervous system (PNS) (Sugerman 2006). The CNS consists of the brain, the control centre for the entire nervous system and the spinal cord. The PNS consists of the nerve networks, which link the CNS with the periphery.

The PNS has two main subdivisions, the somatic nervous system (SNS) and the autonomic nervous system (ANS). Actions carried out by the SNS are both voluntary and involuntary with sensations being perceived consciously, whereas actions carried out by the ANS are involuntary and not usually perceived consciously. The ANS has sympathetic and parasympathetic divisions and is primarily concerned with the innervation and control of visceral organs, smooth muscles and secretory glands. Where there is both sympathetic and parasympathetic nerve innovation their actions have an antagonistic effect, for example sympathetic activity increases the force of contraction of cardiac muscle and the heart rate, whereas parasympathetic activity reduces the force of contraction and decreases the heart rate.

Development of the nervous sytsem

Many neurological problems in infancy may be a result of a malformation that has occurred during embryological development (Padgett 2006). The ectoderm, one of the three primary

DOI: 10.1016/B978-0-7020-3183-0.10033-5

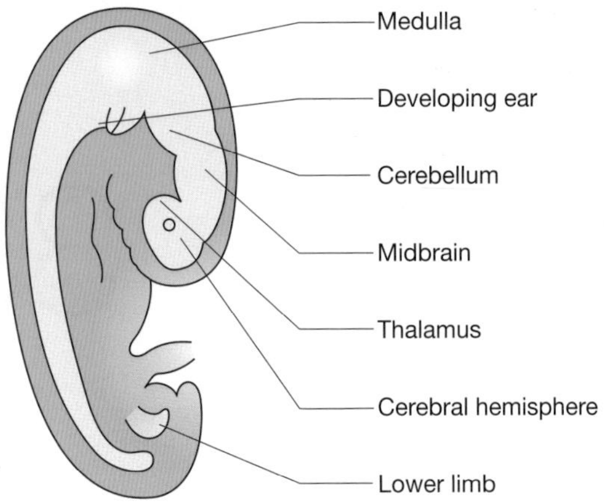

Fig. 33.1 • Representation of the brain and spinal cord at 5 weeks' gestation.

germ layers, forms nervous tissue, the ears, eyes and epidermis. The first obvious sign of nervous system development is during the 3rd week of embryonic life when the dorsal midline of the ectoderm thickens to form the neural plate (Padgett 2006). The lateral margins of the plate become elevated resulting in a midline depression known as the neural groove. Eventually the folds become apposed and fuse together creating the neural tube. The neural tube is completely closed by the end of the 4th week of embryonic development and becomes the CNS (Longstaff 2005). By the 5th week of gestation the rostral portion of the neural tube enlarges and differentiates into the forebrain (cerebrum), midbrain and hindbrain (pons, cerebellum and medulla oblongata) (Fig. 33.1).

In addition to structural developments, neuroepidermal cells increase in numbers. They are the precursors of both the supporting cells and the nerve cells and begin to organise themselves into zones. This results in the typical appearance of the brain: an outer layer of grey matter (cell bodies) and an inner layer of white matter (nerve tracts). Epidermal cells, precursors of both supporting (glial) cells and specialist (nerve) cells, increase in number and migrate through the layers of previously formed cells, adding to the expanding cerebral cortex. During the final stages of specialisation, nerve cells lose the ability to divide, and therefore do not increase in number after birth. Glial cell proliferation and nerve myelination increase the weight and size of the brain, particularly during the 1st year of life. Nerve myelination occurs from 22 weeks of gestation and is probably not complete until adult life (Padgett 2006).

Cells of the nervous system and their function

The two cellular components, the neuralgia (glial cells) and the neuron (nerve cells), are unique to the nervous system. Glial cells form the connective tissue of the nervous system; astrocytes provide mechanical support and help maintain the blood–brain barrier; microglia correspond to brain phagocytes; oligodendroglia and Schwann cells form myelin in the CNS and PNS respectively; and ependymal cells form the epithelial linings.

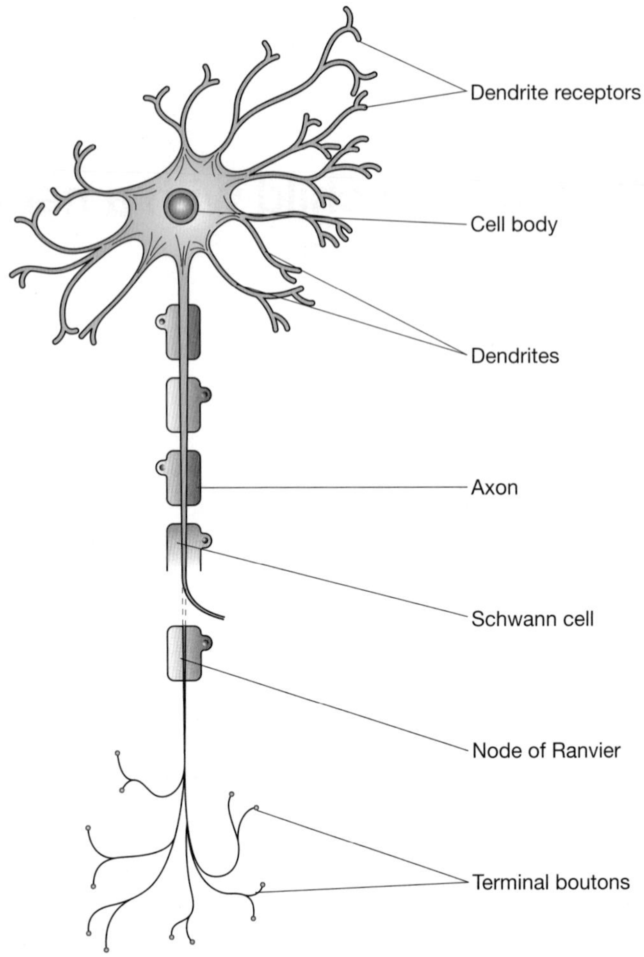

Fig. 33.2 • A typical motor neuron.

The neuron has a specialised structure that facilitates the transmission of electrical impulses (Fig. 33.2). A stimulus of sufficient strength applied to a dendrite receptor site generates a nerve impulse, which is transmitted along the dendrite to the cell body. The impulse exits via the main axonal process (nerve fibre) ending at the terminal boutons. These contain chemical transmitters capable of stimulating adjacent neurons or affector organs. Generating and conducting a nerve impulse is based on the neuron's ability to maintain a difference in the ion concentration outside and inside the cell membrane. Disruption of the ion concentration causes an ionic current flow, which is conducted along the entire neuron, is independent of any further stimulus and is unidirectional. The speed of the nerve impulse increases if (Longstaff 2005):

- body temperature increases
- the diameter of the fibre increases
- myelin is present.

Information passes between neurons at junctions (synapses). When a nerve impulse arrives at the terminal bouton, neurotransmitters such as noradrenaline or acetylcholine are released. These cross the synapse and bind with the receptor site on the adjacent dendrite. Calcium ions are necessary to facilitate this process. Neurotransmitters stimulate or inhibit postsynaptic dendrites, allowing impulses either to proceed or be inhibited.

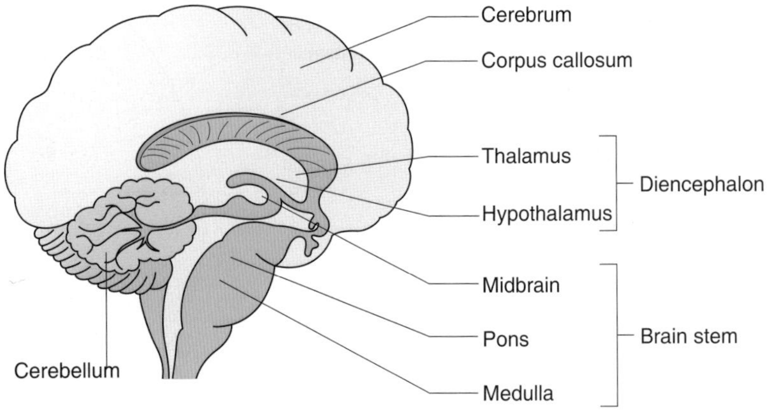

Fig. 33.3 • Cross-sectional view of the brain.

Once the neurotransmitter binds with the receptor site it is rapidly deactivated by enzymes in the postsynaptic junction.

Anatomy of the brain

The brain consists of the cerebrum (two cerebral hemispheres), diencephalon, brainstem and cerebellum (Fig. 33.3). The hemispheres are joined at the base by the corpus callosum (a sheet of nerve fibres allowing communication between the hemispheres).

The cerebrum is by far the largest part of the brain, and is divided into important functional areas (Fig. 33.4). Specific areas of the cortex perform specific functions (Fitzgerald & Folan-Curran 2002):

- The frontal lobe contains the primary motor cortex responsible for controlling movement, the speech area and higher functions including personality and behaviour.
- The parietal lobes contains the primary somatosensory cortex where sensations such as touch, pressure, pain and temperature are consciously perceived.
- The occipital lobe contains the visual cortex.
- The temporal lobes contain the auditory cortex, and areas involved in memory and emotions.

Due to the cross over (decussation) of the nerve fibres at the medulla oblongata each hemisphere communicates with the opposite side of the body.

The diencephalon contains several specialist areas, with the two most important being the thalamus and hypothalamus. The thalamus is a relay and integration centre. The hypothalamus coordinates homeostatic mechanisms and has autonomic, neuroendocrine and limbic functions.

The brainstem collectively describes the midbrain, medulla oblongata and the pons. The midbrain contains part of the auditory system. Most nerve fibres from the body transcend the medulla and midbrain, which function as important relay and integration centres. Although anatomically the brain stem is a relatively small component of the brain, its importance cannot be underestimated. It contains many nuclei and tracts that are essential to key vital body functions, for example the medulla contains nuclei that regulate blood pressure,

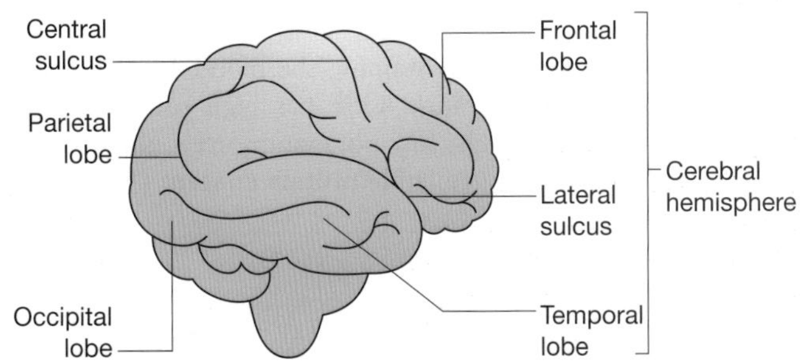

Fig. 33.4 • Major subdivisions of the cerebral hemispheres.

respiration, maintenance of arousal and initiation of sleep. Like the medulla, the pons contains many functional structures but primarily acts as a relay centre between the cerebrum and cerebellum.

The cerebellum sits in the base of the cranial cavity in an area known as the posterior fossa. The cerebellum is important in relation to the coordination of motor activities functions such as tone and posture, and operates at an unconscious level. Unlike the cerebral cortex, responses of the cerebellum affect the same side of the body (ipsilateral).

The ventricular system

The ventricular system is a network of connected chambers or ventricles deep within the brain which contain cerebrospinal fluid (CSF). There are four chambers: two lateral ventricles situated within the cerebral hemispheres, the third ventricle situated in the diencephalon and the fourth ventricle situated between the brainstem and the cerebellum. The fourth ventricle tapers at its base and becomes the very narrow central canal of the spinal cord.

CSF flows constantly beginning in the lateral ventricles before flowing into the third ventricle, and continuing via the aqueduct of Sylvius to the fourth ventricle. CSF leaves the fourth to circulate around the brain and spinal cord via the subarachnoid space (Fig. 33.5). CSF is reabsorbed into the bloodstream via capillaries on the surface of the cerebral hemispheres.

CSF helps maintain the cerebral chemical environment by supplying nutrients and removing toxic substances, is a shock

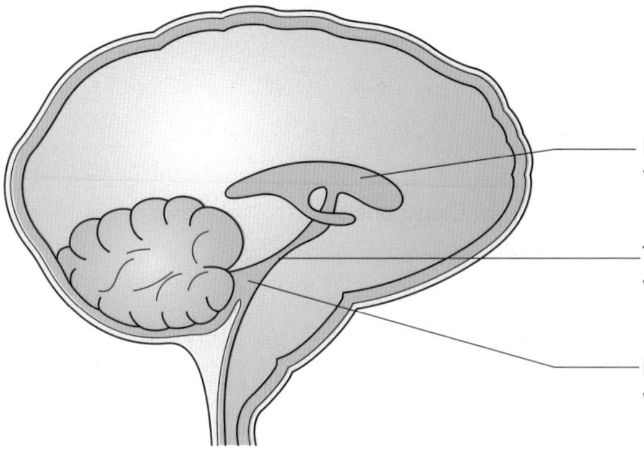

Fig. 33.5 • Cerebrospinal fluid flow through the ventricular system.

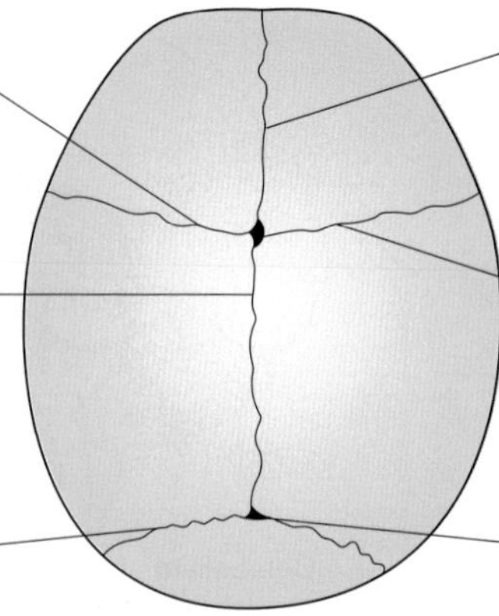

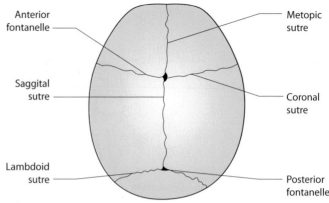

Fig. 33.6 • Sutures of the skull.

absorber, contributes to maintaining the blood–brain barrier, and gives the brain buoyancy. CSF has high sodium, chlorine and bicarbonate levels, low potassium, urea, glucose and amino acid levels, and a negligible protein content (Sugerman 2006).

Blood supply

The brain requires a continual input of glucose and oxygen, with 20% of the total cardiac output reaching the brain each minute (Sugerman 2006). The internal vertebral and carotid arteries, and their subsidiaries ensure the brain has a rich blood supply. These vessels form a system of interconnecting arteries in the base of the brain, known as the circle of Willis. The physiological principle behind the circle of Willis is that in the event of damage to one of the arteries supplying the brain there is the potential for compensation from the communicating arteries thus offering some protection from severe ischaemic damage.

Venous blood primarily returns to the circulation via the superficial veins that drain into the venous sagittal sinus that eventually flows into the internal jugular vein. The deep veins of the cerebral hemispheres drain into the vein of Galen and then into the sagittal sinus.

The composition of the brain's extracellular fluid needs to be regulated because circulatory chemicals are toxic to neurons. This is achieved by the blood–brain barrier, a complex process that is the consequence of specific characteristics of the cerebral capillaries resulting in a highly selective exchange of substances across their endothelial end plates.

Protection and coverings

The brain is supported and protected by the skull and the membranous coverings collectively known as the meninges. The bones of the skull are separated at birth, allowing for brain moulding during delivery and rapid growth within the 1st year of life. Complete ossification occurs at about 8 years of age, and the sutures (Fig. 33.6) cannot be separated even in the presence of raised intracranial pressure after about 12 years of age (Padgett 2006).

Neuron regeneration

The traditional approach to neuroanatomy and physiology associates discrete body functions with specific brain structures (Stephenson 1996). Recent studies suggest latent areas within the brain may be able to assume the functions of damaged areas (Rose et al 1997). In addition, it was presumed that because neuron cell bodies do not have centrioles and the meiotic spindles that are necessary for cell division, there is little capacity to repair and regain function following damage. However, neurons can survive damage, regenerate new axons and form new synaptic connections (Stephenson 1996). The process known as reactive synaptogenesis may result in the recovery of function, but can also result in the development of abnormal connections with abnormal recovery.

Activity

Revisit your knowledge and add more depth by accessing the Evolve website:

- File chapter 9 test your knowledge (brain teasers).
- File chapter 9 PowerPoint teachings (overview of anatomy and physiology of the brain, embryology and cells of the nervous system).

The following textbooks and web sites may be useful

- Crossman AR, Neary D 2000 Neuroanatomy – an illustrated colour text, 2nd edn. Churchill Livingstone, Edinburgh
- Fitzgerald MJT, Folan-Curran J 2002 Clinical neuroanatomy and related neuroscience, 4th edn. WB Saunders, Edinburgh
- Brain source; aimed at sharing neuroscience knowledge http://www.brainsource.com/
- Encyclopedia of Life Sciences; comprehensive coverage of a range of topics including neurosciences http://www.mrw.interscience.wiley.com/

Overview of neurological disorders affecting children

The range of neurological disorders in childhood is vast, terminology is complex and many children who present with a neurological dysfunction may never have a definitive diagnosis.

Table 33.1 Range of childhood neurological diseases

	Features	Example
Congenital malformations	Disruption to normal CNS development, usually occurs early in gestational period Often multifactorial genetic transmission	Hydrocephalus Agenesis of the corpus callosum Microcephaly
Neurocutaneous disorders	Errors occurring in early ectodermal cell proliferation results in a group of disorders, which present with combined CNS, ophthalmic and skin abnormalities	Tuberous sclerosis Sturge–Weber syndrome
Vascular disorders	A diverse group of disorders with various aetiologies from structural anomalies to spontaneous intracranial bleeds	Arteriovenous malformations Intracranial arterial aneurysms Moyamoya disease
CNS infections	Common cause of acute neurological disorders Despite improved preventative programmes through vaccination and improved antimicrobial agents remain a challenge with significant morbidity	Meningitis Intracranial abscesses Encephalitis (measles, herpes simplex, mumps)
Neoplastic disorders	Most common solid tumours in children Often difficult to treat	Medulloblastoma Astrocytoma Brainstem glioma Craniopharyngioma
Progressive degenerative disorders	Includes the many neurometabolic disorders, which although individually rare, collectively are an important group of disorders Most follow an autosomal recessive inheritance pattern Two major groups are the neuronal storage diseases and the leucodystrophies	Tay–Sachs disease Battens disease Niemann–Pick disease Krabbe's disease
Non-progressive brain damage	Persistent disorder as a result of brain insult during early development The underlying problem is static but subsequent development is affected	Cerebral palsy
Neuromuscular disorders	Normal muscle functioning is dependent upon effective muscle and nerve functioning. Children with this group of disorders present with hypotonia and increasing muscle weakness	Duchenne muscular dystrophy Myasthenia gravis Guillain–Barré
Learning disabilities	A wide range of learning disabilities exist from very specific skill deficiencies to complex disorders affecting the ability to carry out activities of living and achieve independent living Aetiology is often due to hereditary and environmental factors	Fragile-X syndrome Down syndrome Autism Asperger's syndrome

A lack of diagnosis is particularly difficult and can be frustrating for the child and family. It is vital for disorders where there is a potential genetic mode of inheritance that the child and family are referred for genetic counselling to assist the parents in decisions relating to planning future children. The outcome of neurological disorders is extremely variable. It is essential the child and family are viewed as unique with individual needs when planning care. The diversity of neurological conditions are presented in Table 33.1.

WWW

Develop your knowledge of these conditions by accessing the following websites:

- Association for Spina Bifida and Hydrocephalus: http://www.asbah.org.uk
- Association for Tuberous Sclerosis: http://www.tuberous-sclerosis.org.uk
- Children's Hemiplegia and Stroke Association: http://www.hemikids.org
- Meningitis Trust UK: http://www.meningitis-trust.org.uk
- Scope (focuses on providing supporting for people with disabilities, primarily with cerebral palsy): http://www.scope.org.uk
- Muscular Dystrophy Campaign: http://www.muscular-dystrophy.org/
- Child Brain Injury Trust: www.cbituk.org/
- Headlines Children with Craniosynostosis: www.headlines.org.uk

Principles of caring for a child with a cerebral dysfunction

Understanding the principles that underpin the management of the child with both acute and long-term neurological dysfunction is essential if care delivery is to be safe and appropriate. Neurological disorders have a unique effect and care must be based on assessment and meeting individual needs. Therefore the general principles of care need to be adapted to each situation, and the child and family's needs. Seizure management is covered in Chapter 23.

Diagnostic procedures

Diagnostic procedures are vital in order to: assist the clinician to establish, where possible, the correct diagnosis; determining the potential prognosis for the child; and to monitor disease progression and/or the effects of treatments.

The child and family require detailed explanation and effective preparation prior to investigative procedures. Consent must be obtained. The type of diagnostic investigations will vary depending on the child's presentation but may include:

- blood profiling, including urea and electrolytes, metabolic and immunological assays, and genetic screening
- lumbar puncture performed to collect CSF samples in order to detect the presence of bacteria or tumour deposits, and the measurement of CSF pressure. Performing a lumbar puncture in a child with a high intracranial pressure may cause brainstem compression with fatal consequences
- neuroimaging; ultrasound, X-rays, computerised axial tomography (CT), magnetic resonance imaging (MRI)
- specialised physiological imaging techniques such as positron emission tomography (PET) and single-photon computed emission tomography (SPECT), assist with evaluating cerebral metabolic functioning and cerebral blood flow
- cerebrovascular studies such as angiography, used to identify cerebrovascular abnormalities such as aneurysms and arteriovenous malformations
- electroencephalogram (EEG) records the electrical activity of the brain and is primarily used to detect changes in brain activity during seizures. Often used as a continuous monitoring procedure with video recording to correlate a child's presentation with EEG changes (video telemetry)
- electromyography (EMG) conduction studies are used to measure electrical activity and velocity times in muscle fibres. Particularly useful in assisting in the diagnosis of neuromuscular and peripheral nerve disorders
- muscle biopsies measure a range of muscle enzymes. Useful in identifying whether a problem is neurogenic or myogenic in origin, assisting in the diagnosis of neuromuscular conditions.

Some of these procedures, such as PET and SPECT, are only available in specialised centres.

Activity

Common imaging techniques are now widely available; therefore all nurses must have appropriate knowledge of these procedures associated care related to these procedures:

Think about the advantages, disadvantages and care needs of the child who requires an X-ray, CT scan or MRI scan.

What strategies would you use to ensure a 2-year-old child successfully undergoes a CT scan?

You might want to add more depth to your knowledge by accessing the Evolve website:

- file chapter 9 imaging techniques.

Raised intracranial pressure

Intracranial pressure (ICP) is the pressure exerted by the cranial contents on the skull. Typical values in older children are 5–15 mmHg and 3–7 mmHg in infants and young children (Chitnavis & Polkey 1998). The rigidity of the skull results in the total intracranial volume being fixed. The intracranial contents (brain, CSF, and blood) must be maintained in a state of equilibrium. Therefore an increase in volume in one component must be reciprocated by a reduction in volume in another component, known as the Monro–Kellie doctrine (Chitnavis & Polkey 1998), which can be represented by the following equation:

$$\text{Intracranial volume} = \text{Brain Volume} + \text{CSF Volume} + \text{Blood Volume}$$

However, there is little ability of the brain to significantly reduce any of these components and an increase in overall volume results in a rise in ICP (Fig. 33.7). Raised intracranial pressure (RICP) is usually described as an ICP above 20 mmHg sustained for 5 minutes or more (Miller & Dearden 1992). Causes include:

- conditions which increase the brain volume:
  - space occupying lesions such as tumour, abscess, haematoma
  - cerebral oedema for example following traumatic brain injury or cerebral infection
- conditions which increase the blood volume or blood flow:
  - obstruction to venous outflow
- conditions which compromise normal CSF levels:
  - blockages within the ventricular system causing hydrocephalus
  - conditions which increase CSF levels are rare but could include tumours of choroid plexus.

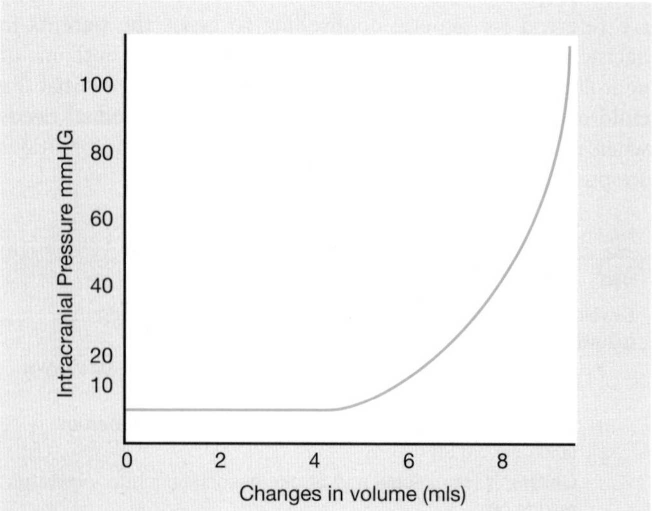

Fig. 33.7 • Volume/pressure curve.

The signs and symptoms of RICP include (Hazinski et al 1999):

- alteration in conscious levels; irritability, lethargy, confusion, decreased responsiveness
- dilated pupils, decreased response to light
- abnormal motor activity or reflexes
- headaches, nausea and vomiting
- Cushing's response (increased blood pressure with a compensatory bradycardia), bradycardia on its own, apnoea. **These are late and ominous signs.**

The signs and symptoms of RICP in an infant, prior to fusion of the skull sutures, usually occur late because increased volume forces the membranes between the skull bones to splay, accommodating pressure changes. There will be more insidious signs such as irritability, poor feeding, general developmental delay, large and tense anterior fontanelle even when the infant is in the sitting position, and increased head circumference (Brett & Harding 1997a).

Once the intracranial pressure starts to rise a cycle of events occurs: ICP increases, cerebral blood flow (CBF) decreases, leading to tissue hypoxia resulting in cerebral vasodilation and oedema, causing further increases in ICP. The brain will shift from the area under pressure to an area of less pressure, resulting in compression, traction and shearing of brain structures. Eventually, downward brain shift occurs, resulting in brainstem herniation with vital centres becoming compressed. Management of RICP is based on the need to prevent cerebral ischaemia by maintaining cerebral perfusion pressure (CPP) between 70 and 80 mmHg (Rosner & Daughton 1990), with care best provided in paediatric intensive care unit.

Evidence-based practice

There are evidence-based guidelines relating to the management of RICP as a consequence of significant brain injury in both children and adults (Adelson et al 2003, Bullock et al 2000). The principles within these guidelines include:

- ventilate and maintain oxygenation, aim for a $PaCO_2$ between 30 and 35 mmHg and PaO_2 between 90 and 100 mmHg. Hyperventilation is not a recommended treatment for TBI but may be of value for brief periods where the $PaCO_2$ is elevated and there is associated acute neurological deterioration, such as acute rises in ICP
- minimising the brain's metabolic needs and preventing activities which normally produce transient rises in ICP by providing adequate sedation, analgesia and paralysis. No specific evidence is currently available relating to the best sedative, analgesia or neuromuscular blocking agent in the management of head injury. Choice will depend on local guidelines and practices. The use of sedation, analgesia and paralysis will limit the ability to perform full neurological assessments
- maintaining an adequate systemic mean arterial pressure, above 75 mmHg for children over 10 years of age and above 65 mmHg for those less than 10 years of age in order to ensure an adequate CPP.
- this is achieved by appropriate fluid resuscitation and the administration of inotropic drugs. An inotrope is an agent which alters the force or energy of cardiac muscular contractions. This group of drugs is useful for resuscitation of seriously ill patients, and for the treatment of hypotension in intensive care settings. In these situations inotropes such as dopamine or dobutamine are administered by continuous infusion. Fluid resuscitation must be judicious due to the potential of increasing cerebral oedema if over hydration occurs
- maintaining CPP above 60 mmHg for children over 10 years of age and above 50 mmHg for those less than 10 years of age. Maintaining an adequate mean arterial pressure will require the use of inotropic support
- maintaining normal electrolyte balance with precise fluid management
- monitoring and record ICP levels and wave patterns; identify 'plateau' waves early. ICP above 20 mmHg will require active treatment such diuretic therapy. Mannitol 20% is the diuretic of choice and the usual dose is 0.25–0.5 g/kg. Monitor serum osmolarity with mannitol use and maintain a level of less than 320 mOmols/L
- decompression surgery may be indicated if the child has an extremely high ICP and high blood pressure due to generalised cerebral oedema but the child's brain is likely to recover
- optimising cerebral venous return by maintaining the head at an angle of 30° and position the head in the midline to prevent constriction of the blood vessels
- maintain normothermia
- monitor EEG in order to detect seizure activity and ensure prompt treatment of seizures.

Neurological assessment

Accurate neurological assessment and skilled observations are essential if changes in neurological function are to be detected. The purpose of a neurological assessment includes (Hickey 2003a):

- identifying the child's normal abilities and developmental stage
- providing a baseline record of the child's neurological status at the time of admission
- identifying the presence and effects of neurological dysfunction
- detecting life-threatening situations
- identifying changes promptly through serial observations
- influencing management decisions by monitoring overall improvements or deteriorations in the child
- assisting in the prediction of the eventual outcome of the neurological insult.

Reflect on your practice

Think about the last time you performed neurological observations on a child:

- Why were the observations being undertaken?
- How frequently were the observations being undertaken? Why?
- How and why did you apply a painful stimuli?
- How and why did you act on any changes in the child's condition?

Neurological observations include: assessment of conscious levels, pupillary reactions, motor functioning and other parameters including the presence of seizures and changes to vital signs. The frequency of undertaking observations will depend on the initial assessment, the stability of the child and the underlying problem. In the acute situation half- to 1-hourly observations seem to be the norm (Ferguson-Clark & Williams 1998). Unless a full assessment is carried out, unconsciousness cannot be distinguished from normal sleep.

Assessment of consciousness

Consciousness is a state of awareness and in general can be thought of as two components – arousal and wakefulness – and is a sensitive indicator of neurological functioning (Hickey 2003a). The first and the most frequently used numerical scale for assessing conscious levels is the Glasgow Coma Scale (GCS) (Teasdale & Jennett 1974). It was developed in the 1970s to reduce the subjectivity and ambiguity when assessing a patient's conscious level. The Glasgow Coma Scale (GCS) assesses three parameters, **eye opening, verbal response and motor response**, with a numerical score given for the best response within each parameter (Table 33.2).

Table 33.2 The Glasgow Coma Scale (Teasdale & Jennett 1974)

Parameter	Score	Components
Eye opening	4	Eyes open spontaneously in response to normal environmental activities
	3	Eyes open in response to direct commands
	2	Eyes open in response to a painful stimulus
	1	Absence of eye opening despite application of a painful stimulus
Verbal response	5	Answers appropriately to questions
	4	Converses but confused
	3	Makes little sense
	2	Incompressible sounds
	1	No verbal response despite the application of a painful stimulus
Motor response	6	Obeys commands
	5	Localisation of a painful stimulus and purposefully moves in an attempt to locate the stimulus and remove it
	4	Withdrawal from the painful stimuli in an attempt to move away from the stimulus but it is not a purposeful movement
	3	Flexion response to a painful stimulus
	2	Extension to a painful stimulus
	1	Flaccidity, there is no detectable movement or change in tone of the limbs despite repeated and varied stimulation

The GCS has undergone several adaptations for use in children, including the James' adaptation (James & Trauner 1985) and the Adelaide Scale (Reilly et al 1988). The National Paediatric Neuroscience Benchmarking group (Tatman et al 1997, Warren 2000) and the National Institute for Clinical Excellence (NICE 2007) advocate using the James' adaptation because it is easy to use, the scoring system (a maximum of 15 and minimum of 3) is internationally recognised and it takes into account the child's developmental stage. The addition of the grimace score makes it suitable for use in intensive care settings (Warren 2000). Spontaneous eye opening in response to normal environmental activities achieves a maximum score of 4, indicating that the arousal mechanisms in the brain stem are functioning. The normal verbal response will depend on the linguistic and cognitive developmental stage of the child and, where possible, should be ascertained from the child or carer prior to undertaking the first assessment (Table 33.3). The final component of the GCS assesses the ability of the child to respond to an instruction that requires the child to undertake a motor action. This requires the child to have an appropriate level of understanding in order to interpret and act on the instructions given. In babies or young infants that do not have the cognitive ability to response to instructions a maximum score of 6 would be recorded if there are normal spontaneous movements.

If a child does not respond to an auditory stimulus or light tactile pressure, and therefore has not achieved the maximum score, the continuation of the assessment requires the application of a painful stimulus. When assessing the motor component of the GCS, it is important to use a central stimulus to ascertain whether the child can locate the site of the stimulus, for example applying pressure over the supraorbital area (Teasdale & Jennett 1974). Sternal rub, although a central stimulus, can potentially damage soft tissues (Hickey 2003a). Nail bed pressure may elicit a flexion reflex response and can be misinterpreted as an attempt to localise to pain. Supraorbital pressure is not appropriate to elicit eye opening because it causes grimacing, and simultaneous eye closing. Under 6 months the normal motor response to painful stimulation is flexion (Brett & Kaiser 1997).

Summation of the three components of the GCS provides a summary of the child's conscious state and can act as a quick reference guide when reviewing the child's condition (Watson et al 1992). The summation ranges in value from 3 to 15, with 15 indicating full consciousness. The score becomes lower as the degree of neurological impairment increases. Coma is usually defined as a score of 8 or less (Kraus et al 1987). Summation of the GCS can conceal the whole picture, and may not be accurate in terms of predicting long-term outcome of the neurological injury particularly following traumatic brain injury (McNett 2007). However, in an acute intracranial catastrophe all three components of the GCS are usually depressed.

Motor function

Evaluating limb responses can assist in determining the site of brain damage; specific deficits will correlate to the specific area of brain damage. Damage to the motor cortex and cerebellum will result in abnormalities in motor function. Assessing motor

Table 33.3 Verbal component of the neurological assessment adapted for use in children (Warren 2000)

Score	Verbal response		
	Infant/young child	**Older child/adult**	**Grimace – all ages**
5	Alert, babbles, coos/uses words or sentences/usually ability	Orientated	Spontaneous normal facial/oro-motor activity
4	Less than usual ability or spontaneous irritable cry	Confused	Less than usual facial/oro-motor spontaneous activity or only response to touch stimuli
3	Cries inappropriately	Inappropriate words	Vigorous grimace to pain
2	Occasional whimpers/moans	Inappropriate sounds	Mild grimace to pain
1	No response	No response	No response

function is not the same as assessing the motor response in the GCS. The assessment of motor function aims to provide an overview of the function of each of the four limbs independently, in terms of muscle strength, muscle tone, posture and the coordination of movements and whether movements are spontaneous or in response to painful stimuli or flaccid (Peters 2007). Abnormal posture and movements should be documented. The neonate's normal response to stimulation is flexion (Brett & Kaiser 1997).

Pupil reactions

Assessment of pupil function provides valuable insights into the physiology of the brainstem. The response of the pupils to light is dependent on intact cranial nerves II and III, which transmit nerve impulses from the retina to the midbrain and from the midbrain to the pupillary muscles, respectively. Assessment of pupils should include size, equality and reactivity to light (Hickey 2003a). The normal response to a direct light stimulus is an immediate brisk constriction of the pupil, and a brisk dilation of the pupil once the light source is removed (Hickey 2003a). Although each eye is examined independently, the response should be observed in both eyes. Light directed into one eye will constrict the pupil in the opposite eye due to the consensual light reflex. The pupillary response is graded and recorded descriptively in terms of brisk, sluggish or non-reactive (fixed). The size of the pupil is either recorded as pinpoint, small, moderate or dilated, or on a scale ratio of 1:8. Pupils are usually between 2 and 6 mm in size, but there may be slight discrepancies between the two pupils.

The assessment of the pupil responses is important because:

- pupil responses can be undertaken on patients who are receiving anaesthetic or paralysing agents
- extremely small pupils can indicate narcotic overdose or direct lower brain stem compression
- a large pupil or unequal pupils usually indicate compression of the midbrain and consequently the oculomotor nerve
- a dilated fixed pupil is an ominous finding and suggestive of a terminal state (Hickey 2003a). **These findings should arouse immediate concern and be reported immediately to medical staff.**
- an irregular or oval pupil may indicate raised intracranial pressure and be the first sign of oculomotor nerve compression due to transtentorial herniation
- drugs that either constrict or dilate the pupils should be accurately recorded.

Vital signs

Alterations in vital signs can indicate pathophysiological changes within the brain, particularly the brainstem. Cardiovascular observations are particularly important because of the relationship between cerebral haemodynamics and cerebral functioning (Hickey 2003a). Compromise to cerebral blood flow will result in a vasomotor response, with blood being diverted from other body systems in order to maintain adequate cerebral perfusion. The resultant rise in arterial blood pressure is known as Cushing's reflex or response (Hickey 2003a). Tachycardia will initially occur as a result of mild hypoxia. Significant compromises to cerebral blood flow cause further increases in blood pressure resulting in a compensatory bradycardia, suggestive of a dangerously high intracranial pressure and usually denotes an intracranial catastrophe is impending.

Changes in respiratory rate and rhythm can occur with neurological dysfunction. Alterations to normal respirations such as hyperventilation, shallow breathing or irregular breathing should raise concerns. Rapidly expanding lesions such as intracranial haemorrhage, direct medulla damage or brainstem herniation are likely to cause respiratory arrest (Hickey 2003a).

Alterations in body temperature, both hypo- and hyperthermia, can be manifestations of neurological impairments. Hyperthermia is probably more common (Hickey 2003a) and can be due to infective and non-infective conditions. Central fever due to neurogenic aetiologies are typically associated with brain tumours, trauma and following neurosurgery.

Additional components of the neurological assessment should include observation of the adequacy of the cough and gag reflex, which can become depressed following widespread brain damage. Brain insults have the potential to cause seizures requiring appropriate monitoring and management because of the resultant hypoxia, which will compound existing problems.

Care of the unconscious child

Unconsciousness is a lack of awareness of one's self, the environment, an impairment of cognitive functioning and an inability to respond to sensory stimuli (Hickey 2003b). There is a myriad of neurological conditions that result in unconsciousness, with the depth and duration lasting for seconds, for example during a seizure, to months, for example following major head trauma.

Activity

Sally is 14 years old and has suffered a cerebrovascular accident necessitating emergency craniotomy and resulting in a prolonged period in paediatric intensive care. She is now stable and able to maintain her own airway. Her nutrition is primarily maintained via gastrostomy feeding. She remains unresponsive and dependent on carers for all her needs. Her family, primarily her mother, although not resident, is actively involved in Sally's care.

- Identify Sally's actual and potential problems.
- Write a detailed nursing care plan outlining how Sally's needs will be met.

Children with impaired levels of consciousness and who are unable to maintain their own airway are at risk of hypoxia and hypercarbia, with potential respiratory failure and therefore will require intensive care (Hazinski et al 1999). However, many children who have impaired levels of consciousness do not require intensive care facilities but are dependent on the healthcare team to meet their needs. The aims of caring for these children are: to ensure activities necessary to sustain life are maintained, prevent complications relating to immobility, maximise the restoration of functions and offer support to the family. Table 33.4 outlines the needs of the child with impaired conscious levels in relation to maintaining essential activities of daily living and preventing complications.

Nursing care of the child undergoing neurosurgery

The principles that apply to every child requiring surgery are also important for the child undergoing cranial surgery. The main goals of care are to minimise potential complications of the surgical procedure and effects of the anaesthetic by ensuring the child and family are prepared appropriately and safely for surgery and recovery needs are met. Surgery and anaesthesia disrupt normal functioning and homeostatic mechanisms and are potentially life threatening.

In general there are few specific preoperative requirements. The child will require preoperative blood sampling, including cross-match, because of the potential for blood loss during surgery. The child and family must be prepared for the immediate postoperative period, including the possibility of being nursed in intensive care, the child's appearance including descriptions of the wound/bandages, drains, facial swelling, and the range and function of monitoring equipment. It is usual practice to undertake skin preparation and hair removal after induction of the anaesthetic. However, it is essential the child and family are prepared for hair removal.

Activity

Jamie is 6 months old and has been admitted for insertion of a ventricular shunt.

- Write a care plan outlining the principles of the pre- and postoperative care Jamie and his family will require.

The postoperative needs of the child following cranial surgery should focus on the prompt detection of complications of both the anaesthesia and the surgical procedure including cerebral haemorrhage (subdural, epidural, intracerebral and intraventricular), RICP, seizures, cerebrospinal fluid leakage, pneumocephalus, hydrocephalus, meningitis, metabolic imbalances and a range of neurosurgical deficits (diminished levels of consciousness, communication difficulties, motor and sensory deficits, diminished swallow and gag reflexes, and visual disturbances) (Hickey 2003c). The immediate postoperative needs of the child following neurosurgery are outlined in Table 33.5.

Pain following neurosurgical procedures occurs as a consequence of muscle and soft tissue damage at the site of the surgical incision. The severity of the pain experienced is linked to the site of surgery – frontal lobe surgery is associated with lower pain intensity compared to occipital and posterior fossa approaches (Thibault et al 2007). Clinical practice guidelines relating to the recognition and assessment of acute pain in children are available, and applicable for children undergoing neurosurgical procedures Royal College of Nursing (RCN 2009). For the child with a neurological problem additional communication problems and an inability to express pain because of nerve and/or muscle damage may exist and there may be associated cognitive, behavioural and emotional difficulties (Hunt et al 2003); therefore it is vital to consider individual requirements for these children because pain assessment is more challenging and these children are likely to receive less analgesia than their able counterpart (Twycross et al 1999). Despite morphine being used widely in the majority of surgical specialities, its use following major neurosurgery is variable (Roberts 2005). Side effects such as respiratory depression can be detected early if the child is regularly assessed and oxygen saturation levels are monitored continuously because respiratory slowing occurs well before there is severe respiratory depression.

Neurological deficits that occur as a result of surgery may require the child's care to shift in focus from managing acute surgical needs to a programme of rehabilitation.

Preparation for discharge must consider the advice the child and parent will require, specific advice to the neurosurgical procedure and, where appropriate, a clear indication of subsequent healthcare interventions.

Rehabilitation

Traditional models of care focusing on disease and treatments are not always appropriate for a child with a neurological problem. The philosophy of rehabilitation focuses on enabling an

Table 33.4 Caring for the unconscious child

Actual/potential problems	Nursing interventions
Altered neurological functioning due to cerebral dysfunction	Monitor neurological functioning through regular assessment Manage alterations in sleep patterns and periods of irritability through structuring activities appropriately, having planned rest periods, using relaxation techniques such as aromatherapy and massage Drugs such as melatonin may be prescribed for sleep disturbances – review their use regularly Ensure stimulation activities are planned and appropriate for the child's age and condition Assess and manage pain appropriately
Risk of altered respiratory function due to underlying cerebral dysfunction, inability to maintain airway and immobility Potential problem of atelectasis and chest infection	Assess respiratory function and identify risk of airway obstruction, ensure position does not compromise the airway, use airway aids and suctioning as appropriate Appropriate monitoring such as respiratory rate and effort, colour, peripheral perfusion and pulse oximetry Assess gag and swallow reflexes, in conjunction with a speech and language therapist, keep the child 'nil by mouth' until these reflexes have returned Ensure regular chest physiotherapy, ensure position changes and passive movements are incorporated into care activities Monitoring for signs of chest infection by recording temperature and changes in the amount and colour of secretions
Unable to maintain nutrition and hydration Potential problems of malnutrition, anaemia, electrolyte disturbances and gastric ulcers	Assess nutritional status, including monitoring of the child's weight Provide a good nutritional intake by appropriate methods that meet the needs of the child, enteral feeding via a naso-gastric/jejunal tube may be necessary. A gastrostomy tube may be more appropriate if long-term enteral feeding is required Ensure nutritional intake reflects increased calorific intake, liaise with the dietician to ensure the correct composition and volume of feed Monitoring intake and output, observing for signs of under/over-nourishment and dehydration If gag and swallow reflex have been assessed to be adequate and there are no other contraindications oral food and fluids should be encouraged. The re-introduction of oral feeding may need to be supplemented by enteral feeding because neurological problems may result in oral-motor difficulties, reduced alertness and increased fatigability contributing to inadequate nutritional intake Consider the child's needs in relation to positioning and supportive seating, taste and textures, likes and dislikes, choice of utensils, and effective age appropriate communication
Unable to maintain self-care needs	Ensure care is appropriate in meeting individual needs and consider usual family practices in relation to maintaining hygiene needs There needs to be particular emphasis on the assessment of the mucous membranes of the eyes and oral cavity for dryness, take appropriate action to keep clean and moist: • corneal dryness will require instillation of artificial tear drops or gels such as hypromellose drops • protecting the eyes by the use of patching if the child is unable to completely close the eyes Assessing oral hygiene needs and involvement of dental hygienist/dentist as appropriate, ensure frequent teeth brushing, consider the need to use suction techniques to prevent aspiration
Potential complications of immobility including:	
1. Skin breakdown	Assess pressure areas using a recognised child-appropriate assessment tool. Implement preventative measure based on the assessment to ensure the integrity of the skin is maintained
2. Muscular skeletal deformities; muscle wasting, muscle contractures, peripheral nerve impairment and poor muscle tone	Liaise with the therapy team to establish individual positioning regimens. Principles include maintaining the child's head in neutral position, with the spine and hips positioning in alignment with the head, maintaining flexion of the limbs and preventing extension of the ankles Ensure staff and child safety by used appropriate moving and handling equipment and techniques Ensure correct positioning is used at all times and use splints where appropriate
3. Poor circulation and inadequate lung functioning	Undertake passive exercises and regular position changes in order to improve circulation, relieve pressure, facilitate lung expansion, prevent urinary stasis, improve gut mobility and minimise muscle atrophy Anti-coagulant therapy and anti-embolism stockings will be necessary in older children

Continued

Table 33.4 Caring for the unconscious child—cont'd

Actual/potential problems	Nursing interventions
4. Infections particularly chest and urine infections	Ensure regular chest physiotherapy, ensure position changes and passive movements are incorporated into care activities Monitoring for signs of chest infection by recording temperature and changes in the amount and colour of secretions Minimising the risk of urine infection; where appropriate nurse the infant child in nappies and older child in pads; ensure meticulous skin care. An indwelling catheter is a potential sources of infection, if required maintain local policies in relation to the care of indwelling catheters and apply the principles of universal infection precautions Assess for the risk of infection by observing colour, smell and concentration of urine and measurement of body temperature
5. Constipation	Monitor bowel motions and manage constipation appropriately including high-fibre diet or supplements, adequate hydration and use of suppositories as necessary

Table 33.5 Immediate postoperative care following cranial surgery

Actual/potential problems	Nursing interventions
Potential airway obstruction and inadequate oxygenation due to depressed conscious levels and the effects of prolonged anaesthesia	Maintain the child's airway by positioning in the recovery position/use airway aids Assess and monitor respiratory effort and oxygen saturation levels Maintain oxygen therapy, ventilatory support may be necessary Assess the child's neurological status
Potential cardiac and respiratory instability due to neurological depression and effect of prolonged anaesthetic, particularly following surgery to the posterior fossa area, which contains vital control centres	Assess and monitor the child's respiratory effort, oxygen saturation levels and vital signs Ventilatory support and invasive blood pressure monitoring may be necessary Assess and report changes in the child's neurological status
Altered neurological functioning due to potential risk of intracranial pressure increases as a result of generalised cerebral oedema and haemorrhage	Regular neurological assessment in order to detect neurological changes, which may indicate a rise in ICP Management of RICP Monitor for signs of haemorrhage including observing wound bandages and drains, if present, for excessive blood loss, changes in conscious levels, raised pulse, falling blood pressure, changes in peripheral perfusion The child may require blood transfusion therapy and/or surgical control of bleeding/removal of haematoma if bleeding is excessive The position of the child's head is important and usually dependent on the procedure and surgeon's preference. In general nursing a child with the head elevated at 30°C and head in the midline is the norm which facilitates good venous return. However, in some surgical procedures for example certain types of shunts, nursing the child upright may result in the development of a subdural haematoma due to rapid drainage of the cerebrospinal fluid
Potential fluid and electrolyte disturbances due to an inability to take oral fluids	The child's fluid intake and output must be monitored In the early postoperative period the child will have an intravenous infusion Unless there is potential damage to the ninth and tenth cranial nerves, which may affect swallowing, the child may begin oral fluids as soon as consciousness is regained. It may be necessary for the child to undergo assessment by a speech and language therapist prior to commencing oral fluids
Maintaining fluid and electrolytes in children who have undergone cranial surgery is a balance between ensuring adequate circulatory blood volume in order to maintain good cerebral perfusion and preventing over-hydration, which will add to cerebral oedema	The management of fluids will be influenced by the type of surgery and tolerance of oral fluids, with the type and amount of fluids administered specific to each child's needs and urea and electrolyte profile Where prolonged intravenous fluid are required the child will need regular blood sampling (including serum osmolality) and circulatory assessment (pulse, blood pressure, capillary refill, temperature gradient difference between core and periphery)
Potential problem of inappropriate antidiuretic secretion or diabetes insipidus following surgery to the posterior fossa area	Measure and monitor urine output, test and record specific gravity Samples will be required in order to measure urine and blood osmolarity
Potential inability to maintain normal thermoregulation	Monitor the child's temperature regularly

Table 33.5 Immediate postoperative care following cranial surgery

Actual/potential problems	Nursing interventions
Hyperpyrexia can be a result of hypothalamus dysfunction and/or irritation of cerebral tissues for example the direct contact of blood with cerebral tissues	Manage pyrexia appropriately because any increase in core temperature increases cerebral metabolic rate, increases cerebral perfusion and potentially adds to any rises in intracranial pressure
Vomiting, as a direct result of RICP and potential side effects of anaesthetic agents	Administer anti-emetics. If vomiting persists the child will require continuation of intravenous fluids and a detailed nutritional assessment Ranitidine may be prescribed to prevent gastric irritation
Pain as a result of wound incision, positioning in theatre, stretching of the meninges and RICP	Assess pain and administer regular analgesia Intravenous opioids may further compromise respiratory effort, oral or rectal codeine may be a suitable alternative Unresolved pain may hinder the ability to undertake an effective neurological assessment
Potential for the development of seizures due to cerebral inflammation/irritation	Observe the child for signs of seizure activity In the unconscious child this may require continuous EEG monitoring Follow seizure management guidelines
Promote wound healing following surgical incision Potential wound infection	Maintain universal infection control measures Wound bandages are usually present for the first 24–48 hours and assist in reducing swelling at the wound site and help secure any drains that may be present Prophylactic antibiotics are rarely recommended Observe wound for redness, hardness and presence of exudate, which may indicate presence of infection and leakage of CSF Monitor the child's temperature Clips are often used to secure the wound and usually removed 7–10 days postoperatively

individual to circumvent impairments in order to minimise disability (Neumann 1995). Programmes of care must be individually designed and strongly influenced at encouraging the child to reach his or her full potential, working within a developmental context to integrate the children back into the family, school and community (Roffe 1989). This can only be achieved through a structured, caring and safe environment with all members of the multidisciplinary team adopting a child- and family-orientated approach to care. The care given will be provided for by a variety of disciplines, the team must have common goals which are integrated into the child's daily routines.

Nurses are a vital component of the multidisciplinary team and their roles include: assessment of the child, particularly in relation to actual or potential problems relating to activities of living; coordination of care and maintaining effective links with all team members; providing technical and physical care; integrating therapies initiated by other professionals into every day care; providing emotional support; and involving the family in care (Long et al 2002). If the child is to be successfully integrated back into the family, the family must be involved in and understand the process of rehabilitation, goal setting and monitoring of their child's progress.

Seminar discussion topic

Donna is a third-year nursing student undertaking a specialist placement on a neurosciences ward. She is enjoying her placement and has been learning to care for children with complex needs, particularly enhancing her practical skills in areas such as tracheostomy and gastrostomy care.

Donna has been caring for Amy, 14 months old, who has a progressive degenerative disease. Amy's development has always been slow and she did not achieve independent sitting. Recently, her condition has deteriorated, with a loss of abilities, recurrent seizures and increased spasticity.

Donna feels able to care for Amy in relation to ensuring all physical needs are met. However, she is finding it difficult to accept that Amy has an undiagnosed condition, with a short life expectancy. She finds it hard to communicate with Amy's parents.

- What issues do you think are important to discuss in relation to this scenario within Donna's learning set?

Emotional and psychological needs of the child and family

The diagnosis of a neurological disorder is devastating for the child and family, having far-reaching effects that can potentially affect physical, cognitive and affective (behaviour, personality) functions (Hickey 2003d). Changes in cognitive and affective functions can be particularly difficult for the family to accept, having the potential to alter all dimensions of family life and changing the anticipated expectations parents may have for their child. It is vital that the emotional and psychological needs of the child and family are considered and incorporated into care because normal coping abilities may become ineffective. The presence of nurses over the 24-hour care period often results in emotional and psychological care becoming a nursing responsibility. Depending on the diagnosis, the child and family will need to adjust to a range of situations and issues, including (Hickey 2003d):

- threat to the survival of the child
- threat to quality of life of the child:
  - motor paralysis
  - bowel and bladder dysfunction
  - communication difficulties
  - sensory deficits
- behavioural problems
- future ability of the child to live independently
- future ability of the child to form relationships
- future education and career prospects
- a dependent child may require the parents to review current care arrangements, which may result in a reduction of income and alteration in lifestyles
- meeting siblings needs.

The family will have many questions in relation to the child's condition, why and how it has happened, and they may be experiencing feelings of guilt. These feelings may be compounded in situations when there is no definitive diagnosis or the child's condition is life threatening; parents my feel frustrated and isolated. Extensive investigations and unpleasant treatments will add to the general despair. The family may be angry that vague signs and symptoms have gone unnoticed. There will be fears in relation to the prognosis and long-term outcomes. The family may be experiencing difficulty in accepting the changes in their child and grieving for the child they know, love and who has been an integral part of their lives. These emotions will affect the family's ability to comprehend information given to them.

It is essential to establish the usual coping strategies and support systems used by the child and family. Long-term support should be aimed at supporting and developing existing mechanisms. Nursing interventions, which form an integral part of everyday practice in supporting the emotional and psychological needs of the child and family, include:

- ensuring the family is given enough opportunity to ask questions and that responses are clear, accurate and honest
- providing and reinforcing information regularly, keeping the family updated. Essential information should be communicated effectively between the whole multidisciplinary team, to ensure a consistent approach to care
- including the child in discussions at a level appropriate to their age and stage of development
- providing support by listening to the family's anxieties and concerns
- ensuring a non-judgemental approach to care respecting the cultural, religious and spiritual beliefs of the family
- assisting the family to make realistic goals in relation to their child's care
- ensuring care is family centred, all aspects of care are discussed and care planning is negotiated with family, and child where appropriate
- recognising that there will be extreme anxiety if a child requires care in different settings; ensure systems allow for smooth transfers
- recognising when there is a need to refer to other members of the multidisciplinary team.

Overview and principles of managing selected neurological conditions in childhood

This section will provide an overview of selected neurological conditions. Meningitis is covered in Chapter 40, abnormalities in physical development including cerebral palsy in Chapter 24 and learning disabilities, including Down syndrome, in Chapter 47.

Brain tumours

Brain tumours are the most common solid tumour and the second most common malignancy in children (leukaemia being more prevalent). In the UK, approximately 350 children are diagnosed with a brain tumour every year (CancerBACUP 2005). Progress in the management of these children has reduced the overall mortality but morbidity, in terms of physical and intellectual sequelae, remains significant (Duffner et al 1993, Stewart & Cohen 1998). Tumours in general are divided into malignant or benign, referring to the ability of the tumour to spread and the sensitivity to treatment. With brain tumours, factors that determine outcome are less clear and influenced by the anatomical position of the tumour and age of presentation. The accessibility of the tumour for surgical treatment influences management options, therefore potential outcomes.

Aetiology

The causes of brain tumours are unclear; contributing factors include (Strother et al 2002):

- exposure to ionising radiation
- association with other cancers, or their treatments
- underlying immunosuppression disorders
- a family history of brain tumours, bone cancer, leukaemia and lymphoma
- familial clustering of embryonal tumours
- potential link to environmental carcinogens.

Pathophysiology and classification of brain tumours

Figure 33.8 shows the anatomical position of the common brain tumours in children:

- Medulloblastomas: part of a group of embryonic tumours collectively known as primitive neuroectodermal tumours (PNETs), which arise from neuroepithelial cells

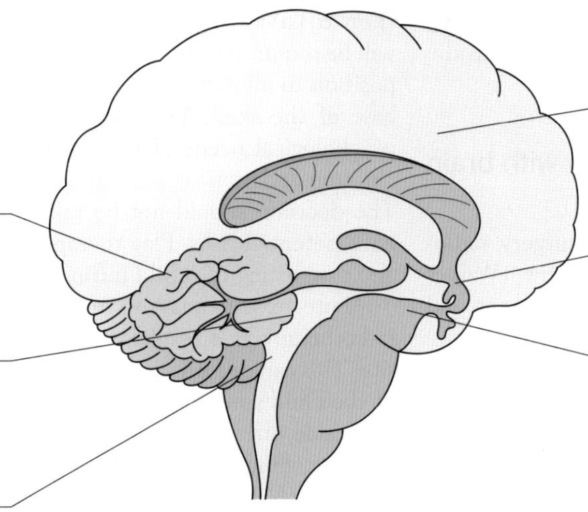

Fig. 33.8 • Common brain tumours: position and frequency (adapted from Vernon-Levett & Geller 1997).

and usually occur within the posterior fossa. The tumour cells have no clear line of demarcation from normal tissue (Brett & Harding 1997b) and often permeate along the CSF pathways resulting in spinal cord deposits (Halperin et al 1994).

- Astrocytomas: found throughout the brain, arising from glial astrocyte cells (Ryan-Murray & Petriccione 2002) and have a tendency to form large cysts. Astrocytomas are graded from I to IV, grade I indicates a benign slow growing lesion and grade IV a highly malignant tumour. The majority in children are graded I or II.
- Ependymomas: originate from the ependymal tissue within the ventricular system (Shiminski-Maher & Shields 1995). The histology varies from benign through to highly malignant. There are many similarities with medulloblastomas, including a tendency to metastasise along the CSF pathways (Brett & Harding 1997b).
- Brainstem gliomas: have varied histology. A definitive diagnosis is not always possible because the position of the tumour within the brainstem may not be conducive to obtaining a biopsy (Brett & Harding 1997b). Most are high-grade astrocytomas, fast growing, diffuse and highly malignant, with extensive branching and a poor response to treatment (Ryan-Murray & Petriccione 2002).
- Craniopharyngiomas: benign, slow-growing tumours arising from epithelial cells within the pituitary gland. Diagnosis can be time consuming and often delayed because signs and symptoms are vague and insidious (Greenwood 1992). The effects are significant because the tumour is difficult to treat due to the anatomical location and the abnormal tissue adhering to surrounding tissues, preventing normal function and resulting in associated endocrine dysfunctions (Strother et al 2002).

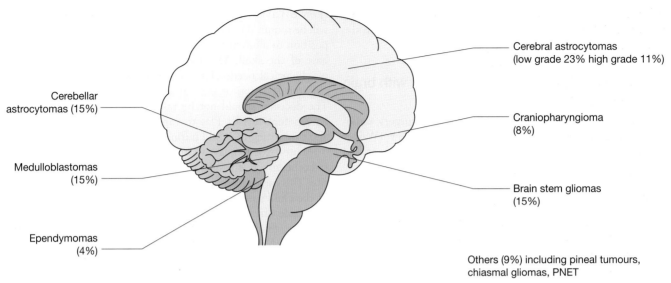

Presentation

Symptoms occurring within a short time span indicate a rapidly growing or aggressive tumour, with gradual symptoms more likely to be caused by a low grade or benign tumour (Stewart & Cohen 1998). Most childhood brain tumours are associated with signs of raised intracranial pressure. In addition there will be specific signs and symptoms related to the altered function/compression of structures within the direct vicinity of the tumour. Children with a medulloblastoma, cerebellar astrocytoma or brainstem ependymoma typically present with cerebellar signs such as ataxia, coordination and gait disturbance (Fenichel 1997a, Worrall 1999). Tumours within the posterior fossa can obstruct CSF flow resulting in hydrocephalus. Any spinal cord involvement may result in neck stiffness. The symptoms of craniopharyngiomas are insidious, the child may suffer visual field defects as a result of compression on the optic nerve discs, a low basal metabolic rate resulting in fatigability, a low blood pressure, disruption to pituitary functioning causing delayed skeletal growth and sexual maturation, and hypothalamic disturbances causing obesity and diabetes insipidus (Brett & Harding 1997b). The specific presentation of supratentorial tumours is directly related to function of the cerebral cortex where the tumour is located (Strother et al 2002) (see Fig. 33.4).

Diagnosis

Diagnosis is often difficult because the presenting symptoms can be vague and non-specific or similar to those of more common childhood illnesses (Stewart & Cohen 1998). Guidelines are available to assist primary healthcare professionals in making prompt and appropriate referrals when a child presents with vague signs and symptoms and a brain tumour is a possible diagnosis (NICE 2005). Diagnosis will be made following a detailed neurological examination and confirmed by a MRI or CT scan. Children with medulloblastoma will require imaging to determine spinal metastasis and a lumbar puncture may be performed in order to ascertain if tumour cells are within the CSF.

Treatment and management of children with brain tumours

Many children will require multimodal therapy: surgery, radiotherapy, chemotherapy and symptom management (Walker et al 1999). Surgery is usually the definitive treatment and aims to (Turini & Redaelli 2001):

- remove the tumour and provide a cure wherever possible
- remove as much tumour as possible
- obtain a biopsy of the tumour so that a definitive diagnosis can be made
- manage raised intracranial pressure
- provide access for other treatments, e.g. chemotherapy.

The general care of the child requiring neurosurgery has been outlined earlier within this chapter. Posterior fossa syndrome is a potential complication following posterior fossa tumour resection, with the symptoms causing additional anxieties for the child and family (Kirk et al 1995). Symptoms usually present 72 hours postoperatively and include cranial nerve palsies, dysphagia, motor weakness, mutism or speech disturbances and emotional liability (Dailey et al 1995, Kirk et al 1995).

Radiotherapy targets and disrupts the action of deoxyribonucleic acid, which is essential for cell division (Shiminski-Maher & Shields 1995). Radiation primarily affects cells during division; therefore rapidly growing tumour cells are especially sensitive to radiation exposure. The aim is to deliver therapeutic doses of radiation that cause tumour cell destruction and inhibit cell division but minimise toxic effects to surrounding healthy tissue. Linear accelerators and computer-assisted equipment have made radiotherapy more precise by ensuring accurate delivery to the tumour site (Lew & LaVally 1995, Moore 1995). Radiotherapy is inappropriate for children less than 3 years of age because of the high susceptibility of the immature developing brain to radiation damage resulting in growth failure and cognitive dysfunction (Lew & LaVally 1995).

Ideally radiotherapy is administered five times a week for approximately 6 weeks, 2–3 weeks following surgery or diagnosis (Walker et al 1999). Radiotherapy is used (Turini & Redaelli 2001):

- for inoperable tumours
- to treat tumours only partially removed at surgery
- to destroy any remaining tumour seeds post-surgery
- to reduce the tumour size in order to relieve acute symptoms prior to surgery
- to treat secondary brain metastasis.

Treatment planning is vital because the child requires immobilising within an individually constructed mould which is essential for ensuring precise and consistent positioning of the treatment area during every radiotherapy session (Lew & LaVally 1995). Children with posterior fossa tumours will be required to lie face down and be immobilised in a prone position to allow the radiation to be directed to the posterior base of the skull. This can be distressing for the child. The psychological needs of the child are important and for some children sedation or general anaesthesia are the only option. The decision should not be taken lightly as both procedures have potential risks. Play therapists are invaluable in preparing and supporting the child during radiotherapy.

Acute toxicity may occur during or immediately following radiotherapy as a result of acute inflammation at the tumour site. This can cause a significant rise in ICP, requiring monitoring of the child's neurological status (Moore 1995). Other immediate side effects include nausea, vomiting, headaches, loss of appetite, fluid and electrolyte disturbances and localised skin irritation (Moore 1995). Children receiving radiotherapy are at risk of developing radiotherapy somnolence weeks to months after the completion of treatment, characterised by excessive lethargy, up to 20 hours a day, and general malaise (Moore 1995), but radiotherapy somnolence is usually self-limiting.

Chemotherapy alone rarely provides a cure but is being used increasingly as an important adjunct therapy (Vernon-Levett & Geller 1997) and in young children chemotherapy offers an opportunity to limit tumour expansion until radiotherapy can be delivered (Duffner et al 1993). Chemotherapy has increased the long-term survival rates of children with brain tumours (Shiminski-Maher & Shields 1995). The difficulty in using chemotherapy for the treatment of brain tumours is poor drug penetration across the blood–brain barrier, due to the tight junction between endothelial cells in the brain capillaries. This impermeability can be overcome by (Turini & Redaelli 2001):

- multidrug combinations
- disruption of the junctions between brain capillaries or endothelial cells by the administration of drugs such as mannitol
- administrating high doses of chemotherapeutic agents such as methotrexate in combination with a rescue therapy such as folinic acid rescue therapy which reverses the excessive drug.

All children receiving chemotherapy should be cared for in a Children's Cancer and Leukaemia Group (CCLG) accredited centre, where treatment protocols are adapted to incorporate the current evidence, and outcomes can be monitored.

In addition to the knowledge and skills required to ensure both the physiological and psychological needs of the child with a brain tumour are being met, the principles of caring for a child having chemotherapy must be applied. The nurse will need to be proactive in minimising the risk of and treating the side effects of chemotherapy including vomiting, sore mouth, pain, bone marrow suppression and increased risk of infection (Vernon-Levett & Geller 1997). Good communication between differing specialties and understanding an overview of all the treatment modalities are essential in order to meet the needs of the child and family.

Symptom management will be necessary to reduce the side effects of treatments and where palliation is the main aim of care (Walker at al 1999). Corticosteriods, primarily dexamethasone, usually prescribed as a short course of treatment, may reduce cerebral swelling and provide temporary relief from symptoms at diagnosis and where there is acute radiotherapy-induced inflammatory response (Walker et al 1999). Low-dose steroids may help to reduce the symptoms of radiotherapy somnolence (Walker et al 1999). Persistent symptomatic hydrocephalus may require the insertion of a ventricular shunt.

Long-term outcomes

Long-term survival for children following the diagnosis of a brain tumour is often accompanied by deficits of motor and sensory functions, delays in neurobehavioural function, cognitive and learning disabilities, visual and hearing deficits, and chronic endocrine deficiencies (Lew & LaVally 1995). Many children will require special educational assistance (Mulhern et al 1998). Radiotherapy in particular has been linked to long-term developmental deficits (Stewart & Cohen 1998) and can cause subcortical white-matter degeneration, ophthalmic and auditory damage, and is linked to alterations in intellectual functioning (Moore 1995). Endocrine dysfunction, particularly growth hormone deficiency and hypothyroidism necessitating hormone replacement therapy, may occur as a result of pituitary and hypothalamic damage following irradiation to the posterior fossa area (Cullen et al 2002). Radiotherapy can cause premature closure of growth plates resulting in precocious puberty (Stewart & Cohen 1998). Neurological disabilities as a result of the effects of the tumour and/or treatments will require the child to have a thorough assessment involving all members of the multidisciplinary team and early initiation of a rehabilitative programme. It is vital that the emotional and psychological needs of the child and family are met.

Craniosynostosis

Craniosynostosis is a condition of premature fusion of the skull sutures affecting approximately 1 in 2000 children (Child Neurology 2002). Simple craniosynostosis is a synostosis of a single suture with no involvement of the facial skeleton. Complex craniosynostosis is a synostosis of one or more sutures with involvement of the facial skeleton, and includes a plethora of crainiosynostotic syndromes; Apert's and Crouzon's being the most well known.

Aetiology

Most cases are sporadic, with the cause unknown. However, craniosynostosis syndromes probably have a genetic mode of inheritance:

- Primary craniosynostosis may be due to a single gene defect (Boyadjiev 2007).
- If a parent and child have craniosynostosis, or two siblings have craniosynostosis with unaffected parents, the risk of another child developing the disorder increases.
- There may be an X-linked mode of inheritance, particularly with sagittal synostosis which is much more common in males.

Craniosynostosis is more likely to occur in:

- boys
- multiple births
- older maternal and/or paternal age
- low birthweight babies
- caucasian ethnic group
- if there have been complications with labour.

Although not substantiated craniosynostosis has been linked with (Hockley 1993):

- drug teratogenicity, particularly the anticonvulsant phenytoin
- maternal excesses of vitamin A and D and ethanol
- intrauterine compression
- pesticides, lead and pollution.

Presentation

In the newborn the cranial sutures are separated by membranous spaces several millimetres wide (see Fig. 33.6). Early closure of a suture inhibits normal perpendicular brain expansion and the skull is forced to grow in a direction parallel to the fused suture (Sarnat & Menkes 2000). The cranial bones remain small and underdeveloped at the site of fusion, while the unaffected bones enlarge to compensate, thus allowing brain growth (May 1992). The characteristic head shape that results depends on which suture or sutures fuse (Fig. 33.9). Craniosynostosis may be apparent at birth but the deformity is usually diagnosed in early infancy when the abnormally shaped head becomes more pronounced (Panchal & Uttchin 2003). Diagnosis is usually made by visual inspection of the skull and palpitation of the sutures. Skull X-rays will show a band of increased bone density at the site of the prematurely closed suture (Fenichel 1997b) and a CT scan will reveal the extent of the premature fusion.

Premature closure of all the cranial sutures can occur. This is referred to as craniostenosis or oxycephaly. Of all types of craniosynostosis, this can produce the most severe central nervous system involvement because total brain growth is restricted and increased intracranial pressure is likely. This may lead to impaired mental and motor functions, optic nerve atrophy and death.

Treatment and management options

Operative correction of the deformity is the treatment of choice (Moos & Hide 1993) and the general consensus of opinion is that it should be undertaken early, preferably within the first year of life (Johnston 2001, Kapp-Simon 1998, Panchal et al 2001). Within this time frame the deformity will not have progressed, the bones will be more malleable and the growing brain will promote a normal head shape, resulting in greater cosmetic improvements. Early treatment potentially minimises later complications such as visual, nasal, phonetic, dental problems, psychological dysfunctions and learning disabilities (Panchal & Uttchin 2003). If left untreated, skull deformities become

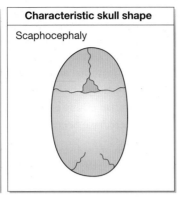

Type of synostosis	Characteristic skull shape
Sagittal synostosis: - fusion of the sagittal suture - most common form of craniosynostosis - accounts for 50–55% of cases	Scaphocephaly 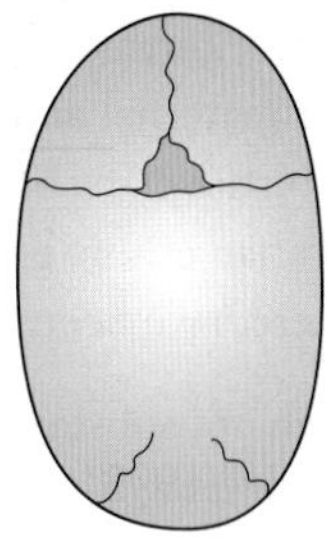
Coronal synostosis: - fusion of one or both of the coronal sutures - accounts for 20–25% of cases	Brachycephaly 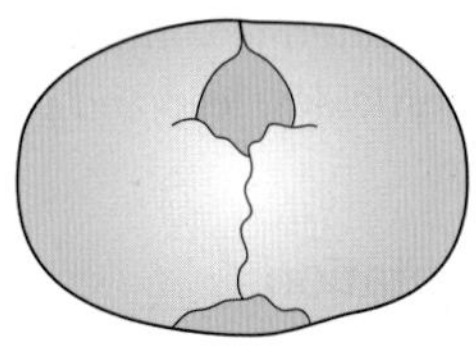
Metopic synostosis: - fusion of the metopic suture - accounts for approximately 10% of cases	Trigoncephaly 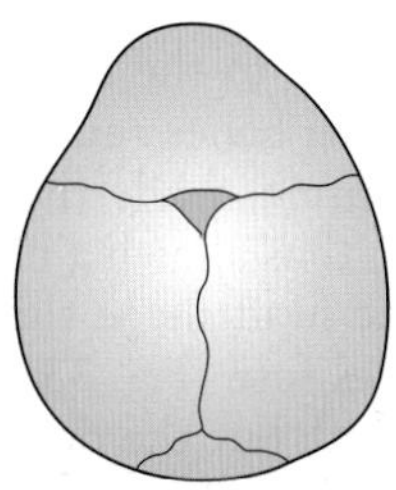
Lambdoid synostosis: - fusion of one or both of the lambdoid suture - rare, accounting for 3–5% of cases	Plagiocephaly 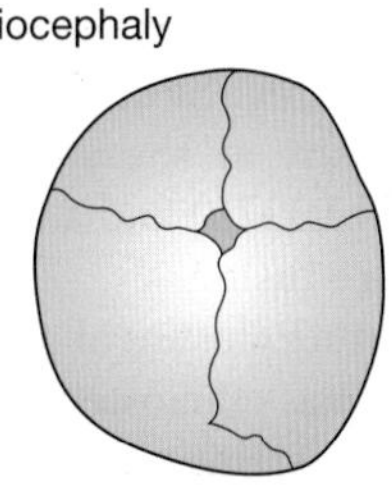

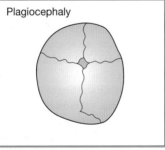

Fig. 33.9 • Types of craniosynostosis and characteristic features (adapted from Johnston 2001, May 2001, Panchal & Uttchin 2003).

permanent and there is increased risk of raised intracranial pressure (Moos & Hide 1993). Prior to surgery, neurodevelopmental assessment is necessary to establish if there are any developmental problems which will aid in predicting the long-term outcomes of surgery and will enable clinicians to offer realistic expectations (Panchal & Uttchin 2003).

Surgery can range from excision of the fused suture, for example in sagittal synostosis, to complex craniofacial surgery involving the repositioning and reshaping of the skull and facial bones (Kershner & Claussen 1986, Polley et al 1998). Correction of craniofacial syndromes requires surgery throughout childhood, with future procedures determined by alterations to cranial-facial structures as the child grows (Panchal & Uttchin 2003). Although, paediatric neuroscience is regarded as a specialist field of practice (Chumas et al 2002, DoH 2002), the complexities involved in craniofacial surgery have resulted in this type of surgery being further identified as a sub-speciality (Child Neurology 2002, Society of British Neurological Surgeons 2001). The management of these children must occur within designated centres, with care delivered by an experienced team of healthcare professionals.

Parents should be given realistic expectations of their child's appearance post-surgery (Drew 1990). They need to be informed that the child's head shape may appear fairly normal immediately after surgery but significant postoperative swelling will occur within a few hours and the child may not be able to open his or her eyes. Blood loss may be significant and the child must be monitored for cardiac instability. The amount of blood loss and circulating fluid volumes must be regularly assessed through repeated blood sampling to monitor full blood count, urea and electrolyte, clotting factors and serum osmolality. The child must be monitored for signs of haemorrhage including observing bandages and drains for excessive blood loss, changes in conscious levels, raised pulse, falling blood pressure and changes in peripheral perfusion (May 2001). An elevated temperature could indicate a wound infection, however hyperpyrexia is common during the first 3–4 days postoperatively, usually as a result of irritation of cerebral tissues by the presence of blood (Panchal & Uttchin 2003). Parents will require support and advice in positioning and handling their child post surgery. The child should be nursed at a 45° head tilt to reduce cerebral oedema.

Long-term outcomes

The extent of the child's long-term care needs and resultant deficits depends on a range of factors including:

- the presence of an associated syndrome
- the severity of craniosynostosis
- damage caused by raised intracranial pressure
- repeated infections where a shunt is present.

The child may have physical problems including visual and hearing deficits, facial dysostosis and prognathism (Drew 1990), and there is great variability in the level of cognitive and psychomotor function (Sarnat & Menkes 2000). For many children and their families, body image is a significant issue and the child and family will require psychological support to assist and support them in dealing with their emotional stress. The follow-up care for children with craniosynostosis will vary depending on the extent of the individual child's needs; for children with complex needs follow-up care is life-long.

Epilepsy

Epilepsy is one of the most common neurological conditions in both adults and children. It has been estimated 1 person in 2000 is diagnosed with epilepsy each year, but the risk increases to 1 in 500 in children less than 1 year of age, and the estimated prevalence rate in children is 1 in 200 (Heaney

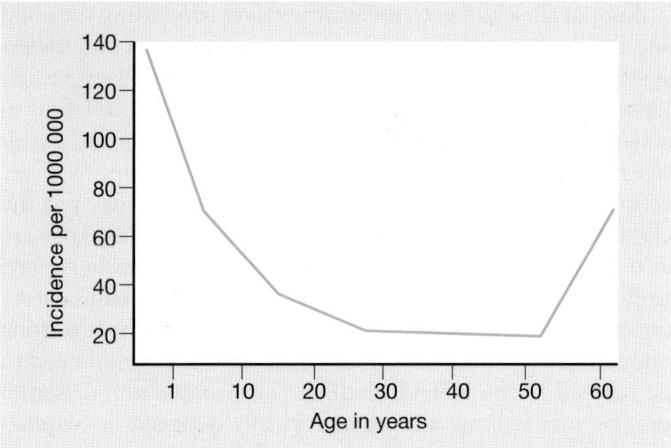

Fig. 33.10 • Incidence per 100,000 people related to age (Appleton 1995).

et al 2002, Royal College of Paediatrics and Child Health 2000) (Fig. 33.10). Although there is no uniform definition, epilepsy can be thought of as an umbrella term used to describe a range of a condition characterised by recurrent, unprovoked seizures (Panayiotopoulos 2005). An epileptic seizure is an episode of excessive neuronal activity that interrupts cerebral function.

Aetiology

Although a range of causes can potentially result in the development of epilepsy in children, aetiology is broadly divided into genetic and congenital malformations that occur during cerebral development, and irreversible brain damage (trauma brain injury, CNS infections, perinatal hypoxia, perinatal intraventricular haemorrhage, tumours) (Appleton 1995, Sander & Shorvon 1996). Epilepsy is also associated with neurodegenerative disorders. However, for the majority of children with epilepsy there is no known cause (idiopathic epilepsy) but it is likely that there is a genetic origin and therefore are best termed cryptogenic (Sander & Shorvon 1996). Epilepsy is more prevalent in families who are socioeconomically disadvantaged (Heaney et al 2002).

Classification

The current classification of epilepsy is based on the 2001 International League Against Epilepsy (ILAE) system (Panayiotopoulos 2005):

- Focal or local seizures; where seizure activity is generated within a localised area of the brain and seizure presentation depends on the specific function at the site of the abnormal activity
- Generalised seizures, where there is widespread nervous disruption across both hemispheres that can result in a range of seizure manifestations
- Unclassified epileptic seizures
- Prolonged seizures, such as status epilepticus.

In addition to the outlined classification system for epilepsy, many epileptic syndromes exist. These syndromes have characteristic seizure patterns, signs and symptoms, which are suggestive of a particular condition; examples include infantile spasms (West syndrome), Lennox–Gaustaut syndrome and juvenile myoclonic epilepsy. Rare types of epilepsy include sleep seizures and photosensitive epilepsies.

Presentation

A diagnosis of epilepsy is usually only made if two or more seizures have occurred. Accurate diagnosis is dependent on a good history and detailed description of the seizure activity (Appleton 1995). Classifying the type of epilepsy needs to consider the age of onset of the first seizure, the types of seizure activity, presence of underlying neurological problems, family history and EEG findings. Epilepsy can present in a range of seizure types; the common terms used to describe seizure types include:

- absence; sudden and usually brief loss of awareness of the surroundings and the child may appear to be staring or have rapid eye blinking
- atonic; sudden and brief loss of muscle tone resulting in the child falling to the ground, often referred to as a drop attack
- aura; abnormal sensations as a result of stimulation of a specific area within the brain, such as visual hallucinations or illusions, auditory, taste or smell hallucinations; may precede other seizure types
- automatism: involuntary repetitive motor activity such as lip smacking
- clonic; limb jerking caused by the muscles contracting and relaxing in quick succession
- myoclonic; a sudden contraction of the muscles that can affect the trunk or be restricted to one or both arms or legs
- tonic; increased muscle tone resulting in stiffness
- tonic-clonic; increased muscle tone that results in rigidity followed by the clonic phase where there is rhythmical jerking movements. The jerking movements last for a variable period of time and there may be reflux emptying of the bladder and bowels. The tonic clonic phase may be preceded by an aura, there may be confusion and lethargy once the seizure activity has ceased
- versive movements; tonic or clonic head and eye deviations which are involuntary and result in sustained unnatural positioning of the head and eyes.

Treatment and management options

The first-line treatment for epilepsy is antiepileptic drugs, with the aim being to use a single drug in the lowest possible dose to control seizures while minimising side effects. A wide range of antiepileptic drugs are now available and choice will depend on the type of seizures and underlying diagnosis, with monotherapy being successful in the majority of children (Camfield et al 1997). Traditionally, sodium valproate has been the first choice for generalised seizures and carbamazepine for partial seizures (Marson et al 2003, 2007a). However, newer antiepileptic drugs such as vigabatrin and lamotrigine are becoming more established (Marson et al 2007b). Parents need to understand the action of the drugs, side effects, drug toxicity monitoring and possible drug interactions (including over the counter drugs).

Activity

Martin, a young person of 16 years, has been diagnosed as having juvenile myoclonic epilepsy within the last 12 months. He has frequent absence seizures where he loses consciousness for between 5 and 30 seconds from which he recovers spontaneously, and is able to continue previous activities. He also has occasional tonic-clonic seizures, which have lasted between 2 and 5 minutes.

How would you assist Martin if you witnessed him having a tonic-clonic seizure in the school grounds?

Think about what you would and would not do.

- You may wish to check your answer on the Epilepsy Action (British Epilepsy Association) web site: http://www.epilepsy.org.uk [search for seizure-first aid]

Intractable epilepsy occurs in 4% of children with epilepsy (Camfield et al 1997). It is difficult to manage even with multiple drug therapy and occurs primarily in children with complex neurological problems (Camfield et al 1997). Additional treatment options, which may offer opportunity to reduce seizure activities in these children, include:

- ketogenic diet: a diet high in fat but low in carbohydrate, thus fat is the main energy source rather than glucose. The metabolism of fats results in the production of ketones, which are thought to have antiepileptic properties (Levy & Cooper 2003)
- surgery: procedures include corpus callosotomy, which aims to prevent seizure activity affecting both hemispheres, and cerebral resections (focal or unilateral hemispherectomy), which aims to remove the site of the seizure activity in uncontrolled localised epilepsy . Surgery requires accurate diagnosis and a focal site for seizure activity
- vagal nerve stimulation: a stimulator is surgically placed under the skin in the left upper chest. It is connected to the vagal nerve by electrodes which are then programmed to stimulate the nerve. The exact reasons for a reduction in seizure activity remain unclear (Kirse et al 2002).

There is no reliable evidence to support these treatments but they appear successful for some children.

Evidence-based practice

The Cochrane Library has a range of systematic reviews relating to treatment options for epilepsy. The Cochrane Library can be accessed at the following:

- http://www.cochrane.co.uk

or via the National Electronic Library for Health:

- http://www.nelh.nhs.uk

Evidence-based guidelines relating to the diagnosis and management of epilepsy in children and adults were published in 2004 by NICE:

- http://www.nice.org.uk

Care of the child with epilepsy involves supporting the child and family during diagnosis and in the management and understanding of treatment modalities. For children with severe epilepsy the family may require additional support in relation to activities of daily living and to promote social, motor and cognitive function of the child. Increased metabolism during frequent seizures and disruption to normal eating patterns may put the child at risk of undernourishment. Children with epilepsy are at risk of injury; parents, other carers and schoolteachers need to be taught the skills required to maintain the child's safety during a seizure and ensure a safe environment without putting undue restrictions on the child. Healthcare advice will need to be tailored to the individual child. For example immunisation programmes will need to be individually designed in conjunction with appropriate government guidelines.

The normal challenges of adolescence will be increased for the young person with epilepsy. The young person will need support and advice about lifestyle choices such as independent living, career opportunities, learning to drive, insurance issues, the need to continue medication, contraception and planning a family (NICE 2004).

www

A wealth of lifestyle and practical advice relating to epilepsy is readily available on the following web sites:

- Epilepsy Action (British Epilepsy Association): http://www.epilepsy.org.uk [search for seizure-first aid]
- National Society for Epilepsy: http://www.epilepsynse.org.uk [search for first aid for epilepsy]

Evidence-based practice

Current immunisation information is available at the following websites:

- http://www.immunisation.nhs.uk
- http://www.doh.gov.uk/greenbook/index.htm

Long-term outcomes

The risk of premature death is 2–3 times higher for people with epilepsy compared to the general population (Hanna et al 2002), with the most common reason being sudden unexpected death associated with seizures (DoH 2003). The effectiveness of antiepileptic drugs achieves protracted remission in 70% of people with epilepsy; the remaining 30% will have an intractable and disabling condition (Hanna et al 2002). Many of these children will have complex care needs and will require physical, emotional and social support in order to maximise their potential.

Hydrocephalus

Hydrocephalus comprises of a highly diverse group of disorders that have little in common except the increased volume of CSF within the intracranial fluid spaces. The overall incidence of hydrocephalus is 0.2–4.2 per 1000 live births (Blackburn & Fineman 1994, Carey et al 1994).

Aetiology

The majority of children with hydrocephalus have an identifiable cause, predictably a result of congenital malformations for example aqueduct stenosis, Arnold–Chiari malformations and Dandy–Walker syndrome. Aqueduct stenosis accounts for about 15% of all cases of hydrocephalus (Brett & Harding 1997a). Other causes of hydrocephalus include:

- tumours that obstruct the flow of CSF
- infections such as meningitis can cause adhesion between the epithelial linings of the CSF spaces, obstructing CSF flow
- intraventricular haemorrhage in premature infants causing an initial blockage within the ventricles and secondary obstruction due to scarring
- associated with spina bifida
- rare causes include arteriovenous malformations, obstruction of venous sinuses (intracranial hypertension), craniosynostosis or hypersecretion of CSF.

Classification

Hydrocephalus is usually classified as:

- communicating hydrocephalus, where the blockage of CSF flow occurs outside the ventricular system
- non-communicating hydrocephalus, where the blockage of CSF flow occurs within the ventricular system.

Presentation

The age hydrocephalus develops is important because the presentation is different between the infant and older child (Kirkpatrick et al 1989). In newborn babies and infants the skull is expandable because the skull sutures have not yet fused, and a rise in CSF levels will not cause a rapid rise in ICP as in older children and adolescents (Brett & Harding 1997a). Hydrocephalus in an infant will result in a rapidly increasing head circumference, tense anterior fontanelle, splayed skull sutures, scalp vein distension, loss of upward gaze and neck rigidity (Kirkpatrick et al 1989). The infant often has a characteristic appearance with a small face in comparison to head size and the eyes have a typical sun-setting appearance (the sclera is not visible below the iris). Nystagmus with vomiting and irritability are important additional symptoms (Kirkpatrick et al 1989). Older children may display the more classic signs of RICP. Age of presentation is important because the causes of hydrocephalus are different across the age span – age influences management options and functional outcomes (Mori et al 1995).

Diagnosis

Fetal hydrocephalus can be diagnosed as early as the 13th week of gestation by ultrasound scan, where ventricular enlargement can be detected. However, accurate diagnosis will require amniocentesis in order to obtain samples for alpha-fetoprotein levels and to identify chromosomal abnormalities. If severe brain dysfunction is suspected termination may be offered. Postnatal diagnosis is usually made following an increase in head circumference (in infants) and neurological examination, with CT scanning confirming the diagnosis.

Treatment and management

The management of hydrocephalus will depend on the cause and severity of the CSF obstruction. Very rarely hydrocephalus can arrest of its own accord. However, the risk of delaying treatment must be balanced with the potential of compromising normal development. Conservative management is rarely a long-term option and is generally reserved for the premature infant post-intraventricular haemorrhage (Chumas et al 2001). Ventricular shunts in these acutely sick infants are difficult to place and often become dysfunctional (possibly due to high CSF protein levels) and infections are common (Pikus et al 1997). Drug therapy has traditionally included the use of diuretics (furosemide and acetazolamide), which are known to decrease CFS production. However, the International PHVD Drug Trial Group (1998) does not advocate the use of diuretics, which are associated with increased neurological morbidity.

The two main surgical procedures used to treat hydrocephalus are endoscopic third ventriculostomy, where an opening is made through the third ventricle and chiasmatic cistern, facilitating cerebrospinal fluid drainage, and the insertion of a ventricular shunt. Endoscopic third ventriculostomy has an advantage in that unlike ventricular shunts there is no need for a permanent implant (Cinalli et al 1998). Success rates following third ventriculostomy are variable because there may be associated problems contributing to the hydrocephalus such as poor CSF absorption (Chumas et al 2001, Siomin et al 2002).

The vast majority of children with hydrocephalus are managed by the surgical insertion of a shunt that diverts excess CSF from the ventricles into another body cavity. A catheter is inserted into the ventricles (the proximal catheter) through a burr hole made in the temporal bone of the skull, just behind the ear. This catheter is attached to a unidirectional valve system situated over the skull. The valve is attached to a second catheter (the distal catheter), which is placed into a body cavity such as the peritoneum (ventriculoperitoneal shunts) or the left atrium (ventriculoatrial shunts). Ventriculoperitoneal shunts (Fig. 33.11) are usually the first choice because they are easier to insert, catheters can be of sufficient length to allow for growth, good absorption of CSF occurs across the peritoneum and there is not the added potential of septicaemia, bacterial endocarditis and shunt nephritis, associated with ventriculoatrial shunts (Keucher & Mealey 1979).

Shunts operate on the same principle; the valve has a threshold pressure, below which the valve remains closed and above which the valve opens allowing CSF to flow through the shunt system. Different valve systems have different resistant pressures: low pressure (5 cmH_2O), medium pressure (10 cmH_2O) and high pressure (15 mmH_2O) (Drake & Kestle 1996). One of the major functional problems with shunt valves is CSF flow increases when the child is upright due to the effects of gravity resulting in over-drainage of the ventricles

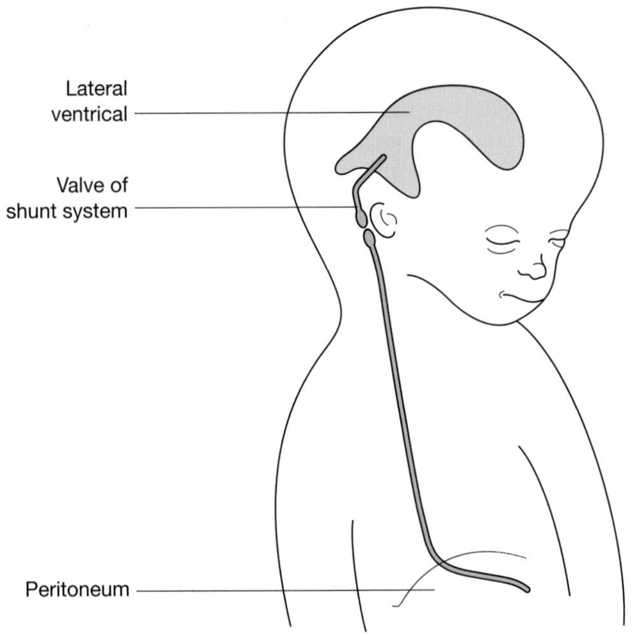

Fig. 33.11 • Position of a ventriculoperitoneal shunt.

Table 33.6 Main complications of ventricular shunts

Complication	Examples
Infection causes colonisation of the shunt system by bacteria causing blockage	Meningitis Wound infection Peritonitis (ventriculoperitoneal shunts) Septicaemia (ventriculoatrial shunts)
Mechanical failure can result in malfunction or blockage of system	Proximal obstruction: the catheter becomes lodged in tissue such as choroid plexus, brain tissue Distal obstruction: the development of intra-abdominal cysts, CSF ascites Catheter misplacement: intracranial, intra-abdominal, intravascular Fractures and disconnections of the catheter Migration of catheter into hollow viscera such as bladder or inguinal canal
Functional failure	Over-drainage Under-drainage Miscellaneous problems affecting shunt function: Intracranial hypotension Post-shunt pericerebral collections Slit ventricle syndrome

(Pudenz & Foltz 1991). This occurs because when in an upright position a larger pressure differential exists between the head and abdomen, resulting in CSF flowing at a higher rate than when a child is lying flat.

A trouble-free shunt is a desirable but elusive goal and unfortunately there are numerous potential complications with intraventricular shunts (Chumas et al 2001). Shunt failure is a major issue with reported failure rates of 40% during the first year following insertion and a further 14% during the second year following insertion (Drake et al 1998). Complications can be broadly divided into three groups: infection, mechanical failure and functional problems (Table 33.6).

The care of the child and family must be specific to current health needs. Initially, the emphasis of care will be directed towards assisting the parents (and older child) to understand and come to terms with the condition and supporting them to care for their child while waiting for surgery. For an infant this may include supporting parents to comfort an irritable child, assisting with feeding and positioning techniques.

The principles of care for the child requiring emergency insertion or revision of a ventricular shunt are centred on managing an acutely ill child with RICP. The sudden rise in intracranial pressure is due to rapidly increasing CSF levels within the ventricles with the risk of cerebral herniation and life-threatening consequences. Neurological changes must be detected promptly, through systematic neurological assessment and observations. In addition care will be primarily aimed at preparing the child for investigations (CT scan) and theatre in an organised and structured manner, while offering support to the child and family. The child who has been vomiting as a result of RICP will require intravenous fluids to correct dehydration.

The immediate potential postoperative complications following insertion of a shunt include intraventricular haemorrhage, blockage of the shunt and subdural haemorrhage, due to rapid overdrainage of the ventricles. Positioning of the child is an important consideration and will be influenced by the type of shunt inserted; nursing staff must ensure they have clear postoperative instructions.

There is no specific care relating to the shunt once inserted; avoiding lying on the shunt site may prevent skin breakdown, particularly in the immediate postoperative period. The child and family will require detailed advice and support in relation to detecting signs and symptoms of shunt failure. The Association of Spina Bifida and Hydrocephalus (ASBAH) offers an effective support network and a range of information for children and their families.

WWW

A wealth of lifestyle and practical advice relating to hydrocephalus is readily available on the following website:

- Association of Spina Bifida and Hydrocephalus (ASBAH): http://www.asbah.org.uk

Long-term outcomes

The child's long-term care needs depend on the reasons for hydrocephalus and the presence of associated conditions such as epilepsy. The majority of children with hydrocephalus will attend mainstream school. However, 40–60% of children will have neurological deficits such as physical, cognitive and behavioural difficulties (Casey et al 1997, Hoppe-Hirsch et al 1998). These children will require appropriate multidisciplinary team input to ensure they reach their full potential.

Traumatic brain injury

Acquired brain injury can result from both traumatic and non-traumatic insults to the brain. Trauma is the main cause of acquired brain injury, due to an external force, which may produce a diminished or altered state of consciousness. The survival rate following traumatic brain injury has increased due to medical and technological advances.

Aetiology

Traumatic brain injury is the leading cause of mortality and morbidity in children and accounts for one-third of accidental deaths in children (Kraus et al 1987, Mahoney et al 1983). The dramatic increase in the number of children sustaining a head injury over the last 30 years is primarily due to increased road traffic use (Mahoney et al 1983, Kraus et al 1987, McMillan & Greenwood 1993). Causes of traumatic brain injury in children include (Durkin et al 1998, Henry et al 1992, Parslow et al 2005):

- Road traffic accidents: account for 40–60% of head injuries, with the majority resulting from a child pedestrian hit by a moving car.
- Falls: account for 20–30% of head injuries; severe head trauma is rare in home accidents.
- Non-accidental injury: the most common cause of severe head injury in children under 1 year.

Associated factors include (Durkin et al 1998, Kraus et al 1987, Henry et al 1992, Parslow et al 2005):

- higher incidence in boys because they develop distance and spatial interpretation later than girls and are more likely to participate in risk-taking behaviours
- seasonal, with the peak incidence occurring during spring and summer and between 2pm and 10pm
- other variables that influence a child's vulnerability to traumatic brain injury include the presence of visual or hearing deficits, learning deficits, low socioeconomic status, urban residence and previous head injury.

Classification

Traumatic brain injury is usually defined as an insult to the brain, not of a degenerative or congenital nature, caused by an external force that results in a diminished or altered state of consciousness (Brain Injury Association of America 2004, Kraus 1987).

Presentation

Minor traumatic brain injury result in transient symptoms such as concussion, no abnormal neurological signs, GCS above 13, and transient symptoms such as dizziness, confusion, headaches and vomiting (Satz et al 2001). Major traumatic brain injury results in unconsciousness, potentially compromising vital functions and an inability to maintain the airway, which threatens life.

Major traumatic brain injury can be described as having two phases:

- Primary injury occurring at the time of injury and can result in:
  - closed head injury due to rapid acceleration or deceleration forces
  - diffuse axonal brain injury as a result of stretching, twisting and tearing of nerve fibres
  - shearing and compression of tissues on the bony ridges inside the skull can result in damage to arteries and veins causing haemorrhage
  - rotational forces add to the shearing effect, particularly where structures are mobile such as the brainstem and corpus callosum – common in shaken babies
  - open or penetrating injuries involve the brain becoming exposed and damaged
  - skull fractures can be linear, comminuted and depressed. Basal skull fractures are particularly important due to the danger of secondary CSF infection
  - localised contusions often occur on the crest of the gyri of the cerebral cortex, and although they may produce dramatic focal neurological signs, tend to have a good overall progress, scarring may result in post traumatic seizures
- Secondary injury occurs after the initial impact as a result of:
  - cerebral hypoxia and ischaemic damage
  - ongoing haemorrhage
  - oedema, which usually peaks 24–48 hours after the injury
  - seizures and the development of CNS infection further may compound secondary injury.

Treatment and management

Minor head injury is common in children (Satz et al 2001). Admission to hospital is not always necessary but is often a precaution if there has been a seizure, a skull facture, an unstable GCS or the cause is suggestive of serious injuries, and to manage persistent symptoms such as vomiting (NICE 2007). The focus of care must be the detection of neurological changes by undertaking a thorough assessment and ongoing observations. The child and family will require appropriate support and detailed discharge advice.

Activity

Danny is 2 years old and has fallen in the playground at nursery. He vomited twice and is irritable. He is currently in the A&E department with his mother. His Glasgow Coma Score is 15 and after a thorough examination he is able to go home. His mother is happy with the decision but is anxious about the possible consequences of Danny's fall.

What advice would you give her in relation to observing Danny over the following 48 hours and long-term complications?

- You may wish to check your answer by referring to NICE (2007) guidelines relating to triage, assessment and management of head injuries in infants, children and adults are available on the NICE website: http://www.nice.org.uk

The NICE (2007) guidelines relating to the triage, assessment and management of head injuries in infants, children and adults outlines the initial priorities of care as: assessment and stabilisation of the airway, breathing and circulation, assessment of neurological status and ascertaining the degree of injury to initiate appropriate levels of care. All children with a GCS less than 8 after stabilisation, will require transfer to a tertiary paediatric intensive care facility. Once the child has been stabilised, the child and family progresses through four distinct phases following major traumatic brain injury (Singer 1996).

Phase 1

Traumatic brain injury is a sudden unwanted event and the initial impact of the injury is life threatening. There is immediate disruption to family life. At this stage the outcome of the injury is unpredictable. The aim of care is to stabilise the child, prevent secondary ischaemic damage, begin the rehabilitation process and support the child and family.

Phase 2

The duration of life support systems and time in a coma is variable, with fluctuating responses and ongoing uncertainty. The agitated child is often difficult to manage and may be distressing for parents. Often parents feel hopeless during this phase. Additional stresses occur as the family attempts to maintain some degree of normal family life.

Phase 3

The child's level of awareness returns and there may be early motor and cognitive recovery. The full extent of injuries becomes more apparent and the enormity of the changes may become overwhelming for the child and family.

Phase 4

Although there may be continued physical and cognitive recovery, emotional recovery can result in changes in personality and behaviour which can be difficult to cope with. Discharge from hospital is a difficult time for the family and transition to community care needs to be well planned if the child and family are to adjust to the effects of the injury. Issues relating to the child's future education require detailed assessment and advanced planning. After major traumatic brain injury, children require detailed continual assessment to monitor development because later milestones may not be achieved or the child may grow into deficits.

WWW

Practical advice relating to head injury is available on the Headway National Head Injuries Association website:

- http://www.headway.org.uk

Evidence-based practice

The NICE (2007) guidelines relating to triage, assessment and management of head injuries in infants, children and adults are available on the NICE website:

- http://www.nice.org.uk

Long-term outcomes

The outcome following minor head injury is favourable and in general there are no long-term effects in relation to cognitive and psychosocial functioning (Satz et al 1997). Deficits associated with mild to moderate head injury include social disinhibition, intellectual impairment, psychiatric disorders, perceptual distortion, learning problems, sensory impairment, neuromotor deficits and severe economic implications.

Both the short- and long-term impact on the child and family following a child sustaining a significant TBI are substantial (Wade et al 2006, Youngbult & Brooten 2006). The long-term impact following a TBI for the child includes difficulties in relation to performing daily living skills, poor communication skills, and general adaptation (Stancin et al 2002). Cognitive, behavioural and psychological recovery (and future development) may not necessarily correlate with physical improvements. Overall the health related quality of life in relation to mental and general health is poor for children who have suffered a severe TBI (Stancin et al 2002). Factors affecting the outcome of major traumatic brain injury include: age (with poorest outcome is in infancy, possibly due to age-specific response to trauma), severity and type of injury, extent of secondary damage, disruption of normal development and pre-existing conditions (Crouchman 1998).

Summary

Caring for the child and family where the child has a neurological problem can be particularly challenging but highly rewarding. The challenges relate to a lack of exposure to caring for children with rare disorders, the uncertain outcome of many conditions, and the potential of many conditions to cause dramatic changes in function for the child, both cognitively and physically. This chapter has outlined the nervous system and general principles of care required for a child with a neurological problem. It is not a comprehensive guide to the management of the wide range of neurological conditions of childhood but does provide insight into the common conditions. There has been an emphasis on an interdisciplinary approach to care delivery, and the need to ensure care delivery is individually designed and strongly influenced by encouraging the child to reach their full potential. Links have been made with other chapters where appropriate.

References

Adelson, P.D., Bratton, P.D., Carney, N.A., et al., 2003. Guidelines for the acute medical management of severe traumatic brain injury in infants, children and adolescents. Pediatric Critical Care Medicine 4 (3), 1–76.

Appleton R 1995 Epilepsy in childhood. Aspects of Epilepsy Issue 1.

Blackburn, B.L., Fineman, R.M., 1994. Epidemiology of congenital hydrocephalus in Utah 1940-1979: report of an iatrogenically related 'epidemic'. American Journal of Medical Genetics 52, 123–129.

Boyadjiev, S.A., 2007. Genetic analysis of non-syndromic craniosynostosis. Orthodontics and Craniofacial Research 10 (3), 129–137.

Brain Injury Association of America 2005 Facts about traumatic brain injury. www.biausa.org [Accessed January 2007].

Brett, E.M., Harding, B.N., 1997a. Hydrocephalus and congenital anomalies of the nervous system other than myelomeningocele. In: Brett EM (Ed.), Paediatric neurology, 3rd edn. Churchill Livingstone, London.

Brett, E.M., Harding, B.N., 1997b. Intracranial and spinal cord tumours. In: Brett EM (ed) Paediatric neurology, 3rd edn. Churchill Livingstone, London.

Brett, E.M., Kaiser, A.M., 1997. Neurology of the newborn. In: Brett, E.M. (Ed.), Paediatric neurology, 3rd edn. Churchill Livingstone, London.

Bullock, R., Chestnut, R.M., Clifton, G., et al., 2000. Guidelines for the management of severe traumatic brain injury. Journal of Neurotrauma 17 (6/7), 451–553.

Camfield, P.R., Camfield, C.S., Gordon, K., et al., 1997. If a first antiepileptic drug fails to control a child's epilepsy, what are the chances of success in a second? The Journal of Pediatrics 131 (6), 821–824.

CancerBACUP, 2005. Children's cancers - brain tumours in children. CancerBACUP, London.

Carey, C.M., Tullous, M.W., Walker, M.L., 1994. Hydrocephalus, etiology, pathological effects, diagnosis and natural history. In: Check, W.R. (Ed.), Pediatric neurosurgery: surgery of the developing nervous system, 3rd edn. WB Saunders, Philadelphia.

Casey, A.T., Kimmings, E.J., Kleinlugtebeld, A.D., et al., 1997. The long-term outlook for hydrocephalus in childhood. A ten-year cohort study of 155 patients. Pediatric Neurosurgery 27, 63–70.

Child Neurology, 2002. Craniosynostosis. Fact Sheet. Available: www.child-neuro.org.uk/neurotext/93html. [Accessed October 2007].

Chitnavis, B.C., Polkey, C.E., 1998. Intracranial pressure monitoring. Care of the Critically Ill Child 14 (3), 80–84.

Chumas, P., Hardy, D., Hockley, A., et al., 2002. Safe paediatric neurosurgery 2001. British Journal of Neurosurgery 16 (3), 208–210.

Chumas, P., Tyagi, A., Livingston, J., 2001. Hydrocephalus - what's new? Archives of Disease in Childhood. Fetal and Neonatal Edition 85 (3), 149–154.

Cinalli, G., Salazar, C., Mallucci, C., et al., 1998. The role of third ventriculostomy in the management of shunt malfunction. Neurosurgery 43 (6), 1323–1327.

Crossman, A.R., Neary, D., 2000. Neuroanatomy - an illustrated colour text, 2nd edn. Churchill Livingstone, Edinburgh.

Crouchman, M., 1998. Traumatic brain injury. In: Ward Platt, M.P., Little, R.A. (Eds.), Injury in the young child. Cambridge University Press, Cambridge.

Cullen, P.M., Derrickson, J.D., Potter, J.A., 2002. Radiation therapy. In: Baggott, C.R., Kelly, K.P., Fochtman et al (Eds.), Association of Pediatric Oncology Nurses. Nursing care of children and adolescents with cancer, 3rd edn. WB Saunders, Philadelphia.

Dailey, A.T., McKhann, G.M., Berger, M.S., 1995. The pathophysiology of oral pharyngeal apraxia and mutism following posterior fossa tumor resection in children. Journal of Neurosurgery 83 (3), 467–475.

Department of Health (DOH), 2002 Specialised services for children - definitions. No.23. Online. Available at:www.dh.gov.uk/en/managingyourorganisation/commissioningspecialisedservices/specialisedservicesdefinition/DH_4001699. [Accessed February 2008].

Department of Health (DOH), 2003. Improving Services for People with Epilepsy. DoH, London.

Drake, J.M., Kestle, J.R.W., 1996. Determining the best cerebrospinal fluid shunt valve design: the pediatric valve design trial. Neurosurgery 38 (3), 604–607.

Drake, J.M., Kestle, J.R.W., Milner, R., et al., 1998. Randomized trial of cerebrospinal fluid shunt valve design in pediatric hydrocephalus. Neurosurgery 43 (2), 294–305.

Drew, A., 1990. A Parents Perspective. Paediatric Nursing 2 (6), 22–24.

Duffner, P.K., Horowitz, M.E., Krischer, J.P., et al., 1993. Postoperative chemotherapy and delayed radiation in children less than three years of age with malignant brain tumors. New England Journal of Medicine 328 (24), 1725–1731.

Durkin, M., Olsen, S., Barlow, B., et al., 1998. The epidemiology of urban pediatric neurological trauma: evaluation of, and implications for, injury prevention programs. Neurosurgery 42 (2), 300–310.

Fenichel, G.M., 1997a. Ataxia. In: Fenichel, G.M., (Ed.), Clinical pediatric neurology. A signs and symptoms approach, 3rd edn. WB Saunders, Philadelphia.

Fenichel, G.M., 1997b. Disorders of cranial volume and shape. In: Fenichel, G.M. (Ed.) Clinical pediatric neurology. A signs and symptoms approach, 3rd edn. WB Saunders, Philadelphia

Ferguson Clark, L., Williams, C., 1998. Neurological assessment in children. Paediatric Nursing 10 (4), 29–35.

Fitzgerald, M.J.T., Folan-Curran, J., 2002. Clinical neuroanatomy and related neuroscience, 4th edn. WB Saunders, Edinburgh.

Greenwood, I., 1992. A benign tumour with lifelong effects. Treatment and management of craniopharyngioma. Professional Nurse 7 (6), 360, 361–358.

Halperin, E.C., Constine, I.S., Tarbell, N.J., et al., 1994. Tumors of the posterior fossa of the brain and the spinal canal. In: Halperin, E.C., Constine, I.S., Tarbell, N.J. (Eds.), Pediatric radiation oncology, 2nd edn. Raven Press, New York.

Hanna, N.J., Black, M., Sander, J.W.S., et al., 2002. The National Sentinel Clinical Audit of Epilepsy-Related Deaths. Epilepsy - death in the shadows. The Stationery Office, London.

Hazinski, M.F., Headrick, C., Bruce, D., 1999. Neurological disorders. In: Hazinski, M.F. (Ed.), Manual of pediatric critical care. Mosby, St Louis.

Heaney, D.C., MacDonald, B.K., Everitt, A., et al., 2002. Socioeconomic variation in incidence of epilepsy: a prospective community based study in south east England. British Medical Journal 325, 1013–1016.

Henry, P.C., Hauber, R.P., Price, M., 1992. Factors associated with closed head injury in a pediatric population. Journal of Neuroscience Nursing 24 (6), 311–316.

Hickey, J.V., 2003a. Neurological assessment. In: Hickey JV (Ed.), The clinical practice of neurological and neurosurgical nursing, 5th edn. Lippincott, Philadelphia.

Hickey, J.V., 2003b. Management of the unconscious neurological patient. In: Hickey JV (Ed.), The clinical practice of neurological and neurosurgical nursing, 5th edn. Lippincott, Philadelphia.

Hickey, J.V., 2003c. Management of patients undergoing neurosurgical procedures. In: Hickey JV (Ed.), The clinical practice of neurological and neurosurgical nursing, 5th edn. Lippincott, Philadelphia.

Hickey, J.V., 2003d. Behavioural and psychological responses in neurological illness. In: Hickey JV (Ed.), The clinical practice of neurological and neurosurgical nursing, 5th edn. Lippincott, Philadelphia.

Hockley, A.D., 1993. Craniosynostosis. Lancet 342, 189–190.

Hoppe-Hirsch, E., Laroussinie, F., Brunet, L., et al., 1998. Late outcome of the surgical treatment of hydrocephalus. Child's Nervous System 14, 97–99.

Hunt, A., Mastroyannopoulou, K., Goldman, A., et al., 2003. Not knowing - the problem of pain in children with severe neurological impairment. International Journal of Nursing Studies 40, 171–183.

International PHVD Drug Trial Group, 1998. International randomised controlled trial of acetazolamide and furosemide in post-haemorrhagic ventricular dilation in infancy. Lancet 352, 433–440.

James, H.E., Trauner, D.A., 1985. The Glasgow Coma Scale. In: James, H.E., Anas, N.G., Perkin, R.M. (Eds.), Brain insults in infants and children. Grune and Stratton, Orlando, FL.

Johnston, S.A., 2001. Calvarial vault remodelling for sagittal synostosis. AORN Journal (Official Journal of the Association of Operating Room Nurses) 74 (5), 623, 634–647.

Kapp-Simon, K.A., 1998. Mental development and learning disorders in children with single suture craniosynostosis. Cleft Palate-Craniofacial Journal 35 (3), 197–203.

Kershner, D.D., Claussen, J.A., 1986. Craniofacial reconstruction. Perioperative care of the craniosynostosis patient. AORN Journal (Official Journal of the Association of Operating Room Nurses) 44 (4), 554–562.

Keucher, T.R., Mealey, J., 1979. Long-term results after ventriculoatrial and ventriculoperitoneal shunting for infantile hydrocephalus. Journal of Neurosurgery 50, 179–186.

Kirk, E.A., Howard, V.C., Scott, C.A., 1995. Description of posterior fossa syndrome in children after posterior fossa tumor surgery. Journal of Pediatric Oncology Nursing 12 (4), 181–187.

Kirkpatrick, M., Engleman, H., Minns, R.A., 1989. Symptoms and signs of progressive hydrocephalus. Archives of Disease in Childhood 64, 124–128.

Kirse, D.J., Werle, A.H., Murphy, J.V., et al., 2002. Vagus nerve stimulation implantation in children. Archives Otolaryngology – Head and Neck Surgery 128 (11), 1263–1268.

Kraus, J.F., Fife, D., Conroy, C., 1987. Pediatric brain injuries: the nature, clinical course and early outcomes in a defined United States' population. Pediatrics 79 (4), 501–507.

Lashford, L.S., Walker, D.A., 1997. Improved care for central nervous system tumours: a mood for change. Archives of Diseases in Childhood 76 (2), 88–90.

Levy, R., Cooper, P., 2003. Ketogenic diet for epilepsy (Cochrane Review). The Cochrane Library. Issue 4. John Wiley and Sons, Chichester.

Lew, C.M., LaVally, B., 1995. The role of stereotactic radiation therapy in management of children with brain tumors. Journal of Pediatric Oncology Nursing 12 (4), 212–222.

Long, A.F., Kneafsey, R., Ryan, J., et al., 2002. The role of the nurse within the multi-professional rehabilitation team. Journal of Advanced Nursing 37 (1), 70–78.

Longstaff, A., 2005. Instant notes – neuroscience. BIOS Scientific Publications, Oxford.

Mahoney, W.J., D'Souza, B.J., Haller, J.A., et al., 1983. Long-term outcome of children with severe head trauma and prolonged coma. Pediatrics 71 (5), 756–762.

Marson, A.G., Al-Kharusi, Alwaidh, M. et al., 2007a The SANAD Study of effectiveness of Valproate, lamotrigine or topiramate for generalise and unclassifiable epilepsy: an unblinded randomised controlled trial. Lancet 369:1016–1026

Marson, A.G., Al-Kharusi, Alwaidh, M. et al., 2007b The SANAD Study of effectiveness of Carbamazepine, gabapentin, lamotrigine, oxcarbazepine or topiramate for the treatment of partial epilepsy: an unblinded randomised controlled trial. Lancet 369:1000–1015

Marson, A.G., Williamson, P.R., Hutton, J.L. et al., on behalf of the Epilepsy Monotherapy Trialists 2003 Carbamazepine versus valproate monotherapy for epilepsy (Cochrane Review). In: The Cochrane Library, issue 4. John Wiley and Sons. Chichester

May, L., 1992. Craniosynostosis – corrective surgery for a cosmetic defect. Professional Nurse 8 (3), 176–178.

May, L., 2001. Craniosynostosis. In: May, L. (Ed.), Paediatric neurosurgery: a handbook for the multidisciplinary team. Whurr Publishers, London.

McMillan, T.M., Greenwood, R.J., 1993. Models of rehabilitation programmes for the brain injured adult: services and suggestions for change in the UK. Clinical Rehabilitation 7, 346–355.

McNett, M., 2007. A review of the predictive ability of Glasgow Coma Scale Scores in head-injury patients. Journal Neuroscience Nursing 39 (2), 68–75.

Miller, J.D., Dearden, N.M., 1992. Measurement, analysis and the management of raised intracranial pressure. In: Teasdale, G.M., Miller, J.D. (Eds.), Current neurosurgery. Churchill Livingstone, Edinburgh.

Moore, I.M., 1995. Central nervous system toxicity of cancer therapy in children. Journal of Pediatric Oncology Nursing 12 (4), 203–211.

Moos, K.F., Hide, R., 1993. Craniofacial surgery - surgical correction of congenital deformities. Surgery 11 (8), 457–465.

Mori, K., Shimada, J., Kurisaka, M., Sato, K., Watanabe, K., 1995. Classification of hydrocephalus and outcome of treatment. Brain and Development 17, 338–344.

Mulhern, R.K., Kepner, J.L., Thomas, P.R., et al., 1998. Neuropsychologic functioning of survivors of childhood medulloblastoma randomized to receive conventional or reduced-dose craniospinal irradiation: a Pediatric Oncology Group study. Journal of Clinical Oncology 16 (5), 1723–1728.

Neumann, V.C., 1995. Principles and practices of treatment. In: Chamberlain, M.A., Neumann, V.C., Tennant, A. (Eds.), Traumatic brain injury rehabilitation services, treatment and outcomes. Chapman and Hall, London.

National Institute for Clinical Excellence (NICE), 2004. The epilepsies: The diagnosis and management of epilepsy in children and adults in primary and secondary care. NICE, London.

National Institute for Clinical Excellence (NICE), 2005. Referral guidelines for suspected cancer. Clinical Guideline 27. HMSO, London.

National Institute for Clinical Excellence (NICE), 2007. Head injury. Triage, assessment, investigation and early management of head injury in infants, children and adults, 2nd edn. NICE, London.

Padgett, K., 2006. Alterations of neurological function in children. In: McCance, K.L., Huether, S.E. (Eds.), Pathophysiology: the biological basis for disease in adults and children, 5th edn. St Louis Mosby.

Panayiotopoulos, C.P., 2005. The epilepsies: seizures, syndromes and management. Bladon Medical Publishing, Chipping Norton.

Panchal, J., Amirsheybani, H., Gurwitch, R., et al., 2001. Neurodevelopment in children with single-suture craniosynostosis and plagiocephaly without synostosis. Plastic and Reconstructive Surgery 108 (6), 1492–1498.

Panchal, J., Uttchin, V., 2003. Management of craniosynostois. Plastic and Reconstructive Surgery 111 (6), 2032–2049.

Parslow, R.C., Morris, K.P., Tasker, R.C., et al., 2005. Epidemiology of traumatic brain injury in children receiving intensive care in the UK. Archives of Disease in Childhood 90, 1182–1187.

Peters, A., 2007. Neurological observations. In: Glasper, E.A., McEwing, G., Richardson, J. (Eds.), Oxford handbook of children's and young peoples nursing. Oxford University Press, Oxford.

Pikus, H.J., Levy, M.L., Gans, W., Mendel, E., McComb, J.G., 1997. Outcome, cost analysis and long-term follow up in preterm infants with massive grade IV germinal matrix haemorrhage and progressive hydrocephalus. Neurosurgery 40 (5), 983–989.

Polley, J., Charbel, F., Kim, D., MaFee, M.F., 1998. Nonsyndromal craniosynostosis: longitudinal outcome following cranio-orbital reconstruction in infancy. Plastic and Reconstructive Surgery 102 (3), 619–628.

Pudenz, R.H., Foltz, E.L., 1991. Hydrocephalus: over drainage by ventricular shunts - a review and recommendations. Surgical Neurology 35, 200–202.

Reilly, P., Simpson, D.A., Sprod, R., et al., 1988. Assessing the conscious levels of infants and young children: a paediatric version of the Glasgow Coma Scale. Children's Nervous System 4, 30–33.

Roberts, G.C., 2005. post-craniotomy analgesia: current practices in British neurosurgical centres – a survey of post-craniotomy analgesic practices. European Journal of Anaesthesiology 22, 328–332.

Roffe, J., 1989. The role of the nurse in paediatric rehabilitation. Paediatric Nursing 1, 11–13.

Rose, F.D., Johnson, D.A., Attree, E.A., 1997. Rehabilitation of the head injured child: basic research and new technology. Pediatric Rehabilitation 1 (1), 3–7.

Rosner, M.J., Daughton, S., 1990. Cerebral perfusion pressures, management in head injury. Journal of Trauma 30, 933–940.

Royal College of Nursing (RCN), 2009. Updated full guidelines: the recognition and assessment of acute pain in children. RCN, London.

Royal College of Paediatrics and Child Health (RCPCH), 2000. A national approach to epilepsy management in children and adults. RCPCH, London.

Ryan-Murray, J., Petriccione, M.M., 2002. Central nervous system tumors. In: Baggott, C.R., Kelly, K.P., Fochtman, D. (Eds.), Association of Pediatric Oncology Nurses. Nursing care of children and adolescents with cancer, 3rd edn. WB Saunders, Philadelphia.

Sander, J., Shorvon, S., 1996. Epidemiology of the epilepsies. Journal of Neurology. Neurosurgery and Psychiatry 61 (5), 433–443.

Sarnat, H.B., Menkes, J.H., 2000. Neuroembryology, genetic programming and malformations of the nervous system. In: Menkes, J.H., Sarnat, H.B. (Eds.), Child neurology. Lippincott, Williams and Wilkins, Philadelphia.

Satz, P., Zaucher, K., McCleary, et al., 2001. Mild head injury in children and adolescents: a review of studies 1970–1995. Psychological Bulletin 122 (2), 107–131.

Shiminski-Maher, T., Shields, M., 1995. Pediatric brain tumors: diagnosis and management. Journal of Pediatric Oncology Nursing 12 (4), 188–198.

Singer, G.H.S., 1996. Constructing supports. In: Singer, G.H.S., Glang, A., Williams, J.M. (Eds.), Children with acquired brain injury. Paul H Brookes, Publishing, Baltimore.

Siomin, V., Cinalli, G., Grotenhuis, A., et al., 2002. Endoscopic third ventriculostomy in patients with cerebrospinal fluid infection and/or hemorrhage. Journal of Neurosurgery 97 (3), 519–524.

Society of British Neurological Surgeons, 2001. Safe paediatric neurosurgery 2001. Society of British Neurological Surgeons, London.

Stancin, T., Drotar, D., Taylor, G., et al., 2002. Health-related quality of life of children and adolescents after traumatic brain injury. Pediatrics 109 (2), 34–42.

Stephenson, R.C., 1996. Therapeutic consistency following brain lesions. Professional Nurse 11 (11), 738–740.

Stewart, E.S., Cohen, D.G., 1998. Central nervous system tumors in children. Seminars in Oncology Nursing 14 (1), 34–42.

Strother, D.R., Pollack, I.F., Fisher, P.G., et al., 2002. Tumors of the central nervous system. In: Pizzo, P.A., Poplack, D.G. (Eds.), Principles and practice of pediatric oncology, 4th edn. Lippincott Williams and Wilkins, Philadelphia.

Sugerman, R.A., 2006. Structure and function of the neurological system. In: McCance, K.L., Huether, S.E. (Eds.), Pathophysiology: the biological basis for disease in adults and children, 5th ed. St Louis Mosby.

Tatman, A., Warren, A., Williams, A., et al., 1997. Development of a modified paediatric coma scale in intensive care clinical practice. Archives of Diseases in Childhood 77 (6), 519–521.

Teasdale, G., Jennett, B., 1974. Assessment of coma and impaired consciousness - a practical scale. Lancet 2, 81–83.

Thibault, M., Girard, F., Moumdjian, R., et al., 2007. Craniotomy site influences post-operative pain following neurosurgical procedures: a retrospective study. Canadian Journal of Anaesthesiology 54 (7), 544–548.

Turini, M., Redaelli, A., 2001. Primary brain tumours: a review of research and management. International Journal of Clinical Practice 55 (7), 471–475.

Twycross, A., Mayfield, C., Savory, J., 1999. Pain management for children with special needs: a neglected area? Paediatric Nursing 11 (6), 43–45.

Vernon-Levett, P., Geller, M., 1997. Posterior fossa tumors in children: a case study. American Association of Critical Care Nurses (AACN) Clinical Issues 8 (2), 214–226, 285–286.

Wade, S.L., Taylor, H.G., Yeates, K.O., 2006. Long-term parental and family adaptation following pediatric brain injury. Journal of Pediatric Psychology 31 (10), 1072–1083.

Walker, D.A., Punt, J.A.G., Sokal, M., 1999. Clinical management of brain stem glioma. Archives of Diseases in Childhood 80 (6), 558–564.

Warren, A., 2000. Paediatric coma scoring researched and benchmarked. Paediatric Nursing 12 (3), 14–18.

Warren, S.M., Greenwald, J.A., Spector, J.A., et al., 2001. New developments in cranial suture research. Cranial Suture Research 107 (2), 523–540.

Watson, M., Horn, S., Curl, J., 1992. Searching for signs of revival: uses and abuses of the Glasgow Coma Scale. Professional Nurse 7 (10), 670–673.

Worrall, L., 1999. Medulloblastoma. In: Miaskowski, C., Buchel, P. (Eds.), Oncology nursing – assessment and clinical care. Mosby, St Louis.

Youngbult, J.M., Brooten, D., 2006. Pediatric head trauma: parent, parent-child, and family functioning 2 weeks after hospital discharge. Journal of Pediatric Psychology Journal 31 (6), 608–618.

Caring for children with diabetes and other endocrine disorders

34

Philomena Morrow Sue Courtman Liz Gormley-Fleming

ABSTRACT

This chapter aims to review the range of problems that may present for the child and family as a result of hormone dysfunction. Care of the child and family with reference to health promotion/education will be significantly addressed in relation to the endocrine disorders presented. Active participation is encouraged throughout to increase and further develop knowledge and understanding. The Evolve website will provide an opportunity for revision of the production and function of hormones in the body and their effect on the growth and development of the child.

LEARNING OUTCOMES

- Understand the role and function of the endocrine system.
- Appreciate how disordered function affects the child.
- Understand the care requirements of the child and family in relation to specific endocrine disorders.
- Understand the specialist nature of caring for a child with diabetes.
- Recognise the importance of health promotion/education in the care of the child and family with an endocrine disorder.
- Appreciate the need for continuing care and support required by the child and family with an endocrine disorder.

Endocrine system

The endocrine system is a chemical communication system that provides the means to control a number of physiological processes within the body. As it is a communication network, the endocrine system contains transmitters, signals and receivers that are called hormone-producing cells, hormones and receptors. The endocrine system consists of a number of distinct glands and some tissues in other organs. The endocrine glands (Fig. 34.1) are:

- pituitary gland
- thyroid gland
- four parathyroid glands
- two adrenal glands
- pancreatic islets (also known as the islets of Langerhans)
- pineal gland
- thymus gland
- two ovaries in the female
- two testes in the male.

Endocrine glands secrete hormones directly into the bloodstream, whereas exocrine glands pass their secretions directly into body cavities. The hormones released by endocrine glands are carried in the bloodstream to their target organ, where they are active. The activity of a number of endocrine glands is regulated through the activity of the hypothalamus.

The hypothalamus

Nine different substances have been identified as hypothalamic hormones that either stimulate or inhibit the release of anterior and posterior hormones (Table 34.1). These hormones are formed in the median eminence of the hypothalamus (the area that is connected to the pituitary gland by the pituitary stalk).

PowerPoint

Access the companion PowerPoint presentation and revise your knowledge in relation to hormone structure, action of hormones, regulation and synthesis and metabolism and excretion of hormones.

DOI: 10.1016/B978-0-7020-3183-0.10034-7

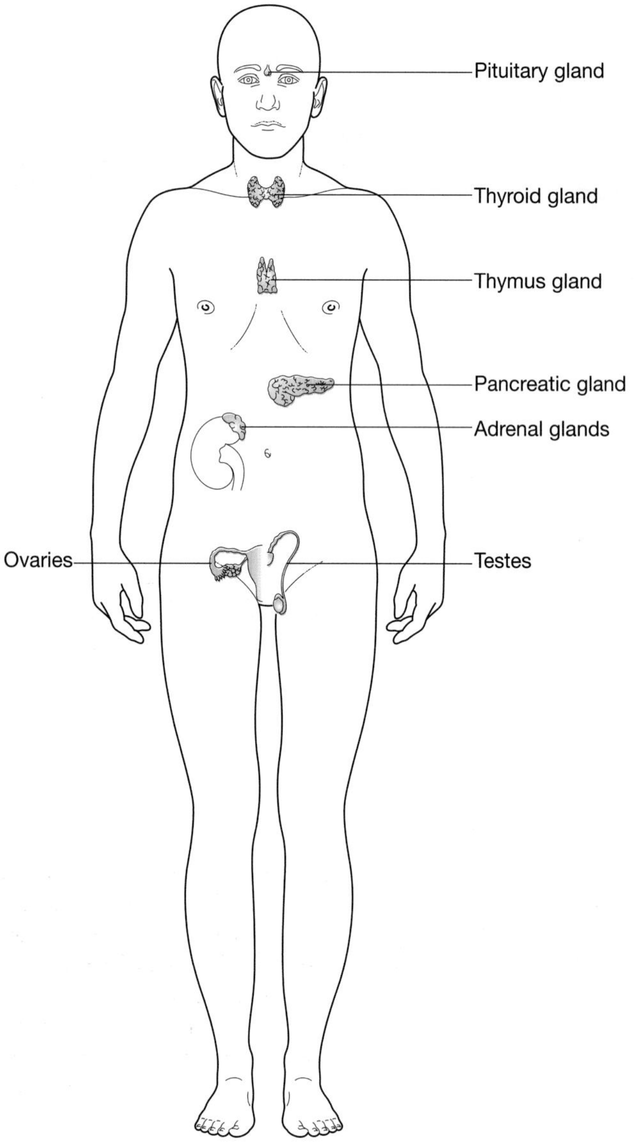

Fig. 34.1 • The glands within the body.

Table 34.1 The hypothalamic hormones

Hypothalamus		
Synthesis of posterior pituitary hormones and transport via nerve axons	Hypothalamic hormones carried in hypothalamo-hypophyseal portal system	
Pituitary gland		
Posterior pituitary (neurohypophysis)	*Middle lobe*	*Anterior lobe (adenohypophysis)*
Oxytocin	Melanocyte-stimulating hormones	Trophic hormones: ACTH, adrenal cortex hormone
Vasopressin (antidiuretic hormone)		
Thyroid stimulating hormone (TSH)		
Growth hormone (GH)		
Follicle stimulating hormone (FSH)		
Luteinising hormone (LH)		
Prolactin (PRL)		

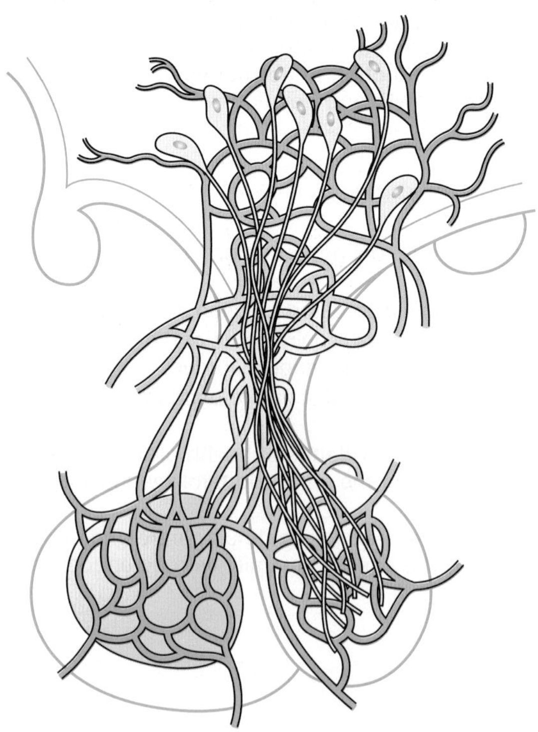

Fig. 34.2 • The pituitary gland.

PowerPoint

Access the companion PowerPoint presentation and look at the discussion on hypopituitarism and hyperpituitarism including pituitary tumours to enhance your knowledge.

You are also advised to revise the section on growth hormone production, regulation and synthesis before proceeding to the next section of this chapter on growth hormone deficiencies.

Pituitary gland

The gland develops from the merging of different tissues (Fig. 34.2).

Anterior pituitary gland

Originates from an upgrowth of glandular epithelium from the pharynx and is known as the adenohypophysis. This is only linked to the brain via the venous hypothalamohypophyseal portal system. This network transports blood from the hypothalamus to the anterior pituitary, thereby transporting releasing and inhibiting hormones secreted by the hypothalamus.

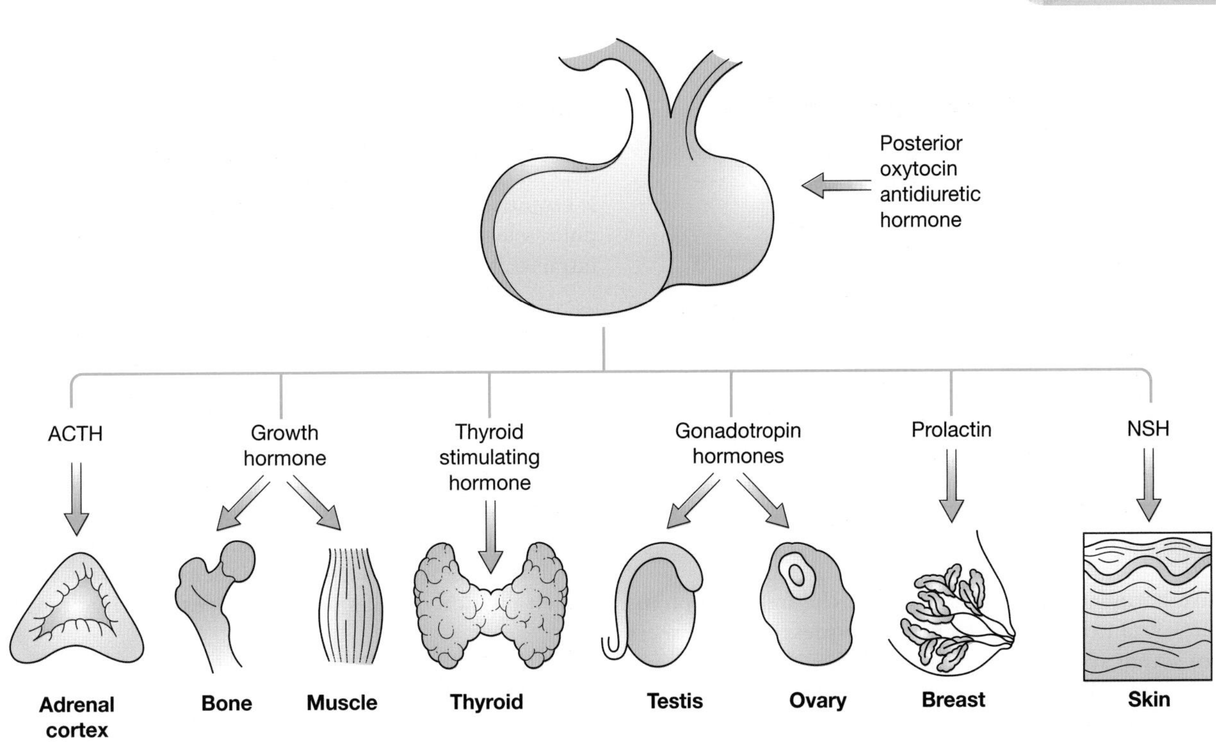

Fig. 34.3 • Anterior pituitary hormones.

These hormones influence secretion and release of other hormones formed in the anterior pituitary (Fig. 34.3):

- Corticotrophin-releasing hormone: controls release of tropic hormones, such as adrenocorticotrophic hormone (ACTH)
- Thyrotrophin-releasing hormone (also known as thyroid-stimulating hormone)
- Growth-hormone-releasing factor
- Gonadotrophin-releasing hormone
- Somatostatin-releasing hormone (also known as growth-hormone-release inhibiting factor)
- Prolactin-inhibiting factor
- Melanocyte-stimulating hormone (MSH).

Posterior pituitary gland

This is derived from a downgrowth of nervous tissue from the base of the brain and is known as the neurohypophysis. It has nervous connections with the hypothalamus, down which the antidiuretic hormone (ADH) and oxytocin pass. ADH and oxytocin are synthesised in the nerve cell bodies of the hypothalamus, transported along the axons, and then stored and secreted by vesicles within the axon terminals. Their release is triggered by nerve impulses from the hypothalamus.

Disorders affecting the pituitary gland

Disorders affecting the pituitary gland result in disruption in regulation of hormone secretion. Symptoms vary depending on the location of the disorder, and are related to a disturbance in production of a specific hormone or group of hormones and relate to the role they play in maintaining health and development.

Hypopituitarism

This term denotes subnormal pituitary hormone production (Parks 2002). It is generally a result of disorders of the anterior pituitary and may involve one or more of the hormones produced (Table 34.2). Deficiencies of anterior hormone production are due to primary disease or disorder of the anterior pituitary. Secondary hypopituitarism, which is attributed to dysfunction of the hypothalamus, affects the synthesis and release of releasing hormones and release inhibiting hormones.

PowerPoint

Access the companion PowerPoint presentation and refer to the discussion on growth hormone for detailed information on assessment and diagnosis in relation to family history, child's history, radiographic and imaging findings, and laboratory findings.

Factors contributing to pituitary hyposecretion include congenital hypopituitarism due to genetic abnormalities or other developmental defects. Congenital hypopituitarism is mainly related to growth hormone deficiency. Disordered pituitary hormone secretion that develops after birth is referred to as acquired hypopituitarism (Parks 2002). This may have resulted from central nervous system trauma, meningitis or encephalitis, vascular abnormalities or haemorrhage, brain tumours, pituitary tumours and/or radiation therapy.

Hyperpituitarism

Hyperpituitarism is a disorder in which excessive secretion of growth hormone increases the growth rate. Pituitary tumours that secrete hormones produce characteristic symptoms of

Table 34.2 Disorders of pituitary hormones

Hypopituitarism	Hypopituitarism
Growth hormone: somatic growth retardation	Somatic growth acceleration Adrenal hyperfunction
Adrenocorticotrophic hormone (ACTH): adrenal hypofunction	Hyperthyroidism Precocious puberty/retarded sexual development
Thyroid hormone: hypothyroidism	
Follicle stimulating and luteinising hormone: absence/regression of secondary sexual characteristics	Prolactin: stops menstruation
Prolactin	

excessive hormone levels. This is rare in children. Symptoms may range from complaints such as listlessness or restlessness to more severe symptoms such as headaches, vomiting or dizziness. In addition, problems due to an increase in any of the hormones produced may give rise to growth, adrenal or sexual dysfunction (see Table 34.2).

Hormonal abnormalities occurring as a result of pituitary tumours or defects will be discussed under specific headings. Oversecretion of growth hormone is usually caused by a pituitary adenoma.

Precocious puberty

Precocious puberty is defined as the onset of secondary sex characteristics by the age of 8.5 years in females and 9.5 years in males (Rudolf & Levene 2006). It is either gonadotrophin dependant or gonadotrophin independent. It is more likely to occur in females and may be idiopathic in origin and is likely to be due to the premature onset of normal puberty. It is recognised today that pubertal development has started to occur earlier due to improvements in nutrition and socio-economic conditions. While it is rare it males, it is far more likely to be due to organic causes. The causes of precocious puberty may be:

- idiopathic/familial tendency
- CNS abnormalities
- acquired – following surgery, trauma, irradiation
- congenital abnormalities – hydrocephalus
- tumours
- adrenal – congenital adrenal hyperplasia, tumours
- ovarian tumours
- testicular tumours
- exogenous sex steroids
- hypothyroidism.

Diagnosis

Diagnosis is based on physical examination, blood analysis, bone age measurements, ultrasonography and radiological imaging – MRI or CT scanning.

Treatment

This is dependent on the cause and may necessitate surgery, chemotherapy or irritation if a tumour is diagnosed. For the female with idiopathic precocious puberty treatment will depend on the age of diagnosis. Monitoring of growth patterns is essential. Treatment is usually administration of gonadotrophin releasing hormone subcutaneously, intramuscularly or intranasally for those cases that are gonadotrophin dependent.

Role of the nurse

The aim of nursing care should focus on the education of the child and parent about the condition, medication administration and to provide emotional support for the family. There may be psychological and behavioural difficulties associated with the early progression into puberty. It must be emphasised to the family that the child is achieving their other developmental milestones – cognition, emotional development and social development – according to their chronological age even if their physical development and appearance is advanced.

Growth hormone deficiencies

Growth hormone deficiency exists when growth hormone is absent or is produced in inadequate amounts to support normal growth. If growth hormone deficiency occurs in combination with one or more other pituitary hormone deficiencies the condition is related to hypopituitarism, as described earlier.

Growth hormone deficiency can be congenital, resulting from deficiency of hypothalamic growth hormone releasing hormone that may be associated with defects such as septo-optic dysplasia or primary pituitary disorders such as defects in the growth hormone gene. Most congenital cases of growth hormone deficiency are currently considered idiopathic (Cutler 2002), which is the most common form, accounting for approximately 50–70% of cases (NICE 2002). Fetal growth is growth hormone independent and therefore infants with congenital growth hormone deficiency are born normal size and weight. However, growth hormone deficiency may present in the newborn period with hypoglycaemia, and prolonged jaundice. These symptoms are often significant early diagnostic features. Growth hormone deficiency becomes evident only during the first years of life, when linear growth begins to slow and is the 3rd percentile or less by the age of 1 year.

Acquired growth hormone deficiency may be the result of injury, infection, inflammatory and granulomatous disease, radiation or tumours of the pituitary gland and/or the hypothalamus; it may become evident during infancy or childhood. Failure to grow normally may also be a key feature of other underlying medical conditions, e.g. chronic renal insufficiency, Turner syndrome, Prader–Willi syndrome, Down syndrome, neurofibromatosis and as a result of chronic disease. Among children who are of very short stature (i.e. at least 3 standard deviations below the population mean), 25% have growth hormone deficiency (NICE 2002).

Principles of nursing care and management

Care and management will be based on the assessment of individual needs of the child and in collaboration with the child and family (Table 34.3). The deficiency is identified

Table 34.3 Nursing care and management of growth hormone deficiencies

Characteristics of child with growth hormone deficiency	Nursing considerations
Short stature	Accurate assessment and monitoring of height and weight
Delayed growth of all body parts	Accurate recording/plotting height and weight on appropriate growth chart
Delayed skeletal maturation	Early recognition of deviation in height and weight pattern
Immature facial appearance	Accurate detailed assessment of child's health and health problems
Increased subcutaneous fat	Assessment of family history
In prolonged growth failure the child will be shorter than children of the same age	Referral for medical consultation and assisting and supporting the child/family during medical examination, radiological surveys and endocrine studies
Hypoglycaemia may be present particularly in young children	

by serum analysis of growth hormones. Brain imaging is also required to identify underlying pathology. A detailed history of the child's physical status and social situation needs to be ascertained.

In children with growth hormone insufficiency, exogenous (biosynthetic) growth hormone (somatropin) is administered by subcutaneous injection; the dose is increased during the period of adolescence. It is continued until the child attains their final height (Rudolf & Levene 2006). The recommended dose varies according to the child's condition and is self-administered at home 6–7 times a week. Biosynthetic human growth hormone has been licensed for use in the UK for long-term treatment of children who have growth failure due to inadequate secretion of normal endogenous growth hormone (NICE 2002). A variety of growth hormone preparations and devices are available, knowledge of which is important if the nurse is to help the child and family choose the most suitable product and device. Although treatment enables many children to reach their adult height potential, this may mean many years of treatment for the child.

Establishing and maintaining optimum therapy both at the outset and over what may be a long period of time may be extremely challenging for many families (Nairn & Moore 2002). The initial and ongoing education of the child and family and the monitoring and maintenance of long-term compliance to achieve the best possible outcomes are important aspects within the role of the children's nurse. In the presence of secondary growth hormone deficiencies the underlying lesion needs to be treated and prognosis is related to the underlying lesion.

Side effects of growth hormone therapy are rare but can include headache, visual problems, nausea and vomiting, fluid retention (peripheral oedema), arthralgia, myalgia, paraesthesia, antibody formation, hypothyroidism and reactions at injection site. Particular attention should be paid to treating children with risk factors associated with diabetes mellitus and slipped capital epiphyses.

Storage and preparation of medication, as well as choosing and alternating the injection site are important aspects of the education process. Timing of administration of growth hormone may be dependent on family routines. The evening is usually the recommended time as this mimics the pattern of normal production of growth hormone. (Hockenberry et al 2003). Compliance to treatment may be enhanced by enabling the child to take control over administration of growth hormone, which may be achieved by the use of the pen injector. The best results are seen in those that are treated early before psychological effects occur.

Evidence-based practice

Growth hormone therapy can increase short-term growth and improve (near) final height (Bryant et al 2004).

Reflect on your practice

- Explain to a parent the technique required to administer a subcutaneous injection.
- Review the advice regarding proper injecting technique for growth hormone at: http://www.heightmatters.org.uk

Activity

Children and parents need to understand the importance of complying with treatment regimes and to be competent in administration. This requires that the child and family are educated regarding the rationale for treatment and adverse effects.

Activity

Review a growth chart for a boy and a girl from birth to 18 years. Identify the nurse's responsibilities in relation to the assessment of the following:

- Weight
- Standing height
- Supine length
- Head circumference.

Review the PowerPoint presentation for measurement technique for standing height (Hall 2000).

Child and family resources

Raising awareness of the guidance on the use of human growth hormone in children with growth failure (NICE 2002; website: http://www.nhsdirect.nhs.uk) and encouraging parents to discuss this guidance with their doctor will provide further

Table 34.4 Normal growth rates for height in children (Desrosiers 2002)

Age	Growth in height
0–6 months	18–26 cm per year
6–12 months	15–28 cm per year
1–2 years	10–13 cm per year
2–3 years	7–10 cm per year
3–4 years	5–8 cm per year
4–5 years	5 cm per year

encouragement to comply with treatment. The Human Growth Foundation is a national organisation of parents who provide education and guidance on the physical, psychological and social development of children with growth problems. This resource may be beneficial in providing parents and children with additional support and advice. Good nutrition and adequate rest is vital when promoting growth. A well-balanced diet with appropriate calorie and protein intake needs to be encouraged.

Children's nurses have a significant role in the routine monitoring of growth and the assessment of growth disorders. The development of good history-taking skills and an accurate, repeatable measurement are central to the success of growth assessment and evaluation. Measuring height is subject to error as a result of poor technique, variations between instruments and observers and diurnal variation (Hall 2000). The child should be measured by the same observer using the same measuring instrument if possible to maintain accuracy and consistency. Parental height should also be measured with the mid parental centile and target height plotted on the percentile chart (Drake & Kelnar 2006).

During therapy, the child's growth needs to be monitored against expected growth on standard growth charts to assess ongoing response to treatment (Table 34.4). Explain to the parents that developmental expectations are the same for a child with growth hormone deficiencies as they are for a child who is developing normally. Expected growth may be based on parental height. It is recommended that treatment should be discontinued if the child's growth velocity is less than 50% from baseline in the first year of therapy, i.e. if extra height gain is not at least half the height gain in the year before treatment began. Persistent problems with adherence to treatment should also be taken into account as part of the re-evaluation process (NICE 2002).

Evidence-based practice

Height is greatest on getting up in the morning – up to 2 cm can be lost over the whole day. Measurements made at different times of the day can significantly affect the measured height and, thus, the estimated rate of growth (Hall 2000).

Activity

Review Chapter 46 on caring for a child requiring palliative care:

- Discuss how this information may be relevant to the care of the child and family in the above situation in relation to bereavement and loss.

Recognition of the complexity of problems experienced by the child and family in relation to growth deficiency and/or short stature is necessary if physical and psychosocial dilemmas are to be overcome. Children who are small for their age may have problems with friends, teachers and parents, who tend to treat them as though they were younger and have reduced expectations of them. In turn, children may not act their age because it is not expected from them and thus experience problems with self-esteem and ability to interact appropriately with others. The child or young person should be encouraged to dress age appropriate rather than size and treated in an age-appropriate manner. Those involved in the care of these children should be aware of the importance of emphasising abilities and strengths rather than physical size.

PowerPoint

Access the companion PowerPoint presentation and revise your knowledge on the production and regulation of secretion of the thyroid hormones before proceeding to the next section of this chapter on disorders of thyroid function.

Disorders of thyroid function

The function of the thyroid gland is to regulate the cellular metabolism. Thyroxine T4, tri-iodothyronine T3 and calcitonin are hormones secreted by the thyroid. These hormones are responsible for normal development of the muscular, skeletal and nervous systems. Disturbance in the secretory pathway of the thyroid hormones may result in an increase or decrease in production. Some of the most common endocrine disorders are disorders of the thyroid gland. The two main disorders are hypothyroidism and hyperthyroidism.

Hypothyroidism

Hypothyroidism is either congenital or acquired (juvenile hypothyroidism). It is due to a deficiency in the secretion of thyroid hormones. Congenital hypothyroidism is relatively common and occurs in approximately 1 in 4000 births (Lissauer & Clayden 2007). Early detection is imperative as this is one of the few preventable causes of severe learning difficulties. This is achieved by neonatal screening. Treatment is lifelong with oral replacement of thyroxine. Cause of congenital hypothyroidism are:

- aplasia or hypoplasia of the thyroid gland (Fig. 34.4)
- hereditary defects in thyroid hormone synthesis that may be associated with maternal administration of

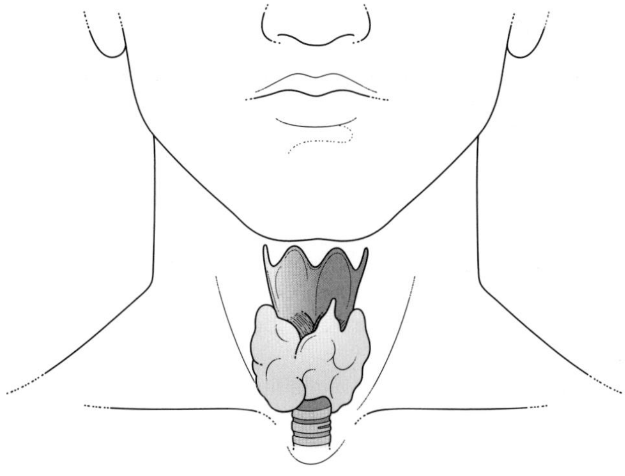

Thyroid gland

Fig. 34.4 • The thyroid gland.

antithyroid drugs during pregnancy (McCance & Huether 2006)
- iodine deficiency – common worldwide but rare in the UK; preventable by iodination of salt in the maternal diet
- thyroid stimulating hormone (TSH) deficiency.

Acquired juvenile hypothyroidism

Juvenile hypothyroidism may be primary or secondary. This is more common in females (Ball & Bindler 2006). Primary causes include:

- defective hormone synthesis resulting from acute thyroiditis caused by bacterial infection
- subacute non-bacterial inflammation associated with viral infections
- autoimmune (circulating antithyroid antibodies) thyroiditis occurring as a result of Hashimoto disease is the most common cause of juvenile hypothyroidism in children (Roth et al 1997)
- an endemic of iodine deficiency or antithyroid drugs, or loss of thyroid tissue can be contributory factors in hypothyroidism.

Secondary hypothyroidism is due to insufficient stimulation of the thyroid gland by thyroid stimulating hormone as a result of hypothalamic or pituitary disorders.

Other autoimmune disorders may develop, e.g. type 1 diabetes mellitus. This is more common in children with Down and Turner syndrome. Addison's disease may also occur in some families (Lissauer & Clayden 2006).

WWW

Review the UK process measures, standards and supporting implementation guidelines for newborn blood spot screening. These are available on the website of the UK Newborn Screening Programme Centre at:

- http://www.ich.uc/.ac.uk

WWW

Obtain further information on thyroxine and recommended dosages at:

- http://emc.medicines.org.uk

Parent information is available at:

- http://www.ivillage.co.uk

Information for children is available at:

- http://www.childrenfirst. nhs.uk/kids/health/illness/thyroid problemss.html

Nursing assessment and diagnosis

Routine neonatal biochemical screening, blood spot test, must be performed on all infants either prior to discharge from hospital or in the community. This will identify most infants that are affected by this disorder.

In children under the age of 2 the symptoms may not be as clear as those associated with hypothyroidism therefore nursing assessment and ongoing monitoring of the neonate with presenting problems is vital to ensure early diagnosis of the condition. Serial measurement of weight, length and head circumference is an important aspect of assessment. Presenting symptoms depend on extent of dysfunction and age at onset. However, if undetected and left untreated in early childhood, permanent defects can arise, for example, mental retardation, deafness, deceleration in growth and other nervous system disorders. At birth there may be difficulty in identifying hypothyroidism. Hypothermia, delay in passing meconium and neonatal jaundice may be significant signs and require to be investigated immediately.

Clinical manifestations of hypothyroidism may not be evident until after 4 months of age. Signs and symptoms may include:

- failure to thrive and feeding problems
- a hoarse cry and protruding tongue caused by myxoedema of oral tissue and vocal cords
- the child may present with constipation and abdominal distension due to hypotonia of abdominal muscles
- umbilical hernia may also be present
- a subnormal temperature, excessive sleeping, slow pulse and a cold, mottled skin may be present
- puffy eyes and loss of the eyebrows may be present

Often the baby is seen as being a 'good' baby, as the baby is often quiet. Skeletal growth may be decelerated due to impaired synthesis of protein, poor absorption of nutrients and lack of bone mineralisation. Enlargement of the thyroid gland, known as goitre, may be evident, particularly in older children. Puberty may be delayed and obesity is often present. If the condition remains undiagnosed and untreated, the child will be dwarfed with short limbs (cretinism) as well as presenting with delayed intellectual development.

Care and management

Once diagnosis is confirmed, treatment is replacement therapy, which is prescribed according to the child's hormonal levels. Treatment is required on a life-long basis. Regular estimates of hormone levels are essential to prevent development of hyperthyroidism. In addition, regular monitoring of growth is necessary throughout childhood. Assessment of cognitive development should also be undertaken. Parental education (and the child depending on their age) is essential as they need to demonstrate an understanding of the disorder and treatment required.

Scenario

June, a 12-year-old who presented with a history of weight loss, anxiety, disturbance in sleep and mood changes, was diagnosed as having Graves' disease:

- When undertaking June's nursing assessment, what specific information would you be required to obtain?
- What specific requirements would need to be considered when planning June's care?

A discussion of this scenario appears at the end of the chapter.

PowerPoint

Access the companion PowerPoint presentation and review regulation of adrenal and renal function before proceeding with the next section of this chapter on disorders of adrenal function.

Activity

Review Chapter 45 on caring for a critically ill child:

- Discuss how this information is relevant to the care of the child with acute adrenal insufficiency.

Hyperthyroidism

Hyperthyroidism is a condition in which the thyroid hormones exert greater than normal responses. Generally there is excess secretion of thyroid hormones, which might be associated with acute, subacute or chronic thyroiditis, tumours of the thyroid, or other tumours of the pituitary (which secretes thyroid-stimulating hormone). This leads to an increase in basal metabolic rate, cardiac function, gastrointestinal function, weight loss, and metabolism of fats, proteins and carbohydrates. While rare in childhood it is most common in teenage girls. Specific diseases that cause hyperthyroidism include Graves' disease and toxic multinodular goitre.

Graves' disease is the most common cause of hyperthyroidism in children. Although the exact cause is unknown, it is thought to be associated with autoimmune abnormalities that cause enlargement and thus hyperfunction of the thyroid gland.

Congenital hyperthyroidism may occur in infants of mothers who have Graves' disease as a result of transplacental transfer of immunoglobulins (Ball & Bindler 2006)

Assessment and diagnosis

Hyperthyroidism is four times more common in girls than boys and most frequently presents in childhood between ages of 12 and 14 years. The condition usually presents with a history in deterioration in school performance.

The other clinical features of hypothyroidism will vary according to the amount and length of hypersecretion. The onset is subtle thus diagnosis may not be reached for a length of time. Weight loss, diarrhoea, rapid growth in height, tachycardia, tremors, increase in appetite, anxiety, learning difficulties/behaviour problems and goitre may be present. Eye signs are uncommon in children but exophthalmos may be evident (Lissaeur & Clayden 2007).

Diagnosis is achieved by laboratory analysis of thyroxine and tri-iodthyronine levels. A thyroid scan will also be performed. Antithyroid antibodies may also be identified in laboratory analysis.

The aim of treatment is to inhibit excessive secretion of the thyroid hormones. First-line treatment is oral medication and this is generally for a 2-year period. Adjunct therapy may also be required, e.g. beta-blockers. Radio-iodine treatment may follow oral medication. Surgery may also be considered if other treatment modalities are unsuccessful.

Nursing care

The aim of nursing care of the child with hyperthyroidism should focus on the education of the child and their parents. They need to be aware of the need to promote rest, the importance of compliance with treatment to avoid relapse and to provide emotional support. Pre- and postoperative care for the child undergoing subtotal or total thyroidectomy is very specific but the general principles of pre- and postoperative care still apply.

Disorders of adrenal function

Disorders of the adrenal cortex (Fig. 34.5) are related to either hyperfunction or hypofunction (Table 34.5).

Evidence-based practice

Puberty imposes greater difficulty in achieving and maintaining adrenal suppression despite optimal doses of substitution therapy (Charmandari et al 2002):

- Discuss.

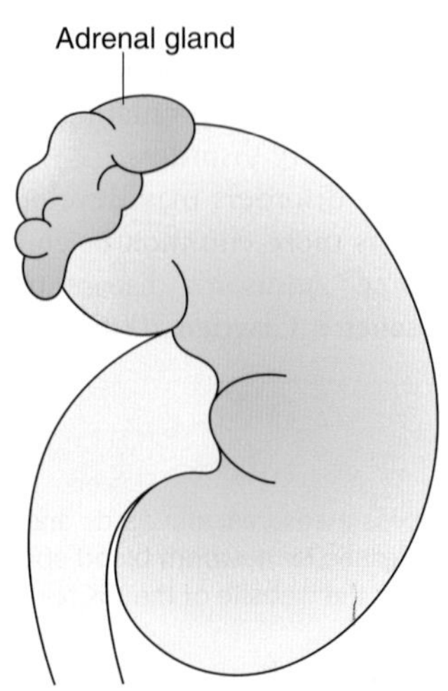

Fig. 34.5 • The adrenal gland.

Table 34.5 Disorders of adrenal function

Hyperfunction of adrenal cortex	Hypofunction
Cushing's syndrome: increased levels of circulating cortisol	Acute adrenocortical insufficiency
	Chronic adrenocortical insufficiency: Addison's disease
Congenital adrenal hyperplasia: increased secretion of adrenal androgens and oestrogens leading to virilisation or feminisation Primary hyperaldosteronism Hyperfunction of adrenal medulla Phaeochromocytoma: increased secretion of catecholamines	

Activity

Review stages of needle play at:

- http://www.nahps.org.uk/needle.htm

Congenital adrenal hyperplasia

This is a group of disorders of adrenal steroid synthesis. Excessive secretion of androgens by the adrenal cortex may occur as a result of a number of conditions of the adrenal gland. However, the most common disorder affecting children is congenital adrenogenital hyperplasia, an inborn deficiency of various enzymes necessary for the biosynthesis of adrenal steroidogenesis (Hockenberry et al 2003). It is an autosomal recessive disorder. Interference with the biosynthesis of glucocorticoids in fetal life results in cortisol secretion being diminished and an increased production of adrenocorticotrophic hormone, which stimulates hyperplasia of the adrenal gland. There is an increased production of various adrenal hormone precursors, including androgens. Deficiency of enzymes necessary for biosynthesis of mineralocorticoids may result in diminished secretion of aldosterone.

In its severe form, excess adrenal androgen production beginning in the first trimester of fetal development results in virilisation of the female infant and life-threatening hypovolaemic and hyponatraemic shock (adrenal crisis) in the newborn.

Assessment and diagnosis

Due to the block in the adrenal production of corticosteroids a build up of androgenic precursors occur and this may lead to ambiguous genitalia in the newborn baby. This is rare. In the female with potentially normal ovaries and uterus, virilisation occurs and sexual development is therefore along heterosexual lines. The abnormality of the external genitalia may vary from mild enlargement of the clitoris to complete fusion of the labioscrotal folds, forming a scrotum, a penile urethra, a penile shaft, and enlargement of the clitoris to form a normal-sized gland.

Signs of adrenal insufficiency (salt loss) may be present during the first days of life. This is an acute presentation with hyponatraemia, hyperkalaemia, hypoglycaemia, dehydration, hypotension and circulatory collapse. In the older child, presentation is usually when the enzyme defect is milder, salt loss may not occur – this accounts for approximately 25% of cases (Ball & Bindler 2006). If untreated, growth rate and skeletal maturation are accelerated. Pubic hair appears early, acne may be excessive and voice may deepen. Excessive pigmentation may develop as a result of melanocyte stimulation by excessive production of adrenocorticotrophic hormone (Kappy et al 2003).

In males, sexual development proceeds normally. Male infants may appear normal at birth but present with salt-losing crisis in the first 2–4 weeks. The infant may present with vomiting, poor weight gain, poor feeding and electrolyte imbalance. The older male child who was not losing sodium may present with rapid growth and precocious sexual development.

Hormonal studies are essential for accurate diagnosis. Adrenal ultrasonography, CT scanning, and MRI may define pelvic anatomy or enlarged adrenals or indicate the presence of an adrenal tumour. Pelvic ultrasonography may help in delineating the internal anatomy of a newborn with ambiguous genitalia.

Nursing care and treatment

Initially, the recognition of ambiguous genitalia in the newborn requires to be attended to immediately in relation to informing the parents and commencing investigations to confirm sexual identity. Early diagnosis and treatment is crucial. Aims of treatment consist of normalising growth velocity and skeletal maturation using the smallest dose of glucocorticoids that will suppress adrenal function. Mineralocorticoid replacement helps to sustain normal electrolyte homeostasis, although excessive use may result in hypertension.

Patient education is necessary as has been described for other endocrine disorders. Parents should understand the child's need for life-long therapy and the side effects, as well as signs of underdosage and requirements during illness. The need for compliance requires to be stressed and the importance of the child carrying appropriate identification. Surgical intervention may be necessary for reconstruction of the female genitalia as soon as possible during infancy in an effort to support ongoing physical and psychological development. Multiple surgical procedures may be necessary, which will require ongoing psychological support for the child and parents. They require ongoing support as they come to terms with the sex of the baby and decisions that they may have to make regarding the need for surgical interventions. Reassurance regarding surgical interventions and the future care and treatment, which will be a life-long commitment, need to be discussed.

Ambiguity in relation to the sex of the newborn can have a devastating effect on parents and other siblings. At this time, anticipation of parental reaction, which may be likened to the process of bereavement and loss, may enhance the nurse's ability to engage in a more therapeutic way at this time. Parents need to have information in relation to the infant's condition reinforced while at the same time being provided with the opportunity to express their own sorrow, loss and disappointment. A decision regarding gender should only be made once all investigations are completed and naming the baby should also be delayed until gender determination is made. Their beliefs and values on gender need to be explored. The healthcare professional should avoid referring to the baby as 'your son' or 'your daughter' and instead refer to the baby as 'your baby'. Genetic counselling should be provided for the child when they reach adolescence and supportive counselling should be organised for the parents along with genetic screening for any future pregnancies.

As the hereditary form of adrenogenital hyperplasia is an autosomal-recessive disorder, parents should be referred for genetic counselling.

Activity

Review Chapters 44 and 45:

- How does the knowledge of both chapters relate to the care of the child with diabetes?

Chronic adrenocortical insufficiency (Addison's disease)

Primary adrenal cortical insufficiency is rare in children. Adrenal insufficiency (Table 34.6) may be the result of:

- hereditary enzymatic defects (congenital adrenal hyperplasia)
- loss of adrenal function due to autoimmune destruction of the gland (Addison's disease)
- pituitary hypothalamic tumours
- irradiation of the hypothalamus.
- haemorrhage/infraction – neonatal, meningococcal septicaemia
- adrenoleucodystrophy – a neurodegenerative disorder
- tuberculosis.

Chronic adrenal insufficiency typically occurs when 90% of adrenal function is lost (Miller 2002).

Acute adrenocortical insufficiency (adrenal crisis)

Acute adrenal insufficiency (adrenal crisis) is most common in the child with undiagnosed chronic adrenal insufficiency who is exposed to additional severe stress, such as major illness, trauma or surgery. Some of the aetiological factors include haemorrhage into the gland from trauma, which may be caused by a prolonged, difficult labour; fulminating infections, such as meningococcaemia, which results in haemorrhage; and necrosis (Waterhouse–Friderichsen syndrome). Other factors include abrupt withdrawal of exogenous sources of cortisone or failure to increase dosage during stress such as surgery or burns and during stressful periods: injury or cold for example (Ball & Bindler 2006).

This condition is rapid in onset. All symptoms as identified in chronic adrenocortical insufficiency are exaggerated. The child may present with circulation collapse, confusion or coma and therefore require emergency interventions. Nursing care is focused on:

- fluid and electrolyte resuscitation
- intravenous administration of glucocorticoids until oral therapy becomes possible
- administration of mineralocorticoids when oral intake is tolerated
- treatment of the underlying illness.

WWW

Review the Department of Health's Guidelines in good practice in consent at:

- http://www.doh.gov.uk/publications

Prolonged care and treatment, as for the child with chronic adrenocortical insufficiency, will be required.

Table 34.6 Causes of adrenal insufficiency

Characteristics of glucocorticoid deficiency	Characteristics of mineralocorticoid deficiency	Nursing considerations
Poor weight gain, weight loss, anorexia Hypoglycaemia Weakness/fatigue Increased levels of adrenocorticotrophic hormone and melanocyte stimulating hormone give rise to hyperpigmentation of skin and mucous membrane	Hyponatremia Hyperkalemia Nausea Gastrointestinal complaints Hypotension Tachycardia	Assessment of dietary intake to avoid obesity Prevent episodes of hypoglycaemia Ensure additional sodium intake (as in table salt) – increase intake in event of sweating, vomiting, diarrhoea Assessment and ongoing monitoring of cardiovascular status Frequent monitoring of vital signs, blood pressure Monitor compliance to treatment of replacement therapy of glucocorticoid and mineralocorticoids on long-term basis Assessment and monitoring for signs of overtreatment: • monitor growth and development and observe for signs of Cushingoid features • regular follow-up and provision of ongoing support and education • encourage child to wear medic alert bracelet

Cushing syndrome

Cushing syndrome results from prolonged exposure of the tissues to glucocorticoids. It may be caused by primary dysfunction as a result of neoplasm or adenoma of the adrenal cortex, or by hypersecretion of adrenocorticotrophic hormone as a result of a pituitary tumour. In addition, Cushing-like syndrome may be an adverse effect from long-term exogenous administration of cortisone used in the treatment of allergic, autoimmune, neoplastic, haematologic, skin and other diseases.

Clinical manifestations

Cushing syndrome is an uncommon syndrome in children and young people (Boscaro et al 2002). However, the resulting hypercortisol causes considerable morbidity in childhood and adolescence (Storr et al 2003). The earliest and most common signs in almost all presenting with the condition are:

- generalised obesity, which is characterised by facial rounding (moon face) and 'buffalo hump' (Fig. 34.6). These result from accumulation of adipose tissue in the trunk, facial and cervical areas
- transient weight gain from sodium and water retention may occur due to the mineralocorticoid effects of cortisol
- growth retardation or complete arrest of growth is present in all but 10% of affected children (Chrousos 2002)
- other clinical manifestations include sleep disturbance, irritability and depression
- muscle weakness and fatigue, due to protein wasting is caused by the catabolic effects of cortisol

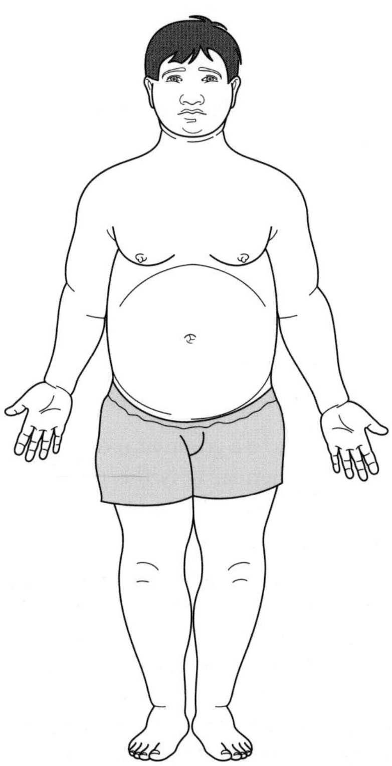

Fig. 34.6 • Cushing syndrome.

- loss of protein matrix leads to osteoporosis, with pathological fractures
- loss of collagen also causes weakening and thinning of the skin through which capillaries become visible. These changes, together with fluid retention, account for the characteristic purple striae
- loss of collagenous support makes blood vessels more susceptible to rupture, leading to bruising. Thin atrophied skin is easily damaged and leads to skin breaks and ulceration (McCance & Huether 1998)
- hyperpigmentation is associated with high serum levels of adrenocorticotrophic hormone, which is thought to increase melanotropic activity. Thus skin, mucous membrane and hair acquire a characteristic bronze colour
- hypertension due to increased vascular sensitivity to catecholamines, which are increased as a result of increased levels of cortisol
- elevated levels of cortisol also cause suppression of the immune system, which increases the child's susceptibility to infection and poor wound healing
- amenorrhoea, advancement or arrest of pubertal development may be encountered.

Glucose intolerance occurs because of cortisol-induced insulin resistance and increased gluconeogenesis and glycogen in the liver.

Assessment and diagnosis

Confirmation of excess cortisol levels may be obtained indirectly by ascertaining fasting blood glucose levels for hyperglycaemia, and serum electrolyte levels for hypokalaemia and alkalosis (Campbell & Glasper 1995). Elevated levels of urinary free cortisol and plasma cortisol obtained in the evening will further aid confirmation of diagnosis.

A dexamethasone (cortisone) test may be used to confirm the diagnosis and confirm the cause. Administration of exogenous cortisone normally suppresses production of adrenocorticotrophic hormone. Cortisol levels remain elevated in children with Cushing syndrome. This helps differentiate between children who are obese and those who appear to have Cushingoid features (Campbell & Glasper 1995).

Computed tomography (CT) or magnetic resonance imaging (MRI) may be carried out when an adrenocorticotrophic hormone-secreting adenoma of the pituitary is suspected.

Care and management

Treatment is specific according to the cause for hyperadrenocorticosteroid levels. Therefore differentiation among pituitary, adrenal and other causes is essential for effective treatment. For adrenal and pituitary causes, treatment generally involves surgical, irradiation and postoperative replacement of cortical hormones.

When Cushingoid features are a result of steroid therapy, the effects may be lessened by administration of the drug in the morning, as this maintains the normal diurnal pattern of cortisol secretion. In addition, an alternate day schedule allows the anterior pituitary an opportunity to maintain more normal hypothalamic–pituitary–adrenal control mechanisms (Campbell & Glasper 1995).

Primary hyperaldosteronism

Primary hyperaldosteronism may be caused by a benign adrenal tumour or by adrenal hyperplasia. This condition results in increased sodium levels with water retention, and potassium depletion. Thus the condition is characterised by paraesthesia, tetany, weakness, polyuria, nocturnal enuresis, periodic paralysis, low serum potassium, elevated sodium levels, hypertension, metabolic acidosis and production of a large volume of urine with a low specific gravity. Plasma and aldosterone levels are elevated, but other steroid levels are variable.

Treatment is with glucocorticoids or spironolactone, which blocks the effects of aldosterone, thereby promoting the excretion of sodium and water and preserving potassium (Hockenberry et al 2003). Subtotal or total adrenalectomy for hyperplasia may be necessary, and surgical removal of a tumour, if present.

The role of the nurse in relation to providing holistic care and treatment from the stage of diagnosis to long-term management of primary hyperaldosteronism is similar to that for other endocrine disorders. When surgery is indicated then involvement in pre- and postoperative care becomes the priority.

Phaeochromocytoma

Phaeochromocytoma is a tumour of the adrenal medulla but may be located wherever chromaffin tissue is present, e.g. sympathetic ganglia and carotid body. Physical manifestations are generally caused by excess secretion of catecholamines. Symptoms may include:

- increased anxiety, such as perspiration and headaches, palpitations tachycardia, hypertension and hyperglycaemia
- dizziness, weakness, nausea and vomiting with diarrhoea
- weight loss and anorexia
- blurring of vision and dilated pupils
- papilloedema, retinopathy and enlargement of the heart
- in severe cases, signs of congestive heart failure may be evident nervousness, excitability and overactivity.

Nursing assessment and diagnosis

A careful history of the onset of symptoms and association with stressful events is helpful in distinguishing between an organic and a psychological cause for the problem (Wong & Wilson 1995). Serum catecholamines are elevated, particularly when the child is symptomatic. Urinary excretion of catecholamines parallels serum levels. The tumour may be identified on CT scan or MRI.

Nursing care and management

Surgical removal of the tumour is the treatment of choice. Prior to surgery, the child's physical condition must be adequately stabilised. Manipulation of the tumour may cause sudden and profound, potentially fatal changes in blood pressure. Hypertension with associated tachycardia may be the result of excessive release of catecholamines during removal of the tumour. Hypotension may occur as a result of catecholamine withdrawal. A preoperative preparation requirement involves the administration of medication, aimed at inhibiting the effects of catecholamines. The major group of drugs used is the adrenergic blocking agents. β-adrenergic blocking agents may be required when α-adrenergic blocking agents are ineffective in controlling release of catecholamines alone. The wanted effect of preoperative drug administration is to lower the blood pressure and minimise the symptoms the child has previously presented with.

During the preoperative period, frequent recordings of clinical observations are required to monitor blood pressure and heart and respiratory rate in an effort to detect hypertensive episodes and observe for signs of congestive heart failure. Daily blood glucose monitoring is required to observe for signs of hyperglycaemia.

The child is likely to remain in hospital in the weeks prior to surgery because of the necessary preoperative preparation and monitoring. The effects of prolonged hospitalisation may increase emotional distress for the child and thus aggravate symptoms. Parental presence and involvement in the child's care must be encouraged. Parents must be fully informed about the child's condition so that they can promote an environment for the child that is as restful and as stress free as possible. They require detailed information regarding the child's surgery and complications that may arise as a result. The child may require admission to the intensive care unit following surgery until the condition is stable postoperatively.

The gonads: ovaries and testes

A variety of abnormalities in chromosomal distribution, gonadal differentiation, gonadal function, testosterone synthesis and action, or adrenal function can lead to aberrant development of internal or external genital structures as described under the section congenital adrenal hyperplasia.

PowerPoint

Access the companion PowerPoint presentation and review:

- abnormalities in female pubertal development and ovarian function.

Before proceeding with the next section of this chapter, on diabetes mellitus, review:

- endocrine regulation of blood glucose.

Diabetes mellitus

Diabetes mellitus refers to a group of metabolic disorders characterised by hyperglycaemia. It is the result of a lack of the hormone insulin and/or an inability to respond to insulin. This interference has varying degrees of disruption of carbohydrate and fat metabolism and storage, excessive gluconeogenesis from protein catabolism, water and electrolyte imbalance.

In childhood, the incidence of type 1 diabetes mellitus (T1DM) is greater than type 2 diabetes (T2DM) and is therefore more likely to be encountered in practice. However, the incidence of T2DM is increasing in all age groups and across races, and may now account for between one-fifth and one-third of all new cases of diabetes. Monogenic diabetes accounts for a small percentage of diabetes in children and results from the inheritance of mutation or mutations in a single gene most often those that regulate beta cell function.

Pathophysiology

Insulin is a hormone secreted by the beta cells located in the islets of Langerhans within the pancreas. It functions to maintain homeostasis and is secreted in response to a rise in the blood glucose level. Insulin acts on cell membranes stimulating the uptake of glucose, amino acids and fats. In addition it is associated with conversion of glucose to glycogen in the liver and muscles, storage of fat in adipose tissue and prevention of gluconeogenesis and the breakdown of protein and fat.

Glugagon is secreted in the alpha cells of the islets of Langerhans and is released when the blood glucose level is low, causing the liver to convert stored glycogen into glucose and release into the blood stream. Insulin and glucagon influence the blood glucose level, each balancing the effects of the other maintaining normoglycaemia (blood glucose levels of 4–8 mmol/L).

In the diabetic patient, the diminishing level of insulin secretion (type 1 diabetes) or when insulin secretion is inadequate to meet the increasing demand posed by insulin resistance (type 2 diabetes), an inability to utilise available glucose causes elevated blood glucose levels and catabolic breakdown of fat with the ensuing production of ketones.

Type 1 diabetes

Type 1 diabetes is characterised by an absolute insulin deficiency resulting in hyperglycaemia and the possible development of diabetic ketoacidosis. Most cases result from a cell-mediated autoimmune response of the insulin producing cells of the pancreatic islets (Fig 34.7). This response results in recruitment of cytotoxic lymphocytes and production of anti-insulin and anti-islet cell antibodies, which progressively destroy the beta cells of the islets of Langerhans in the pancreas. Susceptibility to immunological damage has been associated with strong genetic determinants in combination with environmental factors. Environmental triggers of this immune process that have been proposed include viruses, cows' milk proteins and chemical toxins. Signs and symptoms are:

- polyuria
- dehydration
- polydipsia
- weight loss
- lethargy.

Late characteristics include:

- vomiting due to the ketonaemia
- abdominal pain
- hypovolaemic shock
- hyperventilation due to acidosis
- drowsiness and coma.

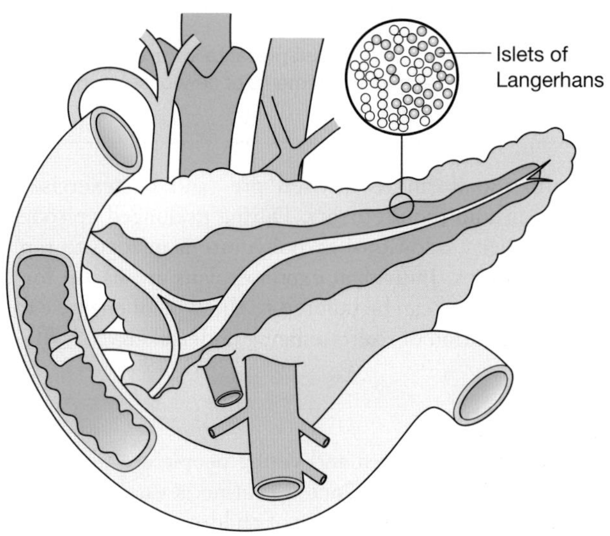

Fig. 34.7 • The pancreas.

Diagnosis

Onset may be acute, precipitated by the stress of an acute illness or insidious over weeks and months. The classic presenting symptoms are thirst, polydipsia, polyuria, weight loss and a recent history of recurrent infections. Diagnosis is made in the symptomatic child by a random plasma glucose level > 11.1 mmol/l (WHO 1999). Children suspected of type 1 diabetes should be referred to a multidisciplinary paediatric diabetes team immediately for assessment. However, in the absence of definitive symptoms or a mild presentation, diagnosis should not be based on a single plasma glucose result. Continued monitoring of fasting and post-prandial blood glucose levels may give a clearer picture. An oral glucose tolerance test (OGTT) may be required to confirm diagnosis though is rarely indicated. If doubt remains as to the type of diabetes, periodic re-testing should be carried out until the diagnosis can be confirmed or refuted.

Initial care and management

The initial management will depend on the child's clinical condition. Those in advanced diabetic ketoacidosis require urgent hospitalisation for emergency treatment. Most newly presenting children can be managed on subcutaneous insulin, but intravenous fluids and an insulin infusion is required if the child is vomiting or dehydrated. Newly presenting children not requiring intravenous therapy should have the choice of in-patient management or home-based care depending on clinical need and in consideration of the family's preference. A child presenting with moderate hyperglycaemia without acidaemia, who is clinically stable and is tolerating oral fluids, may be successfully managed at home with the support of medical and nursing diabetes specialists. The goals of treatment are:

- minimise the frequency and severity of extreme variation in blood glucose levels

- education for the child and family in how to competently manage their diabetes
- achieve normal growth and development
- good general health and well-being
- full participation in school and social activities
- normal socialisation with peer groups
- prevention of long-term complications.

Establishing the correct dosage of daily insulin requires adjustments to be made based on food intake and forthcoming exercise in addition to blood glucose levels. In adolescence, due to insulin resistance, insulin requirements increase. These higher doses are reduced at the end of growth and puberty.

The choice of insulin regimen is determined in consideration of the child's age, family circumstances, lifestyle and individual preferences. Twice daily injection therapy consists of a mixture of long-acting and fast-acting insulin administered before breakfast and evening meal. Premixed pens are available in different percentage ratios of long-acting to rapid-acting insulin. Children on multiple daily injection therapy (MDI) administer a dose of fast-acting insulin before each meal based on the carbohydrate content of the meal and a long-acting insulin, generally given before bed. Insulin therapy is part of the care package given to families at diagnosis which also includes:

- on-going education and management strategies
- practical instruction in injection therapy and blood glucose monitoring
- dietary management
- liaison with nurseries, schools and other secondary care settings
- psychosocial support.

Diet

Nutritional recommendations are the same for all healthy children with or without diabetes. Children with diabetes need sufficient calories to satisfy the requirements for growth and development, as well as achieving the best possible blood glucose control. The intake of calories and nutrients needs to be balanced with the amount of insulin given at a particular time and in consideration of the amount of activity undertaken during the day. NICE (2004a) recommends that the total daily energy intake should be distributed as:

$$\text{Carbohydrate : more than } 50\%$$
$$\text{Protein : } 10-15\%$$
$$\text{Fat : } 30-35\%$$

The type of insulin regime will affect the advice given. It is essential to consider the whole family's customary food habits. Asking the child or parents to keep a food diary for a week is a useful way of understanding meal routines, content and food combinations. Dietetic input is an integral part of diabetes management and review of personal eating patterns, likes and dislikes, different cultures and religions need to be discussed on an individual basis.

A twice daily insulin regimen requires a regular meal pattern of consistent content interspersed with snacks to prevent blood glucose levels dropping between meals. This regimen does not respond well to high glucose foods, which should be kept to a minimum as they will generate swinging blood glucose levels. More flexible meal planning is an option for those receiving multiple injections or on insulin pump therapy.

Exercise

Exercise is for everyone and should be enjoyable. Young children tend to expend energy in a more consistent manner through play, but older children may be involved in more strenuous sporting activities that require more individual planning. The effects of exercise are that:

- the uptake of glucose to the muscles will increase without increasing the need for insulin
- absorption of insulin will be accelerated if an active part of the body is used for the injection site prior to exercise
- insulin must be available during exercise, however, or the uptake of blood glucose will be impeded. In the absence of adequate circulating insulin there will be a lack of glucose inside the cells resulting in an exaggerated response from counter-regulatory hormones leading to hyperglycaemia and the likelihood of ketosis (Riddell & Iscoe 2004)
- hypoglycaemia may become evident hours afterwards as the liver replenishes its stores of glycogen.

Exercise needs both glucose and insulin. If there is insufficient glucose available for the muscles cells, there is an increased risk of hypoglycaemia during exercise. If there is too little circulating insulin, then the available glucose cannot be transported to the muscles and is likely to result in elevated blood glucose levels and the risk of developing ketoacidosis. After exercise the muscles are more sensitive to circulating insulin as glycogen stores within the muscle cells are replenished, leading to an increased risk of hypoglycaemia 8–10 hours after the event (Rodbard 2008).

PowerPoint

Access the companion PowerPoint presentation and review the section on insulin therapy: requirements of new-onset diabetes for more detailed information.

Careful monitoring is advised pre- and postexercise and review of insulin requirements. During prolonged episodes of vigorous activity, additional carbohydrate is needed to replenish energy stores. Individual exercise plans are useful for the serious athlete and can be tailored to the type of energy expenditure and duration of exercise being undertaken.

Needle phobia

Newly diagnosed children and young people are often fearful of the injection process. Once a routine is established in the home environment, the majority of children settle into the pattern of diabetes management and accept that it is a necessary

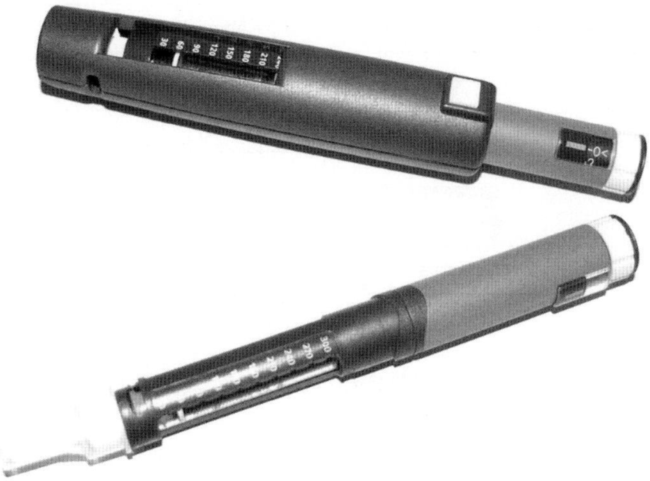

Fig. 34.8 • The Penmate (top) with needle hidden; the NovoPen (bottom) has a 6-mm needle.

procedure. However, a few can present with symptoms of needle phobia. If not resolved, it may affect treatment and diabetes control as the child or young person may adopt strategies such as insufficient blood glucose monitoring or omitting insulin injections, in an attempt to minimise the number of invasive procedures they might have in day. Identifying needle phobia as distinct from objecting to injections is difficult. Close observation of the injection process, looking for signs of extreme anxiety in the child, will alert the children's nurse to needle phobia that may need the support of a clinical psychologist.

Blood glucose monitoring

Self-monitoring of blood glucose (SMBG) is one of the main management tools used to optimise diabetes control. It gives insight into the child's immediate blood glucose status and an opportunity to treat as well as avoid out-of-range values. In type 1 diabetic patients, frequent blood glucose monitoring is associated with an improved HbA1c and is linked to better insulin adjustment for food and a more rapid response to elevated blood glucose levels being treated with additional insulin. The aims of self-monitoring blood glucose are to:

- monitor daily blood glucose fluctuations
- assist with daily insulin dose adjustments
- identify hypoglycaemia and monitor during recovery
- identify hyperglycaemia and monitor during resolution.

Children and young people are encouraged to perform regular blood glucose monitoring, 4+ times per day, particularly before meals. There is a wide variety of excellent blood glucose meters available for home use. The diabetes care team will give advice on the most suitable monitors available and give education in how to use and interpret results.

Activity

Review Chapter 46:

- Discuss how this information may relate to the care of the child with hyperthyroidism or hyperthyroidism.

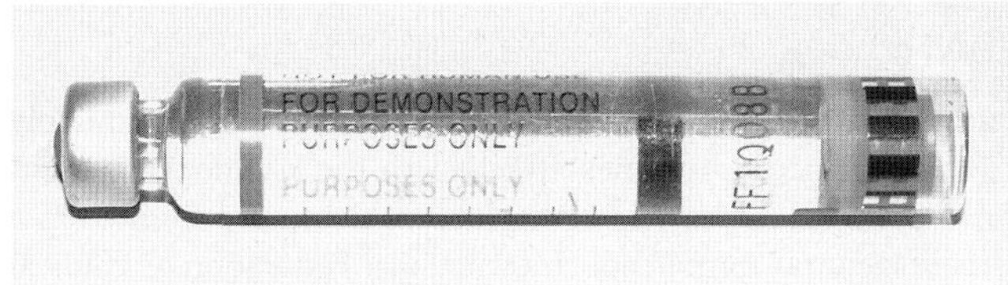

Fig. 34.9 • An insulin cartridge.

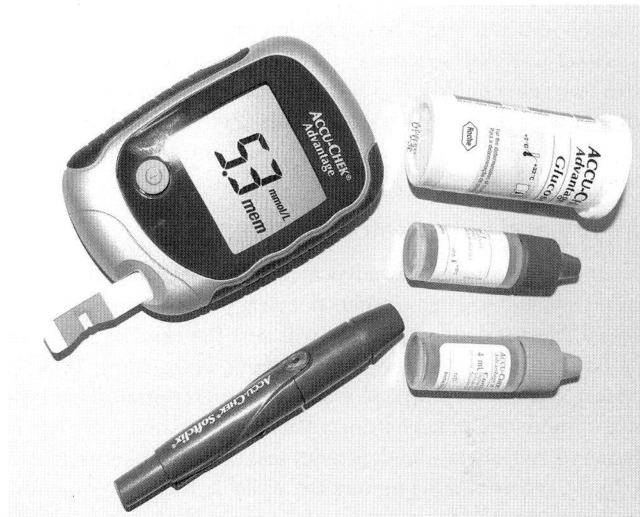

Fig. 34.10 • Blood glucose monitoring equipment.

Evidence-based practice

To ensure the most reliable and consistent absorption of insulin, injections should be made into subcutaneous adipose tissue. There is a difference in absorption rate and duration of different insulins when injected into subcutaneous fat and muscle. Intramuscular injection speeds up absorption and can lead to unexpected hypoglycaemia (King 2003, Polak et al 1996, Strauss et al 2002, Thow & Home 1990).

Additional testing at different times during the day is advised:

- In association with exercise in order to optimise insulin to carbohydrate adjustment.
- During bouts of illness when blood glucose levels are fluctuating and additional doses of insulin are required to prevent hyperglycaemia and the risk of developing DKA
- To confirm hypoglycaemia and monitor recovery
- During periods of rapid growth when insulin requirement is increasing.

It is important to reassure the child or young person that SMBG is a positive tool in managing their diabetes whatever the blood glucose results may be. Each result is just a piece of information that can be used to improve overall control and is not a reflection of them as an individual (Hanas 2007).

WWW

Visit Diabetes UK website for nutritional guidelines for diabetes healthcare professionals at:

- http://www.diabetes.org.uk

HbA1c

During the life cycle of the red blood cell (approximately 120 days) glucose becomes attached to the haemoglobin molecule and forms glycated haemoglobin which is represented as a percentage or as mmol/mol (International Federation of Clinical Chemistry (IFCC) unit of reporting). Known as the HbA1c, it is a reflection of the general blood glucose levels in the previous 2–3 months. Ideally the test is carried out during an outpatient consultation so that it might be used to inform ongoing management.

NICE (2004b) recommends the long-term target for an HbA1c level should be 7.5% (58 mmol/mol) and below without frequent disabling hypoglycaemia, and the child's individual management plan for diabetes should aim to achieve this.

Urinary and blood ketone testing

Urinary ketone testing is advocated during periods of uncontrolled hyperglycaemia, insulin deficiency and during bouts of illness. Their early identification will alert the child or parent to the heightened risk of developing diabetic ketoacidosis (DKA). Urinary ketone test strips are available on prescription. The presence of moderate or large urinary ketones associated with hyperglycaemia reflects insulin deficiency and the risk of ketoacidosis.

Blood ketone testing meters are available for home monitoring but are currently expensive. It is a more acceptable means of testing for the presence of ketones than urine ketone testing and may be of benefit in the younger child and more importantly in insulin pump patients as they have only a small reserve of residual subcutaneous insulin.

Diabetic ketoacidosis

DKA is caused by a relative or absolute deficiency of insulin. It is a medical emergency requiring treatment in hospital with intravenous rehydration and insulin infusion. There are a number of risk factors for the potential development of DKA:

- The newly diagnosed. An improvement in the recognition of symptoms within primary care services has led to a reduction of DKA, though this is variable from one country to another.
- Infection/trauma. Infection or trauma can result in acute stress producing an elevation in counter-regulatory hormones that increase levels of circulating glucose.
- Growth spurt/puberty. The demand for insulin during a growth spurt or puberty requires a corresponding increase in insulin doses.
- Poor control/missed injections. Missed insulin injections coupled with dietary indiscretions will increase the risk of developing DKA and in consequence, recurrent episodes of DKA may be a reflection of mismanagement and will need psychological support to break the cycle of repetition.
- Insulin pump therapy. Insulin pump therapy uses only rapid- or short-acting insulin and therefore the reserve of circulating insulin is small when compared to injection therapy. If delivery of insulin is interrupted from the pump, DKA can develop very quickly.

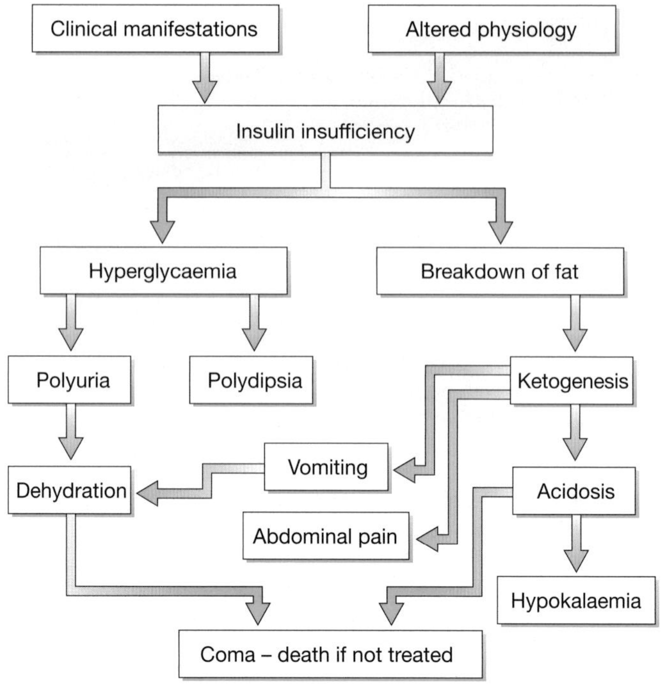

Fig. 34.11 • Diabetic ketoacidosis.

It is important to establish the cause of DKA so that strategies can be employed to reduce the risk of further episodes. An understanding of the altered physiology that occurs when insulin is insufficient is required by the nurse and this is outlined in Figure 34.11.

Characteristics of diabetic ketoacidosis

Presenting signs and symptoms include:

- hyperglycaemia
- polyuria
- polydipsia
- abdominal pain
- nausea and vomiting
- general weakness
- altered consciousness
- weight loss
- Kussmaul breathing (deep sighing respirations)
- acetone smell on breath.

However, not all these symptoms may be present.

Diagnosis of diabetic ketoacidosis

Diagnosis is based on presenting signs and symptoms, clinical assessment of dehydration, abdominal pain/vomiting and neurological status. Hyperglycaemia is found on bedside blood glucose testing initially and acidosis confirmed by venous/arterial blood gas analysis. Ketonuria is detected by urine dipstick testing.

WWW

Topics to be covered in an educational programme have been included in the National Service Framework for Diabetes: Delivery Strategy (DoH 2003):

- http://www.goh.gov/planning2003-2006/index.htm

Familiarise yourself with the four main areas of this programme: nature of diabetes, day-to-day management of diabetes, specific issues in relation to diabetes, living with diabetes.

Goals of management of diabetic ketoacidosis

- Restoration of fluid volume. Normal saline is given gradually over 24–48 hours as rapid fluid replacement has been indicated as a risk factor for cerebral oedema.
- Inhibition of lipolysis. Intravenous insulin is given to suppress the production of ketone bodies and restore normal glucose utilisation and resolve acidosis
- Replacement of electrolytes. As potassium is drawn out of the cells by hypertonicity and lost through osmotic diuresis, there is a substantial depletion of total body potassium. Once circulatory function has been restored, it must be replaced by adding to the intravenous infusion. However, potassium replacement should be delayed until urinary output is documented.

The extent of specific deficits in each patient determines the severity of the ketoacidosis.

Nursing care

Nursing care requires ongoing assessment with particular attention to:

- maintaining accurate fluid balance
- all urine samples being tested for presence of ketones
- hourly BP and basic observations
- hourly or more frequent neurological observations for signs and symptoms of cerebral oedema
- hourly blood glucose measurements (using bedside blood glucose meter)
- cardiac monitoring: presence of a flat T-wave may indicate hypokalaemia.

The child's condition should be monitored until blood glucose returns to normal, ketonuria is resolving and oral feeding has been re-established. All nursing interventions must be accurately reported on and recorded. All interventions should be explained to the child and family as they will need support and reassurance during both the acute and recovery phase of management.

Cerebral oedema

Cerebral oedema is a complication of diabetic ketoacidosis and is the most common cause of death in children with type 1 diabetes (Edge et al 2006). Children's nurses need to be alert for the signs and symptoms of cerebral oedema and report immediately to a senior medical clinician if the patient reports a headache or shows signs of confusion, irritability or reduced level of consciousness, or indeed any change in their neurological status. Prompt recognition and treatment may prevent long-term neurological problems.

Table 34.7 Characteristics of hypoglycaemia

Characteristics	Nursing considerations
Blood glucose < 3.3 mmol/L Hunger, weakness, shaking, sweating Drowsiness at unusual times Headache, behavioural changes Loss of consciousness Convulsions	Requires immediate administration of fast-acting sugar to raise blood glucose If a meal is not anticipated within the next hour a snack – carbohydrate, fat and protein is recommended (Finberg & Kleinman 2002) Check blood glucose level after 30 minutes Assess the need for additional carbohydrate or possibility of hyperglycaemia If child presents with seizure or in a coma administer subcutaneous glucagon as directed – may cause nausea and vomiting so need to administer oral carbohydrate when child is awake Check consistency in routine Check that correct insulin dosage is being administered Encourage regular blood glucose monitoring Encourage controlled snacking Encourage child/family compliance Ensure all involved with the child on a daily basis are educated and trained in recognition and treatment of hypoglycaemia

Hypoglycaemia

Hypoglycaemia is an acute complication of diabetes and is due to a mismatch between insulin administered, food consumed and recent exercise. The symptoms are unpleasant and potentially dangerous causing fear and anxiety in the child and their families. With the drive to achieve tight glycaemic control, the incidence of hypoglycaemia is almost inevitable.

Signs and symptoms

Hypoglycaemia is generally accompanied by signs and symptoms that are in response to the body's attempt to raise the blood glucose level known as autonomic activation and symptoms originating in the brain related to glucose deficiency in the nervous system referred to as neurological dysfunction (neuroglycopenia). Hypoglycaemia is considered to be a recorded plasma blood glucose level of ≤ 3.9 mmol/l.

Activity

Review Chapters 18, 45 and 46:

- Discuss how this information is relevant to the care of the child with Cushing syndrome.

Table 34.8 Signs and symptoms of hypoglycaemia

Autonomic signs and symptoms of hypoglycaemia	Neuroglycopenic signs and symptoms of hypoglycaemia
Irritability	Weakness, dizziness
Trembling	Odd behaviour, poor judgment
Heart palpitation	Unsteady gait
Pallor	Difficulty concentrating
Feeling hungry	Difficulty hearing
Cold sweatiness	Blurred vision
	Loss of consciousness
	Seizures

Table 34.9 Treatment of hypoglycaemia

Mild/moderate hypoglycaemia	Severe hypoglycaemia
The child or parent/caregiver is aware of hypoglycaemic episode and is able to take appropriate action to resolve	Symptoms of hypoglycaemia temporarily disable the child and assistance is required by parent or caregiver Oral glucose is given providing swallow reflex is present; an injection of intramuscular glucagon if no swallow reflex In the hospital setting, intravenous glucose

WWW

Review calculations for fluid and insulin requirements in the guidelines produced by Diabetes UK (Guidelines for the management of diabetic ketoacidosis) and the British Society of Paediatric Endocrinology and Diabetes at:

- http://www.diabetes.org.uk
- http://www.bsped.org.uk/dka.htm

The aim is to restore blood glucose level to within normal limits (4–8 mmol/L):

- Take immediate action and give fast-acting carbohydrate, such as dextrose tablets or a glucose drink (e.g. 10–20 g), by mouth.
- The blood glucose level should start to rise and symptoms improve in 10–15 minutes. Re-test blood glucose level to confirm return of normoglycaemia.
- With normoglycaemia restored, long-acting carbohydrate should be given to maintain blood glucose level.

NB: Patients using insulin pump therapy do not require additional long-acting carbohydrate after a hypoglycaemic episode.

Treatment of mild/moderate hypoglycaemia

For severe hypoglycaemia, urgent treatment is required. If the child is unconscious or fitting, they should be taken to hospital for treatment with glucagon either IM or IV. If recovery is inadequate, IV glucose is administered. Hypoglycaemic events should be evaluated and the cause determined in an effort to avoid similar episodes.

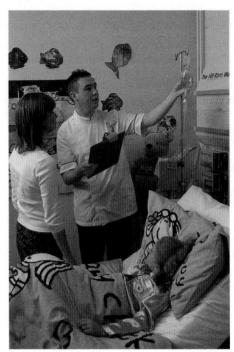

Fig. 34.12 • An 8-year-old girl requiring intravenous therapy.

Evidence-based practice

Structured programmes of lifestyle change which emphasise weight loss (5–7% of body weight) by reduced energy and fat intake and increased physical activity can reduce the risk of overweight people with impaired glucose intolerance developing type 2 diabetes (Diabetes UK 2003b).

Type 2 diabetes

The incidence of type 2 diabetes is rising in children as the prevalence of childhood obesity continues to rise. It is associated with obesity, insulin resistance and metabolic syndrome and is seen in both the paediatric and adolescent population (Peterson et al 2007). Type 2 diabetes occurs when there is insufficient insulin secretion to meet the demand created by insulin resistance. A lack of exercise and a sedentary lifestyle, coupled with excessive calorie intake, are recognised risk factors for obesity and type 2 diabetes. This presents society with a major public health issue with profound implications for the health of future generations and will inevitably place a significant financial burden on our healthcare system (Rodbard 2008). Although there are limited data on the future health outcomes in children with type 2 diabetes, it is expected that the progressive nature of the condition will mirror that seen in the adult population but occur at a much younger age.

Clinical findings may be similar to T1DM in childhood presenting as milder symptoms developing slowly; however, the presence of insulin resistance is a strong indicator of T2DM. A diagnosis of T2DM is made when the presence of elevated plasma blood glucose levels are not thought to be T1DM or monogenic diabetes or

Table 34.10 Clinical characteristics between type 1 and type 2 diabetes

Characteristics	T1DM	T2DM
Age	Throughout childhood	Usually pubertal, however becoming more common in childhood
Onset	Often acute	Insidious
Obesity	Not typically present, often thin	Typically present
Family history of T2DM	Uncommon	Common
Polyuria	Symptomatic	Mild or absent
Polydipsia	Symptomatic	Mild or absent
Ketonuria	Common	Rare

any other underlying cause of hyperglycaemia; however, the levels are sufficient to put the individual at risk of cardiovascular complications. Diagnosis is confirmed if fasting blood glucose concentrations are > 7.0 mmol/l on two separate days, or if random glucose concentrations of 11.1 mmol/l or above on two separate occasions (Resenbloom et al 2008).

Management strategies

The goals of treatment are:

- to encourage weight loss
- to increase physical activity
- to achieve normoglycaemia
- to adopt a healthier lifestyle
- reduction in the rate of complications.

A child with type 2 diabetes is likely to have a 1 in 5 chance of having a parent with type 2 diabetes. This is particularly challenging for healthcare professionals as it requires a greater emphasis on changing behaviour and eating patterns that are often deep seated in the child's lifestyle and success is dependent on the whole family's ability to modify their way of life and eating practices.

Oral or insulin therapy may be necessary when lifestyle changes alone fail to maintain normal glycaemic levels. The aim is to reduce insulin resistance, increase the secretion of endogenous insulin or slow post prandial glucose absorption.

Monogenic diabetes

Monogenic diabetes results from one or more mutations in a single gene which may be dominantly or recessively inherited or may simply be a spontaneous occurrence. The clinical spectrum is broad, ranging from asymptomatic hyperglycaemia to a severe acute presentation. Monogenic diabetes has been reported in all races and ethnicities. The characteristics of monogenic diabetes are:

- presentation of diabetes before 6 months of age
- it can run in families through several generations
- children don't produce enough insulin – which differs from type 2 diabetes, where the individual produces sufficient insulin but are unable to utilise it
- children with monogenic diabetes may not need insulin treatment and can often be treated with oral glycaemic therapy or diet modification alone.

In children, most cases of monogenic diabetes are associated with mutations in genes that regulate β-cell function (Hattersley et al 2006). Diagnosis is based on molecular genetics. As these tests are expensive, only those with a high likelihood of a positive result should be tested. Otherwise the child should be treated as having the type of diabetes that best fits their clinical picture. A diagnosis of monogenic diabetes will have implications for other family members who may have been misdiagnosed with type 1 or type 2 diabetes.

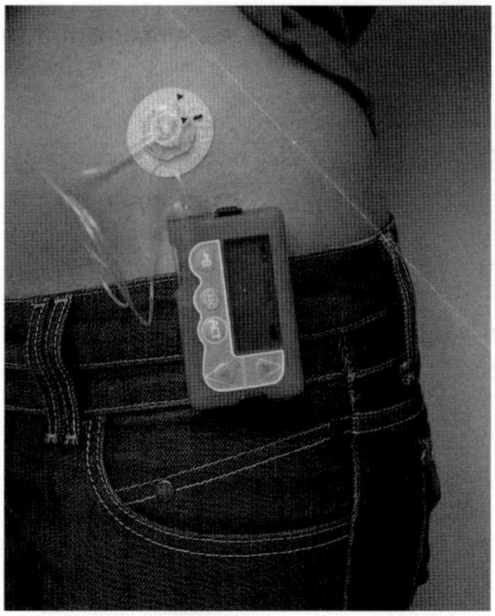

Fig. 34.13 • Insulin pump therapy.

Insulin pump therapy

Insulin pump therapy also known as continuous subcutaneous insulin infusion (CSII) has been used to treat diabetes since the late 1970s but has only become more readily available in the UK over the past few years. It has been successfully used in all age groups and offers a more flexible approach to diabetes management. The advantage of insulin pump therapy is its ability to mimic physiological insulin release by continuously delivering rapid (or short) insulin into subcutaneous tissue (Fig. 34.13).

The pump has a refillable reservoir connected via tubing to a subcutaneously placed catheter that is changed every few days. The pump is programmed to deliver a basal (background) rate of insulin throughout the day and calculated bolus doses are given at the push of a button for meal carbohydrate intake. Current pump technology allows for variable hourly rates of insulin that are set according to the individual child's basal requirement and mealtime bolus insulin doses can be adjusted in speed and duration of delivery based on the composition of a meal and its anticipated glycaemic effects (Roberts & Walsh, 2006).

Suitability for continuous subcutaneous insulin infusion

For patients with type 1 diabetes who are:

- unable to achieve target HbA1c and who experience disabling hypoglycaemia despite multiple daily injection therapy

OR

- have elevated HbA1c (8.5% or above) on multiple daily injections despite high levels of motivation.

In addition:

- for children under 12 years of age CSII may be a treatment option for type 1 diabetes provided MDI is impractical or inappropriate. However, a trial on injection therapy would be expected during teenage years (NICE 2008).

The child's basal requirement and mealtime bolus insulin doses can be adjusted in speed and duration of delivery based on the composition of a meal and its anticipated glycaemic affects. Initiation of therapy should be carried out by trained professionals in CSII and ongoing care by a diabetes team experienced in pump therapy.

CSII is expensive compared to conventional therapy and its use in the UK is dependent on clinical need. Comparative studies between the efficacy of CSII and MDI from a clinical perspective are inconclusive; however, of note is the reduction in frequency and severity of hypoglycaemic episodes reported in patients using CSII. Families describe high levels of satisfaction, a more spontaneous approach to food, fewer glycaemic excursions and increased independence for the older child and adolescent (Plotnick et al 2003).

Insulin injections are commonly given via an insulin pen, though using a syringe and needle is still a practice used in some areas when specific combinations of long- and short-acting insulins are not available as a pre-mixture. Before mixing insulin in the same syringe, there is a need to establish that this procedure does not change the pharmokinetics of both types of insulin, otherwise the practice should be avoided.

Long-term complication of type 1 diabetes mellitus

There are four major long-term complications associated with type 1 diabetes:

- Retinopathy
- Nephropathy
- Neuropathy
- Cardiac disease.

The outcomes from these are presented in Table 34.11. While these complications are uncommon in childhood and may not be clinically visible, early functional and structural abnormalities may be evident in the microvascular systems after a few years following diagnosis. Evidence has indicated that meticulous treatment and control of type 1 diabetes will reduce the risk of microvascular complication significantly (Diabetic Control and Complication Trial 2003). This research also demonstrated that the progression of retinopathy may be slowed with improved control.

Table 34.11 Long-term vascular complications

Complications	Outcomes
Retinopathy	Visual impairment – cataracts, blindness
Nephropathy	Renal failure, hypertension
Neuropathy	Pain, paraesthesia, muscle weakness, autonomic dysfunction
Cardiac disease	Atherosclerosis, hypertension, cardiovascular disease

Retinopathy is the commonest cause of blindness in developed countries. Adolescents have a higher risk of developing retinopathy compared to adults diagnosed with type 1 diabetes and this may rapidly progress towards visual impairment (Donaghue et al 2007). Hence, screening is imperative to detect the early stages of retinopathy in the adolescent. Other complications of type 1 diabetes include:

- delayed growth
- delayed onset of puberty
- associated autoimmune conditions – coeliac disease, hypothyroidism, hyperthyroidism, vitiligo and primary adrenal insufficiency
- lipohypertrophy
- skin ulceration
- limited joint mobility.

Monitoring of growth and development is essential. There may be an increase in height at the time of diagnosis, however, poor weight gain, decrease in the attainment of height and late pubertal development have been reported in those who have poor glycaemic control (Kordonouri et al 2007). After the initial diagnosis and the child's weight is satisfactory they need to be monitored for excessive weight gain. This may occur due to a high energy intake and excessive exogenous insulin. It is more common during puberty especially in females thus necessitating a reduction in their insulin dose towards the end of puberty (Lissauer & Clayden 2006). Obesity will also increase the risk of cardiovascular defects. Girls with type 1 diabetes are more at risk of being obese and developing eating disorders along with the risk of having polycystic ovary syndrome.

Diabetes UK (2000) and the Department of Health National Service Framework (2001) identify that foot problems is the most frequent problem of diabetic neuropathy leading eventually to lower limb amputation for up to 15% of the associated diabetic population. As glycaemic control is difficult to maintain around and during puberty, it has been recognised that this is when microvascular problems are likely to occur. Compliance with treatment and monitoring is not always congruent with the adolescent lifestyle, hence the need for early education of the parents and the child. Diabetes UK (2000) guidelines advise examination of the feet on diagnosis and then annually. Education is also required about correctly fitting shoes and socks, and toe nail cutting.

Thus to minimise the long-term impact of type 1 diabetes and with a view to maximisation of the quality of life of the child, regular surveillance for and the effective management of complications need to occur. Screening should be carried out in accordance with recommendations from NICE 2004. Integrated health and social care should also be provided to those adolescents requiring it (DoH 2003).

Adolescence and type I diabetes

Normal adolescent physical, psychosexual and developmental maturation is affected by diabetes (Lissauer & Clayden 2006). During adolescence, the child will move from dependence to a more autonomous lifestyle and are expected to take increasing responsibility for their care and health needs. Cognitive changes occur as the adolescent moves from concrete thinking to more abstract thinking. They are unable to comprehend the long-term and unseen consequences of their actions. The adolescent with diabetes may become lost to the health services and it is recognised that attendance rates at diabetic clinics drop around the age of 16 years (DoH 2007). The healthcare professional must be alert to the health needs and social issues that may affect the adolescent during this developmental phase.

In addition, diabetes is often more difficult to control due to hormonal changes of puberty as well as the emotional difficulties associated with adolescence. For some, this stage of development will present with behavioural changes such as denial, indifference or depression about their illness. In addition, there may be an unwillingness to conform to treatment regimes, which may give rise to conflict with family and health professionals. There may be a tendency to avoid aspects of their diabetic management, e.g. omit insulin injections or manipulate the regime, and ignore dietary needs. Blood glucose monitoring may not be carried out or results may be falsified. Many teenage girls experiment with crash diets at some time, which is likely to cause major problems in diabetic control. Low adherence rates increases mortality and morbidity thus affecting quality of life in the long term and may necessitate additional healthcare resources.

This is a time when the young person should be encouraged to take increasing control for their diabetes. Evaluation of adherence is an essential role of the healthcare practitioner and this is best achieved by asking the young person about their management of their diabetes (Taddeo et al 2008). Low adherence rates may also test the limits of acceptable behaviour. It may be helpful to identify short-term goals for them and ensure that effort to improve their control is communicated promptly and enthusiastically. A united team approach, with agreement of the essentials they wish to promote and clear, unambiguous guidelines for health and diabetic management is necessary. Repeated information has been identified as a method of improving adherence (Osterberg & Blaschke 2005). Consideration must also be given to the appropriate management of any mental-health issues if adherence to treatment is to be achieved. Peer group pressure may be utilised to promote health, especially in relation to smoking and alcohol consumption. Holiday camps provide opportunities for young diabetics to meet and learn about their diabetic management.

Transition to adult services

The adolescent with type 1 diabetes will experience a smooth transition of care from children's diabetic services to adult diabetic services (Standard 6, DoH 2003). While the adolescent faces unique challenges during this period, the transition between services should not be another challenge. Transition is a multifaceted process and it must acknowledge the medical, psychosocial and educational needs of the young person – it is a purposeful and planned process (DoH 2007). Best practice advocates that transition from children's service to adult services is best undertaken during a period of stability and is planned on an individual basis. The young person and their families must be provided with knowledge, skills and confidence about the transition process and the services they will be accessing in the future. Transition should be based on the emotional development of the individual and not on chronological age. Local protocols for transition to adult services should be in place (NICE 2004). The practical aspects of transition of care for young people with diabetes needs to be made clear to them such as the glycaemic levels required, screening process and any unfamiliar terminology.

Child and family education

The primary goal in caring for children and young people with diabetes is to enable them and their families to manage their own lifestyle and condition, by providing support and structured education as well as drugs and treatment (DoH 2001). Therefore, a coordinated, multidisciplinary team approach to care and management in partnership with the child and family is essential if the following long-term outcomes are to be achieved:

- normal growth and development
- maintaining as normal a home and school life as possible
- good diabetic control, appropriate knowledge, good technique and self-reliance
- avoidance of hypoglycaemia
- prevention of long-term complications.

This will be reflected in the child's personal record that contains the clinical record of care, treatment and management. A personal diabetes record should include the following:

- an agreed care plan, including education and the personal goals of the child and family in relation to care and treatment
- information as to how the child's diabetes is to be managed until the next review to foster greater understanding and ownership of the goals of diabetes care
- identification of social and educational needs, how they will be met and who will be responsible
- identification of the named contact (DoH 2003).

Central role of the nurse

Care of the child with type 1 diabetes requires a multidisciplinary approach through collaboration with paediatricians, endocrinologist, general practitioners, dieticians, psychology services and education providers. The nurse, particularly the community children nurse, plays a central role in the assessment and planning of care for the child and family. The management of diabetes is a complex process and the aim of nursing care should be to meet the holistic needs of the child and family from diagnosis through to the long-term care required with a view to maintaining a good quality of life. This is achieved through education of the child, parents and siblings. Good facilitation of the child's and families care needs will enable a family-centred care approach to be adopted. Effective management of diabetes and increases life expectancy and reduces the risk of complications developing (Diabetes UK 2003a). As this is a lifelong condition, the nurse must consider the developmental stage the child is at when planning care. The timing and giving of information are very important in the initial period after diagnosis and it should be remembered that this will need revisiting at a later time.

Initial teaching for the child and parents/carers will focus on the skills necessary for discharge from hospital, injection technique, home glucose monitoring, recognition of hypoglycaemic episode and hyperglycaemia, dietary management, exercise and recording of information. The child and parents/carer should also be informed of what action to take during normal expected illnesses.

Ongoing nursing assessment is required with the focus on the child's physiological status, psychological state and family's response to diagnosis and treatment constantly being revisited. This will necessitate the nurse accessing other members of the multidisciplinary team as required to support the child and family. The nurse is the central contact point for accessing the multidisciplinary team on behalf of the child and family. Parental guilt may be present at the time of diagnosis and for a period of time after diagnosis. Education requirements should be adopted to suit the needs of the child and family and provided at a rate that suits them (McEvilly 2003).

Coping mechanisms need to be assessed and understood by the nurse so that the plan of care for the child and parents will correctly reflect their educational needs. Individual plans of care should be developed by the child, parent, diabetic nurse and team to address their specific needs in terms of normal life activities, i.e. school, social clubs. The provision of education for school staff and others involved in the school day has been identified as one of the key interventions in the National Service Framework for Standards in Diabetes (DoH 2001).

Home management at the time of diagnosis provides immediate opportunities for the children's nurse to educate the child, parents and others in relation to diabetes. Books, teaching aids and website addresses might enhance the learning process and provide guidance for child and parent in the absence of the nurse (Fig. 34.14). Opportunities should be made for child and family to explore their perceptions of the impact of diabetes on their lives and the implications of care required by the child, and the immediate problems they envisage. Meeting with other parents and children with diabetes may provide additional support.

Parents need to understand the positive support their child will need throughout childhood and into adolescence to optimise physical, psychological, intellectual, educational and social development. This must include a period of independence so that the young person may be enabled to take on the responsibility and develop the confidence to be self-caring (McEvilly 2003).

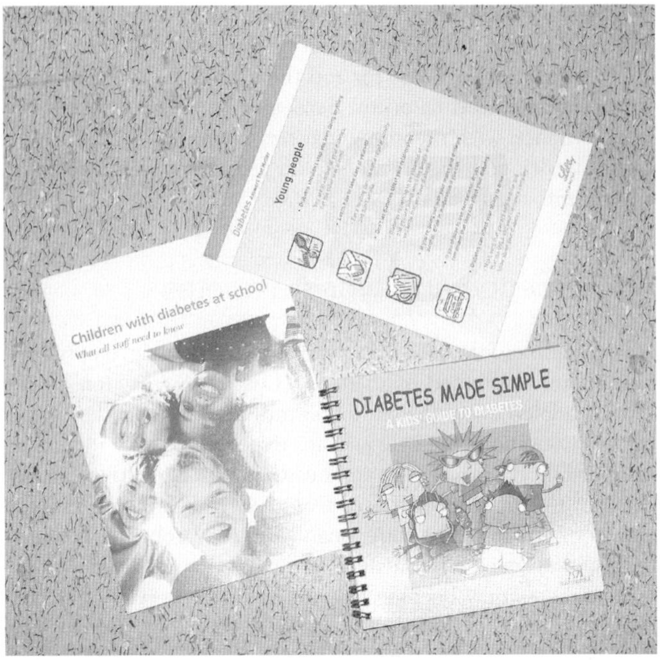

Fig. 34.14 • Examples of information available for child, family and others.

Discussion of the scenarios

June: Graves' disease

Observations necessary to assess June's need to plan her nursing interventions include:

- vital signs of temperature, pulse and blood pressure may be elevated and June may complain of palpitations due to hyperthyroid state
- observation of skin for warmth, moistness and flushed appearance
- respiratory difficulties may present as a result of hypervascularity and enlargement of the thyroid gland
- enlargement of the thyroid gland may be evident
- enlargement and protrusion of the eye balls leading to irritation, pain, lacrimation, photophobia and blurred vision
- monitoring of height may indicate a degree of accelerated growth and development
- monitoring weight may indicate a loss despite having an increased appetite
- june may complain of excessive weakness and lack of ability to engage in usual activities
- observation of her emotional state, nervous excitability and mood stability is necessary as there may be associated hyperactivity of the sympathetic division of the autonomic nervous system.

June's specific care requirements

The symptoms of hyperthyroidism may fluctuate with spontaneous remissions and exacerbations. Mild cases may require no treatment. The condition is generally treated with medical interventions and/or radiation therapy.

Bed rest is advisable at the beginning of medical treatment. This treatment is aimed at controlling symptoms of nervous instability, tachycardia and hypertension that may require the administration of β-adrenergic blocking agents (propranolol, atenolol). Continual monitoring of vital signs is necessary to evaluate effectiveness of interventions and monitor for early signs of complications.

Drugs that interfere with thyroid hormone synthesis, namely carbimazole or propylthiouracil may be prescribed according to the individual needs of the child. Treatment with antithyroid drugs must be continued for at least 2–3 years, with the smallest drug dosage that will produce a symptom-free state in the child.

When response to medical treatment is not achieved then radiation therapy with radioactive iodine may be considered. In some cases, radioiodine is the initial treatment of choice considered (Kappy et al 2003).

In hypothyroidism and hyperthyroidism, the aim of care is to achieve an optimal level of thyroxine that will enable growth and development, including enhancement of intellectual ability. June and her parents need to understand the nature of the condition, the aims and different types of treatment, including dosages of prescribed medication and repeat prescriptions, as well as the signs of under- and overtreatment The consequences of non-compliance needs to be discussed. As with all other conditions the provision of literature and appropriate website addresses as identified may enhance understanding.

Attendance at clinics is essential to:

- monitor June's response to medication
- assess growth and development
- provide the opportunity for June and her family to discuss their fears or problems associated with the care and management of the condition
- enable them to meet other families who have been caring for their children with similar problems which for some may prove beneficial.

The children's nurse can remain as the named contact person and through assessment in collaboration and negotiation with the child and family can plan the education and ongoing support required.

Summary

This chapter has presented an overview of the endocrine system and associated problems that may present for the child and family. Care of the child and family with reference to health promotion and education has been significantly addressed.

Development of knowledge and understanding has been enhanced through active participation and the companion PowerPoint presentation.

Acknowledgements

Thanks to James Davis, Graphic Designer, Media Services, Queen's University Belfast for his work in producing diagrams of the endocrine system and outline of a child with Cushing syndrome. Thanks to Paul Morris, Clinical Skills Technician, School of Nursing, Queen's University Belfast for photographic support and also for allowing his daughter to be involved.

Thanks also to my colleague Patricia McNeilly, Teaching Fellow, and Michael Ward, student nurse, for involvement in photographic evidence. Finally, thanks to Kevin Campbell, Clinical Skills Technician, School of Nursing, Queen's University Belfast for allowing his daughter to participate.

References

Ball, J.W., Bindler, R.C., 2006. Child health nursing partnering with children and families. Prentice Hall, Englewood Cliffs, New Jersey.

Boscaro, M., Nicoletta, S., Scarda, A., et al., 2002. Anticoagulant prophylaxis markedly reduces thromboembolic complications in Cushing's syndrome. Journal of Clinical Endocrinology and Metabolism 87 (8), 3662–3666.

Bryant, J., Care, C., Milne, R., 2004. Recombinant growth hormone for idiopathic short stature in children and adolescence (Cochrane Review). HMSO, London.

Campbell, S., Glasper, E.A., 1995. Whaley and Wong's children's nursing. Mosby, London.

Charmandari, E., Brook, C.G.D., Hindmarsh, P.C., 2002. Why is management of patients with classical congenital adrenal hyperplasia more difficult at puberty? Archives of Diseases in Childhood 86 (4), 266–269.

Chrousos, G.P., 2002. In: Finberg, L., Kleinman, R.E. (Eds.), Saunders manual of pediatric practice, 2nd edn. WB Saunders, London.

Cuttler, L., 2002. In: Finberg, L., Kleinman, R.E. (Eds.), Saunders manual of pediatric practice, 2nd edn. WB Saunders, London.

Department of Health (DoH), 2001. National Service Framework for Diabetes: Standards. Department of Health, London.

Department of Health (DoH), 2003. National Service Framework for Diabetes: delivery strategy. Department of Health, London.

Department of Health (DOH), 2007. Making every young person with diabetes matter. DoH, London.

Desrosiers, P. 2002, Online. Available at: http://www.magicfoundation.org/divisions/ftt.htm.

Diabetes, U.K., 2000. What diabetes care to except. Diabetes UK, Bristol.

Diabetes, U.K., 2003. Guidelines for the management of diabetic ketoacidosis in children and adolescents. Diabetic Medicine 20:786–807. Available at: http://www.diabetes.org.uk.

Donaghue, K., Chiareilli, F., Trotta, D., Allgrove, J., Dahl-Jorgensen, K., 2007. Microvascular and macrovascular complications. Pediatric Diabetes 8, 163–170.

Drake, A., Kelnar, C., 2006. The evaluation of growth and the identification of hormone deficiency. Archives of Disease of Childhood 91, 61–67.

Edge, J.A., Jakes, R.W., Roy, Y., et al., 2006. The UK case-control study of cerebral oedema complicating diabetic ketoacidosis in children. Diabetologia 49, 2002–2009.

Hall, D.M.B., 2000. Growth monitoring. Archives of Diseases in Children 82, 10–15.

Hanas, R., 2007. Type 1 diabetes in children, adolescents and young adults, 3rd edn. Class Publishing, London.

Hattersley, A., Bruining, J., Shield, J., Njolstad, P., Donaghue, K., 2006. ISPAD Clinical Practice Consensus Guidelines 2006-2007. The diagnosis and management of monogenic diabetes in children. Pediatric Diabetes 7, 352–360.

Hockenberry, M.J., Wilson, D., Winkelstein, M.L., Kline, N.E., 2003. Wong's nursing care of infants and children, 7th edn. Mosby, London.

Kappy, M.S., Steelman, J.W., Travers, S.H., Zeitler, P.S., 2003. In: Hay, W.W., Hayward, A.R., Levin, M.J., Sondheimer, J.M. (Eds.), Current pediatric diagnosis and treatment, 16th edn. McGraw-Hill, London.

King, L., 2003. Subcutaneous insulin injection technique. Nursing Standard 17 (34), 45–51.

Kordonouri, O., Maguire, A., Knip, M., et al., 2007. Other complications and associated conditions. Pediatric Diabetes 8, 171–176.

Lissauer, T., Clayden, G., 2007. Illustrated textbook of paediatrics, 3rd edn. Mosby, Edinburgh.

McCance, A., Huether, B., 2006. Pathophysiology: the biological basis for disease in adults and children, 5th edn. Mosby, St Louis.

McEvilly, A., 2003. In: Barnes, K. (Ed.), Paediatrics: a clinical guide for nurse practitioners, Butterworth Heinemann, London.

Miller, W.L., 2002. In: Finberg, L., Kleinman, R.E. (Eds.), Saunders manual of pediatric practice, 2nd edn. WB Saunders, London.

Nairn, J., Moore, B.J., 2002. The role of nurses in providing educational support to growth hormone deficient children, adolescents and their families. Neonatal,. Paediatric and Child Health Nursing 5 (1), 10–13.

NICE, 2002. Guidance on the use of human growth hormone (somatropin) in children with growth failure. NICE, London.

NICE, 2004a. Type 1 diabetes: diagnosis and management of type 1diabetes in children and young people (updated June 2009). NICE, London. http://www.nice.org.uk/nicemedia/pdf/CG015ChildrenFullGuidelineUpdate.pdf (accessed June 20 2009).

NICE, 2004b. Type 2 diabetes: diagnosis and management of type 2 diabetes in children and young people. NICE, London http://www.nice.org.uk/nicemedia/pdf/CG66FullGuideline0509.pdf (accessed June 20 2009).

NICE, 2008. Continuous subcutaneous insulin for the treatment of diabetes mellitus. Review of technology appraisal guidance 57. NICE Technology Appraisal Guidance 151. NICE, London.

Osterberg, L., Blaschke, T., 2005. Adherence to medication. New England Journal of Medicine 353, 487–497.

Parks, J.S., 2002. In: Finberg, L., Kleinman, R.E. (Eds.), Saunders manual of pediatric practice. WB Saunders, London.

Peterson, K., Silverstein, J., Kaufman, F., Warren-Boulton, E., 2007. Management of type 2 diabetes in youth: an update. American Family Physician 76 (5), 658–664.

Plotnick, L.P., Clark, L.M., Brancati, F.L., Erlinger, T., 2003. Safety and effectiveness of insulin pump therapy in children and adolescents with type 1 diabetes. Diabetes Care 26 (4), 1142–1146.

Polak, S., et al., 1996. Subcutaneous or intramuscular injections of insulin in children. Are we injecting where we think we are? Diabetes Care 19 (12), 1434–1436.

Riddell, M.C., Iscoe, K.E., 2006. Physical activity, sport and pediatric diabetes. Pediatric Diabetes 7, 60–70.

Roberts, R., Walsh, J., 2006. Pumping insulin, 4th edn. Torrey Pines Press, California.

Rodbard, H., 2008. Diabetes screening, diagnosis and therapy in paediatrics patients with type 2 diabetes. Diabetes Care 10 (8), 184.

Rosenbloom, A.L., Silverstein, J.H., Amemiya, S., Zeitler, P., Klingersmith, G., 2009. ISPAD Clinical Practice Consensus Guidelines 2009 Compendium. Type 2 diabetes in children and adolescents. Pediatric Diabetes 10 (suppl. 12), 17–32.

Roth, C., Scortea, M., Stubbe, P., et al., 1997. Autoimmune thyroiditis in childhood. Experimental and Clinical Endocrinology and Diabetes 105 (4), 66–69.

Rudolf, M., Levene, M., 2006. Paediatrics and child health, 2nd edn. Blackwell Publishing, Oxford.

Storr, H.L., Plowman, P.N., Caroll, P.V., et al., 2003. Clinical and endocrine responses to pituitary radiotherapy in paediatric Cushing's disease. An effective second line treatment. Journal of Clinical Endocrinology and Metabolism 88 (1), 34–37.

Strauss, K., et al., 2002. A pan-European epidemiologic study of insulin technique in patients with diabetes. Practical Diabetes International 19 (3), 71–76.

Taddeo, D., Egedy, M., Frappier, J.Y., 2008. Adherence to treatment in adolescents. Paediatric Child Health 13 (1), 19–24.

Thow, J., Home, P., 1990. Insulin injection technique: depth of injection is important. British Medical Journal 301 (22), 3–4.

Wong, D.L., Wilson, D., 1995. Whaley's and Wong's Nursing care of infants and children. Mosby, St Louis.

World Health Organization (WHO), 1999. Definition, diagnosis and classification of diabetes mellitus and its complications. Report of a WHO consultation: Part 1: diagnosis and classification of diabetes mellitus. WHO, Department of Noncommunicable Disease Surveillance, Geneva. Online. Available at: http://www.staff.ncl.ac.uk/philip.home/who_dmc.htm.

Useful Websites

ACTH Association: http://www.cushingsacth.co.uk
British Thyroid Foundation: http://www.btf-thyroid.org
British Society of Paediatric Endocrinology and Diabetes: http://www.bsped.org.uk
CREST website: http://www.crestni.org.uk
Diabetes Nursing: http://www.diabetesnursing.com
Diabetes UK: http://www.diabetes.org.uk
Diabetes National Service Framework: http://www.doh.gov./nsf/diabetes
National Institute of Child Health and Human Development: http://www.nichd.nih.gov/publications/pubs/pit.htm
The Endocrine Society: http://www.endo-society.org
The Hormone Foundation: http://www.hormone.org
Child Growth Foundation: http://www.heightmatters.org.uk

Caring for children with orthopaedic disorders

35

Brian Silverwood

ABSTRACT

The aim of this chapter is to give the reader a basic introduction to the specialty of orthopaedics in relation to the child with common bony injuries/disorders and the medical and nursing care they may receive. The word 'orthopaedic' is derived from the Greek 'orthos pais' and means 'straight child'. The specialty has expanded from correcting disorders in children to include all areas of musculoskeletal surgery and conservative management (Danby & Edwards 1999).

Caring for children with an orthopaedic injury provides the nurse with a challenging and rewarding experience. Unlike most other paediatric specialties, the child admitted to the orthopaedic ward is usually well and active and requires, apart from attention to the bony injury/surgery, planning and interaction to provide him or her with play and distraction to prevent boredom. Many children's and emergency nurses care daily for children with bony injury and therefore require a sound knowledge base both to deal with the injury and to reassure the anxious child and parent.

LEARNING OUTCOMES

- Describe bone structure, formation and resorption and the core functions of the skeleton, joints and muscles.
- Outline common childhood fractures and methods of management.
- Understand the pathophysiology of common childhood conditions and the medical/surgical treatments available.
- Devise an individualised plan of nursing care for a child who faces a period of immobility.
- Discuss the importance of discharge planning.

Glossary

Abduction: Moving a body part away from the body.
Adduction: Moving a body part towards the body.
Artho: Prefix meaning relating to a joint.
Congenital: Present at birth.
Distal: Situated further away from the area of consideration.
Dorsiflexion: Movement of hand or foot towards the dorsal surface.
Dysplasia: Abnormal development of skin, bone or other tissues.
Entonox: A self-administered inhaled pain relieving agent consisting of 50% nitrous oxide and 50% oxygen.
Equinovarus: The foot points downwards and inwards.
Equinus: The foot points downwards.
Extension: Straightening a joint.
Flexion: Bending a joint.
Hyperextension: Excessive extension.
Intramedullary: Within the medullary (inner) cavity of a long bone.
Inversion: Downwards and inwards movement of the foot.
Lateral: Situated away from the midline of the body.
Macrophage: A large scavenger cell that wanders between cells and removes bacteria and other foreign bodies from blood and tissues.
Medial: Near to the midline of the body.
Proximal: Situated close to the point of origin or attachment.
Osteoblast: A bone-forming cell.
Osteoclast: A large cell that resorbs bone.
Osteocyte: A basic bone cell.
Osteomyelitis: Inflammation of the bone due to infection.
Osteotomy: A surgical cut across the bone.
Rotation: Turning about an axis.
Sclera: Whites of the eyes.
Subluxation: Partial dislocation.
Valgus: A limb deformity in which the extremity is more away from the body's midline.
Varus: Opposite of valgus.

Bone biology

The function of the skeletal system

The musculoskeletal system consists of 206 bones with their surrounding muscles. The main functions of the bones of the skeleton are to support and give shape to the body, to protect vital organs and to provide a system of levers that enables the

DOI: 10.1016/B978-0-7020-3183-0.10035-9

body to make movements. In addition, bone serves as storage sites for certain minerals such as calcium and is also responsible for the production of red and white blood cells, a function performed by the red bone marrow. Yellow bone marrow acts as a storage site for lipids.

Activity

Using a suitable anatomy and physiology textbook, or suitable online source, identify and name the different bones of the body. Examine the relative significance of each bone in relation to its main function and location within the human skeleton.

Bone structure

Bones are extremely strong and can withstand considerable forces. Bone is very resilient and can return to its normal shape after the removal of the force that caused it to become misshapen. This tensile strength and resilience is due to the framework of interwoven fibres within bone called collagen, which is a tough, white, slightly flexible material. Bones are made up of two types of tissue (Fig. 35.1):

- Compact or cortical bone: is the dense and hard part of the bone that gives the bone its shape and strength. It is made up of many rods, known as the Haversian system. These have a central canal, which contains blood vessels and nerve fibres, and is surrounded by several sheets of bone tissue called lamellae. The Haversian canals branch and interweave, giving bone great strength along lines of stress.
- Cancellous or spongy bone: is composed of fine bars of bony tissue that interlace with one another to give a honeycomb appearance. These bars of tissue are known as the trabecular bone and are strong, light and provide an excellent structure to absorb stress. The space within the trabeculae is filled by the red blood marrow.

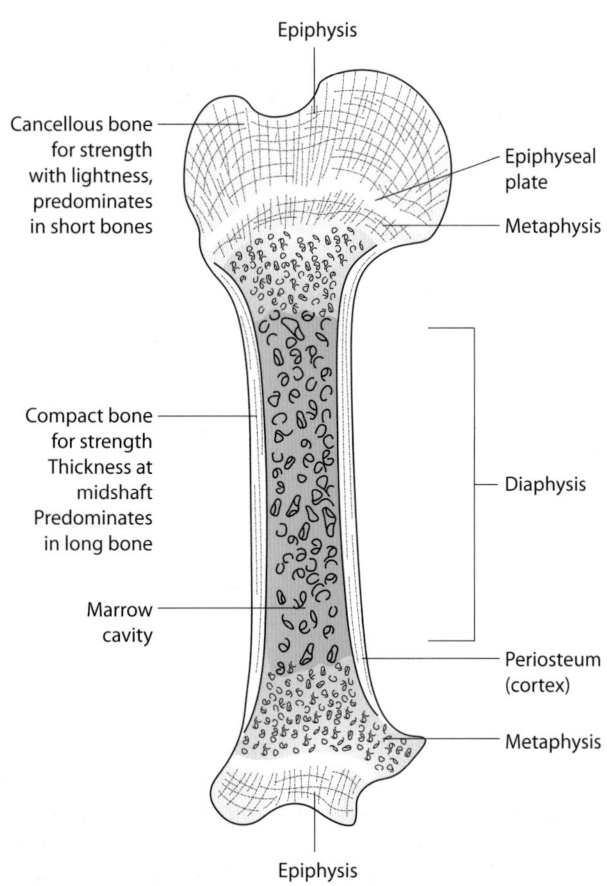

Fig. 35.1 • Cross-section of bone.

All bones are covered by a layer of fibrous tissue called periosteum, which protects the bone and allows the circumference of the bone to grow.

Bone growth, formation and resorption

Bone is constantly remodelling and adapting to the daily stresses placed on our skeleton (Silverwood 2003) (Fig. 35.2). From infancy through to adolescence, bones are actively growing in length, width and density (Table 35.1). Bone remodelling is regulated by several factors including:

- mechanical loads arising from muscle forces regulate the process of bone formation and resorption. For example, a tennis player's racket arm is typically stronger and wider than a non-player's arm because the remodelling bone has adapted to the increased daily strain and loading experienced when serving the ball
- calcium: this is the most abundant mineral found within the body. It is arranged around the matrix of collagen, which gives bone its strength and rigidity. Calcium is stored in the bone and released when serum calcium levels are low. A normal serum calcium level is required to allow adequate muscle contraction, transmission of impulses across nerve cells, activities of some enzymes and the building of strong bones
- parathyroid hormone (PTH): controls distribution of calcium. When serum calcium concentrations are low the hormone causes increased calcium absorption from the intestines, calcium reabsorption by the kidneys and increased bone resorption. Parathyroid hormone also regulates the synthesis of the active metabolites of vitamin D, which also enhance absorption of calcium from the intestine.
- sex hormones: oestrogen and testosterone provide a 'control' over bone resorption and keeps bone remodelling in homeostasis.

Fracture repair and bone healing

The fractured ends of the bone bleed and form a clot. The inflammatory healing process commences and the dead tissue and clot is removed by macrophages. The initial strands from the blood clot begin to change into osteoid tissue, which develops and forms callus around the fracture site; osteoclasts remove necrotic bone and osteoblasts develop new bone (Apley & Solomon 2001). Between 6 and 12 weeks, as the

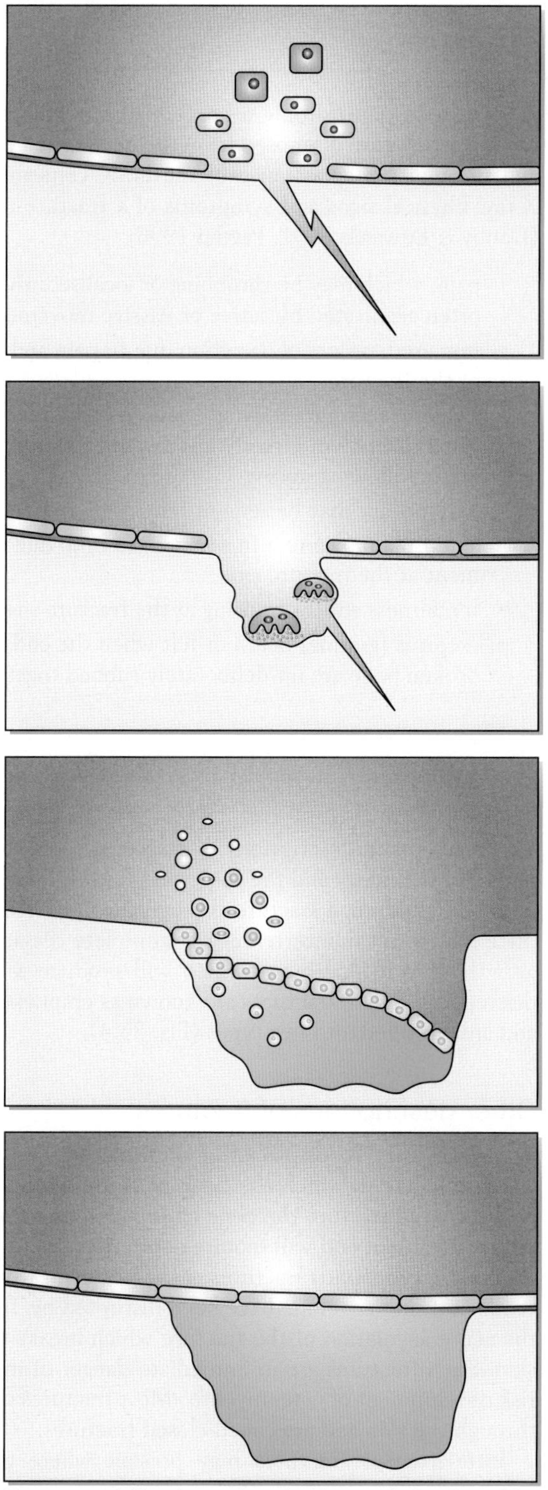

Bone resorption
At random the lining cells of bone become activated by substances including PTH & calcitriol, change from a pancake shape to a cubiod shape. The cells then secrete ODF (osteoclast differentiating factor) which allows the cells to fuse and differentiate into mature multinucleated osteoclasts (bone eating cells).

The osteoclast resorb (munch) away at the bone. New osteoclasts are activated and start resorption as the remodelling moves across the area of bone requiring repair. This resorption lasts around 2 weeks then the osteoclasts undergo apoptosis (programmed cell death).

Bone formation
Osteoblasts (bone forming cells) are derived from marrow stromal cells. They are attracted by bone derived growth factors and the remains of the self destructed osteoclasts.

The secreting osteoblasts then make layers of osteoid and slowly refill the cavity. The osteoblasts secrete a range of growth factors including osteocalcin and other proteins. The osteiod mineralises as the cavity fills.

Over a period of around 3–4 months the crystals of mineral become closely packed together and the density of the new bone increases. The final osteoblasts turn into lining cells which participate in the release of calcium from the bone. Some osteoblasts turns into osteocytes (bone cell) which remain in the new bone and are connected by long cell processes which can sense mechanical stresses to the bones

Fig. 35.2 • Bone remodelling (reproduced with permission from Silverwood 2003.)

callus hardens, the bone regains some mechanical strength. Further callus maturity occurs between 12 and 26 weeks. By 1–2 years bone remodelling has occurred (see Fig. 35.2) and normal bone shape has been restored. Unlike adults, children can restore bony deformity resulting from a significant (up to 30°) malalignment through bone remodelling (Danby & Edwards 2001).

Joints

A joint or articulation is where two or more bones are in close contact with each other. Joints are classified according to their mobility and structure into fibrous, cartilaginous or synovial. Fibrous joints exist between bone and cartilage. The surfaces are simply joined by fibrous tissue and there is little or no

Table 35.1 skeletal development (Gallo 1996)

Infancy	Rapid growth in proportion and size as calcium is added to cartilage-like bones
	Calcium content in relation to body size increases faster than any other stage of life
Childhood	Growth continues
	Bone density and thickness increase
	Bone formation outpaces resorption
Adolescence	Growth accelerates
	Bone growth peaks around ages 12–17 in boys and ages 11–15 in girls
	Bone density and thickness increase
	Bone formation outpaces resorption
Age 20	90% of peak bone mass achieved
Age 35	Peak bone mass achieved
	Note: Peak bone mass is about 30% higher in men than women
Age 40	Bone resorption begins to outpace formation
	Adult bone loss occurs at a rate of 6–8% per decade

movement. Cartilaginous joints allow a small degree of movement and are covered by layers of cartilage linked by a thick pad of tissue, for example, between vertebral bones. Synovial joints, which include all limb joints, permit a great deal of movement and are the most common type of joint. Hyaline cartilage covers the articulating surfaces to prevent friction and a fibrous capsule encloses the joint and helps hold the bones in place. A synovial membrane lines the capsule, which secretes synovial fluid to lubricate the structure.

Activity

Identify the differing types of joint within the human skeleton and justify the joint type in relation to its function and location.

Skeletal muscle

The skeletal muscles are known as voluntary muscles because they produce movement under voluntary control. These muscles are composed of large elongated cells known as muscle fibres, which are bound together by connective tissue into small bundles and are further bound into larger bundles forming the muscle. Each muscle is enveloped in a sheet of fibrous tissue known as the fascia, which is continuous with the tendon. Tendons are composed of bands of fibrous tissue, which attach muscles to bones.

Muscle activity is coordinated and most muscles work in pairs or groups; muscle tissue is capable of contraction and relaxation and may be stimulated by nervous, chemical, electrical or thermal stimulation.

Fractures

A fracture is quite simply a break in the continuity of bone. Most fractures are diagnosed from the description of the injury and the physical appearance of the limb, confirmed by plain X-ray. Physical signs and symptoms of a fracture may include (Danby & Edwards 2001, Pagdin 1996):

- pain, which may be throbbing or localised: the pain is often aggravated by active or passive movement
- impaired, or loss of, function due to pain and the nature of the fracture
- swelling at the fracture site caused by oedema/haematoma formation. Usually increases in the first 12–24 hours following injury
- a deformity may be seen or felt
- abnormal movement in a particular limb due to movement at the fracture site
- tenderness and/or bruising at the fracture site
- crepitus (grating) heard or felt when the ends of the broken bone are un-deliberately rubbed together.

Types of fracture

There are many descriptions of fractures, depending on the nature of the injury and the force that causes the fracture (Fig. 35.3). In children, a fracture through the epiphyseal (growth) plate may result in interference or complete cessation of bone growth of that long bone, which will produce a limb-length discrepancy. These fractures are known as epiphyseal fractures and are classified into five types (Fig. 35.4).

Other descriptions of fractures

A fracture may be displaced or undisplaced. An undisplaced fracture is one in which the bone ends are lined up, whereas in a displaced fracture the bone ends or fracture fragments are out of alignment and will require correction.

Open (compound) fractures are fractures in which the soft tissue and skin envelope have been disrupted by, for example, the acute angulation of the fracture which breaks through the skin. Such fractures are in immediate danger of infection and risk development of osteomyelitis. Most fractures do not break through the skin and are called closed fractures.

Intra-articular fractures may present where the fracture involves the joint surface. If there is a step or gap in the joint surface this may need surgery to correct it.

Fracture complications

There are many potential associated complications with fractures including the following:

- Infection: in open fractures, a wound infection may spread from the skin and soft tissues and infect the underlying

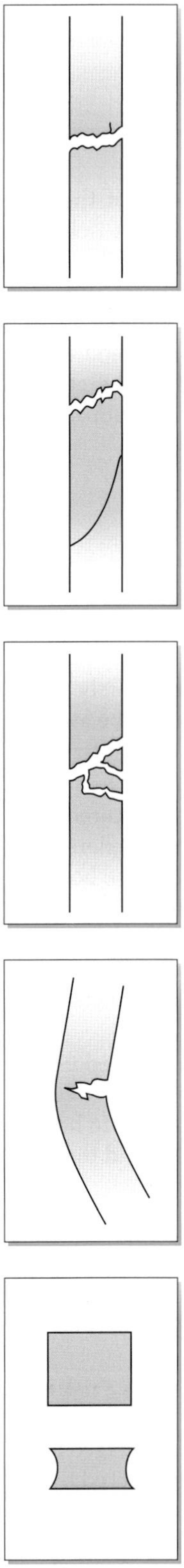

Transverse

Usually the result of a bending injury caused by direct impact and the fracture lies across the shaft of the long bone.

Oblique

Usually the result of a combination of a bending and twisting injury and lies across the shaft of the bone.

Spiral

Usually the result of a pure twisting injury. The fracture line spirals around the shaft of the bone.

Comminuted

Occurs when the bone is broken into more than two fragments. Usually the result of severe force.

Greenstick fractures

Greenstick fractures are only found in children where the bone has not completely calcified and is more elastic. Therefore, a direct blow to the bone will cause it to bend but not completely break. The bone is said to resemble a green twig which never breaks cleanly.

Crush fractures

Examples of crush fractures may be seen when the bone is pathologically weak due to disease. For example, children with moderate/severe osteogenesis imperfecta will have several crush fractured vertebrae.

Fig. 35.3 • Types of fracture.

bone. Often, children are at increased risk due to the activity at the time of fracture, which may involve dirt, grit or grass. The child with an open wound should have the wound cleaned and be commenced on systemic antibiotic therapy. If the wound is very dirty it will be left open, dressed appropriately and then closed later on.

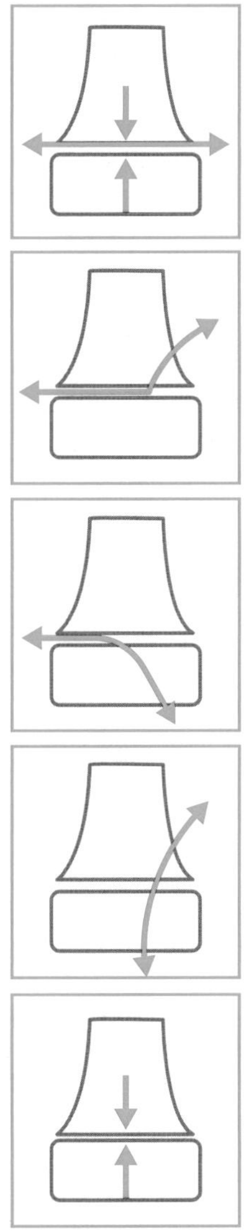

Type I
Injuries occur when the fracture line is along the plane of the growth plate. If the fracture is undisplaced it may be missed due to the absence of a fracture line on X-ray. Pain on weight bearing will be the main symptom.

Type II
Injuries occur when the fracture line is along the plane of the growth plate but extends into the metaphysis (the growing portion of a long bone) on one side. This gives the appearance of the 'triangle sign' on X-rays

Type III
Injuries occur when the fracture line is along the plane of the growth plate, but extends into the epiphysis (bone end) on one side.

Type IV
Injuries occur when the fracture extends from the epiphysis through the growth plate into the metaphysis.

Type V
Injuries involve a crush injury to the growth plate. This may not be obvious on X-ray but the clinical signs will suggest a serious injury

Fig. 35.4 • Epiphyseal fractures.

- Malunion: this is when the fracture heals in the wrong position/alignment. This may be due to poor reduction or the result of an unstable fracture that slips following reduction. It is important that all children with fractures are seen afterwards as frequently as needed to ensure the bone heals in the right position.
- Delayed union: this complication occurs for a variety of reasons. It may be because the blood supply to the fracture is poor or the fracture is inadequately immobilised. The fracture heals but takes longer than expected.
- Non-union: the fracture fails to heal. This may be due to infection, trapped soft tissues or local bone necrosis.
- Avascular necrosis: the blood supply becomes disturbed to the bone fragments causing failure to heal. It may not present until some time following the injury.
- Fat embolism: a fat deposit originating from the bone marrow at the fracture site may enter the blood stream and block a blood vessel. This may have potential fatal consequences if the blockage is caused in a major organ, for example, the lungs.

- Damage to structures: in severe fractures other structures may be affected, for example, ischaemia to blood vessels, nerves, organs.
- Compartment syndrome: the fascial compartments within the upper and lower limbs are at risk when bleeding occurs into them from the fracture. The closed non-elastic space fills with blood and increases the pressure on the venous drainage, thereby raising the pressure in the compartment. This starves the muscle cells of oxygen and they die. The circulation can also be disturbed by a bone fragment or very tight plaster cast. The signs and symptoms of compartment syndrome in an upper limb may include:
  - painful clawing of the fingers with increasing pain on passive extension of the fingers
  - altered sensation, including a burning sensation or patchy loss of sensation
  - the pulse is weak, intermittent or absent
  - the fingers are cold and bluish
  - weak ability to flex the fingers.

Many texts describe these signs of compartment syndrome as the five Ps:

- Pallor
- Paraesthesia
- Paralysis
- Pain
- Pulselessness.

The main symptom to note is pain, which is out of proportion to the injury and which is intractable. This condition needs to be recognised early because it is limb-threatening and prompt surgical attention can save the limb.

Neurovascular observations

When a child enters the hospital with a fracture, the neurovascular status should be assessed initially, then half-hourly for 4 hours, then hourly for 12–24 hours prior to and following repair of the fracture. This involves assessing colour, sensation, temperature, pulse and movement of the limb. Any alteration of these observations should be reported immediately to the orthopaedic team.

PROFESSIONAL CONVERSATION

Rebecca is a newly qualified registered children's nurse on Part 15 of the NMC register.

Yesterday we had a young boy who had a supracondylar fracture to his left elbow. I observed when checking neurovascular observations that his fingers were very dusky and when I tried to extend his fingers he was screaming out in pain. I was very concerned but didn't really feel very confident so I went to ask the ward manager but she was busy with a parent. I remembered what my preceptor had told me so I contacted the orthopaedic registrar. He came to the ward immediately and within 20 minutes the child was being escorted to theatre for a fasciotomy to release the pressure on his brachial artery. Later the registrar came and thanked me. He said I had probably saved the boy from developing Volkmann's ischaemia or losing his arm. I am really glad I listened to my preceptor and now really do realise the importance of neurovascular observations.

Failure to recognise a compartment syndrome of the forearm may result in the child developing Volkmann's ischaemic contracture caused by progressive muscle necrosis. The muscle is replaced by scar tissue leading to flexion contractures and clawing of the fingers. The result of this condition involves operations to release forearm flexors, muscle slide and tendon lengthening. Prevention through diagnosis would be attained by restoration of blood flow through reduction of compartmental pressure.

Treatment of fractures

The five Rs summarise the five main aims of fracture treatment:

1. Resuscitation: the child with a fracture should rarely require fluid resuscitation, but the nurse should be aware of the signs and treatment necessary for shock. In fractures, shock may be related to pain and blood loss.
2. Reduction: describes the realignment of the fractured bone ends. The best reduction will take place under general anaesthesia where the surgeon can manipulate the bone and observe the correction using an image intensifier. This is especially relevant to children in whom it would not be acceptable to attempt reduction using sedation in the casualty department. Alignment may be acceptable in children with greenstick fractures.
3. Restriction: after the fracture has been manipulated into a good position it needs to be held until bony union occurs (usually 6 weeks in children). The methods used to hold the fracture will depend on the bone affected and the nature of the injury and will include one of:
   - plaster cast
   - traction
   - internal or external fixation.

   The aim of restriction is to prevent any deformity and allow bone growth to proceed normally.
4. Restoration: when a limb is immobilised there is a risk that the muscles and joints will stiffen and lose some function. Therefore it is important that the child is encouraged to exercise all joints and muscles except those affected by the injury. For example, a child with a fractured distal radius who has an above-elbow cast can be encouraged to exercise all digits, which keeps the fingers nimble, encourages the muscle to move within the cast and promotes venous return.
5. Rehabilitation: when the method of restriction has been removed the limb must be exercised to restore normal ranges of movement. Children are quick to return to normal activity but may require the help of a physiotherapist.

Activity

A child presents with head injury and an open fractured femur following a road traffic accident.

- What immediate nursing and medical approach should be taken to resuscitate this 7-year-old child who has deteriorating consciousness and in hypovolaemic shock?
- Prioritise and analyse each intervention in relation to how it will stabilise the child's condition.

Methods of holding fractures

Plaster casts

Plaster casts hold a number of advantages for the child with a fracture, including:

- allowing the child to mobilise and perform most activities of daily living
- low cost and readily available
- light and porous, which allows the skin to breathe
- relatively easy to use and apply
- strong, providing protection
- permeable to X-rays.

Disadvantages include:

- it may cause discomfort including itching and feel heavy and warm and a child will be tempted to push toys and small objects down the cast leading to pressure sores
- it may hide developing problems:
  - a poorly applied cast may cause pressure on the skin and encourage the development of a pressure ulcer
  - a surgical wound following an open reduction may develop sepsis
- it is not waterproof.

Reflect on your practice

Consider what education and skills you need to be competent in the application of a plaster cast.

In what way does this relate to your professional accountability and the recommendations of the British Orthopaedic Association (BOA)?

Plaster casts – nursing care

Prior & Miles (1999) considered the following when caring for an inpatient with a plaster cast:

- Care should be taken not to apply pressure to the cast during the drying period to avoid causing dents in the cast (plaster of Paris takes 24–48 hours to dry; synthetic, fibreglass casts take around 30–60 minutes). The limb should be supported on a pillow to provide even pressure along the cast which prevents undue pressure on bony prominences.
- Elevation of the limb may be necessary to help reduce the amount of swelling which, within a cast, may cause constriction and neurovascular impairment.

Plaster casts – observations

- The cast should be observed regularly for cracking, softening or breakdown.
- If a child has had an open reduction, the cast should be observed for blood loss, which will stain the cast. A line drawn around the cast illustrates any further blood loss.
- Neurovascular observations should be performed, see p 530.
- When the child has recovered and appears stable the cast may need trimming to improve comfort. Hip spica casts will need protection around the edges to prevent contamination by urine and faeces.

Before a child is discharged home, the parent and child should receive advice regarding care of the plaster (sample discharge advice in companion PowerPoint presentation). See p 538–9 for nursing and discharge care for a hip spica cast.

Activity

Examine your hospital's plaster care advice sheet given to the patient on discharge.

- Can you think of ways of improving the information provided and could it be made more child friendly?

Plaster casts – cast bracing

Cast bracing is commonly used following internal fixation of a femoral or tibial fracture. The cast brace comprises plaster casts on the upper and lower limb, which are connected by hinges. These allow a greater degree of mobility to help prevent joint stiffness and allow the child to mobilise with partial weight-bearing, which encourages bone healing.

Traction

Traction is a pulling force. It is used to reduce and maintain alignment of fractures, to immobilise inflamed or injured joints, relieve pain, correct mild deformities and reduce muscle spasm. Traction is either fixed or balanced:

- Fixed traction is achieved by exerting a pulling force on the point splinted between two fixed points.
- Balanced traction exerts a pulling force on the part held between two mobile points, and works by using the patient's weight against the applied load.

Common forms of balanced and skin traction used with children include:

- Thomas splint traction: fixed traction that works against the force of the body (Fig. 35.5). It is used in the treatment of femoral fractures usually as a means to hold and pull the fracture until the swelling subsides before internal or external fixation.
- Gallows traction: works by the body's weight being balanced by an applied load. Is frequently used in babies and infants with femoral fractures to allow the swelling to subside prior to the application of a hip spica (Fig. 35.6).

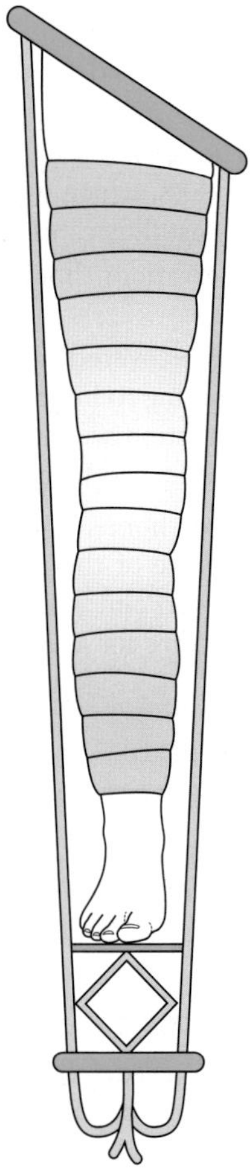

Fig. 35.5 • Thomas splint traction.

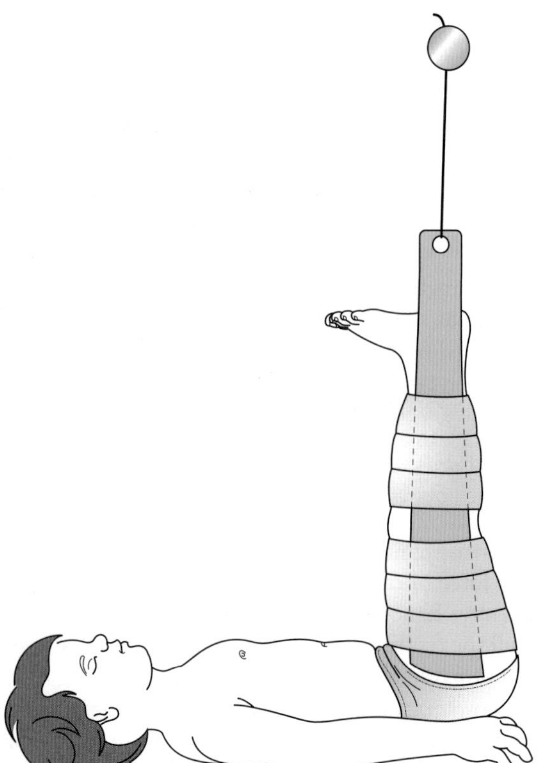

Fig. 35.6 • Gallows traction.

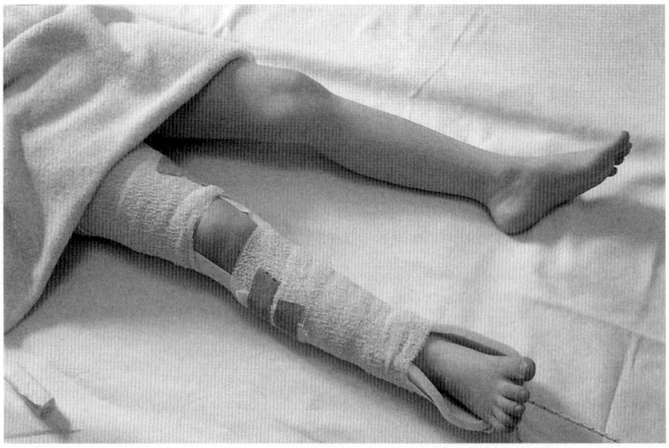

Fig. 35.7 • Simple skin traction.

- Simple skin traction (Fig. 35.7): commonly used to rest the affected limb or joint prior to surgery and to reduce pain/muscle spasm. It involves applying adhesive strips of material to either side of the affected limb. The limb is then bandaged, taking care to leave the knee free. The cord allows a pull to be exerted on the strips, which is transmitted from the material and skin to the underlying tissues and bone. Only a moderate amount of pull can be exerted using weights and the bed end is then elevated to provide counter traction.
- Skeletal traction: now rarely used in paediatrics because of the advances in surgical techniques. It may be used if the alignment of the fracture is difficult to achieve and maintain and internal fixation is not possible. It involves the insertion of a sterile pin through an area of strong bone, such as the femoral condyles, tibial tuberosity or calcaneum. A metal stirrup is then attached to the pin ends and cord fastened to it. Weights are attached to the stirrup and hang over a pulley; they are then left free hanging over the elevated bed end. Skeletal traction is also used following trauma, such as when the integrity of the skin is damaged and the application of skin traction would be difficult.
- Slings traction: used for children with hip conditions who require a combination of bed rest and allows the physiotherapist to teach the child a range of exercises performed on the hip and lower limbs.

Nursing care of the child on traction

Once traction has been applied, the child's pain and discomfort is usually relieved but analgesia may still be required. The nurse should be aware of the following observations and care when nursing children on traction.

The position of the patient

Often, the position required for successful traction will cause difficulty with the activities of daily living including eating, drinking, washing, elimination and learning. Assistance with these activities are essential, as well as maintaining the privacy and independence of the patient.

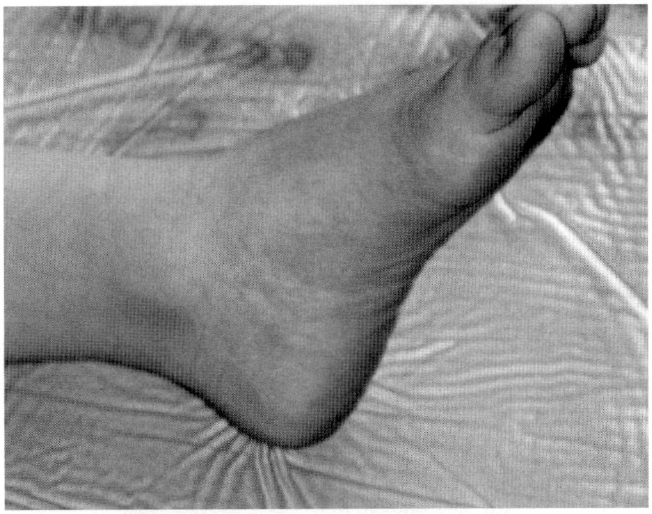

Fig. 35.8 • Polymer gel pad.

Once over the initial discomfort of an injury, the child will become frustrated and bored due to loss of mobility. The school-age child may display poor behaviour. This should be dealt with sensitively but firmly to prevent general disruption to the ward. The nurse should employ the full skills of the play specialist and ward teacher, and encourage full parental participation in their child's care. Once adjustment, has been made the child will quickly establish a rapport with the ward team.

The child is at risk from the usual complications of bed rest:

- Pressure ulcers: bony prominences, including the buttocks and heels, are at risk of pressure ulcers as the result of the constant pressure between the skin surface and the hard mattress. Frequent cleansing, minor alterations in position and the use of pressure-reducing mattresses or polymer gel pads (Fig. 35.8) will lessen the risk of pressure sore development.
- Kidneys: urinary stasis may result in kidney stones or a urinary tract infection leading to difficulty passing urine, therefore the child should be encouraged to drink plenty of fluids.
- Bowel: significantly reduced exercise and the decrease of roughage can lead to constipation, therefore the child's diet should include increased fibre and fluid. Laxatives may be prescribed.

Reflect on your practice

Look at the National Institute for Clinical Excellence (NICE) guidelines on the use of pressure-relieving devices at:

- http://www.nice.org.uk

What sort of pressure-relieving devices do you have in your area and do they meet the needs of your patients?

Bandages

Constriction of the limb by bandages used with traction may cause disturbance to the circulatory system, muscles, joints and nerve supply. Bandages should be applied firmly, but not tightly, and removed each span of duty to check skin integrity/sensitivity due to adhesive skin traction (Box 35.1).

Box 35.1

Application of skin traction (Silverwood 2006)

- Skin traction can be a painful procedure for a child and careful preparation must therefore be given, including a detailed explanation and appropriate analgesia, before the procedure is commenced, to gain the child's cooperation and trust.
- Privacy should be maintained throughout the procedure.
- The limb should be cleaned prior to applying the adhesive skin traction, to prevent the risk of infection.
- The ankle joint is kept free allowing normal movement of that joint.
- The patella is left free and the leg placed in slight flexion, thus preventing deformity and stiffness.
- Pressure on bony prominence should be avoided or pressure sores may occur.
- Folds and creases in the strapping should be avoided to prevent discomfort or sores.
- The temperature and colour of the limb is checked to ensure the tension of strapping is correct.

PowerPoint

Access the PowerPoint presentation for a detailed description of the mechanics of traction and a step-by-step guide on applying skin traction.

Internal fixation

The many types of internal fixation devices include plates, screws and intramedullary nails/rods. Internal fixation (Fig. 35.9) allows accurate reduction of the fracture and stabilisation of the reduced position. It allows the child to mobilise and avoids joint stiffness by encouraging prompt rehabilitation. It encourages good bone union and reduces the time spent in hospital. Complications include the risks associated with a general anaesthetic, the potential of infection and other postoperative complications. Further surgery is required to remove the device. When possible, the surgeon will remove the fixation device at 6–12 months, although removal may not always be possible and the device may be safely left in situ.

External fixation

A fracture may be held by transfixing screws, which pass through the bone above and below the fracture. The screws are held together with a rigid frame or lockable sliding bar. External fixation is particularly useful for fractures with severe soft tissue damage, fractures with nerve or blood vessel damage, unstable comminuted fractures that can be held to length until bone healing occurs and infected fractures where internal fixation may be unwise (Apley & Solomon 2001). The fixation device is left in place until bone healing occurs. Older children may remove the

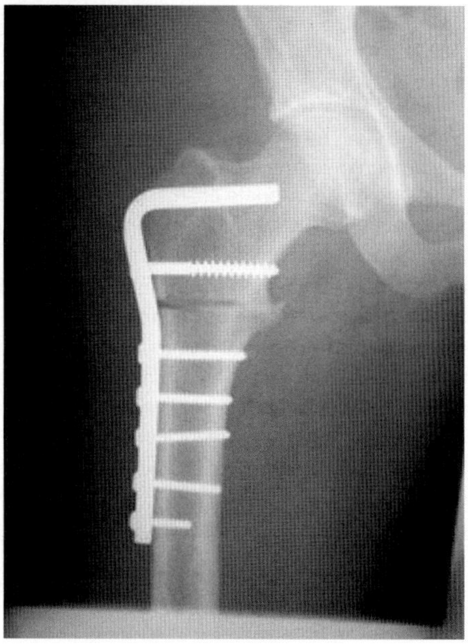

Fig. 35.9 • Internal fixation.

screws themselves by using Entonox in outpatients (Pickup & Pagdin 2000), avoiding further general anaesthesia. Complications occurring from external fixation are pin-site infections and occasionally delayed union. Occasionally a stress fracture may occur at the site of one of the screws following removal. External devices (Fig. 35.10) are used in limb reconstruction and leg-lengthening treatments throughout the UK.

Evidence-based practice

Skeletal pin site care

There remains little consensus regarding the correct management of skeletal pin sites (Bernardo 2001, Rowe 1997, Sims & Whiting 2000, RCN 2009). Surgical literature tends to focus on the prevalence of pin-site infections whilst nursing literature usually describes pin-care techniques as measures to minimise complications. Lee-Smith et al (2001a b) previously published summary guidelines and a Cochrane review was undertaken and published during 2004 (Temple et al 2004). Until evidence-based practice based on a significant multicentre trial is published, individual centres should review the literature themselves to reach local multidisciplinary consensus.

Scenario

Charlotte is a second-year adult branch student nurse who is on allocation within the local general hospital A&E department.

A 4-year-old boy is brought to the A&E department by emergency ambulance and is taken immediately to the resuscitation room. The child appeared pale, was immobilised with a hard collar around the neck and had a splint around his leg with a large blood-stained dressing.

Later, after the child is transferred to the nearest children's hospital, Charlotte asks her mentor why aspects of the child's assessment and stabilisation were different and why the child was rushed to another hospital when all the 'hard work' had been done. The mentor responded by explaining how the management of polytrauma (multiple injuries) is different between children and adults.

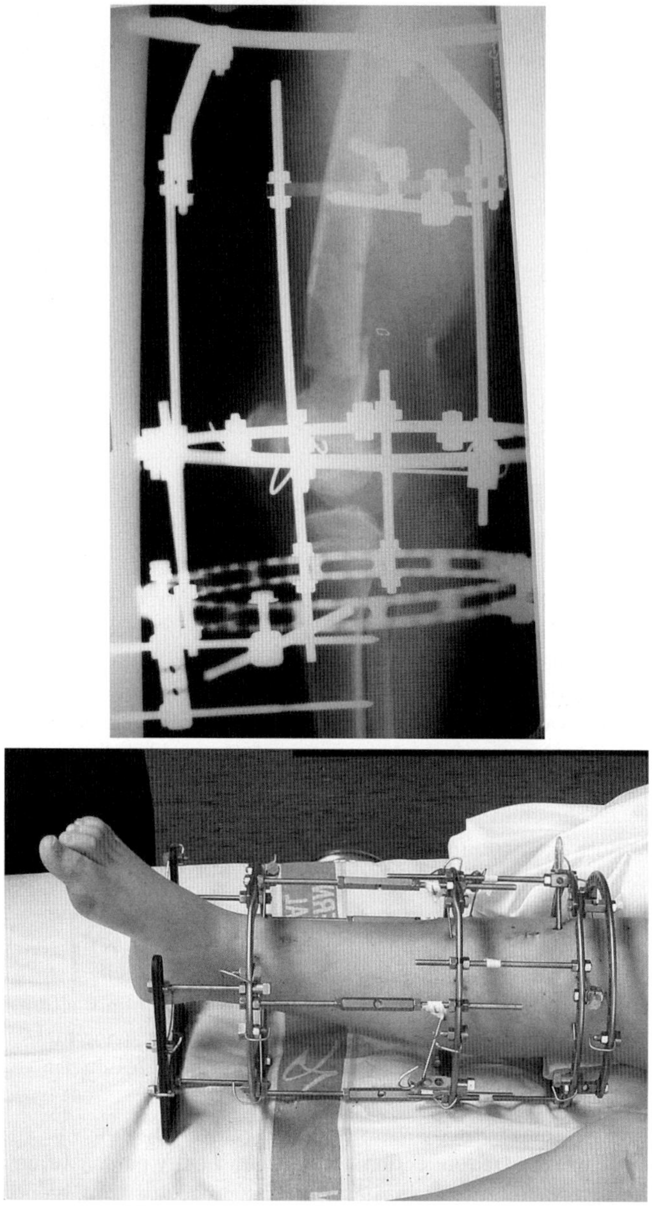

Fig. 35.10 • External fixation (Ilizarov frame).

Polytrauma

Trauma is the most common cause of death in childhood. The most common causes of multiple trauma in children include road traffic accidents, falls from height and physical child abuse. Initial assessment and management of children with multiple injuries should be carried out within a dedicated resuscitation room according to the guidelines of advanced paediatric life support (APLS) and advanced trauma life support (ATLS) as recommended by the Royal College of Surgeons (Bell 2002, Glasgow & Kerr Graham 1997). Initial stabilisation should be followed by transfer to a specialist paediatric centre with the necessary paediatric intensive care unit, specialist neurological, anaesthetic, orthopaedic, radiological and medical teams.

Within an adult-orientated centre it is important to remember that during initial assessment children present specific anatomical differences from the adult:

- The head and tongue are large whereas the face and oral cavity are small. This may present difficulties with endotracheal intubation and the large head increases the risk of cervical spine injuries during the time of the accident.
- Regarding the airway, infants are obligate nose breathers, nasal passages are narrow and therefore easily obstructed and children between the ages of 3 and 8 years commonly present with adenotonsillar hypertrophy. The differences in the anatomy of the epiglottis and larynx require a different intubation technique. Ribs are more horizontal in appearance, elastic in structure and breathing diaphragmatic, leading to considerable lung injury without fracture.
- Blood volume varies according to age. Bearing in mind the smaller circulating blood volume in relation to age and size a femoral fracture may produce enough blood loss to lead to haemorrhagic shock/cardiac decompensation. The pulse rate of children is higher and blood pressure lower and is more prone to the effects of anxiety. Cardiac output is largely dependent on the heart rate as the stroke volume is small and fixed meaning bradycardia is poorly tolerated.
- Abdominal organs are more vulnerable as the abdominal wall is thin and the diaphragm more horizontal.
- Children's bones have growth plates, injury to which may cause permanent growth arrest of that bone leading to short limbs.

Structured APLS and ATLS approach

On arrival in the casualty department, ATLS advises four steps in the management of the child presenting with polytrauma:

1. Initial assessment
2. Resuscitation
3. Secondary survey
4. Definitive care.

Steps 1 and 2 are performed simultaneously.

Initial assessment (primary survey) and resuscitation

Assesses vital functions and consists of five steps:

A = Airway patency and cervical spine control: if the gag reflex is absent or in doubt the child's airway will be maintained by utilising an oropharyngeal (Guedel) airway or endotracheal intubation. The trauma team will assume that cervical spine injury will have occurred so a rigid collar will be applied.

B = Breathing adequately to maintain oxygenation: assessment will be made of reduced respiratory effort and for potential life-threatening emergencies such as tension pneumothorax, haemopneumothorax and pericardial tamponade.

Table 35.2 Recognition of stages of shock

	Assessment of % blood loss		
Sign	**<25**	**25–40**	**>40**
Heart rate	Tachycardia	Tachycardia	Tachycardia or bradycardia
Systolic blood pressure	Normal	Normal or decreasing	Decreasing
Pulse volume	Normal/reduced	Reduced	Reduced
Capillary refill time (normal < 2 seconds)	Normal/increased	Increased	Increased
Skin	Cool, pale	Cold, mottled	Cold, pale
Respiratory rate	Tachypnoea	Tachypnoea	Sighing
Mental state	Mild agitation	Lethargic, Uncooperative	Reacts only to pain

C = Circulation and control of bleeding: the aim here is to detect the presence of circulatory shock (Table 35.2) and sites of blood loss which, where possible, should be controlled. Intravenous access is paramount; however, access is often difficult in children due to peripheral shutdown. Intraosseous needles (special needles designed to be screwed into the lumen of the bone) may used until a central line is accessed later. Shock is managed by rapid fluid bolus/replacement and administration of high concentration oxygen through bag and mask or reservoir mask.

D = Disability (neurological assessment): the central nervous system is examined only after completion of ABC and resuscitation. Initial assessment will determine if the child is:

- A = alert
- V = responds to voice
- P = responds to pain
- U = unresponsive.

During the secondary survey the child will be scored using the Glasgow Coma Score.

E = Exposure: to fully examine front and back; secondary survey.

Secondary survey

Following the initial assessment and resuscitation, strong analgesia such as morphine will be considered to lessen pain. The child will undergo radiological examination of the cervical spine, pelvis and chest (other X-rays may depend on the history and initial assessment) and a thorough head to toe, front and back examination. Vital signs of ABCD will be continually checked and interventions made to deal with other, less life-threatening injuries. For example, a nasogastric tube may be passed to relieve gastric dilatation and a urinary catheter passed to prevent urinary retention and allow accurate recording of fluid balance. The secondary survey may take place within the

Table 35.3 Classification of open fractures (Bell 2002)

Type I	An open fracture with a wound <1 cm long and clean
Type II	An open fracture with a laceration >1 cm long without excessive soft tissue damage, flaps or avulsions
Type III	Massive soft tissue damage, compromised vascularity, severe wound contamination, marked fracture instability
Type IIIA	Adequate soft tissue coverage of a fractured bone despite extensive soft tissue laceration or flaps or high-energy trauma irrespective of the size of the wound
Type IIIB	Extensive soft tissue injury loss with periosteal stripping and bone exposure; usually associated with massive contamination
Type IIIC	Open fracture associated with arterial injury requiring repair

secure environment of a paediatric intensive care unit where definitive care will commence.

Orthopaedic definitive care in polytrauma

- Bone is more elastic in children than in adults, pelvic fractures require increased high-energy trauma to occur. Most pelvic fractures rarely cause difficulties and unite well with minimal intervention.
- Children are at increased risk of spinal cord injury. The cervical spine area must be protected with a hard collar and the child log-rolled until detailed examination and investigation has ruled out spinal cord injury.
- Fractures of the long bones should be stabilised as soon as possible. In the short term, a femoral fracture will be stabilised using splintage; however, it is preferable to stabilise all long bone fractures through internal or external fixation (see Fig. 35.10) because it aids nursing care and provides secure stabilisation. Neurovascular assessment should take place as soon as the child's initial resuscitation as the risk of compartment syndrome is increased in children with multiple injuries.
- Most compound or open fractures are caused by high-energy road traffic accidents. The presence of an open fracture often suggests other injuries. Open fractures are classified as shown in Table 35.3.

Open fractures may require immediate intervention through an operative procedure to stabilise, clean and close the wound to prevent the development of sepsis. The injury will require copious irrigation to clean the wound. Vascular repair may be performed immediately following stabilisation of the fracture. A plastic surgeon may be required to perform complex free flap skin grafts in the most serious cases. The child will be commenced on broad-spectrum intravenous antibiotics.

Advances in paediatric medical and surgical management ensure the child with multiple injuries often makes a full recovery. However, every attempt should be made to reduce the risk of potential fatal injury through education, car safety, traffic calming and suitable children's play areas.

WWW

Visit the resuscitation council UK for the latest advanced paediatric resuscitation guidelines at:

- http://www.resus.org.uk

Osteogenesis imperfecta

Description

Osteogenesis imperfecta (OI), commonly known as 'brittle bone disease', is a hereditary disorder characterised by bones that break easily (Silverwood 2001). The defective gene affects the body's collagen in one of two ways, underproduction of otherwise normal collagen fibres (mild OI; type I) or abnormal or 'bent' collagen fibres, giving more severe forms. The defect interferes with bone turnover, leading to an inability to accumulate bone as healthy children would (Hill et al 2003). The characteristic features of osteogenesis imperfecta vary immensely between each child. The classification now in general use was proposed by Sillence et al in 1979 and is based on genetic, clinical and radiological features (Table 35.4).

The incidence of osteogenesis imperfecta in the UK population is estimated to be around 6000, based on a prevalence of 1:10,000. Around 1200 of these are children, with around 200 children severely affected (Bishop 1999a). Children with severe osteogenesis imperfecta may be diagnosed in utero using ultrasound, or at birth when the baby presents with 'classic' features including a triangular face and several new and healing fractures of long bones. However, children with milder forms may face a long road towards diagnosis. Many parents have to endure investigation by the authorities of suspected child abuse (Mahoney 2000).

Treatment

The management of OI focuses on minimising fractures and maximising function and independence. This is achieved through a combination of coordinated surgical and medical management with physiotherapy and occupational therapy (Silverwood 2001).

Medical management

This includes the administration of a bisphosphonate (intravenous pamidronate or oral risedronate). They are based on the chemical structure of a naturally occurring substance within the body called pyrophosphate (Bishop 1999b) and bind very strongly to bone reducing the actions of osteoclasts. The beneficial effects of pamidronate include:

- a substantial increase in bone mass
- a reduction in fracture frequency
- increase in height of previous crush-fractured vertebrae
- a reduction of chronic bone pain and fatigue
- improved mobility and reduced dependence on mobility aids
- increase in thickness in the tube walls of long bones.

Table 35.4 Classification of osteogenesis imperfecta (OI)

Type	Description
I	Most common and mildest form of OI
	Fractures occur occasionally, especially before puberty
	Normal or near normal stature
	Sclera often blue
	Bone deformity is minimal or absent
	Brittle teeth (dentinogenesis imperfecta); hearing loss
	Collagen structure is normal but the amount is less than normal
II	Most severe form
	Lethal at birth, or shortly following birth, due to complex respiratory problems
	Growth retardation in utero
	Numerous fractures, long bones crumpled and bowed, ribs appear beaded
	Collagen abnormal
III	Bones fracture easily. Fractures often present at birth, plain X-rays may show partially healed fractures.
	Several crush fractured vertebrae
	Short stature
	Sclera may be blue, but may lighten with age
	Brittle teeth and hearing loss common
	Barrel shaped rib cage. Respiratory problems possible
	Triangular face
	Bone deformity severe. Spinal curvature present
	Collagen abnormal
IV	Bones fracture easily, especially in infants and children
	Shorter than average stature. Crush fractured vertebrae
	May have bowing of long bones and develop spinal curvature
	White sclera. Brittle teeth and hearing loss possible
	Collagen abnormal

The treatment is given in combination with multidisciplinary care. The physiotherapist deals with improving mobility and physical function and the occupational therapist maximises the child's independence of performing the activities of daily living.

Surgical management

The mainstay of surgical management is intramedullary rod fixation. The aim of rodding long bones is to correct and prevent bony disorders. Rods are either fixed length or expanding. Expanding rods are telescopic and expand as the bone grows in length. These hold a number of advantages over fixed rods, not least because the child requires less frequent change of the rod and when the rod requires revision; only the expanding part of the rod is changed (Stockley et al 1989). Complications may include infection, migration or separation of the rod and a bent rod following fracture (Wilkinson et al 1998). Although the operation may appear complicated, the average length of the admission lasts only 3–4 days. The perioperative period lasts around 1–2 hours, the child returns to the ward with an intravenous infusion (until diet and fluids are re-established) and a patient-controlled analgesia (PCA) to ensure adequate pain control. A lightweight cast or a cotton/crepe bandage will protect the limb for 4–6 weeks.

Table 35.5 Nursing care of osteogenesis imperfecta (OI)

Parents	Listen to what the parents have to say about the handling of their child. Regard them as colleagues because they are experts in their child's routine care
Babies and infants	Toys should be soft and easy to handle
Lifting	Head, trunks and buttocks should be evenly supported when the baby is lifted Make your movements slow, methodical and gentle
Changing nappies	Avoid lifting by the ankles. Change the nappy by lifting under the buttocks and place the nappy with the other hand
Dressing	May suffer excessive sweating. Use cotton clothing Position/set out clothes next to the baby Openings should be generous. Slip your hand up the sleeve and pull the baby's arm through
Positioning	Babies with OI can develop flattening of the head Reposition frequently on alternate sides and supine Support the position with soft rolled sheets
Feeding	Often a poor feeder Small, frequent feeds Hold the child to give comfort, utilising a soft pillow
Constipation	Ensure adequate hydration Advice on diet, including fibre and fruit
Transporting around hospital	Traditional methods, i.e. in the cot, are satisfactory. Consider using a car seat, which provides a comfortable protective environment
Older children	Very independent Regarded as above normal intelligence (Wacaster 1996) and appreciate normal adult conversation

Nursing care

The nursing care of osteogenesis imperfecta is outlined in Table 35.5.

WWW

For further information regarding osteogenesis imperfecta visit:

- http://www.oif.org/site/PageServer
- http://www.brittlebone.org

Developmental dysplasia of the hip

Description

Developmental dysplasia of the hip (DDH) is a recent term used to describe a dislocation of the hip joint occurring at birth (congenital) or during the first year of life (Benson & Macnicol 2002). The head (ball) of the femur does not sit true in the acetabulum (socket). There are varying degrees of dislocation including the following:

- Unstable: the shape of the head of the femur and acetabulum are normal or near normal. Using manipulation the head of the femur may be moved in and out of the acetabulum.
- Subluxed: the head of the femur is only in partial contact with the acetabulum. The acetabulum is not of a normal shape.
- Dislocated: the head of the femur lies completely out of the joint. Usually the shape and size of the joint is abnormal and will deteriorate further if left out of the joint.

Incidence varies between different countries but is estimated to be 1.5 per 1000 in European countries (Danby & Edwards 2001). Incidence is higher in girls than boys, and in first-born babies. The cause of DDH is unclear but it is believed that there may be a genetic factor because it tends to run in families. Other examples of contributory factors include lax ligaments, which is caused by increased levels of oestrogen during pregnancy, overdue pregnancies and breech deliveries. Environmental causative factors have been shown in the North American Indian and Eskimo population where babies are carried with their legs straight.

The classic signs of DDH may include the paediatrician observing a 'hip click' during routine postnatal checks. Other signs may include: the thigh showing a partial lateral rotation, flexion and abduction, asymmetry of the hips and a flattening of the buttock. The baby will be referred to a paediatric orthopaedic surgeon who will perform ultrasound scanning to establish the severity of the condition.

Treatment

Treatment will depend on the time of diagnosis, but may be divided into conservative and surgical treatments.

Conservative

The aim is to hold the legs abducted and flexed so that the head of the femur falls naturally into the acetabulum. The constant pressure of the ball of the femur helps to mould the acetabulum and therefore stabilise the hip. This may be achieved in a young baby by the wearing of double nappies or the wearing of a special splint shaped in the form of an 'X' or 'H'. This fits around the thighs of the legs and wraps over the shoulders to maintain position. Examples include the Cambridge splint, Pavlik harness and von Rosen splint. The splint will be worn constantly for a minimum of 12 weeks and is removed only for examination.

Traction was, until a few years ago, the treatment of choice for babies whose treatment had failed with splints or for a baby diagnosed later. The hip is reduced by gradually abducting the hips over a 4–6-week period before being held in plaster. A popular example was the Japanese frame. Plaster fixation is commonly used following manipulation of the hips under anaesthesia. The types of plaster casts used include a double hip spica or a frog plaster. The baby is reviewed in clinic at 6 weeks where the hips are reassessed for hip stability. Plaster treatment may last for 6–9 months and the family requires support and advice during this period.

Surgical

Surgical treatments are used when either conservative method has failed or the diagnosis is made late. Common procedures include the following:

- Tenotomy: the groin tendon is lengthened. This releases a tight tendon that had prevented satisfactory reduction of the hip.
- Open reduction: allows the femoral head to be surgically placed in the acetabulum. The position is maintained by plaster cast.
- Femoral derotation osteotomy: a surgical break of the bone used to return the femur to a normal anatomical position following open reduction of the hip. The break is held in place by a blade plate until bone healing has occurred and the plate is removed between 6 and 12 months. A hip spica cast is used to maintain position during the first 6–8 weeks.
- Salter's osteotomy: may be performed in a late diagnosis where poor development of the acetabulum has occurred. This involves surgical reconstruction of the acetabulum to prevent further dislocation.

Nursing care of a child with a hip spica cast

Hip spicas are cumbersome and uncomfortable for the child and parents, who have to carry a largely immobile child in a heavy cast, although young children soon learn to drag themselves around the floor despite the hip spica. Parents must be taught how to lift and carry the child before discharge. Parents should be made aware of the signs of wound infection under the plaster – usually identified by an unpleasant smell from the plaster combined with a pyrexia. If this occurs, or if the cast cracks or softens, the parent should contact the hospital promptly.

Hygiene

The plaster edges must be examined for rough edges, which can cause skin breakdown. A daily sponge-down replaces bathing. Talcum powder should be used sparingly around the plaster because it can cause excessive irritation to the skin under the cast. Hair washing can be a problem and usually requires two people, one to hold the child over the bath, the other to wash. Nappy care requires some thought. A larger disposable nappy is usually required; nappies should not be tucked under the cast, which could result in the risk of pressure ulcers and excessive dampening.

Sleeping

Younger children are less likely to be affected by the plaster, although wind can be troublesome, therefore winding after feeding is important. Children in casts may sleep for only short periods and often become restless. Disturbed nights can result from itching and an inability to turn over. A child in a spica takes up much more room than one without therefore the width of the bed may require thought; placing the mattress on the floor can be useful and also removes the fear of the child falling out of bed. Supporting the child in a comfortable position can be done with foam or pillows but care must be taken to prevent pressure points or strain on the cast. The child may require fewer bed clothes – the plaster acts as insulation.

Transport

This is often a major problem for the family with a child in a hip spica cast but the ability to get out of the home is important for the parent and child. Smaller babies will often fit into a push chair with some extra support from pillows. Transporting a child in a cast by car is difficult, as children cannot be safely strapped into car seats; special harnesses are sometimes available. An occupational therapist will advise the parent regarding safe transport.

Eating and drinking

Some children are able to eat and drink lying on their tummies, others require support in an upright position either strapped in a normal high chair or using a bean bag. There are also designs available of specific 'hip spica' chairs. A closed cup or straw is the best method of drinking and preventing too many accidents.

Clothing

Usually larger sizes are required, these can be split and then applied using tapes, poppers, velcro or zips.

Play

Play and activity should be encouraged as much possible to allow the child to develop as normal and to provide him or her with a means of releasing the tension experienced while in plaster. Physical and very active play will be almost impossible. The child will have to rely on imaginative or 'craft' types of play. A child in a plaster can become isolated from friends and peers. Contact should therefore be encouraged, although games should not be allowed to become too boisterous.

Activity

Devise some play activities for the following children on the ward:

- A 10-month-old on gallows traction.
- Two 8-year-old boys with Thomas splint traction.
- A 14-year-old girl on bilateral skin traction.

Talipes (clubfoot)

Description

Congenital (present at birth) talipes (ankle and foot) equinovarus (pointing downwards and inwards) is the most common congenital abnormality of the feet, which are malformed and irregularly positioned. It varies in type and severity. The cause is unknown, although there may be a hereditary or genetic component. It has been associated with other congenital conditions and it may be caused by the position of the foot in utero. Incidence is 1 per 1000 births (Catteral 2002). Diagnosis is usually made at birth but increasingly through prenatal ultrasound scanning. The aims of treatment are to have a functional, pain-free, plantigrade foot and able to get into normal footwear.

Treatment

Conservative treatment

This includes physiotherapy on newborn babies: the parent is taught to stretch the ligaments and tendons. Adhesive strapping is applied around the foot, up the sides of the legs and anchored around the knee in an overcorrected position. Plaster cast fixation involves the foot being manipulated by the surgeon into an overcorrected position, with the knee flexed to prevent the cast slipping off. The cast is changed regularly due to rapid growth of baby and the foot is re-manipulated. This acts by stretching the soft tissues. A more recent treatment known as the Ponseti technique involves serial progressive casting with tendo-achilles tenotomy.

Surgical treatments

These vary widely in type and will depend on the severity of the talipes and the child's age. Surgical intervention is usually started at 9 months, with the aim of achieving correction in time for walking. Examples include soft tissue releases followed by a period in plaster through to bony procedures of the foot. An increasingly popular treatment is to correct the abnormality by using an external circular frame (Ilizarov frame), which allows the position of the foot to be altered slowly by both stretching the soft tissues and distracting osteotomies in the bones of the foot. When a normal position is achieved the frame is 'locked' until bone healing has occurred. The whole period of treatment may take around 6 months followed by a period in plaster.

Perthes' disease

Perthes' disease, also known as Legg–Calvé–Perthes' disease, after Legg (an American), Calvé (a Frenchman) and Perthes (a German), was first described around 1910. It is characterised by a loss of circulation to the head of the femur leading to avascular necrosis. This is followed by a period of revascularisation lasting 18 months to 2 years. During this period the bone is soft and revascularisation often results in fracture and or collapse of the femoral head. The resulting non-spherical shape causes the child to have stiffness and pain. The cause of Perthes' disease is unknown; statistics show that it is more common in boys than girls around ages 3 to 8.

The child often presents with an acutely painful hip due to inflammation of the hip joint. There is often a painful obvious limp that has appeared merely over a few hours. The condition is usually diagnosed through X-ray following other investigations to rule out conditions that cause similar symptoms, for example, epiphyseal dysplasia.

Treatment

Conservative/surgical treatment

Traditionally, these children were placed on periods of prolonged bed rest and non-weight-bearing on the affected hip because it was thought weight bearing caused the head to collapse. Treatment approaches now suggest maintaining the head within the acetabulum. These is achieved conservatively through casting and bracing or surgically by a femoral rotational osteotomy or pelvic osteotomy. If the hip shows tightness on examination the child may already have flattening of the femoral head and the outcome will be less favourable. In such cases a period of traction and physiotherapy is given to release tightness usually followed by surgical hip adductor releases.

It is known that diagnosis before the age of 4 years leads to a good outcome irrespective of treatment, and in all ages at least 70% of affected children do well with no long-term disability.

Discharge planning

Effective discharge planning for the child who undergoes orthopaedic surgery should begin at preadmission clinic or on admission to the ward. The family should receive information about care of a plaster cast and or the importance of cleansing pin sites daily for external fixators. They need to be able to recognise potential complications of surgery, including the signs of infection and the difference between 'routine' discomfort and severe pain. Parents should be encouraged to follow the exercises given by the physiotherapist to maintain joint mobility. The nurse must act as the coordinator to ensure the family receives multidisciplinary ongoing care in the community, including the community nursing team, social services, occupational therapy and physiotherapy. For example, an older child going home with a broomstick or spica cast may require home assessment by the occupational therapist, who will need to arrange for the child to have a urinal, bed pan or even a hoist to enable transfer from the bed to a wheelchair. A number of support groups supply advice, support and information for families of children with specific conditions.

It is outside the scope of this chapter to provide a detailed review of the many childhood orthopaedic conditions. Review the references and further reading sections of this chapter or use the many online sources.

WWW

For further information about support groups, visit:
- http://www.steps-charity.org.uk/

WWW

Read about common childhood orthopaedic conditions online at:
- http://www.orthoseek.com

and/or:
- http://www.orthoteers.org

References

Apley, B., Solomon, A., 2001. Concise system of orthopaedics and fractures, 2nd edn. Arnold, London.

Benson, M.K.D., Macnicol, M.F., 2002. Developmental dysplasia of the hip. In: Benson, M.K.D. et al (Eds.), Children's orthopaedics and fractures, 2nd edn. Churchill Livingstone, Edinburgh, pp. 359–383.

Bell, M.J., 2002. Polytrauma in children. In: Benson, M.K.D. et al (Eds.), Children's orthopaedics and fractures, 2nd edn. Churchill Livingstone, Edinburgh, pp. 579–586.

Bernado, L.M., 2001. Evidence based practice for pin site care in injured children. Orthopaedic Nursing 20 (5), 29–34.

Bishop, N.J., 1999a. Osteogenesis imperfecta: current perspectives and Treatment. European Calcified Tissue Society

Bishop, N.J., 1999b. Drug treatment of children with OI. Brittle Bone Society Newsletter. Issue 70, November.

Catteral, A., 2002. Early assessment and management of the club foot. In: Benson, M.K.D. et al (Eds.), Children's orthopaedics and fractures, 2nd edn. Churchill Livingstone, Edinburgh, pp. 464–477.

Danby, D.J., Edwards, D.J., 2001. Essential orthopaedics and trauma, 3rd edn. Churchill Livingstone, Edinburgh.

Gallo, A.M., 1996. Building strong bones in childhood & adolescence: reducing the risk of fractures in later life. Pediatric Nursing 22 (5), 369–374.

Glasgow, J.F.T., Kerr Graham, H., 1997. Management of injuries in children. BMJ Publishing, London.

Hill, C., Hampshire, D., Silverwood, B., Bishop, N.J., 2003. Recent advances in the management of osteogenesis imperfecta. Current Paediatrics 13, 151–157.

Lee-Smith et al, 2001a. Pinsite management. Toward a consensus: part 1. Journal of Orthopaedic nursing 5:37-42

Lee-Smith et al, 2001b. Pinsite management. Toward a consensus: part 2. Journal of Orthopaedic nursing 5:125-130

Mahoney, C., 2000. Handle with care. Nursing Times 96 (1), 24–26.

Pagdin, J., 1996. The musculoskeletal system. In: McQuaid, L. et al (Eds.), Children's nursing. Churchill Livingstone, Edinburgh, pp. 239–262.

Pickup, S., Pagdin, J., 2000. Procedural pain: Entonox can help. Paediatric Nursing 12 (10), 33–36.

Prior, M.A., Miles, S., 1999. Casting: part one. Nursing Standard 13 (28), 49–53.

RCN 2009 http://www.rcn.org.uk/development/researchanddevelopment/networks/clinical_focus_or_field_of_research2/NEBPOT/pin_site_are_project [Accessed: 2 March 2009]

Rowe, S., 1997. A review of the literature on the nursing care of skeletal pins in the paediatric and adolescent setting. Journal of Orthopaedic Nursing 1, 26–29.

Sillence, D.O., et al., 1979. Genetic heterogeneity in osteogenesis Imperfecta. Journal of Medical Genetics 16, 101–116.

Silverwood, B., 2001. Osteogenesis imperfecta: care & management. Paediatric Nursing 13 (3), 38–42.

Silverwood, B., 2003. Building healthy bones in children. Paediatric Nursing 15 (5), 27–29.

Silverwood, B., 2006. Practice 34: Traction. In: Twigg & Mohammed (Eds.) Practices in children's nursing: guidelines for hospital and community, 2nd edn. Churchill Livingstone, Edinburgh, pp. 411–420.

Sims, M., Whiting, J., 2000. Pin-site care. Current evidence for best practice in preventing infection when using external fixators to stabilise bones. Nursing Times 96 (48), 46.

Stockley, I., et al., 1989. The role of expanding intermedullary rods in osteogenesis imperfecta. Journal of Bone & Joint Surgery 71-B:3.

Temple, J., et al., 2004. Pin site care for preventing infections associated external bone fixators and pins (Cochrane review). Issue 1. Wiley, Chichester.

Wilkinson, J.M., et al., 1998. Surgical stabilisation of the lower limb in osteogenesis imperfecta using the Sheffield telescopic intramedullary rod system. Journal of Bone & Joint Surgery 80-B:6.

Wacaster, P., 1996. Managing osteogenesis imperfecta: a medical manual. Osteogenesis Imperfecta Foundation, Gaithersburg, USA.

Further Reading

Benson, M.K.D., et al., 2002. Children's orthopaedics and fractures, 2nd edn. Churchill Livingstone, Edinburgh p 464–477.

Glorieux, F.H., Bishop, N.J., et al., 1998. Cyclic administration of pamidronate in children with severe osteogenesis imperfecta. New England Journal of Medicine 339 (14), 947–952.

Kanis, K.A., 1996. Textbook of osteoporosis. Blackwell Science, London p 74–78.

McCarthy, G.T., 1992. Physical disability in childhood. An interdisciplinary approach to management. Churchill Livingstone, Edinburgh.

McRae, R., Esser, M., 2002. Practical fracture treatment, 4th edn. Churchill Livingstone, Edinburgh.

Miller, M., Glover, C., 1999. Wound management: theory and practice. NTBooks, London.

Miller, M., Miller, J.H., 1985. Orthopaedics and accidents illustrated. Hodder & Stoughton, London.

Royal College of Nursing, 1992. A practical guide to casting. Royal College of Nursing Society of Orthopaedic Nursing and Smith & Nephew, London.

Saleh, M., Scott, B.W., 1992. Pitfalls and complications in leg lengthening: the Sheffield experience. Seminars in Orthopaedics 7 (3), 207–222.

Staheli, L.L., 2003. Fundamentals of pediatric orthopedics, 3rd edn. Lippincott Williams Wilkins, Philadelphia.

Young, I.D., 2002. Genetics for orthopaedic surgeons. Remedica Publishing, London.

Section 3

Health problems and health promotion

Prevention of childhood injuries

36

Jo Sibert Donna Mead Jim Richardson

ABSTRACT

The primary aim of this chapter and its companion PowerPoint presentation is to explore accidents in childhood. This will include consideration of mechanisms of injury and risk factors. The specific risks for children and causes of their vulnerability in this respect will be examined. Finally, a full analysis of measures that children's nurses can take to reduce morbidity and mortality will be made. The significance of this can be seen in the fact that accidents remain the single most frequent cause of death in children over the age of 1 year.

LEARNING OUTCOMES

- Explore strategies for reducing the incidence and severity of childhood accidents.
- Describe and evaluate effective health education and promotion measures in relation to accident prevention.
- Examine specific accidents, their associated aetiology and their incidence.

Introduction

The prevention of injuries is an important issue for all those working with children because of the scale of the morbidity and mortality they cause. Injuries are unlikely to be prevented by campaigns covering all types of injury: the aetiology and preventative solutions are far too complex for that. However, a well-researched multidisciplinary action on individual types of accidents can be successful.

WWW

You can find information and tables about the scale of the problem of accidents in childhood at:

- http://www.dti.gov.uk/ccp/topics1/pdf1/hass032002 data.pdf

In preventing a particular injury, a methodological approach is needed: looking first at the size and nature of the problem, then deciding what preventive solutions are possible, implementing them on a small scale and then introducing them more widely when they have proved to be effective. There are three main strategies for injury control:

- Education of children and parents
- Changing the environment
- Enforcing changes in the environment by law.

This approach of education, environment and enforcement has become known as the 3 E's strategy. The introduction of child-resistant containers for medicines and household products is an example of a change in the environment that has reduced the incidence of accidental poisoning. Likewise, the reduction of the speed limit through enforcing local speed management strategies (particularly around schools, town centres and residential areas) has reduced both the incidence and severity of road traffic accidents. Teaching children to swim is an example of an education intervention that can reduce death from drowning. However, whereas all three strategies have had some success in reducing the incidence of childhood accidents, most successes have followed environmental changes. Educational campaigns by themselves are of only limited value. However, they do have a role and this is explored in detail further in the chapter.

What can a practitioner do?

Possible roles of the practitioner in injury prevention are:

- as an advocate for children
- through working with local authorities and non-governmental organisations on safe community activities
- through working with families to ensure that the safety focus is firmly on the individual child

DOI: 10.1016/B978-0-7020-3183-0.10036-0

- through encouraging a safe environment for children during the child surveillance programme
- through opportunistic education
- through responding to local issues.

Activity

Children's nurses working in the trauma area of an inner city hospital have noted that, in the summer months, many more children are admitted with serious trauma following road traffic accidents with the child as pedestrian:

- Using the 3 E's approach outlined above, make a list of proposals for action that might reduce the number and seriousness of the accidents.

As an advocate for children

Before environmental measures are introduced by legislation, campaigns are needed to encourage the voluntary uptake so that ergonomic and effectiveness evaluation can be undertaken. Education can result in a change in public opinion, and the nurse can act as advocate and empower parents to lobby for environmental change. For instance, parents can be educated that safe playground equipment is needed for their children. They can then pressure the local authority to act.

In 1977, the Child Accident Prevention Trust (CAPT) was formed in England. The Trust brings many disciplines together to foster research and action on accidents involving children. There are similar, but less well funded, groups in Wales (Child Safe Wales; Diogelu Plant Cymru), Scotland (Child Safe Scotland) and in other parts of the world. Similar groups exist throughout the word, e.g. Kidsafe in Australia – which claims to have halved childhood accidents since its inception in 1979.

www

For details on Kidsafe, go to:

- http://www.greenweb.com.au/kidsafe/

For details on CAPT, which includes Child Safe Wales:

- http://www.capt.org.uk/Publications/default.htm

Encouraging a safe environment for children during the child surveillance programme

A number of studies (Schlesinger et al 1966, Sibert & Williams 1983) have shown that, by themselves, mass education campaigns to prevent accidents to children are ineffective. However, there is evidence to suggest that health visitors visiting the home and giving specific one-to-one attention to accident prevention can make a difference in the way that families behave, in particular with regard to the installation of safety equipment (Roberts et al 1996).

Activity

A health visitor is undertaking a safety review for a family comprising a single, unsupported mother with three children aged 6 months, 18 months and 2.5 years:

- Consider each child's characteristics and stage of development together with the physical layout of the home and social determinants.
- Make notes on the areas that the health visitor and mother will look into and proposals for improving safety in each of those areas.

One of the problems is that it is extremely difficulty to establish firm cause and effect between safety interventions and reduction in incidence of severity of accidents. For example, a paper by Kendrick & Marsh (1997) reports on a randomised controlled trial of an intervention package of safety education in primary care assessed by the frequency of minor injuries. The intervention package was not effective in reducing the frequency of minor unintentional injuries in children at home. This is perhaps not surprising with such a difficult outcome measure where attendance in A & E is dependent on so many factors apart from the severity of the injury and when severe injuries (the ones we want to prevent) are not common enough to assess in this way.

The Child Surveillance Programme is an excellent example of an initiative that stresses injury prevention through the various editions of 'Health for all children'. This has become the basis for work with children in primary care. It stresses injury prevention.

www

More information on the Child Surveillance Programme can be found at:

- http://www.healthforallchildren.co.uk

Working with local authorities and non-governmental organisations on safe community activities

The least effective way, in the long-term, of tackling the problem of childhood accidents is for locally derived actions to develop haphazardly. Strategies need to be within a national strategy, which encompasses epidemiology, legislation and evaluation, and with appropriate resource allocation. Once the overall strategy is in place, coordinated local activities can set the direction. In 1996, a public health team from the Karolinska Institute in Stockholm developed the concept of local action through safe communities. The first World Injury Control Conference (1989) approved a manifesto for safe communities: 'Safety – a universal concern for all'. The second World Conference in Atlanta, Georgia, confirmed this.

www

For details of road safety strategies in Wales and Scotland, visit:

- http://www.wales.gov.uk/subitransport/content/ consultation/saferoads/index.htm#top
- http://www.scotland.gov.uk/cru/kd01/blue/r-acc00.htm

Experience with Safe Child Penarth (Sibert & Stone 1998) showed that safe community projects on an individual child basis are possible but difficult to assess. Problems in demonstrating causal relationships between preventative intervention and outcomes such as reduction in overall injury presentation are problematic. It is very difficult to establish with any certainty whether the change that is observed was brought about by an intervention or by some other factor in the child's life and experience. Similarly, an increase in presentation at A & E departments does not necessarily mean a failed intervention. However, a paper by Sibert et al (1999), looking at preventing injuries in public playgrounds, showed that there has been some success with limited projects involving one type of injury such as playground injury. Throughout the UK there are small groups undertaking community projects.

Much is done on a low budget or voluntary level. One should not expect too much from community projects and it is not reasonable to expect them not only to show that an injury prevention method works but also that the method of applying the method works. One of the problems of small-scale community projects is sustainability, in that interest often lapses over time. It is essential that sustainability is incorporated into the design of initiatives.

Overall, practitioners should take the opportunity for opportunistic safety education. A randomised trial by Clamp & Kendrick in 1998 showed that GP advice coupled with access to low-cost equipment for low-income families resulted in increased use of safety equipment and other safe practices. These findings are encouraging for provision of injury prevention in primary care.

Scenario

Children and families in some communities have a tradition of cooking with an open fire. The following factors are important:

- flammable clothing
- young women and female children undertaking cooking wearing loose clothing
- the high incidence of accidents resulting in burn injuries.

Activity

Propose a set of information which could be used to give to these families that would help them to reduce the risk of burn injuries in this situation.

Risk factors for injury

Social gradients

Among children aged 0–14 in England and Wales, fires are the second leading cause of accidental death. There is a steep social class gradient in the risk of fire-related death, due in part to social class differences in the prevalence of risk factors for residential fires, such as lone parenthood, financial difficulties and living in rental accommodation or poor quality housing.

Difference in smoke alarm ownership might also help to explain this social class gradient. Households least likely to have alarms include lone parent and low-income households and rental accommodation.

Activity

Consider the advantages and disadvantages of fire alarm giveaway schemes, targeted at high-risk households in a densely populated, multicultural, materially deprived community.

Social factors are important in childhood injuries. Road traffic injuries to children are five times more common and deaths in house fires 16 times more common in materially disadvantaged families. Similar social class gradients are seen in other injuries to children, with the disadvantaged children having more injuries. The reasons are complex. Poorer families usually live in more dangerous environments, for example, it is much easier for a child to have a road accident if the house opens straight onto a main road in the inner city than if it is a detached house with a garden. Psychosocial stress factors are also involved in the aetiology of many childhood injuries, particularly road traffic injuries and accidental childhood poisoning.

Personality

The question of personality in childhood accidents and whether children can be injury prone is difficult. It is much more likely that injury proneness is related to the environment, both physical and social, rather than to personality factors. It is probably more correct to speak of an injury-prone community than an injury-prone child. Nevertheless, the characteristics of the child as a person will have a role to play. For example, adolescence is a particularly vulnerable time because children of this age are striving to become independent, are inclined to ignore rules and are prone to thrill-seeking and risk-taking behaviour.

www

For details of the European Parliament's Injury Prevention Programme, go to:

- http://europa.eu.int/comm/health/ph_determinants/environment/IPP/ipp_en.htm

Details of British activity in this field can be found at

- http://www.rospa.com/CMS/index.asp

Specific accident types

Road traffic accidents

Pedestrian road traffic injuries

Pedestrian road traffic injuries are particularly common in the inner city and in children from socially deprived families. Fatality rates are correlated with the prosperity of the area. Psychosocial stress is an important factor in road traffic injuries and the interaction of a poor environment with stress is probably involved in many injuries.

Children, particularly boys under 10 years, are particularly at risk from pedestrian road traffic injuries. Parents may overestimate the ability of their children to handle traffic and let them go out on the road unsupervised. Sharples et al (1990), looking at deaths from head injuries in the northern region, found that 72% of these deaths occurred between 3 pm and 9 pm and mostly to boys playing after school.

Environmental change and child pedestrian road traffic injuries

The most effective means of preventing pedestrian road traffic accidents is by modifying the environment. Residential areas can be redesigned to give priority to pedestrians and to separate them from traffic. The speed of traffic can be reduced by speed humps and safe crossings can be provided. There is now good evidence that area-wide engineering schemes and traffic-calming schemes reduce injuries (Towner et al 2001). The provision of play areas will reduce the number of children on dangerous streets. The Safe Community approach is a way of introducing traffic calming.

Education and child pedestrian road traffic injuries

It is possible to teach some children pedestrian skills. One approach is designating safer routes to school. Two randomised trials (Thomson et al 1992, Thomson & Whelan 1997) have showed improvements in children's finding safe places to cross the road. However, there is little evidence that these programmes have actually gone on to prevent injuries. Roberts (1994) concluded that safety and traffic education are unlikely by themselves to prevent road traffic injuries. School-based traffic clubs have not been shown to be effective.

Passenger accidents

The protection of children in cars from serious injury and death must be an important part of any child safety programme. A major part of such protection is the development of child-restraint systems and seat belts. The campaign group Belt Up School Kids (BUSK) has been campaigning since 1993 for the introduction of seatbelts on minibuses and other vehicles used by school children.

WWW

For details on BUSK go to:

- http://www.ldv.co.uk/main_site/busk_about.htm

Much of the research on seat belts has been on adult passengers. There is good evidence that seat belts are effective in preventing death and serious injury. The Transport and Road Research Laboratory found that no child died in a 2-year period when in a restraint whereas 264 non-restrained children were killed in that period. Child-restraint systems have the unexpected bonus of improving children's behaviour and this probably improves driving standards. The problem is getting children to use them.

In young children and babies the barrier to the use of child restraints has in many cases been cost, and child-restraint loan schemes have been developed to help poorer families. They appear to be an effective strategy to increase the number of children safely transported in cars (Towner et al 2001). However, a randomised controlled trial demonstrating restraint use did not appear to increase correct use (Christopherson et al 1985).

Educational campaigns used to persuade children to wear seat belts have had mixed results. Miller & Pless (1977) found no significant differences in seat belt use, although Macknin et al (1987) found a campaign effective in the short term. Most countries have believed that legislation is needed to ensure seat belt usage. Serious injuries fell by 20% following the 1983 legislation in the UK compelling the wearing of seat belts in front seats. A systematic review (Towner et al 2001) of nine studies in the US evaluating seat belt legislation concluded that it was associated with reductions of injuries and death and increases the numbers of children using restraints. Many children remain unrestrained, however.

Cycle helmets

The story of cycle helmets illustrates the international evolution of an environmental solution to a problem. Analysis by Clarke & Sibert (1986) of accident and emergency admissions shows that a significant number of children sustained severe head injuries after a cycle accident. Research-based evidence includes at least five case control studies (Malmaris et al 1994, McDermott et al 1993, Spaite et al 1991, Thomas et al 1994, Thompson et al 1989) that show the effectiveness of cycle helmets in preventing head injury. Work from Seattle (Rivara et al 1994) found that cyclists had an 85% reduction in their risk of head injury by wearing helmets. In addition to this compelling evidence there is also evidence in papers by Cameron et al (1994) and Pitt et al (1994), of a reduction in injuries following increases in cycle helmet use. These studies followed the introduction of safety legislation. State legislation regarding cycle helmets has been introduced sporadically in Australia and USA. Its effect continues to be monitored. No such action has been taken in the UK and, despite the research evidence, arguments continue as to whether cycle helmets are the solution to the problem. One centre, in Reading (cited in Lee et al 2000), has had some success in getting older children to use helmets but elsewhere experience is much less encouraging.

It is likely that the optimum way to reduce cycle injuries to children consists of a combination of designated cycle tracks, cycle proficiency education and cycle helmet legislation. The government's THINK website offers further advice.

WWW

For details on THINK go to:
- http://www.thinkroadsafety.gov.uk/

Smoke detectors and house fires

Fires and flames are a significant cause of accidental death in childhood – second only to road traffic accidents in many countries in Europe. The majority of children die in conflagrations in private dwellings, often in conditions of poverty. Many children die from gas and smoke inhalation rather than from direct heat. There have been striking changes in the number of children who have died from fire in recent years. Despite this, the death rate from fires is unacceptably high. A major component of the reduction has been the fall in the number of deaths from the ignition of clothing following flame proofing regulations and the reduction of open fires. House fires are a particular problem in poor families and are 16 times more common in social class V than social class I.

Smoke detectors are widely used in several countries. Reports by the US Fire Administration (1980) and the Council for Scientific Affairs (1987) found them to be effective, particularly for children, as shown in DiGuiseppi et al (1998). Roberts (1994) indicates that they are becoming more established in the UK. They have an important role in the prevention of conflagrations and their use should be enforced both in public and private housing.

The effectiveness of education programmes to use smoke alarms has been less clearly established. In a recent systematic review of controlled trial interventions to promote smoke alarms, DiGuiseppi & Higgins (2000) suggest only modest potential benefits from education to promote smoke alarms. Smoke alarm promotion through the child surveillance programme may be more effective. Most effective of all would be regulations to have wired alarms in all housing, particularly in housing for the poor. This is because a major problem is that neither giving away smoke alarms nor enacting legislation will necessarily increase the prevalence of functioning alarms (Roberts & DiGuiseppi 1999).

Seminar discussion topic

Every family receiving state benefits should receive free smoke alarms, assistance to fit them and 6-monthly checks to ensure that they are working satisfactorily.

Scalds

Scalds are among the most distressing injuries a child can receive. They do not often cause death but they do cause considerable pain, they often need prolonged treatment and they often result in life-long scarring. This scarring and deformity may result in considerable emotional difficulties that can affect the child's whole life. Clearly it would be much better if we could prevent these concerning injuries rather than have to treat them. Sadly, evidence from Wales (Eadie et al 1995, Green et al 1984) suggests that there had been no reduction in the numbers of scalds to children since 1956. There has been a change in the pattern of these injuries. Hot water from teapots caused a fifth of the injuries in 1956. This has declined to very few cases in 1991. However, hot liquids from cups now cause almost half the scald injuries compared with less than one case in ten 35 years ago. People are now making hot drinks with instant coffee and tea bags in the cup rather than in the pot.

The most common cause of scalds – those from the cup – presents particular difficulties for prevention. It is difficult to see how an environmental solution such as an especially designed cup would be practicable or acceptable. More encouragingly, there may be preventive solutions to these injuries that involve environmental modification that may be successful with kettle and bath scalds. The usual mechanism of a scald from a kettle is the child pulling the flex that overhangs the work surface. A preventive answer to this has been the use of coiled or short flexes. Recently there has been a change in European Consumer Standards. Flexes (coiled or otherwise) should now be no longer than 80 mm. This hopefully will result in a reduction in scalds.

The majority of bath scalds are caused when the child falls in the water (Yeoh et al 1994). A reduction in the temperature of tap water entering the bath should prevent these scalds. Although standards for gas and electricity recommend 60°C maximum for thermostats, many households have water temperatures above 60°C (Murray 1988). Even at this temperature, a partial thickness burn to a child will result in 10 seconds (Lawrence & Bull 1976). There may be considerable consumer resistance to the altering of thermostats. A study in New Zealand (Waller et al 1993) evaluated an educational programme to reduce the temperature of hot tap water in homes. They found that there were significant decreases in tap water temperature in their study population but that the majority of households still had a temperature above 55°C. A more easily acceptable solution should be the use of thermostatic mixer taps for the bath set at 43°C. This is the answer that is now accepted practice in the NHS Estates (Health Guidance Note 1982). High cost is at present a key factor in their more widespread introduction.

WWW

Further details on scalding can be found at the Department for Trade and Industry's website:
- http://www.cst.gov.uk/homesafetynetwork/bs_intro.htm

Drowning

Drowning is the third most common cause of accidental death in children in the UK and in Europe. When the problem was reviewed in 1992 (Kemp & Sibert 1992), each site of drowning incident has a definite age range and corresponds to a stage in child development:

- Babies who cannot protect themselves when they fall in bath water.
- Toddlers who wander off and drown in accessible water (garden ponds in the UK, drainage ditches in the Netherlands and domestic swimming pools in southern Europe)
- Older children who die when swimming unsupervised.

Drowning deaths in the UK were again reviewed for 1998–99 (Sibert et al 2002). There was a reduction by one-third in deaths over the 10 years (however, garden ponds were a particular problem).

Prevention of drowning

- **Supervision**: there is evidence that supervision of swimming and water activity should prevent drowning. In the UK only one child dies a year in municipal pools where there is clear observation of swimming enforced by the Health and Safety Executive, whereas many die in rivers, lakes and canals where there is no supervision. Certainly, there has been an overall fall in the number of deaths of children from drowning, which has coincided with better supervision. Some European countries have a clear emphasis on the supervision of swimming.
- **Drowning in hotel pools**: there is clear evidence from work by consumer organisations and from press reports that children drown in hotel pools while on holiday. These deaths are likely to be preventable if these pools could be supervised. Progress could be achieved by action by tour operators.
- **Provision of safety fences in domestic pools**: in affluent, warm countries, drowning in swimming pools is a common cause of death in toddlers. There is evidence from Australia that fencing domestic pools can prevent drowning. Pearn & Nixon (1977) compared drownings in private swimming pools in Brisbane and in Canberra. Fencing has been introduced by regulation in parts of Australia, South Africa, New Zealand and parts of the United States (Langley 1983, Orlowski 1989, Pearn & Nixon 1977).
- **Garden ponds**: just as Australian toddlers drown in swimming pools, British children drown in garden ponds. The numbers are small but they are preventable deaths. No home with children under five should have an open garden pond. This should be clearly stated in the Child Surveillance Programme.

WWW

Advice on water safety can be found at:

- http://www.lifesavers.org.uk/

Activity

Devise a leaflet to give new parents information aimed towards preventing babies drowning in baths.

Falls

Falls cause some deaths in childhood but are also the most common cause of presentation to the A & E department. They have a varied aetiology. They may be on one level, such as falling on the pavement, at home or in the school playground. Younger children may be dropped, fall from furniture or fall down the stairs. Older children fall from trees, cliffs and mountains, play equipment and buildings. Poor window catches and design allow a number of accidents, particularly in high-rise flats. The introduction of safety catches or window guards will reduce these. In New York City a programme providing free window guards (the 'Children Can't Fly' programme) has been successful in preventing window falls in a poor area of New York (Spiegal & Lindaman 1977).

Falls downstairs are a particular problem for toddlers. Much can be done to prevent them, by better stair design and stair gates. The use of stair gates can be encouraged by the health visitor, and a Safe Community programme. Open stairs with wide gaps between balustrades may be aesthetically beautiful but are dangerous for young children. In 1985, UK building regulations were changed to make certain that a 100 mm sphere could not be passed through any opening or guard to a flight of stairs.

Baby walkers

The danger of falls from baby walkers has been highlighted by a number of studies throughout the European Union:

- In Greece, Petridou et al (1996) identified the incidence of baby walkers' injuries as 3.5/1000 per year. They also identified that these do not have any benefit for child development.
- In the UK, Glendill et al (1987) identified baby walkers as a major hazard without benefit. Kendrick & Marsh (1998) identified baby walker use as common across all social groups and as being associated with other unsafe practices such as not using stair gates or fireguards. They believed that health professionals should support campaigns to limit the sale of baby walkers but, in addition, they should ascertain each family's reasons for walker use and try to find acceptable alternatives. They should also make the family aware of the importance of properly fitted stair gates and fireguards, and help the family to obtain and use such items of safety equipment.

Baby walkers offer risks of injury but no benefit to children. There are EU regulations on baby walkers but many do not comply with them. There is a clear argument that they should be banned. They should be discouraged in any health promotion programme with families with young people.

Activity

Using the 3 E's approach, introduced earlier, plan health education strategies to discourage the use of baby walkers.

Farm injuries

Agriculture is an essential part of the work of the UK within the European Union. Recently, much attention has been paid to bovine spongioform encephalitis, however many more people have died from agricultural injuries than from new variant CJD.

Agriculture is unique in that a significant component of the work force is made up from children under the age of 16, especially at times of peak activity in the farming year. For children, the most significant feature in considering farm-related accidents is that the farm is perceived as a place of excitement and adventure. For many, the farm is often also the home, or the place where holidays are taken. There have been a number of studies:

- In 1989, Doyle & Conray in Ireland reviewed farm injuries. They also found significant unrecognised problems.
- Schelp (1992) in Sweden found that the dominant types of injuries were falls, crushes and eye injuries.
- In the UK, Cameron et al (1992) reviewed the problem of farm accidents among children by a 12-month prospective study of farm accidents involving children in the county of Dyfed and found that one child in 50 living on a farm presents with a farm-related accident in a year. None of these non-fatal cases had been reported to Health and Safety Executive, although they should have been by law. There is also legislation to prohibit the driving of tractors by children under the age of 13 and to prohibit the riding of any persons as passengers on tractors, trailers, or other field implements. This has been in place for many years but is often ignored. A safe community approach is being tried in some places, for example Ceredigion, Wales.
- In the USA, a study from 1990 to 2003 into fatal and non-fatal injuries, found 8 deaths per 100,000 child farm residents per year.

Farm safety should be an integral part of the Child Surveillance Programme in rural areas.

Playground injuries

Play is vital for children in their physical development and their ability to make social relationships. Although children play at home and in organised groups, many play in playgrounds provided by local authorities and private organisations. Playgrounds provide an alternative to playing in dangerous places such as the road and need to be as safe as possible. Professionals will wish to influence playground safety in their districts by lobbying the local authority. There has been much work developing safer equipment and surfaces and producing acceptable safety standards. This has been done in Europe, America and Australia. These standards and safety features in modern playgrounds have been developed in the laboratory using road crash adult cadaver data on head injury. They include safety surfaces, modifying equipment and maintenance.

Injuries to children in playgrounds are a complex subject. They are influenced by many factors, including the environment of the playground, the behaviour of the child and the frequency of use. There is a potential conflict between safety and play value. The quality of the literature is not high and there are few intervention studies. Many of the studies that have investigated playground injuries have described overall injuries. This may have resulted in insufficient focus on the injuries that really matter: those to the head and fractures. A historical review implies that there were serious head injuries before the introduction of modernisation and safety surfacing. Indeed, the prevention of head injuries was the reason why safety surfacing was introduced. There are very few serious head injuries now in modern playgrounds. We believe that safety surfacing is important to prevent head injuries and should be continued. These and other safety measures such as swing design should not prevent children getting play value out of equipment in modern playgrounds. Play can be exciting but not unnecessarily dangerous.

WWW

The Royal Society for Prevention of Accidents has factsheets on playgrounds at:

- http://www.rospa.co.uk/cms/

There is also evidence that safety surfacing has prevented overall injuries, although there is no evidence that fractures of the arm have been prevented by safety surfacing; indeed, the rate of fractures is remarkably constant of all presentations throughout the literature. There are biomechanical reasons for this. We need now to be developing surfaces that are protective against fractures while not compromising safety against head injury. There are difficulties in implementing intervention studies to prevent playground injuries. Despite these difficulties we really must be looking to perform more of these studies if safety is going to progress. The key to this is ongoing surveillance in partnership between health professionals and the local authority.

Poisoning

Accidental poisoning is predominantly seen in children under the age of 5 years but older children may be involved if they are developmentally delayed. The peak age is between 1 and 4 years. This is a key area because of the preventive value of child-resistant containers and packaging.

Children may take a variety of substances accidentally. These are conveniently divided into medicines (prescribed and non-prescribed), household products and plants. The majority of children who take poisons do not have serious symptoms. Medicines may be of low toxicity, e.g. the oral contraceptive pill or antibiotics, intermediate toxicity, which may cause symptoms in young children, or of potential high toxicity (Sibert & Routledge 1991). Many of the household products children take may be relatively non-toxic, however a few, such as caustic soda, soldering flux and paint stripper may cause serious harm.

Child-resistant containers and packaging

Dr Jay Arena in Durham, North Carolina, first suggested child-resistant containers (CRCs) in 1959. These containers were evaluated in a community in the US by Scherz (1970) and found to be successful. They were then introduced with successful results into the US for aspirin preparations (Walton 1982). Following this work in the US, child-resistant closures were progressively introduced in some countries in Europe. There have been few studies evaluating these changes.

In the UK, CRCs were introduced by regulation in 1976 for junior aspirin and paracetamol preparations. This resulted in a fall in admissions of children younger than 5 years after salicylate poisoning (Jackson et al 1985, Sibert et al 1977). In 1982, a voluntary agreement between the British government and the Royal Pharmaceutical Society ensured that all prescribable solid dose medication would be placed in CRCs or safety packaging with exceptions only for the elderly and infirm. In 1985 Department of Trade and Industry regulated for a number of household products to be sold in CRCs. Now many medicines are dispensed in opaque unit packaging.

Information on child-resistant container and packaging regulations from the 15 countries in the European Union has been collected. Some countries appear to have no regulations at all, some have regulations for some household products and some have regulations for some medicines and some household products. There is good evidence that child-resistant containers and packaging prevent childhood poisoning. There is also evidence that their use is very variable across the European Union. Regulations that involve consumer products should be harmonised throughout the European Union.

Summary

The range and mechanisms of the most common accidents to children as well as the changes in incidence of different forms of accident over time offers a good range of insights. Strategies for keeping children safe can be discerned and action planned following a framework such as:

- education
- environment
- enforcement.

The field of child safety and accident prevention provides examples of how health education can be delivered opportunistically. This is an area where children's nurses can help families to improve the safety and well-being of children. Every encounter between nurse and family is an opportunity to give useful information.

References

Arena, J.M., 1959. Safety closure caps. Journal of the American Medical Association 169, 1187–1188.

Cameron, D., Bishop, C., Sibert, J.R., 1992. Farm accidents in children. British Medical Journal 305, 23–25.

Cameron, M.H., Vulcan, A.P., Finch, C.F., 1994. Mandatory bicycle helmet use: an evaluation. Accident Analysis and Prevention 26, 325–327.

Christopherson, E., Sosland-Edelman, D., LeClaire, S., 1985. Evaluation of two comprehensive infant car seat loaner programs with one-year follow-up. Pediatrics 76, 36–42.

Clamp, M., Kendrick, D., 1998. A randomised controlled trial of general practitioner safety advice for families with children under 5 years. British Medical Journal 316, 1576–1579.

Clarke, A.J., Sibert, J.R., 1986. Why child cyclists should wear helmets. Practitioner 230, 513–514.

Council for Scientific Affairs, 1987. Preventing death and injury from fires with automatic sprinklers and smoke detectors. Journal of the American Medical Association 257, 1618–1620.

DiGuiseppi, C., Higgins, J.P., 2000. Systematic review of controlled trials of interventions to promote smoke alarms. Archives of Diseases of Childhood 82, 341–348.

DiGuiseppi, C., Roberts, I., 1998. Smoke alarm ownership and house fire death rates in children. Journal of Epidemiology and Community Health 52, 760–761.

Doyle, Y., Conroy, R., 1989. Childhood farm accidents; a continuing cause for concern. Journal of the Society of Occupational Medicine 39, 35–37.

Eadie, P.A., Williams, R., Dickson, W.A., 1995. Thirty-five years of paediatric scalds: are lessons being learned?. British Journal of Plastic Surgery 48, 103–105.

First World Conference on Accident and Injury Prevention (Stockholm), 1989. Manifesto for safe communities. World Health Organization, Geneva.

Glendill, D.N.S., Robson, W.V., Cudmore, R.E., Tavistock, R.R., 1987. Baby walkers – time to take a stand. Archives of Diseases of Childhood 62, 491–494.

Green, A.R., Fairclough, J., Sykes, P.J., 1984. Epidemiology of burns in childhood. Burns 10, 368–371.

Health Guidance Note, 1982. Safe hot water and surface temperatures. NHS Estates. HMSO, London.

Jackson, R.H., Craft, A.W., Lawson, G.R., Sibert, J.R., 1985. Changing pattern of poisoning in children. British Medical Journal 287, 1468.

Kemp, A., Sibert, J.R., 1992. Drowning and near drowning in children in the United Kingdom. Lessons for prevention. British Medical Journal 304, 1143–1146.

Kendrick, D., Marsh, P., 1997. Injury prevention programmes in primary care: a high risk group or a whole population approach. Injury Prevention 3, 170–175.

Kendrick, D., Marsh, P., 1998. Baby walkers: prevalence of use and relationship with other safety practices. Injury Prevention 4, 295–298.

Langley, J., 1983. Fencing of private swimming pools in New Zealand. Community Health Studies 7, 285–289.

Lawrence, J.C., Bull, J.P., 1976. Thermal conditions which cause skin burns. Engineering in Medicine 5, 61–63.

Lee, A., Mann, N.P., Takriti, R., 2000. A hospital-based promotion campaign aimed to increase bicycle helmet wearing among children aged 11–15 living in West Berkshire 1992-98. Injury Prevention 6, 151–153.

Macknin, M., Gustafson, C., Gassman, J., Barich, D., 1987. Office education by pediatricians to increase seat belt use. American Journal of Diseases in Children 141, 1305–1307.

Malmaris, C., Summers, C.L., Browning, C., Palmer, C.R., 1994. Injury patterns in cyclists attending an accident and emergency department: a comparison of helmet wearers and non-wearers. British Medical Journal 308, 1537–1540.

McDermott, F.T., Lane, J.C., Brazenor, G.A., Debney, E.A., 1993. The effectiveness of bicycle helmets: a study of 1710 casualties. Journal of Trauma 34, 834–844.

Miller, J., Pless, I., 1977. Child automobile restraints: evaluation of health education. Pediatrics 59, 907–911.

Murray, J.P., 1988. A study of the prevention of hot tap water burns. Burns 14, 185–193.

Norton, C., Rolfe, K., Morris, S., et al., 2004. Head injury and limb fracture in modern playgrounds. Archives of Diseases in Childhood 89 (2), 152–153.

Orlowski, J.P., 1989. It's time for pediatricians to 'rally round the pool fence'. Pediatrics 83, 1065–1066.

Pearn, J.H., Nixon, J., 1977. Are swimming pools becoming more dangerous? Medical Journal of Australia 2 (21), 702–704.

Petridou, E., Simou, E., Skondras, C., et al., 1996. Hazards of baby walkers in a European context. Injury Prevention 2, 118–120.

Pitt, R.W., Thomas, S., Nixon, J., et al., 1994. Trends in head injuries amongst cyclists. British Medical Journal 308, 177.

Rivara, F.P., Thompson, D.C., Thompson, R.S., 1994. The Seattle children's bicycle helmet campaign: changes in helmet use and head injury admissions. Pediatrics 93, 567–569.

Rivers, R.P., Boyd, R.D., Baderman, H., 1978. Falls from equipment as a cause of playground injury. Community Health 9, 178–179.

Roberts, I., 1994. Smoke alarm use: prevalence and household predictors. Injury Prevention 2, 263–265.

Roberts, I., DiGuiseppi, C., 1999. Smoke alarms, fire deaths and randomised controlled trials. Injury Prevention 5, 244–246.

Roberts, I., Kramer, M., Suisa, S., 1996. Does home visiting prevent childhood injury? A systematic review of randomised control trials. British Medical Journal 312, 29–34.

Schelp, L., 1992. The occurrence of farm-environmental injuries in a Swedish municipality. Accident Analysis and Prevention 24, 161–166.

Scherz, R.G., 1970. Prevention of childhood poisoning. Pediatric Clinics of North America 17, 713.

Schlesinger, E.R., Dickson, D.G., Westaby, J., et al., 1966. A controlled study of health education in accident prevention: the Rockland County child injury project. American Journal of Diseases in Children 111, 490 –4-96.

Sharples, P.M., Storey, A., Aynsley-Green, A., Eyre, J.A., 1990. Causes of fatal childhood accidents involving head injury in northern region, 1979–86. British Medical Journal 301, 1193–1197.

Sibert, J.R., Craft, A.W., Jackson, R.H., 1977. Child resistant packaging and accidental child poisoning. Lancet ii, 289–290.

Sibert, J.R., Lyons, R.A., Smith, B.A., et al., 2002. Safe water information monitor collaboration. Preventing deaths by drowning in children in the United Kingdom: have we made progress in 10 years? Population-based incidence study. British Medical Journal 324 (7345), 1070–1071.

Sibert, J.R., Mott, A., Rolfe, K., et al., 1999. Preventing injuries in public playgrounds through partnership between health services and local authority: community intervention study. British Medical Journal 318, 1595.

Sibert, J.R., Routledge, P., 1991. Accidental child poisoning – can we admit fewer children with safety? Archives of Diseases in Childhood 66, 263–266.

Sibert, J.R., Stone, D., 1998. Injury prevention in the UK – the European dimension. Injury Prevention 4 (Suppl), S34–S41.

Sibert, J.R., Williams, H., 1983. Medicine and the media. British Medical Journal 286, 1893.

Spaite, D.W., Murphy, M., Criss, E.A., et al., 1991. A prospective analysis of injury severity among helmeted and non helmeted bicyclists involved in collisions with motor vehicles. Journal of Trauma 31, 1510–1516.

Spiegal, C.N., Lindaman, F.C., 1977. Children can't fly: a program to prevent childhood morbidity and mortality from window falls. American Journal of Public Health 67, 1143–1147.

Thomas, S., Acton, C., Nixon, J., et al., 1994. Effectiveness of bicycle helmets in preventing injury in children: a case control study. British Medical Journal 308, 173–176.

Thompson, R., Rivara, F.P., Thompson, D.C.A., 1989. case control study on the effectiveness of bicycle safety helmets. New England Journal of Medicine 320, 1361–1367.

Thomson, J., Ampofo-Boeteng, K., Pitcairn, T., Grieve, R., 1992. Behavioural group training of children to find safe routes to school. British Journal of Educational Psychology 62, 173–183.

Thomson, J., Whelan, K., 1997. A community approach to road safety education using practical training methods. The Drumchapel Project. Road Safety Report No. 3. Department of Transport, London.

Towner, E., Dowswell, T., Mackereth, C., Jarvis, S., 2001. What works in preventing unintentional injuries in children and young adolescents? An updated systematic review. NHS Health Development Agency, London.

US Fire Administration, 1980. An evaluation of residential smoke detectors under actual field conditions. Final report, EMW-C-002. US Fire Administration, Washington DC.

Waller, A.E., Clarke, J.A., Langley, J.D., 1993. An evaluation of a program to reduce home hot tap water temperatures. Australian Journal of Public Health 17, 116–123.

Walton, W.W., 1982. An evaluation of the poison prevention act. Pediatrics 69, 363–370.

Yeoh, C., Nixon, J., Dickson, W., et al., 1994. Patterns of scald injuries to children in the bath. Archives of Diseases in Childhood 71, 156–158.

Information is the key to empowerment

37

E Alan Glasper Cathryn Battrick Tom CA Hain

ABSTRACT

The primary aim of this chapter and its companion PowerPoint presentation is to consider the role of all types of information in empowering children and their families in health care. Key background documents are discussed, the role of the children's nurse in providing information is considered, and issues explored around ensuring such information is accurate, relevant and communicated clearly for the child and his family.

LEARNING OUTCOMES

- Define empowerment in the context of health promotion.
- Consider the importance of providing information to support family-centred and self-care.
- Understand key issues raised in the Bristol Inquiry related to information giving.
- Review current initiatives in the field of consumer health information.
- Identify quality criteria for health information.
- Appreciate the role of NHS Direct Online.

Introduction

There is growing recognition in the UK of the need for healthcare professionals to improve the way they communicate with patients and the public. There is also acknowledgement that written and other information resources play an increasingly important role in modern health care, with a focus on empowering service users. Such information needs to be developed with service users and, where possible, with children themselves, and needs to be of the highest standards. The report of the Bristol Inquiry (Department of Health (DoH) 2001), which is perhaps the most in-depth analysis of a modern health service and its systems, made a number of key recommendations for improving communication. As a consequence, many national initiatives have emerged.

Empowerment

The term 'empowerment' has become somewhat of a buzz word, yet it is often misunderstood or used as a euphemism for any strategy that saves nursing time. The term stems from the Latin word *potere*, meaning 'to be able' and is also linked to the word *potent*, meaning 'powerful, cogent, persuasive and having or exercising a great influence'.

However, the rhetoric of empowerment is somewhat different from the concreteness of strategies of empowerment that purport to enable people to make health-related decisions. Although the pursuit of empowerment strategies by nurses is a relatively recent phenomenon, it has become an integral component of advocacy. The term 'empowerment' is appealing perhaps because it conjures up images of power and independence. The nursing profession has embraced advocacy as a method of promoting family-centred care but the methods of achieving its implementation have changed considerably over the years. From a position of interceding or pleading a case for families, children's nurses now act as guardians for their rights to autonomy and free choice. Indeed, current health promotion ideology accepts empowerment as enabling and supporting people to set their own health agendas and to take control of their health status through skills development and critical consciousness-raising (Glasper & McWilliams 1998).

Although there have been many innovations in patient advocacy, and empowerment is a real force within the field of child care, it has to be stressed that patients and families are sometimes passive bystanders in the process and this results in inequalities in the healthcare professional–family relationship. Gann (1991) has stated that information giving is the key to empowerment and, if this is true, the provision of information will enhance the relationship between the professional and the family.

DOI: 10.1016/B978-0-7020-3183-0.10037-2

Patient-centred care

When considering the role of health information, it is important to place this in context within a framework for patient-centred care. In the late 1970s, the Planetree organisation, based in Connecticut, USA, pioneered a model for patient-centred care that is widely used today (Planetree 2003). Planetree states that its model is holistic and considers healing in all dimensions – mental, emotional, spiritual and social, as well as physical. It aims to maximise healthcare outcomes by integrating complementary medical therapies such as mind/body medicine and therapeutic massage with conventional medical therapies. Within the Planetree model a strand has developed that focuses on empowering patients through information and education. This is achieved through a variety of initiatives, including production of information tailored for the individual, collaborative conferences for patients and experts and the development of patient-care pathways. Many similar initiatives based on Planetree have since emerged in the UK.

The Bristol Royal Infirmary Inquiry (2000)

Close to 200 recommendations were made following the national, public 'Bristol Inquiry' (DoH 2000a). Many of the key recommendations relate to the means through which information is obtained and communicated to children and their families (Box 37.1). It is important to consider these in context. The main issues leading to the national public inquiry are clarified in the summary document itself.

Box 37.1

Key messages from the Bristol Inquiry

- Patients must be involved in decisions about their treatment and care, wherever possible (recommendation 1)
- Health professionals must adopt the notion of partnership, where the patient and professional meet as equals with different expertise (recommendation 3)
- Information about treatment and care should be given in a variety of forms, be given in stages and be reinforced over time (recommendation 4)
- Information should be tailored to the needs, circumstances and wishes of the individual (recommendation 5)
- Information should be based on the current available evidence and include a summary of the evidence and data, in a form which is comprehensible to patients (recommendation 6)
- Various modes of conveying information, whether leaflets, tapes, videos or CDs, should be regularly updated, and developed and piloted with the help of patients (recommendation 7)
- The public should receive guidance on those sources of information about health and health care on the internet which are reliable and of good quality: a kitemarking system should be developed (recommendation 9)
- Patients must be given such information as enables them to participate in their care (recommendation 12)
- Before embarking on any procedure, patients should be given an explanation of what is going to happen and, after the procedure, should be given the opportunity to review what has happened (recommendations 13, 16).

WWW

Read the summary of the Bristol Inquiry Report online at:

- http://www.bristol-inquiry.org.uk/final_report/Summary.pdf

In the summary report, specific references are made to characteristics of the information made available to the families represented in the inquiry:

> Such information as was given to parents was often partial, confusing and unclear ... Patients should be able to gain access to information about relative performance of a hospital, or a particular service or consultant.

This illustrates the need for healthcare professionals to ensure all information is complete and clearly communicated. Nurses should be in a position to respond appropriately when asked by families for details of a hospital's performance (such information may be provided within a Commission for Health Improvement report) as well as details related to clinicians' performance.

Another key issue raised in the Bristol report is whether staff have the skills to communicate effectively:

> All healthcare staff who treat children should be trained in communicating with young people and parents.

This statement implies that the content of basic and postgraduate training courses for many healthcare staff should be reviewed in light of the findings from the Bristol Inquiry. A number of communication-related training initiatives have since emerged. For example, the new NHS University is developing a communication skills module within its induction programme for all new NHS staff (NHSU 2004).

The Bristol Inquiry recommendations suggest that a range of information is usually required by the child and family, not only information about treatment and care, but also information that supports the child and family to deliver care for themselves. All information should be discussed face-to-face and information supporting such discussion should be made available, at least in written format. Where multimedia resources exist, these may add considerably to the usefulness of the resource (for example, a video/DVD demonstrating the use of a piece of equipment such as an inhaler can be a very useful aid).

Following the Bristol Inquiry report, other key initiatives illustrate the stronger focus for information provision in the context of empowerment and advocacy. Included are the Children's National Service framework (DoH 2003) and the Welsh Children's Commissioner's report 'Telling concerns' (Children's Commissioner for Wales 2003).

Children's National Service Framework (2003)

In April 2003, the DoH published the Children's National Service Framework for hospital standards (DoH 2003). This is one of a range of Millenium child health polices which pertain to children's nursing. It is recognised within this seminal document that children and their parents should be given support and information to enable them to understand and cope with the illness or injury, and the treatment needed. The document indicates that there will be a greater focus on delivering better information: for children, young people and their parents on health and health services, and how to access them; about children receiving care, through support of an integrated care pathway; to support clinical practice; and for monitoring and continual improvement of services. Coles et al (2007) have however demonstrated that compliance by hospitals to policy recommendations varies enormously. Perhaps child health policy is only as good as the children's nurse who delivers the standards of care embodied within them.

Children's Commissioner for Wales report (2003)

The 'Telling concerns' report (Children's Commissioner for Wales 2003) considers how far systems for complaints, whistle blowing and advocacy are effective in safeguarding and promoting the rights and welfare of children in Wales. Relating to complaints and representation of children, the report recommends that local authority social services should continue to involve children and young people in the review and future design of information material (recommendation 3.7). In relation to advocacy, the report states that local authority social services, in partnership with the advocacy provider, should continue to involve children and young people in the production of any publicity materials (recommendation 5.17).

The growth of consumer health information as a specialism

Patient organisations have in many ways been leading the development of health information services for a number of years, responding particularly to information needs unmet by the NHS. Sophisticated information services will provide a range of information in a variety of formats and often in different languages. A number of national information services have developed rapidly over the last decade. When supporting the child and family in obtaining current information to support health needs, the nurse is now able to draw upon a number of services available nationally. Examples of these services are summarised in this chapter and NHS Direct Online (http://www.nhsdirect.nhs.uk), is now considered by many to be the lead organisation in the field of consumer health information.

Patient organisations and self-help groups

Patient organisations and self-help groups have a rich history of providing combined information services for specific target audiences. For example, people with cancer can use specialist telephone advice services provided by CancerBacup (http://www.cancerbacup.org.uk) or Macmillan Cancer Relief (http://www.macmillan.org.uk). Through such services, users can access further information in leaflet format or via the internet. However, although the aforementioned services are recognised as leaders in their field, the quality of similar services can be variable and the nurse should take time to review exactly what is being provided before recommending such services to families. Some hospitals such as the Oxford children's hospital have established sophisticated mechanisms for involving children and young people in developing information-giving strategies. Their young people's executive known as yippee (http://www.oxfordradcliffe.nhs.uk/getinvolved/YiPpEe/yippee_home.aspx) have developed an information booklet for children and young people in hospital called 'Young Voices'. The booklet includes personal stories of children who have been patients and information about the hospital and the staff who work there.

The Commission for Patient and Public Involvement in Health (CPPIH) was established in January 2003 to set up and support Patients' Forums. This was abolished on the 31 March 2008 when Patients' Forums were replaced by Local Involvement Networks (LINks) (Glasper 2008). LINks are designed to give citizens a stronger voice in how their health and social care services are delivered. They are run by local individuals and groups and their role is to ascertain what people want from their local health services. Each local authority (that provides social services) has been given funding and is under a legal duty to make contractual arrangements that enable LINk activities to take place. Evidence relating to the consultation activities of patient organisations with children and their families is evaluated during audits of compliance to healthcare policies.

Telephone services

The telephone, mainly through NHS Direct, now plays a very significant role in healthcare provision throughout the UK. Nurses can develop telephone skills that will allow them to give information, communicated clearly to a client at the other end. There are currently 22 NHS Direct call centres across the UK, providing a round-the-clock national telephone advice service. Some 6 million calls are taken through this service each year, a figure that is expected to rise to around 15 million.

Internet services

NHS Direct Online was launched by the Prime Minister in December 1999. A range of databases covering health topics is available 24 hours a day, and receives more than 450,000 visitors each month. Users of NHS Direct Online are able to access a number of databases to obtain information about health and health services and current health news items. In the future, users will also be able to develop personal space for information.

WWW

Visit the NHS Direct Online website and consider how the information available may be of use to a child (and the family) that you are currently looking after:

- http://www.nhsdirect.nhs.uk

NHS direct online (http://www.nhsdirect.nhs.uk)

NHS Direct Online is a website providing high-quality health information and advice for the people of England. It is unique in being supported by a 24-hour nurse advice and information helpline. NHS Direct Online is viewed as the public interface with the NHS, providing health information, advice and appropriate use of NHS resources (Jenkins & Gann 2002).

NHS Direct Online has become one of the most popular websites in the UK, with around half a million people now visiting the website each month. It has established itself as Europe's leading health website (Jenkins & Gann 2003). This was recognised in May 2003 when it won the eHealth Europe award for empowering citizens in management of health and well-being at the European Commission in Brussels.

History

The government introduced 'The NHS Plan' as a plan for investment with sustained increase in funding to reform the NHS. The vision was to give the people of Britain a health service fit for the 21st century: a health service built around the needs of the patient (DoH 2000b). The need for a knowledge (information)-based NHS is a political imperative. The national strategic programme (DoH 2000c) is concerned with major developments in the use of information technology within the NHS, including development of services using electronic communications. The government's vision is for information and IT to connect delivery of 'The NHS Plan' with the capabilities of modern information technologies. As a result, December 1999 saw further diversification of the services provided by NHS Direct with the launch of NHS Direct Online (http://www.nhsdirect.nhs.uk). The aim of this site is to provide a gateway to high-quality and reliable health information and advice (for clients and public in England) on the internet (Nicholas et al 2002). NHS Direct Online provides multichannel access and is made up of several components, which aim to deliver information with a high level of user involvement.

NHS Direct Online provides public access to a variety of topics and users can benefit from information services including the following:

- Online encyclopaedia: this is a comprehensive guide to over 600 common medical conditions. The encyclopaedia contains sections on diagnosis and treatments along with explanatory diagrams and images.
- Self-help guide: an interactive, easy-to-use guide to treating common health problems at home. A 'body key' helps you identify your symptoms, then by answering simple step questions, you will be advised what to do next. The guide is also available in book form and is distributed through a variety of routes including pharmacies, doctors' surgeries, supermarkets and 'new mother' packs.
- Local NHS services: a searchable database of hospitals and community health services, GPs, dentists, opticians and pharmacies in England. Addresses, telephone numbers, opening times and location maps are just some of the details provided. There are also contact details for all Health Authorities and NHS Trusts in England.
- Other links: this section hosts a directory of links to selected websites and other resources for a range of medical conditions where the user can seek further advice and information.
- Audio clips: for users who would like to listen to information, there is a selection of the College of Health's audio files in RealAudio format. To access this type 'audio clip' into the search box.
- Hot topics: this section offers up-to-date information on the latest health issues. NHS Direct Online provides an important role in disseminating information to the public in the event of a health scare.
- Health information enquiry service: this is a very practical and popular health information enquiry service. The user completes a simple form, which is then researched by a health information professional. To maintain confidentiality, the user is allocated a password and, within 5 working days, is notified by e-mail that the information is ready. The user can access the information they requested by entering their previously allocated password.
- FAQs: this section contains the site's most frequently asked questions about health and health care. The most frequently asked questions and answers on child health include:
  - feeding/weaning
  - childhood vaccinations
  - how to reduce the risk of cot death.
- HealthSpace: this is a personal 'health organiser' created in a secure environment on the internet, in which users can record key personal health information (e.g. blood group, medication, allergies, appointments) and care wishes (e.g. organ donation, birth plans). HealthSpace can act as a 'postbox' for health news of interest to the user and for responses to health information requests submitted to the website's online enquiry service. Password permission to a user's HealthSpace could be shared with a partner, carer or doctor if they wished. NHS Direct Online is now working with the national programme for IT to develop HealthSpace as a web portal through which patients can access their electronic NHS records (Gann 2003).
- NHS Direct digital TV: this health information service in the interactive area on digital TV became available at the end of 2004. It offers information about:
  - the NHS Direct services, details of local NHS services, national bodies, voluntary organisations and patient groups
  - health information on illnesses and conditions, tests, treatments and operations, self-care advice and medicines
  - healthy living
  - hot topics on current health issues.
- The NHS Direct digital TV service will continue to develop and expand over time, and subject to successful piloting, may offer transactional services such as ordering repeat prescriptions.

Activity

Explore the NHS Direct Online 'body key'. Do you find it easy to use?

Clinical governance

To maintain the information on the site, topics are regularly reviewed and updated. The NHS Direct Online Editorial Board acts as a single editorial board for NHS Direct Online content whether in a web, information point, digital TV or print format. The editorial board is responsible for:

- a consistent editorial policy across NHS Direct Online
- prioritising content development
- commissioning content from third parties
- quality assurance of content
- reviewing users' suggestions for new content
- ensuring consistency with other NHS websites
- ensuring synergy with the NHS Direct telephone service.

The 21st-century patient

Nurses have a long history of 'being there' for people who are in need of health care (Cudney & Weinert 2000) and there is an opportunity for nurses to reach those people who may be isolated. Although the internet is not a new medium, it can be considered contemporary for the delivery of nursing/health care and is an innovative way of providing support, education and reassurance. There are many websites and chat environments where people exchange ideas and opinions on health related issues; however, their validity and reliability could be open to question and depends on the 'ownership' of the chat platform. As NHS Direct and NHS Direct Online are extensions of the NHS, they can instil confidence and trust.

Activity

Access the NHS Direct Online site and challenge it with a number of child-health-related questions. Discuss how efficient you thought the system was in your learning group.

Television services

In 2001, the DoH piloted information services, delivered by television, to explore the use of new interactive technologies (Dick 2001, Hain 2001). The pilot services included the following:

- Appointment booking: where viewers can book appointments with their GP via the TV
- Text service: where thousands of pages of health information can be accessed, working in a similar way to a conventional teletext service
- Health videos: seven half-hour programmes for pregnant women and new mothers are all screened daily. Each programme deals with a different stage of pregnancy. The viewer is able to see the video relevant to her specific period of pregnancy
- Online consultation: where a viewer can see and talk with a NHS Direct nurse. The nurse can then display multimedia information to support the consultation.

All of the pilot TV services underwent extensive evaluation and the DoH began rolling-out a national service in 2004 (DoH 2000b).

Information kiosks

An increasing number of information kiosks are available to the public. These are located in public areas, often libraries or hospital waiting areas. Kiosks allow the user access to health information databases through a user-friendly interface.

Commercially produced information

Some excellent health information resources are produced commercially, in print and electronic format. However, there is also much that is of dubious quality and the nurse should review each on an individual basis. Information to look out for is that which carries an NHS logo, but even these can be subject to abuse and no information should be taken at face value.

PROFESSIONAL CONVERSATION

John, a registered children's nurse on Part 15 of the professional Nursing and Midwifery Council Register, is discussing information-giving with a recently qualified colleague

Getting better information to parents

Until recently, I had been uncertain how to go about guiding parents to good information. I had heard a great deal about information on the internet not being trustworthy. I got some good advice from one of the staff in my PALS service, which is rather like a Citizen's Advice Bureau specifically for health issues. I also discovered that there is an organisation called CHIQ (the Centre for Health Information Quality) that tests health information to ensure that it is accurate, clear and relevant for patients and the public.

I know there are a number of producers of health information who work with CHIQ and carry their mark of quality – the TriangleMark. Now when parents and children need health information, I suggest they look out for the TriangleMark. The CHIQ website is at http://www.chiq.org/chiq and NHS Direct Online (http://www.nhsdirect.nhs.uk) also has some good information.

Face-to-face with families

Patient and public involvement forums

It is not yet clear how children will be involved in LINks. However, there is no doubt that involving certain patient groups, such as children and young people, will be challenging. Although the Bristol Inquiry catalogued a whole series of misdemeanours that resulted in a climate of poor practice, there has been a paucity of advice on how to capture the views of children and young people. Children's nurses will have to explore every opportunity to give children and young people a strong voice in determining the future of their health service.

The need to liaise with families is exemplified in the review of Birmingham Children's Hospital in 2002, in which one of the key areas highlighted was the need to consult adequately on the patient and public involvement strategy and to engage staff and stakeholders in the development of the long-term strategic vision for its services. This is a powerful message of what is to come, and individual Trusts will ignore children and young people at their peril.

Although there is intense pressure on healthcare professionals to include the voice of the child in all aspects of care, it should be remembered that the views of parents need to be sought in their own right. However, parental views are but one facet of family satisfaction with health care and reliable and valid instruments need to be developed to optimise the voice of the child and young person. Children's nurses are in a unique position with their overarching philosophy of family-centred care to help in eliciting the voice of all families in the health service.

Patient advice and liaison services (PALS) (www.doh.gov.uk/patientadviceandliaisonservices)

In responding to increasing demand for information, the development of new information services should be seen as significant. One major and rapidly emerging service is that provided by the Patient Advice and Liaison Services (PALS), which provides service users with access to skilled information-giving staff.

The NHS Plan announced the commitment to establish PALS in every trust by 2002. PALS are central to the new system of patient and public involvement. They are complementary to existing services, such as mental health and learning disability advocacy. In providing information and on the spot help for patients, their families and carers, they will be a powerful lever for change and improvement. PALS aim to:

- advise and support patients, their families and carers
- provide information on NHS services
- listen to concerns, suggestions or queries
- help sort problems quickly on behalf of patients and the public.

PALS act independently when handling patient and family concerns, liaising with staff, managers and, where appropriate, relevant organisations, to negotiate immediate solutions and to bring about changes to the way that services are delivered. If necessary, they can also refer patients and families to specific local or national support agencies. Some children's hospitals have combined their PALS services with that of family information services.

Providing information to families

The exchange of information takes place during any and almost every interaction between a health professional, the child and a member of the child's family. The children's nurse has a critical role in ensuring the child and his or her family has access to adequate, high-quality information. Children's nurses are among the best communicators in health-care, ideally experienced to inform, educate and advise.

There are information points at each stage of the child's journey through the healthcare system. The nurse should be aware of these, and be in a position to provide additional information as required. Whereas some parents prefer not to have any information, the majority expect to have as much as can be made available. The four main information points in the journey for the family with a hospitalised child are: preadmission, on admission, during the hospital stay and after discharge.

Preadmission

Information provided before the child arrives in hospital should cover details about how to get to the hospital; travel issues, such as parking and cost of parking (often a significant concern to parents); how to get to the relevant department once inside the hospital; and details of key members of hospital staff. There should be a standard introductory leaflet to cover these issues, to accompany personalised information. The hospital's web address should be included. Some hospitals offer preadmission programmes and such provision features in standards set by the National Service Framework. Rice et al (2008) suggest that children prepared for hospital admission through a preadmission programme may have less stressful healthcare journeys.

On admission

The nurse admitting the child is likely to be using a standardised admission sheet, which, if set out well, will provide an ideal framework for exploring the immediate information needs of the family. It is particularly important here to explain the hospital's own signage system. For example, colour-coded directional signs and long place names such as 'paediatric rheumatology clinic', can be confusing.

During the hospital stay

Leaflets giving details of any investigations should be read through with the child and family. The nurse should explain any unfamiliar terms. The family should be given the opportunity to think about and write down any questions they may need answering. In addition to discussing these issues with appropriate staff, the family may require back-up with leaflets, or printed information from the hospital's own information systems or the internet (local hospital policy on internet usage should be checked; some hospitals do not allow staff access to the internet). When internet usage is permitted, the nurse will ideally have an opportunity to take the family through some of the most common NHS-approved websites for health information. Children First For Health (http://www.childrenfirst.nhs.uk/about/index.html) is a kite-marked website designed for children and their families who use health services such as hospitals. Although the site is hosted by Great Ormond Street hospital all children's units can 'piggy back' onto it via their own hospital websites. One of the aspirations of the National

Service Framework is that all families in hospital have access to high-quality information via the hospital website.

Activity

Does your children's unit have a website? Can families access the children first website as a hypertext link?

The children's nurse should be appropriately trained in knowing where to get hold of useful information, and how to be critical of its quality. Additionally the nurse should be aware of others inside and outwith the clinical team who can help in the sourcing of information. There are always key informants within the hospital team with whom the nurse may need to liaise with to ensure that the most useful and appropriate information is obtained: the PALS lead and/or the local healthcare librarian. The local healthcare librarian is often only too willing to help find and source relevant information for families. The clinical governance lead and the clinical effectiveness lead will also be responsible for ensuring that a range of reliable information is readily available. These and other key information leads are identified in Box 37.2.

Activity

Identify your hospital's policy dealing with internet usage.

Are there any issues to be resolved if you want to be able to use the internet to get information for your families?

After discharge

When a child is discharged from hospital, some nurses now provide business cards that give the telephone number on which the nurse can be reached. When 24-hour nursing advice service is not available, a telephone linked to voice-mail is now standard practice to ensure calls can be followed up. In addition, written information should be provided and the family should be aware of who to contact once the child is back at home. This is likely to include the relevant member of the multidisciplinary team but additional details of patient support groups and organisations should also be given. An increasing number of excellent support services are available to families, although families should be encouraged to scrutinise these carefully before giving any personal details. In addition, the family will have a variety of services that they can access through the telephone, internet, information kiosks and TV, etc. However, it is possible for families to drown in a sea of information and not actually access the key facts they need to continue to care for their sick children.

The children's nurse is in an ideal position to ensure information is provided at a rate and volume appropriate to the needs of the family. Often, family members will ask when they need to know something but the nurse should get into the habit of checking that information needs are being met. It is also important to check that the family understands the information that is given; levels of illiteracy and low adult reading ages should not be underestimated. The child will not always ask for information and neither will the child's parents/carers. A key service where face-to-face consultation and the provision of written and other resources are combined are Centres for Health Information and Promotion (CHIPs), such as the Southampton Family Information Service, the Family Information Centre at The Hospital For Sick Children, Great Ormond Street and the 'Rolls Royce service' provided at 'Sick Kids' hospital in Toronto, Canada.

Box 37.2

Key information needs:

- Patient Advice and Liaison Service (PALS) manager
- communications director
- clinical directors
- clinical governance/effectiveness leads
- healthcare librarian
- information management and technology team
- family information nurse.

WWW

Go to the Sick Kids website and visit health information for parents. Select an information leaflet and discuss its features in your learning group:

- http://www.sickkids.on.ca/chip/

The family information service

Hospitals such as the University Hospital of Southampton provide information to many families attending with sick children. This ranges from preadmission information to specific information related to illness (Glasper et al 1995).

The wide variety of clinics offered within the outpatient department at Southampton, coupled with a busy A&E department, catering for large numbers of children, generates an increased need for family-centred information. In addition, this hospital like many others, such as Aberdeen children's hospital and Great Ormond Street in London, provides a range of inpatient information services for children.

The introduction of the Patient's Charter, the findings of the Bristol Inquiry, and the bench mark standards of child health polices such as the NSF have highlighted the responsibility of hospitals to provide health information to families, not only to meet their needs but also to promote family involvement in care. In addition, the shift of resources from tertiary to primary health care increasingly encourages hospitals to focus more broadly on health promotion. In Southampton, for example, there has been a proliferation of materials provided to families attending the hospital, and all members of the multidisciplinary team have been involved. As part of a move towards a coordinated strategy, a specialised information service was developed. The Family Information coordinator provides information for families for sick children throughout all areas where children are cared for.

The aim of any CHIP is to provide specialist materials for carers and children to help them understand and cope with health and health- and illness-related family concerns. Currently they are located in large tertiary hospitals and concentrate on families with sick children, although they also promote healthy lifestyles for all. The role of a CHIP is to augment and support information provided by healthcare staff to families. In many ways a CHIP is similar to a PALS and, in some hospitals (such as the Hospital for Sick Children, Great Ormond Street), they are combined within one structure. Increasingly the recognition that CHIPs are valuable to families is beginning to accelerate their adoption in even smaller children's units.

Activity

Access the companion PowerPoint presentation to see photographs of family information centres

The fundamental component of a CHIP philosophy is the sharing of complete and unbiased information to families in an appropriate and supportive manner. This is a response to the increasing reality that parents seek out health information as a way of coping positively with new or difficult child health situations.

The provision of a CHIP within a busy area of the hospital allows nurses to be much more assertive in the promotion of health information and opportunistically involve even those families who, under normal circumstances, would prove passive in the pursuit of health information. Most parents want to understand their children's medical condition and give appropriate explanations to their children.

CHIPs employ a number of strategies to achieve their aims. These are:

- the organisation of materials designed to provide families with information appropriate to the care of children
- the promotion of partnership in care
- the creation of an infrastructure that allows members of the multidisciplinary team to communicate with one another and individual families through the utilisation of appropriate technologies.

Producing local information

Prewritten leaflets are unlikely to satisfy all potential clients and staff may wish to develop their own. Writing a family information leaflet may, on the surface, appear easy but the reality is that they cannot be generated one evening at home. Although they can be designed and produced using easily available desktop publishing software, the actual contents require rather more skill.

Reflect on your practice

You are keen to develop a leaflet for a child you are looking after:

- How can you find out if such a leaflet already exists?
- Who should be involved with the development of the leaflet?
- Where and how could they meet together?
- What issues should they be made aware of in relation to national/local information policy?

Improving the quality of health information

Readability formulae

Readability formulae can help the writers of family information leaflets to assess how well their writing can be understood by the reader. However, such formulae are not a panacea to correct the inadequacies of badly written information (Glasper & Burge 1992).

Many tools are available to help writers and editors improve the way their messages are presented. The Flesch index (Flesch 1948) and Fog index (Gunning 1952, 1968) use mathematical formulae to test how easy writing is to understand. Similarly, the SMOG (Standard Measure of Gobbledegook; McGlaughlin 1969) can be used to measure the readability of information leaflets, for example for patients with asthma (Smith et al 1998).

Activity

Access the companion PowerPoint presentation to read more about SMOG. Read Smith et al 1998 online at:

- http://www.pubmedcentral.nih.gov/articlerender.fcgi?article=28620

Services such as the Write Stuff (http://www.writestuff.com) provide a range of tools, guides and tips. One of earliest and most celebrated tools is the Ten Principles of Clear Statement (Box 37.3), which was developed in America (Gunning 1952).

Writing patient information leaflets

Family information leaflets should be:

- comprehensible: does the reader understand the text?
- usable/readable: can the reader apply the information?

Box 37.3

Ten principles of clear writing

(CHIQ 2003 – after Gunning's Ten Principles of Clear Statement):

1. Keep sentences short
2. Use simple rather than complex explanations
3. Use familiar words where possible
4. Avoid unnecessary words
5. Put action into verbs used
6. Write like you talk
7. Use terms your reader can picture
8. Link in with your readers' experience
9. Use a wide variety of writing techniques
10. Write to express, not impress.

- accessible: can the reader find the information easily (or is it lost in a sea of ambiguous text)?

Before rushing to your computer to produce your patient information leaflet:

- know your purpose: what is it you want to achieve?
- know your target audience: who are you writing for? (the child or carer or both?)
- know your subject: do you have the knowledge to write the material?
- know the setting under which the target audience will read the leaflet.

When writing information leaflets, make sure that they contain:

- awareness information: which allows the reader to relate to the contents of the information leaflet
- how to information: which allows the reader to optimise the purpose of the leaflet
- principles information: which gives real concrete information on why, for example, certain drugs actually work.

Healthcare professionals are not always the best people to write the information leaflets and, skilled as they are, may not have the particular skills to write for different patient groups. Seeking advice from organisations such as the Help for Health Trust and librarians will help to ensure that the final product is useful.

What style to use for patient information leaflets

- Use informative not descriptive headings: for example, 'Commuter disease' (not very inspiring), 'What is commuter disease?' (better), 'Living with commuter disease' (best of all).
- Try to personalise the leaflet by using personal pronouns such as 'I', 'we', 'us' or 'you'.
- Use decisive language, which is clear and unambiguous.
- Describe actions positively. For example, 'Do not administer unless the patient is developing a temperature' (bad), 'Give only when the patient has a temperature above 38 degrees centigrade' (much clearer).
- Use familiar words: 'Your child has fractured his or her leg' (not good), 'Your child has broken his or her leg' (better). Do not assume that the general public understands medical jargon.
- Use short paragraphs with strong topic sentences.
- Use simple visual images.
- Use at least 12-point type (larger if possible) for younger readers.

Activity

Access the companion PowerPoint presentation to see examples of patient information leaflets

Making sure information is relevant

Involving families

Families and children should be involved at some stage during the production of good-quality health information to ensure information is relevant and accessible. Families should be involved to identify relevant issues, provide balance against professional opinion and encourage family consumer ownership. The involvement of families and their children in producing health information may also avoid wasting resources. Families might choose to become involved for a variety of reasons, for example, to improve information, to be able to influence services and to identify areas of need. Three key ways in which families can be involved in the production of health information are: consultation, collaboration and user control:

- **Consultation**: Families are asked for their views, which may or may not be adopted in full. It is important that all contributions are acknowledged so consumers do not feel their time has been wasted.
- **Collaboration**: Collaboration involves a more active, ongoing partnership between the family and the producers of information media. This can increase the likelihood that outcome measurements, assessment criteria and evaluation have greater relevance.
- **User control**: Here, families design and undertake the project. This results in increased consumer involvement throughout the project and is likely to address questions that may not have been considered important by the producers. Families should be involved before, during and after the information has been produced. It is important to build feedback mechanisms into resources so that consumers can continue to feed in their comments and suggestions. It is also important to ask families to evaluate information, in order to measure how effective it is.

Some useful websites for more information on consumer involvement are:

- involve (formerly Consumers in NHS Research): http://www.invo.org.uk/
- the Patients Forum: http://www.thepatientsforum.org.uk/default.asp

Making sure information is clear

Communicating clearly

Communicating health messages clearly is an essential principle for producing consumer health information. Well-presented and easy-to-read information is vital for everyone. Three key areas of communication can be identified: format, content and language:

- Format: is the information communicated via an appropriate and accessible medium?

- Content: is the message clearly communicated?
- Language: is the choice and style of language appropriate?

Format

Information should be made available in the most appropriate format to meet the user's needs. You can use multiple formats, for example a leaflet supported by online resources. If you use a variety of formats, make sure they complement each other, for example an online resource can offer direct links to other sources of information.

Think about translating information into different languages so that ethnic minorities can access it. Consider any cultural implications this may have.

It is also important to consider how easy it is for the users to find their way around the information, i.e. is the navigation method clear? For example, does it have a glossary and clearly defined headings, is there a contents list, etc.?

For improved legibility of printed materials, use at least 12-point type. Dark type on a pale background is recommended, as is a basic font such as Arial. For further advice on legibility see:

- Plain English Campaign: http://www.plainenglish.co.uk
- RNIB clear print guidelines: http://www.rnib.org.uk
- Basic Skills Agency website: http://www.basic-skills.co.uk

Content

The content should be relevant to the target audience. The material should state who it is aimed at and the source of the information should be made clear to the consumer, as should the name of the author, the date and the copyright owner. It should also be clear if the publication has been sponsored by a commercial company. The information should be balanced and up-to-date, giving clear signposting to other references and links.

Repetition should be used to good effect, to reinforce the most important parts of the information.

Language

The pitch, tone and choice of language should be considered. Language should be pitched at a level that will be familiar to your target audience. Give advice rather than orders. Use 'we' and 'our' and address the reader as 'you'. Absolute statements should also be avoided. So, for example, instead of saying 'You will experience particular symptoms', say 'You may experience…'. Avoid using jargon or abbreviations that people may not recognise, or make sure that they are clearly explained. Language should be non-discriminatory (for gender and race).

It is recommended that any organisation producing consumer health information develops a house style (grammar, abbreviations, font, titles, colours, etc.) to ensure consistency across all publications, and also a list of preferred terms, again to ensure consistency and to avoid causing offence.

It is important to note that many of the clearest and easy-to-use information resources emerge from the field of child health.

Activity

Pick up a patient information and test it against the CHIQ checklist for quality. Can you identify good and bad examples of practice?

- What issues around *accuracy* have and have not been addressed?
- What issues around *clarity* have and have not been addressed?
- What issues around *relevance* have and have not been addressed?

Making national information available

A number of key national resources should be made available to families.

- Discovery Health: provides a range of services, including games and features, news headlines, and a TV guide that complements an interactive TV service. There are different sections, including those for men's health, and women's health (see: http://www.discoveryhealth.co.uk).
- StartHere: this system provides a range of health and social care information. Of particular note is a user-friendly interface, where text on the screen is kept to a minimum and navigation is assisted with large icons representing buttons (see: http://www.starthere.co.uk).
- Patient.co.uk: this website has more than 500 leaflets available online, covering a range of health and disease topic areas. Most GPs in the UK have access to these same leaflets to print out for patients and carers (see: http://www.patient.co.uk).
- The Brain and Spine Foundation: has published 27 booklets on a variety of neurological conditions and procedures. A related helpline service was launched in 1998 and has since responded to more than 18,000 calls; a website receives more than 3000 users a month (see: http://www.brainandspine.org.uk).
- Midirs (Midwives Information and Resource Service): produces a series of leaflets called 'Informed Choice', which provides fully referenced content for consumers and health professionals on a range of health issues around pregnancy and birth (see: http://www.midirs.org).
- EIDO Healthcare: produces procedure-specific, medico-legal documents to support the consent process. Recent research indicates that patients find these very easy to understand (see: http://www.eidohealthcare.com).
- BUPA (British United Provident Association): produces a range of health information resources, including fact-sheets, healthy-living articles and news items (see: http://www.bupa.co.uk).
- National Knowledge Service (NKS): with many databases supporting health care in the UK produced nationally, the DoH is developing the NKS to coordinate development and provide access to these through one website. The NKS is piloting quality assurance techniques. Probably the best-known component of NKS is NHS Direct Online, which provides a

range of online health services, including a health encyclopaedia.

- The Child Health Specialist Library: an indispensable resource that is now available from the National Electronic Library for Health (see: http://www.nelh.nhs.uk/childhealth).

Activity

Take a virtual tour of the Child Health Specialist Library:

- *http://www.nelh.nhs.uk/childhealth*

Linking local information strategy to national strategy

A key responsibility on the part of whoever leads on patient information is to ensure that local strategy fits with national strategy. Much of this may be achieved by working closely with those staff identified in Box 37.2. Patient information leads within an organisation should identify a lead and meet regularly, taking forward and developing local strategy with the support from the highest level. A nurse with a patient information role must have an appreciation of the current national strategy documents including National Service Frameworks, the Clinical Negligence Scheme for Trusts and review instruments from the Commission for Health Audit and Inspection

National Service Frameworks

- National Service Frameworks: set national standards and identify key interventions for a defined service or care group
- National Service Frameworks: put in place strategies to support implementation
- National Service Frameworks: establish ways to ensure progress within an agreed timescale
- National Service Frameworks: form one of a range of measures to raise quality and decrease variations in service.

The Healthcare Commission

The Commission for Health Audit and Inspection (CHAI), commonly referred to as the Healthcare Commission, is the independent inspection body for the NHS. CHAI publishes reports on NHS organisations in England and Wales. It highlights where the NHS is working well and the areas that need improvement. CHAI reviewers inspect healthcare services against national standards; this includes assessment of information services (Sweeting & Hain 2002).

Clinical negligence scheme for trusts

You can find out about the information requirements under the Clinical Negligence Scheme for Trusts (CNST) from the NHS Litigation Authority's website (http://www.nhsla.com).

Making sure information is accurate

Working with evidence

Evidence-based health care is a particular focus for the UK government: 'The government is determined that the services and treatment that patients receive across the NHS should be based upon the best evidence of what does and does not work' (DoH 1998). This same principle applies to health information in that all health information should be based upon the best, reliable evidence. It is essential to appraise critically the evidence on which health information is based.

There are three broad bands of originators of evidence: the State, the commercial sector and non-State or voluntary organisations. These different originators are motivated by different factors to produce the evidence that informs patient information. The State is motivated by political demands, a public-service ethos, professional interest and cost efficiency. The commercial sector is motivated by competition, the direct influence on consumers and sales/profit. The non-State and voluntary sectors are motivated by the service to their members, competition for funding, profile and income. It is therefore very important to recognise the motivation behind the evidence.

All evidence is of value, whether it comes from systematic research or individual opinion. Therefore the most important issue of including the evidence base in patient information is always to state where the information comes from so that consumers can make their own objective decisions. It is recommended that a five-point checklist for objectivity is used when researching the evidence base:

1. Where does the evidence come from?
2. Is it up-to-date?
3. Is it relevant to your target audience?
4. Does it detail other options?
5. Does it detail the risks and benefits?

In addition, there are three basic principles for producing evidence-based patient information:

1. Always specify the evidence source.
2. Always balance the evidence: use a combination of patient opinion and expert research/opinion.
3. Always ensure evidence is up-to-date and current.

Summary

There is a growing recognition of the importance of providing information to the child and his or her family throughout all phases of the child's healthcare journey. A number of key national initiatives directly support children and their families with their information needs. A number of different services are available to support healthcare professionals to meet these information needs. The information needs to be accurate, relevant and communicated well, and reinforced over time. The children's nurse plays a crucial role in ensuring family understanding of key health messages, both through face-to-face communication and by providing appropriate guidance on where to access high-quality health information resources when face-to-face consultation is not practical.

Acknowledgements

The section on NHS Direct Online was contributed by Aideen M Tarpey, Clinical Adviser (Nursing), NHS Direct Online.

References

Centre for Health Information Quality (CHIQ), 2003. Guidelines for producers and reviewers of health information. Online. Available at: http://www.hfht.org/chiq/guidelines.htm [accessed 31 December 2003].

Children's Commissioner for Wales, 2003. Telling concerns: report of the Children's Commissioner for Wales' review of the operation of complaints and representations and whistleblowing procedures and arrangements for the provision of children's advocacy services. Online. Available at: http://www.childpolicy.org.uk/Document/DocumentDownload.cfm/Telling%20Concerns.pdf?DType=DocumentItem&Document=Telling%20Concerns%2Epdf [accessed 31 December 2003].

Coles, L., Glasper, E.A., Fitzgerald, C., Le fluffy, T., Turner, S., Wilkes Holmes, C., 2007. Measuring compliance to the NSF for children and young people in one strategic health authority. JCYPN 1, 7–15.

Cudney, S., Weinert, C., 2000. Computer-based support groups, nursing in cyberspace. Computers in Nursing 18 (1), 35–43.

Department of Health, 1998. The new NHS: modern and dependable. DoH, London.

Department of Health (DoH), 2000a. Final report of the Bristol Royal Infirmary inquiry. Online. Available at: http://www.bristol-inquiry.org.uk/final_report/index.htm [accessed 31 December 2003].

Department of Health (DoH), 2000b. NHS Plan: a plan for investment, a plan for reform. DoH, London.

Department of Health (DoH), 2000c. Delivering 21st century IT support for the NHS. National strategic programme. The Stationery Office, London.

Department of Health (DoH), 2001. The patient's charter. DoH, London.

Department of Health (DoH), 2003. Getting the right start: National Service Framework for Children. Online. Available at: http://www.doh.gov.uk/nsf/children/index.htm [accessed 31 December 2003].

Dick, P., 2001. Towards NHS Direct TV. British Journal of Healthcare Computing & Information Management 18 (9), 22–24.

Flesch, P., 1948. A new readability yardstick. Journal of Applied Psychology 32, 221–233.

Gann, R., 1991. Consumer health information: the growth of an information specialism. Journal of Documentation 47 (3), 284–308.

Gann, B., 2003. Enabling patient access and expertise. In: Dean, K. (Ed.), Connected health thought leaders: essays from health innovators. Premium Publishing, London, pp. 8–15.

Glasper, A., Burge, D., 1992. Developing family information leaflets. Nursing Standard 6 (25), 24–27.

Glasper, E.A., Lowson, S., Manger, R., Phillips, L., 1995. Developing a centre for health information and promotion. British Journal of Nursing 4 (12), 693–697.

Glasper, E.A., McWilliams, R., 1998. Developing a Centre for Health Information and Promotion. In: Glasper, E.A., Lowson, S. (Eds.), Innovations in paediatric ambulatory care. Macmillan, Basingstoke.

Glasper, E.A., 2008. Turning up the volume on youth participation. British Journal of Nursing 17 (8), 495.

Gunning, R., 1952. The technique of clear writing. McGraw-Hill, New York.

Gunning, R., 1968. The Fog Index after twenty years. The Journal of Business Communications 6, 3–13.

Hain, T., 2001. A quality assurance programme for NHS Digital TV services. Health Expectations 4 (4), 260–262.

Help for Health Trust, 1997. Health information service, central support 1997-1998. Summary of contract with NHS Executive. Online. Available at: http://www.hfht.org [accessed 31 December 2003].

Help for Health Trust 2003 Online. Available at: http://www.hfht.org [accessed 31 December 2003].

Jenkins, P., Gann, B., 2002. Developing NHS Direct as a multichannel service. British Journal of Healthcare Computing and Information Management 19 (4), 20–21.

Jenkins, P., Gann, B., 2003. NHS Direct Online in 2003. British Journal of Healthcare Computing and Information Management 20 (6), 25–27.

McLaughlin, G.H., 1969. SMOG grading: a new readability formula. Journal of Reading 12, 639–646.

NHS Executive, (NHSE). 1996. Patient partnership: building a collaborative strategy. NHSE, Leeds.

NHS Executive(NHSE), 1998. Information for health: an information strategy for the modern NHS. NHSE, Leeds.

NHS University (NHSU) 2004 Online. Available at: http://www.nhsu.nhs.uk/learning/progcat.html [accessed 17 February 2004].

Nicholas, D., Huntington, P., Williams, P., et al., 2002. NHS Direct Online: its users and their concerns. Journal of Information Science 28 (4), 305–319.

Planetree, 2003. Creating patient-centered care in healing environments. Online. Available at: http://www.planetree.org/PDF/brochure.pdf [accessed 31 December 2003].

Rice, M., Glasper, A., Keeton, D., Spargo, P., 2008. The effect of a pre-operative education programme on pre-operative anxiety in children: an observational study. Paediatric Anaesthesia 18, 426–430.

Smith H, Gooding S, Brown R, Frew A 1998 Evaluation of readability and accuracy of information leaflets in general practice for patients with asthma. Online. Available at: http://bmj. bmjjournals.com/cgi/content/full/317/7153/264 [accessed 31 December 2003].

Sweeting, A., Hain, T., 2003. Monitoring health information services: a new tool for information quality review. Health Expectations 6, 182–186.

38

Inherited conditions and the family

Maggie Kirk Emer Parker

ABSTRACT

This chapter and its companion PowerPoint presentation aim to help you in your understanding of the impact of genetic conditions on family life and to gain an awareness of the implications of advances in genetics for children and their families.

LEARNING OUTCOMES

- Appreciate the impact that a genetic illness may have on family life.
- Apply basic genetic principles to understand how genetic conditions can be passed on in families.
- Evaluate the role of the children's nurse in helping families to access genetic information and supporting their decision making based on this.
- Appreciate some of the ethical issues surrounding the application of genetic technologies of relevance to children and their families.

Glossary

Alleles: The different forms that a gene may have at one particular position (or locus) on a chromosome.

Autosome: An 'ordinary' or non-sex chromosome.

Carrier: An individual who has a copy of a disease-causing gene, but does not have the disease. Such individuals are usually heterozygous for a recessive condition.

Dominant: A characteristic that is evident in an individual even when there is only one altered copy of a particular gene present.

Expressivity: The severity or extent to which a disease or condition is expressed.

Gene: The functional unit of inheritance, composed of a sequence of DNA.

Genome: All of the genetic information contained in the 23,000 or so genes carried on an individual's chromosomes. The normal human genome comprises 22 pairs of autosomes, and one pair of sex chromosomes, as well as mitochondrial DNA.

Genotype: The genetic make-up of a person.

Hemizygous: Having just a single copy of a gene or DNA sequence, rather than the usual two. Men are normally hemizygous for most genes on the sex chromosomes.

Heterozygote: An individual who has two different forms of a particular gene.

Homozygote: An individual who has the same form of an allele on both chromosomes.

Karyotype: The chromosome make-up of an individual.

Multifactorial: Traits or conditions that are the result of interactions between different genes, and between genes and the environment.

Penetrance: The proportion of a population with a particular genotype that actually express that genotype. A condition that is not always expressed, even though the individual has the associated genotype, is said to have reduced penetrance.

Pharmacogenetics: The study of how different people respond to drugs due to their genetic make-up, in order to identify new, more specific and more effective drug targets with fewer side effects.

Phenotype: The observed characteristics of an individual.

Recessive: A characteristic that is apparent in an individual only when it is not masked by a dominant allele. Thus it is seen in the homozygous state (i.e. when both copies of the particular allele have been inherited), or in the hemizygous state.

Sex chromosomes: The X and Y chromosomes in humans.

Introduction: the genetics revolution

The interest that we have in how characteristics are passed down through the generations is demonstrated at a typical family gathering following the birth of a new baby. We like to identify who the baby most resembles, what features he or she may have inherited from a particular 'side' of the family. As the child grows and develops, the attribution of characteristics may be broadened from the mainly physical (he has his mother's eyes) to include aspects of temperament (she has her father's quick temper). With the advances in knowledge and understanding of the role that inheritance plays in our health and

DOI: 10.1016/B978-0-7020-3183-0.10038-4

development, we have the potential to become more specific about the contribution of each parent to the features observed in their children. The range of features for which we can identify a genetic component will also increase, such as musicality, reading ability or sports performance. Of course parents (and grandparents) take pride in the positive attributes but how do they feel when a child has inherited a less desirable characteristic, such as an illness?

With the 'genetics revolution' we are beginning to appreciate far more the extent of the role that genes play in health and illness – and it is far more extensive than most people imagined, and more complex. Genes and environment interact along a continuum, with relatively rare disorders at the one end where genes alone will dictate the existence of disease, and at the other end, a few diseases in which environmental factors only play a part (Fig. 38.1). Most diseases, though, represent the outcome of the interactions between different genes, and between genes and the environment. Alongside our growing understanding of the nature and function of these genes and their interactions, we are also gaining knowledge of the role of some genes in protecting against disease, and of others in influencing our responses to medicines.

What is behind the genetics revolution is the Human Genome Project, the first phase of which was completed in 2003, 2 years ahead of schedule. This ambitious international project has deciphered the sequence of the chemicals that make up the DNA within the human blueprint (genome), paving the way for the next phase as our 23,000 or so genes are identified. Such advances in knowledge will have a profound impact on health care, with an increasing focus on individualised preventive medicine based on genetic risk, informed by environmental risk assessment. Bell (1998) outlined how genetics research would lead to the following:

- **A new disease classification:** based on the molecular mechanisms that cause disease rather than the clinical manifestation, e.g. in type 2 diabetes with the identification in particular of the maturity onset diabetes of the young (MODY) subtypes, based on the particular gene involved. There is also now a range of subsets of childhood leukaemia based on gene expression, chromosomal and molecular abnormalities. This will go alongside a better understanding of the pathological mechanisms of disease, and of the influence of environmental factors.
- **The possibility of earlier detection of disease, with an increasing range of genetic tests:** currently there are tests for around 200 of the 10,000 or so single gene disorders, and this number will grow as more and more genes are identified that account for these conditions. Genetic tests are also being developed to identify the genetic component of common diseases, and these will help identify people who may be at greater risk. Some genetic tests may become available commercially, as is already seen for example, for cystic fibrosis.
- **Greater opportunities for prevention:** by identifying individuals and sub-populations who might be more at risk, and identifying ways of modifying or preventing this risk.
- **Better targeted and more effective treatments:** using genotype to identify subtypes of populations who are more likely to display an enhanced response or increased toxicity. Those with the MODY subset $HNF1\alpha$ mutation are very sensitive to sulfonylureas for example.
- **New types of treatment:** with rational drug development based on an understanding of the pathogenesis, with a longer-term focus on gene therapy. Gene therapy trials are already being conducted worldwide for a range of conditions, including cystic fibrosis, inherited childhood blindness and leukaemia.

The implications of all these for individuals, families and professionals are far-reaching. Iredale (2000) reminds us that with earlier genetic testing and more prompt, targeted and improved treatments, including the potential for gene therapy, some diseases that were once fatal are being considered more as chronic. Thus children with such conditions are being seen not only by nurses in paediatric intensive care but in ambulatory paediatric and adolescent care settings.

The potential for misuse of new knowledge and technologies has also to be considered. We are in a unique position of knowing ahead of time the potential impact and in the UK new initiatives are already underway to help the health professional workforce to prepare for these advances.

The genetics White Paper

The UK government's genetics White Paper 'Our inheritance, our future' detailed how the NHS should prepare for and respond to scientific advances to maximise the opportunities presented by genetics and meet the challenges it poses (Department of Health (DoH) 2003):

> The new genetics knowledge and technology has the potential to bring enormous benefits for patients: more personalised prediction of risk, more accurate diagnosis, safer use of medicines and new treatment options
>
> (DoH 2003 p 22).

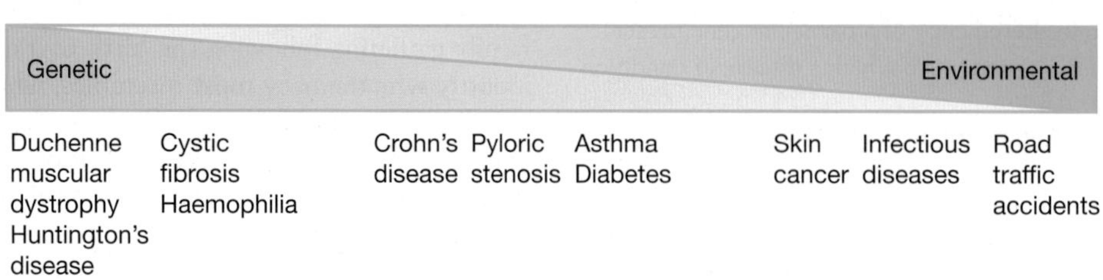

Fig. 38.1 • The contribution of genetic and environmental factors to health and disease.

The paper outlined that existing specialist genetics centres would continue to play a leading role in maximising the benefits of new genetics knowledge, and would be strengthened to cope with the increasing demand through capacity-building investment. In recognition of the need to prepare other (non-genetic) healthcare professionals as the impact of genetics moves across all areas of the NHS, the NHS National Genetics Education and Development Centre was established in 2004. Its role is to act as a catalyst in driving and coordinating activity to boost capability of the NHS workforce to incorporate genetics into healthcare practice.

WWW

Read the genetics White Paper on line:

- http://www.doh.gov.uk/genetics/whitepaper.htm

What are the four key action strands? Which do you think has the potential to impact most on your professional practice?

The White Paper acknowledged that the exact timing of the different advances is uncertain and this was echoed in the progress review of the White Paper (DoH 2008). The review outlined progress against a number of initiatives, including gene therapy and newborn screening, also reiterating that genetic testing will become increasingly widespread and useful, facilitating more accurate diagnosis. This will affect not only children and families with new conditions, but also those with pre-existing conditions where previously no diagnosis was available. What will this mean for families and what do we know already about how genetic diseases can affect family life?

The impact of genetic disease on family life

Family functioning is affected when a child becomes ill because of the usual stresses and practical problems associated with this. If the illness becomes prolonged, or if the child has a chronic condition, in particular one that is degenerative, these stresses are exacerbated. What part might the fact that a disease is 'genetic' play in this? Does it make any difference to the family?

The question of whether genetic conditions bring added stresses is an important one. Over the next 10–15 years there will be an increase in the number of children for whom a genetic diagnosis becomes possible, not only for children newly affected by a condition but also for those with existing, previously undiagnosed conditions, as genetic discoveries are made. Depending on the current policies surrounding the testing of children, there could also be an increase in the number of children for whom predictive testing would reveal a high risk of developing a condition, such as cardiomyopathy.

A mother's account of her experiences following the diagnosis of two of her sons with adrenoleucodystrophy offers a powerful insight into how genetic diseases can impact on family life (McGowan 1999). Adrenoleucodystrophy is a degenerative metabolic disorder inherited as an X-linked condition; the variable range of symptoms is associated with a build up of fatty acids. McGowan says: 'The diagnosis of an inherited condition can drop a bombshell into family relationships' (p 197). She states earlier that: 'We now take nothing for granted, such as the simple hopes that our sons will become teenagers or adult men' (p 195).

Two mothers tell their stories of the impact of a genetic disease on family life on the website Telling Stories, Understanding Real Life Genetics (www.geneticseducation.nhs.uk/telling stories). Sarah talks movingly of how she felt on being told her son's diagnosis of Niemann–Pick disease, a lipid storage condition:

> It's such an overwhelming thing to be told that your son's got a genetic disorder because your children's lives are mapped out and you have hopes and dreams for them and to be told that things are going to be different for one of your children – it's very hard.

Rachel has two children with cystic fibrosis. She writes:

> How has it changed our life? In every way imaginable. Not expecting grandchildren. Spend a lot of time at the hospital. Daily routine is EXTREMELY different from that of parents of healthy children, we spend 2–2½ hours a day doing physio, three hours a day giving intravenous medicine at the moment, and have to give my son a total of 26 doses of oral medications per day, and my daughter a total of 11 doses of oral medications per day.
>
> My marriage has been put under intense strain from all the emotional stress involved in caring for our children. Our children can't live a normal life, and we can't be normal parents. We don't think the thoughts that normal parents would. We don't take their health or life expectancy for granted. We try to make every moment count for them, because we don't know how many they have. We take tons of photos, to remember as much as we can of them growing up.

Whyte (1992) studied four families caring for children with cystic fibrosis. As well as describing the stresses associated with the 'chronic burden of care', she analyses the part that the genetic nature of the illness plays and concluded that it has a profound effect. The assault on self-image and self-esteem of parents who feel they are unable to produce healthy children can be devastating, and the implications of this for future childbearing are keenly felt. Related to this are the tough decisions that parents may have to face about their reproductive options. This is especially challenging when parents may be considering an option to terminate a pregnancy following prenatal diagnosis. If they have an existing child with the condition, there may be worries that this could devalue that child, and explanations to the child could be difficult.

Activity

What circumstances can you think of where genetics will have an impact on family life? Make a list of the instances and compare these with those shown in the companion PowerPoint presentation. Read Rachel's story in full at www.geneticseducation.nhs.uk/tellingstories/stories.asp?id=20 for the direct link.

So how do families with children affected by, or at risk of, genetic conditions adapt to the situation? Canam (1993) describes the tasks that parents have to face in adapting to chronic childhood illness:

- Accept the child's condition
- Manage the condition on a day-to-day basis

- Meet the normal developmental needs of the child
- Meet the developmental needs of other family members
- Cope with continuous stress and periodic crises
- Assist family members to manage their feelings
- Educate others about the child's condition
- Establish a support system.

We will consider each of the stages in relation to genetic diseases.

Accepting the condition

Canam (1993) identifies acceptance as the first phase in the process. Seeking answers and a reduction of uncertainty are integral to this but a definitive diagnosis is not always available, particularly if the condition is rare. If the condition is one that is already 'in the family' the difficulties can vary. Many families may be accepting, with an established support system, but other parents have to cope with accusations of 'irresponsibility'.

One factor that can have an impact on accepting a condition is its visibility. The shock of a major physical abnormality can be profound and the reactions of others on first meeting the child serve as a reminder of this. Lack of visibility can also make it more difficult for the family and others to accept. When the condition is associated with behavioural problems (such as autism or Tourette syndrome) its physical invisibility frequently presents problems with tolerance and understanding from others, both within and outside the family.

Fanos (1999) reported how acceptance by siblings may be influenced by the visibility of a condition in an affected brother or sister. She noted that the visibility of ataxia telangiectasia (a recessive condition characterised by unsteady gait and involuntary movements) caused less resentment of the time given to the child, less guilt and less tendency to idealise the affected sibling, than children with cystic fibrosis. However, it was associated with more embarrassment and shame.

Manage the condition on a day-to-day basis

The problems of coping with the practical matters of everyday living when a child (or any family member) has a chronic illness have been widely reviewed (see Chapter 44). A crucial factor in dealing with the problems are resources, including time, energy, money and social support systems, and the availability of all of these over an extended time. The extent of the resources needed will vary according to the specific condition. With a condition such as cystic fibrosis, for example, the child will need daily physiotherapy, regular visits to clinics, careful supervision of diet and may require frequent periods of hospitalisation. Medication will need to be given and regular supplies maintained. The extra workload may make full- or even part-time employment impractical for one parent. In managing the condition on a day-to-day basis, then, the parent may have to adjust to reduced career prospects, loss of role and problems with self-esteem. The latter may be a factor of the feelings of guilt at having passed on a condition to the child.

Meet the normal developmental needs of the child

The nature of the condition and how debilitating it is will clearly be a significant factor in how well the developmental needs of the child can be met. The instinctive desire to protect the child can be further fuelled by feelings of guilt, predisposing to 'spoiling' and children may take advantage of this. Labelling of the child by the family or by others can further compromise the situation.

PROFESSIONAL CONVERSATION

I was enjoying my placement with the community paediatric team. I enjoyed meeting the families and seeing their care from another perspective, it is so different to the hospital setting. This particular visit was to see Lucy and her son Gareth. I knew them from previous admissions to the ward. Gareth is 7 years old and he has multiple problems - developmental delay, some autistic features and feeding problems. The reason for today's visit was to discuss the genetic test results that Lucy was to have been given at the genetic clinic earlier that week.

The nurse spent the first few minutes catching up with Gareth's progress, his feeding and his toilet training. Then she asked about the test results. *Lucy started to cry as she explained that all the tests had come back negative. I did not understand why she was crying - surely this was good news to hear Gareth does not have a genetic condition. I listened while she talked about the guilt that she is responsible for Gareth's problems, her description of her pregnancy, wondering if she had done something during this time that caused it all. I tried to reassure her reminding her that the geneticist had told her that it was not her fault. She turned to me and said 'How can they say that if they do not know what did cause his problems?'*

I did not know what to say.

Reflecting on this visit later I realised that my response to Lucy had been very naive. I had not thought about her position and that a positive result showing that her son had a serious genetic condition could be preferable to a negative one which left her with so many unanswered questions and a guilt that seemed could only be erased if she could replace it with certainty.

Meet the developmental needs of other family members

Fanos (1997) reminds us that the accessibility of a parent for the psychosocial support of a child is a crucial factor in his or her well-being. If the condition is an autosomal dominant one, a parent may already be trying to cope with his or her own illness, or that of the partner. With one (or more) child affected by a condition, the accessibility of the parents will be compromised – more so when they are grieving the death of an affected child. With frequent hospital stays, the availability of a parent on a day-to-day basis will also be severely limited. In a later study of the impact on siblings of boys with severe combined immunodeficiency disorder, most expressed distress over the prolonged absence of the mother during hospitalisation of the ill brother (Fanos & Puck 2001). They concluded that parents need help in balancing the needs of well siblings with those of an affected one.

PROFESSIONAL CONVERSATION

The Bradley family was well known to me – various members had been back and forth to the cystic fibrosis clinic over the years. Teresa was just 15 when she came and asked me about carrier testing for cystic fibrosis. Her cousin has the condition and her mum, older sister and another cousin are carriers, as well as her aunt and uncle of course. The family has always talked openly about cystic fibrosis and Teresa said she felt it was now her turn to be tested. I was a bit concerned because of her age, although she is quite mature and sensible, but also because I wondered how she might feel if she turned out not to have the gene. With so many of her family being carriers (in fact, all of the older females and the uncle) a negative result might exclude her from 'the gang'. I don't think the family had registered this and I know they would not knowingly exclude her but the potential for her to feel left out needed to be raised.

Cope with continuous stress and periodic crises

Sickle-cell disease and cystic fibrosis (both autosomal recessive conditions) are typical examples of how the pattern of the illness is one of continuous stress, managing the condition on a daily basis with a regime of medication and other therapy, interspersed with crises, both familial and medical. A child in sickle-cell crisis (where the abnormally shaped red blood cells can cause infarction and necrosis) and a chest infection in a child with cystic fibrosis require prompt hospitalisation and aggressive clinical intervention. The gradual deterioration of a child with a degenerative condition such as Duchenne muscular dystrophy (X-linked) as he becomes increasingly dependent on his family, also provokes continuous stress.

The day-to-day fluctuations in condition and the uncertainty this brings make a major contribution to stress (Locker 1991, Nereo et al 2003). To this symptomatic uncertainty is added the trajectory uncertainty of being able to predict the course and outcome of the disease. This is not only because of individual variation in gene expression, but also because of advances in management in a fast-moving research field, underpinning hopes for more effective treatments or even cure (through gene or stem cell therapy) in the future.

Activity

Read Merry France-Dawson's story about her experiences of living with sickle-cell disease in 'The troubled helix' (France-Dawson 1996). She recalls overhearing her father being told she would not survive the night as a young girl in ITU over 30 years ago, and describes how she then 'lived by instalments'.

Managing the family's feelings

It is important to acknowledge the positive contribution that the child makes to the family, irrespective of the nature of the condition. Kearney & Griffin (2001) conceptualise the experiences of parents of children with developmental disability as being a dynamic between joy and sorrow. Although there are undoubtedly negative experiences, these can be balanced by positive feelings such as hope and humour. As McGowan expresses it: 'My sons are special people, beyond their genetic flaw…' (McGowan 1999 p 199).

Nonetheless, the sorrows can be profound and long-lasting, and other feelings such as guilt, blame, anger, fear, anxiety and depression can also be difficult to cope with. One factor that may be more apparent in families with a child affected by a genetic condition is the feeling of guilt. This can take the form of 'survivor guilt' in unaffected family members, including children. In one study examining the long-term psychological effects of genetic testing for a hereditary colorectal cancer, some children with a negative result and a positive-testing sibling demonstrated an increase in symptoms of anxiety at follow-up (Codori et al 2003).

The guilt that parents can feel can be overwhelming. In his book about his daughter Alex, Frank Deford recounts eloquently the impact of genetic disease on family life (Deford 1983). Alex had cystic fibrosis, and she lived until she was 8 years old. The story of Alex's life, of the family's struggle with her disease, and of her death is indescribably moving and essential reading for any children's nurse. Deford captures some of the feelings that many parents may experience in this situation:

> Ultimately, whether in my dealings with Carol [his wife], with Alex herself, with anyone involved with the disease – or with myself, for that matter – the major emotion pressing upon me was the feeling of inadequacy … And I could not explain how I felt, because of the shame, nor could I ever escape, because of the guilt.
>
> (Deford 1983 p 96)

He goes on to say:

> When our child was dying – when she was dying because of the genes we passed on to her – no matter how irrational it may have been to flagellate ourselves, there were times, in the mustiest corners of self-awareness, when we had to. Had to. I could not forgive Carol any more than I could forgive myself. After all, we quickly enough assume credit for the genes that make our children attractive and bright – she takes after me. It's only human nature, then, that we also accept the responsibility when we pass on genes of destruction.
>
> (Deford 1983 p 94)

Of course, such feelings are not the prerogative of parents in this situation. Many parents will blame themselves for contributing in some way to their child's condition. However, with genetic disease, particularly the single gene disorders and chromosomal conditions, the cause may be clearly attributable to one or both parents. Furthermore, as the condition may be passed on to future generations, this may be accompanied by ongoing guilt and fear that subsequent children will also inherit it.

Educate others

There are thousands of single gene disorders and chromosome abnormalities and most are rare. However, even the more common ones are unfamiliar to most health professionals outside the specialist genetics service. The aetiology of multifactorial conditions such as asthma, cleft lip and palate, and autism is also complex and the genetic component often unclear. The families tend to become the experts, demonstrating knowledge and understanding of the condition and using this to educate others involved in the care of the child. Many contribute to the work of support groups such as Contact a Family (www.caf.org.uk), and their websites can provide a valuable education resource for other families. The Telling Stories website (www.geneticseducation.nhs.uk/tellingstories) is developed with patients and carers, using family stories primarily as an education resource for health professionals.

Establish a support system

With any chronic illness, the healthcare system becomes a major part of the family's environment and they need to become socialised into it. The success of this depends in part on the quality of information available and on accessible and effective multi-agency communication. Support groups can thus be life savers.

Seminar discussion topic

Read online about the Human Fertilisation and Embryology Bill, introduced in the House of Lords in 2007, at:

- http://www.parliament.uk/documents/upload/HLHumFertEmbrBill.pdf

The Bill seeks to update current regulation of assisted reproduction and embryo research in the light of developments in technology. Clause 14(4)(9) of the Bill states that when using assisted reproduction (such as pre-implantation genetic diagnosis), embryos that are known to be at risk of developing 'serious physical or mental disability' or 'serious illness' must not be preferred to 'normal' embryos. The explanatory notes to the Bill define deafness as a serious disability, thus the Bill will prevent the selection of embryos for deafness. This clause generated considerable debate and controversy, particularly among groups such as the British Deaf Association.

Read the notes of the Bill and consider some of the following issues:

- Do you consider deafness as a serious disability?
- Is deliberately selecting embryos with deafness immoral?
- Is the Bill preventing reproductive freedom?

The phases of adaptation we have described can be 'worked through' by families, with time and support. However, it is important to note that individuals within a family will progress at different rates, and the progress itself may not be linear as individuals move back and forth between the stages. Whyte (1992) identifies that a crucial aspect of the process is the synchrony with which partners move through these phases.

Many of the challenges facing families that we have outlined so far apply to other diseases, and not just genetic disease, but the distinction between these is becoming blurred as advances in genetics research increasingly are revealing the genetic component of common diseases. The next section explains how genes can be passed on through the generations and how 'faulty' genes may lead to disease and ill health.

It runs in the family: the role of genetic factors in disease

There are over 4000 simply inherited serious genetic disorders, such as cystic fibrosis, sickle-cell disease and Duchenne muscular dystrophy. Together with the chromosomal abnormalities such as Down syndrome, they account for about 10 to 20 cases of genetic disease per 1000 population. However, by the age of 60, about 60% of the population is likely to have been affected by a disease that is partially genetically determined. Our genes, at least in part, determine nearly all of our characteristics, including how we respond to infection, and so they play a fundamental role in our health. But what are genes and how can they lead to ill health that can be passed on through the generations?

Genes

Almost every cell of the body contains a complete set of genes, each one representing a chemical instruction to make one or more proteins, protein sub-units or RNA molecules, for different cell functions, guiding development from embryo to adult. It is estimated that we have about 23,000 genes, which direct the development, growth and function of every cell in the body, its tissues and organ systems. There are genes that control other genes, switching them on or off according to the cell type and the functions it performs. For example, in the pancreas, the gene providing the instructions for the manufacture of insulin might be turned on, whereas genes for making keratin, a structural protein found in hair and nails, would be switched off. There are also genes that control cell growth and division; faults in these genes can lead to different types of cancers.

Genes are made up of DNA

The genes themselves are located on the chromosomes, each chromosome being made up of two enormously long strands of DNA, joined together and tightly coiled into a double helix. The genes are spaced along the DNA molecule, and are an integral part of it.

DNA molecules consists of four different chemical bases (nucleotides), A, C, G and T. A gene has thousands of these bases, some, like the dystrophin gene (associated with Duchenne muscular dystrophy), have millions. Each chromosome is made up 100s-1000s of genes. If the DNA molecule that comprises one chromosome was likened to a tower of Lego®, then the tower could be built using only four colours of Lego® blocks – but the tower could be about 100 million blocks high!

It is the order or sequence of the four nucleotides within a gene along the length of a DNA molecule that contains the instructions to make specific proteins or protein sub-units, in the form of a chemical code. A block of three nucleotides (a triplet) represents the code for one amino acid, the building blocks of proteins. Essentially, each gene is made up of a series of three-letter words (using a four-letter alphabet), which, when deciphered, gives us a sequence of amino acids.

Alterations to the genetic make-up

The sequence of the chemical bases that make up the DNA in each of the 23 pairs of chromosomes is the same in every person for about 99% of the human genome. However, there are variations in the remaining genetic material and it is these variations that make us unique.

Some of the variations occur by chance, and although many such mutations are repaired, some are not. Of these, some may confer an advantage to the genome but others may be harmful, particularly if the number of mutations increases with increasing age and exposure to environmental hazards. These mutations are effectively gene errors. Mutations that occur in the sex cells can be passed on to future generations.

The nature of the gene error can also vary. Some arise when a single nucleotide from an entire gene sequence is accidentally replaced by a different nucleotide. The mutation associated with sickle-cell disease is a classic example of this type of 'point' mutation. Sickle-cell disease is the most common of the haemoglobinopathies, affecting about 1 in 300 people of Afro-Caribbean origin, with about 1 in 10 being carriers of the disease. The mutation can be advantageous for some carriers, providing resistance to malaria for a short time.

Haemoglobin is formed from four chains of amino acids, two α chains, and two β chains, each of which is associated with a haem group that binds with oxygen. In sickle-cell disease there is a mutation in the gene on chromosome 11 that provides the code for the β chains. A single base (A) within the gene is replaced by a different base (T). This alters the code so that the amino acid valine is assembled instead of glutamine, and this single alteration is sufficient to change the normal β-globin structure of haemoglobin (Fig. 38.2). The result is that the red blood cells become abnormally shaped in conditions of reduced oxygen levels, such as during an infectious illness. The sickle-shaped cells can block capillaries, causing painful infarctions at times of such crises, and the disturbances to blood flow can also cause leg ulcers. Internal organs are compromised, and splenomegaly may be apparent. Premature destruction of the abnormally shaped cells also leads to anaemia, and a loss of immune function predisposes the child to infection.

If the mutation has an effect that is so marked that it is always seen in the phenotype, the phenotype is said to be dominant, and the phenotype provided by the allele on the other chromosome is masked by it. On the other hand, if the effect is apparent only when both alleles of a chromosome pair are the altered version, the mutation is said to be recessive. Sickle-cell disease has a recessive phenotype, although people with one altered gene ('carriers') may show some signs of the disease under extreme conditions of low oxygen.

An analogy can be drawn with a fluorescent light containing two tubes. When functioning normally, the tubes together provide a steady illumination. If one tube is faulty, so that it flickers constantly, the effect can be so irritating as to 'override' the light from the other tube. On the other hand, if the fault resulted in the tube being unable to function, so long as the other tube worked effectively, the light itself would still be functional, albeit with a reduced intensity; this is analogous to a recessive mutation. If both tubes have the same fault, the light will not work.

How genes are passed on through families

Mutations that occur within a gene (known as the single gene disorders) show characteristic patterns of inheritance some times referred to as Mendelian patterns, as they are passed on through generations, depending on whether the associated phenotypes are dominant or recessive, and located on an autosome or the sex chromosomes (Table 38.1).

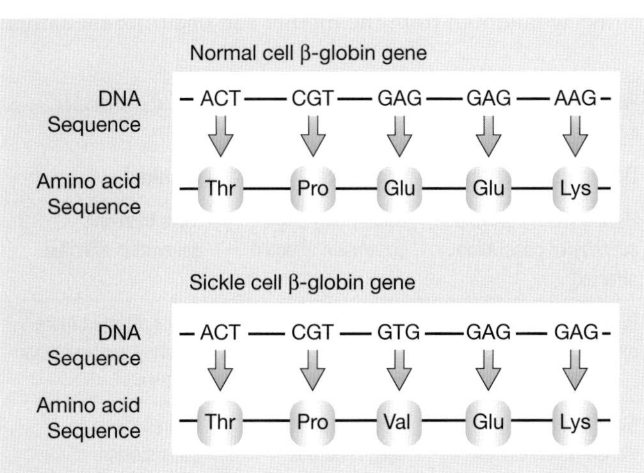

Fig. 38.2 • The sickle-cell mutation.

Table 38.1 Examples of single gene conditions seen in childhood

Autosomal dominant	Autosomal recessive	X-linked recessive
Achondroplasia	Cystic fibrosis	Haemophilia A and B
Marfan syndrome	Sickle-cell disease	Alport syndrome
Osteogenesis imperfecta	Thalassaemia	Fragile X
Tuberous sclerosis	Phenylketonuria	Red–green colour blindness
Neurofibromatosis type 1	Spinal muscular atrophy (Werdnig–Hoffman disease)	Duchenne muscular dystrophy
Gilles de la Tourette syndrome (Tourette's)	Congenital deafness	Glucose-6-phosphate dehydrogenase deficiency

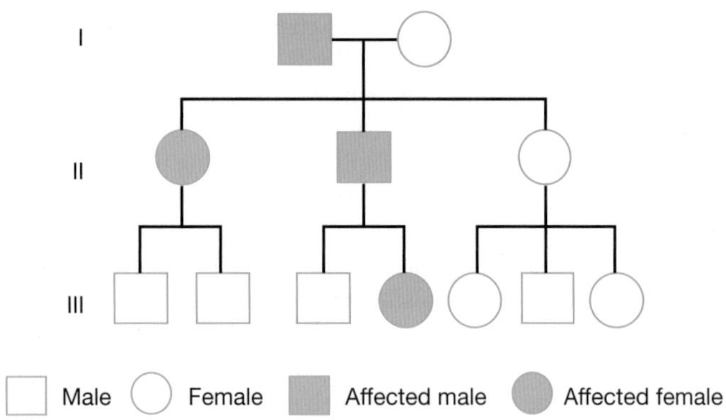

Fig. 38.3 • Family tree for an autosomal dominant condition.

Because an autosomal dominant trait is invariably manifest in the affected person, the family tree will typically show someone affected with the condition in each generation, and with both sexes affected in similar numbers (Fig. 38.3). Each child of an affected parent has a 1 in 2 or 50% chance of inheriting the altered gene but unaffected parents do not transmit it.

Activity

Visit the NHS National Genetics Education & Development Centre website to read the Family History Series and test your knowledge by completing the puzzle on p.23. Browse the other resources in this section of the website, such as the worksheets to practice drawing family trees.

- http://www.geneticseducation.nhs.uk/family_history/Family_History_Series.pdf

In contrast, an autosomal recessive trait can be carried through generations 'hidden' from view, because carriers show no symptoms. Often, the first indication of the condition being 'in the family' is when an affected baby is born of parents who are both carriers. The chances of this happening are usually quite rare, but higher when parents are related – such as first cousins. Some conditions are associated with a higher carrier frequency in particular populations, such as cystic fibrosis in white northern Europeans (in the UK, this frequency is approximately 1 in 25). When parents are both carriers, with each conception there is a 1 in 4 or 25% chance that the baby will be affected by the condition, and a 1 in 2 or 50% chance that the baby will be a carrier.

When the gene under question is located on the X chromosome, the pattern (known as X-linked inheritance) is somewhat different. As males have only one X chromosome, genes located on that chromosome will always be expressed even if recessive, as they do not have the partner chromosome to compensate. Males are thus said to be hemizygous for X-linked genes. X-linked inheritance can be either recessive or dominant, although the latter is much rarer. Male-to-male transmission is not seen but all daughters of affected males will inherit the faulty gene (Fig. 38.4). Women who are carriers have a 50% chance of passing on the altered gene to their sons (who will then be affected) and their daughters will have a 50% chance of being carriers themselves. The characteristic features of

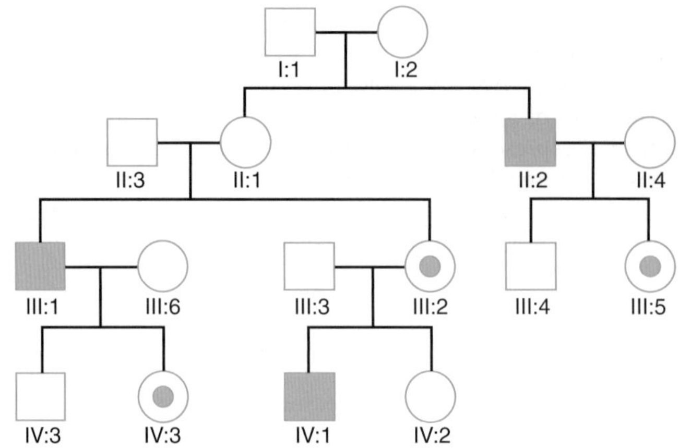

Fig. 38.4 • X-linked inheritance.

the three types of inheritance can be summarised as shown in Table 38.2.

There are occasions when a family history does not seem to follow the typical pattern. Alterations to mitochondrial DNA show a mother-to-child inheritance. New mutations in the sex cells of a parent can account for the appearance of a dominant trait in a family even though neither parent is affected. Some dominant traits can also be affected by penetrance and expressivity. Traits associated with a reduced penetrance may not be expressed in an individual, and when they are expressed, the severity of expression may also vary. Neurofibromatosis is a dominant condition with variable expression such that it may have gone undetected in an individual at first and thus appear to 'skip' a generation in affected families. However, closer examination would reveal, for example, some of the characteristic pigmented patches (café-au-lait spots) on the skin. Finally, non-paternity can also account for an otherwise puzzling family tree, and this situation has to be dealt with sensitively.

DNA is packaged into chromosomes

Chromosomes are the more visible elements of inheritance, seen under the microscope as tightly packed coils of DNA. Cells have 23 pairs of chromosomes, one member of each pair being inherited from the mother and one from the father.

Table 38.2 The family tree: characteristic features of classically inherited diseases

Dominant inheritance	Recessive	X-linked
Usually more than one successive generation affected	Usually only one generation affected	More than one generation affected
People of both sexes affected	People of both sexes affected	Males affected more severely generally than females
Male to male transmission evident	Offspring of two healthy parents affected	No male to male transmission

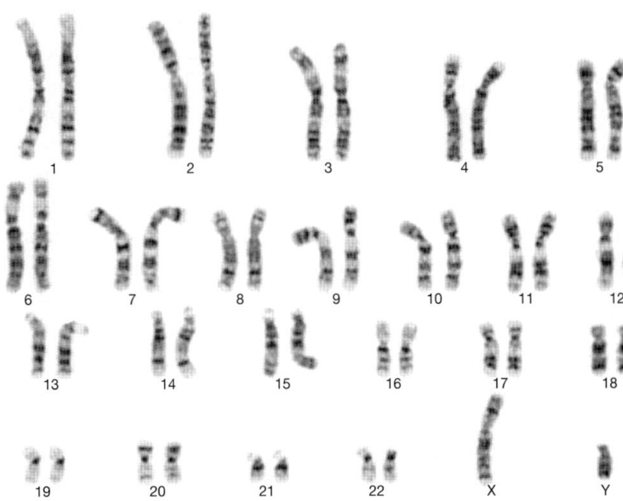

Fig. 38.5 • A normal male karyotype.

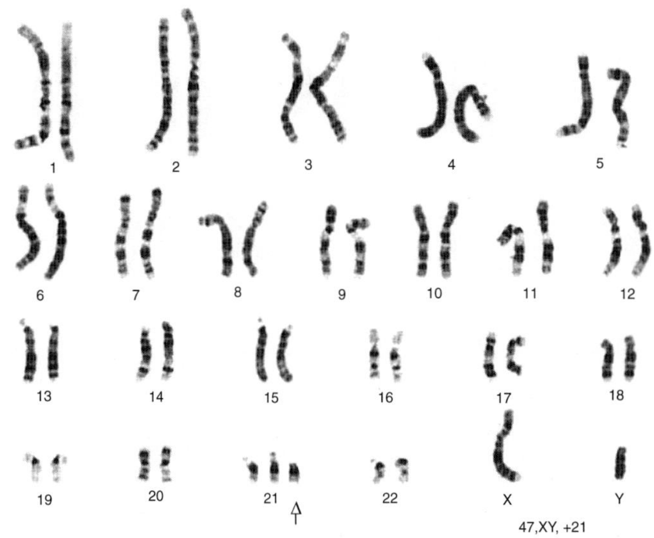

Fig. 38.6 • Trisomy 21 karyotype (Down syndrome).

We inherit one set of 23 chromosomes, and thus one set of genes, from each parent, passed on through the egg and sperm cells. The total chromosome number of 46 is restored with the fusion of the egg and sperm to form the embryo.

When the chromosomes are examined in the laboratory, they are set out in a systematic way, according to their matched pairs, arranged in order of size, and aligned with the shorter arm of the chromosome (designated p) above the longer one (q). This arrangement is the karyotype (Fig. 38.5).

Members of a pair of chromosomes are referred to as being homologous, and each member of the pair will have the same genes in the same order. However, the form of a particular gene may be a little different on each chromosome – these different forms are known as alleles. For example, a gene that provides instructions for making eye pigments occurs at the same position (locus) on each chromosome of the pair. If both chromosomes have identical alleles (e.g. brown eye pigment) the person is homozygous at that locus. If the alleles are different (e.g. one brown and the other blue) the person is heterozygous at that locus.

As well as errors that occur in the DNA sequence, at 'gene level', we can also have errors at the level of the chromosome, involving part or whole chromosomes. Such errors account for more than 50% of all spontaneous first trimester losses, 20% of second trimester losses, and occur in about 1 in 160 live births. The errors involve alterations either to the number or structure of chromosomes.

Alterations to chromosome number are the most common. Polyploidy is the term given to cells that contain a multiple of 23 chromosomes. In humans, triploid (69 chromosomes) and tetraploid (92 chromosomes) conceptions can occur, but are incompatible with survival. An embryo that is aneuploid has missing or additional chromosomes, most commonly one additional chromosome (trisomy). The general rule is that we can tolerate additional genetic material more readily than a loss, so monosomy (loss of one chromosome) is not compatible with life. The exception to this is Turner syndrome, a condition seen only in girls where there is a loss of one X chromosome.

The most common form of aneuploidy is trisomy and whilst most trisomic fetuses are spontaneously aborted, some survive to term and beyond. Down syndrome, and its association with increased maternal age, is the most well known (Fig. 38.6). Trisomies of the sex chromosomes (XXX female, XYY male, or XXY Klinefelter male) have much less severe consequences, and many people with this condition may be undiagnosed until after puberty, or at fertility clinics.

Structural alterations occur when chromosome material becomes rearranged following breakage and abnormal reconstitution. Parts of a chromosome may become detached and lost, duplicated, or rearranged (Table 38.3). Breaks can be caused spontaneously, or by certain viruses, drugs or radiation. The effects of these depend on the nature of the rearrangement and whether there is an overall loss or gain of genetic material.

A translocation occurs when there is an exchange of material between two different (non-homologous) chromosomes

Table 38.3 Some examples of chromosome rearrangements

	Example	Karyotype
Numerical		
Gain of a whole chromosome	Down syndrome (Trisomy 21) Klinefelter syndrome	47,XX (or XY) +21 Gain of an autosome (Chr 21) 47,XXY Gain of a sex chromosome
Loss of a whole chromosome	Turner syndrome	45, X Loss of a sex chromosome
Structural		
Translocation	Balanced Robertsonian translocation	45,XY t(14;21) Chr 14 and 21 have fused to form one chromosome
Deletion	Cri du chat	46,XX (or XY)5p–Partial deletion on short arm of Chr 5
Microdeletion	22q	46,XX (or XY)22q–Microdeletion on long arm of Chr 22

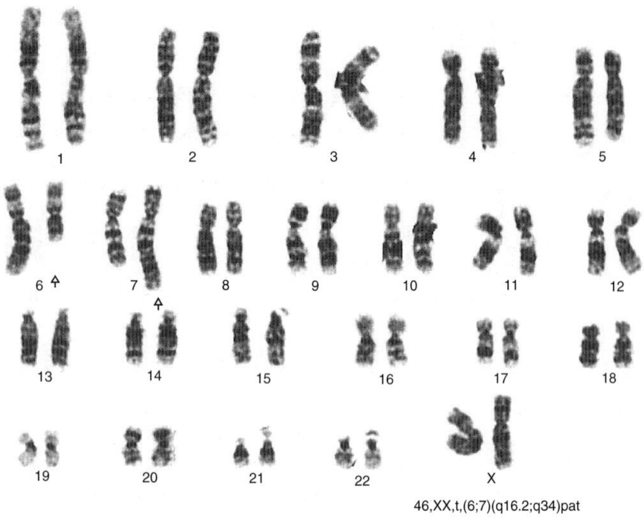

Fig. 38.7 • Karyotype of a reciprocal translocation. Genetic material has been exchanged between one of each pair of chromosomes 6 and 7 (arrowed).

(Fig. 38.7). These are the most clinically significant of the structural chromosome rearrangements. In most cases, there is no net loss or gain of chromosomal material during the exchange process, and the translocation is thus said to be 'balanced'. It is estimated that 1 in 500 individuals has a balanced translocation, usually with no health consequences for the individual. However, problems arise during the formation of the egg or sperm cells, and some may carry unbalanced chromosomes, often causing early pregnancy loss or multiple abnormalities in the infant.

Genetic testing

Genetic testing refers to the analysis of a specific gene, its product or function, or other DNA and chromosome analysis to detect or exclude an alteration likely to be associated with a genetic disorder (Harper & Clarke 1997). Different types of genetic tests include:

a. Diagnostic: carried out on individuals who either have, or are suspected of having, a particular condition because of clinical signs or symptoms.

b. Predictive tests, carried out on asymptomatic people, and can be of two types:

- Presymptomatic, carried out on individuals at high risk of an adult-onset condition, where an abnormal test result indicates that development of the condition is almost inevitable, e.g. Huntington disease.
- Predispositional testing, aimed at identifying susceptible individuals at increased risk of developing a condition, where the increased risk of the condition developing may be substantial but is not necessarily certain, e.g. breast cancer.

c. Carrier: identifies healthy individuals at risk of having a child affected by a genetic condition.

The term 'genetic laboratory' test could be applied where the test involves the direct analysis of genetic material (nucleic acid or chromosomes, e.g. Figs 38.5, 38.6, 38.7) or the analysis of biochemical parameters, such as the concentration of metabolites or the activity of enzymes, to diagnose a genetic condition or make predictions about the genetic make-up of a person. Genetics information can also be obtained from clinical examination, imaging and family history. For instance a sigmoidoscopy in a young person at risk of inherited bowel cancer through familial adenomatous polyposis (FAP) could be defined as a genetic test in that it gives 'genetic information.'

Cystic fibrosis provides a useful example to illustrate how 'finding' the gene can help in understanding the underlying disease mechanism and in providing a direct genetic test. Children with cystic fibrosis generally fail to thrive and are prone to recurrent respiratory infections, amongst other problems. When the gene associated with CF was identified in 1989, it was found to be one that codes for a transmembrane regulator protein (known as CFTR). The normal protein helps to control the flow of chloride ions across cell membranes and so produces good-quality mucus secretions. If this flow is compromised, sodium and water balance will be affected leading to abnormal secretions and a build up of thick mucus. Most mutations in Europe (70%) show a deletion of three bases at a specific position of the CFTR gene. This results in the loss of the amino acid phenylalanine from the protein product and this deletion may be detected using direct analysis of DNA.

Understanding how genes that contribute to ill health can be inherited, how they can then be detected to inform a diagnosis and then communicating this and other information to parents and children is part of the role of professionals within the genetics service. However, with the integration of genetics into mainstream services and increasing demand for genetic information, there is a growing need for all health professionals to develop competence in this area. The next section looks at the role of the children's nurse in relation to this.

Genetic counselling and the family journey: the role of the children's nurse

Genetic counselling is:

> a communication process between the counsellor and the individual or family which deals with the medical and other implications associated with the occurrence, or the risk of occurrence, of a genetic disorder in a family
>
> (DoH 2003 p 91).

In the UK, families are referred to the specialist genetics service most commonly by their GP or paediatrician. Nurses have a crucial role in alerting colleagues to a possible need for referral through their awareness of family history. Patients are seen by a clinical geneticist and/or a genetic counsellor at outpatient clinics, although home visits are sometimes made.

Barr & Millar (2003) argue that genetic counselling should be seen as an integral part of the adaptation process that parents and other family members journey through. The role of the children's nurse is then to journey with the family, helping family members 'prepare for, engage in and move on' irrespective of the information provided at the genetic clinic. To do so effectively, the nurse has to be equipped with sufficient knowledge and understanding of genetics to be able to support the family, placing genetics information into context as a part of that journey.

The extent of the knowledge and skills required in genetics by all nurses in the UK has been set into a competence framework and described in a report (Kirk et al 2003). The authors worked with stakeholders (including professional and client groups) to identify the knowledge, skills and attitudes in genetics that nurses should demonstrate.

WWW

Read the report online:

http://www.geneticseducation.nhs.uk/teaching/downloads/FitforPractice_FinalReport.pdf

Discuss in your learning group if you think the competences are relevant for children's nurses.

Seven competence standard statements were constructed, representing the minimum standard that should be achieved by nurses at the point of registration (Box 38.1). Identifying people who might benefit from genetic services and information was acknowledged as the key competence, and requires all nurses to have some skills in family history taking. The report also suggests learning outcomes and practice indicators for each competence statement, and indicates how the competency framework may be adapted for more experienced practitioners.

Reflect on your practice

- Do you think you could demonstrate these competences in your practice?
- How can you address any deficit you identify in your skills?

Although the competences apply to all nursing professionals, the situations in which children's nurses in particular need to use genetic knowledge and skills have been outlined by the Association of Genetic Nurses and Counsellors (2002). These include where the children's nurse would need to:

- provide supportive, informed communication at the time of diagnosis or receipt of definitive results
- act as a trusted and informed carer for children growing up with genetic conditions (such as muscular dystrophy or cystic fibrosis), as they may be probing increasingly for information about the condition, its prognosis and effect on life plans
- help parents deal with feelings of anger, guilt or blame as they acknowledge their own genetic contribution to the child's illness or consider prenatal diagnosis in a future pregnancy
- enhance awareness of conditions which may mimic non-accidental injury or abuse, such as osteogenesis imperfecta or conditions that result in failure to thrive
- facilitate referral to local genetic services when appropriate.

The need for clear and accurate information, delivered sensitively and at a pace and level appropriate to the understanding and needs of family members is fundamental, but this is not always achieved (Chapple et al 1997, Fallowfield & Jenkins 2004, McGowan 1999). The family nurse can help in 'going over' information with the family, working with them at their own pace – and is in the ideal position to recognise that individuals within the family may be at different stages of adaptation. Preparing families for genetic counselling, helping them

Box 38.1

The seven core competence standard statements

All nurses, midwives and health visitors, at the point of registration, should be able to:

1. Identify clients who might benefit from genetic services and information:
   - through an understanding of the importance of family history in assessing predisposition to disease
   - seeking assistance from and referring to appropriate genetics experts and peer support resources
   - based on an understanding of the components of the current genetic counselling process.
2. Appreciate the importance of sensitivity in tailoring genetic information and services to clients' culture, knowledge and language level:
   - recognising that ethnicity, culture, religion and ethical perspectives may influence the clients' ability to utilise these.
3. Uphold the rights of all clients to informed decision making and voluntary action:
   - based on an awareness of the history of misuse of human genetic information
   - understanding the importance of delivering genetic education and counselling fairly, accurately and without coercion or personal bias
   - recognising that personal values and beliefs may influence the care and support provided to clients during decision-making.
4. Demonstrate a knowledge and understanding of the role of genetic and other factors in maintaining health and in the manifestation, modification and prevention of disease expression, to underpin effective practice.
5. Demonstrate a knowledge and understanding of the utility and limitations of genetic testing and information:
   - including the ethical, legal and social issues related to testing and recording of genetic information
   - the potential physical and/or psychosocial consequences of genetic information for individuals, family members, and communities.
6. Recognise the limitations of one's own genetics expertise:
   - based on an understanding of one's professional role in the referral, provision or follow-up to genetics services.
7. Obtain and communicate credible, current information about genetics, for self, clients and colleagues:
   - using information technologies effectively to do so.

to have realistic expectations, is an important aspect of placing genetic information into context.

Evidence-based practice

Barr & Millar (2003) describe the expectations and experiences of parents of children with learning disabilities in relation to genetic counselling. They found that parents largely felt unprepared for their appointment with the genetic consultant and that this could mean that parents hold unrealistic expectations about the appointment. The authors recommend that priority should be given to gaining an understanding of the expectations of clients prior to the first appointment.

Skirton (2001) stresses the importance of certainty in the family's quest for a diagnosis, but there will be many times when a diagnosis is not available. It is worth noting here that as more genetic tests become available, there will also be circumstances where families who had not previously been given a diagnosis will be recalled, and a definitive diagnosis may become possible. These families may well experience a readaptation, particularly where a genetic cause can now be attributed to one or both parents.

Part of giving reliable information includes the need to avoid false reassurance, but at the same time provide a balanced perspective, helping the family to maintain hope. Support groups can be particularly helpful, but information about these needs to be delivered at an appropriate time, and the nurse needs to be aware of the type and quality of information available.

Evidence-based practice

The importance of providing good-quality information for parents and families is widely acknowledged, but how is this defined? Mitchell & Sloper (2002) used four focus groups of parents and one of professionals to explore how parents preferred to receive information, and their views on best practice. They propose a model that takes a three-dimensional approach, combining good-quality information that offers a review of local resources and more in-depth material, with personal guidance from a 'key worker' such as a community-based professional.

Reflect on your practice

- Do you think you provide 'three-dimensional information' for your families? Are you confident that you do not over-rely on one source, such as leaflets?
- How do you check that your families have understood the information you have provided?

At the heart of effective communication is the relationship that the nurse has with the family. Trust is central to this, developed through open, honest communication and practice within an ethical framework as indicated by the competence standard statements. Some of the ethical issues surrounding the application of genetic technologies are of particular relevance to children's nurses.

PROFESSIONAL CONVERSATION

Geraldine is a registered children's nurse

Recognise the limitations of one's own genetics expertise

For me, the most important competency is knowing when to say I don't know and then getting help from someone who does! I think this was brought home to me last year. I'd been talking to a mum who had brought her daughter to clinic for an unrelated problem. She was obviously a bit down and told me that she'd had a termination of pregnancy a few weeks earlier after an abnormality (a neural tube defect) was picked up on scan. She and her husband wanted to try for another baby, but were scared of the same thing happening again. I told her the chances of it recurring were a million to one. And then without really thinking it through, I reassured her that as well, she could have an earlier genetic test by chorionic villus sampling. She asked what that would show. Of course at that point I realised I was out of my depth and said I'd check it out and get back to her. When I contacted our local genetics nurse, she was very helpful but I was embarrassed when I learnt that in fact the mum's chance of a recurrence was actually 1 in 20 (5%). Maybe I shouldn't have said anything, but it's natural to want to reassure families. I was able to liaise with the genetics nurse though about getting back to the mum, and I am more careful now about what I say.

- Whose role was it to provide information for this mother? Should it be the role of any one professional group?

Ethical issues for children's nurses

Although the benefits that new genetic technologies may bring to help people with or at risk of a genetic disease are to be welcomed, there are also concerns about potential harms. An increase in genetic testing may challenge personal privacy, undermining the 'right not to know'. Some authors voice concern that it has the potential to promote discrimination, and devalues the existence of people with a disability (see, for example, Ward 2002). Newell (2000) claims that the prediction that an embryo is at risk of an increasing number of 'defects' is regarded as a standard basis for a decision to terminate the pregnancy on 'therapeutic' grounds.

The application of new genetic technology in reproductive decision-making provokes fierce debate on occasion. One aspect of this is the selection of embryos during in vitro fertilisation, on the basis of its genotype, for the purposes of helping an existing child. This could potentially help families such as McGowan's, where a bone-marrow transplant from a sibling with appropriate genotype could help her sons. She states that:

> At this stage, my husband and I have rejected such options as we feel it is not right for us to have a child for such reasons … I really believe that people should be valued for more than just their genes.
>
> (McGowan 1999 p 197).

Activity

Yasmin and Michael have a happy, stable relationship. They are about to decide whether to start a family. Draw a decision tree (like a flow diagram) for the couple, starting with the question 'shall we have children?' and assuming that their initial decision is that they will. Work through all the subsequent decisions they have to make, up until the final decision of 'shall we have another child?'

Try and include all possible options, incorporating your knowledge of current reproductive technologies. What decisions might they have to make in the pre-conceptual and antenatal periods? What decisions might they face in the immediate postnatal period? Which do you think might be the most difficult?

Once you have done this, you might like to draw another decision tree, but this time think of a couple facing this decision back in the 1950s. How has the nature of reproductive decision-making changed? Does increased choice bring greater freedom?

Certainly, a common concern is about whether and where a line should be drawn between using genetic information to prevent harm (negative eugenics) and to promote desirable characteristics (positive eugenics). Iredale (2000) reviews these issues and concludes that nurses need to play an active role in promoting good genetic health, underpinned by an appreciation of the history of genetics and the eugenics movement. Professional practice also has to incorporate the ethical principles of privacy, confidentiality, informed consent and non-discrimination.

Seminar discussion topic

Read 'Stamping out short people' by Gregory Stock, accessed online at:

•http://www.com/wired/archive/11.11/view_pr.html

Describing the 'official recognition' by the Food and Drug Administration (FDA) agency in the US of the use of growth hormone for healthy but short children, the author supports the use of enhancement technology to make us 'stronger, smarter and faster'. He argues that 'The biggest risk isn't that we'll make mistakes or create a race of superhumans. It's that we'll proceed too cautiously with health enhancements that would benefit us all.'

- Is it a fundamental human right to be able to access new technologies to improve our inherited characteristics?
- Do parents have the right to enhance the characteristics of their children?
- What about unborn children? Do they have a right to inherit an 'un-enhanced' genome?

One of the key ethical issues for children's nurses is the genetic testing of children, in particular predictive testing for conditions of early and later adult onset, and carrier testing. Early identification of at-risk children might facilitate earlier surveillance and treatment, and would remove uncertainty (Carmichael et al 1999) but there are potential disadvantages. This issue is reviewed by Clarke (1997), who notes that many professional groups recommend caution. He outlines grounds for caution in carrying out predictive testing of healthy children for late-onset disorders on four counts:

- The child loses its autonomy as an adult to make its own decisions.
- Loss of confidentiality because the child's genetic status is known to its parents.
- The psychosocial consequences for the child, which might include labelling, fatalism, damage to self-esteem, and alteration to family dynamics.
- Although the parents may make the decision they feel will be best for the child, they will do so from a hypothetical perspective. The child, faced with the reality, may see things differently. Clarke uses Huntington disease as an example to illustrate this. Ahead of the gene being identified, the majority of at-risk families stated that they would seek testing once this became possible. In reality, when the gene was found, the majority of at-risk adults chose not to be tested, preferring to retain uncertainty.

Fanos (1997 p 27) makes a further point when she states that:

> The very children and adolescents most at risk for being tested for genetic disorders are those who have grown up in a world where the illness has already made a very real appearance. Parents may not be emotionally available to help their children with the impact of testing procedures or results because of their own illness or guilt over issues of inheritance.

PROFESSIONAL CONVERSATION

"I was asked to go and see Rebecca at home because the neonatal screening test on her baby George had revealed her son to have Duchenne muscular dystrophy. Of course, this meant there were quite a few implications for the family. Rebecca could be a carrier of the condition, and her siblings could also, so it would be important to make sure that Rebecca understood this, and understood how she might want to take this into account for further reproductive decisions. I would also need to make sure that Rebecca understood what being a carrier would mean for herself in terms of her own health. Lots to tell her – lots to ensure she understands. The headache for me is that Rebecca is only 13 years old herself."

This issue came to the forefront once again when the UK government commissioned an examination of the potential for genetic profiling at birth. The conclusion was that it was unlikely to be practical or acceptable for the foreseeable future (Human Genetics Commission 2005). However, in its progress review, the DoH raised concerns about the ethical issues that may be raised by analysis of free fetal DNA from maternal blood samples (DoH 2008). The role of the children's nurse, acting as an advocate, is central to upholding the rights of children in relation to genetic testing.

Summary

The advance in genetics knowledge and related technology is transforming health care, moving a hitherto specialist subject, with its focus on rare conditions, into mainstream services. Understanding how genetics can affect families is increasingly important for children's nurses as they support families in their care. Being able to interpret and communicate information about genetics accurately, honestly and sensitively is a central feature of the role. A wider appreciation of the ethical issues that may arise, not only for children and their families, but also for wider society, is also important.

References

Association of Genetic Nurses and Counsellors (AGNC) Education Working Group, 2002. Education in genetics for health professionals not working in specialist genetic units. Report E, Reports for the Genetics Policy Unit Department of Health. AGNC, Birmingham.

Barr, O., Millar, R., 2003. Parents of children with intellectual disabilities: their expectations and experience of genetic counselling. Journal of Applied Research in Intellectual Disabilities 16, 189–204.

Bell, J., 1998. The new genetics in clinical practice. British Medical Journal 316, 618–620.

Canam, C., 1993. Common adaptive tasks facing parents of children with chronic conditions. Journal of Advanced Nursing 18, 46–53.

Carmichael, B., Pembrey, M., Turner, G., Barnicoat, A., 1999. Diagnosis of fragile-X syndrome: the experience of parents. Journal of Intellectual Disability Research 43 (1), 47–53.

Chapple, A., Campion, P., May, C., 1997. Clinical terminology: anxiety and confusion amongst families undergoing genetic counselling. Patient Education and Counseling 32, 81–91.

Clarke, A.J., 1997. The genetic testing of children. In: Harper, P.S., Clarke, A.J. (Eds.), Genetics, society and clinical practice. BIOS, Oxford, pp. 15–29.

Codori, A.M., Zawacki, K.L., Petersen, G., et al., 2003. Genetic testing for hereditary colorectal cancer in children: long-term psychological effects. American Journal of Medical Genetics 116A, 117–128.

Deford, F., 1983. Alex. The life of a child. Viking Press, New York.

Department of Health (DoH), 2003. Our inheritance, our future. Realising the potential of genetics in the NHS. The Stationery Office, London.

Department of Health (DoH), 2008. Our inheritance, our future. Realising the potential of genetics in the NHS. Progress Review. The Stationery Office, London.

Fallowfield, L., Jenkins, V., 2004. Communicating sad, bad and difficult news in medicine. Lancet 363, 312–319.

Fanos, J., 1997. Developmental tasks of childhood and adolescence: implications for genetic testing. American Journal of Medical Genetics 71, 22–28.

Fanos, J., 1999. 'My crooked vision': the well sib views ataxia telangiectasia. American Journal of Medical Genetics 87 (5), 420–425.

Fanos, J., Puck, J., 2001. Family pictures: growing up with a brother with X-linked severe combined immunodeficiency. American Journal of Medical Genetics 98 (1), 57–63.

France-Dawson, M., 1996. Some observations about my life with a sickle cell condition. In: Marteau, T., Richards, M. (Eds.), The troubled helix. Cambridge University Press, Cambridge, pp. 47–50.

Harper, P.S., Clarke, A.J., 1997. Genetics, society and clinical practice. BIOS, Oxford.

Humans Genetics Commission, 2005. Profiling the newborn: A prospective gene technology? Human Genetics Commission, London.

Iredale, R., 2000. Eugenics and its relevance to contemporary health care. Nursing Ethics 7 (3), 205–214.

Kearney, P.M., Griffin, T., 2001. Between joy and sorrow: being a parent of a child with developmental disability. Journal of Advanced Nursing 34 (5), 582–592.

Kirk, M., McDonald, K., Anstey, S., et al., 2003. Fit for practice in the genetics era: a competence-based education framework for nurses, midwives and health visitors. University of Glamorgan, Pontypridd.

Locker, D., 1991. Living with chronic illness. In: Scambler, G. (Ed.), Sociology as applied to medicine. Baillière-Tindall, London, pp. 81–92.

McGowan, R., 1999. Beyond the disorder: one parent's reflection on genetic counselling. Journal of Medical Ethics 25, 195–199.

Mitchell W, Sloper P 2002 Information that informs rather than alienates families with disabled

Nereo, N., Fee, R., Hinton, V., 2003. Parental stress in mothers of boys with Duchenne muscular dystrophy. Journal of Pediatric Psychology 28 (7), 473–484.

Newell, C., 2000. Biomedicine, genetics and disability: reflections on nursing and a philosophy of holism. Nursing Ethics 7 (3), 227–236.

Skirton, H., 2001. The client's perspective of genetic counselling – a grounded theory study. Journal of Genetic Counselling 10 (4), 311–329.

Ward, L., 2002. Whose right to choose? The new genetics, prenatal testing and people with learning difficulties. Critical Public Health 12 (2), 187–200.

Whyte, D., 1992. A family nursing approach to the care of a child with a chronic illness. Journal of Advanced Nursing 17, 317–327.

Further Reading

Marteau, T., Richards, M. (Eds.), 1996. The troubled helix: social and psychological implications of the new human genetics, Cambridge University Press, Cambridge.

Skirton, H., Patch, C., 2009. Genetics for healthcare professionals. A lifestage approach, 2nd edn. Scion Publishing Ltd, Oxon.

Useful Websites

The NHS National Genetics Education Development Centre: education website with an array of different resources including a link to the Telling Stories pages: http://www.geneticseducation.nhs.uk

Essentially an online textbook on genetics: http://www.usd.edu/med/som/genetics/curriculum/TableofContents.htm

Public Health Genetics Foundation, Cambridge: a good all-round resource with a regular 'round up' of current papers and events: http://www.phgfoundation.org.uk

The GeneTests website offers detailed information about particular conditions and tests with an illustrated glossary: http://www.genetests.org

This Genetics Home Reference site provides clear information and a good glossary: http://ghr.nlm.nih.gov/

The Genesense website provides a useful resource for health professionals that seeks to demystify genetics: http://www.genesense.org.uk

The Genetics Education Program for Nurses developed at the Cincinnati Children's Hospital provides a number of free resources: http://www.cincinnatichildrens.org/ed/clinical/gpnf/default.htm

Health problems of the neonate

39

Sandie Skinner Mary Brophy Clare Barrow

ABSTRACT

The primary aim of this chapter and its companion PowerPoint presentation is to provide insight into the health problems of the neonate. Although it is not possible to cover every problem or potential problem the most pertinent problems to nursing management are addressed. Main areas to be covered are hypothermia, hypoglycaemia, neonatal nutrition, neonatal infection, pain, jaundice, respiratory illness and attachment.

LEARNING OUTCOMES

- Recognise a potentially ill neonate.
- Understand the rationale for interventions.
- Apply knowledge of potential problems to minimise distress of neonate and their parents.
- Evaluate and assess the care provided for an ill neonate.

Glossary

Extremely low birth weight (ELBW): An infant with a birth weight below 1 kg.

Intrauterine growth retarded (IUGR): An infant with a symmetrical low birth weight below the 10th percentile.

Low birth weight (LBW): An infant with a birth weight below 2.5 kg.

Nasogastric feeding: The practice of feeding an infant via a tube which is inserted through the nose and advanced to the stomach and normally left indwelling for up to a week.

Neonate: Describes an infant from birth to 28 days.

Orogastric: As with nasogastric but sited via the mouth.

Post-term: An infant born after 42 weeks.

Preterm: An infant born before 37 weeks' gestation.

Small for gestational age (SGA): An infant with an asymmetrical birth weight below the 10th percentile.

Very low birth weight (VLBW): An infant with a birth weight below 1.5 kg.

Introduction

The history of neonatology began with French midwives and obstetricians. Even after specialised neonatal care began to develop in the USA in the 1950s and 1960s, the approach to care was primarily from an obstetric and anaesthetic viewpoint. Specialist neonatologists and neonatal nurses have evolved to care for the most vulnerable of the paediatric population.

Specialised neonatal units often in large university hospitals have evolved over the last 40 years to offer highly technological support to care for ill neonates. Preterm infants as young as 23 weeks' gestation, and weighing <500 g, to term neonates with respiratory, surgical or cardiac problems are cared for on these neonatal units. Environmental adaptation is necessary for survival (Warren 2002). Recently, the focus of care has been the relationship between neonatal nursing practice and long-term developmental outcomes (Turrill 2003). Studies have shown that developmental outcomes are influenced by both the infant's physiological stability and by the neonatal environment. This has implications for nursing practice.

WWW

Read National Service Framework documents at:

- http://www.doh.gov.uk/nsf/neonatal.htm

Neonatal hypothermia

Hypothermia is a significant cause of morbidity and mortality in the neonate (Roberton & Rennie 2001). Humans attempt to maintain their body temperature within a certain range to maintain metabolic functions. The normal temperature range

DOI: 10.1016/B978-0-7020-3183-0.10039-6

for term neonates is 36.5–37.5°C per axilla and in preterm neonates 36.4–37.1°C (Mertenstein 2002).

Definition of hypothermia

Hypothermia is the cooling of the body's core temperature to below 35°C (Campbell & Glasper 1999). Neonates are at risk of hypothermia primarily because of their size because, although small, they have a large surface area in proportion to body weight, a large head size (through which heat is lost) in relation to the rest of the body and an immature hypothalamus resulting in poor vasomotor control. Those neonates primarily at risk of cold stress are (Crawford & Morris 1994):

- preterm infants (born less than 36 weeks)
- infants who are small for gestational age or with intrauterine growth restriction
- infants with respiratory distress
- infants in shock
- infants with congenital anomalies
- infants with convulsions
- infants with bleeding problems.

Temperature regulation

Temperature regulation is a complex process. The hypothalamus, which is located at the base of the brain, is responsible for temperature regulation. Receptors in the skin, abdomen, spinal cord and internal organs provide the hypothalamus with information to maintain temperature balance. The hypothalamus produces hormones in response to temperature imbalance and, together with the autonomic and sympathetic nervous systems, regulates temperature (Hackman 2001). For example, if the neonate is subject to reduction in body temperature, cold stress stimulates thermoreceptors to send impulses to the heat-promoting control centre in the hypothalamus, which in turn triggers responses to retain body heat. Vasoconstriction reduces heat loss through the skin. The adrenal medulla releases hormones that increase cellular metabolism and the thyroid gland releases thyroid hormone, which increases metabolic rate. Significantly, this requires an intact central nervous system. Furthermore, temperature regulation requires oxygen because it is an aerobic process. Glucose is also needed to carry out this aerobic process for heat production.

Non-shivering thermogenesis is a significant and unique form of heat production in the neonate (Klaus & Fanaroff 1993). Neonates generate most of their heat from the breakdown of brown fat. 'Brown fat' refers to the deeply red, highly vascularised areas surrounding an infant's scapular, clavicular and sternal areas. It is rich in fats and glycogen. The full-term infant has sufficient storage of brown fat to maintain temperature for up to 4 days. Heat is generated by hydrolysis of triglycerides in brown fat utilising oxygen in the process. The responses to cold of neonates in a hypoxic state will be jeopardised. Non-shivering thermogenesis is inhibited by drugs, intracranial haemorrhage and hypoglycaemic states.

Heat loss

There are four main routes of heat loss: evaporation, convection, conduction and radiation (Avery 1987). Evaporative heat loss occurs when water is converted to water vapour during perspiration or respiration. Neonates, wet from amniotic fluid and delivered into a cool labour ward can lose heat at a rate 0.25°C/minute (Roberton 1992). It is therefore important to dry the neonate thoroughly with warmed towels and dress him or her promptly. Convective heat loss occurs when the infant's heat is lost to surrounding cooler air, which is why it is important to dress infants and to keep them out of draughts.

Conductive heat loss occurs when the infant comes into direct contact with a cool surface. One way to prevent this would be to prewarm anything in contact with the neonates skin. Finally, radiative heat losses occur when the infant radiates heat to a cold exposed surface such as a window. In this case the neonate should be nursed away from windows and a constant environmental temperature maintained (Sheeran 1996).

Effects of cold stress

The effect of cold stress is well documented. Constriction of skin blood vessels occurs in response to cold in neonates. The effect of peripheral vasoconstriction is to increase the core skin temperature gradient. Increased metabolic rate leads to increased oxygen consumption, lactic acid production, hypoglycaemia, and in very low birthweight infants decreased surfactant synthesis and secretion. Blood coagulopathies also occur leading to increased capillary permeability and haemorrhage.

WWW

Up-to-date reviews of comparative thermal care are available at:

- http://www.nichd.hih.gov/cochrane/cochrane.htm

Neutral thermal environment

The neutral thermal environment (NTE) is the provision of an environmental temperature that minimises oxygen consumption. The neutral thermal environment varies according to the maturity of the neonate and whether the infant is nursed in an incubator or a radiant heater and is dressed or not. Optimal weight gain and normal physical development occur when a neonate is cared for in a neutral thermal environment appropriate to his or her age and weight. Neonates should be nursed in a neutral thermal environment that maintains the neonate's peripheral temperature at 36.5°C.

Nursing management

Initially, a thorough assessment of the neonate and history are required. Does the neonate look pale? How does the infant feel? Is the infant cool to touch? Is there a difference between central and peripheral temperatures? A hypothermic infant may appear pale and is cool to touch. This is primarily due to vasoconstriction. Is there associated acrocyanosis, a blueish discoloration around the mouth? Is the infant tachypneoic or in respiratory distress? A hypothermic infant may develop respiratory distress secondary to the bodies attempt to maintain a normal temperature consuming oxygen in the process. How does the infant handle? Is the infant irritable or lethargic? Behavioural changes may occur as cold stress continues.

A history should be taken to assist with assessment. Maternal history is important because infants of diabetic mothers are at higher risk of hypothermia due to rapid depletion of glycogen stores. Drugs that mother have received during labour may affect the infant after birth. Side effects of sedatives include hypothermia, hypoglycaemia, lethargy and respiratory depression.

An unstable temperature may indicate infection. If infection is present a full blood count with differential will reveal elevated white cells and a positive result on blood culture analysis. Neurological sequelae, such as absent or poor temperature control and fitting may be significant and a head scan may reveal an intraventricular haemorrhage.

Neonates requiring specialist care should be initially nursed in a prewarmed incubator (38°C). Incubators prevent heat loss through radiation and convection. Radiant warmers similarly prevent heat loss and allow easier access. Care to prevent overheating is vital as hyperthermia can lead to dehydration, hypernatraemia, hyperbilirubinaemia and increased metabolic demands.

Preventive measures are initiated to maintain a normothermic state from delivery onwards. Neonates are initially dried with a warm towel and placed on the mother's abdomen, or dried and dressed. However, ill neonates less than 32 weeks' gestation are placed immediately in a plastic bag to reduce heat loss. A hat is applied prior to transferral to a neonatal unit in an incubator. Minimal handling of an ill hypothermic neonate is important to minimise cold stress.

Rewarming

Slow rewarming of a mildly hypothermic neonate is advocated at about 1°C/hour. However, in neonates with extreme hypothermia, defined as a core temperature less than 35°C, rapid warming is advised to avoid the deleterious effects of metabolic acidosis and prolonged asymptomatic hypoglycaemia.

Temperature measurement

Although rectal temperature recording has been described as the gold standard for core temperature assessment, there are potential problems with this method for example, bowel perforation and cross-infection (Roberton 1992). Intermittent axillary measurement is the most commonly and frequently used method in neonatal care. Accuracy depends on consistent and universal measurement for a duration of 3 minutes at the same site (Sheeran 1996). Continuous skin and core temperature measurements are recorded in critically ill neonates. A temperature gradient is significant determining tissue perfusion.

Activity

On your ward placement at the neonatal unit describe measures taken to:

- prevent cold stress
- warm up a cold infant.

www

Read the following report:

- http://www.neonatology.org.classics/mj1980/ch03.html

Neonatal hypoglycaemia

Hypoglycaemia in the neonate is one of the most common clinical care issues facing the paediatric nurse. Increasing evidence suggests that neonatal hypoglycaemia may have long-term neurological effects (Cowett & Loughead 2002). Care is complicated by inconsistent definitive laboratory values of hypoglycaemia and by variable clinical signs and symptoms in term and preterm neonates.

Definition of hypoglycaemia

Hypoglycaemia is described as a low blood sugar. Neonatal values for low plasma blood sugars vary from below 1.7 mmol/L to below 2.6 mmol/L (Fleming et al 1991). Significant hypoglycaemia depends on the infant's age, weight and clinical status. Neonates are at risk of hypoglycaemia because of a lack of glycogen and fat stores.

Gluconeogenesis

In response to adaptation to extrauterine life, the healthy neonate creates fuel from glycogen and fat. While postnatal hormones mediate this response certain conditions predispose the neonate to hypoglycaemia. There are two main reasons for hypoglycaemia in neonates, the increased utilisation of glucose and the decreased production of glucose stores.

Glucose is obtained from two sources: glycogenolysis and gluconeogenesis. Initially, hepatic and muscle glycogen stores are broken down to form glucose and are rapidly utilised in the first 24 hours. The process of converting glycogen back into glucose is known as glycogenolysis (Tortora & Gabrowski 1993).

In gluconeogenesis, glucose is formed from the breakdown of fats and proteins. Glucocorticoid hormones of the adrenal cortex mobilise proteins and thyroid hormones mobilise proteins and fats thus making glycerol available (Tortora & Gabrowski 1993). Gluconeogenesis is regulated by changes in insulin and glucose ratios, catecholamine release, fatty acid oxidation and activation of liver enzyme production (Stables 1999). Prior to stabilisation at an average blood glucose level of 3.6 mmol/L, neonatal blood glucose levels fall to their lowest level between 2 and 6 hours old (Stables 1999).

Neonates at risk of hypoglycaemia

- Small for gestational age (intrauterine growth retarded)
- Preterm infants
- Hypoxic infants
- Infected infants
- Infants of diabetic mothers
- Hypothermic infants
- Infants with congenital heart disease.

Infants primarily at risk of hypoglycaemia are small for gestational age (SGA) neonates. Reduced glycogen stores combined with increased glucose utilisation account for hypoglycaemic states. Preterm infants are also at risk of hypoglycaemia. In the low birthweight infant, reduced enteral or parenteral intake may explain low plasma glucose levels. Immature hepatocytes, impaired gluconeogenesis and glucogenolytic enzyme activity suggest that preterm neonates are dependent on continuous exogenous nutrition. Hypoxic neonates utilise glucose at an increased rate and are therefore at risk of hypoglycaemia. The main problem is the reduced rate at which glucose is formed during anaerobic glycolysis. The problem is compounded by the fact that the neonate is unable to feed in the regular way due to hypoxic state (Brooks 1997).

Hypothermic infants are also at risk of hypoglycaemia. In an attempt to maintain temperature with normal levels the neonate utilises glycogen and plasma glucose levels fall. Therefore early recognition of the effects of cold stress should involve consideration for administration of glucose intravenous infusion. Infants of diabetic mothers are one of the most common groups of neonates to experience hypoglycaemia. This is due to impaired glucose production and excessive insulin levels from prolonged intrauterine exposure to elevated blood sugar levels.

Infected infants frequently present with hypoglycaemia. Although this could be associated with inadequate calorie intake it is mainly as a result of sepsis-induced increased metabolic rate. Inborn errors of metabolism may give rise to a defective gluconeogenesis.

Clinical signs and symptoms of hypoglycaemia

- Abnormal cry
- Apnoea
- Cardiac arrest
- Coma
- Convulsions
- Cyanosis
- Hypothermia
- Hypotonia
- Jitteriness
- Lethargy
- Tachypnoea
- Tremors.

Sequelae of hypoglycaemia

A significant feature of neonatal hypoglycaemia is that an infant can have extremely low blood sugars without any signs or symptom. Although short-term neonatal hypoglycaemia will not cause CNS damage, prolonged neonatal hypoglycaemia has serious consequences. Neuroglycopenia, the CNS depletion of glucose, can develop with apnoea leading to depression of consciousness and/or convulsions. In the long term, severe hypoglycaemia can lead to severe developmental abnormalities (Roberton & Rennie 2001).

Nursing management of the hypoglycaemic infant

Nursing management is dependent on a thorough assessment of the potentially hypoglycaemic neonate. Knowledge of the causes of hypoglycaemia (hypothermia, poor feeding history), a thorough history to include maternal risk factors (infant of a diabetic) and difficulties during or after delivery (prolonged labour, birth asphyxia), signs (intrauterine growth retarded infant) and symptoms, and a plasma glucose level are important. Care centres on prevention of hypoglycaemia. Avoidance of risk factors is essential. The greatest risk factors are cold stress and poor feeding. Therefore it is important to nurse an infant in a neutral thermal environment. Unless contraindicated due to respiratory illness or birth asphyxia, early feeding is advocated.

Infants at risk of hypoglycaemia should have blood glucose levels monitored 4–6-hourly. If a Haemacue reading is less than 3.0 mmol/L, or YSI of below 2.6, a plasma glucose sample is obtained for analysis. If this result is lower than 2.6 mmol/L, the neonate is fed smaller amounts of milk more frequently by bolus intermittently or continuously via a nasogastric or orogastric tube. Fluid volumes are increased accordingly, usually calculated a day ahead of requirements. A hypoglycaemic neonate should be nursed in a warmed incubator or on a radiant warmer. Hypoglycaemic neonates with an apparently normal temperature may be working excessively to maintain their temperature within normal limits, thereby utilising glucose stores. Therefore it is important to monitor the infant's temperature closely. The neonate is monitored for symptomatic hypoglycaemia and for signs of respiratory distress. A repeat blood sugar level within an hour will indicate the need for further treatment. If the readings are consistently low, intravenous therapy is commenced.

Activity

Amy is an intrauterine growth retarded infant with a plasma glucose of 2.2 mmol/L. Her mother is an insulin-dependent diabetic:

- Describe how you would explain to Amy's breastfeeding mum the importance of feeding Amy via nasogastric tube and nursing her in an incubator.

Neonatal nutrition

Meeting the nutritional needs of a sick and/or premature neonate is vital to his or her recovery and growth. Oral feeding is the desired outcome, however, depending on the age and severity of illness of the neonate, parenteral and enteral routes may have to be considered. An essential component of nursing management is to individualise nutritional requirements.

Growth and development

Physically growth of the intestine and maturation of intestinal absorption continue to develop. At birth, the intestine is approximately 250 cm long and the stomach has a capacity of 90 mL (Kanneh & Davies 2000). Neonates tolerate small amounts of milk and feed frequently. There is a well coordinated suck and swallow reflex. This suck and swallow reflex develops from 34 weeks' gestation onwards. This has implications for feeding preterm infants, although some preterm infants can develop this reflex earlier. In terms of intestinal absorption, pancreatic function is immature hence there are limited enzymes for fat and carbohydrate breakdown. Therefore neonates are at risk of malabsorption characterised by intolerance to feeds. Inadequate liver enzymes can lead to physiological jaundice a common treatable illness of infanthood. Intestinal mucosal immunoglobulin levels are low and neonates are at increased risk of infection, therefore care of feeding equipment is essential. Glycogen stores are depleted in periods of extreme stress of hypoglycaemia and hypothermia. In neonates gluconeogenesis is impaired thereby limiting compensatory responses to adverse conditions of illness. This highlights the importance of adequate nutritional support. In addition to intestinal growth and maturation, the motility function of the gut continues to develop. A measure of gastrointestinal motility is the passage of stools in the first 24 hours of life, however, the more premature the infant the greater the delay in defaecation. Enteral feeding promotes gastric emptying and the release of hormones that can stimulate peristalsis in term and preterm infants (Mertenstein 2002). In neonates, however, the rate of gastric emptying is prolonged.

Nutritional requirements

Ideally, the healthy preterm neonate should gain 15 g/kg/day in weight, 1 cm in length per week and 1 cm in head circumference per week, whereas the term neonate is expected to gain 20–30 g/day (Berseth 2002). Accurate calculation of feeds is essential to ensure the correct volume fluid, on average 150 mL/kg/day and calorific intake, on average 115 mL/kg/day (Kanneh & Davies 2000). Insensible losses are taken into account. Neonates are weighed on admission and twice weekly thereafter, depending on clinical stability and diagnosis. Weights and head circumferences are plotted on graphs called percentile charts. For example, infants on the 10th percentile or graph line means that 10% of the population of infants are smaller and 90% are bigger. Typically, neonates lose 5–10% of their bodyweight in the first week of life. Preterm infants have a higher body water content so may appear to lose more. Infants should have regained their birth weight by 2 weeks of age.

Feeding

The way in which adequate nutritional intake is achieved depends primarily on neonatal well-being and level of maturity. In a well neonate, oral feeding – by breast or bottle – is initiated as soon as possible after delivery and infants are fed on demand. Healthy, low birthweight infants should have a nasogastric tube passed and feeding commenced. Breastfeeding is recommended nutritionally because human milk provides easily digestible protein, fat, carbohydrate and water for normal growth in the term infant (Mertenstein 2002). In terms of anti-infection, breast milk provides immunoglobulins (IgA), leucocytes, complement, lactoferrin and lysozome, which protect the infant from neonatal infections and reduces the incidence of necrotising enterocolitis (Yeo 1998). Breast milk also contains growth hormones and minerals and trace elements necessary for organ maturation and growth. Apart from the nutritional benefits of breastfeeding, the physical and emotional benefits have been well documented, especially for ill or preterm infants. Mothers are encouraged to express breast milk for ill neonates. Expression of breast milk will initiate and maintain lactation. Successful breast expression depends on thoughtful patience and guidance. Breast pumps (electrical or hand) and a breastfeeding room are widely available on neonatal units. Initially, mothers are encouraged to express every 3 hours to stimulate milk production. Breast milk can be frozen for up to 3 months. Once defrosted, it should be used within 4 hours.

Although breast milk is the preferred source of neonatal nutrition, it should be noted that infections such as cytomegalovirus, herpes, hepatitis B and HIV can be transmitted through breast milk. Expressed breast milk samples are routinely sent for culture and sensitivity to detect contamination. Furthermore, certain drugs are excreted in breast milk and women taking these drugs should therefore not express milk. Breast milk given to very low birthweight infants will need to be supplemented because infants weighing less than 1.5 kg require a higher protein and calorific intake. These infants are also at risk of hyponatraemia and therefore need sodium supplements. Calcium and phosphorous supplements reduce the risk of bone growth disorders of prematurity such as metabolic bone disease. Iron stores of infants born at 32–34 weeks or less are deficient and therefore supplemental iron is given with feeds. Folic acid and vitamins are given also (Roberton & Rennie 2001).

Standard infant formulae have been modified to imitate breast milk. Special preterm formulae have been developed to meet high protein and mineral requirements of low birthweight infants. Accurate calculation of fluid requirements is essential to promote infant well-being. In terms of the need for iron and vitamins, new formula feeds compensate this so these may be needed but not necessarily.

WWW

Read about the Department of Health (DoH) infant feeding report at:

- http://www.doh.gov.uk/pdfs/infantfeedingreport.htm

Problems with oral feeding

Prolonged oral ventilation can interfere with the normal function of the mouth and swallowing. Speech therapists play an important role in assisting infants to develop a suck and swallow technique. Oral disorders can interfere with feeding. The normal negative pressure of feeding is impaired in infants with unilateral and bilateral cleft lip and palate; a prosthetic palate will alleviate feeding difficulties. Pierre–Robin syndrome is characterised by poor muscular development and retromicronathia. Feeding is problematic but this can be overcome with the use of soft, elongated teats. Tongue-tie can prevent breastfeeding and therefore may require surgical intervention.

Enteral nutrition

Infants who have difficulties with sucking or who are unable to suck can be fed into the stomach orogastrically, nasogastrically or transpylorically into the small intestine. Gastric feeding may be continuous via syringe pump or intermittently by hourly to 4-hourly bolus feeds. Assessment for complications is essential. Feeds should be discontinued:

- if gastric aspirate every 3–4 hours is greater than the volume of feed
- if there are signs of intestinal obstruction for example, abdominal distension, the presence of bile-stained aspirates or vomitus and failure to pass faeces or passage of blood-stained stools
- if feeding triggers apnoeic attacks
- if the infant has necrotising enterocolitis
- postoperatively.

Non-nutritive sucking is the practice of giving the neonate a dummy during feeding to help the infant associate sucking with the feeling of having a full stomach and improves the sucking reflex.

Parenteral nutrition

Total parenteral nutrition is the administration of total nutritional requirements intravenously to the infant unable to feed for more than 3 days. It is characterised by the gradual increase in fluid, proteins, fats and glucose concentrations to promote normal growth (Table 39.1). Electrolytes are monitored on a daily basis and adjusted accordingly. Light-sensitive vitamins and trace elements are also added to the intravenous solution. Total parenteral nutrition can be given via a peripheral venous line, however, due to the vein sclerosing nature of highly concentrated solutions central venous lines are the preferred method of administration.

Table 39.1 Intravenous feeding guidelines for the neonatal unit (University Hospital of Wales)

	Total daily fluid intake (mL/kg per 24 h)			
Day	Weight <1.5 kg	Weight >1.5 kg	Nitrogen	Intralipid 20% (mL)
1	90	60	–	–
2	110	90	–	–
3	130	110	0.06	–
4	150	140	0.12	2.5
5	170	150	0.18	5.0
6	180	160	0.24	7.5
7	190	170	0.30	10.0
8	200	180	0.30	12.5
9	200	180	0.30	15.0

Reproduced from Yeo (1998).

Reflect on your practice

What feeding related advice would you give to a first-time mother of a severely ill neonate?

Infection in the neonate

Neonates are susceptible to infection due to an immature immune system. Infection of the neonate can be contracted prenatally such as seen in congenital infections, during delivery due to prolonged rupture of membranes (> 24 hours) or maternal infection for example and in the neonatal period either as superficial (umbilical) or systemic infections.

Immunity

There are two types of lymphocyte-mediated immunity in the neonate:

- Cellular immunity, produced by B cell and T cell lymphocytes, enables the infant to produce some antigens in response to infections.
- Humoral immunity, produced by immunoglobulins, offers protection from viruses and bacteria.

Initially, the neonate is protected by maternal immunoglobulins that cross the placenta in utero. Immunoglobulin G (IgG), which is present at birth, carries specific antigens to diseases that the mother has encountered and therefore the infant can produce antibodies in response. IgG potentially offers protection against tetanus, diphtheria, measles, rubella, mumps, as well as common strains of streptococci (Yeo 1998). IgM produced by the fetus offers protection from Gram-negative bacteria such as *Escherichia coli*. IgA is present in breast milk and protects the infant from gut infection.

Nursing care

Nursing care centres on prevention of infection and assessment and early diagnosis of sepsis. Ways to prevent infection are adherence to strict hand washing techniques and wearing gloves (Ramsey & Moules 1998). Infected infants should be nursed in isolation. Equipment should be cleaned regularly. Mothers should be encouraged to provide breast milk for their infant and parental education on the importance of prevention of infection is advocated.

Frequent assessment of the neonate is vital to identify early signs of infection. Signs of infection in the neonate are often subtle. Is the infant quiet? How does the infant look: pale, mottled, jaundiced, presence of a rash? How does the infant handle: irritable, lethargic? How does the infant feel: hot, cool? How is the infant's breathing: fast, slow, using accessory muscles of respiration, nasal flaring? How does the infant feed: slowly, disinterested, vomiting, large aspirates? A septic infant's condition can deteriorate rapidly due to limited compensatory mechanisms.

Pain in the neonate

For paediatric nurses, one of the most challenging situations is managing pain in the patient who cannot speak. It is well established that the neonate can feel pain (Franck 2002). Compared with older children neonates are more sensitive to pain and vulnerable to its long-term effects (Anand 2001).

Physiology of pain

Nociception, i.e. pain perception, is transmitted via pathways in the peripheral and central nervous systems and is fully established by 37 weeks. Research has shown that pain inhibitory pathways are immature at birth, suggesting a developmental hypersensitivity to pain (Franck et al 2000). This means that preterm infants may be at greater risk of pain than the term infant. Behavioural and physiological responses to pain are observed to determine levels of pain in the neonate.

Facially, an infant in pain has a furrowed brow, eyes are closed tightly, nostrils flare, a mouth is unnaturally opened and a grey pallor to face. In terms of movement, an infant in pain will initially display sharp, tense movements and will withdraw the affected limb. As pain intensifies or is prolonged, the infant will lie still with clenched fists, altered breathing and little eye movement. Fingers and toes will be held tightly curled and the infant will cry almost all of the time. The nature of the cry is important. A prolonged, intense, high-pitched cry indicates severe pain. The severity of pain may compromise the infant's respiratory status. A mewing pitiful cry together with apnoea indicates a pre-respiratory failure state. Physiologically, there is increased heart rate, blood pressure is also raised, oxygen saturations fall and there is evidence of palmar sweating (Kanneh & Davies 2000).

Activity

During your placement on the neonatal unit, make a list of the painful procedures that you have observed. Note the infant's response and how the pain was controlled.

Nursing care

The aim of nursing care is to prevent pain and to minimise discomfort in neonates. Therefore infants should be assessed using an appropriate neonatal pain scale, for example the Liverpool Infant Distress Scale (Horgan & Choonara 1998). Currently, audit of pain tools are advocated (Royal College of Nursing (RCN) 2002). Non-pharmaceutical methods are incorporated into the nursing care plan to minimise environment-induced distress. For example, the care of neonates should be consolidated to avoid continuous disturbance. Infants should be handled gently with pre-warmed hands and equipment, and offered gentle reassurance. Minimal handling of ill infants is advocated. Quiet periods during the day should be observed to promote rest. A daytime/night-time pattern should be established. Infants should be shielded from bright lights. Noise levels should be kept to a minimum and alarms attended to promptly. Infants should be contained within soft boundaries to promote a sense of security. Thoughtful use of electrodes and tape is important. Physical pain during blood sampling or intravenous cannulation can be minimised with the administration of oral sucrose via pacifier (Boyd 2002). Also, breastfeeding effectively reduces pain in term neonates undergoing minor invasive procedures (Carbajal 2003). In terms of pharmaceutical management of pain, effective pain relief is essential if indicated. Fentanyl or morphine is administered frequently; paracetamol is also administered. Regular administration of analgesia is important in pain management.

WWW

For further definitive reading, see:

- http://www.cirp.org/library/pain/anand

For guidelines for recognition and assessment of pain in neonates, see:

- http://www.rcn.org.uk

For prevention and management of pain stress in the neonate, see:

- http://www.guideline.gov/summary/ summary.aspx?doc_id=2597&nbr=1823

Neonatal respiratory problems

The most common reason for admission to a neonatal unit is for respiratory difficulties. Respiratory difficulties can be present at delivery, requiring prompt resuscitation and admission to the neonatal unit for further treatment, but they can also occur during the postnatal period.

Clinical signs of respiratory dysfunction

- Cyanosis: the infant becomes 'blue' due to lack of circulating oxygen.
- Tachypnoea: the breathing rate is in excess of 60 breaths per minute.
- Sternal and intercostal recession: this becomes evident as the work of breathing becomes harder. It is more pronounced in preterm infants who have a more pliable rib cage.
- Grunting: infants expel air explosively over a partially closed glottis to attempt to retain some function residual volume so as to maintain alveolar distension.

Activity

Discover how neonatal staff monitor infants for these signs of respiratory difficulties.

Respiratory distress syndrome

The most common respiratory difficulty in preterm infants is respiratory distress syndrome. The more preterm an infant is, the worse the condition is likely to be. In the very preterm infant, the disease is usually present at delivery and needs immediate treatment. In infants of greater gestational age, the disease can be seen to worsen gradually over a period of several hours. All of the clinical signs of respiratory distress are seen.

Respiratory distress syndrome is a disease directly resulting from the fact that the lungs are underdeveloped and the normal system of gaseous exchange is disturbed. One of the main problems is that the squamous epithelial type 2 cells producing surfactant are too immature and so insufficient amounts of surfactant are produced. Surfactant is necessary to reduce the surface tension of the alveoli, allowing continuous partial distension, and thus maintenance of functional residual capacity.

Diagnosis is usually assumed when an X-ray, performed when the infant is at least 4 hours of age, shows a typical 'ground glass' appearance. Duration of this disease is usually 5–7 days.

Treatment

- The severity of the disease can be reduced significantly by the use of antenatal steroids.
- Artificial surfactant is given to any infant with respiratory distress syndrome who is intubated.
- Inspired oxygen is given to maintain oxygen saturations between 85 and 93%.
- Continuous positive airways pressure (CPAP) or intermittent positive pressure ventilation (IPPV) can be used to maintain functional residual volume and to ensure that adequate gaseous exchange is maintained.

Activity

Discover how continuous positive airways pressure works and how it is administered.

Transient tachypnoea of the newborn

The most common condition causing respiratory difficulties in the term infant is transient tachypnoea of the newborn (TTN). This condition is most often seen in infants who are delivered by Caesarean section. The infant absorbs pulmonary alveolar fluid during labour and delivery. This loss of physiological function with Caesarean section is thought to be very significant because the presumed aetiology of tachypnoea of the newborn is transient pulmonary oedema (Kenner et al 1993). All five clinical signs of respiratory distress may be seen, depending on the severity of the condition.

The chest radiograph may show increased perihilar interstitial markings and increased plural fluid, especially in the minor fissure. The duration of the condition is usually 1–3 days.

Treatment

- Inspired oxygen to maintain oxygen saturations above 95%.
- Continuous positive airways pressure or intermittent positive pressure ventilation if maximal inspired oxygen fails to maintain adequate gaseous exchange.

Neonatal pneumonia

Pneumonias may occur at any gestational age. They may be congenital, i.e. onset from birth to 48 hours or age, or nosocomial, i.e. onset after 48 hours of age. They are usually caused by bacteria or a virus. The poorly developed immune system of the neonate makes them more prone first to contracting pneumonia and second to a rapid acceleration of the condition. Pneumonias are even more likely to occur in ventilated neonates (Roberton 1992).

The chest radiograph may show consolidation, interstitial infiltration or, particularly in group B streptococcus pneumonia, a 'ground glass' appearance. The diagnosis of pneumonia is also made by blood cultures, white blood cell count and C-reactive protein count. The duration of the disease is likely to be 5–7 days but may occasionally be prolonged – up to 3 weeks.

Treatment

- Broad-spectrum antibiotics for all infants with any clinical signs of respiratory difficulties: usually benzylpenicillin, gentamicin and/or cefotaxime.
- Specific antibiotic treatment once the organism/sensitivity is known.
- Inspired oxygen to maintain oxygen saturations appropriately.

- Continuous positive airways pressure or intermittent positive pressure ventilation may be used if maximal oxygen fails to maintain adequate gaseous exchange.

Activity

- Name two bacteria and two viruses that cause neonatal pneumonia.
- What is a normal white cell count from birth to 1 week of age?

Principles of nursing management for infant with respiratory distress

- Ensure continuous positive airways pressure or ventilation endotracheal tubes are in the correct position to promote effective ventilation. Secure tubes to minimise trauma to the infant's face.
- Observe for signs of deterioration in condition and report to medical team promptly.
- Maintain oxygen saturations between 90 and 93% in preterm infants and greater than 95% in term neonates.
- Administer analgesia as prescribed; observe for signs of pain.
- Reposition the infant 6-hourly.
- Ensure minimal handling of infants.
- Educate parents to care for their infant.

Persistent pulmonary hypertension of the newborn (PPHN)

- Prolonged constriction of pulmonary blood vessels causes pulmonary hypertension.
- Idiopathic or secondary to:
  - meconium aspiration
  - congenital diaphragmatic hernia
  - sepsis
  - acidosis.
- Treatment:
  - ventilation and oxygen
  - inotropes
  - nitric oxide
  - ECMO.

Meconium aspiration syndrome

- Meconium passed at or before delivery and inhaled in the presence of hypoxia
- Chemical pneumonitis:
  - interstitial oedema
  - small airway obstruction
  - concomitant persistent pulmonary hypertension of the newborn
- Treatment:
  - ventilation and oxygen
  - antibiotics
  - surfactant
  - treatment for persistent pulmonary hypertension of the newborn.

Jaundice

Physiological jaundice

Red blood cells have a lifespan of approximately 120 days. As the life of these red blood cells ends, they need to be destroyed. When red blood cells are destroyed in the liver and the spleen via the reticuloendothelial system, the globin is preserved for reuse and the haem is further broken down. This process produces bilirubin in a fat-soluble, water-insoluble form called unconjugated bilirubin. It cannot be excreted in bile or urine and must be further converted in the liver so that a conjugated, water-soluble bilirubin is produced that can be excreted by the body (Kelner & Harvey 1987).

The bilirubin is carried to the liver for conjugation in the circulating blood. Binding sites are located on the albumin carried in the plasma and the bilirubin binds to these sites until it is passed into the liver cells (the hepatocytes). Once in the hepatocyte, uridine diphosphate-glucoronal transferase joins the bilirubin with a water-soluble glucuronide to create bilirubin monoglucuronide. This is called conjugated bilirubin; this structure is water soluble. It is transferred into the bile for excretion in the stool. In the neonate, several factors combine to overload this normal function.

In utero the fetus has a high haemoglobin level of 18–22 mg/dL as a result of the high number of circulating red blood cells. This allows sufficient transport of oxygen from maternal to fetal cells. At birth these cells are no longer required and must be destroyed. This is helped by fetal red blood cells having a lifespan of 80–100 days. The increased number of red blood cells being broken down means that there are increased amounts of unconjugated bilirubin.

The mechanisms for the transfer and breakdown of bilirubin, ex utero, can take several days to become fully activated. The more preterm the infant, the longer this process can be delayed. This adds to the amount of unconjugated bilirubin.

Once bilirubin has been conjugated and transferred to the intestine, it can be broken down by bilirubin gluconidase, an enzyme found in the small intestine. In the neonate, the passage of stool is slow for the first few days of life and this allows more breakdown by the enzyme. Normal gut flora inhibits this process but it is several days before normal gut flora is present. Also, in breastfed infants there is a continued lack of normal gut flora, which also allows more breakdown. This often causes what is known as 'breast milk jaundice'.

These combined factors result in more unconjugated bilirubin than there are binding sites. Some of this bilirubin can be stored in the skin, which is what gives the infant their yellow colour. There is a limit to how much can be stored in the skin and the excess is carried in the circulating blood with nothing to bind to. This is called 'free' bilirubin. Free bilirubin passes easily through the blood–brain barrier, where it is transferred into the brain cells. This can result in 'kernicterus', which causes brain damage. It is for this reason that it is necessary to provide treatment to restrict the amount of free bilirubin in the circulating blood.

Activity

- Find out which method of assessing for treatment is used in your local neonatal unit.
- What kinds of problem are associated with kernicterus?

Any infant who appears jaundiced will have a blood test taken to measure the serum bilirubin level. If the level is high, treatment will be given. The serum bilirubin level will be tested regularly. Once it falls to low levels, treatment will be discontinued. Assessing whether the levels are high enough for treatment can be done by plotting the level against a universal chart.

Treatment with phototherapy is invariably successful. This is the use of a specific wavelength of light onto the skin. This light wavelength causes a chemical reaction in the bilirubin stored in the skin. This reaction changes the stored unconjugated bilirubin into conjugated bilirubin, which can be excreted.

One of the side effects of phototherapy treatment is that it accelerates the digestive process, resulting in diarrhoea. This actually enhances the reduction of bilirubin because it allows less time for bilirubin gluconidase to breakdown the conjugated bilirubin. The light can be delivered by a lightbox placed over the cot or incubator. This means that the infant must be naked for the light to fall on the skin. Infants may need to be transferred to an incubator if they are unable to maintain their core temperature when naked. Phototherapy can also be given via a 'biliblanket': a fibreoptic light source is used to provide the appropriate wavelength of light into a specially developed small rectangular 'blanket', which can be wrapped around the infant's torso and used underneath the clothes. This causes less disruption to the infant and is more acceptable to parents. Treatment usually lasts for 3–7 days.

Non-physiological jaundice

The most common cause of non-physiological jaundice is incompatibility of blood groups. This problem used to be more common than it is now because the Rhesus blood proteins are highly antigenic, causing severe jaundice. The introduction of anti-D for any antenatal event and post-delivery for women whose partner has a different blood group has reduced the incidence of this condition significantly.

ABO incompatibility is probably more common than Rhesus incompatibility but is usually mild and does not require treatment other than phototherapy. However, in some instances the condition is very severe and requires prompt and efficacious management.

The best treatment commences antenatally with all pregnant women being screened for blood group and for antibodies. Sometimes there is no indication of problems until hydrops is seen on scan. It is possible for some fetuses to have in utero transfusions to maintain the pregnancy until viability. Fetuses are affected to varying degrees. In the most severe cases, there is fetal anaemia, cardiac failure, oedema and hydrops. The prognosis is poor and only immediate exchange transfusions provide any hope of survival.

In less severe cases, the infant may appear normal at birth but signs of clinical jaundice become apparent within hours of delivery. Jaundice is never a normal finding before 24 hours of age and if there is any doubt a serum bilirubin level must be measured. If there is any indication of problems blood for a Coombs test should be taken at delivery.

Phototherapy will be given in the first instance. There is no evidence to support the theory that double phototherapy is more effective as this process is rate-limited. If the level rises too high then an exchange transfusion will be given. This procedure aims to remove the affected blood and replace it with blood that has normal erythrocytes and a normal bilirubin level. Thus it will relieve anaemia and help to prevent kernicterus. Assessing whether an exchange transfusion is required can be done by plotting the serum bilirubin level against a universal chart. If the serum bilirubin level is above this number then an exchange transfusion should be given.

In severe cases, several exchange transfusion may be required before the infant's condition becomes stabilised.

www

For current British Neonatal Practice, see:

- http://www.neonatal-nursing.co.uk

Activity

- Describe what a Coombs test is and why it is helpful?
- What other tests can be used?
- What are the principles of undertaking an exchange transfusion?

Nursing care issues

- Undressing infants can lead to hypothermia, requiring incubator care.
- The use of the phototherapy lamp can increase the ambient temperature surrounding the infant. The set incubator temp should be reduced by 1°C for all infants already being nursed in an incubator.
- Care should be taken that infants are changed regularly to avoid skin problems.
- Nappies should be used to ensure gonads are protected at all times.
- Eye shields must be used at all times to prevent the slight risk of retinal damage.

- Feeding and interaction with parents should be actively encouraged. Up to 4 hours in 24 hours out from under the phototherapy lamp does not affect treatment levels as treatment is rate-limited.
- Attention to good nutrition and adequate fluids are essential to avoid dehydration and/or weight loss.
- Constant reassurance of family members is usually required.

Parents

Parents feel a sense of loss for the interrupted pregnancy or an unexpected outcome. They may feel a sense of isolation from others and each other. The inability to produce a healthy infant, coupled with the inability to protect an ill neonate from invasive and sometimes painful procedures, leaves the parents feeling inadequate. In essence, parents are not only the mourning the loss of their perfect infant but anticipate the grief for the potential loss of their newborn. The birth of an ill or premature neonate has an overwhelming destabilising effect on parents. Many parents of newborns go through identifiable behaviours similar to a grief response. Parents' initial reaction to the birth of an ill infant is one of acute shock, characterised by irrational behaviour, feelings of despair and crying. Parents may feel guilty and blame themselves or each other for the unexpected outcome. Feelings of guilt are followed by feelings of anger and resentment, which can be internalised or directed towards healthcare professionals. With empathetic care parents can learn to cope and adapt as they are taught how to care and become increasingly involved in their infant's life. Psychosocial meetings provide a forum to discuss current and anticipated problems that may arise during provision of neonatal care. Healthcare professionals endeavour to promote attachment between the infant and family in a supportive and nurturing environment.

Attachment

Since the 1970s it has been acknowledged that the interaction between newborn infants and their families is essential in establishing good family dynamics. However, it has taken a long time to break down the barriers to interaction and integration, and the art of promoting family interaction is still one of the most challenging areas of neonatal nursing today. Often, the neonatal nurses can be the greatest barrier to parenting in the neonatal intensive care unit because they are seen as the gatekeepers to the infants (Griffin 1990).

Currently, most neonatal units encourage parents to visit their infant/infants whenever they choose. However, any indication by the staff that parents are interfering with the routine of the unit or that the nurses are too busy to speak to them will result in parents staying for a minimum of time and they will be reluctant to return. When families are given restricted visiting times or have restrictions on who may visit without good explanations, this can make the whole family, including the parents, feel unwanted and unwelcome in the unit.

Neonatal units are busy, noisy, bustling places, caring for a range of infants, some of whom are very ill and require constant, highly technical care. This environment is very frightening for parents and can make them reluctant to visit their infant at all and reluctant to touch or cuddle their infant, because they are frightened that this may make their condition worsen. In fact, research has shown that positive touch is essential to good developmental outcomes. It is therefore imperative that neonatal nurses are proactive in ensuring that contact and interaction are initiated as soon as possible after admission and are sustained until discharge (Harrison et al 1996).

Being welcoming and making as much time for parents as they want or need seems very simple but it is important because it allows parents to relax and spend time getting to know their new infant. One of the most important aspects of this care is to include parents in plans and decisions about the care of their infant, by ensuring that they are fully informed and that their views are sought. As much written information as possible should also be given as verbal information is soon forgotten in stressful situations. Recognition of the mother by the infant is said to occur after eye contact over a 72-hour period. In infants without health problems, mothers spend many hours cuddling and gazing at their infant. This recognition is established within a few days but is delayed when an infant is ill. Therefore the neonatal nurse should encourage cuddling and gazing whenever possible to establish early recognition.

Kangaroo care, where parents spend extended time cuddling their infant with skin-to-skin contact, has been proven to improve the condition of the infant in the short term and to improve developmental outcomes in the long term and should be encouraged.

WWW

For information on neonatal death see:

- http://www.uk-sands.org

Summary

Neonatal nursing is as challenging as it is rewarding. As neonatal care continues to evolve it is important for paediatric nurses to develop evidence-based practice and to keep abreast with changes. A neonate's outcome rests in nurses' hands.

References

Anand, J.K.S., 2001. Consensus statement for the prevention and management of pain in the newborn. Archives of Pediatrics and Adolescent Medicine 155, 297–303.

Avery, G.B., 1987. Neonatology. Pathophysiology and management of the newborn, 3rd edn. Lippincott, Philadelphia.

Berseth, C.L., 2001. Feeding methods for the preterm infant. Seminars in Neonatology 6, 417–424.

Boyd, S., 2002. Sucrose analgesia: a realistic alternative to conventional pharmacology for pain relief in neonates. Journal of Neonatal Nursing 8 (6), 184–190.

Brooks, C., 1997. Neonatal hypoglycaemia. Neonatal Network 16 (2), 15–21.

Campbell, S., Glasper, E.A. (Eds.), 1999. Whaley and Wong's nursing care of infants and children, 6th edn. Mosby, St Louis.

Carbajal, R., 2003. Analgesic effect of breastfeeding in term neonates: randomised controlled trial. British Medical Journal 326, 13–15.

Cowett, R.M., Loughead, J.L., 2002. Neonatal glucose metabolism: differential diagnosis, evaluation and treatment. Neonatal Network 21 (4), 9–18.

Crawford, D., Morris, M., 1994. Neonatal nursing. Chapman and Hall, Bury St Edmunds.

Fleming, P.J., Speidel, B.D., Marlow, N., 1991. A neonatal vade mecum, 2nd edn. Edward Arnold, London.

Franck, L.S., 2002. Some pain, some gain: reflections on the past two decades of neonatal pain research and treatment. Neonatal Network 21 (5), 37–41.

Franck, L.S., Greenberg, C.S., Stevens, B., 2000. Pain assessment in infants and children. Pediatric Clinics of North America 47 (3), 487–512.

Griffin, T., 1990. Nurse barriers to parenting the special care nursery. Journal of Perinatal Neonatal Nursing 4 (2), 56–57.

Hackman, P.S., 2001. Recognising and understanding the cold-stressed term infant. Neonatal Network 20 (8), 35–41.

Harrison, L., Olivet, L., Cunningham, K., et al., 1996. Effects of gentle human touch on preterm infants: pilot study results. Neonatal Network 15 (26), 35–42.

Horgan, M.F., Choonara, S., 1998. The Liverpool infant distress scale. Paediatric and Perinatal Drug Therapy 2, 14–16.

Kanneh, A., Davies, F., 2000. Physical characteristics and physiological features of the full term neonate: theory, practice integration. Part 1. Journal of Neonatal Nursing 6 (1), 4–8.

Kelner, J.H., Harvey, D., 1987. The sick newborn baby, 2nd edn. Baillière Tindall, London.

Kenner, C., Brueggemeyer, A., Gunderson, L.P. (Eds.), 1993. Comprehensive neonatal nursing: a physiologic perspective. WB Saunders, Philadelphia.

Klaus, M.H., Fanaroff, A.A., 1993. Care of the high-risk neonate, 4th edn. WB Saunders, Philadelphia.

Mertenstein, G.B.M., 2002. Handbook of neonatal intensive care, 5th edn. Mosby Year Book, St Louis.

Ramsey, T., Moules, J., 1998. The textbook of children's nursing. Stanley Thornes, Cheltenham.

Roberton, N.R.C. (Ed.), 1992. Textbook of neonatology, 2nd edn. Edward Arnold, London.

Roberton, N.R.C., Rennie, J., 2001. Neonatal intensive care, 4th edn. Edward Arnold, London.

Royal College of Nursing (RCN), 2002. Clinical practice guidelines. The recognition and assessment of acute pain in children. Audit protocol. Royal College of Nursing, London.

Sheeran, M.S., 1996. Thermoregulation in neonates. Journal of Neonatal Nursing 2 (4), 6–9.

Stables, D., 1999. Physiology in childbearing with anatomy and related biosciences. Ballière Tindall, Edinburgh.

Tortora, G.J., Grabowski, S.R., 1993. Principles of anatomy and physiology, 7th edn. Harper Collins, New York.

Turrill, S., 2003. A focus of care for neonatal nursing: the relationship between neonatal nursing. Practice and outcomes. Paediatric Nursing 15 (5), 30–34.

Warren, I., 2002. Facilitating infant adaptation: the nursery environment. Seminars in Neonatology 7, 459–467.

Yeo, H., 1998. Nursing the neonate, 1st edn. Blackwell Science, Oxford.

Further Reading

BAPM, 1996. Standards for hospitals providing neonatal intensive care. BAPM, London.

Health problems during infancy

40

Kathy Scanlon Anna-Lisa Sorrentino Maureen Harrison
Terri Fletcher Gill Prudhoe

ABSTRACT

Infancy is a period of remarkable growth and development. Between 1 month and 12 months of age the infant will undergo major changes in physical development. Motor skills, cognition and social skills develop at a rapid pace during this period. The roles of nature and nurture contribute to the growth and development of the infant in both positive and negative ways. Nature, or heredity, has significant influence on general growth and development correlating around related family size and patterns of maturation. Nurture, or the environment, including diet, again plays a significant role for the developing infant. The infant remains dependent on adults to identify health needs and detect health problems. This chapter will focus on the following four significant areas that influence the growth and development of the infant: nutrition, skin (and specifically atopic eczema), sleep and immunisation. These topics have been identified as significant because problems in these areas can impair the growth and development of the infant both in the short term and long term into later life.

LEARNING OUTCOMES

- Discuss the effects of nutrition on growth and development.
- Explain how skin conditions (e.g. atopic eczema) can affect the developing infant.
- Outline the role of sleep in an infant's development.
- Discuss the role of immunisation for infant health.

Nutrition

Nutrition in the first year of life plays an important role in a child's development and energy intake has been shown to positively correlate with weight gain in the first year of life (Heinig et al 1993). An infant grows more in the first 6 months of life than at any other time. The early period of infancy is where important changes in diet and nutritional needs occur, e.g. weaning onto solid food. The importance of nutrition and how good nutrition can determine the growth and development of the child is clearly recognised. Research by Barker (1990), Barker et al (2002) and Eriksson et al (2001) suggests that nutritional status in infancy can be linked to ill health in adult life. Periods of nutritional deficiency during infancy have been linked with ischaemic heart disease, stroke, hypertension and non-insulin diabetes mellitus in middle age (Department of Health (DoH) 2003). Adequate nutrition is also essential for intellectual development (Richards et al 1998, Singhal et al 2001).

Milk feeds

The DoH (2003) clearly identifies that breastfeeding is the optimum form of nutrition for infants in the first 6 months of life as breast milk provides all the balanced nutrients an infant needs.

The National Institute for Clinical Excellence (NICE 2008) recommends the promotion of breastfeeding for all women during antenatal consultations and midwives should particularly encourage women with a family history of allergy, young

TABLE 40.1 Breast milk is the best form of nutrition for infants

Benefits to infant	Benefits to mother
Less likely to develop gastrointestinal, respiratory and urinary infections	Reduced risk of developing pre-menopausal breast cancer
Less likely to develop obesity in later childhood	Increased likelihood of returning to pre-pregnancy weight
Less likely to develop type 1 diabetes	Delayed resumption of the menstrual cycle
Less likely to develop atopic disease	
Promotes gut development and function	

Adapted from Infant Feeding Recommendation (DoH 2003)

DOI: 10.1016/B978-0-7020-3183-0.10040-2

women, those who have low educational achievement and those from disadvantaged groups.

Mothers should be supported in their choice of infant feeding, however should it be their choice to formula feed a commercial iron-fortified formula should be substituted. All mothers who choose to use infant formula should be shown how to make up a feed before leaving hospital or before the mother is left after a home birth (NICE 2008).

Current legislation provides strict controls on the advertising and labelling of all types of formula feeds to ensure that breast-feeding rates are not affected by the promotion of such products. In addition formula milks must show clear differentiation between infant formula (0–6 months) and follow-on formula (after 6 months) (DoH 2009a). 'Follow-on' milks have higher protein and mineral content than standard infant formula. Unmodified cow's milk should not be given as a main drink before 1 year of age (DoH 1994) because it is low in iron and vitamin C.

WWW

Read the DoH guidelines on breastfeeding at:

- http://www.doh.gov.uk

Milk calculations

To calculate the correct quantity of milk feed for an infant who is full-term, and developing within normal parameters, it is important to consider expected weight gains and losses. Weight gain is expected to be in the region of 200 g per week during the first 3 months of life, although, as the infant first adapts to the environment, there is an expected weight loss within the first 2 weeks of life. This usually constitutes a loss of approximately 10% of body weight, i.e. if an infant weighs 3.5 kg at birth, there will be an estimated loss of 350 g.

Achieving weight gain

To achieve weight gain, the infant is offered 150 mL/kg of body weight every 24 hours, i.e. if the infant weighs 3.5 kg:

$$150\,\text{mL} \times 3.5 = 525\,\text{mL}/24\,\text{hours}$$

It is then necessary to divide this overall quantity into a set number of feeds. Under normal circumstances, an infant in the first month of life will be offered feeds approximately every 4 hours, which equates to six feeds in 24 hours:

$$525\,\text{mL}/6 = 87.5\,\text{mL}$$

Therefore one needs to prepare 90 mL of feed in each bottle (Hubbard & Trigg 2000).

Activity

- Use the above formula to calculate the quantity of feed an infant weighing 4 kg needs in 24 hours.
- Then calculate the amount required for each feed if six feeds are required per day.

Activity

- Identify the constituents of commercial iron fortified formula milk.
- Compare and contrast those constituents with breast milk.

Weaning

Weaning is the process of gradually changing an infant's diet from milk alone to a combination of milk and solids (DoH 1994, DoH 2008). This also involves the process of giving up one method of feeding for another, which for infants usually refers to relinquishing the breast or bottle for a cup and spoon. It is a psychologically significant period because the infant is required to give up a major source of oral pleasure and gratification. Weaning is generally regarded as a major task for infants with the development of independence involving participation in the social activity of meal times. The major change in feeding is the addition of solid foods to the infant's diet.

When to start weaning

Weaning should start when the infant reaches 6 months of age (DoH 2003, DoH 2008). Many parents according to Foote et al (2003), Hamlyn et al (2000) and Fewtrell (2003) choose to give solid foods before 6 months. However, parents should be encouraged to continue milk feeds until at least 4 months (17 weeks). Weaning should not commence before 4 months because the immature digestive and renal systems cannot cope with solid foods (DoH 1994, Scientific Advisory Committee on Nutrition 2003). Parents should be encouraged to view 4 months (17 weeks) as the earliest time to commence weaning.

It is imperative that individual circumstances are considered when health professionals are giving advice on the age for the introduction of solid foods. At 6 months of age infants reach a transition period. By this time the gastrointestinal tract has matured sufficiently to handle more complex nutrients and is less sensitive to potentially allergenic foods. Tooth eruption is beginning, which facilitates biting and chewing (DoH 1994, Hockenberry 2003).

Activity

- With the advent of the primary dentition which teeth appear first?
- Which other aspect of infant development does the development of chewing aid?

Eating a weaning diet requires the infant to have a level of neuromuscular coordination that may not be achieved prior to 6 months, e.g. holding the head in an upright position, sitting up. Around 6 months of age, the tongue-thrust reflex, which causes food to be pushed out of the mouth, is reducing. Chewing motions and the ability to move food to the back of the mouth and swallow are developing (DoH 1994, DoH 2003, Hockenberry 2003). Therefore, developmentally, the infant becomes ready to move into the weaning stage.

Table 40.2 The weaning period

Age	Suggested diet	Developmental tasks
6 months	Start weaning with bland foods The DoH (2003) recommends iron-enriched infant rice cereal as a starter food, e.g. baby rice. Smooth purées of vegetables, e.g. potato, swede, parsnip and fruit purées, e.g. pear, banana	Accustom infant to taking food from a spoon
From 7 months to 8–9 months	Introducing a variety of textures Purées of increasing variety of vegetables, meats, fruits Thicker purees gradually progressing to a lumpy texture, e.g. mashed vegetables As the infant progresses then move on to minced chicken, meat, fish or lentils and pulses like kidney beans Lumpier finger foods including chopped hard-boiled eggs, cubed or grated hard cheese, raw soft fruit and vegetables, e.g. tomato, banana	Expose to different textures and different tastes Develop ability to chew and swallow Start 'finger' feeding Introduce cup
Around 9–12 months	Continue progression with textures Wholemeal breads, cereals and pasta Chopped meats, chicken, fish and live Lightly cooked or raw vegetables and fruits A variety of textures for potatoes, noodles, and puddings, e.g. rice pudding Unsweetened orange juice as a drink with meals	Progress to a mature diet of 3 main meals with 2 or 3 snacks during the day
1 year	Adult texture Family meals: take the infant's portion out before adding salt and leave as adult texture, chop to bite size if needed Whole milk as a drink	Progress to self-feeding by continuing with finger foods Developing social skills by participating in family meals

The weaning diet should consist of foods from all main food groups: carbohydrates, proteins, fats and oils, and sugars as well as fruit and vegetables (Table 40.2). However, when preparing foods for the infant, additional salt and sugar should be avoided due to the immaturity of kidneys and liver (DoH 1994).

New foods should be added to the infant diet one at a time. Infant cereal may be given mixed with modified formula milk in a bowl. If the infant is breast fed the cereal can be mixed with expressed breast milk or water. Fruit juices can be mixed with the dry cereal – the vitamin C content of the juice enhances the absorption of iron. Vitamin C is destroyed by heat and juice should therefore not be warmed. Offer fruit juice from a cup rather than a bottle to prevent the development of dental caries.

WWW

Visit the DoH website and read the report on infant feeding:

- http://www.doh.gov.uk/public/infantfeedingreport.htm

Food intolerance

The terms 'food intolerance' and 'food allergy' are often used interchangeably. However, the conditions are very different.

Foods to avoid

Common foods such as milk, eggs, soya, wheat, peanuts, tree nuts (e.g. hazelnuts), sesame seeds and, in older children, fish and shellfish, which form about 90% of cases of food allergy should be avoided.

Cow's milk intolerance

According to Fiocchi et al (2003), cow's milk intolerance is a multifaceted disorder representing adverse systemic and local gastrointestinal reactions to cow's milk protein. The hypersensitivity may be manifest through a variety of signs and symptoms. These may appear within 45 minutes of milk ingestion or after a period of several days, e.g. cow's milk intolerance may be manifest as colic or sleeplessness in an otherwise healthy infant. The diagnosis is made after careful history taking.

Cow's milk allergy

Allergy to cow's milk affects 2–7% of infants under 1 year old. It is the most common food allergy in childhood (David 1993, Williams 1999). Children usually grow out of milk allergy by the age of 3, but about 20% of these children will still be allergic to milk as adults.

Cow's milk allergy is caused by a reaction to a number of allergens in cow's milk. The protein in milk can be broken down into curds (casein), which form when milk sours. Whey is the watery part that is left when the curd is removed. A reaction can also be triggered by small amounts of milk received through the mother's breast milk from dairy products she has eaten, or, from feeding cow's milk to the infant.

The symptoms of milk allergy are often mild and can affect any part of the body. In more severe episodes symptoms can include rashes, diarrhoea, vomiting, stomach cramps and difficulty in breathing. In a very few cases, milk allergy can cause anaphylaxis.

Table 40.3 Cow's milk intolerance: generalised signs and symptoms

Digestive	Respiratory	Dermatological	Behaviour	Generalised
Diarrhoea	Sneezing	Eczema	Excessive crying	Failure to thrive
Vomiting	Coughing	Urticaria	Sleeplessness	Retarded growth
Colic	Chronic nasal discharge	Vascular	Hyperactivity	Malnutrition
Abdominal pain	Asthma	Facial pallor	Lethargy	
Haematochezia (bloody stools)	Bronchitis	Infraorbital oedema (swelling under the eyes)		
Malabsorption	Recurrent croup			
Enteropathy	Otitis media			
Constipation				
Anorexia				

Process of diagnosis

- A good history: including family allergic predisposition.
- Diagnostic tests: stool analysis for blood (frank and occult bleeding can occur from colitis), serum levels of immunoglobulin E (IgE) and skin-prick testing.
- Milk elimination: the most definitive diagnostic strategy is elimination of milk, followed by challenge testing after improvement of symptoms.

Therapeutic management

- Simple exclusion diet: eliminate a single food or food constituent.
- Multiple food exclusion diet: elimination of all dairy products.

Infants fed cow's milk formula are managed primarily by changing the formula to a casein or whey hydrolysate milk formula in which the protein has been broken down (or predigested) into its amino acids through enzymatic hydrolysis.

Soya-based formula is not recommended because as many as 20% of these infants are also allergic to soya (Fiocchi et al 2003). Goat milk and sheep milk are not appropriate substitutes either plus they are deficient in folic acid.

Infants who are breast fed but have symptoms of cow's milk hypersensitivity (Table 40.3) are treated by eliminating all dairy products from the lactating mother's diet. These mothers need vitamin D and calcium supplementation. Infants are maintained on the dairy-free diet for 1–2 years, after which time very small quantities of milk are reintroduced.

Differences between food allergy and food intolerance

The differences between food allergy and food intolerance are shown in Table 40.4.

Activity

- How would you explain cow's milk allergy to a parent/caregiver?

Table 40.4 Food allergy and food intolerance

Food allergy	Food intolerance
An immediate reaction	Often delayed reaction – from hours to days
Reaction is local	May affect remote organs
Usually IgE-mediated	Rarely IgE-mediated
Cause is normally easily detected	Often has multiple food causes Cause may be evident only after a period of avoidance

Implications for nursing

The principle nursing objectives are assessment and identification of potential milk allergy and appropriate health education advice and counselling of parents regarding substitute milk feeds.

The protein-hydrolysed formulae are less palatable than milk-based formulae. Consequently, reluctance to accept the new formula by the infant may be a problem. This can be overcome by introducing the formula gradually over a period of days. Parents also need to be reassured that the infant will receive complete nutrition from the new formula and will suffer no ill effects from the absence of cow's milk.

Once solid foods are started, parents require guidance in avoiding all associated milk products during weaning. This requires carefully reading all food labels to avoid potential addition of milk products to the prepared food.

Activity

When you next go shopping examine food labels for inclusion of milk products:

- Discuss your findings with your mentor.
- What information can you now give to parents following this activity?

Lactose intolerance

Lactose intolerance is the reduced ability to digest milk sugars due to insufficient production of the enzyme lactase, which breaks down the sugar lactose for digestion. The resulting intolerance causes symptoms such as bloating, abdominal pain and diarrhoea shortly after ingesting milk products:

- Congenital lactose intolerance: appears soon after birth when the diet contains lactose from milk.
- Late-onset lactose intolerance: is similar to the congenital type but manifests later in life.

Milk from mammals including cows, goats, sheep and humans, contains lactose. This means that goat and sheep milk are not suitable alternatives to cow's milk for infants and children with this condition.

Management

There is no medical treatment (Food Standards Agency (FSA) 2003) for lactose intolerance but the symptoms can be avoided by controlling the amount of lactose in the diet. This requires elimination of dairy products in the diet. In infants, a soya-based formula can be substituted for cow's milk formula or human milk. As dairy products are a major source of calcium and vitamin D, supplementation of these nutrients is needed to prevent any deficiency.

Identification of sources of lactose is required, e.g. especially hidden sources such as bulk agents in certain medications. Check with the pharmacist regarding this possibility when ordering medications of any sort.

Vegetarian diets

The potential for nutritional deficiencies in vegetarian diets for infants cannot be overemphasised. Achieving a nutritionally adequate vegetarian diet is not difficult but requires careful planning and knowledge of nutrient sources.

The major nutrient deficiencies (Table 40.5) that may occur in the stricter vegetarian diets are inadequate protein required for growth, inadequate calories for energy and growth, poor digestibility of many of the natural, unprocessed foods, especially for infants. Deficiencies of vitamin B12, niacin, thiamine, riboflavin, vitamin D, iron, calcium and zinc also occur (Hamlyn et al 2000, Savoie & Rioux 2002, Shaw & Pal 2002).

When solid foods are introduced, the safety and digestibility of the foods should be reviewed. Raw fruits with seeds and nuts are dangerous for infants because of the risk of aspiration. Beans, grain cereals and vegetables should be served well cooked and pureed or mashed to aid digestibility during infancy.

Activity

- Plan a healthy, nutritious diet for a lactovegetarian infant who has started weaning. Provide a rationale for your choices.

Ensuring the right foods

To ensure sufficient protein in the vegetarian diet, foods with incomplete proteins (those that do not have all of the essential amino acids) must be eaten at the same meal with other foods that supply the missing amino acids. The three basic combinations of foods consumed by vegetarians that generally provide the appropriate amounts of essential amino acids are:

- grains (cereal, rice, pasta) and legumes (beans, peas, lentils, peanuts)
- grains and dairy products (milk, cheese, yoghurt)
- seeds (sesame, sunflower) and legumes.

The best assurance of nutritional adequacy is to eat a variety of foods. Families need guidelines for selecting foods that provide essential nutrients without exceeding energy requirements. Nurses and health visitors involved in the care of infants play an important part in the health education process. By understanding the factors such as cultural and religious dietary needs that may influence the decisions parents make concerning weaning, health professionals can adapt recommended weaning guidelines appropriately for individual families (Shaw & Pal 2002).

Activity

- Plan an appropriate weaning diet for an infant of the Islamic faith. Include halal meat in the diet.

Growth and failure to thrive

Altered growth, or failure to thrive (FTT), refers to a state of inadequate growth from inability to obtain and or use calories required for growth. It is a symptom not a disease. Thorough assessment of nutritional intake, physiological growth parameters and family needs are necessary to develop plans of care to promote nutritional intake for growth and development (Wells 2002). There are two general categories of failure to thrive:

- Organic failure to thrive: can occur as a result of a physical cause. Examples of physical causes include congenital

Table 40.5 Vegetarian diets

Types of vegetarian diet	Foods included/excluded	Potential nutrient deficiencies
Lacto-ovovegetarian	Exclude meat from their diet but include milk, eggs and sometimes fish	Protein intake needs monitoring
Lactovegetarian	Exclude meat and eggs but include and drink milk	Low in protein as well as iron
Vegan	Eliminate any food of animal origin, including milk and eggs	Low in protein, minerals, calcium
Macrobiotic	More restrictive than pure vegetarian diet. Cereals, especially brown or polished rice, are the mainstay of the diet	Low in protein, minerals, calcium

heart defects, neurological conditions, chronic renal failure, malabsorption syndrome, endocrine dysfunction, disease processes (as in cystic fibrosis and AIDS).

- Non-organic failure to thrive: most often the result of psychosocial factors unrelated to physical disease. Factors may include inadequate knowledge of nutritional needs of infants, stressors affecting the family, social problems (Krugman & Dubowitz 2003).

Assessment

Growth measurements alone are not used to diagnose children with failure to thrive. The finding of persistent deviation from an established growth curve is cause for concern. Percentile charts should be used for all infants. If weight and height measurements fall off the percentile indicated by birth weight for that percentile then failure to thrive should be considered.

Activity

- Examine a variety of assessment tools used to assess growth and development of infants.

Reflect on your practice

- How were the growth and development charts used for the assessment of an infant with poor growth that you have nursed?
- Did the assessment tools provide all the necessary information needed to develop an appropriate plan of care?
- What other information was required?

Factors leading to inadequate feeding

- Health education: i.e. inadequate nutritional health education for parents.
- Attachment disturbance: with maternal–child attachment relationships.
- Health beliefs: concerning the constituents of a healthy diet.
- Family stress: which may include financial worries, substance misuse, marital problems, mental health problems, e.g. depression.

The above factors require assessment and the infant may require hospitalisation for an assessment of physiological status. The needs of the family will also need to be assessed. The multidisciplinary team, including social workers, health visitors, dietitians, will play an important role in the assessment and planning of appropriate interventions to support the family in providing for the nutritional needs of the infant.

Eczema

Atopic eczema

Infantile eczema is also known as atopic dermatitis or atopic eczema; the terms are often used synonymously. The term atopic eczema will used here.

Atopic eczema is an inflammation of a genetically sensitive skin (Cork 1999). Eczema is a symptom rather than a disorder. The condition is multifactorial and indicates that the infant is oversensitive to certain substances, called allergens, which can gain entry to the body via four methods:

- Digestive tract: in foods
- Inhalation: dust, pollen
- Direct contact: wool, soap, strong sunlight
- Injections: insect bites, vaccines.

Atopic eczema is rarely seen in breastfed babies until they begin to get additional food. The condition appears to have a definite familial tendency and emotional factors are often involved. Atopic eczema usually begins around 2–6 months of age and generally undergoes spontaneous remission by 3 years of age. The infant has a greater than normal risk of developing dry skin and eczema later in life.

Eczema may occur later in childhood at 2–3 years and in most cases the skin heals by age 5 years (Cork 1997). Preadolescent and adolescent eczema begins at about 12 years of age and may continue into adulthood. Some children develop the triad of atopic eczema, asthma and hay fever. The 2007 NICE guidelines confirm that the assessment of any child presenting with eczema-type symptoms should ascertain a family history of asthma or hay fever.

Location and development of atopic eczema

When atopic eczema occurs during infancy it affects each infant differently in terms of both onset and severity of signs and symptoms. A rash may first appear in patches around the cheeks and chin, combined with local vasodilation, which gives the rash a red appearance. This can progress to spongiosis (the breakdown of the dermal skin cells and the development of intradermal vesicles) (Spagnola & Korb 2002). This can be seen as red, scaling, oozing skin. Scratching can eventually produce a weeping skin. The skin may then become infected. Chronic scratching produces lichenification or coarsening of the skin folds. Aycliffe (2009) in a comprehensive review of the management of eczema confirms that more girls than boys are affected by the disease.

Once the infant becomes more mobile and begins crawling, exposed areas, such as the inner and outer parts of the arms and legs, may also be affected. Atopic eczema may also affect the skin around the eyes, the eyelids, and the eyebrows and lashes. Scratching and rubbing the eye area can cause the skin to redden and swell. Rubbing also causes patchy loss of eyebrows and eyelashes. Over time, atopic eczema may lead to development of an extra fold of skin under the eyes.

An infant with atopic eczema may be restless and irritable because of the itching and discomfort of the disease (Table 40.6). Difficulty in sleeping can occur due to the nature of pruritus.

Activity

- Access the companion PowerPoint presentation. You will find a diagram of the skin: identify the areas of altered physiology as described below.

Table 40.6 Atopic eczema

Feature	Dermatological description
Red and inflamed area	Erythema
Intense itching sensation	Pruritus
Hives (red, raised bumps) that may occur after exposure to an allergen, at the beginning of flares, or after exercise or a hot bath	Urticaria
Breakdown of dermal cells and the formation of intradermal vesicles	Spongiosis
Small raised bumps that may open when scratched and become crusty and infected	Papules
Small, rough bumps, generally on the face, upper arms, and thighs	Keratosis pilaris
Thick, leathery skin resulting from constant scratching and rubbing	Lichenification
An extra fold of skin that develops under the eye	Atopic pleat (Dennie-Morgan fold)
Eyelids that have become darker in colour from inflammation or hay fever	Hyperpigmented eyelids
Inflammation of the skin on and	Cheilitis around the lips
Dry, rectangular scales on the skin	Ichthyosis
Increased number of skin creases on the palms	Hyperlinear palms

Altered physiology

Researchers including Cork (1997) have observed differences in the skin of those with atopic eczema that may contribute to the symptoms of the disease.

The outer layer of skin, the epidermal layer, is divided into two parts: an inner part containing moist, living cells, and an outer part, known as the horny layer or stratum corneum, containing dry, flattened, dead cells. Under normal conditions, the stratum corneum acts as a barrier, keeping the rest of the skin from drying out and protecting other layers of skin from damage caused by irritants and infections. When this barrier is damaged, irritants act more intensely on the skin.

The skin of an infant with atopic eczema loses moisture from the epidermal layer, allowing the skin to become very dry and reducing its protective abilities. Thus, when combined with the abnormal skin immune system, the infant's skin is more likely to become infected by viruses (e.g. herpes simplex) or bacteria (e.g. *Staphylococcus* and *Streptococcus* spp.).

Immunoglobulin E (IgE) is a type of antibody that controls the immune system's allergic response. An antibody is a protein produced by the immune system that recognises and helps fight and destroy viruses, bacteria, and other foreign substances that invade the body. Normally, IgE is present in very small amounts but levels are high in 80–90% of people with atopic eczema (Hanifin & Rajka 1980, Hoare et al 2000).

Box 40.1

Signs and symptoms of atopic eczema

Signs of atopic eczema

- Erythema
- Vesicles that weep
- Development of a dry crust
- Scaling
- Worse in winter
- Lesions easily infected by bacterial or viral agents
- Periods of temporary remission
- Laboratory studies may show an increase in IgE and eosinophil levels
- Extremes of temperature, humidity and sunlight can aggravate

Symptoms of atopic eczema

- Intense itching (pruritus)
- Scratching
- Irritable
- Unable to sleep
- May flare up following immunisations

Assessment

Atopic eczema can present with a variety of symptoms. The symptoms can vary in intensity and also over time. Assessment of general health, past medical history, familial history plus specific assessment of skin should be carried out. In infancy, lesions are located on the:

- cheeks
- scalp
- trunk
- outer aspects of hands and feet
- skin folds.

Lesions can also be generalised, i.e. they can cover the entire body. The signs and symptoms of atopic eczema are shown in Box 40.1.

Exploration of any family history of allergies is necessary. Although atopic eczema runs in families, the role of genetics or inheritance is still not clear. It does appear that more than one gene is involved in the disease. Studies suggest that genetics play an important part in the inheritance of the disease (Spagnola & Korb 2002). Infants and children are at increased risk for developing the eczema if there is a family history of other atopic disease, such as hay fever or asthma. The risk is significantly higher if both parents have an atopic disease. In addition, studies of identical twins, who have the same genes, show that in an estimated 80–90% of cases, atopic disease appears in both twins. Fraternal (non-identical) twins are no more likely than two non-related people in a general population to both have an atopic eczema.

Aycliffe (2009) has discussed the use of scoring tools to ascertain the presence of eczema in an affected child. The National Eczema Society provides information on the optimum method of doing this: www.eczema.org/professionals.html.

Major and minor features of atopic eczema

A preliminary diagnosis of atopic eczema can be made if the patient has three or more features from each of two categories: major features and minor features (Hanifin & Rajka 1980, National Eczema Society 2003).

Major features

- Intense itching.
- Characteristic rash in locations typical of the disease.
- Chronic or repeatedly occurring symptoms.
- Personal or family history of atopic disorders (eczema, hay fever, asthma).

Minor features

- Early age of onset.
- Dry skin that may also have patchy scales or rough bumps.
- High levels of immunoglobulin E (IgE).
- Numerous skin creases on the palms.
- Hand or foot involvement.

Allergic sensitivity

Allergens are substances from foods, plants, animals or the air (e.g. dust mites, pollens, moulds). They inflame the skin by causing the immune system to overreact. Inflammation occurs even when the infant is exposed to small amounts of the substance for a limited time. It is not yet certain whether inhaling these allergens or their actual penetration of the skin causes the problem. When infants with atopic eczema come into contact with an irritant or allergen they are sensitive to, inflammation-producing cells become active. These cells release chemicals – histamines – that cause itching and redness. As the infant responds by scratching and rubbing the skin, further skin damage occurs (Spagnola & Korb 2002).

Food allergy

The most common allergenic (allergy-causing) foods are eggs, milk, peanuts, wheat, soy and fish. A recent analysis (Spagnola & Korb 2002) of a large number of studies on allergies and breastfeeding indicated that breastfeeding an infant for at least 4 months may protect the infant from developing allergies. Mothers with a family history of atopic conditions should be advised to avoid eating common allergenic foods during late pregnancy and breastfeeding.

Elimination diets

A basic diet of hypoallergenic food is given to the infant initially. One new food at a time is added to determine the infant's reaction to it:

- If the infant is allergic to cow's milk, a substitute such as soya bean milk can be used.
- Vitamin supplements may be needed, particularly if the infant is not taking fruit and vegetables.

Irritants

Irritants are substances that affect the skin directly, causing it to become red and itchy or to burn. The substances that irritate and the effects of these irritants vary from one person to another. Over time, family members learn to identify the irritants causing infants the most trouble. Wool or synthetic fibres and rough or poorly fitting clothing can rub the skin, trigger inflammation, and cause the itch–scratch cycle to begin. Soaps and detergents may have a drying effect and worsen itching, and some perfumes and cosmetics may irritate the skin. Exposure to certain substances, such as solvents, dust, or sand, may also make the condition worse. Cigarette smoke can irritate the eyelids (Hockenberry 2003).

Managing the infant with atopic eczema

The management of black skin is generally the same as white skin (National Eczema Society 2003). However, some differences in skin structure can lead to some specific problems. Changes in skin colour can occur when the pigment layer of the skin is disturbed by the disease process. Thickening of the skin (lichenification) is more likely in black skin. Once inflammation processes reduce, the skin will return to a normal colour, although this can take several months. Often, no explanation can be found for a particular flare-up of the condition, and many factors are probably working in combination at all times.

Family needs

When an infant has atopic eczema, the family may have to cope with the stress and frustration associated with the disease and nurses undertaking an assessment should ascertain how the condition is impacting the family; for example, if it is adversely affecting the child's ability to form and sustain friendships (Aycliffe 2009). The infant may be fussy and irritable and unable to keep from scratching and rubbing the skin. Sleepless nights also cause irritation to both infant and family. Distracting the child and providing activities that keep the hands busy are helpful but require much effort on the part of the parents or caregivers. Another issue family's face is the social and emotional stress associated with changes in appearance caused by atopic eczema.

Activity

Reflect on your experiences caring for an infant who has atopic eczema:

- What were the contributory factors causing an exacerbation of the condition for that particular infant?

www

A wide variety of information for both adults and children/young people is available on the National Eczema Society website:

- http://www.eczema.org

Principles of care: controlling atopic eczema

- Hydrate the skin
- Relieve pruritus
- Reduce inflammation and flare-ups
- Prevent secondary infection.

Hydrate the skin

- Give lukewarm, not hot, baths.
- Use emollient bath treatments.
- Apply emollient immediately after the bath to assist in trapping moisture and preventing moisture loss. If an emollient is not applied within 3 minutes of leaving the bath, evaporation causes excess drying of the skin (Spagnola & Korb 2002).
- *Safety point:* emollients can make surfaces slippery. Remain with the infant all times while in bath to prevent accidents, e.g. drowning.
- Avoid bubble baths and harsh soaps, which can cause irritation. Remember emollients are available in a range of preparations including shower and bath products (Aycliffe 2009).
- Pat, do not rub the skin, dry.

Relieve pruritus

- Prevent scratching or rubbing whenever possible.
- Attempt to distract the infant with activities to keep him or her from scratching.
- Keep fingernails cut short.
- Gloves and/or cotton socks may need to be placed over hands.
- Avoid fibres such as wool.
- Consider the use of prescribed sedating antihistamines to promote sleep and reduce scratching at night.

Reduce inflammation and flare-ups

- Protect skin from excessive moisture, irritants and rough clothing.
- Avoid situations where overheating occurs.
- Consider potential irritants with toys.
- Select soft cotton fabrics when choosing clothing.
- Limit exposure to dust, cigarette smoke, pollens and animal dander.
- Recognise and limit emotional stress.
- Occasional flare-ups: may require the use of prescribed topical steroids to diminish inflammation.
- Acute flare-ups: may require the use of wet wraps.

Prevent secondary infection

- Learn to recognise skin infections and seek treatment promptly.
- Secondary skin infections can be managed with prescribed systemic antibiotics.

Emollients

Soaps and detergents are drying because they remove natural lipids from the skin surface. Emollients provide a barrier to prevent water evaporating from the skin and also foreign irritants from entering. Emollients can be applied in liberal amounts twice a day and whenever the skin feels dry and itchy.

Emollients are available in various forms, including creams, ointments, lotions, soap substitutes and bath additives. Twitchen & Lowe (1998) describe the action of emollients as hydrating, soothing and smoothing of the scales on the skin.

Medical treatments

Corticosteroids

These can be administered locally or systemically. Topical corticosteroid creams and ointments are effective in suppressing inflammation and providing symptomatic relief (Cork 1999). Topical steroids should be applied sparingly and only to affected skin. Side effects of repeated or long-term use of topical corticosteroids can include thinning of the skin, infections, growth suppression in children, and stretch marks on the skin.

When topical corticosteroids are not effective, a systemic corticosteroid may be prescribed. This is taken orally instead of being applied directly to the skin. An example of a commonly prescribed corticosteroid is prednisone. This medication is only prescribed for short periods of time. The side effects of systemic corticosteroids can include skin damage, thinned or weakened bones, high blood pressure, high blood sugar and infections (Devilliers et al 2002). Corticosteroids should not be suddenly stopped. It is very important that the doctor and family work together when reducing and completing the corticosteroid treatment.

Antibiotics

Antibiotics to treat skin infections may be applied directly to the skin in an ointment, as well as taken orally. If viral or fungal infections are present, the doctor may also prescribe specific medications to treat those infections.

Antihistamines

Antihistamines can reduce night-time scratching and allow more restful sleep when taken at bedtime. This effect can be particularly helpful for infants whose night-time scratching makes the skin lesions worse (NICE 2007).

Wet-wrap dressings

Wet-wrap dressings (Box 40.2) can be used when the atopic eczema does not respond to the first-line treatments of emollients and topical steroids. Wet-wrap dressings are an effective means of rehydrating and cooling the skin and reducing inflammation. The wet-wrap can also involve use of topical steroids for increased absorption, which in turn reduces the itch–scratch cycle (Hanifin et al 2003).

This treatment is usually commenced in the hospital setting. The technique can easily be taught for use at home (Twitchen & Lowe 1998).

By participating in making the decision to use wet-wraps, families with an infant with atopic eczema may feel they have gained some control over this condition. There are benefits to

Box 40.2

Wet-wrap dressings

A water-based emollient is applied all over the body. The emollients are covered with a double layer of wrapping of tubular bandages. The innermost wrapping is moistened with warm water. The outer layer is a dry layer of tubular bandage.

The benefits include the evaporation of water gradually from the wet layer causing a slight cooling of the skin, which partly relieves the itching. The moisture in the dressing helps to soften the skin, allowing better penetration of the topical corticosteroid, while the two layers of dressing can act as a mechanical barrier to scratching (Pei et al 2001).

children of rehydrating the skin in this way, such as improvements seen in reduction of pruritus and improvements in sleeping patterns following the use of wet wrap dressings. Aycliffe (2009) reminds nurses of the National Patient Safety Agency (NPSA) warnings about the fire hazards associated with paraffin-based skin products, especially near naked flames.

Frequency of use

The bandages are usually left in place for up to 24 hours and the process is repeated daily until the skin is clear. However, as Donald (1997) found wet-wraps are most effective during the first 8 hours of application and so are best used at night. This may prove a more acceptable way of incorporating the treatment into daily activities.

Once the skin state has responded to treatment, a maintenance regimen of bandaging may be required. Prolonged positive effects on the skin are achieved when occlusion is continued for a further 2 weeks to prevent skin dryness. Application of the wet-wraps may then be reduced to alternate nights, and further reduced until the skin state is maintained without occlusion. Twitchen & Lowe (1998) found the itch-scratch cycle seems to be broken more effectively this way.

Allergy

Some patients have allergic reactions to either the emollients, the topical steroids or the tubular bandaging used. Allergy may present as increased pruritus and exacerbation of the eczema. Treatment should be discontinued and reviewed for alternative management methods.

Temperature

Wet-wraps may cause the infant to feel very cold, resulting in shivering. Reducing the time wet-wraps are in situ, ensuring the home or hospital environment is warm, applying the treatment to localised areas only may surmount this difficulty. Alternatively, the bandaging may cause overheating, which can exacerbate pruritus. In such cases, it may have to be accepted that wet-wrap bandaging is simply not appropriate.

Other methods of treatment

Hoare et al (2000), in a systematic review of research into atopic eczema treatments, found there was insufficient evidence to make recommendations on treatments such as Chinese herbs, homeopathy, massage therapy, hypnotherapy and evening primrose oil.

WWW

Access the systematic review into atopic eczema treatments. The report is available on the DoH health technology assessment website:

- http://www.ncchta.org

Sleep and rest

Sleep patterns are regulated by both biological and psychological processes (Jenni & O'Connor 2005). Sleep is created by the brain and it is vital for brain health and development; it is a complex natural phenomenon, common to all human beings (Bennett (2003). Infants and children have different needs for sleep and rest; the amount depends on their age and development. Bangura (1998) acknowledged that throughout the process of sleep maturation occurs, the pattern of sleep changes from frequent brief periods of sleep to a single prolonged uninterrupted sleep. An infant may expect to sleep for a period of 16 hours a day, compared with an older child who requires 9–12 hours sleep per 24 hours.

Sleep is known to be a part of a circadian rhythm. Each circadian rhythm ensures a 24-hour cycle regulated by physiological and behavioural responses (Braine 2009) and disruption of this cycle or 'body clock' can influence health significantly. This body clock is thought to be located in the anterior hypothalamus in the suprachiasmatic nuclei (SCN) (Young et al 2008). Melatonin, a hormone produced by the pineal gland released in response to signals from the SCN, works with serotonin, both being important in maintaining sleep. Melotonin levels are influenced by the number of daylight hours with more melotonin produced when there is longer exposure to daylight. High levels of melotonin also result in the lowering of the body temperature at night (Braine 2009).

As well as the sleep–wake circadian rhythym, there is also a temperature circadian rhythym. McGraw et al (1999) identified that the temperature circadian rhythm appears first followed by the wake cycle and finally sleep, with a clear wake–sleep cycle being developed by 3 months of age (Miano et al 2009). In older children and adults there is a high correlation with a drop in the body temperature followed by the onset of sleep, and conversely, a rising in the body temperature brings increased arousal and wakefulness. Wright et al (2002) also identified the close link between a higher state of arousal and better performance and the body's temperature reaching its peak during the normal circadian range. This feature of increased arousal during the time of peak body temperature in the evening can be seen in many infants from 6 weeks of age; parents often mention the problems of managing an infant who simply will not settle. However, later in the evening as the body temperature drops, the infant will soon settle into sleep. In older children it is known (Wright et al 2002) that working memory, subjective alertness and visual attention are increased when the body temperature is higher, for example in the hours from waking until midday, but after lunch when the body temperature drops, concentration falls with it and many children are very sleepy, a feature called the 'postprandial dip'.

Physiology of sleep

The wake–sleep cycle is influenced by the hormone melatonin, the production of which is related to daylight, and preliminary evidence (McGraw et al 1999) suggests that exposing infants to sunlight, rather than artificial light is important in the early development of this rythym.

Bennett (2003) identified that studies using electroencephalography (EEG) discovered that there are distinct sleep patterns and levels. These are described as rapid eye movement (REM) sleep and non-rapid eye movement (NREM) sleep. Sleep commences with NREM, followed by REM, and this cycle continues throughout, alternating from one to the other; each cycle may eventually last up to 90 minutes (Finlay 1991).

In infancy, REM tends to control a baby's sleep pattern. During REM sleep significant brain organisation takes place with neurons in the brain cortex becoming inter-linked and connections to and from the thalamus being established. Parents may notice increased motor activity during sleep such as facial grimaces and hand stretching as these interconnections in the brain are made (Horne 1988).

Overall a lot of physiological development occurs during sleep (Bangura 1998, Bennett 2003) and sleep has significant restorative properties. Gronfier et al (1996) clearly demonstrates the correlation between secretion of growth hormone (a principle hormone involved in healing) and delta (slow) wave sleep. It has been demonstrated that sleep deprivation decreases the activity and response of the immune system, therefore compromising healing processes (Dinges et al 1995). Human studies directed at determining clinically important relationships between sleep loss and illness trajectories are currently lacking, but studies with well subjects have clearly demonstrated that sleep is important to the recovery process as an integral homeostatic mechanism and therefore should be promoted (Weinhouse & Schwab 2006).

Routines and barriers to sleep

By 3 weeks of age, most infants have established a pattern of sleep and have apportioned the times of sleep equally between day and night. At 3 months of age, most infants tend to sleep for 12 hours at night, i.e. 19:00 hours to 07:00 hours. Colic, crying and sleep disturbance have been suggested to be associated with the melatonin production, which codes the day length. Regular sleep patterns need to be promoted otherwise the infant may be at a disadvantage and fail to distinguish appropriate signals for sleep.

Psychological factors that influence sleep patterns include cognitions, cultural norms and behavioural aspects. Behavioural aspects (i.e., learned behaviours) of the wave–sleep cycle is relevant for the understanding of children's sleep patterns and the management of their sleep disorders.

The beneficial effects of the sleep pattern

A bedtime routine is effective in promoting sleep patterns. A separate area for sleeping and allowing children to fall asleep by themselves should be encouraged. Established positive sleep behaviour may prevent the development of irregular sleep in later life, and it will almost certainly reduce the possible effects of a tired and irritable child. It has been demonstrated that children can become over-reactive without sleep (Minde et al 1994) and behavioural difficulties are three times more likely in children with sleep problems (Sadeh et al 2003). In addition, a parent who has had little sleep may feel vulnerable and overreact in stressful situations. Hence, the quality of family life may be reduced.

Establishing routines

As soon as it is possible, it is beneficial to establish a routine with a set bedtime, to enable the infant to differentiate between day and night. For example, a bath, bedtime story and darkening the room may induce sleep. A routine like this has a definite end-point – sleeping – therefore for the child to associate this routine with sleep onset is a very positive reinforcement to trigger the desired behaviour.

Reorganising areas for day activities is another way to promote rest and may be advantageous. If space is restricted, part of the room may be partitioned, enabling the cot to be visually separated from the rest of the living quarters. Parents need to establish whether the infant is too warm or too cold; if uncomfortable the baby is unlikely to sleep.

If routines are not established, the most commonly reported difficulties with sleep patterns (Table 40.7) are managed well using the following behavioural modifications.

Behaviour modification

- Minimal check: a system used to modify sleep patterns in infancy has been referred to as the 'minimal check programme'. This permits the parents to observe the infant briefly at regular intervals during the period if an infant is crying. The period of time between checking has ranged from 5 to 20 minutes; infant sleep patterns have been found to improve with this system.
- Parental presence programme: this is based on the concept that sleep disturbance in young children is due to

Table 40.7 Common childhood sleep problems

Sleeplessness problem	How it is manifest
Inappropriate sleep onset association	The child will not fall asleep without a set of demanding conditions being met, for example the parents getting into the bed with the child
Limit setting sleep disorder	The parent has been unable to set the limits for the child, for example a regular bed time

Adapted from (Wiggs 2009)

the child's separation anxiety. Parents remain with the child during the first week of the programme, sleeping in the same room but in a separate bed, so that if the child wakes during the night interaction and involvement is withheld. After the allocated period the parent returns to a different room. Withdrawal of the parent can be done gradually, as above, or abruptly. Abrupt removal is likely to result in a temporary increase in undesired behaviour, such as crying and refusing to stay in bed, but this is eventually followed by a decrease in this type of behaviour. Parents must be warned of the sequence of unexpected behaviour patterns so that they do not abandon attempts to establish a more positive routine. Parents may also need to modify their own behaviour; they may not be able to cope with the child's upset and may re-enter the child's area to ease their own mind before the child has become used to the new routine without them. This would then reinforce the child's negative behaviour (Wiggs 2009).
- Graduated extinction and fading: this approach involves reducing the intensity of the parental response that is sustaining the undesirable behaviour. Graduated extinction involves in increasing the time before responding to bedtime crying (incremental graduated extinction) or decreasing the time spent with the infant on settling or on night awakening (decremental graduated extinction). Studies that have incorporated this method have resulted in marked improvements within the infant's sleep pattern.

The success of any modification programme depends on parental agreement and, where applicable, both parents need to have discussed the subject and are both prepared to undertake the chosen method. Behavioural interventions can be used successfully to manage child sleeplessness (Wiggs 2009) and are favoured above the use of medication. Ensuring that families can access appropriate support and help when sleeping problems are reported is vital to avoid long-term problems for all family members.

Activity

- Reflect on your practice when nursing infants and preparation for sleep.
- Explore the rituals attached to preparation for sleep and consider the positive and negative aspects of the rituals you have observed.

Sudden infant death syndrome

Fleming 2000 defines sudden unexpected death in infancy as: 'The sudden death of an infant which was not anticipated by any professionals or carers involved with the child 24 hours prior to the event that led to death.' Fleming et al (2000) describe sudden infant death syndrome as the unexpected and sudden death of an apparently normal and healthy infant that occurs during sleep and without evidence to suggest a disease. Fleming et al (2000) state that some sudden and unexpected infant deaths can often be explained following thorough post-mortem examination and other investigations. Cot deaths that remain unexplained after a thorough examination are usually registered as sudden infant death syndrome (SIDS). Sometimes other terms like sudden unexpected death in infancy (SUDI) or unascertained may be used. It is currently one cause of death in children between 2 weeks and 1 year of age. At present, statistical evidence suggests that the incidences are 1:300–350 live births. The origin is unknown but causative factors have been proposed, including inadequate biotin in the diet, mechanical suffocation, a defect in the respiratory mucosa, extensive apnoeas, a virus and immunoglobulin abnormalities. Sudden infant death syndrome occurs more often in infants aged 10–14 weeks, especially those born prematurely, in boys more than girls and more often during the winter months. Evidence suggests that those infants who have experienced an upper respiratory tract infection may be predisposed to sudden infant death syndrome. The syndrome is neither infectious nor hereditary, although there may be a higher possibility of it occurring within the same family, which may imply genetic factors are involved.

Epidemiology of sudden infant death syndrome

Table 40.8 looks at the determinants of sudden infant death syndrome.

Activity

- Examine Table 40.8. Discuss how and why the identified factors may cause a higher prevalence of sudden infant death syndrome

Table 40.8 Sudden infant death syndrome (adapted from Wong 2001)

Determinant	Incidence
Frequency	0.6 per 1000 live births (1998)
Sleep patterns	Prone, soft bedding, overheating, co-sleeping with adults
Peak periods	2–4 months, 95% occur by 6 months
Feeding habits	Lower incidence in breast-fed infants
Males to females	Higher percentage of males affected
Siblings	Possibly greater
Maternal	Young age, cigarette smoker, poor prenatal care, alcohol and drug dependency
Time of death	During sleep
Socio-economic factors	Increased occurrence in lower-socio-economic classes
Birth	Higher incidence in preterm infants, low birthweight infants Multiple births Neonates with low Apgar scores Infants with respiratory disorders

Children at greater risk

In view of the research findings, some children are more at risk than others are. These include:

- infants with a life-threatening condition needing cardiopulmonary resuscitation (CPR)
- preterm infants who continue to experience apnoeic episodes at the time of hospital discharge
- siblings of two or more sudden infant death syndrome victims
- infants with complex disorders or conditions, e.g. hypoventilation.

Equipment for monitoring within the home environment is recommended for these children, providing parents are aware of cardiopulmonary resuscitation techniques. At present there are no diagnostic tools to indicate which infants will live or die, but monitoring infants may alleviate parental anxiety.

Preventive strategies are directed at decreasing known risk factors, such as mothers requiring prenatal care, avoiding cigarette smoking and substance misuse both before and after the child's birth. The bedroom being at a suitable temperature (18°C) and the infant wearing suitable clothing helps to prevent sudden infant death syndrome.

There are recommended health education messages to reduce the risk of cot death (these are available online at: http:// www.sids.org.uk/fsid):

- Place your baby on his or her back to sleep.
- Place your baby with his or her feet to the foot of the cot, to prevent wriggling down under the covers.
- Do not let anyone smoke in the same room as your baby.
- Do not let your baby get too hot.
- Keep your baby's head uncovered.
- If your baby is unwell, seek medical advice promptly.

Whether subsequent siblings are at risk of sudden infant death syndrome remains unclear, but if home monitoring is an option this needs to be discussed with paediatricians, health visitors and nurses.

Ramifications for nursing

Campbell & Glasper (2001) acknowledge that the loss of a child from sudden infant death syndrome presents the parents with a serious emotional matter, with which they must cope. In addition to grieving, the parents must face a catastrophic situation that was sudden, incomprehensible and unexpected.

Entering the room and finding the child

It is usually one of the parents who discovers the child dead in the cot, with bedclothes disarranged and the blankets over the child's head. Often the parent can be alone in the house and must deal with the situation while coping with the emotional turmoil of shock, panic and grief.

The first of the personnel to arrive on the scene may be either the police or the paramedics. It is important to ask only essential questions in a non-judgemental manner when providing support and comfort for members of the family. Ambulance attendants should be educated to recognise the characteristic signs of sudden infant death syndrome and be able to inform the parents that the possible cause was sudden infant death syndrome, but that this cannot be predetermined. The compassion demonstrated by the ambulance attendants/police/health professionals in the first few minutes may help the parents to cope with the guilt and despair that accompany these types of situations.

Arriving at the hospital

On arrival to the A & E department, the nursing staff usually has first contact with the family and the infant is attended to by the doctor to certify death. As this period is emotionally charged, it is important to extract factual information from parents. This may include:

- What time was the infant found?
- How did the infant look?
- What position was the infant in?
- What assistance was provided?

Any questions that suggest responsibility should be avoided, such as was there any jealousy from other siblings?

It is necessary to determine the actual events: what happened when the parent/carer entered the infant's room, what resuscitation was attempted (this might have given rise to fractured ribs, internal bleeding and bruising, which will need clarification). During this discussion, the doctor or nurse needs to approach the subject of a post-mortem, as the actual diagnosis of sudden infant death syndrome cannot be determined until this has been completed. Verbal and written information needs to be given regarding the post-mortem and funeral arrangements. Lawrence (1989) advised that mothers who were breastfeeding required accurate information regarding cessation of lactation.

Compassion towards the parents may consist of enabling them to say goodbye to their child, in privacy. Before this happens, the nurse needs to ensure that the infant appears tidy and the room is in order. As this may be the last time the parents wish to see their child, they should be given as much time as needed, in peace and quiet.

The child's belongings needed to be returned to the parents. Contacting relatives or friends to take the parents home or a nurse escorting them to their car may be advisable.

At home

Parents may receive a visit from their GP and health visitor, whereby issues of coming to terms with the infant's death may be explored. This may take more than one visit and consideration may need to address siblings and their grieving. A referral (and contact) details maybe given to the Foundation for Sudden Infant Death (FSID).

Dedicated charities, support groups and associations, can provide advice and help to families affected by sudden infant death syndrome. FSID provides information and a 24-hour helpline.

WWW

Access more information on the Foundation for the Study of Infant Deaths (FSID) website at:

- http://www.sids.org.uk

Activity

- Describe the grieving process.
- How can the primary healthcare team help the bereaved parents after the loss of an infant?

An important issue for many parents is later pregnancies, and concerns related to recurrent sudden infant death syndrome. Some parents may wish to re-establish their family within 12 months or so. One possibility of a subsequent child is that the infant may be a replacement for the previous one. If the pregnancy is a success, further anxiety may arise, especially near the time of the other infant's death, which may be characterised by the parents being overprotective.

The health visitor can support the family in their decision for another child. The Care of the Next Infant (CONI) scheme allows the health visitor to provide effective support to prepare families for the birth of the next child.

The law requires that a coroner investigates all sudden and unexpected deaths in infants to certify the cause of death. The coroner's representative, usually a police officer, will ask the parents for information. The police are authorised to investigate unexpected deaths; they usually visit the home, and may sometimes take photographs and remove items such as bedding.

Chapter 8 of Working Together to Safeguard Children (DfES 2006) identifies the process of Serious Case Reviews (SCRs). SCRs are undertaken when a child dies (including suicide), and abuse or neglect is known or suspected to be a factor in the death.

Chapter 7 of Working Together to Safeguard Children (DfES 2006) sets out the procedures to be followed when a child dies. There are two interrelated processes for reviewing child deaths (either of which can trigger a serious case review):

- a rapid response by a group of key professionals who come together for the purpose of enquiring into and evaluating each unexpected death of a child
- an overview of all child deaths (under 18 years) in the Local Safeguarding Children Board (LSCB) area(s), undertaken by a panel.

The purpose of a Child Death Review (DfES 2006 Chapter 7) is to collect and analyse information about each death with a view to identifying (Pearson 2008, Sidebotham et al 2008):

- any case giving rise to the need for a serious case review
- any matters of concern affecting the safety and welfare of children in the area of the authority.
- any wider public health or safety concerns arising from a particular death or from a pattern of deaths in that area.

www

Access more information on the Care of Next Infant (CONI) website at:

- http://www.sids.org.uk/fsid/coni

Apnoea of infancy

Apnoeic episodes can be defined as one of the following:

- central: absence of airflow and respiratory effort
- obstructive: absence of airflow but respiratory effort
- mixed: absence of airflow and respiratory effort followed by resumption of respiratory effort.

Short periods of central apnoea (15 seconds) are normal at any age. Pathological apnoea refers to a respiratory pause that is prolonged and may be accompanied with cyanosis, pallor, hypotonia and bradycardia. Apnoea of infancy (AOI) occurs in infants greater than 37 weeks' gestation. The clinical appearance of this disorder may be classified as life threatening. Apnoea of infancy may be associated with many other disorders such as sepsis, convulsions, upper airway abnormalities metabolic disorders and impaired regulation of breathing during sleep or feeding.

Diagnosis

- Electroencephalogram (EEG)
- Electrocardiogram (ECG)
- Blood chemistry
- Chest radiograph
- pH study: to determine gastro-oesophageal reflux

Ramifications for nursing practice

Confirmation of diagnosis needs to be discussed with parents before the provision of home monitoring. If monitoring is decided on, this may cause additional stress and members of the nursing team are an ideal source of support for the family. Parents need to be educated on the equipment, observation of the infant and immediate care in relation to cardiopulmonary resuscitation (CPR).

There are several types of home monitoring which are available, however monitors will be provided based upon local resources and policy. Monitors will be provided that are suitable for use within the home environment.

Guidelines for the use of the apnoea monitors (adapted from Campbell & Glasper 2001) are:

- Apnoea monitors have limitations, i.e. false alarms, however they should continue to be utilised.
- Do not adjust any settings to eliminate false alarms, this may reduce effectiveness.
- Place the monitors on an appropriate surface and not covered by sheets and blankets.
- Do not sleep in the same bed as a monitored infant, movement may reduce effectiveness.
- Pets and other children should be kept away from the monitor.
- Check the monitor several times a day to ensure that it is working, i.e. batteries and cord.
- Ensure that the caregiver can reach the infant in less than 10 seconds.

- Read the monitor's manual for usage carefully and report problems promptly.
- Prepare in advance for the event of an emergency by having telephone numbers next to the telephone.
- Health education is required in relation to recognising signs and symptoms of health problems and the need to communicate with health professionals.
- Education on when to initiate cardiopulmonary resuscitation.

Activity

- Design and develop written guidelines as supporting material for parents using an apnoeic monitor for home monitoring.

Immunisation

McCarthy (2001) suggested that immunisation programmes within both the underdeveloped and developed world have a significant and beneficial effect on children's health. Vaccines are the products of the advancement with biotechnological techniques and ongoing research. Immunisations need to be administered safely by professionals who are competent and knowledgeable.

The importance of immunisation

In 1998, the Health Education Authority (now the Health Protection Agency) defined immunisation as the process by which immunity is produced against a variety of bacterial and viral infections.

In England, epidemiological studies demonstrated that outbreaks of measles, mumps and rubella would occur if education was not effective and not targeted at the most vulnerable groups in society.

The World Health Organization (WHO 1984) adopted the goal of eliminating measles, poliomyelitis, neonatal tetanus, diphtheria and rubella by the year 2000. For this to be achieved in England, a primary objective of a 90% primary immunisation rate for all children under the age of 2 years had to be attained by 1995. This was met and, in 1992, a new target of 95% was introduced. Bedford (2003) supported these findings by acknowledging that for the vaccination programme to be effective, high levels of immunity are needed, to reduce and prevent the circulation of these illnesses.

The DoH (2003) released the statistics shown in Table 40.9 pertaining to measles. The figures suggest that there are still not enough children being vaccinated in the age group 1–4 years. This should be of concern to parents, the National Health Service and other allied organisations. Bedford (2003) acknowledged that to be given the equivalent of two injections of measles, mumps and rubella in the form of two separate injections takes at least 5 years, which leaves the child unprotected for an unnecessarily long period and might pose a risk to other individuals because herd immunity will fall, posing a risk to the community at large. Those who cannot be immunised, such as the immunosuppressed, neonates and pregnant women, will be at an increased risk of the disease.

Further reasons that contribute towards the high rate of notifications between 1 and 4 years may reflect the transient population, as well as mothers returning to work before the completion of the immunisation programme. Tudor-Hart (1971) suggested the inverse care law: that those who needed health care the most received the least and that those who would most benefit from the service are often less likely to use it, although children from the higher socioeconomic classes were readily accepting the need for immunisation.

During the 1990s, concerns developed as to the efficacy and safety of the measles, mumps and rubella (MMR) vaccine. The government stated that this would be investigated, by reliable sources – predominantly the Health Protection Agency. If the threats to health were considered of significance action would be taken. In 2002, Uhlmann et al highlighted concerns about the combined vaccine resulting in autism and inflammatory bowel problems; by contrast, Dales et al (2001) demonstrated that the MMR vaccine continues to be used extensively in the US, and had been in use since 1972 without a correlation between use and the recently observed increase in autism. Bedford (2003) indicated that after a single-antigen vaccine had been advocated and used for a sustainable period of time, many countries changed their strategy for controlling measles and began using the combined MMR vaccine so that children were protected from three of the most harmful infections. The aim was to eradicate measles, mumps and rubella; this was the first time that children had been offered protection from mumps. Bedford (2003) suggested that no vaccine was 100% effective. Ramsay et al (1994) indicated that following the initial injection of the combined MMR vaccine, approximately 10% of children within the population are not protected, suggesting that measles will occur amongst children who have been immunised. Following an outbreak of measles that occurred in Quebec in 1989, De Serres et al (1995) considered 62 siblings who developed measles: 41 had been vaccinated. This indicated that the vaccine had not been effective. However, further analysis demonstrated different findings: all 17 unvaccinated siblings acquired measles, whereas only 41 of 441 vaccinated siblings developed the disease. The results indicate that

Table 40.9 Notification of measles by age group (2001–03)

Year	<12 months	1–4 years	5–9 years	10–14 years	15 years	Unknown	Total
2001	575	1127	298	86	140	24	2378
2002	751	1631	435	106	210	54	3187
2003	528	1275	429	111	164	22	2529

the vaccine has an efficacy of 91%; if the children had not been immunised, there would have been a further 400 cases.

Healthcare professionals whose specialty involves the administration of immunisations need to pursue non-attendees and actively involve parents in their decision to immunise. Nevertheless, parents in all socioeconomic classes have their own justifications for not having their children immunised. Aston (1998) suggested that the reasons may be because of practical problems, or indifference. Crawford (1995) found the single most important factor that influenced most parents in favour of immunisation were the knowledge, enthusiasm and confidence of the healthcare professional.

The presenting of information to parents by healthcare professionals needs to be undertaken impartially and the parents need to understand the importance of making the appropriate decision in the best interest of the child.

Activity

- You are a student nurse. A parent tells you: 'I have read in the national press that there are risks associated with immunisations. My friend has refused the MMR vaccination for her child and I'm worried about what to do for my child.'
- What would you advise?

Activity

- A parent asks: 'Should my children be vaccinated? My daughter is 2 months old and my son is 5 years old and has just started school'. Explain the advantages and disadvantages of vaccinations to this mother. Identify the evidence to support your answer. Refer to:
- http://www.doh.gov.uk/policyandguidance
- http://www.hpa.org.uk/infections/topics

Health promotion

Health promotion and education contribute to providing parents and members of the public with information relating to immunisations for children. The importance of health promotion and education has been greatly emphasised over the past decade. 'The health of the nation' (DoH 1992) and 'Our healthier nation' (DoH 1998) emphasise the importance of good health for everyone from the young to the old. These documents recognise that individuals need to promote activities that have a beneficial consequence, and lessen those that cause significant harm and induce ill health.

The contribution of the nurse, the midwife and the health visitor has been extensive (DoH 2002, Hall 1996, Lindsey & Hartrick 1996). However, for health promotion programmes to be successful, it is important to consider the choice of target population so that the best possible results can be achieved. To improve health, communities need to gain more control over these systems through their full involvement in decision making. In order for this to be achieved health professionals need to empower, collaborate and provide resources to promote health.

Table 40.10 Childhood immunisations

Age	Immunisation	Notes
2 months: 1st dose	Diphtheria, pertussis, tetanus and polio	Three doses needed – primary course
3 months: 2nd dose	Hib	
4 months: 3rd dose	Measles, mumps and rubella	
12–15 months and 3–5 years	Booster: diphtheria, tetanus and polio Second dose: measles, mumps and rubella	Administered over the age of 12 months Three years after completion of primary course

Adapted from: http://www.doh.gov.uk/Policy/AndGuidance

Premature infants

It is essential that premature infants receive their immunisations according to the immunisation schedule at the appropriate chronological age. The first and second immunisation of an extremely premature infant (less than 28 weeks' gestation) should be administered in hospital (DoH 2009).

The ages at which the different immunisations should be given are shown in Table 40.10.

The immune response

Immunity may be either active or passive and involves the stimulation of antibodies. Active immunisation is provided by the stimulation of the host's antibodies, whereas passive immunisation involves the administration of antibodies. Passive immunity may be short term, whereas active immunity may be life-long. (Further detail can be found in Chapter 31).

Passive immunity

Passive naturally acquired immunity

This method of immunity is acquired prior to birth, by the transfer of antibodies across the placenta to the fetus, and eventually to the baby in the form of breast milk. The variety of antibodies depends upon the mother's active immunity. The baby's lymphocytes are not effectual and the effects of the immunity are transitory.

Passive artificially acquired immunity

In this form of immunity, the antibodies have been prepared, either by animal or human serum and are injected into the recipient. The source of the antibodies may be derived from an individual who is recovering from the infection or from animals – usually horses – that have been artificially actively immunised.

The immunoglobulins that have been obtained may be given prophylactically, to prevent the infection, or therapeutically after the infection has started. The proteins within the serum may cause the lymphocytes to be damaged most notably on subsequent occasions, which, according to Waugh and Grant (2003), may cause a severe reaction.

Active immunity

Active immunity is created when an adjusted form of the infecting agent is administered, stimulating the production of antibodies. Active immunity is preferable to passive immunisation because of its duration. The manufacturing of vaccines is complex and requires a great degree of skill and knowledge. There is a fine line between ensuring that the antibody is effective and deactivating the antigen.

Active naturally acquired immunity

Individuals can produce their own antibodies by the following:

- Having acquired the infection: Waugh & Grant (2003) suggested that during the illness B lymphocytes in the plasma cells produce antibodies in adequate quantities to engulf the infection. After recovery, the memory B cells maintain a specific ability to produce the specific antibodies to respond to a future infection by the same organism therefore immunity is bestowed.
- Having a subclinical infection for example a microbial infection, insufficient to cause a clinical disease but the memory B cells may be produced to create immunity.

Active artificially acquired immunity

This form of immunity develops as a result of a response to the administration of dead or live artificially weakened microbes (Waugh & Grant 2003). These are referred to as vaccines or toxoids, they retain antigenic properties that stimulate immunity, but cannot cause the disease. These vaccines can prevent microbial diseases.

Activity

An infant has been admitted onto your ward for investigations. The mother informs you that she is pregnant, and one of her friends has told her that children do not require immunisations. To rectify misconceptions:

- What advice would you offer?
- Identify the literature that would provide the evidence base for the advice given to the parent.

Immunisation against certain diseases produces lifelong immunity. In other contractable diseases the immunity may last either years or weeks before a further vaccination is necessary. The loss of immunity may be as a result of a different strain of the same microbe, which causes the same clinical illness, e.g. the virus that causes the common cold.

Diphtheria

Pathology

The 'Immunisation against infectious diseases' (The Green Book) (DoH 2009) characterises this very rare condition in the UK as an acute infectious disease caused by the bacterium *Corynebacterium diphtheriae*. It causes the production of a systemic toxin and an adherent false membrane (pseudomembrane) to the lining of the throat. The toxin that is produced is harmful to the tissues of the heart and central nervous system. The false lining to the throat can interfere with eating, breathing and verbal communications. The lymph glands within the neck swell and the neck becomes oedematous. If it remains untreated, the condition is fatal due to respiratory obstruction, heart or renal failure.

Children who are hospitalised are nursed in isolation, and given the diphtheria antitoxin (Box 40.3), antibiotics, bed rest and fluids plus additional supportive measures as required.

Pertussis (whooping cough)

The 'Immunisation against infectious diseases' (The Green Book) (DoH 2009b) has characterised pertussis as an acute infectious disease caused by *Bordetella pertussis*.

Before the start of immunisation in the 1950s, the average number of notifications in England and Wales was in excess of 100,000 (Health Protection Agency 2003). In 1972, immunisation approval was over 80% and, during that year, there were only 2069 notifications of whooping cough. Public anxiety increased regarding the safety of the vaccine after a report was published connecting a group of children who had been vaccinated with brain damage. By 1975, immunisation had fallen to 30%, which subsequently lead to epidemics in 1977 and 1981–83.

Box 40.3

History of the diphtheria antitoxin

Baker & Katz (2004) suggested that during the 1870s and 1880s diphtheria was one of the major diseases of childhood. The mortality rate was high, especially within cities. Baker & Katz (2004) identified that in New York fatalities ranged from 42 to 49%. Medical practitioners usually encountered a child experiencing difficulty breathing and who was asphyxiating, apart from surgical intervention and intubation by the 1880s there was little in the way of resources.

Emil von Behring was one of the first scientists to explore a vaccine to combat diphtheria; he combined an extract of the deadly disease toxins with antitoxins taken from healthy animals. In 1913, clinical trials established that children had conferred immunity without harmful side effects. Parish (1965) indicated that Bela Shick of the University of Vienna, in the same year had also identified a simple skin test that could determine whether an individual was immune to diphtheria.

These achievements were suddenly curtailed due to the First World War and proving the efficacy of the toxin-antitoxin became the responsibility of the Director of Hygiene Services – WH Park – who recruited more than 100,000 children within the American public school system for research, which eventually gave him acclaim as one of the leading advocates of this vaccine.

However, some countries did not advocate the use of toxin-antitoxin. In France, an effective vaccine was developed at the Pasteur Institute in the 1920s. The French Academy of Medicine approved this for children in 1927 and it begin to be used in France during the 1930s. This has become the preferred method of vaccination of children in developed countries.

This caused an extra 200,000 cases to be reported and 100 deaths. In the 1990s, public confidence in the pertussis vaccine steadily rose, due to professionals advocating the advantages, reaching 93% in 2002–03.

Despite the levels of vaccination being high, international reports suggest that there is reappearance of whooping cough. The Public Health Laboratory Service (PHLS) has been monitoring the condition and analysis of the information for 1995–97 indicates that the proportion of whooping cough in younger unvaccinated people is growing. The PHLS suggest that to cause a reduction within the condition in older age groups and reduce the spread of the communicable disease to infants too young to be fully protected may be achieved by introducing a booster before starting school; this was commenced in 2001.

Pertussis is commonly spread by droplet infection and the incubation period is usually 7–10 days (but see http://www.immunisation.org.uk, where it is suggested that the period of infection could be from 7–21 days after the initial onset of the paroxysms).

Although there has been a reduction in the numbers of notifications since the introduction of the vaccine, pertussis remains a significant cause of illness and death in the very young. Those infants admitted to hospital under 6 months of age often require admission to paediatric intensive care. It must also be recognised that pertussis is often not diagnosed as presentations can be atypical and unsuspected.

Signs and symptoms

- Paroxysms of coughing
- Loud whoop on inspiration
- Viscid mucus may be produced following the cough
- Fever
- Sneezing
- Watery eyes
- Vomiting.

Nursing care

- Assess vital signs, temperature, respiratory rate, heart rate, blood pressure, oxygen saturation levels and record
- Observe for any signs of cyanosis: administer prescribed oxygen as condition dictates
- Promote rest – provide suitable toys and games
- Encourage family-centred care/partnership in care
- Provide oral fluids and diet as tolerated
- Provide vomit bowls, tissues and encourage oral hygiene
- Administer antibiotics as prescribed – although does not reduce the duration of the illness, stops the spread of the illness.

Potential complications

(as determined by http://www.immunisation.org.uk):

- Bronchopneumonia
- Weight loss: possibly related to nutritional intake
- Brain damage: related to poor cerebral perfusion
- Death

Tetanus

Steimle et al (2002) and Department of Health (2009b) defined tetanus as being caused by the bacterium *Clostridium tetani*. Although tetanus is preventable by the administration of a vaccine, tetanus is unique for it is not spread from person to person but by entering the body through a wound. The bacterium associated with tetanus is found in environmental sources, which include soil, dust or faecal matter from animals with spores in their intestine. In the neonatal period tetanus is aquired due to an infection of the umbilical stump (DoH 2009b).

Steimle et al (2002) suggested that minor wounds have led to higher rates of tetanus cases, primarily due to the fact that a severe wound is usually treated within a healthcare setting, as opposed to a smaller wound being viewed as less harmful and consequently not requiring treatment. Tetanus may also occur following surgery, dental infection and termination of pregnancies in an unhygienic setting.

Clinical signs and symptoms

There are several forms of the infection; localised, generalised, cephalic and tetanus neonatorum. However, Behrman & Kliegman (2002) indicated that the clinical examination of the wounds do not appear any different to an uninfected wound:

- Localised tetanus: uncommon in children, but causes pain, rigidity and spasms close to the wound site. The symptoms may last for weeks but resolve without complications.
- Generalised tetanus: this particular one causes gradual muscle rigidity, especially within the jaw, which may result in difficulty in swallowing. Convulsions may also be seen and contractions of various muscles. The airway may suddenly be compromised and as a result lead to respiratory insufficiency. The individual may be conscious but experience a great deal of pain. The duration of the illness may be from 2 to 6 weeks.
- Cephalic tetanus: this form may precede the former or be 1–2 days after otitis media, trauma to the face and head or due to the presence of a nasal foreign body according to Behrman & Kliegman (2002).
- Neonatorum tetanus: this usually starts 3–10 days after birth. Signs and symptoms include difficulty in sucking, swallowing, stiffness, excessive crying and contractions.

Pathology

The disease is as a result of exotoxins, tetanus toxin, or tetanospasmin and tetatanolysin, which may cause the tetanus toxin and result in muscle contraction, spasm and rigidity (Behrman & Kliegman 2002). The disease may also affect the neuromuscular junctions and cause paralysis. The toxins may proliferate, which may be characterised by tissues being inadequately oxygenated.

Signs and symptoms

- Headache
- Muscular stiffness in the jaw
- Dysphagia
- Stiffness in the neck
- Rigidity in the chest, back and abdominal muscles
- Sweating and fever.

Symptoms may start between 5 and 10 days after infection, but can range from 2 to 50 days (Steimle et al 2002).

Management of care (Steimle et al 2002)

- It may involve an admission to intensive care unit (for respiratory management)
- Treatment of sepsis
- Neutralising toxin before reaching the central nervous system
- Cardiac instability may need to be treated
- Determining urea and electrolyte and administering appropriate intravenous hydration
- Treatment to entry or wound site – by debriding and irrigation
- Monitoring pressure areas
- Analgesia.

Complications

- Rigidity of the muscles of the face, neck and jaw
- Muscle tears
- Vertebral fractures
- Respiratory problems: airway obstruction
- Pneumonia
- Septicaemia
- Cardiovascular instability.

PowerPoint

Access the companion PowerPoint presentation.

Eradicating tetanus

In industrialised countries, as the result of childhood immunisation programmes, the advancement of wound care, and improved farming practices, incidences of tetanus are infrequent. The PHLS (2000) suggests that the incidence is low in the UK; on average 6 cases were notified each year between 1990 and 1999.

The WHO (2001) identified that neonatal tetanus is a significant health issue in developing countries; in 1989 the World Health Assembly set an objective to eradicate the disease by 1995. However, most countries within the African region missed the goal. In 2001, WHO estimated that 124,000 cases and 93,000 deaths per year are principally due to tetanus in the African regions. A revised goal to eradicate neonatal and maternal tetanus globally was set for 2005. To achieve this aim, support was given to the member states in the region to:

- achieve elimination of maternal and neonatal tetanus
- validate the achieved status of elimination
- implement strategies for maintaining the situation.

The planned implementation of national immunisation programme resulted in the African region being divided into two categories:

- Category 1: countries that had eliminated or were close to eliminating neonatal tetanus and needed ongoing programmes.
- Category 2: countries with a high disease burden.

Steimle et al (2002) suggested that herd immunity is not a significant factor in the prevention of tetanus because it is an organism within the environment, which cannot be transferred from individual to individual. Therefore persons exposed to the bacteria need to have the antibodies in their blood at the time. Unless immunised they remain at risk of infection; contracting the infection does not provide immunity.

Poliomyelitis (POLIO)

This name comes from the Greek words *polio* (meaning grey) and *myelon* (meaning narrow – suggesting the spinal column). Polio has been described as an infectious disease, caused by a virus. Although the virus can cause an effect at any age, it predominantly affects children under 3 years of age (over 50% of cases) (see http://www.polioeradication.org). One of the most significant effects of the disease is paralysis, which is almost always permanent. In severe cases the disease may lead to death by asphyxiation.

PowerPoint

Access the companion PowerPoint presentation for some historical information about polio.

The WHO (2002b) declared that 51 countries within the European region had been free of polio for over 3 years. A global initiative was set out to eradicate polio by 2005. A coalition of four agencies includes:

- WHO
- Rotary International
- Centers for Disease Control and Prevention (CDC)
- The United Nations Children's Fund (UNICEF).

The objectives are:

- To stop the spread of the wild poliovirus as soon as possible and declare all WHO areas free by the end of 2005.
- To implement policies, include containment of the wild poliovirus and the development of post immunisation policies.
- To organise systems, including strengthening routine immunisations and surveillance for communicable diseases.

The countries mainly affected by the poliovirus are in the developing world: Africa, south Asia, and areas which are affected by conflict with reduced healthcare systems and poor sanitation. To stop the transmission of the poliovirus will involve:

- providing immunisation coverage to infants in the first year of life with four doses of the oral vaccine
- providing additional doses of the oral polio vaccine to children under the age of 5 years during national immunisation days
- surveillance for wild poliovirus through reporting mechanisms and laboratory testing, for children under the age of 15 years
- targeting a specific area when the wild poliovirus is within that area.

Pathology

The Centers for Disease Control and Prevention (2002) described the poliovirus as a member of the enterovirus subgroup. This particular type of virus is found within the digestive system and is stable at an acid pH. There are three serotypes – P1, P2 and P3 – within the poliovirus group. Immunity to one serotype may not produce considerable immunity to the others. The poliovirus is inactivated by heat, chlorine and ultraviolet light.

The virus enters the gastrointestinal system via the oral cavity and establishes itself within the pharynx and gastrointestinal tract. The virus may spread from the throat to be excreted via faeces; this may occur for several weeks after the onset of the illness. The poliovirus replicates in the gastrointestinal tract, attacks the local lymphoid tissue, penetrates the bloodstream and then, as it has a high affinity to nervous tissue, it infiltrates the nerve fibres and causes widespread destruction of the motor neurons (DoH 2009b).

Signs and symptoms

- The intubation period is usually 6–20 days but may range from 3 to 35 days.
- May be asymptomatic but there is still a risk of emitting the virus to others.
- Non-specific illness: characterised by sore throat and fever nausea, vomiting and abdominal pain, influenza.
- Non-paralytic aseptic meningitis: rigidity within the neck, back and/or legs, abnormal sensation. Symptoms may last up to 10 days and there is a full recovery.
- Flaccid paralysis: paralysis generally begins 1–10 days after initial symptoms and continues for 2–3 days, although there is usually no further paralysis. When the temperature is within an acceptable range, sufferers may also experience loss of superficial reflexes, severe muscle pain and spasms. Strength returns and patients do not experience permanent loss of sensation or changes within levels of understanding.
- Paralytic polio: three classifications:
  - spinal polio: asymmetric paralysis; often the legs are affected
  - bulbar polio: weakness of muscles supplying the cranial nerves
  - bulbospinal polio: combination of both bulbar and spinal paralysis.

WWW

Find out more about the signs and symptoms of polio from the following websites:

- http://www.polioeradication.org/vaccines
- http://www.immunisation.org.uk

Epidemiology

The following may transmit the poliovirus infection according to the polio eradication programme:

- human: person to person
- faecal to oral.

In children who have not yet established urinary and bowel control, food or drink contaminated by faeces are ready sources of transmission. At first the disease circulates quietly, because of the way it affects the central nervous system, and the onset is insidious.

The vaccine

The polio vaccine was developed during the 1950s and 1960s; the inactivated version was licensed in 1955 and was used until the 1960s. In 1963 the trivalent oral vaccine was permitted and licensed. The oral polio vaccine contains antibiotics and following administration the virus may be passed in faeces for up to 6 weeks. To acquire immunity against polio the schedule needs to be undertaken.

Until the introduction of the first vaccine in the 1950s, the poliovirus affected many young children. Polio remains endemic in a small number of developing countries, with a number of cases reported in Africa (BMJ 2004) and subsequent cases reported in polio-free countries in 2005/2006 (DoH 2009b). To ensure that countries remain clear of polio and its effects, healthcare professionals need to educate parents of the benefits of the vaccination and public health measures need to be monitored to maintain effective methods of cleanliness.

Activity

You are a student nurse assisting with the care of a 7-week-old girl. The child's mother readily acknowledges that she will be having her daughter vaccinated within the near future but she has read that there are two types of vaccines – inactivated and a live version – and requests your advice on which one would be most suitable. What do you advise her?

To aid development of your knowledge, access the following:

- http://www.cdc.gov/nip/publications

Haemophilus influenza

During the 1930s a prominent scientist – Margaret Pittman – demonstrated that haemophilus influenza could be isolated, and identified six forms or capsular types: a, b, c, d, e and f. Within the blood and cerebrospinal fluid, it was also found that almost all the cases examined revealed capsular type b.

Before the advent of effective vaccines, the WHO (2003) suggested that haemophilus influenza type b (Hib) predominantly causes meningitis and pneumonia in children under 5 years of age and was a cause of concern both in developed and developing countries. Hib can be carried without symptoms and prior to the development of a vaccination programme approximately 4 in every 100 children carried the organism (DoH 2009b). In developing countries, Hib would mainly cause pneumonia, whereas in developed countries the primary cause would be bacterial meningitis. To reduce the incidence of these infections, a vaccination programme was required because antibiotics are essential for the treatment but resistance to antibiotics may result, therefore prevention was required and vaccination is the most effective public health strategy in reducing the spread of Hib.

Pathology

The WHO (2003) defined haemophilus influenza as a Gram-negative bacterium. The infection is attributed to strains carrying a polysaccharide capsule. Type b causes nearly all-systemic infections, 15% of children in non-vaccinated populations carry Hib in their nasopharynx. However, from this perspective a small percentage will develop the disease. The transmission of the infection is by droplet and, as a result, those individuals who are symptomatic are important in the distribution of the organism. In the USA, the Centers for Disease Control and Prevention (see http://www.cdc.gov) stated that the exact mode of causing a systemic infection is unknown but that a previous infection such as a viral or an upper respiratory tract may be a contributory factor.

Epidemiology

The prime periods for infections before the establishment of a vaccine were between September and December, and between March and May. Factors that may predispose the individual to exposure of the infection are overcrowding within the household, the size of dwellings, schools, children's nurseries, older siblings attending school and socioeconomic influence. Other factors may include whether or the not the individual has a chronic disease, may cause susceptibility to other infections.

Diagnosis

This is usually confirmed by laboratory testing and infected bodily fluid may show Gram-negative coccobacilli suggestive of haemophilus influenza.

Signs and symptoms

- Meningitis: an infection that affects the meninges within the brain. Meningitis caused up to 65% of cases before the pre-vaccine era. An elevated temperature, altered conscious level and neck rigidity, are common clinical signs.
- Epiglottitis: this is as a result of an infection that causes swelling of the epiglottis, the tissue that prevents food entering the lungs. Epiglottitis affects the throat and causes airway obstruction, leading to a high risk of mortality if untreated.
- Septic arthritis (joint infections), cellulitis (an infection that may affect the skin) and pneumonia are clinical signs of a severe infection.
- Osteomyelitis: an infection that affects the skeletal system.

Medical management

Haemophilus influenza type (b) requires the individual to be hospitalised and treated with intravenous antibiotics from the cephalosporin group (see http://www.cdc.gov). A 10-day course is usually required.

The vaccine

The vaccine was developed and licensed in the USA in 1985. Initially it was not effective in children younger than 18 months. According to the WHO (see http://www.who.int), the vaccine in current usage is based on Hib polysaccharide conjugated to a protein carrier, such as the diphtheria toxoid-like protein (PRP-HbOC) tetanus toxoid (PRP-T) or meningococcal outer membrane (PRP-OMP). The conjugation of the PRP to the relevant protein causes a T cell response to the Hib polysaccharide.

The immunisation is usually given in infancy (minimum age 6 weeks) at intervals of 1 month. A booster dose is usually given at 12–18 months of age but in developing countries the disease usually occurs before this age.

Activity

A staff nurse tells you that he has been approached by a parent whose infant is to be discharged from the children's medical ward today. However, the mother has disclosed that her son has not received his primary course of immunisations because she was unsure of how to proceed with the amount of literature pertaining to the subject, of the advantages and disadvantages.

The staff nurse poses the following questions to you:

- What information would you offer?
- Which resources would you provide to support your verbal information?
- How would you explain the method of administration of the Hib vaccine?
- Finally, where should vaccines be stored on the ward and at what temperature?

What do you reply?

Measles

Measles is a viral illness that can be spread by droplet infection; the virus is referred to as the paramyxovirus (DoH 2009b). Richardson (2001) suggested the initial symptoms appear after an incubation period of 6–19 days. The first signs before a rash include irritability, elevated temperature, cough, feeling generally unwell and conjunctivitis. Over the next few days, Koplik's spots develop (small red spots within the oral cavity) approximately 1–2 days before the rash. Bedford (2003) described the rash as being maculopapular (red and blotchy). It usually starts at the hairline and spreads to other areas of the body over a period of 3 days. After 3 or 4 days, the rash may become brownish in appearance and then become less evident. The fever that accompanies the illness usually subsides before the rash diminishes.

Affected infants experience a fever and tend to feel uncomfortable and irritable. Davies et al (2001) identified that infants may have loss of appetite, cough, cold and conjunctivitis. The period for which an individual remains infectious is unknown, although it is acknowledged that the 1–2 days before the rash develops the patient is infectious.

Within the general population, where immunisation has not been undertaken there is a higher threat of transmission. Measles is a notifiable disease once diagnosed.

Epidemiology

According to the WHO (2002a), in 2001 there were 745,000 deaths from measles, and 30–40 million cases. The WHO suggested that many of the deaths could have been prevented by the use of a vaccine. The infection is more prevalent in areas where the population are disadvantaged, this usually applies to the developing countries.

Bedford (2003) suggests that in the UK before the routine administration of the vaccine in 1968, 90–95% of children under the age of 10 years had been infected. After 1968, the incidence of measles fell by 98%.

Diagnosis

The illness is usually construed by clinical examination. Bedford (2003) implied that the PHLS has increased monitoring and provided the NHS with equipment to test saliva for measles-specific IgM from cases notified to the Office for National Statistics, thus providing actual confirmation.

Treatment

Children who do not experience complications can be managed within the home environment. The treatment of measles is symptomatic, which includes providing medication to alleviate distress and reduce discomfort, which may be in the form of paracetamol or brufen elixir, and the encouragement of oral fluids to prevent dehydration. Some children may develop photophobia and need to be nursed in a darkened room with minimal light.

Complications

The complications that may result tend to be seen in individuals who are malnourished or immunosuppressed. Bedford (2003) indicated that concerns are as a result of ear infections (otitis media), pneumonia, croup, seizures and encephalitis. Atypical complications include idiopathic thrombocytopenia. During pregnancy, measles may result in premature labour.

Prevention

The first vaccine to be successful against the virus that caused measles was made available in the USA in 1963, and in the UK in 1968. It stimulated the production of antibodies.

In 1988, the British government had a change of policy in relation to single-antigen vaccines, and began to use the combined measles, mumps and rubella (MMR) vaccine a single injection, which provides greater protection against the three diseases. For the first time there was a vaccine for mumps and a single immunisation for rubella, which enabled prepubescent girls to be vaccinated, thus reducing the transmission of the virus during pregnancy to the unborn fetus. Since the advent of this strategy the number of cases of rubella has fallen.

The aim of this programme is to eliminate the diseases and 95% of the public need to be vaccinated to stop the spread of measles (Bedford 2003). The initial dose of the vaccine is given at the age of 12–15 months, and this is followed by a second dose before starting school.

Side effects

The MMR is a live vaccine, which means that side effects are possible. These include fever, irritability, cough or cold, and drowsiness. Side effects are less common with the second dose.

The MMR vaccine contains a small quantity of egg; as a result there has been concern whether or not children who have an allergy to egg should be given the vaccine because of the risk of an acute reaction. Although there is evidence to suggest it is safe, the DoH (1996) issued guidelines for safe practice, suggesting that it may be advisable to undertake the procedure in a hospital setting. Bedford (2003) indicated that most professionals would advise this course of action providing that the child had experienced an anaphylactic reaction, but those who had not experienced this type of reaction could be immunised without any specific precautions.

Despite this programme of vaccination, recent reports from the Health Protection Agency (2008a) indicate a steep rise in the numbers of confirmed cases of measles. The controversy surrounding the publication of research by Dr Andrew Wakefield (Wakefield et al 1998) that suggested the vaccine was responsible for the development of enterocolitis and autism, although it was later refuted (Cole 2005), has led to public reluctance to immunise.

Mumps

Moses (2004a) defined mumps as being caused by a paramyovirus, which affects the parotid glands. In 2008a, the Health Protection Agency stated that '... humans are the

Activity

Access the companion PowerPoint presentation for information on the debate concerning MMR vaccine:

- Explore the controversial issues surrounding the MMR vaccine and make notes.
- Examine and discuss the concerns surrounding single vaccines.

www

Refer to the WHO (2002b) initiative for vaccine research:

- http://www.who.int/vaccine research/diseases/measles/en

only known host of the mumps virus, and that it is a notifiable disease', suggesting that when it is suspected by law, it has to be reported (see the HPA website at: http://www.hpa.org.uk).

Mumps is a common childhood infection and may occur at any age. The disease is transmitted either by direct patient-to-patient contact or is airborne, by infected droplets of saliva. The highest rate of occurrence is late winter and early spring. The virus is prevalent where there are a large number of children, for example, preschools and schools. According to the Health Protection Agency (2008b), mumps was the cause of 1200 hospital admissions each year in England and Wales before the development of the MMR vaccine. Mumps was made a notifiable disease in 1988. In the year 2000 there were 2162 cases of mumps, with one of the last outbreaks being in the North of England mainly affecting secondary school children, who had either not received the MMR vaccine or had not completed the course and had received only one dose.

Signs and symptoms

- Usually starts with a headache and an elevated temperature.
- Characterised by a swelling of the parotid glands, which may either be uni- or bilateral. However, the Health Protection Agency (2008a) suggested that 30% of cases in children did not show any of the symptoms.
- The intubation period varies from 14 to 21 days.
- Can be transmitted several days before and after the swelling of the parotid glands.
- Individuals who have been exposed to the virus should consider themselves infectious from 12 to 25 days after contact.

Moses (2004a) suggested that patients also experience general malaise and anorexia. This is thought to be as a result of the pain and discomfort experienced when eating and drinking due to tenderness at the mandibular angle, and redness within the oral cavity at the opening of the parotid duct.

Treatment

The treatment of mumps is symptomatic and most people improve after 10 days (Health Protection Agency 2008b).

Complications

Complications comprise (Health Protection Agency 2008b):

- aseptic meningitis: 15%
- orchitis usually unilateral: in up to 20% of postpubertal males; infertility rarely occurs
- oophritis in 5% of postpubertal females; rarely infertility
- deafness: 1:15000 cases, usually affects one ear
- encephalitis
- pancreatitis
- arthritis
- nephritis
- pericarditis.

Although there is no evidence to suggest that mumps may cause any fetal abnormalities, if infected during the first 3 months of pregnancy there is an increased possibility of a spontaneous abortion.

Prevention

Since the development of the MMR vaccine in 1988, the 3-yearly sequences associated with mumps have ended. No single vaccine that is effective against mumps is licensed in the UK.

The immunisation schedule involves administering a vaccine at 12–15 months of age and a further one at 4–5 years. However, the Health Protection Agency (2008b) states that '... there is not an age limit' and, when necessary, the two doses can be given 1 month apart. The initial dose will give approximately 61–91% protection, therefore two doses will be required to provide more effective immunity (DoH 2009b).

Activity

With the aid of a diagram of the human body, illustrate the possible complications that may result from mumps. The following might help:

- http://www.hpa.org.uk/infections/topics_az/mumps/gen_info.htm

Rubella

Rubella was initially thought to be a variant of measles and scarlet fever, and was referred to as the third disease. It was first described as a separate disease in Germany, in the mid 1800s, and consequently became known as 'German measles' (Cherry 2003). An epidemic occurred in 1940 and the following year an Australian ophthalmologist – Norman Gregg – described 78 cases of infants acquiring congenital cataracts, following maternal exposure to the virus in early pregnancy. The virus was first isolated in 1962, and classified as a rubivrus (Cherry 2003).

Pathology of the illness

The Centers for Disease Control and Prevention (2003) suggested that the virus may replicate within the nasopharynx and regional lymph nodes. After 5–7 days, it proliferates to the tissues; it is at this stage that the fetus may become infected.

Epidemiology

The disease occurs throughout the world and is an infection that affects only humans. As it is not transferred by an animal source, infants who have contracted congenital rubella may continue to shed the virus for a considerable length of time; a true carrier state has not yet been confirmed.

The infection is transmitted via human contact, either by airborne transmission or secretions from the respiratory system of an infected individual. The Centers for Disease Control and Prevention (2003) state that it is not communicated to humans by insects. The infection is more prevalent during the late winter and early spring.

Since 1997, the Centers for Disease Control and Prevention (2003) has reported that the greatest number of infants born with congenital rubella syndrome in America were to women of Hispanic origins, mostly in Latin America or the Caribbean countries where the vaccine was not routinely used or the immunisation programme has only just been fully implemented.

Clinical manifestations

Acquired rubella

The period of incubation for rubella varies from 12 to 23 days (DoH 2009b). The symptoms are frequently mild involving low grade fever and generally may be non-apparent (Centers for Disease Control 2003). Moses (2004b) suggested that in children, a rash may cover the soft palate and face. Older children may experience a mild fever, general feeling of being unwell, lymphadenopathy and an upper respiratory tract infection, prior to the rash. Both the Centers for Disease Control and Prevention (2003) and Moses (2004b) indicate that the rash starts on the face and generally spreads to all parts of the body. It usually lasts for 3 days and may be pruritic. A maculopapular rash may be evident for 2 weeks. Complications arising from the infection are rare in children but comprise:

- Arthritis: which may affect up to 70% of adult women who contract rubella.
- Encephalitis: may affect more adults. Mortality statistic varies from 0 to 50%.
- Disorders affecting the blood: e.g. thrombocytopenia, which is characterised by a low platelet count, causing gastrointestinal or cerebral haemorrhaging.

The duration of these complications varies from days to months, but most individuals recover (DoH 2009b).

Congenital rubella

Due to vaccine development, initially as a single vaccine and then incorporated as part of the triple vaccine MMR (Box 40.4), the objective is to prevent congenital rubella.

Box 40.4

The rubella vaccine

The rubella vaccine is a live attenuated virus. The vaccine was first developed in 1965 at the Wistar Institute. It is available in three sources: the single antigen, combined with the mumps vaccine or with the measles and mumps vaccine (MMR). In clinical investigations, the vaccine has proved to be 95% effective in persons aged 12 months or over after a single dose. The Centers for Disease Control and Prevention (2003) established that the vaccine is effective for at least 15 years against both to rubella and viraemia. Further studies have provided evidence suggest that one dose of the immunisation, provides long-term immunity, which is probably life long.

Vertical transmission, i.e. from the maternal blood to the fetus, may cause catastrophic effects, especially during the first trimester. The infection may affect all the organs and cause a variety of congenital defects. During this period the virus may cause spontaneous abortion (miscarriage) or premature labour.

The risk of congenital problems decreases as the pregnancy progresses between 11 and 16 weeks, with fetal damage rare after 16 weeks (DoH 2009b).

Activity

Explore the effects that congenital rubella syndrome has on:

- the infant
- the family
- the National Health Service
- the Social Services department
- the education system.

Initially, the following websites may help your search:

- http://www.cdc. gov/nip/publications/pink/rubella.pdf
- http://www.who. int/vaccines/en/rubella.shtml

When you have found the necessary information pertaining to this subject, share the information with your colleagues and identify services in your area for an infant who has complex developmental needs.

Diagnosis

The key to diagnosis is initially by taking a detailed history, however confirmed diagnosis may be determined from nasal secretions, blood, urine and cerebrospinal fluid (Cherry 2003). Acute rubella virus may be confirmed by a significant elevation in rubella antibody titre in acute and recovery stages, by the serum specimens or by the level of serum rubella IgM (Centers for Disease Control and Prevention 2003). The serum needs to be obtained as soon as possible, which may be defined as 7–10 days, following the onset of the infection and 2–3 weeks later.

Rarely other tests that might assist in confirmation of the diagnosis include:

- enzyme-linked immunosorbent assays
- haemagglutination inhibition test
- immunofluorescent antibody.

Treatment

The treatment of rubella depends upon a number of factors, including the severity and whether the woman is pregnant.

The mild cases may just need to be advised upon encouraging oral fluids, rest and analgesia with antipyretic properties to alleviate discomfort and fever. More severe cases may acquire hospitalisation and treated accordingly if complications arise, for example encephalitis may require treatment within an intensive care unit, for monitoring vital signs to initiating ventilatory support, in addition to intravenous medication.

References

Aston, R., 1998. Who wouldn't protect children? The Practitioner 242, 503.

Aycliffe, V., 2009. Clinical features and management of atopic eczema in children. Paediatric Nursing 21 (9), 35–43.

Baker, J.P., Katz, S.L., 2004. Childhood vaccine development: an overview. Paediatric Research 55 (2), 347–356.

Bangura, K., 1998. Dying for a snooze. Nursing Times 94 (21), 29–30.

Barker, D.J., 1990. The foetal and infant origins of adult disease. British Medical Journal 301, 1111.

Barker, D.J.P., Eriksson, J.G., Forsen, T., Osmond, C., 2002. Fetal origins of adult disease, strength of effects and biological basis. International Journal of Epidemiology 31, 1235–1239.

Bedford, H., 2003. Measles: the disease and its prevention. Nursing Standard 17 (24), 46–55.

Behrman, R.E., Kliegman, R.M., 2002. Nelson's essentials of pediatrics, 4th edn. WB Saunders, Philadelphia.

Bennett, M., 2003. Sleep and rest in PICU. Paediatric Nursing: Critical Care 15 (1), 3–6.

Braine, M.E., 2009. The role of the hypothalamus, part 2: regulation of sleep–wake cycles and effect on pain. British Journal of Neuroscience Nursing 9 (2), 113–119.

Campbell, S., Glasper, E.A. (Eds.), 2001. Whaley and Wong's children's nursing, 6th edn. Mosby, St Louis.

Centers for Disease Control and Prevention (CDC), 2002. Epidemiology and prevention of vaccine preventable diseases, 7th edn. CDC, Atlanta, GA.

Centers for Disease Control and Prevention (CDC) 2003 Rubella and rubella vaccine. Online. Available at: http://www.cdc.gov/nip/publications/pink/rubella.pdf

Cherry, J.D., 2003. Rubella virus. In: Feigin, R.S., Cherry, J.D., Demmler-Harrison, G.J., Kaplan, S.L. (Eds.), Textbook of pediatric infectious disease, 5th edn. Elsevier, USA.

Cork, M.J., 1997. The importance of skin barrier function. Journal of Dermatological Treatment 8, S7–S13.

Cork, M.J., 1999. Taking the itch out of eczema: how the careful use of emollients can break the itch-scratch cycle. Asthma Journal 4, 116–120.

Crawford, J., 1995. Winning the fight against disease: a review of childhood immunisation. Child Health 2 (5), 187–191.

Dales, L., Hammer, S.J., Smith, N.J., 2001. Time trends in autism and in MMR immunization, coverage in California. Journal of the American Medical Association 285, 1183–1185.

David, T.J., 1993. Food and food additive intolerance in childhood. Blackwell Scientific, Oxford.

Davies, E., et al., 2001. Manual of childhood infections. Cited in: Bedford H 2003 Measles: the disease and its prevention. Nursing Standard 17 (24), 46–55.

Department for Education and Skills (DfES), 2006. Working together to safeguard children. HMSO, London.

Department of Health (DoH), 1992. Health of the nation: a strategy for health in England. HMSO, London.

Department of Health (DoH), 1994. COMA report on weaning and the weaning diet. HMSO, London.

Department of Health (DoH) 1996 Immunisation against infectious diseases. Online. Available at: http://www.greenbook/index.htm

Department of Health (DoH), 1998. Our healthier nation. HMSO, London.

Department of Health (DoH), 2002. About pertussis (whooping cough). Online. Available at: http://www.immunisation.org.uk

Department of Health. (DoH), 2003. NHS immunisation statistics. Online. Available at: http://www.dh.gov.uk/Policy/ions/topics

Department of Health, (DoH), 2008. Weaning: starting solid food. HMSO, London.

Department of Health, (DoH), 2009a. Guidance and legislation on powdered infant milk. 14 May 2009. Online. Available at: http://www.dh.gov.uk/en/Healthcare/Children/Maternity/Maternalandinfantnutrition/DH_081924

Department of Health, (DoH), 2009b. Immunisation against infectious diseases. Online. Available at: http://www.greenbook/index/htm.

De Serres, G., et al., 1995. Measles vaccine efficacy during an outbreak in a highly vaccinated population: incremental increase in protection with age at vaccination up to 18 months. Cited in: Bedford H 2003 Measles: the disease and its prevention. Nursing Standard 17 (24), 46–55.

Devilliers, A.C., de Waard-van der Spek, F.B., Mulder, P.G., Oranje, A.P., 2002. Treatment of refractory atopic dermatitis using 'wet wrap' dressings and diluted corticosteroids: results of standardised treatment in both children and adults. Dermatology 204 (1), 50–55.

Dinges, D., Douglas, S.D., Hamarman, S., Zaugg, L., Kapoor, S., 1995. Sleep deprivation and human immune function. Advances in Neuroimmunology 5, 97–110.

Donald, S., 1997. Know how: wet wraps in atopic eczema. Nursing Times 93 (44), 67–68.

Eriksson, J.G., Forsen, T., Osmond, C., Barker, D.J.P., 2001. Early growth and coronary heart disease in later life: longitudinal study. British Medical Journal 322, 949–953.

Fewtrell, M., Lucas, A., Morgan, J.B., 2003. Factors associated with weaning in full term and preterm infants. Archives of Disease in Childhood. Neonatal edition F296, F301 Ed 88.

Finlay, G., 1991. Sleep and intensive care. Intensive Care Nursing 7, 61–68.

Fiocchi, A., Restani, P., Gualtiero, L., Martelli, A., 2003. Clinical tolerance to lactose in children with cow's milk allergy. Pediatrics 112 (2), 359.

Fleming, P.J., Diar, P.S., Bacon, C., Berry, P.J., 2000. Sudden unexpected death in infancy. The CESDI SUDI Studies, 1993–1996.

Food Standards Agency (FSA) 2003 Food intolerance. Online. Available at: http://www.foodstandards.gov.uk

Foote, K.D., Marriott, L.D., 2003. Weaning of infants. Archives of Diseases in Childhood 88, 488–492.

Gronfier, C., Luthringer, R., Follenius, M., Schaltenbrand, N., Macher, J.P., Muzet, A., Brandenberger, G., 1996. A quantitative evaluation of the relationships between growth hormone secretion and delta wave electroencephalographic activity during normal sleep and after enrichment in delta waves. Sleep 19, 817–824.

Hall, M., 1996. Health for all children. Oxford University Press, Oxford.

Hamlyn B, Brooker S, Oleinikova K, Wands S 2000. Infant feeding survey 2000. BMRB International, London. Online. Available at: http://www.doh.gov.uk/public/infantfeedingreport.htm

Hanifin, J.M., Rajka, G., 1980. Diagnostic features of atopic dermatitis. Acta Dermatologica Venereologica 92, 44–47.

Health Protection Agency (HPA) 2003 Infections. Fact sheet for schools: wired for health. Online. Available at: http://www.hpa.org.uk/infections/topics

Health Protection Agency (HPA), 2008a. Measles figures soar. Press release. Online. Available at: http://www.hpa.org.uk/webw/HPAweb & HPAwebStandard/HPAweb_C/1227774034336?p=1204186170287

Health Protection Agency (HPA), 2008b. General information: mumps. Online. Available at: http://www.hpa.org.uk/HPA/Topics/Infectiousdiseases/InfectionsAZ/1191942172901/

Heinig, M.J., Nommsen, L.A., Pearson, J.M., Lennerdal, G., Deney, K.G., 1993. Energy and protein intakes of breast fed and formula fed infants during the first year of life and their association with growth velocity: the DARLING study. The American Journal of Clinical Nutrition 58, 152–161.

Hoare, C., Li Wan Po, A., Williams, H., 2000. Systematic review of treatments of atopic eczema. Health Technology and Assessment 4 (37), 1–191.

Hockenberry, M.J., 2003. Wong's Nursing care of infants and children, 7th edn. Mosby, St Louis.

Horne, J., 1988. Why we sleep. Oxford University Press, New York.

Hubbard, S., Trigg, E., 2000. Practices in children's nursing. Guidelines for hospital and community. Churchill Livingstone, London.

Jenni, O.G., O'Connor, B., 2005. Children's sleep: an interplay between culture and biology. Pediatrics 115, 204–216.

Krugman, S., Dubowitz, H., 2003. Failure to thrive. American Family Physician 68 (5), 879–884.

Lawrence, R.A., 1989. Breastfeeding: a guide for the medical professional, 3rd edn. Mosby Yearbook, St Louis.

Lindsey, E., Hartrick, G., 1996. health promoting nursing practice: the demise of the nursing process? Journal of Advanced Nursing 23 (1), 106–112.

McCarthy, H., 2001. Childhood immunisation. Nursing Standard 15 (44), 39–44.

McGraw, K., Hoffman, R., Harker, C., Herman, J.H., 1999. The development of circadian rhythms in a human infant. Sleep 22, 303–310.

Miano, S., Villa, M.P., Blanco, D., Zamera, M.D., Rodriquez, R., Ferri, R., Bruni, O., Peraita-Adrados, R., 2009. Development of NREM sleep instability–continuity (cyclic alternating pattern) in healthy term infants aged 1–4 months. Sleep 32 (1), 83–90.

Minde, K., Faucon, A., Faulkner, S., 1994. Sleep problems in toddlers: effects of treatment on their daytime behaviour. Journal of the American Academy of Child and Adolescent Psychiatry 33, 1114–1121.

Moses, S. 2004a. Mumps. Practice notebook.com, a family medicine resource. Online. Available at: http://www.fpnotebook.com/ID233.htm

Moses, S. 2004b. Rubella. Practice notebook.com, a family medicine resource. Online. Available at: http:www.fpnotebook.com/ID233.htm

National Eczema Society (2003) Online. Available at: http://www.eczema.org

National Institute for Clinical Excellence (NICE), 2007. Atopic eczema in children. Management of atopic eczema in children from birth up to the age of 12 years. Clinical Guideline 57. NICE, London.

Parish, H.J., 1965. A history of immunisation. E and S Livingstone, Edinburgh.

Pewson, G., 2008. Why children die: a pilot study 2006; England (North East, South West and West Midlands), Wales and Northern Ireland. CEMACH, London.

Pei, A.Y.S., Chan, H.H.L., Ho, K.M., 2001. The effectiveness of wet wrap dressings using 0.1% mometasone furoate and 0.005% fluticasone proprionate ointments in the treatment of moderate to severe atopic dermatitis in children. Pediatric Dermatology 18 (4), 343–348.

Public Health Laboratory Service (PHLS) 2000. Cited In: Steimle, D., Aston, R., Van Damme, P. (Eds.), Tetanus and diphtheria. Nursing Standard, 16 (22), 33–35.

Ramsay, M., et al., 1994. Measles vaccine: a 27-year follow up. Cited in: Bedford H 2003 Measles: the disease and its prevention. Nursing Standard 17 (24), 46–55.

Richards, M., Wadsworth, M., Rahimi-Forashani, A., Hardy, R., Kuh, D., Paul, A., 1998. Infant nutrition and cognitive development in the first offspring of a national UK birth cohort. Developmental Medicine and Child Neurology 40 (3), 163–167.

Richardson, M., et al., 2001. Evidence base of incubation periods, periods of infectiousness and exclusion policies for the control of communicable diseases in schools and preschools. Pediatric Infectious Diseases Journal 20 (4), 380–391.

Sadeh, A., Gruber, R., Raviv, A., 2003. Effects of sleep restriction and extension on school age children: what a difference an hour makes. Child Development 74, 444–445.

Savoie, N., Rioux, F.M., 2002. Impact of maternal anaemia on the infant's iron status at 9 months of age. Canadian Journal of Public Health 93, 203–207.

Scientific Advisory Committee on Nutrition, 2003. Introduction of solid foods. DoH, London.

Shaw, N.J., Pal, B.R., 2002. Vitamin D deficiency in UK Asian families: activating a new concern. Archives of Diseases in Childhood 86, 147–149.

Sidebotham, P., Fox, J., et al., 2008. Preventing childhood deaths: an observational study of child death overview panels in England. Department for Schools and Families, London.

Singhal, A., Cole, T.J., Lucas, A., 2001. Early nutrition in preterm infants and later blood pressure. The Lancet 357, 413–419.

Spagnola, C., Korb, J.D., 2002. Atopic dermatitis. eMedicine Journal 3 (10).

Steimle, D., Aston, R., Van Damme, P., 2002. Tetanus and diphtheria. Nursing Standard 16 (22), 33–35.

Tudor-Hart, J., 1971. The inverse care law. Lancet i, 405–412.

Twitchen, L.J., Lowe, J.A., 1998. Atopic eczema and wet-wrap dressings. Professional Nurse 14 (2), 113–116.

Uhlmann, V., Martin, C.M., Sheils, O., et al., 2002. Potential viral pathogenic mechanism for new variant inflammatory bowel disease. Molecular Pathology 55, 1–6.

Wakefield, A., et al., 1998. Ileal-lymphoid nodular hyperplasia, non-specific colitis and pervasive development disorder in children. Lancet 351 (9103), 637–641.

Waugh, A., Grant, A., 2003. Ross and Wilson anatomy and physiology in health and illness, 9th edn. Churchill Livingstone, London.

Weinhouse, G.L., Schwab, R.B., 2006. Sleep in the critically ill patient. Sleep 29 (5), 707–716.

Wells, J., 2002. Growth and failure to thrive. Paediatric Nursing 14 (3), 37–42.

Wiggs, L., 2009. Behavioural aspects of children's sleep. Archives of Diseases in Childhood 94, 59–62.

Williams, M., 1999. Food intolerance. Nursing Times 95 (21), 68–69.

World Health Organization (WHO), 2001. Vaccines, immunisation and biologicals: neonatal and maternal tetanus. Online. Available at: http://www.who.int/vaccines/en tetanus shtml.

World Health Organization (WHO), 2002a. Child and adolescent health and development. Cited in: Bedford H 2003 Measles: the disease and its prevention. Nursing Standard 17(24):46–55.

World Health Organization (WHO), 2002b. Initiative for vaccine research. Online. Available at: http://www-who.int/vaccine_ research/diseases/measles/en.

World Health Organization (WHO), 2003. Immunization, vaccines, biologicals. Online. Available at: http://www.who.int/vaccines/en/haeflub.shtml.

World Health Organization (WHO), 2006. Position paper on haemophilus influenzae type b conjugate vaccines. Online. Available at: http://www.who.int/immunization/REH_47_8_pages.pdf

Wright, K.P., Hull, J.T., Czeiler, C.A., 2002. Relationship between alertness, performance and body temperature in humans. American Journal of Physiology. Regulatory. Integrative and Comparative Physiology 283, R1370–R1377.

Young, P.A., Young, P.H., Tolbert, D.L., 2008. Basic clinical neuroscience, 2nd edn. Lippincott Williams & Wilkins, Philadelphia.

Useful Websites

Polio eradication initiative: http://www.polioeradication.org/vaccines/polioeradication/all/background/disease/asp

Information in relation to child health issues: http://www.cyh.com/cyh/parentopics/usr-srch 2.stm

Advice for parents regarding childhood illness: http://www.surgerydoor.co.uk

Health problems in early childhood

41

Arija Nikola Parker

ABSTRACT

Early childhood, as a period of growth and development, is a wonderful time in a child's life, characterised by the opportunity to investigate a world that has a lot to offer in terms of exploration and discovery from a preschooler's perspective. Parents will have a similarly rewarding experience, observing through their own eyes the experiences of their offspring. However, the magic and wonder of this period can, in reality, be very different, depending on social, economic and political factors, and the lifestyles we have to pursue living in the 21st century. This might mean that this is a very stressful time for parents and children alike. In addition to the broader societal influences, health problems may occur by the very nature of the developmental stage the child is progressing through. Preschool children are constantly on the move, questioning and reacting to everything around them in the absence of the sophisticated cognitive ability to deal with the potential dangers that seem to be around every corner, even within the child's home itself. It is a period of life when a large percentage of this age group are socialised into nursery schools and see a wider world than that of home and family. As a result, they are influenced by their peer group and other significant adults such as nursery nurses and teachers.

LEARNING OUTCOMES

- Identify the health problems that may specifically affect the early childhood period.
- Link the problems to the preschool developmental stage of childhood.
- Utilise the brief discussions to expand and develop knowledge and understanding in relation to children's nursing practice.
- Acquire a basic understanding of how the Activities of Living (Roper et al 1996) apply to children's nursing practice.

Introduction

This chapter will address the health problems specifically related to preschool children, with the obvious exclusion of issues covered directly in other chapters. Each section, structured by a heading relating to Activities of Living (Box 41.1), will detail the developmental and physiological aspects that relate specifically to the preschool child. This is followed by a brief description of the health-related problem, its management and the implications for the healthcare professional, most usually a practice nurse, children's nurse, health visitor or community children's nurse. These implications relate particularly to the nurse's role in offering parental advice and education, ensuring that this chapter has a health promotion/education focus. The broad range of topics covered means that detailed information will have to be gained by reading the more specifically focused chapters, utilising the companion PowerPoint presentation and consulting the related websites and further reading references evident at the end of the chapter.

Powerpoint

The companion PowerPoint presentation contains supplementary information and answers to questions posed within this chapter.

The overall aim is to take a tour around the child and family's daily life, identifying where health problems may occur that will bring them into contact with healthcare professionals and, more particularly, children's nurses and/or health visitors. In light of the need for a holistic approach to subject coverage and a felt requirement for this chapter to have a structure, the Roper–Logan–Tierney model of Activities of Daily Living (1996) will be used as subheadings to ensure subject coverage. Although this model is not utilised exclusively in the children's nursing world, its influence is evident in any piece of nursing documentation used in paediatric clinical areas. It is generally integrated into a framework to support the philosophy of family-centred care widely cited and utilised in the practice of children's nursing.

The model uses a framework of 12 activities (Box 41.1) of living used within the context of the biological, psychological, sociocultural, environmental and politico-economic factors

DOI: 10.1016/B978-0-7020-3183-0.10041-4

Box 41.1

Activities of living (from Roper et al 1996)

- Maintaining a safe environment
- Communicating
- Controlling body temperature
- Breathing
- Eating and drinking
- Personal cleansing and dressing
- Mobilising
- Working and playing
- Expressing sexuality
- Sleeping
- Dying.

that will impinge and affect an individual's life in society today. The model of living incorporates the idea of lifespan from birth to death, however short or long an individual's life may be. The children's nurse is thus usually involved in her client's care for only one stage of a person's lifespan and has a significant role in assisting child and family to reach adulthood by optimising health potential. The idea of a dependence/independence continuum, which is another element of the model, transfers readily to a children's health and social care setting, although the process of gaining independence is not motivated by the notion of being healthy or being ill but via the process of a developing child making the first steps to doing things on his or her own and gaining independence in activities of living. In the same way as with an adult patient, illness will scupper the drive for independence temporarily, where in a child's case re-learning skills barely learned should be achieved with relative ease. Thus the preschooler's dependence on parents/carers fluctuates as he or she starts learning to perform the activity of living tasks alone, although dependence on parents is high because of the need for constant supervision.

Reflect on your practice

- Are nursing models used in the clinical areas in which you have clinical experience?
- If so, which models are used?
- Do they improve the quality of care children and families receive?

From the perspective of the children's nurse caring for a sick child during a period of illness, regression in skill acquisition may occur, which will cause great frustration to a child who is gaining independence, and confusion may arise in relation to a child's developing independence if, for example, a nurse may take on the caring role without understanding the roles the child is developing, i.e. dressing a child who usually, with minimal assistance, would work through getting dressed in the morning. Insight into the child's developmental stage and an appreciation of the family dynamics gained via questions triggered by such a model give the nurse valuable information regarding her client to then individualise care via the use of the nursing process (Roper et al 1996).

Maintaining a safe environment

The preschool period of development is a time when a child has the opportunity to explore a world, which expands by the minute, hour and day as mobility increases and as, with growth in height and the ability to climb, different objects become more visible and new targets are more readily achievable. The need to climb higher, explore in greater detail and play more exciting games is a necessary stage in learning and developing limits and boundaries in relation to preventing harm and accidents during later years, although at this stage it means little to the person directly involved, namely the child him- or herself. It is the adult who has the responsibility of averting a potential accident seemingly at every minute of the day. This responsibility can be overwhelming and, even with the best intentions and correct interventions, accidents still happen.

The acceleration of gross motor skill acquisition means that a toddler at 20 months of age is throwing and kicking a ball quite effectively, although the direction and purpose of the act itself may be inconsistent. They climb with no fear of falling. At 2 to 3 years they are jumping, running and riding a tricycle with no problems and their abilities, from a fine motor and gross motor skills perspective, are developing at speed. At this time, cognitive abilities mean that, in Piagetian terms, the child is egocentric, i.e. unable to separate his or her own perspective from others: 'You see what I see, you think what I think', which will affect the child's perceptual and communication behaviour (Bukatko & Daehlar 2004). Thus, the ability to predict what might happen as a result of his or her actions is limited. Using Piaget's theoretical terms, during the preoperational (or intuitive) period, language is developing, although intelligence is evident before starting to utilise words, as is evident by observing the way children act and behave in their environment. However, although children can link words together by the age of 2 it is clear that they cannot reason or make sense of the world in a logical way (Sylva & Lunt 1982).

When environmental factors, such as the houses we live in, the toys children play with and the areas children play in – all key components to modern living – are taken into account, it is not surprising that, even with the most safety-conscious and aware parents, accidents happen. In addition, inadequate adult supervision, the influence of stress and the size of the child are factors that contribute to an increased risk of accidents taking place.

These factors account for the fact that 500,000 children under the age of 5 attended A&E departments in 1999, and that in this year 90 children died as a result of accidents in the home in England and Wales. Although perceived as a place of safety, the home actually provides the necessary combination of obstacles and risks to ensure that the 0–4 age group is at a high risk of falls, strikings (i.e. bumping into static objects or being the victim of being hit by moving objects), burns, foreign bodies in eye or other orifices, and so on. The vast majority of these will be dealt with in the A&E department, as minor injuries, with no need for follow-up (Department of Trade and Industry (DTI) 2001). However, this is not to devalue the implications on child health and the important role of nurses in preventing such accidents. Thus the role of health visitors, children's nurses in health education and health promotion are key to preventing the health problems that may result due to accidents. According to information from the Royal Society for the Prevention of Accidents (ROSPA), in conjunction with the above statistics, falls account for the majority of non-fatal accidents and the highest numbers of deaths are due to fire. ROSPA argues that most accidents are preventable through increased awareness, improvements in the home environment and greater product safety. The nursing care of children who have sustained injuries as a result of accidents is discussed in the related chapters. What follows are additional statistics and recommendations with regard to the nursing role as a health educator/promoter in some very specific areas related to the preschool child.

www

The Royal Society for the Prevention of Accident's website contains fact sheets including one dealing with child safety in the home:

- http://www.rospa.com/childsafety/indet.htm

Other links which may be useful include the following:

Health Development Agency (2003) 'Prevention and reduction of accidental injury in children and older people – evidence briefing', which can be accessed at:

- http://www.nice.org.uk/aboutnice/whoweare/aboutthehda/hdapublications/prevention_and_reduction_of_acc

Reflect on your practice

On the link to the ROSPA child safety pages you can access the European Child Safety Alliance (2009), Child Safety Report Card Scotland accessed at:

- http://www.rospa.com/childsafety/actionplan/scotland/report_Card.pdf

This identifies that children and young people from more deprived families of being at higher risk of injury and death from unintentional injury.

Why should this be so?

Accidental poisoning

In the years 2006/07 the National Poisons Information Service (NPIS) received around 500,000 poisons-related enquires. Of these enquiries 35% related to children under 10 years of age and of these 88% related to the under-5 age group (HPA 2007). Cases involve intentional overdose in adults and adolescents, and accidental ingestion in children, which accounts for about 7% of all accidents (Pickford 2000). The most commonly implicated drugs are iron, methadone and tricyclic antidepressants, although, realistically, anything can be accidentally ingested by a child.

Management of the child

The management will depend on the amount of drug ingested and how long it takes the child and parent to seek medical assistance. The care is based on advice offered by the NPIS. If attending A&E, the parents should take the container, packaging or part of plant/fungi with them and have an idea of time it was ingested. In the case of herbicidal poisoning it is important that the brand name as well as manufacturer's name is known so that the active ingredient and solvents can be identified by the poisons centre (Northall & Cullen 1999).

PowerPoint

Access the companion PowerPoint presentation and read the advice offered to parents with regard to preventing accidental ingestion in pre-school age children.

Implications for the healthcare professional

Many strategies can be employed to prevent the accidental ingestion of many substances, which include controlling the child's access to poisons, making the environment safer and/or changing the child's behaviour (Pickford 2000). The main reasons for accidental ingestion are inappropriate storage of medicines, lack of safety awareness and insufficient supervision of children. Liquid preparations, purposely formulated to make them more palatable for children, add to the probability that, when children get access to these medicines, they are more likely to consume large amounts. For example, iron and vitamin preparations generally look attractive and taste good as well. Thus the health message involves ensuring safety of medicines within the home are out of reach and out of sight in child-resistant containers. Any chemicals, i.e. cleaning fluids like bleach, should be stored in their original containers and be out of reach and any unwanted medicines and chemicals should be disposed of accordingly.

Part of the developmental aspect of care involves educating the child with regards to encouraging them not to put things like berries in their mouths, in terms they will understand, as well as encouraging parents not to buy plants with poisonous leaves or berries or those that irritate skin. Toddlers put anything and everything in their mouths, so home safety is of prime importance.

In most localities in England, children presenting in A&E with accidental ingestion are followed up by their health visitor to prevent re-occurrence via a system of post-accident support visits (Cernik 1999a).

Reflect on your practice

Jenny, aged 3, has been admitted to the ward having ingested an unknown quantity of her mum's iron tablets, which she takes because she has iron-deficiency anaemia due to pregnancy. Jenny's mum could not remember how many tablets were left in the bottle and Jenny, wanting to be like mummy, climbed onto a stool and helped herself to the container, which is kept in a kitchen cupboard.

- What are the risks of iron overdose to Jenny?
- What will be the nursing management of Jenny while admitted to the ward?
- What advice should be given to her mother on discharge?

The answers to these questions can be found in the PowerPoint presentation.

Choking

Anatomical aspects, including an obviously smaller airway, contribute to the problems children can experience when playing with certain toys. Children of this age persist in putting all sorts of things in their mouths. It is a problem that has the potential to lead to death, where almost anything can be inhaled including, obviously, food sources. Children aged 3 are more likely to have enlarged tonsils and adenoids, which also increases the risk of choking.

Management of the child

The general advice regarding physical removal of the object from the mouth is to leave well alone unless it is clearly visible and easy to remove. The problem is likely to be exacerbated if the foreign body is pushed further down the airway. Diagnosis is not always very clear but the obvious signs of choking are respiratory compromise, which is accompanied by coughing, gagging and stridor. Evidence-based intervention should follow the Advanced Life Support Group guidance (2005) for managing a choking child, which utilises a basic life support approach, incorporating an algorithm that includes cycles of back blows and chest/abdominal thrusts to relieve the obstruction.

WWW

Look at this BBC interactive resource, which tests your first aid knowledge, as well as being of use for parents:

- http://www.bbc.co.uk/health/first_aid/skills_programme/respiratory_index.shtml

Implications for the healthcare professional

All children's nurses should be trained in basic and advanced paediatric life support and should be able to teach parents about basic life support and how to manage the choking child. Attendance on a first aid course should be encouraged for parents (and nurses) generally. For greater discussion and detail see Chapter 27.

Scenario

Peanuts are seen as the prime suspects in cases of preschool choking episodes. Why do they pose such a risk and what other food and objects could be a cause of concern, particularly for this age group?

WWW

The Ontario Sick Children's Hospital is an excellent resource for information giving for families. It includes a child physiology section, aimed at parents and caregivers, which will help you as a healthcare professional explain visually how and why choking is more likely to occur in this age group as well as discussing the mechanics of breathing more generally:

- http://www.aboutkidshealth.ca/HowTheBodyWorks/default.aspx (the front page of the section)
- http://www.aboutkidshealth.ca/HowTheBodyWorks/Respiratory-System.aspx?articleID=10130&categoryID=XL (this will take you direct to the section on the respiratory system)

Burns and scalds

In 1999, 47,000 children sustained a burn or scald. The most vulnerable group is the under-3s, in whom injury sustained is with hot fluids, steam, hot fat and boiling or hot water (DTI 2001). Other sources of burning are dry heat (contact with a hot surface such as an iron or directly from flames), chemicals, electrical appliances and radiation (i.e. overexposure to sunlight). Again, this age group has a particular vulnerability to physical damage due to physiological aspects, including the fact that they have proportionally more extracellular fluid than adults. As a result fluid loss is higher if burned or scalded. Children under 5 years of age account for nearly 45% of all severe burns and scalds and half of the accidents happen in the kitchen. The most likely suspects are cups of hot drinks, which are inadvertently placed where the child can reach up and pull them over themselves. Other causes include unsupervised children falling or climbing into a bath of hot water and accidents involving kettles, saucepans, fires and chip pans.

This subject area is a topic in its own right and thus is given the attention required in the related chapters. What will suffice here is the first aid advice that may be offered by health visitors, nurses and/or NHS Direct in the case of a child that has sustained a minor burn (i.e. sunburn) or scald in the home situation (Table 41.1).

WWW

Look at the BBC interactive first aid website. Test your first aid knowledge in relation to burns and scalds:

- http://www.bbc.co.uk/health/first_aid/skills_test/burnsandscalds_challenge.shtml

WWW

Look at the NHS Clinical Knowledge Summaries (CKS) guidance for the management of burns and scalds:

- http://cks.library.nhs.uk/burns_and_scalds

Non-accidental injury

The issue of non-accidental injury within this age group is also relevant here. See Chapter 19 for a more in-depth discussion.

Table 41.1 The immediate management of the scalded child and the role of the healthcare professional

Action	Rationale/evidence base	Additional information
Run the affected area under a cold water tap or in a bath for at least 10 minutes	Reduce the risk of further heat damage by cooling the affected area	Cold water should be applied even if a delay occurs
Remove bracelets, rings, watches and any other restrictive objects	Will cause constriction if swelling occurs	
After cooling remove clothing from affected area	To assess the extent of the damage and prevent further damage	Do not do immediately following injury – it may cause further damage and removal of skin
Apply cold compress if further relief needed and/or apply a dressing	To promote comfort and reduce distress to a child who might not want to see the burn/scald To protect the burn/scald from further damage Application of a dressing promotes moist healing	Do not advise application of adhesive, sticky or fluffy dressings The choice of dressing has to be guided by the fact that it should promote the maximum amount of movement of the affected area
Analgesia	To relieve pain In the home the analgesic of choice is paracetamol	
De-roof blisters or not?	The evidence base is unclear as demonstrated by the following comments for and against: The wound assessment process is clearer and joint movement is enhanced if you de-roof the blisters (Bosworth 1997) The blisters have a protective function and should be aspirated (as opposed to de-roofed) to reduce pressure only if necessary (Flanagan & Graham 2001, Gowar & Lawrence 1995)	The guidance from CKS based on best evidence base, recommends leaving the blister intact unless they are very big or in an awkward place where aspirating them would be the treatment of choice

Sources: Taylor (2001), CKS (accessed March 2009)

WWW

The NSPCC website offers information leaflets for parents, which are also relevant to healthcare professionals, identifying how to manage challenging toddler behaviour:

- http://www.nspcc.org.uk/html/home/informationresources/forparentscarers.htm

Mobilising

Again in this chapter we ignore the pre-existing health problems identified pre-, peri- or postnatally. The inquisitive nature of the child in relation to exploring his or her environment means that falls and many other accidents can occur, resulting in a range of injuries from simple bruising and sprains to complex fractures. Chapter 35, on orthopaedics, focuses on conditions that relate directly to this age group and gives detailed information of the nursing interventions and health promotion that should be offered to parents/carers and children.

Communicating

The acquisition of language and the whole process of a child's voyage from preverbal to verbal communication is complex and little understood. It is clear that a child's verbal communication increases with exposure to, and experience of, language. It is a healthy response to environmental stimulation, associated with normal development of hearing, neurological function and intellectual development (Woodfield 1999). The area of developing communication skills encompasses many factors, where the key to development is a healthy parent/child relationship. Again the use of developmental milestones, in the hands of community healthcare professionals working in partnership with parents and carers, will identify the very particular problems within the early childhood experience that can pose obstacles to development of effective communication skills.

During early childhood, the child will progress from speaking single words at 12–18 months to speaking in sentences, with a massive growth in vocabulary and the use of syntax – inflections, negatives, questions and passive voice – by the age of 5. The child also develops a sense of humour and starts to understand the pragmatics of a situation, i.e. the use of voice, form in sentence construction and choice of word in achieving a given end, for example, a favourable response to question by the use of words like 'please' and 'thank you' (Bukatko & Daehlar 2004).

Again, community-nursing staff – especially health visitors – are at the forefront of identifying where potential problems are of issue. Any hearing problems will have been identified ideally within the first year of life via parental concerns and/or the distraction test which is performed by health visitors at 6–9 months via the usual child surveillance screening (Hall & Elliman 2003).

Developmental stages again define when children will display problems in hearing due to language development. The rate of speech and language acquisition varies from child to child and, if English is the child's second language, it can be difficult for an English-speaking healthcare professional to assess how language is developing (Cernik 1999b).

Glue ear

Glue ear (which can also be defined as chronic secretory otitis media or otitis media with effusion) is an inflammation of the mucous membranes that line the middle ear and is associated with malfunction in the drainage mechanism of the middle ear. The result is a build-up of fluid and increased pressure behind the tympanic membrane. The reason children are susceptible to this problem is the anatomically shorter, wider and more nearly horizontal Eustachian tubes and the frequent upper respiratory tract infections they seem to acquire. It is very much a preschool child problem, whereby one in four children under the age of 10 will have an episode of acute otitis media, with a peak incidence of diagnosis between the ages of 3 and 6 (Scottish Intercollegiate Guidelines Network (SIGN) 2003).

Acute otitis media is caused by bacterial or viral infection, as opposed to glue ear, which usually has a non-infectious cause as described above. Glue ear is also associated with perennial and/or seasonal allergic rhinitis, enlarged adenoids, prolonged exposure to cigarette smoke, lack of breastfeeding in infancy and living in a household with many family members (Wong 1997).

PowerPoint

Access the companion PowerPoint presentation and find the diagram of the major parts of the ear. Test your knowledge by completing an unlabelled diagram.

The problem of otitis media is usually diagnosed by parents, perhaps in partnership with health visitors or the GP, because of problems with language development and speech. The child may present with other signs, including tugging at ear lobes due to pain and earache, discharging ears, and general tiredness and fatigue due to having to concentrate to hear, especially in social situations such as nursery. Other signs are deterioration in behaviour, obvious difficulty in hearing – the child asks for the television to be turned up – and speech difficulties generally, i.e. difficulties with pronunciations and shouting inappropriately (Wong 1997). The acute form of the disease will present with the characteristic signs of inflammation including earache, pyrexia and general irritability and may be preceded by a cough or other upper respiratory tract symptoms, whilst a child with glue ear may present only with the signs of hearing loss as discussed earlier (SIGN 2003).

Management of the child

Pain and discomfort is treated with paracetamol and/or other analgesics and the infection, if present as an acute otitis media, may be treated with antibiotics. With recurrent infections, i.e. more than four in 6 months, and in the case of a secretory otitis media, if the child is aged 3 and over and presents with speech and language problems, he or she will be referred to an otolaryngologist (SIGN 2003), which may result with an admission to a local hospital, on a day-case basis, for surgical intervention in the shape of myringotomy and grommet insertion. Surgical intervention remains controversial and the mainstay of glue ear management is the watch and wait approach (or 'watchful waiting'; SIGN 2003), and all forms of glue ear should improve spontaneously (Maw 2000). The National Institute for Heath and Clinical Excellence (NICE) have published guidelines identifying the group of children who will benefit from surgical intervention (2008). An alternative approach to managing glue ear is via autoinflation, which involves blowing a balloon with the nose, resulting in a raise in intranasal pressure, which opens up the Eustachian tubes. The evidence base is yet unclear and conflicting, but there may be some clinical benefit (Reidpath et al 1999). NICE (2008) advise that autoinflation should be considered for children who will cooperate with the procedure.

WWW

Useful website for users of healthcare services:

- http://www.patient.co.uk

More specifically, information about myringotomy and grommet insertion:

- http://www.patient.co.uk/showdoc.asp?doc=23069159

Royal National Institute for the Deaf:

- http://www.rnid.org.uk

The RNID's leaflet relating to insertion of grommets:

- http://www.rnid.org.uk/information_resources/factsheets/healthcare/factsheets_leaflets/glue_ear.htm

Activity

William, aged 2, has been admitted to a day-case ward for insertion of grommets:

- On recording his baseline observations what would you expect the normal ranges of observations be for a preschool age child?

See PowerPoint presentation for answers.

Implications for the healthcare professional

The role of the health visitor, midwife, practice nurse and community nurse in monitoring for problems in communication has already been mentioned. They perform a valuable function in health promotion and illness prevention, via advice to parents to stop smoking and promote breastfeeding.

Breathing

This is the period of time, when starting nursery, attending playgroups or just socialising generally, when a runny nose seems to be a permanent feature of early childhood. It is not a very attractive or helpful addition to a child's development, but a requirement in developing immunity and resistance to infection. Life in the 21st century means that the need for childcare in this preschool age group is on the increase, especially where there is an economic need for the main carer to go out to work. Many studies have shown that care outside the home does contribute to acute respiratory illness in childhood and that these children experience these infections generally at an earlier age but fare better in the long term than children who are exposed to infection only when starting school. It has to be mentioned that there are no clear conclusions as to whether this is a risk or benefit overall (McCutcheon & Fitzgerald 2001). Physiologically, children aged 1–4 are more susceptible to respiratory illness due to immaturity of the respiratory system and, anatomically, they have narrower airways and as a result are more likely to have enlarged adenoids and tonsils.

Upper respiratory tract infections

Around 80% of respiratory infections involve only the nose, throat, ears and sinuses and cover a number of different conditions, such as common cold (coryza), sort throat, acute otitis media and sinusitis (Lissauer & Clayden 2007). Thus a child will typically present with sore throat, fever, nasal blockage and discharge and earache accompanied by a troublesome cough. The discussion at this point is brief and covers minor illness only due to the detailed coverage offered in Chapter 27.

Management of the child

The illness is most likely to be managed at home and affect all the family with maybe only a visit to the GP and/or advice from organisations like NHS Direct as a healthcare intervention. The advice usually consists of the use of antipyretics such as paracetamol, rest and encouraging plenty of fluids, although hospital admissions may occur due to febrile convulsions, wheezy episodes and severe upper respiratory tract infections, which will require greater medical intervention.

WWW

NHS Direct:
- http://www.nhsdirect.nhs.uk/

Implications for the healthcare professional

General advice, if sought, will come from community staff, GPs and NHS Direct and/or primary care centres.

Asthma

Asthma is a chronic condition characterised by hyperresponsiveness of the airway due to inflammation. This results in the narrowing of the airway with associated cough and wheeze. The causative agents include genetic predisposition and environmental factors, including parental smoking, exposure to allergens in infancy and viral infection in infancy (Budd & Gardiner 1999). Chapter 27 provides much greater detail about the ever-increasing incidence of this illness. It will suffice in this section to give a brief introduction in relation to the specific needs of this age group.

WWW

The British Thoracic Society:
- http://www.brit-thoracic.org.uk/

Management of the child

Attaching the diagnosis of asthma to the preschool child is controversial because at least one child in seven will have a wheezing episode before they reach the age of 5. Assessment is difficult, although a diagnosis will require an accurate history of predisposing factors, incidence of wheeziness as well as auscultation and investigation via chest X-ray when a child presents with a wheezy episode initially. Peak expiratory flow rate (PEFR) is not a useful measure in this age group, who are unable cognitively to comply with the complex instructions, thus careful monitoring by parents in the form of a diary, if recurrent wheezing is becoming a problem, is an aid to diagnosis.

The mainstays of treatment and management are through the avoidance of triggers, i.e. allergens and smoking, use of inhalers 'preventers' and 'relievers' using the stepwise approach as advocated by the British Thoracic Society (BTS), which outlines the specific needs of the under-5 age group of children (BTS/SIGN 2008).

Implications for the healthcare professional

Nurses caring for children have a health education role to play, facilitated by the production of evidence-based guidelines that aid a consistent approach to health promotion. The National Asthma Campaign is an excellent source of information for healthcare professionals and parents/children alike. The outpatient clinic and dedicated asthma clinics, in the acute sector and in the community, ensure that very specific needs in relation to symptom management are offered to ensure that a child can live life to the full and not be restricted by the diagnosis of asthma.

WWW

The National Asthma Campaign:
- http://www.asthma.org.uk/

Croup (laryngotracheobronchitis)

Again, the information offered here is supplemented significantly in Chapter 27. Croup has been defined as a 'swelling of the submucosa in the subglottic area' (Webster et al 1998). It can occur at any age, but is particularly common in the

Box 41.2

Signs of acute respiratory distress

- Increased respiratory rate
- Recession: intercostal, subcostal or sternal
- Inspiratory or expiratory noise: stridor or wheeze
- Grunting (usually only seen in infants)
- Accessory muscle use
- Flaring of the alae nasi
- Skin colour, i.e. cyanosis
- Mental status, i.e. agitation and/or drowsiness
- Increased heart rate

6 months to 3 year age group. The infection is usually viral in origin and results in narrowing of the upper airway, presenting as hoarseness of voice, with a barking cough and inspiratory stridor. Any swelling in an already narrow airway will potentially cause respiratory distress (Box 41.2) and this is the case with croup, where the narrowest area, the cricoid cartilage, is affected.

Management of the child

The key to management is careful assessment of respiratory function as per the Advanced Life Support Group guidelines (ALSG 2005), i.e. airway, breathing and circulation (ABC) followed by a detailed examination of respiratory function. This involves ensuring that the child has a patent airway as a matter of emergency intervention, then proceeding to assess the extent of respiratory distress which includes respiratory rate, effort, pattern of breathing and airway resistance. Croup scoring systems are available to facilitate the assessment.

The potential diagnosis attached, due to the presenting symptoms, may be epiglottitis, although, because of the *Haemophilus influenzae* type b vaccination, this is very rarely seen today. The awareness of epiglottitis as a potential cause still has to be evident if planning to carry out throat inspection or take a throat swab especially for unvaccinated children.

Use of humidity is the mainstay of croup management though the evidence base for using this method of management is debatable (D'Amore & Campbell Hewson 2002). Its usefulness as a placebo means that it is still worth giving the advice to parents. All the advice offered on parent information internet sites as well as the leaflets given on discharge from hospital advocate the use of steam to produce humidity, i.e. by placing wet towels on radiators, as useful to alleviate symptoms. Any intervention that reduces stress and promotes relaxation in a child (and parent) who will be very distressed should be seen to be helpful. The use of steroid therapy is the key to manage croup. They reduce the inflammatory response and the steroids most commonly used are budenoside (via nebuliser) or dexamethasone (orally). Both have been found to be equally effective with minimal differences in the onset and duration of action (Chandler 2002). Which one used will largely depend on local guidelines and efficacy of use, i.e. dependent on the age of the child and his or her compliance with treatment.

Nebulised adrenaline is used in extremes cases, although the child must be ECG monitored because of the risk of transient tachycardia. This drug will be used to buy time until the child is transferred to a high-dependency environment (see Chapter 27).

The aims of care are to monitor and facilitate respiratory effort, promote rest, reduce pyrexia, promote intake of oral fluids and educate and support family (Chandler 2002).

Implications for the healthcare professional

The management of the child who comes into contact with A&E and/or paediatric assessment areas, which results in admission to hospital, will have an impact on the role of the children's nurse, who obviously has to have evidence-based guidelines to hand, as well as the nursing skills and competence to care for the child and family. This illness can be very frightening and the key to care is communication and sensitive management with the aim of early discharge and potentially a follow-up visit or phone call from a community children's nursing team.

Eating and drinking

The infant stage of feeding is vital for future development, and the early childhood stage is no less important. A child's energy requirements and need for a consistent supply of protein, vitamins and essential minerals increase with rapid growth and high activity. Capacity for food is limited by the child's anatomy, i.e. size of stomach, so there is a requirement for nutrient-dense foods to meet growth requirements (Flanagan & Kennedy 1999). It is a critical time in relation to nutrition and habits developed now tend to continue through life.

Childhood obesity is of epidemic proportions in the USA and an estimated 17.6 million children under 5 were classed as overweight worldwide (WHO 1997). In response to this epidemic the World Health Organization have produced a global strategy to deal with this serious problem (WHO 2004). Since then the WHO, in 2007 has estimated that 22 million children under the age of 5 years were classed in the overweight category throughout the world, where more than 75% of overweight and obese children live in low- and middle-income countries. The cause of this goes beyond the genetic makeup of an individual. In the UK, the prevalence of obesity in preschool children increased from 5.4% in 1989 to 9.2% in 1998 (Bundred et al 2001). Economic growth, modernisation and urbanisation have had an effect on our calorific intake and the types of foods we eat, which means that generally as a population we eat a diet with a higher proportion of saturated fats and sugars. The 21st-century diet, compared with that of the 1950s, provides children with less iron and fewer starchy foods, and more confectionery and soft drinks (British Nutrition Foundation 2003).

We also have a more sedentary lifestyle and participate in less physically demanding work generally, i.e. children even 20 years ago were walking to school whereas now they are driven everywhere. Today, children no longer play outdoor games, preferring the indoor activities like watching television and using a computer. The physical aspects of obesity will have significant effects on our health, notwithstanding the emotional and psychological effects on the child, who may develop a negative self-image and, as a result, low self-esteem (Strauss 2001) from the teasing and sometimes even bullying from peers and friends. NICE (2006) have also produced a guideline with respect to preventing, identifying, assessing and managing obesity in children and adults with advice and recommendations that have an impact across care settings and in relation to the age group under consideration here – early years settings. The targets identified relate to increasing physical activity and providing a healthy balanced diet whilst working in partnership with parents/carers.

WWW

The British Nutrition Foundation's website contains useful resources for nurses and has a focus on education in primary and secondary schools:

- http://www.nutrition.org.uk/

Healthy eating advice for preschool children includes the advice that children up to the age of 2 should be offered relatively small volumes of food, full-fat versions of dairy products and should not be given starchy foods that are very high in fibre. Children aged 1 and above should be eating three meals a day with two in-between-meal snacks. From the age of 2 there should be a gradual introduction of low-fat dairy products for children who are growing well and eating a varied diet and by the age of 5 should be eating as per 'eating for health' plate model (SIGN 2003), which involves a balanced approach to eating from the five food groups: fruit and vegetables; bread, cereals and potatoes; milk and dairy products; meat, fish and alternatives; foods containing fat and foods containing sugar.

WWW

The British Dietetic Association offers information and resources useful for healthcare professionals, parents/carers and children alike, i.e. Eat 2b fit campaign (2003):

- http://www.bda.uk.com/

Economic factors add to the problems of society today and economically poorer families tend to have poor diets, which include high intakes of salt, sugar and dietary fat. They lack fruit, vegetables and iron. The effect of poverty and the impact of advertising, as well as fads and diets, all add to the increasing problem of obesity. As healthcare professionals, working in partnership with colleagues in education and social services sector, we have a major role to play in ensuring that parents get up-to-date nutritional advice and are aware of resources available to support families in need of financial help to feed their children.

A child may develop an allergy to food at any time during early childhood, i.e. peanut allergy. However, most milk-based allergies are developed during infancy and are discussed in Chapter 40. The focus in this section will be on the particular problem affecting this group of children, which fits into the title of nutritional deficiencies namely iron-deficiency anaemia.

Altered growth or failure to thrive

'Altered growth' or the more recognisable term 'failure to thrive' is attached to a child who is failing to grow adequately – a definition at its most basic. Another definition is that of a child with a weight consistently below the 3rd or 5th percentile for age and/or a child who is failing to maintain a previously established pattern of growth (Wright 2000). This still simplistic definition belies the complexity of the syndrome, which involves not just monitoring nutritional intake but has to take note of the whole context – family and environment, economic, social, emotional and psychological factors. The primary focus is on weight and this, via developmental screening, is monitored closely during infancy and regularly during early childhood, which in itself is controversial, although accepted as standard practice in the UK. The constant monitoring of weight can be a cause of great worry to mothers in particular. The controversy is supported by recent changes in the percentile charts used, which responds to changes in UK reference data, reflecting the changes in our society with regards to whole populations of children, including children from ethnic minority groups, which means that children who are simply small in stature do not end up with a diagnosis of failure to thrive. Generally, the diagnosis is made in infancy so the discussion will stop at this point, though obviously the effects on the child and family will continue into early childhood.

Nutritional deficiencies

As already mentioned, the preschool child may experience nutritional deficiencies of many types and the key one to discuss here is the effect of iron deficiency, which causes anaemia. The particular groups of children affected are those from ethnic minority groups and socioeconomically deprived toddlers (MacDonald 1999). Iron deficiencies impair psychomotor development and cognitive functions. The main causes of iron-deficiency anaemia include prolonged use of breastfeeding. Breast milk is the obvious nutritional source up to 6 months of age; however, the infant needs alternative sources of iron after 6 months. Other reasons include the early introduction of cow's milk before the age of 1, and the fact that toddlers tend to be fussy eaters and eat small portions of food, drink lots of juice and are reluctant to eat meat (MacDonald 1999).

Management of the child with iron-deficiency anaemia

The child will present with pallor, lethargy and impaired cardiopulmonary function (Belton & Hambridge 1991). There is evidence to support the fact that even with mild iron-deficiency anaemia the child will exhibit a decrease in responsiveness, decreased physical activity and attentiveness, thus delaying development. Once identified and diagnosed from history and blood tests the child will be treated with supplemental iron as well as promoting intake of iron-rich foods.

Scenario

A parent asks you to identify the food sources of iron, which her son, Edward, is likely to eat and ways of encouraging Edward to eat them. What is your response?

See the PowerPoint presentation for suggestions.

Implications for the healthcare professional

There have been suggestions, via a working group focused on the nutritional aspect of weaning (Department of Health (DoH) 1991a,b), to introduce screening for preschool children to ensure early treatment and guidance for children and parents experiencing this problem. However, no guidelines exist at present, although these would be very useful for children's nurses and all those involved in caring for children.

Health visitors will have a key role in assessing and monitoring a child's nutritional intake via diet history taken from parents, as well as educating generally about nutritional issues while undertaking other health checks during visits.

Another area to consider is the issue of food fortification, which does happen with the addition of vitamins and iron to foodstuffs such as cereals. There is a lack of accurate data on the utility of this intervention, although the evidence base supporting the use of iron-fortified formula in preventing iron-deficiency anaemia in infants and young children is more conclusive (MacDonald 1999).

As already mentioned, care has to be taken with storing iron preparations and the drug may cause abdominal upset and constipation.

Eliminating

Early childhood is when many new skills are learnt and one of the key areas involves the move from nappies to using the toilet via the process of toilet training. This usually happens between the ages of 2 and 3, with most children achieving full control by the age of 4 (Rogers 2002). It is a complex process, which involves a lot of practice – control of micturition involves coordination between several complex feedback loops running between bladder and the brain. The child needs to be aware of the need to pass urine, which has to take priority over other activities, there being multiple distractions at this age. The child has to perceive the signal correctly to be able to get to the toilet in time. There are also social issues to consider, i.e. sitting or standing as a gender issue. The whole process is complicated by clothing, the need to use toilet paper and then by having hands to wash. For this age group there will be no discussion in relation to encopresis and enuresis – the child is learning and mastering the art during these early years, although this does not mean that a child may have no problems within this activity of living. Health visitors have an important role in health education and support during the toilet training period, which will take place within the child's home in a safe environment. A variety of problems can affect a child in this particular age group, including the intestinal parasites, constipation (which may go hand in hand with the nutritional problems already mentioned) and gastroenteritis. Gastroenteritis serves as an example of a problem that can affect all ages but can have more severe consequences in the preschool child.

PowerPoint

Access the companion PowerPoint presentation for general parenting advice and hints and tips for successful toilet training.

PowerPoint

Access the companion PowerPoint presentation. Study the table summarising common intestinal parasites, including *Giardia*, which causes gastroenteritis. Having studied the table, you will note that not all parasites cause gastroenteritis.

Gastroenteritis

Acute gastroenteritis is characterised by sudden onset of diarrhoea and/or vomiting and includes a variety of symptoms including poor appetite, fever and abdominal cramps and can be defined as an increase in stool frequency and/or change in consistency of the stools (McVerry & Collins 1999). Many cases are caused by rotavirus as the usual suspect, though there can be bacterial and parasitic causes also.

The results of gastroenteritis can be serious in infancy and early childhood because any loss of fluid will affect fluid balance dramatically due to increased metabolic rate and the distribution of intracellular and extracellular fluid, which is different from adult fluid balance (Table 41.2). It is responsible for more than 1 billion cases and at least 4 million deaths per year worldwide. It can occur on average twice annually in child under 5 years of age, or three times if attending child care outside of the home (Prescilla 2003).

Activity

How do you assess the degree of dehydration the preschool child is experiencing on presentation either in the home, A&E or assessment area on a paediatric ward?

Answers on the PowerPoint presentation.

Management of the child

Mild to moderate dehydration should be treated with oral rehydration solution for 3–4 hours with resumption of normal feeding following this. The administration of these solutions can be problematic, because children object to the taste of these solutions. The management of more severe dehydration will be dealt with on the basis of the evidence of the consensus based guidelines developed by Armon et al (2001) and via the NHS Clinical Knowledge Summaries area on gastroenteritis detailed in the 'www' box as well as by following the guidance from WHO (2006).

Table 41.2 Summary of the main causes and effects of gastroenteritis in children

Causative organism	Incubation period	Signs	Transmission	Additional points
Rotavirus	15–30 hours Once infected the illness can last more than a week, though usually 5–7 days	Severe diarrhoea: watery frequent stool Pyrexia Nausea and vomiting	Faecal–oral route with secondary spread via respiratory route	Distinct seasonal pattern, i.e. winter months Mostly occurs in children aged 3–15 months
Adenovirus spp.	5–12 days and the illness usually lasts 5–12 days	Diarrhoea and also linked with an URTI	Person to person Faecal–oral Aerosol	Seasonal pattern, i.e. winter months in cold weather
Hepatitis A	28 days and can last up to 4 weeks	Fever Malaise Nausea Jaundice		Children may have no symptoms Vaccination is available
Campylobacter	2–5 days typically and lasts 2–7 days usually with a spontaneous recovery blood	Pyrexia Abdominal pain Watery, profuse, foul-smelling diarrhoea, which may contain blood	Ingestion of contaminated food and milk (birds pecking milk bottle tops) Undercooked chicken and also carried in domestic animals	Seasonal pattern in that it usually peaks in the early summer
Salmonella spp.	6–72 hours and can last for days or weeks	Rapid onset of symptoms, which include nausea, vomiting and colicky abdominal pain Diarrhoea may contain blood and mucus	Undercooked poultry and eggs are the prime sources responsible Carried by poultry, pets and animals	Incidence increases July–October
Shigella spp.	2–4 days and is self-limiting lasting 3–5 days, though remains communicable for 1–4 weeks	Variable onset with high fever, cramping abdominal pain Watery diarrhoea with mucus and blood	Person-to-person contact indirectly via toilet flush, door knobs, etc.	Frequently affects children and incidence peaks in late summer
Escherichia coli	Variable depending on strain and self-limiting to 10 days	Gradual or sudden onset Diarrhoea is explosive and green and watery Pyrexia and abdominal distension	Personal to person via inanimate objects Undercooked meats	Summer
Escherichia coli 157	1–6 days, although can take 14 days	Haemorrhagic colitis, bloody diarrhoea and severe abdominal cramps		

Sources: Jones (2003), Lowe (2002), McVerry & Collins (1999), Prescilla (2003).

WWW

CKS guidance (NHS Institute for Innovation and Improvement) - gastroenteritis:

- http://cks.library.nhs.uk/gastroenteritis/management/quick_answers/scenario_no_confirmed_cause_children

Patient information leaflet:

- http://cks.library.nhs.uk/patient_information_leaflet/gastroenteritis#360222000

PowerPoint

To feed or not to feed?

Access the companion PowerPoint presentation for more information relating to the management of mild-moderate gastroenteritis.

Implications for the healthcare professional

Health education relates to the issue of fluid management, although most parents realise that the prevention of dehydration is the way of managing the illness. Notifiable illnesses, such as salmonella, will need to be referred to the public health services and the importance of hand hygiene reiterated to all family members and contacts. The nurse working in the community will obviously need to be in possession of the assessment skills which would indicate, via information offered to parents, the point at which a child should be referred to the acute paediatric services for more intensive management, i.e. intravenous fluids.

Many resources are available to help in the process of managing infection control in places such as nurseries and schools, as well as in the home. Teaching children and families how and when to wash their hands is a very basic but highly effective way of reducing the incidence of gastroenteritis.

PowerPoint

Assessing the child presenting with gastroenteritis

Following (or in conjunction) with measurement of baseline observations and general assessment in relation to child's level of dehydration, what questions should you be asking of the parent/carer/child?

www

Many useful resources are available to help teachers in both schools and nurseries to teach infection control to preschool children and parents. Look at the Healthy Schools website at:

- http://www.healthyschools.gov.uk/Default.aspx

The following website link takes you to the 'catch it, bin it,kill it' respiratory and hand hygiene campaign (2008)

- http://www.dh.gov.uk/en/Publicationsandstatistics/Publications/PublicationsPolicyAndGuidance/DH_080839 (Have a look at the section aimed at younger children featuring Dirty Bertie)

Will it appeal to the preschool age group or is it more appropriate for older children?

Will the message be received and understood by children of whatever age?

www

The eMedicine website is a useful resource. It is medically orientated and American in origin, but provides useful information for all healthcare professionals:

- http://emedicine.medscape.com/

www

Health Protection Agency:

- http://www.hpa.org.uk/

Information relating to salmonella infection:

- http://www.hpa.org.uk/webw/HPAweb&HPAwebStandard/HPAweb_C/1195733816528?p=1204013004068

Personal cleansing and dressing

The preschool age child will be learning to wash and dress him- or herself under the supervision of parent or carers. It is an ideal time to check the integrity of the skin and identify any problems that can affect children of this age. This is the time when the child can learn about the importance of hand hygiene and develop good habits that will last a lifetime, i.e. brushing teeth and washing hands, information that will be reinforced at nursery and playgroups.

Dental caries

An important, if often neglected area, is the affect of tooth decay on a child's development and growth. Dental caries are very easy to prevent and healthy teeth are a good indicator for future dental health (Ottley 2002). Generally, the incidence of tooth decay in the UK has decreased markedly, although there is little improvement in children from less advantaged areas. Children from lower social classes and ethnic minority populations are more likely have dental problems (Davies et al 2001). The younger a child is when he or she starts having the teeth brushed, the less the likelihood of decay (Hinds & Gregory 1995).

Activity

The Department of Health NHS Plan (2000) national target was no more than one decayed, missing or filled tooth for 5-year-old children by 2003:

- Has the target been achieved?
- Do we promote dental hygiene in acute inpatient services?

It has been found in many studies that community nurses can be very effective as dental health educators (Blinkhorn & Davies 2001). The recommendation from this study was that dental advice, and a free dental pack, should be given at the 8-month hearing test and follow-up session. The basic and essential advice is to brush teeth twice a day with fluoride toothpaste either with a manual or powered brush. The preschool child should use toothpaste formulated for children, which has a lower fluoride content, because the child is unable to rinse and spit out the toothpaste effectively and will swallow most of it. Children only develop the manual dexterity to brush their own teeth properly at the age of 6, so the parent needs to assist and do the initial brush and maybe allow the child to finish off the process. Bottles are designed for babies not toddlers and, as discussed in the section on iron-deficiency anaemia, taking juice from a bottle put the teeth in danger of prolonged contact with sugar; a feeder cup should be used from 6 months of age. There is no need to dictate what to eat and not eat, and sweet things can be eaten as long as they are confined to eating times. Early visits to the dentist also help the process, so that children do not develop anxieties about going to the dentist (Ottley 2002). These recommendations are supported by the SIGN (2005) guideline where there is also a recommendation that a multi-professional approach is taken with multiple interventions starting during pregnancy and onwards, where oral health promotion programmes, including toothbrushing, for young children should start before the age of 3, ideally in places like nursery settings.

www

British Dental Health Foundation:

- http://www.dentalhealth.org.uk/

Information about the use of fluoride:

- http://www.dentalhealth.org.uk/faqs/leafletdetail.php?LeafletID=17

Eczema

The word eczema has Greek origins and means 'to boil over'. It describes red itchy skin, which develops into a rash of pustules, which eventually break down and leak serous fluid. It usually appears during the first year of life, although it can happen to adults and children at any point in their lives. The term 'atopy' is usually applied to childhood eczema, where the cause is inherited and results due to an immunological response (IgE) to environmental antigens. The areas most commonly affected are neck, flexures of the wrists and ankles, antecubital and popliteal areas (Elliott 1999).

Activity

Define the following dermatology terms, which you will come across in clinical practice: blister, bulla, erythema, excoriation, papule, petechiae, pruritus, purpura, pustule, urticaria and vesicle.

Answers on the PowerPoint presentation.

Management of the child

The basic management is that of easing the itching, maybe with the use of antihistamines, preventing scratching by cutting and filing of the child's nails, preventing infection by regular bathing and, most importantly, keeping the skin well hydrated with the regular use of emollients. Topical steroids can be used to reduce inflammation and as an immunosuppressant. Night-time is particularly problematic, when damage due to scratching can be significant. This is the time when the use of antihistamines is useful as well as the use of wet-wrap bandages, which ensure that as well as cooling the skin affected areas are inaccessible to the child. It has to be noted that antihistamines are being used in this instance for their sedative properties – the itch caused by eczema is not histamine mediated and the antihistamine is therefore unlikely to reduce the itchiness of the skin (RCN 2008). NICE (2007c) and the Royal College of Nursing (RCN 2008) have produced comprehensive guidelines to aid the nurse caring for the complex needs of the child and family. NICE (2007c) advocate the use of a stepped approach to care starting with the mainstay of emollients with other treatments coming into play as flare ups occur as already mentioned above.

PowerPoint

Access the companion PowerPoint presentation for additional information regarding treatment and management of childhood eczema.

The overriding aim is to break the cycle of pruritus and scratching by removing the causative and aggravating factors with care. It has to be noted that special diets used to exclude some of these factors can cause major problems nutritionally and affect the child's growth and development.

Implications for the healthcare professional

The children's nurse will be a key information giver and provider regarding the protective basis of breastfeeding for any future children, and also for managing the effects of the house-dust mite, pollens, moulds and animal fur within the home. Caring for a child with a potentially severe and chronic illness can give the mother (as the usual prime caregiver) a burden of extra physical work. The time spend bathing, dressing and nappy-changing a child who has the overwhelming need to scratch can be extraordinarily difficult. The diagnosis of atopic eczema also brings an extra burden of housework, as well as making meal times more difficult if a restricted diet is indicated (Elliott & Luker 1997).

The nurse needs to develop long-standing and effective partnerships with the child and family, especially in the more severely affected group of children, in whom chronicity is an issue. The nurse will have to be conversant in the arena of complementary medicine, as parents might be seeking to use alternatives such as Chinese herbal medicine, phototherapy and evening primrose oil. The nurse needs to take account of the fact that many of these treatments do not have a robust evidence base, and indeed, neither does the wet-wrapping technique. The nurse will also have a role in directing parents to seek the help and resources that support groups may have to offer and may also be able to help when the child is going through the transition of leaving the home environment and going to nursery and then on to school. The RCN (2008) advocate a supportive, child/family-centred approach aimed at promoting self-care.

www

Visit some websites dealing with eczema and offering further information at:

- http://www.eczema.org/
- http://www.skincarephysicians.com/eczemanet/

The following link offers useful advice for starting school with eczema and is a highly visual and easy site to use generally:

- http://skincareworld.co.uk/libraryscw/Learning/Articles/startingschool.htm

Scabies (*Sarcoptes scabiei*)

This parasite is a mite. Its name, which translated from the Greek is called the 'flesh cutter', sounds very dramatic but this is literally what this mite does as it burrows into the skin. Symptoms occur due to an allergic reaction to the waste products produced by the mite. The female mite will remain under the surface of the skin and lay eggs in the burrow, feeding on nutrients from the cells through which she has chewed. The active larvae will emerge through the burrow to invade the surrounding skin. It is quite difficult to diagnose because the rash displayed does look like an eczema type rash.

Statistically, this parasite affects the school-age child more frequently than the preschooler, although it warrants attention in this section because young children will come into contact with the infection due to family contact and via nursery and play groups.

The burrows are found between the fingers and on the anterior wall of the axilla. Scabies is contagious and spread in children by direct physical contact, although hand-holding needs to be for 10 minutes or more. Mites can only survive a maximum of 3 hours away from the skin and they are difficult to catch from clothing or bed linen. This will hopefully reassure children's nurses that it is not easy to acquire the mite and prevent the over-reaction that many lay people and professionals may have when informed that a client has scabies.

PowerPoint

Access the companion PowerPoint presentation for:
- photographs of the scabies mite
- diagrammatic representation of the life cycle of the mite.

Management of the child

The key symptom is intense itching, most commonly at night time. The itching is localised to the actual burrow sites, is burning in sensation and generalised. It can be mild to severe and occurs 4–6 weeks after infestation.

The treatment for scabies lacks a convincing evidence base and involves the application of scabicide over the whole body (Hadfield-Law 2001, Walker & Johnstone 2003). Permethrin is the treatment of choice in children. It is applied over the entire body surface and left to dry for 8–12 hours. It needs to be applied to cool dry skin, left for the correct time and washed off with plain, cool water followed by a bath. Following treatment, the rash can continue for 3–4 weeks. Sheets, clothes and fabric worn next to the skin should be washed in hot water and dried at high temperatures to kill the parasites.

Implications for the healthcare professional

The nurse needs to know how to treat scabies effectively, based on the limited evidence for efficacy, as well as ensuring that the treatment is undertaken correctly and all family members and close contacts are treated effectively. There is a wider public health issue and role in preventing outbreaks by limiting contacts, early diagnosis and health education. Pains should be taken to avoid scaring other parents and children and to take a reality check in relation to the infection. The infection can cause a lot of embarrassment to the sufferer and family members unnecessarily, and this is avoidable with education and support.

Head lice

Head lice are small, six-legged wingless insects, grey-brown in colour and 1–3 mm long. They feed by sucking blood from the scalp of their host every 3–6 hours. The female louse lays about five eggs a day. These are smaller than pin heads and are laid on the hair shaft 1.5 cm from the scalp surface. The eggs hatch in about 7 days and the egg shells are left empty (nits). The young head lice (nymphs) take about 6–12 days to mature. The best places to find live lice are behind the ears and on the back of the head. The diagnosis can only be made on identifying a living, moving, head louse found in the hair (Blenkinsop 2003). Infestation is wide spread, especially in nurseries and schools. It is very irritating and if left untreated skin infections can occur.

PowerPoint

Access the companion PowerPoint presentation for:
- photographs of nits and head lice
- diagrammatic representation of the life cycle of the head louse
- health promotion and treatment advice.

Management of the child

Treatment is with pediculicides on an individual-patient basis and following a 'structured mosaic' of treatments. This involves using the topical lotion in a structured way checking for effectiveness as you go along. If one fails you try a different class of insecticide from those available. The Cochrane review evaluating the effectiveness of pediculicides and/or wet combing methods was not conclusive (Dodd 2003), although further studies have been undertaken and are ongoing. The idea of 'bug busting' has become popular. This is a physical method of wet-combing using a fine-toothed comb on conditioned hair for 30 minutes every 3rd or 4th day over a 2-week period. The evidence base for the efficacy of all these treatments is questionable, although clinical guidelines do advocate the use of wet combing and, from a common sense point of view, the process does track the life cycle of the head louse, thereby in theory physically removing the infestation and the problem.

PowerPoint

Access the companion PowerPoint presentation for information on bug busting, what it is and how to do it.

Implications for the healthcare professional

There needs to be physical evidence of living lice before starting pediculicide treatment. Close contacts should be identified and treated at the same time. Nurses need to be aware of the local treatment policy because there is resistance to some products. As with the management of scabies, nursing advice will have to take account of the embarrassment and stigma children and families may experience. There is no need to keep children away from nursery because they will have had the lice for several weeks before diagnosis.

WWW

CKS guidance on head-lice infestations is available at:
- http://cks.library.nhs.uk/head_lice/management/quick_answers/scenario_initial_presentation#-252608

Patient information leaflet:
- http://cks.library.nhs.uk/patient_information_leaflet/head_lice

Controlling body temperature

Children have a metabolic rate that is three times faster than that of an adult. The basal metabolic rate is related to the proportion of body surface area in relation to body mass, with obvious changes as body size increases. Thus young children have a higher metabolic rate and smaller body masses thus generating more heat with a smaller surface area from which to lose it (Casey 2000). Add to this the immaturity of temperature regulation centre (the hypothalamus) and it is clear, especially in this particular age group, that the children are particularly susceptible to temperature fluctuations. Thus an increase in body temperature is one of the most common symptoms of illness in children, whether caused by infection or head injury (where damage to the hypothalamus has been sustained). Body temperature is not just altered by environmental temperature but also by crying, playing and emotional upset (Wong 1997).

Febrile convulsions

A fever can be defined as an abnormal rise in body temperature usually above 37.5°C (Porth 1994), although it has to be remembered that child temperatures are higher than adult ones and the evidence base for defining what is 'normal' for a child's temperature is questionable (Mackowiak et al 1997).

Due to the influencing factors already detailed, it is not surprising that 3% children between the ages of 6 months and 3 years experience a febrile convulsion, which is caused by a rapid rise of temperature, most often caused by a bacterial or viral infection. Febrile convulsions can occur up to about the age of 7. There appears to be a genetic predisposition and convulsions can reoccur within the same period of illness or during future illnesses. Although frightening for parents and carers, febrile convulsions are usually benign with little risk of neurological damage, although some parents worry that their child may develop epilepsy in the future. The convulsions themselves usually last 1–2 minutes and are generalised in nature. If they do last longer (i.e. greater than 30 minutes) they may warrant further investigation, especially if the convulsion also has focal features and/or if the seizures recur in the same illness (Lissauer & Clayden 2007).

Management of the child

The child with pyrexia will present with a variety of signs dependent on the stage of fever, i.e. shivering, feeling cold or hot and flushed, and during the diaphoresis phase potentially shocked with cold, mottled extremities and general pallor (Casey 2000).

Although there is evidence to suggest that a fever has a therapeutic purpose (Casey 2000, Tortora & Grabowski 2002), because the high temperature will also restrict the growth and activity of the invading bacterial/viral microorganisms, we do intervene to mechanically reduce temperature – the main aim being to promote comfort and alleviate the distress a high temperature may cause child and parent, as well as to prevent any further convulsions. These methods include the use of antipyretics such as paracetamol and ibuprofen, and the use of environmental interventions such as reducing clothing, making sure that the clothing that remains is loose-fitting and made of cotton, reducing the amount of bedding, using blankets and sheets rather than quilts, reducing room temperature by opening windows, using a fan (ensuring that the fan is directed away from the child and the effects do not cool the child too rapidly) and encouraging cool oral fluids (Trigg & Mohammed 2006).

The use of tepid sponging is still indicated in many textbooks, although the evidence base indicates that it does not significantly reduce temperature and may induce shivering, which will subsequently increase temperature rather than reduce it and may precipitate a crisis inducing a state of shock. A review of a limited number of studies by Watts et al (2003) concluded that there is only minimal clinical benefit from sponging in temperate climates, with the adverse affect of also causing discomfort to the child. The recommended rate of cooling of 0.5°C per hour can be more readily and comfortably achieved with the administration of antipyretics (Blumenthal 2000, Herder 1994). The evidence base supporting the use of antipyretics as a prophylaxis for febrile illness is not conclusive. Pursell (2000), having carried out a literature review of the major studies exploring the effectiveness of paracetamol and ibuprofen in reducing temperature and preventing reoccurrence of a further febrile convulsion, concluded that their usefulness should be considered in terms of promoting comfort alone. He argues that education about supportive care is of greater importance than obsessively administering paracetamol at regular intervals. These approaches taken to managing a child with a pyrexia are supported by the NICE (2007a) guideline, who also advocate that tepid sponging is not used as cooling method, not using antipyretics as a routine or to prevent febrile convulsions, as well as not giving paracetamol and ibuprofen at the same time.

Implications for the healthcare professional

The advice resulting from the evidence base, in relation to the nursing care of a febrile child, is careful observation of the child and avoiding too frequent temperature measurement, which will exacerbate the anxiety of parent and child (Trigg & Mohammed 2006). However, it is generally accepted that temperature will be measured 1 hour after administration of antipyretics to ensure that they are having an effect and temperature reduction is not too dramatic. In supporting parents and carers, they should be advised that reoccurrence may occur and to ensure the safety of the child without restraint, i.e. in pram or chair. After the convulsion the child should be placed in the recovery position or on his or her side and someone should stay with child until he or she recovers. Advice will be offered regarding cooling methods and, in some cases, parents will need to be shown how to administer rectal drugs, i.e. diazepam and paracetamol.

The children's nurse needs to be aware of the normal ranges of temperature, which thermometer to use dependent on age of child and how to use temperature-measuring equipment available in the clinical areas and at home (RCN 2007). She or he should also remember that in the management of a febrile illness other vital signs are also important, i.e. heart rate, respiratory rate and capillary refill time. The nurse will also have to consider what additional nursing interventions will need to be undertaken, i.e. collection of specimens, so that the underlying cause of the febrile illness (e.g. urinary tract infection) can be identified and treated. Urinary tract infection (UTI) is a common bacterial infection causing illness in infants and children, which may be difficult to recognise in children because the presenting symptoms and signs can be non-specific, especially in the under-3 age group (NICE 2007b). It is usual practice in the acute setting to collect a clean catch specimen of urine as a matter of routine to exclude a diagnosis of UTI.

Infectious diseases

Chickenpox

This illness is the classic preschool/early school years childhood illness. Chickenpox (varicella zoster) virus is spread by droplet from respiratory secretions and contact with skin lesions and contaminated objects. The incubation period is 2–3 weeks (typically 14–16 days). Infectivity is high 2 days before eruption of a macula rash and up to 5 days after the rash has become papular and developed into vesicles, where crusts have formed. Some children may display all three stages of the rash at the same time. The rash tends to spread from scalp or trunk to cover the whole of the body. Complications include secondary bacterial infections such as pneumonia, abscesses or cellulitis or even encephalitis with staphylococci or streptococci bacterial infections, although these are unusual in most children (Lissauer & Clayden 2001).

PowerPoint

Access the companion PowerPoint presentation for photographs of a child with chickenpox to aid identification of the rash in clinical practice.

Management of the child

The essential management, usually at home, is to isolate the child from others. Calamine lotion may be applied to alleviate pruritus, the skin should be kept clean and pyrexia managed as discussed above. It is recommended that nails are kept short and children apply pressure to itchy areas rather than scratch them. The child should obviously be isolated from others during the infective stage. The illness will only cause significant complications to the immunocompromised or newborn child.

Implications for the healthcare professional

Health promotion via GP, practice nurse and/or health visitor is to ensure that parents do not give aspirin or any salicylates to treat symptoms because of the risk of Reye's disease and otherwise give basic advice in relation to symptom management.

Measles

It is worth mentioning measles as an illness within this section to reassert the nurse's role in promoting the uptake of MMR vaccination. We are more likely at this period of time to see outbreaks of measles infection where there is low coverage of vaccination. The introduction of the combined MMR vaccine, which was well received in 1988, means that cases of measles were reduced from over 26,000 in 1989 to 2438 in 1999 with only 4.3% of cases confirmed (Public Health Laboratory Service (PHLS) 2002).

Measles, a notifiable disease, is caused by a virus and is spread through airborne droplets. A prodromal period of 2–4 days when the child is feverish, coughing, tired and has conjunctivitis is followed by increases in temperature and sometimes Koplik's spots (white spots on a red background) appear in the buccal mucosa before the rash develops. The rash is maculopapular, starts at the hairline and progresses down the body. Three days later the rash becomes brownish and then fades. Complications include otitis media, pneumonia, croup, convulsions and encephalitis. Needless to say, as with most illnesses, the rate of complication is higher in this age group (Bedford 2003, Lissauer & Clayden 2001).

Diagnosis is confusing, and health professionals are now less experienced in diagnosis. However, the PHLS, to improve data collection, now issues saliva tests to confirm illness in suspected cases of measles, mumps and rubella.

PowerPoint

Access the companion PowerPoint presentation for photographs of a preschool child with measles.

Management of the child

Most children with measles will be managed at home with symptomatic management of temperature (as above). Some children experience photophobia, so the common sense approach of dimming the lights is the best way to manage this situation.

Implications for the healthcare professional

The key area of nursing activity is in providing information about the MMR vaccine and encouraging evidence base discussion surrounding the facts about the safety of the vaccine, a debate no doubt that will continue for many years.

Scenario

A parent asks for your opinion as to whether she should give consent to the MMR vaccination:

- Reflect on your own feelings, beliefs and attitudes to the MMR vaccine.
- What effect has the media had on your role in advising parents to have (or not have) the vaccine?

Playing (and working)

Play is an integral aspect of childhood and children in their early preschool years spend a lot of time engaged in play activities. Play is essential for development, as well as just giving pleasure to child and parent also. One skill learned is another game to be played (Sylva & Lunt 1984). Piaget considered that intelligence is closely linked with play. Through play the child has the opportunity to master and practise skills. The type of play engaged in changes through the developmental stages and thus any problems in development can be observed in play activities, thus stressing the importance of the role hospital play specialists and nursery nurses have when they undertake play and developmental assessments working as part of the multidisciplinary team. We should never undervalue opportunities to play with the children in our care, whether on the hospital ward or in the child's home, because it is a means of identifying in a non-stressful, non-invasive way whether developmental problems are evident.

Inequalities in health were highlighted in the DoH White Paper 'Our healthier nation' (DoH 1999). One of the vehicles introduced by the Labour government to improve health inequalities is the Sure Start programme, which is targeted at disadvantaged children and focuses on improvement in the child's health as well as social and emotional development and ability to learn, which involves the use of play via play groups activity.

WWW

Useful information about Sure Start:

- http://www.surestart.gov.uk/

Expressing sexuality

This is a time when boys and girls are starting to get the idea that boys and girls are somehow different. It is at the age of 2–3 years when children acquire gender identity. According to Kohlberg's cognitive developmental theory gender satiability is developed around their 4th birthday (Bukatko & Daehlar 2004). A child's identification of gender is based on physical features such as length of hair and clothing rather than on differences in genitalia, but in these preschool years they will begin to prefer to play with same-sex children and to enforce gender-role norms. How much this is due to nature and how much to nurture, via the attitudes and behaviour of parents, peers and teachers, is debatable. This will affect their self-esteem and perception of self, as well as other factors relating to socialisation within specific environments. However, for the purposes of this chapter there are no specific health problems to be identified at this point so this brief discussion will suffice.

Sleeping

Sleep is essential for human well-being and functioning. The human circadian rhythm is cyclical, lasting 24 hours and consisting of sleep and wakefulness, which is reflected in periods of related activity and inactivity (Gustafasson 1992). Sleep is a time for growth and renewal and for the body to rest and replenish what has been utilised during the period of activity whilst awake. The activity of growth hormones is especially noteworthy with respect to the client group under consideration.

The sleep requirements of this age group are still substantial and are individually based and consist of a long period of night-time sleep and daytime naps, which is not surprising considering the activity of the child as well as the learning and growth that is taking place. Sleep is governed by our biological clock. While sleeping, growth hormones are actively functioning and developing. Sleep is a complex process that has two phases: rapid eye movement (REM) and non-rapid eye movement (NREM), which are cyclical in nature. REM sleep dominates a baby's sleep when the brain is growing and developing rapidly (Bennett 2003), which supports the theory that REM sleep promotes emotional healing and the growth and repair of brain tissue (Evans & French 1995). The obvious effects of sleep deprivation mean that growth will be affected, as will the other requirements of normal physiological functioning, such as cellular immunity and tissue repair, the reaction times and the attention span.

Whereas a newborn sleeps for 16–20 hours, a 3–18-month-old child will need 15–18 hours, including naps, and a 3-year-old will need approximately 11 hours of sleep, although there are individual variations.

Sleep deprivation leads to behavioural and family problems; it is not just the child who is sleep deprived, which can lead to family problems generally. The amount of sleep a child is getting or not getting is generally a major preoccupation of parents because of the effect it has on their coping ability. It can lead to disruption of family relationships, marital disharmony and to an altered parent/child relationship (Pritchard 1999). Persistent lack of sleep leads to other behavioural problems in this age group. Other sleep problems include night terrors, head banging and rocking and nightmares.

Management of the child

The key is successful interaction between the parent and child. New sleep patterns can be learned, as can other behaviours, by giving the child cues, routine and consistency (Pritchard 1999). The use of 'transitional objects' for children aged 1–3 can help, i.e. blankets, teddies and other comforters. Naps are commonplace for this age group, although nursery and then school put a stop to this. Each situation has to be managed individually, with careful assessment, and will include an assortment of strategies such as developing certain night-time rituals, e.g. bath, stories and drinks. The environment should be calm, dark and at an ambient temperature.

The generic advice on many internet-based parental advice sites is the common sense approach to sleep, i.e. enjoy bedtime and its related routines, not to use going to bed as a punishment or to put the child to bed before he or she is tired. The lighting should be dimmed and everyone should talk in a quiet voice. The advice relating to a crying child is not necessarily to pick him or her up but to stay close. Use of the parental bed is not contraindicated as a short-term strategy for promoting sleep and alternative therapies may aid the process of falling asleep, e.g. lavender oil in the bath and listening to calming music. The use of positive reinforcement can also help, i.e. star charts and rewards.

WWW

Visit a website offering advice to parents and healthcare professionals in relation to sleep problems and management:

- http://www.netdoctor.co.uk/health_advice/facts/childrensleep.htm

The Loughborough Sleep Research Centre:

- http://www.lboro.ac.uk/departments/hu/groups/sleep/pop_articles/children_sleep.html

Implications for the healthcare professional

Although specific disorders have not been discussed in this section, it is useful to consider the effect sleep deprivation can have in the home environment, never mind in the hospital sector, for the child and parent. Thus nursing considerations need to relate to how we ensure that parents and children get a good night's sleep on a hospital ward, as well as identifying and helping out with problems the parent may wish to discuss when the child is first assessed. Sleep generally is given a low priority during the assessment process, the focus being on the presenting problem itself.

Dying

Again this is not something we would associate with this age group. However, the effects of grief and bereavement may be an issue and children's nurses need to develop an understanding of how preschool children express feelings of sadness and happiness in general. Behavioural and emotional disturbances may go hand in hand with any of the health problems identified. We must not assume that in the 21st century, in a Western society, all children have a wonderful experience of early childhood.

Summary

This chapter is not an exhaustive account of the health problems a child may experience during early childhood through all the key areas have been covered at a level aimed to arouse interest and encourage further reading to develop an in-depth knowledge base with regard to this interesting time of life. The focus is not only on a physiological health-problems-based approach, but also on promoting health and well-being to ensure a seamless transition from life at home and at nursery to starting school.

References

Advanced Life Support Group (ALSG), 2005. Advanced paediatric life support. The practical approach, 4th edn. BMJ Publishing, Plymouth.

American Academy of Pediatrics (AAP), 1996. Practice parameter: the management of acute gastroenteritis in young children. Pediatrics 97 (3), 424–435.

Armon, K., Stephenson, T., MacFaul, R., Ecccleston, P., Werneke, U., 2001. An evidence and consensus based guideline for acute diarrhoea management. Archive of Diseases in Childhood 85, 1320142.

Bedford, H., 2003. Measles: the disease and its prevention. Nursing Standard 17 (24), 46–52.

Belton, N., Hambridge, K., 1991. Essential element deficiency and toxicity. In: McLaren, D. (Ed.), Textbook of paediatric nutrition, 3rd edn. Churchill Livingstone, Edinburgh.

Bennett, M., 2003. Sleep and rest in PICU. Paediatric Nursing 15 (1), 3–6.

Blenkinsop, A., 2003. Nurse prescribers: head lice. Primary Health Care 13 (8), 33–34.

Blinkhorn, F., Davies, K., 2001. A role for health visitors in oral health promotion. National Dental Health Education Group Journal Spring, 9–11.

Blumenthal, I., 2000. Fever and the practice nurse: measurement and treatment. Community Practitioner 73 (3), 519–521.

Bosworth, C., 1997. Burns trauma: management and nursing care. Baillière Tindall, London.

British Nutrition Foundation (BNF) 2003 Online. Available at: http://www.nutrition.org.uk/

British Thoracic Society (BTS) and Scottish Intercollegiate Guideline Network, (SIGN), 2008. British guideline on the management of asthma – a national clinical guide. Online. Available at: http://www.brit-thoracic.org.uk

Budd, C., Gardiner, M., 1999. Paediatrics. Mosby, London.

Bukatko, D., Daehlar, M.W., 2004. Child development: a thematic approach, 5th edn. Houghton Mifflin, Boston.

Bundred, P., Kitchiner, D., Buchan, I., 2001. Prevalence of overweight and obese children between 1989 and 1998: population based series of cross-sectional studies. British Medical Journal 322, 1240–1253.

Casey, G., 2000. Fever management in children. Paediatric Nursing 12 (3), 38–42.

Cernik, K., 1999a. The developing child. In: Booth, K., Luker, KA., (Eds.), A practical handbook for community health nurses: working with children and their parents. Blackwell Science, Oxford

Cernik, K., 1999b. Caring within families. In: Booth, K., Luker, K.A., (Eds.), A practical handbook for community health nurses: working with children and their parents. Blackwell Science, Oxford

Chandler, T., 2002. Croup. Paediatric Nursing 14 (7), 41–47.

Cork, M.J., 1997. The importance of skin barrier function. Journal of Dermatological Treatment 8, s7–s13.

D'Amore, A., Campbell Hewson, G., 2002. The management of upper airway obstruction in children. Current Paediatrics 12, 17–21.

Davies, G., et al., 2001. Caries among 3-year-olds in Greater Manchester. British Dental Journal 190, 381–384.

Department of Health (DoH), 1991a. Dietary reference values for food, energy and nutrients for the UK. HMSO, London

Department of Health (DoH), 1991b. Weaning and the weaning diet. HMSO, London

Department of Health (DoH), 1999. Saving lives: our healthier nation. The Stationery Office, London.

Department of Health (DoH), 2000. Modernising dentistry: implementing the NHS plan. HMSO, London.

Department of Trade and Industry(DTI) 2001. Working for a safer world: 23rd annual report of the home and leisure accident surveillance system – 1999 data. HMSO, London.

Dodd, C.S., 2003. Interventions for treating head lice. Cochrane Review. The Cochrane Library, issue 3. Update Software, Oxford.

Elliott, B., 1999. Managing atopic eczema: evidence and issues. In: Booth, K., Luker, K.A. (Eds.), A practical handbook for community health nurses: working with children and their parents. Blackwell Science, Oxford.

Elliott, B., Luker, K., 1997. The experiences of mothers caring for a child with severe atopic eczema. Journal of Clinical Nursing 6, 241–247.

Evans, J., French, D., 1995. Sleep and healing in intensive care settings. Dimensions of Critical Care Nursing 4, 189–199.

Flanagan, C.M., Kennedy, L., 1999. Nutrition in childhood: advice and dilemmas. In: Booth, K., Luker, K.A. (Eds.), A practical handbook for community health nurses: working with children and their parents. Blackwell Science, Oxford.

Flanagan, M., Graham, J., 2001. Should burn blisters be left intact or debrided? Journal of Wound Care 10 (1), 41–45.

Gowar, J., Lawrence, J., 1995. The incidence, causes and treatment of minor burns. Journal of Wound Care 4 (2), 71–74.

Gustafasson, U., et al., 1992. The relevance of sleep, circadian rhythm and lifestyle, related to holistic theory of health. Scandinavian Journal of Caring Sciences 6 (1), 20–23.

Hadfield-Law, L., 2001. Dealing with scabies. Nursing Standard 15 (31), 37–42.

Hall, D.M.B., Elliman, D. (Eds.), 2003. Health for all children, 4th edn. Oxford University Press, Oxford.

Herder, S., 1994. Sponge baths for fever: a waste of nursing time. American Journal of Nursing 94 (10), 55.

Hinds A, Gregory T 1995 National diet and nutrition survey: children aged 1 ½–4½. Vol. 2: report of the dental survey. HMSO, London

Jones, S., 2003. A clinical pathway for pediatric gastroenteritis. Gastroenterology Nursing 26 (1), 7–18.

Laufer, M., 2003. Toxocariasis. eMedicine Journal. Online. Available at: http://www.emedicine.com/ped/topic2270.htm

Lissauer, T., Clayden, G., 2007. Illustrated textbook of paediatrics, 3rd edn. Mosby, London.

Lowe, S., 2002. An overview of gastrointestinal infections. Nursing Standard 16 (49), 47–52.

MacDonald, A., 1999. Iron deficiency in infants and children. Primary Health Care 9 (6), 17–24.

Mackowiak, P.A., et al., 1997. Concepts of fever: recent advances and lingering dogma. Clinical Infectious Diseases 25, 119–138.

Maw, R., 2000. Re-evaluating the ENT procedures. The Practitioner 244, 608–617.

McCutcheon, H., Fitzgerald, M., 2001. The public health problem of acute respiratory illness in childcare. Journal of Clinical Nursing 10, 305–310.

McVerry, M., Collins, J., 1999. Managing the child with gastroenteritis. Nursing Standard 13 (37) 59–53.

National Institute for Health and Clinical Excellence (NICE), 2006. Obesity: guidance on the prevention, identification, assessment and management of overweight and obesity in adults and children, NICE, London

National Institute for Health and Clinical Excellence (NICE), 2007a. Feverish illness in children. Assessment and management in children younger than 5 years. NICE, London

National Institute for Health and Clinical Excellence (NICE), 2007b. Urinary tract infection in children. diagnosis treatment and long term management. NICE, London

National Institute for Health and Clinical Excellence (NICE), 2007c. Atopic eczema in children. Management of atopic eczema in children from birth up to the age of 12 years. NICE, London

National Institute for Health and Clinical Excellence (NICE), 2008. Surgical management of otitis media with effusion in children. NICE, London

Northall, F., Cullen, G., 1999. Pesticide poisoning: herbicides. Emergency Nurse 7 (2), 22–26.

Ottley, C., 2002. Baby tooth care: a forgotten priority? Nursing Standard 16 (18), 40–44.

Pickford, M., 2000. Prevention of poisoning. Primary Health Care 10 (3), 38–41.

Porth, M., 1994. Pathophysiology: concepts of altered health states, 4th edn. Lippincott, Philadelphia.

Prescilla, R.P., 2003 Gastroenteritis. eMedicine Journal. Online. Available at: http://www.emedicine.com/ped/topic834.htm

Pritchard, P., 1999. Sleep disorders in the preschool child: how the health professionals can help. In: Booth, K., Luker, K.A. (Eds.), A practical handbook for community health nurses: working with children and their parents. Blackwell Science, Oxford.

Public Health Laboratory Service (PHLS), 2002. COVER programme: April to June. CDR Weekly 12, 39.

Pursell, E., 2000. The use of antipyretic medications in the prevention of febrile convulsions in children. Journal of Clinical Nursing 9, 473–480.

Reidpath, D.D., Glasziou, P.P., Del Mar, C., 1999. Systematic review of autoinflation for treatment of glue ear in children. British Medical Journal 318, 1177.

Rogers, J., 2002. Managing daytime and night-time enuresis in children. Nursing Standard 16 (32), 45–52.

Roper, N., Logan, W., Tierney, A., 1996. The elements of nursing: a model for nursing based on a model of living, 4th edn. Churchill Livingstone, Edinburgh.

Royal College of Nursing, 2007. Standards for assessing, measuring and monitoring vital signs in infants, children and young people. Guidance for Children's nurses and nurses working with young people. RCN, London.

Royal College of Nursing, 2008. Caring for children and young people with eczema. Guidance for Nurses. RCN, London.

Royal Society for the Prevention of Accidents (ROSPA), 2003. Fact sheet: child safety at home. Online. Available at: http://www.rospa.com.htm

Scottish Intercollegiate Guidelines Network (SIGN), 2003. Diagnosis and management of childhood otitis media in primary care: a national clinical guide, 66. SIGN, Edinburgh.

Scottish Intercollegiate Guidelines Network (SIGN), 2005. Prevention and management of dental decay in the pre-school child: a national clinical guide, 83. SIGN, Edinburgh.

Strauss R 2001 Childhood obesity and self-esteem. Pediatrics 105:e15

Sylva, K., Lunt, I., 1982. Child development: a first course. Basil Blackwell, Oxford.

Taylor, K., 2001. The management of minor burns and scalds in children. Nursing Standard 16 (11), 45–51.

Tortora, G.J., Grabowski, S.R., 2002. Principles of anatomy and physiology, 10th edn. Harper Collins, New York.

Trigg, E., Mohammed, T.A., 2006. Practices in children's nursing; guidelines for hospital and community, 2nd edn. Churchill Livingstone, Edinburgh.

Walker, G.J.A., Johnstone, P.W., 2003. Interventions for treating scabies: Cochrane methodology review. The Cochrane Library, issue 2. John Wiley, Chichester.

Watts, R., Robertson, J., Thomas, G., 2003. Nursing management of fever in children: a systematic review. International Journal of Nursing Practice 9, S1–S8.

Webster, H., et al., 1998. Pulmonary system. In: Slota, M. (Ed.), Core curriculum for pediatric critical care nursing. Saunders, London.

Wong, D., 1997. Whaley and Wong's essentials of pediatric nursing, 5th edn. Mosby, St Louis.

Woodfield, T.A., 1999. The acquisition of speech and language. Journal of Child Health Care 3 (3), 35–38.

World Health Organization (WHO), 1997. Obesity, preventing and managing the global epidemic: report of the WHO consultation of obesity. WHO, Geneva.

World Health Organization 2004 Global strategy on diet, physical activity and health. WHO, Geneva. Can be accessed online at: http://www.who.int/dietphysicalactivity/strategy/eb11344/strategy_english_web.pdf

World Health Organization, 2006. The treatment of diarrhoea: a manual for physicians and other senior healthcare workers. WHO, Geneva.

Wright, C., 2000. Identification and management of failure to thrive: a community perspective. Archives of Diseases in Childhood 82, 5–9.

Bibliography

NHS Centre for Reviews and Dissemination, 1998. Preschool hearing, speech, language and vision screening. Effective Health Care 4(2). Online. Available at: http://www.york.ac.uk/inst/crd/crdpublications.htm

NHS Centre for Reviews and Dissemination, 2002. The prevention and treatment of childhood obesity. Effective Health Care 7(6). Online. Available at: http://www.york.ac.uk/inst/crd/crdpublications.htm

Scottish Intercollegiate Guidelines Network (SIGN), 2003. Management of obesity in children and young people. Quick reference guide: 69. SIGN, Edinburgh. Online. Available at: http://www.sign.ac.uk

Health needs of middle childhood

42

Susan Hooton Diane Scott

ABSTRACT

The purpose of this chapter is to provide the reader with an understanding of the world of the developing school child and the major health issues associated with this age group. For the purposes of this chapter, 'the middle childhood years' are defined as the primary/middle (in those areas of the country that have middle schools) school years: 5–12 years of age.

LEARNING OUTCOMES

- Consider theories of child growth and development.
- Relate common health and social care needs to child development.
- Outline major health promotion strategies and related issues.
- Consider common illnesses, disorders and hospitalisation.
- Consider the needs of the school-aged child in a practice setting (medical assessment unit).
- Enhance understanding of mental health and psychological well-being of the middle-school-aged child.

The social world of the school child

> The health and well being of children are inextricably linked to their parents' physical, emotional and social health, social circumstances and child rearing practices
>
> (American Academy of Pediatrics 2003 p 111)

In considering children's health, the need to consider the child's age, stage of development and social circumstances is of prime importance. The child's developmental stage will influence the way he or she perceives their world, the way that he or she interacts with others and his or her ability to adjust and adapt to changing health and social situations. Knowledge of child development therefore, provides vital clues for those working with children about the biological, psychological and social influences on a child's life, and the threats and dangers to children's health associated with everyday living. The better we understand the particular needs of children at varying developmental stages, the better we can provide care that will be acceptable and less frightening to the child.

Reflect on your practice

Think of a child you have nursed recently and consider how his or her stage of development and understanding helped them to cope with their situation.

The National Service Framework (NSF) for Children (Department of Health (DoH) 2003) contains standards for all groups working with children in health and social care settings and will be central in steering the way that services develop. This document enshrines the basic principle of making services suit the needs of children and states that the care we deliver to children must be genuinely 'child centred', wherever that care is delivered. For this to happen, those working with children across health, education and social care settings must ensure that children's wishes and experiences are taken into account (Smith 2003) and understand that children need very different support and facilities at different developmental stages. These principles are carried forward in an educational context in 'The Children's Plan' (Department for Children, Schools & Families 2007).

Activity

- Placing the school child at the centre, map the range of social contacts that the average child will develop throughout their middle school years.
- What factors might influence the extent of this social network?

DOI: 10.1016/B978-0-7020-3183-0.10042-6

Initially, the major influence on infants and very young children comes through the family members with whom the child most frequently comes into contact (Bukatko & Daehler 1998, Mountain 2002). As the child matures and starts attending nursery and school, the social circle of the child extends, providing new contacts and new challenges to the 'established order' within the child's life. For the middle-school-aged child, this extended social network widens to include school friends and others outside of the family.

Many of these contacts will present new intellectual, cultural and physical interests and challenges for the school child; they may be involved in planning activities to help children perform and acquire new skills. Children will also find that as they mature, they have very different expectations placed on them, which will be formal and informal in nature (Bukatko & Daehler 1998).

The early primary school years see young children develop social skills such as sharing, turn taking and participation in group activities. It is the age where rules and rituals are learnt through play and structured activities; the need for conformity in middle school years being a central characteristic within the games that are so important to children (Bukatko & Daehler 1998, Piaget 1968). The later primary/middle school years are a time of gang membership and club membership with secret passwords and rituals that initiate and regulate the order of membership.

Schaffer (2004) proposes that children's groups usually adopt:

- routines
- customs to which members must conform
- distinct ways of greeting and dressing
- private jokes and verbal play routines
- agreed opinions about public and authoritative figures
- agreed opinions about popular music and sporting teams
- common values about what is right and wrong.

It is easy to see how a peer culture develops and how individual youngsters take on an individuality ascribed by their peers. Shaffer (2004) suggests this may conflict with and differ from the culture shared with adults and questions the assumption that young people acquire knowledge solely from adult family members, as 'peer collaboration' is clearly a central feature of maturity and knowledge acquisition. Ladd et al (2008) studied 5–12-year-olds and found that whereas during periods of rejection, children exhibited negative or negligible growth in school participation, when non-rejected, they manifested confidence and positive growth.

Rules are an important part of everyday life. They make it possible for us to get along with one another. If children do not learn how to behave, they will find it difficult to get on, both with grown-ups and with other children. They will find it hard to learn at school, will misbehave and will probably become unhappy and frustrated (Royal College of Psychiatrists 2008). Discipline is also acquired through group and team play and, increasingly, self-discipline must develop if children are to be included in group activities. Leaders are appointed who direct others and roles and rules are established which the school child will be expected to respect. The child is exposed to umpires, referees, school prefects and monitors and other figures of authority who will control and direct activity with authority.

However, not all school children adapt well to their changing world. Spender et al (2001) warn that many children will experience difficulty with these expectations and that not all school children are able to adapt to the challenges placed on them, often resulting in the child refusing to attend school. School refusal is a common phenomenon, which often presents with physical symptoms such as:

- nausea
- abdominal pains
- headaches
- diarrhoea
- panic attacks.

Interestingly, such symptoms often subside following the decision to allow a child not to attend school (Rutter 1999, Spender et al 2001). The 'peak times' for school refusal are at transition periods and are most commonly seen in 5 and 11 year olds, when children start or change schools.

Spender et al (2001) also noted that up to 5% of school children will present with other disruptive or behaviour problems serious enough to cause dysfunction and referral. Conduct disorder is a well-reported problem for many school children and is diagnosed when the young person can be assessed as displaying different types of misbehaviour, typically three from a prescribed list (Spender et al 2001) and may result, if untreated, in the child being excluded from school. This is an extremely undesirable situation as there are proven links between conduct disorder and childhood truancy which may result in future criminal activity (Mental Health Foundation 1999).

PowerPoint

Access the companion PowerPoint presentation (slide 1: Excellence in schools).

Between 5 and 12 years of age, children rapidly develop strength and balance. Exercise and physical activity is essential for the child's growing sense of coordination and for muscle and bone development. Much of the school child's exercise and physical activity will be experienced through school activities and physical education remains a key component of middle school curriculum. There is, however, much concern that school children in the 21st century engage in less physical activity than children of previous decades.

Activity

Make a list of popular playground games that promote activity. What are schools doing to:

- Promote such games?
- Prevent such games?
- What influences the trends in playground games?

It is suggested that school children are increasingly assessed on cognitive abilities such as numeracy and literacy skills, leaving less time in the curriculum for physical activity (Napier et al 2000). Also, social activity out of school appears to be restricted as school children become more technologically proficient and TV, video and computer games become all consuming. Although these technological games may keep young people occupied for great lengths of time, they certainly result in long periods of inactivity. In fact, obesity and other conditions associated with inactivity such as lethargy and constipation are increasingly prevalent within the middle school population.

The older school child enjoys being creative, enjoying puzzles and quizzes and is able to engage in complex games of fantasy. Stories are enjoyed and reading and numerical skills enable the child to understand more of the world about them. School children also have a developing interest in their bodies and their bodily functions, a factor that has been incorporated into health-enhancing activities. For example, this awareness of the natural interests of children has been successfully applied to teaching about health matters in school as well as leading to the creation of 'clubs' and summer schools for children learning how to cope with conditions such as diabetes and asthma.

Between 5 and 12 years, children have the ability to develop a strong sense of citizenship. This is a natural extension of them becoming able 'navigators' in the world outside of the home; they develop a strong sense of independence and justice and a developing sense of morality. Schaffer (2004) suggests that children develop morally through social and intellectual means and friendships often act as 'peer sociometrics', providing a measure as to how well children are developing moral awareness. However, it should be noted that although some children are naturally shy, prolonged reluctance to go to particular places or to meet particular people may be a sign of bullying or abuse (DoH 2008a). Moral development differs according to how well accepted children are by their peers and how well they engage with those around them. Schaffer (2004) lists characteristics demonstrated by popular children with a strong sense of moral awareness compared with rejected children and children who have suffered neglect and discusses the difficulties children experience internalising and externalising their individual experiences through interaction with their peers. Williams et al (2007) study the developmental course of interpersonal aggression up to and during adolescence. Such interactions are fundamental to the way that children start to formulate ideas about future intentions and career aspirations, largely based on the roles, opinions and expectations of those around them (Schaffer 2004, Piaget 1968, Flatman 2002).

PowerPoint

Access the companion PowerPoint presentation (slide 2: Characteristics of popular children; slide 3: Characteristics of rejected children and slide 4: Characteristics of neglected children).

Napier et al (2000) recognise the ways in which education and play are essential prerequisites to the school child in developing confidence and self-esteem. They adopt a constructivist stance in suggesting that school children play a very active role in their development and oppose views that child development is a passive process, shaped by adults. They assert that children are involved in constantly assessing themselves through their relationships and interactions with others as well as through their own social achievements. There is much evidence that personal attainments and mastery over the environment are important factors in developing confidence and self-reliance in childhood (Bukatko & Daehler 1998 p 255–265, LaMontagne 1984, Napier et al 2000 p 60–65) and that the establishment of self-concept is interrelated with the development of self-esteem in childhood.

Napier et al (2000 p 65) suggest that self-concept and self-esteem are also essential elements in the central task of developing a sense of self-identity. They highlight studies that demonstrate a shift in perspective from the preschool child's (egocentric) emphasis on self-description towards the older school child's descriptions of self as compared with others, which happens at about 7 years of age. The fundamental links between physical, emotional and social development of the school-aged child and how this relates to and influences childhood health will underpin much that follows in this chapter.

The school child and health promotion

The application of theories of child development to the health needs of school-aged children is vitally important to ensure successful implementation of health-promotion strategies (Downie et al 1991).

Reflect on your practice

- What are the major health campaigns aimed at school children?
- How do we decide what to target and what needs to be achieved?
- Who decides what to target?

PowerPoint

For middle-school-aged children, much health promotion activity is directed towards:

- road safety: link to PowerPoint presentation slide 6
- personal safety: link to PowerPoint presentation slide 7
- risks of sun bathing: link to PowerPoint presentation slide 8
- dental health: link to PowerPoint presentation slide 9
- nutrition: link to PowerPoint presentation slide 10.

Those involved in promoting health for the middle-school-aged child range from health advisors at government level and Strategic Health Authorities charged with improving the health of local populations and health economies, to individuals working directly with children such as school nurses, teachers, scout and guide leaders and health promotion specialists who might visit schools and organisations as part of the planned curriculum.

WWW

Learn about successful ways of presenting health promotion messages to children by visiting:

- http://www.comiccompany.co.uk

The government health strategy as outlined in 'Our healthier nation' (DoH 1999) outlined the need to consider child health in the context of healthy families, healthy schools and healthy communities; realising the complex interdependence between children's health and the society in which they live. Schools are often seen to be ideally placed to improve children's health and all schools are expected to have policies for promoting health (World Health Organization (WHO) 2002). A new UK-based Child Health Promotion Programme (CHPP) 'Pregnancy and the first five years of life' sets out the government's intentions to provide greater emphasis on promoting the health and well-being of children in the early stages and support a core programme for all children, with additional services for children and families with particular needs and risks. It is recognised that partnership working between different agencies on local service development will be essential along with a re-focus on changing public health priorities such as obesity, social and emotional development (DoH 2008a).

Healthy living and personal and social education (PSE) are key components of the national curriculum, implemented in all schools. In fact, the concept of the health promoting school is now a key indicator against which schools are monitored.

Reflect on your practice

- Make a list of factors that might identify a school as 'a health-promoting school'.
- How might children's services in hospitals learn from this initiative?

PowerPoint

Access the companion PowerPoint presentation (slide 5: Health-promoting schools).

As they progress through school, children are increasingly able to take on board health promotion messages and to begin to take an active role in looking after themselves. The cognitive development of school children enables them to relate increasingly complex events and mental representations (Bukatko & Daehler 1998, Piaget 1968). They begin to understand cause and effect, which is classed as moving through the stage of 'concrete operations' between 7 and 11 years, towards the formal operational stage of the older school child who is able to reason hypothetically. The cognitive developmental theorist Piaget (1968) further suggests that school children now become less egocentric and better understand how they relate to others. Although Piagetian theories have received criticism over the years (see Shaffer 2004 p 190), many subsequent studies have confirmed his general claims about the sequence of children's developmental acquisitions and have refined and built on Piaget's early work to address weaknesses. According to Piaget, the older school child also has increased ability to classify, sequence, group and sort complex information and understand related concepts. This understanding will help application of health promotion messages for the older school child, as long as the individual abilities of each child are acknowledged within the process.

In agreement with Piaget, the constructivist child theorist Vygotsky proposes that children are active contributors to their own learning and development. Vygotsky stresses the importance of adults needing to understand the motivation behind each individual child's learning and accurately pick up the cues children send out to other individuals as a 'cooperative enterprise' (Shaffer 2004 p 201). Vygotsky places particular emphasis on:

- interactivity between individual adults and children: as opposed to relying on age-related learning, which is the traditional Piagetian approach to understanding cognitive child development
- contextualising a situation and taking into account the social, historical, cultural and environmental factors that influence individual learning
- participation: the child participates and even drives events during learning encounters, as opposed to being a passive recipient.

Vygotsky's theories complement those of Piaget when considering how children might learn about their health and keeping healthy and how adults might more effectively deliver health-promotion messages to children.

The concept of empowering children through health-promotion activities has been prevalent in much of the UK health-promotion literature for the past decade. Many school-aged children take responsibility for managing conditions such as asthma and diabetes, and are fully able to self-manage their conditions, which is especially important in situations where parents are not always around, for example when the child is at school or during leisure activities.

Child health should not be seen as a privilege, afforded to certain groups of children. It is now well recognised, through the UN Convention (United Nations General Assembly 1989), that children have the right to live healthy lives and much work is directed towards addressing ongoing health inequalities in our society.

PowerPoint

Access the companion PowerPoint presentation (slide 11: UN Convention – children's rights).

The links between socioeconomic disadvantage and poor child health are well recognised (Acheson 1999), as is the link between children who live in disadvantaged households and their increased exposure to domestic violence and to childhood accidents. The Children's National Service Framework (NSF)

(DoH 2003), which sets out standards for the health and social care for all children in England, states that:

> The improving picture of child health is marred by stark and persistent inequalities in health between children from advantaged families and those who are poor, across different ethnic groups, and across different parts of the country and different neighbourhoods.

Successful health promotion strategies are multidimensional and must acknowledge the complex interplay of cultural, socio-political, economic and biological factors (Downie et al 1991). To improve the health of school children, the individual child's ability to take on board health messages and the relevance of those messages to the child's everyday 'reality' must be central to any health promotion activity.

The DoH (2003) has recognised the need to understand the nature of children's contact with health services and states that children and young people are frequent users of all types of health care, compared with adults. Children will be seen for routine health checks and immunisations during childhood, and are frequent visitors to A&E departments, but the NSF acknowledges the central caring role of families when it states that '80% of all episodes of illness in childhood are managed by parents'. The pattern of attendance of children to health services is becoming better understood. The NSF states that 'a school child will present at the GPs up to two to three times per year and one-quarter of all older children will attend an Accident and Emergency department'. What is less well understood, is how to optimise health-promoting opportunities for children, to reduce the incidence of childhood accidents and promote healthy growth and development.

Common childhood accidents

The middle-school-aged child has constantly developing and improving capabilities. School children become more adventurous in play, have increased mobility, and are generally allowed more freedom to travel alone (Bukatko & Daehler 1999). As children develop major developmental accomplishments, they come closer to danger and are extremely prone to accidents. In fact, the child's increasing sense of independence can be directly related to many of the major causes of accidents in childhood. Accidents remain the most common cause of death among children over 5 and road traffic accidents account for two-thirds of all fatal accidents among school-aged children (Department of Transport (DoT) 1992, 2000). The major causes of accidents to school children are:

- road traffic accidents
- falls
- head injury
- burns and scalds
- drowning
- poisoning
- bodily injury.

Minor soft tissue injuries, bruising and abrasions due to accidental injury are extremely common in middle childhood but the most common cause of severe injury and death is due to motor vehicle accidents, usually involving the child as a pedestrian. The DoT (2000) figures show that more than 5000 child pedestrians were killed or seriously injured on British roads that year, with many of these accidents being preventable. There is a national road safety target to reduce child deaths by 2010 (Dept for Transport) underpinned with an educational programme 'On the safe side – Local responsibilities for road safety education in schools' strategy which commenced in 2003.

PowerPoint

Access the companion PowerPoint presentation (slides 12 and 13: Department of Transport).

Wilson (1995) states that accident rates in childhood show distinct social class differences. She records that 'the chances of a child of unskilled manual parents being killed in a traffic accident are four times greater than those of a child of professional parents, and for a child of an unemployed head of household, they are seven times greater'. She suggests that lack of supervision, lack of suitable play areas and lack of private transport are contributing factors, all of which are key indicators of social and economic disadvantage. Additional factors are linked to motivational factors, and particularly adherence to responsible social values appear to be important in placing certain children at greater risk of traffic accident than others (DoT 2008).

Trauma and surgery

The major reasons for non-medical admissions to hospital for school children are either associated with trauma, often following an accident, or for planned surgery. Admissions to general surgical units might typically be due to:

- general trauma following accidents/falls
- head injury
- appendicitis
- surgical investigations
- lacerations
- dog bites/wounds
- non-complicated cosmetic surgery.

The Royal College of Nursing (RCN) Paediatric Nurse Manager's Forum report provides valuable information regarding the type of surgical admissions most commonly experienced in childhood (RCN 1999). It shows that the distribution of special surgical services across UK children's services is as follows (RCN 1999):

- orthopaedic (41.7%)
- ENT (38.2%)
- ophthalmology (7.2%)
- plastic surgery (5.5%)
- neurosurgery (2.4%)

- maxillofacial (2.0%)
- urology (2.0%)
- oral surgery (1.1%).

Orthopaedic conditions of middle childhood

Dearmun & Taylor (1995) suggest that there are usually two distinct groups of children admitted to the orthopaedic ward; those with unplanned, emergency admissions, usually following an accident, and those children with congenital or diagnosed mobility problems, who can be well prepared for hospital. However, the most common reason for a child referral to an orthopaedic surgeon is following a fracture.

As the developing child becomes more adventurous in play, more involved in competitive sport and is allowed more freedom, the incidence of musculoskeletal injuries increases dramatically. The 'weak link' in the school child's developing skeleton is described as being the growth plate or the epiphysis, making epiphyseal separations common, along with fractures of the child's long bones. Most fractures are caused by blows applied to the skeleton, which result in breaking of the bone due to the excessive force. Jones states that because children's bones have different biochemical properties from adult bones, bowing, buckle fractures and greenstick fractures, which are incomplete fractures, are all common in childhood. Children's fractures heal more quickly, with quicker recovery of function and, increasingly, children with a fractured femur may find that they can have their traction at home, provided by a Hospital at Home team, to avoid lengthy hospital admissions and separation from family members.

Upper limb fractures of childhood are also common, usually occurring as a result of falling onto an outstretched hand, and most commonly occurring in school playgrounds and play areas. Fractures of the elbow are among the most unstable fractures and often need surgical fixing with plate insertions.

Certain orthopaedic conditions of childhood are more difficult to diagnose, such as the phenomenon of 'growing pains', which is a frequent complaint of school-aged children. It is stated that about 15% of children go through a period where they wake at night due to pains in their legs. Although this condition affects many children and is acknowledged to be a painful condition, there are no specific clinical treatments apart from sympathetic management, involving heat application, simple stretching exercises, massage and reassurance.

Day-case surgery

Many school children will find themselves being admitted to hospital as day patients, as much more childhood surgery is now delivered in day-case units. This is to be applauded because it means that children and their families spend much less time in hospital and children miss less school. Thornes (1991) published a comprehensive report advocating day-case surgery for children and identified 12 quality standards for the care of children undergoing day-case surgery. She upheld the principle of 'keeping children safely within their families, with the parents remaining the principal carers' thus reducing separation anxiety and family disruption.

However, the RCN Nurse Managers Report (1999) found an increasing number of children admitted to adult day-care units with few of Thornes' standards being met. Feasey (2000) undertook a study looking at the quality of care in children's day-case surgical units, across a wide range of ages and surgical procedures. She looked to investigate the experiences of parents taking their child home on the actual day of surgery. Her findings were that:

- attendance at preadmission preparation clinics appeared to help reduce parental anxiety around the time of discharge
- parents responded positively to a follow-up telephone call on the day of discharge
- the possibility of extending telephone follow-up service to medical admissions should be explored
- many families are not invited to preoperative preparation sessions, despite growing evidence of their success
- pain control following discharge requires further study
- families requiring overnight stay were grateful for this service
- information giving (oral and written) for parents and children is improving.

She concluded her study by stating that many more families now expect to take their children home on the day of surgery, placing greater demands than ever on day-case services, and the need to ensure safety for children and their families following discharge from hospital.

Scenario

Jack, aged 7, is to be admitted to the day-case ward for removal of a benign growth. Jack's family live a distance from the hospital and Jack's mum recently had twin daughters:

- Make a list of the advantages of day surgery from Jack's perspective.
- Make a list of the advantages of day surgery to Jack's parents.
- Are there disadvantages from either point of view?

PowerPoint

Access the companion PowerPoint presentation (slide 15: Advantages of day surgery).

Darbyshire's (2003) study of mother's experiences following day surgery confirmed many of the above points outlined by Thornes' earlier work. He concluded that, given the likelihood of even shorter inpatient stays for many children, due to worldwide political and economic factors, the 'reality' of children's and parents' fears following discharge must be sought and taken into account.

Much work has been conducted on the specialist requirements of children in terms of the care they receive, the knowledge and skills of those providing care and the environment in which care is delivered. The Children's NSF (2003) sets out standards for the environment in which children should be nursed.

Reflect on your practice

- Read the NSF Standards. How well does your hospital comply?
- Who has responsibility within the hospital for ensuring the standards are met?
- Have children been asked what they think of the standards?
- Should they be asked?

WWW

Learn about standards for children in hospital from the Getting the Right Start (NSF) website:

- http://www.doh.org.uk

Access the Millennium Charter Standards for all sick children and families on the Action for Sick Children website:

- http://www.actionforsickchildren.org

Standards for children's rights to play and education in hospital are available on the National Association of Play Staff website:

- http://www.nahps.org.uk

The DoH states that 'Care should be delivered in a safe, suitable and child-friendly environment'. Sadly, the RCN (1999) report found that more than 50% of the children admitted to non-paediatric areas are admitted to adult surgical inpatient areas that do not cater for the specific needs of children. The Children's NSF has made a commitment to involve children directly in the care that they receive. This commitment has been followed through and strengthened in the 'Children Bill' (House of Commons 2004). The standards have resulted from consultation with children and respond to what children say they most want from hospitals and, as a result, there are standards on:

- environment
- diet and nutrition
- play and recreation
- education.

All these websites outline aspects of care that are important to children as service users but which may be sadly neglected if children are cared for in adult environments (DoH 2003).

The school child's growing ability to understand complex information and to understand relationships between health, illness and treatment means that they can be involved in decisions regarding their care in quite complex ways.

Evidence-based practice

- Consider your working environment and make a list of the ways in which children are involved in making decisions about the care they receive.
- Can you find evidence that supports the need for children to be more fully involved in care decisions?

PowerPoint

Access the companion PowerPoint presentation (slide 14: Involving children in care).

Franck & Jones (2003) have produced a computer game designed to teach coping techniques for 6–12-year-olds undergoing venepuncture. Venepuncture is known to be one of the most distressing and worrying aspects of treatment for children (Cummings et al 1996, Franck & Jones 2003). In acknowledging that children need to be better involved in decisions regarding their care, Franck & Jones (2003) have built in a series of options for children to help alleviate pain and distress associated with venepuncture. Options range from the type of information the child requires, choice of therapeutic approach, such as whether to use breathing techniques, relaxation techniques or distraction techniques for pain control, and whether the child would like to rehearse the needle procedures in a safe and fun environment. This initiative demonstrates how understanding and matching the needs of school children to reflect their developmental abilities can result in a resource that helps children make decisions about how they want to manage their pain. Further examples of appropriately and directly involving school children in their care include:

- involvement in preadmission clinic activities
- involvement in care planning and goal setting
- choice around bed/cubicle/personal space
- choice around visiting/visitors
- choice around clothes to be worn for theatre
- choice around parents being in anaesthetic rooms
- choice around parents being in recovery rooms
- involvement in patient-controlled analgesia (PCA)
- involvement in completing pain assessment charts.

Reflect on your practice

How well does your clinical area provide the above choices for children and young people?

Assessment of the school child in the medical unit

Due to the expansion of ambulatory care services, many children will now be admitted directly to the Medical Admissions Unit for assessment and treatment. In assessing the school-aged child who presents to the children's medical unit, the need to consider the age and stage of development continues to be highly significant. Obtaining an appropriate history, followed by a physical examination, are vital components in carrying out an accurate assessment and this requires a level of communication and trust not only with the parent or carer but, more importantly, with the child. Assessment should be carried out in a safe, suitable and child-friendly environment (DoH 2003). Increasingly, short-stay assessment and observation facilities are being developed and utilised in children's medical units, with a move to care on an ambulatory basis, where possible. Admission is only usually necessary for very young babies or children with signs of serious acute infection and homecare with support from, for example, Hospital at Home or community nursing teams is recommended.

Activity

You are helping to prepare a hot and anxious 6-year-old for a medical assessment by the consultant nurse. What do you need to consider to help to reassure the child and his father who is accompanying him?

Preparation for assessment

The environment should be prepared according to the condition of the child, avoiding barriers such as desks and with age-appropriate toys or games. Personal details and the reason for assessment are communicated in advance from the referral source and the assessor should familiarise him- or herself with the details, addressing the child by name. Establishing a good rapport with the child and parent/carer from the outset is important. School-aged children generally have had enough contact with healthcare personnel that they can rely on past experiences to guide them (Barnes 2003).

The quality of past experiences may render a child wary or frightened during health assessment. A few minutes spent in determining what the child already knows or expects will happen to them is important. Time taken to reassure and explain to the child what will happen throughout the assessment process will help to overcome the fear of injury or embarrassment. The use of simple diagrams and teaching dolls is advocated to support this (Engel 1997). School-aged children are curious about the use and usefulness of equipment. A simple explanation about the purpose of equipment before using it can be reassuring, for example by telling the child 'I am going to listen to your heart beat through this stethoscope' and then allowing the child to handle and use the equipment.

Establishing a diagnosis rests on a traditional tripod of history, physical examination and investigations, with a carefully taken and properly recorded history as the clinical keystone (Barnes 2003, Engel 1997).

Taking a history from children aged 9–12 years

Increasingly, nurses are involved in undertaking health assessments of children. In some units nurse practitioners are trained to carry out initial assessments and should clarify their roles in the assessment process as they introduce themselves. Reassuring the family about the relevance of the information that they give and who has access to the information recorded is necessary at the start of the consultation. Throughout the assessment, information should be recorded accurately in a chronological order and following local hospital and NMC standards for record keeping. For example, the date and time of the assessment must be recorded, as well as details of who is accompanying the child and who is giving the history; the record should be signed by the assessor.

Activity

What points need to be considered to promote effective communication during a medical assessment?

A broad opening statement such as: 'Tell me why you've come along to see us today', helps to identify what prompted the referral and enables the child or parent/carers to discuss underlying concerns or worries. Open-ended questions used throughout the assessment encourages the child and parent/carer to tell their story and enable a more detailed history to be obtained. Age-appropriate language and the avoidance of jargon is important. School-aged children still think in concrete terms (Bukatko & Daehler 1998) but at a more sophisticated level than younger children, and throughout the assessment clarity should be sought as to whether the child has understood what has been said.

Children of school age are able to give their versions of events with parents' corroboration of certain points. Older children should be able to describe their own symptoms. Gill & O'Brien (2003) give an example of a child's description:

> We saw a bright 10-year-old boy with a proven duodenal ulcer. He described his pain as being 'like a laser beam going through my stomach'. Brilliant.

The history should follow a logical sequence with details of the:

- presenting complaint: this should include the onset and duration of the complaint, any previous episodes, aggravating or relieving factors and associated symptoms (Barnes 2003, Gill & O'Brien 2003)
- previous medical history: previous notes should be obtained and reviewed prior to the assessment enabling a picture of the child's general health state to be obtained, where possible. Knowing the reasons for previous hospitalisation and response to illness helps in planning interventions for the current illness episode
- birth history: more relevant for the younger child but this may be important where the child is experiencing developmental or neurological problems
- feeding history: including details of appetite, likes and dislikes
- growth and development: growth pattern and whether normal milestones have been reached
- allergies: including the type of reactions
- immunisations: checking if the child is fully immunised or reasons for not being immunised
- medication: recording current prescription and non-prescription drugs, dose, frequency and duration of use
- infectious contacts: including anyone else with similar symptoms and exposure including recent travel
- social history: behaviour and temperament and particularly school progress and attainment

- family history: ages and health of immediate family members, family dynamics, familial illnesses and any congenital disorders.

PowerPoint

Access the companion PowerPoint presentation (slide 16: Medical assessment).

In eliciting the history, it is also necessary to establish what action or measures the child and family have already taken to try and cope with the illness. An attentive and empathic approach should be demonstrated during the assessment, the assessor listening carefully and picking up on what is not said as well as what is being said, from the child and parent. A good assessor is able to maintain appropriate eye contact, pick up on non-verbal cues and give encouraging gestures to aid communication. Respect for other cultures and the use of behaviour acceptable to that culture is necessary. Where possible, any underlying worries should be addressed throughout the consultation. An opportunity is provided to establish goals and to educate and support the child and family. When a child is referred for assessment children, parents/carers are concerned and broadly seek four degrees of information, which the assessor should address:

- What is it? What is wrong?
- What caused it? How did it happen?
- What will be the outcome?
- Will it happen again?

Throughout the assessment the assessor should observe the child, without staring or looking too closely, noting whether the child appears sick or generally well and noting particularly the interaction and relationship between the child and the parent/carer.

Physical examination: systems review

The child's age and stage of development must also be considered in the approach to examining each child. Each system of the body should be examined (Barnes 2003, Gill & O'Brien 2003). School-aged children, like younger children, can become suddenly unwell and exhibit acute symptoms. A detailed assessment should be used to detect those with serious illness or progressive signs of severe illness. An orderly systematic head-to-toe approach is advised but may be varied to suit the child.

The school-aged child, if able, should be allowed to stand on his or her own feet for part of the examination and the least distressing aspects of the examination should be performed first. Modesty is an issue and the assessor should have a good examination technique, exposing only the area to be examined and allowing the child to remove his or her own clothes as necessary. A gown should be provided to maintain some privacy. It is important to provide reassurance throughout the examination and when normal findings are made. The child's general appearance should be noted including the nutritional state and a record of the child's height and weight should form part of the assessment process. A standing height should be obtained. A wall-mounted stadiometer is recommended to get an accurate measurement, the child standing with heels, buttocks and shoulders against the wall. Weight should be estimated with the child on a standing scale in light garments, and read to the nearest 0.1 kg (Barnes 2003). The measurements should be plotted on an appropriate growth chart. Interval measurements, over a period of time should be used to establish a growth pattern.

PowerPoint

Access the companion PowerPoint presentation (slide 17: Measurements photograph).

Baseline observations should be recorded as part of the assessment process. Temperature measurement is particularly important in assessing whether the fever correlates with the severity of the illness – for example, when a child presents with a fever, signs of local infection should be assessed.

There is a changing illness pattern in the school-aged child from the young child. As body systems mature, e.g. the immune system becomes more competent, then infection can be localised and a more efficient antibody–antigen response produced (Rudolf & Levene 1999). The older the child, the more specific the symptoms will be and the greater the ability of the child to describe the symptoms, e.g. the site or nature of any pain. Physical signs, e.g. Kernig's sign in neck stiffness, are more specific in older children.

A variety of factors predispose children to develop acute illness, such as the development of common infections when first starting school, on coming into contact with other children. Signs of acute and potentially severe illness in school-aged children include (Rudolf & Levene 1999):

- toxicity: a high fever with marked flushing and possibly confusion
- severe pain: associated with pallor, tachycardia and immobility
- change in conscious level: always a sign of a severe illness
- shortness of breath and difficulty speaking
- dehydration
- any acute difficulty walking or unsteadiness of gait.

Discussion with a more experienced assessor should take place on finding any of the above signs.

Completing the assessment

The child and parent/carer should be informed when the assessment is complete, providing the opportunity for them to ask any questions. Appreciation should be stated for their cooperation and the assessment findings should be shared with the child and family carer. Finally, the child and parent/carer should be informed about what will happen next and, where a treatment plan is commenced, this should be agreed with the child and family carer and recorded in the notes.

The chronically ill school child

Certain groups of children will have prolonged contact with child health services throughout their childhood and into early adulthood. This includes children with chronic or enduring illnesses. The major chronic conditions of middle childhood are:

- asthma
- diabetes
- disability
- neurological conditions
- hyperactivity, attention deficit syndrome
- anaemia and blood disorders.

Early supportive interventions by the primary healthcare team are essential in providing support to children with chronic illnesses and their families. Children with multiple chronic conditions are known to be at increased risk of loneliness and social isolation leading to depression. Children's community nurses are well placed to work with chronically ill children and their families and to prevent unnecessary hospitalisation. Carter (2000) found that community children's nurses were found to employ high degrees of trust, flexibility, support, reflexivity and empowerment in their work with chronically ill school children. They were also found to be a much-valued resource for children and families wanting physical and psychological support. Jackson & Vessey (2000) discuss the impact of a chronic health condition on the general development of the school child. They suggest that a lack of physical stamina and school absences, which are often associated with chronic illness, may prevent children from participating in school and extracurricular activities. Such activities are known to contribute to widening social circles, gaining social skills and developing a sense of accomplishment and skills of self-sufficiency, leaving the chronically ill school child vulnerable in these aspects of development.

Children may also resist activities during which 'deformities' or disabilities may become exposed, to prevent embarrassment and ridicule, leading to withdrawal from mainstream activities and social isolation at school. Jackson & Vessey (2000) further highlight the need for school children with chronic illnesses to be given the skills, resources and opportunities to communicate information about their conditions to other school children, thereby removing the 'mystery and speculation' that often surrounds those who appear to be different.

Factors known to place children at greater psychological risk are:

- having a poor self-concept
- having a dysfunctional family
- living in isolated areas or in poverty
- taking medications that affect the child's psychological state
- enduring long-term mental health problems.

Although there are many risks presented to the chronically ill school child, there is also a growing awareness of how psychological problems in childhood can be alleviated by promoting resilience within the child and their family (Ray & Ritchie 1993, Rutter 1999).

PowerPoint

Access the companion PowerPoint presentation (slides 21 to 26: Risk and resilience factors).

Jackson & Vessey (2000) suggest that this is especially so for children with chronic ill health if 'therapeutic adherence' or compliance is to be achieved. This places particular demands on health professionals to work within the ethos of family-centred care and to communicate openly and honestly to school-aged children about their illnesses and to gradually and increasingly involve them in key decisions regarding their health care (Jackson & Vessey 2000). Parental compliance is, of course, essential because the child's condition will be predominantly managed at home. However, it is acknowledged that problems such as overprotection, parental guilt or despair or feelings of loss for the healthy child might adversely affect the child's adaptation and ability to manage their condition well socially.

Mental health problems in school children

Since the publication of the Health Advisory Services (HAS) report 'Together we stand' (HAS 1995), increased attention has been paid to children's and young people's mental health issues and the services that are provided for children and families. The report highlighted the increased incidence of mental health problems and disorders in children and young people and the need for improved services, and provided a framework to promote the commissioning of integrated and tiered services to cater for young people.

Activity

- What is mental health?

Attempt to write a definition of children's mental health.

The Children's NSF (DoH 2003) acknowledges that in childhood, 'whilst physical health has improved, mental health problems are on the increase'. Spender et al (2001) define mental health in children and young people as:

- a capacity to enter into and sustain mutually satisfying personal relationships
- a continuing progression of psychological development
- an ability to play and to learn so that attainments are appropriate for age and intellectual level
- a developing moral sense of right and wrong
- the degree of psychological distress and maladaptive behaviour being within normal limits for the child's age and context.

This definition has become universally accepted, across varying professions and reflects the HAS definition (1995) and the definition of young people's mental health as presented in the House of Commons report to the Health Select Committee into Child and Adolescent Mental Health (1997). Others have also attempted to define mental health in childhood.

PowerPoint

Access the companion PowerPoint presentation (slides 17 and 18: Department of Education and Skills).

Activity

Which definition do you prefer and why?

Spender et al (2001) state that 2–5% of children seen in primary care settings who are presented by their parents will have mental health problems as the main complaint. They state that hyperactivity, anxiety or behavioural problems are common overriding concerns. They further suggest that many children will initially present with physical problems, leading to a situation where it is difficult to tell whether the physical problems led to the psychological problems or vice versa. They provide the following list of risk factors to help with individual psychological assessment in children:

- Chronic physical illness
- Low intelligence
- Damaged brain
- Parental psychiatric disorder
- Family disruption
- Angry, bitter family relationships
- Rejection by parents
- Rejection by peers.

Activity

- Make a list of individuals who are available to school-aged children with whom children might discuss mental health issues.
- Now rank in order the individuals who young people are most likely to seek out.

PowerPoint

Access the companion PowerPoint presentation (slide 19: Seeking out help and advice).

www

Learn more about children's and young people's mental health at:
- http://www.youngminds.org.uk

This form of assessment can be used very effectively with school children, who are able to engage in discussion, play and other activities which will all inform the initial mental health assessment.

The Children's NSF (DoH 2003) emphasises the need to undertake appropriate mental health assessments on children and young people. It states that it is essential '... to ensure that staff have an understanding of how to assess and address the emotional well being of children, and are able to identify significant mental health problems'. It further states that all hospitals receiving and treating children and young people should have policies and liaison arrangements in place to deal with:

- management of overdoses
- acute psychiatric crisis
- direct clinical work
- complex cases
- child protection cases
- long-term and life-threatening diseases
- the death of a child.

It is therefore essential for those working with children with mental health problems in hospital settings to promote the mental well-being of school-aged children and to understand the social world of the child and the everyday worries and concerns that the child might have.

Bullying: risk and resilience

Many studies describe the harmful psychosocial effects of bullying in schools, identifying indicators of bullying as withdrawal, depression and suicidal ideation. Whitney & Smith (1993) found from their studies that roughly one in four primary school children and one in ten secondary school children are bullied at least once per term. Health-promoting schools will have policies to deal with aggression and bullying and encourage disclosure from children or their friends (WHO 2002).

Children who are different or withdrawn at school are known to be prime targets for bullying, placing school children with illnesses or disabilities at particular risk. Supervision and active promotion of resilience within all children are factors that reduce bullying (Social Services Inspectorate 1998, Whitney & Smith 1993). The Social Services Inspectorate reports highlight the particular social needs of disabled children at school. Few would dispute the move towards integrating children with special needs and disabilities into mainstream education (the benefits to both disabled and non-disabled children have been well discussed), however children with disabilities in mainstream schools need particular support. The Social Services Inspectors report (1998) states that there are 327,000 children under the age of 16 in England and Wales who have one or more disabilities. This figure is likely to rise with the number of infants now receiving early neonatal intervention. It is essential, therefore, that supportive mechanisms are in place for disabled children, children with learning difficulties and chronically ill children at school, and that the rights of all children to protection are upheld whilst children are apart from parents and other carers.

The Mental Health Foundation (1999) has identified a combination of factors that are known to promote resilience in children and have identified the following as 'protective' factors:

- friends
- supportive educational environment
- hobbies and social networks
- sense of humour
- communication skills
- religious and spiritual orientation.

Much of the present work on resilience has been informed by the work of Michael Rutter (1999). Rutter observed that some children seem to cope better with life events than others facing the same challenges. He has conducted extensive research into defining and listing the 'protective factors' that promote resilience in children and young people, and help them cope better with adversity.

PowerPoint

Access the companion PowerPoint presentation (slides 20 to 22: Risk factors and slides 23 to 25: Resilience factors).

Mental health and social disadvantage

There is much evidence linking social disadvantage with mental health problems in childhood, making clear the need for health and social factors to be considered together. However, certain groups of children remain vulnerable and are known to experience poorer physical and mental health outcomes as a direct result of their social circumstances.

Activity

Make a list of children who you consider to be particularly 'vulnerable' in today's society.

Your list will probably have included:

- 'looked after' children in local authority care
- children who have parents with mental illness
- children who care for relatives
- children living with domestic violence
- children living in poor/disadvantaged families
- children living in isolated communities
- children from minority ethnic backgrounds
- 'displaced' children (refugees)
- homeless youngsters.

Many of these youngsters will have additional health needs associated directly with their demanding social circumstances. Practitioners will have to find ways to access and to engage effectively with children and families in disadvantaged and isolated settings and will need particular skills in working with children and families to truly optimise child health for many children. The Children's Society in their 2008 'Good Childhood Inquiry' found that a number of children submitting evidence commented on the importance of being free from stress, pressure and worry. In some cases they explicitly linked pressure to school, the influence of peers, bullying, family expectations and their looks. Interestingly when asked what has the most negative impact on children's well-being generally, adults responding to the GfK NOP poll rated family breakdown and conflict (29%) and peer pressure (23%) highly. Many of the submissions expressed concern about the impact that poverty and social disadvantage has on mental health and well-being, and the report summarises that refugee children, children in trouble with the law, children with disabilities and children at risk on the streets, are most at risk of poor mental health.

Summary

This chapter has attempted to present the major health issues and health problems of school-aged children. Emphasis throughout has been placed on the need to look at the individual child's developmental stage as a key factor to understanding and communicating central messages about health and well-being.

The need to gain an understanding of the child's family and social circumstances has also been stressed, as this so often enables us to gain a clearer picture of the child's everyday experiences and the barriers that many children face to living healthy lives. Thankfully, for the majority of school children, a visit to a health centre will be a pleasant experience and visits to hospital will be unusual and reduced to a minimum, with family and carers playing a central role.

The real challenges for us as a society, are about making the world a healthier and safer place for all children, to protect the most vulnerable of children and to enable families to care for their children in ways that promote physical, social and mental well-being.

References

Acheson, D., 1999. Inequalities in health. HMSO, London.

American Academy of Pediatrics, 2003. Foreword. Pediatrics 111 (6), 1541.

Barnes, K., 2003. Paediatrics. A clinical guide for nurse practitioners. Butterworth Heinemann, London.

Bukatko, D., Daehler, M., 1998. Child development: a thematic approach, 2nd edn. Houghton Mifflin, New York.

Carter, B., 2000. Ways of working: community children's nurses and chronic illness. Journal of Child Health Care 4 (2), 66–72.

Cummings, E.A., Reid, G.J., Finley, G.A., 1996. Prevalence and source of pain in pediatric outpatients. Pain 68 (1), 25–31.

Darbyshire, P., 2003. Mothers' experiences of children's recovery. Journal of Child Health Care 7 (4), 291–312.

Dearmun, A., Taylor, A., 1995. Nursing support and care: meeting the needs of the child and family with altered mobility. In: Carter, B., Dearmun, A.K. (Eds.), Child health care nursing: concepts, theory and practice, Blackwell Science, Oxford, pp. 500–514.

Department for Children, Schools & Families 2007. 'The Children's Plan': Building Brighter Futures. The Stationery Office, London.

Department of Health (DoH), 2003. Getting the right start: National Service Framework for children. Standards for hospital services. The Stationery Office, London.

Department of Health (DoH), 2008a. The child health promotion programme. The Stationery Office, London.

Department of Transport (DoT), 1992. Road accidents: Great Britain. HMSO, London.

Department of Transport (DoT), 2000. The casualty report, UK government statistics service. HMSO, London.

Department of Transport (DoT), 2008. Childhood Accidents and their Relationship with Problem Behaviour. http://www.dft.gov.uk/pgr/roadsafety/research/rsrr/theme1/childhoodaccidentsandtheirre4729?page=1#a1000

Downie, R.S., Fyfe, C., Tannahill, A., 1991. Health promotion models and values. Oxford University Press, Oxford.

Engel, J., 1997. Pediatric assessment, 3rd edn. Mosby, St Louis.

Feasey, S., 2000. Quality counts: auditing day surgery services. Journal of Child Health Care 4 (2), 73–77.

Flatman, D., 2002. Consulting children: are we listening? Paediatric Nursing 12 (7), 28–31.

Franck, L.S., Jones, M., 2003. Computer-taught coping techniques for venepuncture: preliminary findings from usability testing with children, parents and staff. Journal of Child Health Care 7 (1), 41–54.

Gill, D., O'Brien, N., 2003. Paediatric clinical examination made easy, 4th edn. Churchill Livingstone, London.

Health Advisory Services, 1995. Together we stand: child and adolescent mental health services. HAS, London.

Jackson, P.A., Vessey, J.A., 2000. Primary care of the child with a chronic condition, 2nd edn. Mosby, St Louis.

Ladd, G., Herald-Brown, S.L., Reiser, M., 2008. Does chronic classroom peer rejection predict the development of children's classroom participation during the grade school years? Child Development 74 (4), 1001–1015.

LaMontagne, L., 1984. Three coping strategies used by school aged children. Pediatric Nursing 10 (1), 25–28.

Mental Health Foundation, 1999. A bright future for all: promoting mental health in education. MHF, London.

Mountain, G., 2002. Parenting in society: a critical review. In: Smith, L., Coleman, V., Bradshaw, M. (Eds.), Family centred care: concept, theory and practice. Palgrave, Basingstoke.

Napier, N., Banton, R., Medforth, N., 2000. Children and assessment. In: Wyse, D., Hawtin, A. (Eds.), Children: a multi-professional perspective. Arnold, London.

Piaget, J., 1968. A theory of development. International encyclopaedia of the social sciences. Macmillan, New York.

Ray, L.D., Ritchie, J.A., 1993. Caring for chronically ill children at home: factors that influence parent coping. Journal of Pediatric Nursing 8 (4), 217–225.

Royal College of Nursing, 1999. Children's services: acute health care provision. RCN, London.

Royal College of Psychiatrists, 2008. http://www.rcpsych.ac.uk/mentalhealthinfo/mentalhealthandgrowingup/goodparenting.aspx

Rudolf, M., Levene, M., 1999. Paediatrics and child health. Blackwell Science, Oxford.

Rutter, M., 1999. Resilience: concepts and findings. Journal of Family Therapy 21, 119–144.

Schaffer, R., 2004. Introducing child psychology. Blackwell, Oxford.

Smith, F., 2003. Getting the right start: the children's National Service Framework. Paediatric Nursing 15 (4), 20–21.

Social Services Inspectorate, 1998. Inspection of services to disabled children and their families. The Stationery Office, London.

Spender, Q., Salt, N., Dawkins, J., Hill, P., 2001. Child mental health in primary care. Radcliffe Medical Press, Oxford.

The Children Bill, 2004. House of Lords. The Stationery Office, London.

The Children's Society 2008 Good Childhood Inquiry. http://www.childrenssociety.org.uk

Thornes, R., 1991. Just for the day. Caring for children in the health services. British Paediatric Association, London.

United Nations General Assembly, 1989. Convention on the rights of the child. United Nations, New York.

Whitney, I., Smith, P.K., 1993. A survey of the nature and extent of bullying in junior/middle and secondary schools. Education Research 35, 3–5.

Williams, S.T., Jewsbury Conger, K., Blozis, S.A., 2007. The development of interpersonal aggression during adolescence: the importance of parents, siblings and family economics. Child Development 78 (5), 1526–1542.

Wilson, M., 1995. Children, health and families. In: Carter, B., Dearmun, A.K. (Eds.), Child health care nursing: concepts, theory and practice. Blackwell Science, Oxford.

World Health Organization, 2002. A world health report 2002: reducing risks, promoting healthy life. WHO, Geneva.

Child and adolescent mental health: the nursing response

43

Michael Cooper Colman Noctor

ABSTRACT

The aim of this chapter is to explore the issues of mental health in relation to childhood and the adolescent developmental tasks. The challenges facing adolescent health care will be explored with a particular consideration of the nursing response. The assumption is made that nursing is primarily an interpersonal activity and that for the nurse this is a starting point for successful interventions in adolescent health care. There are two central themes for this chapter. First, there is strong and growing evidence for the fundamental inter-relationship between physical mental and social health. Problems in adolescence in any of these areas indicate the likelihood of long-term adverse health and social consequences (Royal College of Paediatrics and Child Health (RCPCH) 2003). Second, is training and skills. In this chapter the case will be made that the children's nurse can make a significant contribution to the care of this client group in terms of physical and mental health. There are consistent and growing calls for better training and the support of specialist practitioners in adolescence and/or mental health.

LEARNING OUTCOMES

- Link childhood mental health and issues in adolescence.
- Review the nature of adolescence.
- Consider the impact of the adolescent developmental tasks on health behaviours.
- Be able to locate the young person in terms of their developmental tasks.
- Review the interpersonal and communication skills required when working with young people.
- Explore the nature of the therapeutic relationship.
- Identify nursing responses to young people with emotional problems and/or mental health issues.
- Locate appropriate resources to inform best practice with young people.

Introduction

This chapter is set within the context of both the 'National Service Framework for children, standards for hospital services' (Department of Health (DoH) 2003), the 'National Service Framework for children, young people and maternity services' (DoH 2004) and the CAMHS Review (DoH 2008). The earlier NSF advocates child-centred services that consider the whole child, not simply the illness. Seeing the whole child also means recognising that health protection and promotion, and disease prevention are integral to the young person's care in any setting. In exploring child-centred care it is recognised that the child exists within the context of a family, school, friends and local community. Further, children and young people have rights, and their treatment is a partnership. Respecting the role of parents is seen as a significant part of providing services for children.

Prevention and health promotion are also seen as a fundamental question of attitude that looks beyond the immediate treatment of the presenting problem. This chapter seeks to explore those strategies involved in the promotion of mental health and opportunities for the prevention of health risk behaviours. The 'National Service Framework for children, young people and maternity services' (DoH 2004) builds and develops the earlier work seeking to ensure that all children and young people get services that are age appropriate, accessible and that recognise that their needs are different. It is a national blueprint to ensure personalised child-centred health and social care services. It recommends that all staff working with children are able to recognise the contribution they can make to children's emotional well-being and that they understand their responsibilities for supporting children in difficulty.

The CAMHS review (2008) stresses the need to integrate CAMHS into all spheres of child health care, therefore emphasising the need for sick children's nurses and other allied

DOI: 10.1016/B978-0-7020-3183-0.10043-8

disciplines to be aware of the mental health needs of children. This review highlights that these needs not only exist for children with predominant mental health problems but also for children who present with a primary physical problem and associated mental health needs. This report highlights how a child with a physical disorder or condition is twice as likely to develop mental health problems as the child without such difficulties (Shooter 2005). Thus emphasising the need for sick children's nurses to be sensitive to and aware of the needs of children to maintain a sense of psychological well-being.

This term 'psychological well-being' is thought to be the most useful description of mental health needs of children and adolescents as too often we limit ourselves to viewing mental health problems as diagnosable, symptom-apparent mental illnesses. There is a shift in mental health now to move away from the predominantly medical models, but not towards a polarised social model. Rather the aim is to view the child or adolescent as psychosocial beings with both psychological and social contributing factors to both their difficulties and possible solutions. The term psychological well-being also incorporates emotional, cognitive and behavioural attributes of well-being (CAMHS Review 2008).

There is also a move to fine tune the general public's view of mental health where incompatible extremes exist. Like the assumption that one needs the criteria of symptoms to be mentally unwell, on the contrary, our view of mental wellness is equally important. Recent refreshing insights into young people's views of mental health indicated that young people realistically do not view being mentally healthy as being happy all the time but rather view it as being able to cope with the potential happiness that accompanies living (CAMHS Review 2008).

Working with adolescents is a task many groups find challenging. In the foreword to the report 'Bridging the gaps' (RCPCH 2003), David Hall reminds us that the British stand accused of 'not liking children'; he suggests perhaps we like adolescents even less. Generally, adolescents are considered to have needs that differ from both adults and children yet they are often nursed in environments that also contain either adults or children. If we add to this issues of emotional distress/mental health, things seem to move beyond the perceived areas of expertise or competence of many children's nurses (Norwich Union 2001). The picture may be complicated further by the nurse having to move quickly from the parents of a child who is seriously physically ill to an emotionally distressed, abusive, swearing, adolescent whose physical health may or may not appear to be seriously compromised. It is these dilemmas that this chapter wishes to address by providing information and educational resources, but more importantly some practical guidance on the interpersonal skills that might be helpful with this client group.

The nature of adolescence

It is commonly accepted that there are some dominant ideas about adolescence. It can be defined as a period in human development linked to biological markers, involving transitions (that can be seen as stages), in which the central task is establishing identity. It is suggested that universal definitions of adolescence should at best be restricted to describing adolescence as a 'period of transition' in which, although no longer seen as a child, the young person is not yet considered an adult. The World Health Organization's (WHO 1995) definition of adolescence states that the stage is commonly associated with physiological changes occurring with the progression from the appearance of secondary sexual characteristics (puberty) to sexual and reproductive maturity. Dehne & Riedner (2001) suggest that these biological markers create problems because the falling age of onset of the menarche attributed to improved health means there is now a widening gap between the age of sexual maturity and the age at which sexual relations become legitimate. A central dilemma of the adolescent experience is that in some cultures physical maturity comes well before legal definitions of adulthood in terms of legal sexual behaviour, the right to vote, join the military, etc.

The combination of young people's relative inexperience in sexual matters and the social stigma attached to them being sexually active creates vulnerability that is only now being recognised and addressed (Dehne & Riedner 2001). However, adolescence is not characterised just a sexual dilemma, there is also vulnerability in relationships with peers, with adults and with organisations. It seems that adults don't know how to take adolescents seriously because they do not find it easy to understand their experience.

Activity

Although the biological triggers for puberty might be universal, how might the cultural ethnic values influence this process? What effect might economic and social factors have?

There is, however, a view that the dilemma of adolescence has been overplayed, in terms of a life stage that, by its very nature involves serious conflict and upheaval. More recent thinking suggests much less necessary difficulty and much more continuity between the child that was, through adolescence to the adult that will be. It is considered that normal adolescents negotiate this period of life transition with relatively little major disruption or sustained high-risk behaviour (Offer 1987, cited in Burt 2002).

Even if the more optimistic view of adolescence is taken, healthcare settings are likely to see more of those children involved in high-risk behaviours. These high-risk behaviours are also linked to the precursors of mental health problems, low self-esteem and dysfunctional families (British Medical Association (BMA) 2003).

The developmental tasks of adolescence

A simple definition for adolescence, which acknowledges the developmental stages, is offered by the Registered Nurses Association of Ontario (RNAO) in its guidelines for nursing practice entitled 'Enhancing healthy adolescence':

> The period of transition from childhood to adulthood that can be divided into early (11–14 years), mid (15–17 years) and late (18–21 years)
>
> (RNAO 2002a)

Individuals will negotiate these stages in their own time but, as a general principle, it is helpful to view adolescence in this way. There seems to be a significant degree of agreement that the stage models of the adolescent journey see personal identity as the focal concern (Kroger 1989, cited in La Voie 1994). These models take a stage approach, starting with the preadolescent, and continue the process of change through to post adolescence (La Voie 1994).

It is helpful to see the key adolescent task as a search for identity, that is, a sense of separate self but, as always, the self in relation to others. Adolescents are in search of an identity that will lead them to adulthood, they make a strong effort to answer the question 'Who am I?'.

Of the stage models, Erickson's psychosocial model is perhaps the best known. Erickson (1963) describes the adolescent task/crisis as identity versus confusion. He notes that the healthy resolution of earlier conflicts can now serve as a foundation for the search for an identity. If an individual has developed a sense of trust and a strong sense of industry then the search for identity will be easier. The adolescent must make a conscious search for identity. This is built on the outcome and resolution to conflict in earlier stages. If the adolescent cannot make deliberate decisions and choices, especially about vocation, sexual orientation and life in general, role confusion becomes a threat.

Activity

How might our unresolved adolescent experiences influence our relationship with troubled young people?

Jacobs (1998) looks at adolescence in three stages:

- early adolescence and sexuality
- middle adolescence: authority and independence
- later adolescence: faith and responsibility.

In this model, early adolescence is linked to puberty and reinitiates issues of sexual identity and attitudes as part of the overall quest for personal identity. The young person may become very self-conscious and also very preoccupied with appearance and dress. The young person's changing physical appearance matters a great deal. This might evoke feelings of pleasure and confidence or strangeness and shame. Rivalry and competition are often important elements at this time as part of the adjustments within peer groups. However, rivalry is not confined to peer groups: just at the time the children are finding their sexual identity, their parents are conscious of imminent or present changes in themselves.

Jacobs talks of how a mother may be entering her menopause at the same time as the daughter achieves her menarche or a father may be aware of his spreading midriff and lack of muscular tone just as his son is reaching his peak of physical fitness. Even if that is not the case, parents in the UK will be made aware of their changing life position in what is a very youth-oriented culture. These changes in life positions for all family members are the context in which the young person's ambivalence towards his or her parents is acted out. On the one hand, the parent is still needed as an object of love and a protector but on the other there is a strong desire to push the parent away to find their own confidence and object of love. To both love and hate parents, who then may respond by being hurt or angry, can be a difficult conflict for the young person to contain and manage.

There is also the consideration of current changes to the adolescent landscape. One must consider that the cultural advances in technology and exposure via mobile technology and the internet mean that our adolescent population is bombarded with dialogue and imagery far beyond their developmental capacity. They are exposed to sexual images and sexual discourse that their emotional development has not the capacity to cope with. This can contribute to the high octane mood swings and outbursts that are understood by an increasing pressure to cope. This mismatch between cultural demand and emotional maturity means that sometimes adolescents resort to toddler-like coping strategies of tantrums, sulking and verbal and physical 'meltdowns'. This can be understood by proposing that this behaviour is symbolic to the return to a primitive manner of coping or regression in a time of increased stress and an inability to cope. The lack of expressive ability inherent in the adolescent means that their feelings are expressed through acting out behaviours like outbursts, rebellious dress sense and/or periods of withdrawal or refusal to communicate.

Implications for the healthcare professional

It is important to be mindful of the young person's need to assert him- or herself and of the adult response of meeting the challenge or setting the boundaries. This must be within a context of an acceptance of the young person and an understanding of what is motivating his or her behaviour. The limits must contain but not crush the young person's emotions and behaviour. It is important to recognise that although we (as nurses) may appear to be the target of their discontent, it is likely that bigger issues are being acted out. These issues relate to their main developmental task of trying to assert who they are, within the context of ill health. Their illness has the potential to undermine their sense of independence directly through their own thoughts and beliefs. This might also be done indirectly and unwittingly through the actions of anxious parents and/or the collusion of nursing and medical staff.

This natural process of adolescence – separating from the parents as a way of increasing independence – may happen without much drama or may be very dramatic. Separation can be made easier if the young person can achieve a degree of financial independence. This might be quite a challenge if the young person is in continuing education, unemployed or unable to work through ill health. In the last stage, Jacobs suggests the concern is for the wider issues of their place in the wider society and their own transition into adulthood. For some there is concern about what is wrong with society and optimism about their proposed solutions. It is this stage that some of the compromises that underpin adult functioning are beginning to be made.

Coleman (1989) developed a 'focal theory' of adolescence, which suggests that at specific ages in adolescence different relationships come into focus, in the sense of being most prominent, or important. In early adolescence the concerns about heterosexual relationships are to the fore. In middle adolescence (15 years) the peer group becomes very important and in late adolescence (peaking at 17 years) conflicts with parents become central. Coleman (1989) added that there may well be overlap between the issues and that none of the issues are tied to a particular age or developmental level. A key idea that arises is that if the young person is able to deal with these issues one at a time it is easier to cope with the complex issues of adolescence. This would be why only a minority of young people are overwhelmed by the transitions of adolescence and might also link with Erikson's assertion that successful transition is linked to the success, or not, of earlier life stages. Therefore the more difficulties there have been earlier in life, the more likely adolescence will be a difficult time. During this process of individuation (separating out one's own identity), adolescents increasingly transfer their emotional attachment from parents to peers. Close peer friendships have a positive influence on adolescents' social and personality development and adolescents who perceive their peer friends as supportive have fewer psychological problems greater confidence and less loneliness (Hay & Ashman 2003).

Activity

How might such knowledge about peer relationships influence our attempts to manage disruptive behaviour in a clinical setting?

Parental relationships remain important in terms of self-worth, particularly for those adolescents whose transition is well adjusted. Those who are more troubled tend to disregard parents and teachers as sources of self-esteem, preferring alternative audiences such as peers, as a change to the negative feedback from parents and school (Hay & Ashman 2003).

What is significant from a nursing point of view is that we should take as much account of the adolescent's developmental stage as we would of the developmental stage of the younger child. If we want to be helpful and respectful, we need to go to where they are. This is the starting point of any helping relationship. As nurses, we can begin to make progress in giving appropriate care only when we begin to understand how even the most undesirable of youthful behaviours usually represent (Burt 2002):

- the attempts of adolescents to complete these developmental tasks
- ambivalence about whether they want to move on to adulthood
- their perception that they may never complete the tasks successfully.

Peer relationships

An understanding of the adolescent's developmental tasks will allow the nurse to focus caregiving in the most effective manner. The most important nursing intervention might be for the nurse to spend time with the young person's key friends, helping them accommodate the changed circumstances of the illness so that supportive peer relationships can be maintained (not sure about this?). This in turn will enhance the young person's self-concept and self-esteem, which will be needed in facing the difficult adjustments ahead. This strategy will also serve as a protective factor against emotional distress and the risk of mental ill health. This would support the idea of moving beyond pure medical thinking and embrace the concept of adolescent health (Bennett & Tonkin 2003).

Lifespan developmental theories tend to support these important ideas (Goosens & Marcoen 1999):

- They see the developing person as an active agent in his or her own development.
- Person and context are related: the individual must be seen within the context of their family, their peer group and their developmental stage.
- Developmental readiness: i.e. adolescents will fare better if they are allowed more time to deal with important issues in their lives.
- 'Arena of comfort': this idea suggests that if adolescents feel comfortable in some environments then discomfort in other areas can be tolerated.

Activity

- How might the young person's sense of agency be influenced by ill health?
- Do the assessment strategies take into account the context of the person and their illness?
- Do the clinical procedures ensure space and the right information is being offered to help the young person accommodate the changes that are happening to them?
- How might the 'arena of comfort' concept be used in the planning of care?

When thinking of a holistic assessment process, it might be helpful to reflect on the interplay between the young person's illness and their transition through the adolescent developmental tasks. You might want to think of some questions you could ask during the assessment phase that might help you locate where the young person is in terms of their adolescent transition.

Issues of sexuality, gender relationships and physical attractiveness

Sexuality might be seen as a taboo subject in that it is often an overlooked issue for those working with children and adolescents. Clearly, the reality is that children are exposed to issues of sexuality extensively within the popular media. Children and adolescents are aware of changes in their own bodies and those of their family and friends. There is a need to be sensitive to the young person's accommodation of his or her own sexuality in earlier adolescence, and their possible uneasiness with themselves in terms of sexuality. In middle adolescence we need to be aware of how younger nurses may be drawn by the young person into their peer network. They may want to see the nurse as a friend or identify with them, compete with them, or even reject them as a peer. The young person might develop intense feelings about individual nurses that may involve love and/or sexual attraction. It is worth noting that the changing attitudes in society to the expression of sexuality mean that we need to be aware of issues of primary sexual orientation, heterosexuality, homosexuality and/or bisexuality.

There is a need to keep the young person safe, and in some situations to keep staff safe as well. The issues arising out of nurses working with patients of the opposite gender are often underplayed, perhaps partly as an unconscious denial of the young person's sexuality. There is a significant trend for young women (led by their role models in popular culture) to suggest that some expression of bisexuality is cool. This could be followed by an increase in children of both sexes having sexual attraction towards nurses in what is a predominately female nursing work force.

Being ill can be a significantly challenge to the individuals confidence about their sexuality, personal appearance and thus self-worth. Studies show that awareness of sexuality and physical attractiveness significantly influenced females' and males' sense of self-worth (Hay & Ashman 2003).

Factors that influence adolescent health and the healthcare response

Key documents in this area (CAMHS Review 2008) are:

- Bridging the gaps: health care for adolescents (RCPCH 2003)
- Adolescent health (BMA 2003)
- National Service Framework for children in hospital (DoH 2003)
- National Service Framework for children, young people and maternity services (DoH 2004).

The factors that contribute towards health risk behaviours in children and young people are closely related to the factors that contribute to emotional distress and mental health problems.

There is strong and growing evidence for the fundamental inter-relationship between physical, mental and social health. Problems in any of these areas indicate the likelihood of long-term adverse health and social consequences (RCPCH 2003). These links mean that young people with health problems are likely to have a greater risk of presenting with mental health problems. It is important to note that most adolescents negotiate this period of life transition with relatively little major disruption or sustained high health-risk behaviour. Those who do experience major disruptions and who persistently engage in problem behaviours now have a significantly higher risk of health problems in later life. Thus successful intervention now has important payoffs in terms of future health problems prevented and future satisfying and productive lifetimes promoted (Burt 2002). There is a strong relationship between adolescent health and other aspects of adolescent life such as education, employment and housing. Interventions therefore should be multiprofessional and involve cooperation between health, education and social services (BMA 2003).

Most reports on adolescent health focus on health interventions in terms of health risks and protective factors. Key health risk factors identified by the BMA report 'Adolescent health' (BMA 2003) include nutrition, exercise and obesity, smoking, drinking and drug use, mental health and sexual health. Similar health outcomes were selected for study in an Australian report, 'Evidence-based health promotion no. 2: adolescent health' (Department of Human Services Victorian Government 2000). This systematic review identified six health outcomes: tobacco use, alcohol and drug use, sexual risk-taking behaviour, crime and antisocial behaviour, depression, and suicidal behaviour. There will be similar patterns in other industrially developed countries, although Australia has not identified obesity. Perhaps with sport and outdoors activity so embedded in the culture, the effects of overeating are mitigated by attitude, activity and exercise.

Research has shown that certain factors mitigate against health-risk behaviours:

- Within the individual: self-esteem, internal locus of control (feeling confident that one's own efforts will produce desired effects).
- Familial: absence of marital discord, family cohesion and a good relationship with at least one parent.
- Environmental: having at least one good relationship with a significant adult figure other than one's parents (Burt 2002).

Activity

How might this information about mitigating factors in health-risk behaviours shape the priorities of nursing actions?

Factors that increase the likelihood of health risk behaviours

The more positive the young person's self-esteem, the greater his or her sense of self-efficacy. Negative self-efficacy is linked with general unhappiness and past worries. The links are stronger for girls than boys but are significant for both. Negative self-efficacy and low self-esteem increase the possibility of health-risk behaviours. Poverty, family dysfunction or lack of parental involvement and support are the risk factors that consistently differentiate the youths most likely to get into serious trouble from those who don't (Burt 2002).

Common antecedents to health-risk behaviours (Catalano & Hawkins 1995, cited in Burt 2002) are:

- extreme economic deprivation
- family conflict
- family history of the problem behaviour
- family management problems
- neighbourhood qualities that offer pervasive opportunities to engage in the problem behaviour (e.g. substance misuse) and that have a structure of disorganisation and low attachment identity.

According to the CAMHS Review (2008) mental health problems are likely to occur in the presence of three or more stressful events. The most common (Audit Commission 1999) are:

- physical illness
- family stressors
- social problems
- education underachievement.

It can be seen that the contemporary health problems of young people occur within the context of the physical, social, cultural and political realities within which they live. Recognition by self-report that most adolescent health concerns were actually social and psychological in nature suggests that the time has come to throw off pure medical thinking and embrace the notion of adolescent health. What is needed is a holistic model of health care highlighting the multiplicity of human needs that may exist beyond and yet create the context of the presenting complaint (Bennett & Tonkin 2003).

Implications for healthcare practice

There are four statutory areas that involve intervention with young people with mental health problems or feelings, thoughts or behaviours that are deemed 'dysfunctional' in some way. These include statutory areas and sectors such as education, health, social care and youth justice. The philosophies of each of these sectors lead to different ways of framing and describing these problems. Therefore it is often problematic when a young person is misplaced in one of these sectors where their needs would be better addressed in another. It is therefore of significant importance that we create an awareness of the needs of young people with mental health problems so that their care can be planned with efficiency. It is often after discharge from a Sick Children's Hospital that the necessary referral will need to occur therefore the issue of sign posting is especially pertinent to that role. There is also a need for CAMHS to become more integrated into other alternative systems and cultures (CAMHS Report 2008).

The above reinforces what has been said before: that the young person has to be seen in the context of his or her relationships with peers and family, and also within his or her social, economic, environmental and cultural parameters. Health risk behaviours are unlikely to decrease just with the production of a health promotion leaflet and advice. However, if this is linked to a nursing style that demonstrates respect and a genuine desire to seek to understand the individual, the impact is likely to be greater. Such a style is likely to promote self-efficacy and self-esteem and a move from a condition-centred to a child-centred approach (Beresford & Sloper 2003).

There are also issues regarding equity of access for children who exist on the margins. Consequently these children present as significantly at risk for developing mental health problems. These children and young people may be vulnerable for a number of reasons, including (CAMHS Report 2008):

- because their problems are hidden from the system – for example, refugees, those seeking asylum, travellers, those who are homeless and young runaways
- because their problems are not recognised or addressed due to discrimination or lack of awareness – for example, children from black and minority ethnic communities
- because of the presence of other serious conditions – as may be the case for children with learning difficulties or disabilities
- because their mental health needs (defined as 'behavioural, emotional and social difficulties' or BESD) result in problems with their educational progress
- because they are experiencing difficulties through abuse or neglect
- because they have needs in a number of areas and are at risk of falling between services – for example, children in care, teenage mothers and fathers, those in contact with the youth justice system, those with complex chronic illness.

Childhood mental health

The idea that our early experiences shape our later lives is not new. The work of Freud and the psychoanalysis movement highlighted the importance of early life, and Bowlby (1988) and others made the link between problems in adolescence and childhood experiences. In early childhood our mental health is mediated in large part by our relationship with our primary caregivers. Recent neurological research is commented on in the CAMHS Review (2008) and reinforces the importance of early intervention to reduce the impact of stress in pregnancy and to promote attachment and acknowledge the long-term effects of attachment disturbances. This is particularly referred to in the case of children from disadvantaged circumstances

Illness can be seen as easier to define than health and is often described in diagnostic manuals. However, the question needs to be asked: what is mental health? The definition in 'Bright futures: promoting children and young people's mental health' (The Mental Health Foundation 1999) offers some indicators. This definition states that a mentally healthy child or young person is one who has the ability to:

- develop psychologically, emotionally, socially, intellectually and spiritually
- initiate, develop and sustain mutually satisfying relationships
- use and enjoy solitude
- become aware of others and empathise with them
- play and learn
- develop a sense of right and wrong
- resolve (face) problems and setbacks satisfactorily and learn from them.

It is as difficult to define mental health as it is health in general, but it is widely agreed that in children, mental health is indicated by (NHS Health Advisory Service 1995 p 15):

- a capacity to enter into and sustain mutually satisfying personal relationships
- continuing progression of psychological development
- an ability to play and to learn so that attainments are appropriate for age and intellectual level

- a developing moral sense of right and wrong
- the degree of psychological distress and maladaptive behaviour being within normal limits for the child's age and context.

Thinking about what makes us mentally healthy

The following is a list of attributes related to being mentally healthy. It might be helpful to spend a little time thinking about how your mental health is maintained and what factors contribute to your maintenance of these attributes:

- Self-esteem
- Physical growth
- Emotional growth
- Resilience
- Ability to make good personal relationships
- A sense of right and wrong
- The motivation to face setbacks and learn from them
- A sense of belonging
- A belief in my ability to cope
- How to solve problems.

A useful definition of mental health (or psychiatric) disorder was given by Rutter & Graham (1968) as:

> An abnormality of emotion, behaviour or relationships which is developmentally inappropriate and of sufficient duration and severity to cause persistent suffering or handicap to the child and/or distress or disturbance to the family or community.

In making a child psychiatric assessment five key questions are asked (Goodman & Scott 1997):

- Symptoms: What sort of problem is it?
- Impact: How much distress or impairment does it cause?
- Risks: What factors have initiated and maintained the problem.
- Strengths: What assets are there to work with?
- Explanatory model: What beliefs and expectations do the family bring?

Strengths can often be seen in terms of protective factors that increase resilience in the face of stressors. Generally the interplay of risk and protective factors determines whether the child overcomes the stressors they face. In some situations the stressors can be so great or so many that they cannot be defended against.

Resilience factors

In the child

- Being female
- More intelligent
- Easy temperament when an infant
- Secure attachment
- Positive attitude, problem solving approach
- Good communication skills
- Planner, belief in control
- Sense of humour
- Strong faith
- Capacity to reflect.

In the family

- At least one good parent–child relationship
- Affection
- Supervision, authoritative discipline
- Support for education
- Supportive relationship/marriage.

In the environment

- Wider supportive network
- Good housing
- High standards of living
- High school/college morale and positive attitudes with policies for behaviour, attitudes and antibullying
- Schools/colleges with strong academic opportunities
- Schools/colleges with non-academic opportunities
- Range of sport, leisure opportunities
- Appropriate relationships with adults.

Mental disorders can include (BMA 2003):

- emotional disorders, such as phobias, anxiety and depression
- conduct disorders
- hyperkinetic disorders, such as attention deficit disorder
- developmental disorders
- habit disorders
- eating disorders
- post-traumatic syndromes
- somatic disorders, such as chronic fatigue syndrome
- psychotic disorders, such as schizophrenia and drug-induced psychosis.

Reflect on your practice

Some factors affecting resilience cannot be influenced directly by nursing care. However, it might be helpful to consider those aspects of the children's ward environment that are likely to contribute to a young person's resilience.

www

For a fuller account of child and adolescent mental disorders and latest evidenced-based findings, go to:

- http://www.focusproject.org.uk/finding-the-evidence

The mental health of adolescents

The mental health of adolescents is extremely important not only in itself but also because of the strong links that it has with adolescent health-risk behaviours, violence and delinquency. In many senses, mental health is at the centre of adolescent health frameworks. Poor mental health can influence exercise patterns, obesity and body image, substance misuse and high-risk sexual behaviour.

Key points

- Early adolescence (11–14): high rates of conduct and emotional disorders
- Mid to late adolescence: peak time for the onset of depressive disorders and schizophrenia
- Depressive symptoms: very common in adolescence. Most depressive disorders at this age are co-morbid with anxiety or slightly less common conduct disorder
- Self-injury and self-harm: there is confusion over terminology with the incidence being given as 1:17 and possibly as high as 1:10. Deliberate self-harm is common in adolescent girls. The peak age for presentation is 15–24 for women and 25–34 for men
- Eating disorders: e.g. bulimia and anorexia nervosa, disproportionately affect young females. This group has one of the highest death rates of all psychiatric illness
- Attempted suicide: the rate of suicide is very low under 14 years old; attempted suicide begins to occur around 11 or 12 and increases rapidly in the early and mid teens. Young men are particularly at risk and are less likely than girls to show their distress beforehand.

Prevalence rates

There is a lack of data indicating the overall psychological well-being of young people in the UK and the prevalence of lower level, subclinical mental health problems. However, there is an indication over an overall increase in prevalence rates since the 1970s. A study in 2004 indicated that 10% of young people between 5 and 15 had a clinically diagnosable mental disorder (Collishaw et al 2004). Prevalence rates varied according to a number of characteristics, in particular:

- gender – higher incidence in boys than girls
- age – more common in 11–15-year-olds than 5–10-year-olds.

A majority fell under the categories of emotional, conduct or hyperkinetic disorders. A sample of children from this survey was followed up over the subsequent 3-year period to investigate the persistence of the disorders (Parry-Langdon 2007):

- Children who experience three or more stressful life events, such as bereavement, divorce or serious illness are three times more likely to develop a mental disorder.
- 3% of those who did not have an emotional or behavioural disorder in 2004 had developed one by 2007. Mental health of the mother was a significant factor in the child's prognosis.
- One-third who were diagnosed in 2004 still had them in 2007 and family, household and social circumstances were also playing a significant role.
- 43% who maintained they still were experiencing problems had significant difficulties showed co-relations in parent's educational attainment and occupation and the number of siblings in the family.

There are some children and young people who are significantly more likely to experience mental health problems in comparison with the general population. Nearly 50% of children in local authority care have a clinically diagnosable mental health disorder compared to 10% of those who live in private homes (Meltzer et al 2003). Children with disabilities are twice as likely to develop psychological problems as those without. Teenage mothers are three times more likely to suffer postnatal depression and mental health problems in the first 3 years of their child's life (Ermisch 2003).

All of these findings form the basis for recommendations to drive cultural change that promotes awareness and 'ownership' of mental health and psychological well-being therefore influencing a more responsive service for all children, young people and families.

Interventions in child and adolescent mental health disorders

Wider interventions

Early intervention in adolescent mental health problems is essential to try and stop the deterioration of mental health, alleviate distress, and minimise the impact of mental health disorders on education and social development (BMA 2003). Such interventions might include:

- education about mental health problems
- first-line services to promote emotional well-being
- social skills training
- antibullying policies.

Child and adolescent mental health services

The Child and Adolescent Mental Health Service (CAMHS) offers four levels, or tiers, of interventions. Tier 1 represents early and preventative interventions through to tier 4, which represents tertiary services.

Tier 1

This primary level includes interventions by GPs, health visitors, school nurses, social services, voluntary agencies, teachers, juvenile justice workers and residential social workers. Non-specialists should:

- identify mental health problems early in their development

- offer general advice and in certain cases treatment of less severe problems
- pursue opportunities for promoting mental health.

Tier 2

Clinical child psychologists, paediatricians (especially community educational psychologists), child psychiatrists, community child psychiatric nurses/nurse specialists should be able to offer:

- training and consultation to other professionals
- consultation for professionals and families
- outreach to families and children requiring more specialist help but are unwilling to use specialist services
- assessment, which may trigger treatment in another tier.

Tier 3

A specialist service for more complex, severe and persistent disorders. It usually comprises a multidisciplinary team or service including child and adolescent psychiatrists, social workers, clinical psychologists, community psychiatric nurses, child psychotherapists, occupational therapists, art, music and drama therapists. The service offers:

- assessment and treatment of child and adolescent mental health disorders
- assessment for referrals to tier 4
- contributions to consultation and training at tiers 1 and 2
- participation in research and development projects.

Tier 4

Access to infrequently used but essential tertiary level services such as day units, highly specialised community teams and inpatients units for older children and adolescents who are severely mentally ill and at suicide risk. Providing:

- adolescent inpatient units
- secure forensic adolescent units
- eating disorder units
- specialist teams for sexual abuse
- specialist teams for neuropsychiatric problems (Department for Health and Department for Education and Employment 1995).

Although there are some challenges to the tiered system and recent moves toward a system of universal, targeted and specialised care systems, the tiered model remains embedded in the healthcare culture. Whether it is to be continued or reformed the CAMHS Review (2008) recommends that the kernal principal of CAMHS healthcare delivery are for services to have equity of access and the capacity to respond to the mental health needs of children more efficiently.

The need for intervention

- The prevalence of disorders is high: 10.4% of children, aged 5–15 years old, in England, Scotland and Wales, have been found to have a diagnosis of mental disorder based not just on symptoms but on evidence of distress or interference with personal function (Meltzer et al 2000).
- A significant rise in the prevalence of psychosocial disorders – depression, eating disorders, substance misuse, suicide and suicidal behaviour, crime and conduct disorders – in young people aged between about 12 and 26 years has been documented in developed Western countries, including Britain, since the end of the Second World War (Rutter & Smith 1995).
- Only a relatively small proportion of children with significant mental health problems and disorders find their way to specialist mental health services. This was found to be around 20% in the UK survey quoted above (Meltzer et al 2003). It is estimated that as many as 60–70% of children and adolescents who experience clinically significant difficulties have not had appropriate interventions at a sufficiently early age.

What works: primary prevention

- The earlier in the child's life the prevention commences, the more likely it is to be effective.
- Prevention needs to be disorder, context and objective specific. Focused, highly structured, proactive programmes targeting risk factors rather than problem behaviours are more efficacious than generic unstructured ones, such as the provision of counselling or group discussion.
- There is good evidence that effective programmes have the following features in common:
  - Comprehensiveness: successful programmes include multiple components because no single programme component can prevent multiple high-risk behaviour.
  - System orientation: interventions should be aimed at changing institutional environments as well as individuals.
  - Relatively high intensity and long duration: successful programmes are rarely brief. Short-term programmes have, at best, time-limited benefits, especially with at-risk groups. Multi-year programmes tend to have an impact on more risk factors and have more lasting effects.
  - Structured curriculum: there is no clear indication as to the 'ideal curriculum' for preventive interventions, but proactive interventions should be directed at risk and protective factors rather than problem behaviours. In this way, multiple adverse outcomes may be addressed within a single programme.
  - Early commencement: this has been shown to be essential, and intervention during pregnancy brings additional benefits.

- Specific to particular risk factors: it is unrealistic to hope that a generic preventive intervention will be able to reduce the risk for all psychological disorders. Prevention needs to be disorder, context and objective specific.
- Specific training: there is less consistency in the literature on the qualifications required to carry out preventive work. Most studies in the UK use health visitors who have a statutory obligation to visit young children and their carers.
- Attention to maintaining attendance: those families most in need of early prevention programmes are likely to need high levels of support to engage in an intervention, and continued assistance to maintain attendance. In experimental programmes, they are the most likely to drop out.

WWW

For a more detailed exploration see 'What works in promoting children's mental health: the evidence and the implications for Sure Start programmes' at:

- http://www.surestart.gov.uk.doc/0-34D33E.pdf

Promoting emotional well-being

It has been suggested that everyone in contact with young people should take the symptoms of emotional distress, behavioural difficulties and hyperactivity seriously, because they impair function and development and are unlikely to be transient. It was identified earlier that a significant number of professionals find working with adolescents difficult (BMA 2003). However, a key point of this chapter is that nurses can make a difference. In general, caring and protective relationships are potent protective factors against adverse outcomes: 'to hug is to buffer'. Connections with prosocial adults or mentors can be an important protective factor for young people at risk (Department of Human Services Victorian Government 2002). It is imperative to the promotion of child and adolescent health that nurses develop the skills that will enable them to successfully engage with the young person and ensure a nursing interaction that is rewarding both for the young person and the nurse.

Nurses often think they have not got the skills to work with young people with mental health problems or indeed any adolescents. There is sometimes confusion about what the task is. Clearly it is not therapy or counselling – that is for skilled therapists. However, there is a duty to promote health (physical and mental) by enhancing protective factors and intervening to reduce health risk behaviours. The therapeutic relationship the nurse enacts with the young person is the key intervention strategy.

What do young people want?

When asked what they want, each time the feedback is similar: young people want more say and more prominent involvement in the main action (Bennett & Tonkin 2003). Young people have identified barriers to their effective use of services (RCPCH 2003):

- Lack of information
- Management of confidential issues
- Lack of expertise and continuity of care
- Failure to respect the validity of the young person's views
- Being cared for alongside younger children or with a population they regard as elderly
- Particular issues of access to services, disability, poverty, ethnicity, being looked after (in care) and sexual orientation.

The Healthcare Commission's first national survey of the young patient's experience was encouraging in that over 90% of respondents rated their care from excellent to good (Healthcare Commission 2004). Communication with staff was highly rated. The main concern was that young people wanted to be more involved in the decisions about their care. There was also a feeling that explanations about procedures, risks and benefits could be improved, and this supports previous work.

A consistent concern of young people is that they are not really listened to or taken seriously. There is a need for respect, a word that has strong currency with young people – particularly the idea of being disrespectful. Respect is related to the young person feeling empowered in the relationship, being listened to and what they say being acted upon if appropriate (Ahmad et al 2003).

Implications for practice

As a starting point, we must be able to work with the young person within the context of his or her developmental stage, i.e. in terms of their transition and what matters most to that individual right now: assessing the issues and the relationships that are in focus currently. A second important consideration might be the beliefs we bring to this relationship. What are our thoughts and feelings about adolescents generally and this young person in particular? When we are thinking about the young person we need to place him or her within the context of family and peers. Lastly, there is a need for an understanding of the nature of their illness and its unique interaction with their personhood.

Young people have identified certain key characteristics in adults who are approachable. The approachable adult (Lightfoot & Sloper 2002):

- is welcoming, and so makes the young person feel comfortable
- is interested in the young patient as a person, not just in the illness, and so is someone a young person can have an 'ordinary chat' with
- explains things in a straightforward way
- can help the young person express his or her opinions
- will not patronise or judge the young person, but will take him or her seriously
- will take forward issues raised, with the relevant staff
- will mediate where there is conflict between patients and staff.

Young people can define their sense of well-being in terms of a continuum where feeling good and getting stressed are polarities of experience. In the report 'Listening to children and young people' (Ahmad et al 2003), young people identified what made them feel good. Significant factors contributing to feelings of emotional well-being included: having people to talk to, personal achievement, being praised and generally feeling positive about oneself. Relationships with family or peers could contribute either positively or negatively to the sense of well-being.

Recent research into the child and adolescent mental health services ('The Good Childhood Inquiry'; Children's Society 2008) indicated that service users had the following expectations of staff who came in contact with them:

- A clear understanding of child development and mental health.
- An ability to actively promote mental health and psychological well-being.
- The use of language and communication that young people and their families understand.
- An ability to identify the mental health needs of young people early and direct them towards appropriate support services.

Some of the identified barriers to effective intervention included:

- the use of over complicated terminology and unclear interpretations
- the presence of stigma around mental health problems and those seeking services
- there was evidence of mismatched expectations between young people and families and service providers.

Interpersonal skills in the helping relationship with young people

There is a powerful case for the provision of specialist units (Viner & Keane 1998) and/or specialist nurses (Needam 2000). Children's nurses often feel they do not have the skills to work with adolescents in general (Norwich Union 2001), let alone those with additional emotional or mental health problems. Some would go further and suggest that working with adolescents should be supported by a nurse specialist role in adolescent mental health. In 'Bridging the gap' (RCPCH 2003) the RCPCH calls for additional training in adolescent health. The difficulty in this approach is that for each new problem or contemporary issue there are often the twin calls for more resources and more training. Although not arguing against specialist support or additional training, it could be suggested that there is a danger of deskilling the existing nurses. It could be suggested that it would be better to think of key, core transferable skills, first, before considering the need of specialist skills.

If the description of the approachable adult outlined above is linked to what young people say they need to feel good, it could be argued that specialist skills are not required for most interactions. However, the professional nurse should have skills that go beyond lay care both in terms of the quality of their interactions and in terms of intentionality. Intentionality refers to the conscious and deliberate use of interpersonal skills to enhance the therapeutic nature of the interaction (Heron 2001).

Furthermore, children's nurses are already well acquainted with developmental stages so extending this concept into adolescence should not mean further extensive training. Whereas it is totally appropriate for children's nurses to be supported by adolescent health/mental health specialists, it is suggested that children's nurses can develop a therapeutic style that does allow meaningful engagement but that is not specialist or a specific therapy.

The therapeutic style of the nurse

Nurses need to find a way of interacting that is more than 'having a chat' or the collecting of information for assessment but does not go as far as 'doing therapy'. Cooper & Glasper (2001 p 35) described such a process as a 'therapeutic encounter', describing it as:

> A dynamic and sensitive interaction between what is known (professional knowledge) and what is 'yet to be known' (the young person's story).

Two key elements are identified:

1. The nurse's ability to have an internal ongoing reflective conversation (reflection in action).
2. The interaction is influenced by the belief systems of the nurse and the 'tribal stories' present in their working environment.

The reflective conversation will be monitoring the potential impact of the nurse's personal beliefs and the collective 'tribal stories' on the relationship they are forming with the young person. Cooper & Glasper (2001) give this example of extracts from tribal stories related to young people who self-harm:

> Working with young people who self-harm often feels like it is a waste of time.
>
> Our skills could be better used looking after someone who has a 'real illness'.
>
> We are very busy here; there is not the time to give these people what they need.
>
> They should be looked after somewhere else; this is not the place for them.
>
> They are always manipulative; they tell lies.
>
> We came into nursing to look after people with real illnesses, not these people.
>
> Anyway, even if we had the time what could we say? If they are going to do it they will do it anyway!
>
> Even if you do speak with her she won't answer, bet she will be back!

An example of a reflective 'self-conversation' when confronted by a young person who is rejecting care, swearing and being abusive might be:

> *Initial thoughts*: I find adolescents difficult when they are like this. They are so self-centred. I am having a hard shift. I don't need this. What about the other children and parents? They don't deserve this either.
>
> *Initial formulation*: This young person needs to be told what the limits are.

This preliminary assessment is likely to be reinforced by the tribal story (collective staff belief) that this young person is disruptive and either needs 'sorting out' or shouldn't be there in the first place. There is a tendency to see adolescents as being disruptive in an environment aimed at younger children (Norwich Union 2001). These collective beliefs might reflect the difficulty nurses have in finding the appropriate way to relate to these young people. Further reinforcement for this formulation might come from other parents and children's disapproval of the young person's behaviour. Another thing that might support this initial position is that, as a principle, it is good to set boundaries. The issue here, however, is the timing of such an intervention and whether it will inflame or calm the situation. The nurse needs to hold back the response and ask:

> *Reflective question*: What else should I be paying attention to in this situation?

The first internal conversation is focused primarily on the nurse. There is a need to re-focus on the young person and to try and assess what is motivating their behaviour by exploring the following issues:

- What is the young person's underlying emotional state?
- What does he or she need?
- Is he or she trying to assert his- or herself?
- Is he or she feeling vulnerable and dependent, not grown up?
- Is he or she fearful for the future?
- How is the young person viewing me, my approach, my non-verbal communication?

This should lead to a reformulation:

> *Reformulation* – new hypothesis: This young person is scared. He/she is going for surgery tomorrow and wants help but is fearful about appearing childlike. He/she is probably angry about being ill, being with little children, and is not sure if we can be trusted. This uncertainty might be influenced by his/her previous attachment history and how reliable adults have been in the past. Has he/she had a secure base in times of trouble? Other factors influencing his/her behaviour will be his/her level of self-esteem and feelings of self-efficacy.

Specific core communication skills

Key communication skills make it more likely that the nurse will arrive at this more sensitive formulation. One of the key qualities central to all therapeutic communication is the ability to truly 'attend' to the other person. This is referred to as giving 'free attention'; this is the essential precursor of a second important quality 'active listening' (Egan 1990).

Free attention

Heron (1975) describes giving free attention as:

> A subtle and intense activity of being present for the client; it involves gaze, posture, facial expression, maybe touch. It has the qualities of:
>
> – being supportive: out there with the client
>
> – being expectant: waiting for the human being to emerge in ways that are meaningful to him or her and his or her fulfilment
>
> – being non-anxious: the practitioner is free of claims and demands, of any harrying attitude towards the client.
>
> It is always wider and deeper than the qualities of the client's speech, being attuned to his emerging potential as well as his actual behaviour.

Further, Heron (1975) suggests giving free attention is the *sine qua non* of all other sorts of interventions if they are to be truly and effectively human. Egan (1990) identifies the following questions that nurses should ask when 'attending' a client:

- What are my attitudes towards this client?
- How would I rate the quality of my presence to the client?
- To what degree does my non-verbal behaviour indicate a willingness to work with the client?
- What attitudes am I expressing in my non-verbal behaviour?
- What attitudes am I expressing in my verbal behaviour?
- To what degree does my non-verbal behaviour reinforce my internal attitudes?
- In what ways am I distracted from giving my full attention to this client?
- What am I doing to handle these distractions?
- How might I be more effectively present for this person?

One of the tribal stories that have a basis in fact is that of the 'busy nurse'. It is certainly true that there are many demands on a nurse's time. Student nurses will often prefer to be busy because then they feel more 'nurse like'. So 'attending' is a skill that requires some practice and, more significantly, a belief that it is an important thing to do. However, once the skill is acquired it takes up far less time than might be at first imagined.

Active listening

The second core skill is active listening. Egan (1990) suggests that listening carefully to what the client has to say seems:

> ... to be a concept so simple to grasp and so easy to do that one may wonder why it is given such explicit treatment here.

He suggests that it is amazing how often people fail to listen to one another. Certainly, young people often complain that they are not being listened to. Complete active listening involves four things:

1. Observing and reading the client's non-verbal behaviour: posture, facial expressions, movement, tone of voice, etc.
2. Listening to and understanding the client's verbal messages.
3. Listening to the whole person in the context of the social settings of life.
4. Tough-minded listening.

Points 1 and 2 can be understood from our life experience but it might be helpful to enlarge on what Egan means by items 3 and 4.

He refers to a 'people in systems' framework, which is the need to understand each client not just in terms of a specific illness or problem but also with careful attention to his or her life setting, personal values, and biological and sociopsychological characteristics.

Tough-minded listening is about accepting that the client's feelings and visions of themselves, others and the world are real and need to be understood. However, clients' perceptions of themselves and their worlds are sometimes distorted. This does not mean that helpers challenge clients as soon as they hear any kind of distortion. Rather, they note gaps and distortions and challenge them if and when it is appropriate to do so.

Most communication theory will give lists of the factors that prevent effective listening. Egan (1990) identifies obstacles to listening and understanding clients:

- Inadequate listening: distracted, not giving our full attention.
- Evaluative listening: judging the merits of what is being said, comparing it to our own value system.
- Filtered listening: it is impossible to listen to others in an unbiased way, therefore the more self-knowledge we have the more we will recognise our particular filters.
- Knowledge as a filter, especially professional knowledge: we might be listening to validate a theory, maybe a diagnosis, rather than listening to the person.
- Fact-centred rather than person-centred listening: some assessment strategies might put us into a fact-centred approach.

Attending and active listening are the key vehicles for conveying respect to others. Studies show that young people work best with professionals who convey respect for them (Amhad et al 2003).

The importance of listening to the story

Narrative theory is based on the supposition that, in large measure, people are the stories they tell themselves and that are told about them. Narratives can occur at different levels of social functioning. There are social and cultural narratives, interpersonal narratives and intrapersonal narratives. The narrative approach rests on the assumption that narratives are not representations of reflections of identities, lives and problems. Rather, narratives constitute identities, lives and problems. According to this position, the process of therapeutic re-authoring of personal narratives changes lives, problems and identities because personal narratives are constitutive of identity (Carr 1998). In short, this approach suggests we are the stories we tell about ourselves, and are told about us. Further, our stories are embedded in and influenced by a wider social and cultural context.

Such an approach can have a number of implications for nursing practice. Within the context of these ideas we can explore nursing in terms of dominant discourses or stories. A discourse can be described in terms of:

> Historically, socially, and institutionally specific structure of statements, terms, categories and beliefs that are embedded in institutions, social relationships and texts
>
> (Carr 1998).

If the assessment process reflected narrative theory, the approach would first seek the meaning the young person and his or her family gives to the events, rather than a professional system that seeks to impose meaning and explain behaviour.

Reflect on your practice

How much is the nursing task to explain, to inform, to understand, or to help the young person, make sense of things?

Implications for the healthcare professional

Nurses, when faced with the complex lives and backgrounds of young people with emotional disturbances, often feel powerless and think the situation is hopeless. Young people who come in with a history of repeated self-harm often provoke these feelings, accompanied sometimes by a degree of resentment. This may occur because the nurses fail to understand what the therapeutic task is. Clearly a life that has become so complex is hardly going to be turned around by an inpatient stay on a children's ward.

What we do know is that if the nurse can offer a secure, accepting base to the young person that is a positive experience. The other main therapeutic strategy is to listen nonjudgementally and with care and compassion to the young person's unfolding story. This may not seem very active but it could be life enhancing for the young person.

One of the key ideas of narrative theory is the notion of 'repositioning', that is, taking up a different position in relation to the young person and or the problem. When we interact with young people and their families we are heavily influenced by a number of professional, personal and cultural discourses (tribal stories). A discourse is a dominant social and cultural story that can set the context in which an interaction takes place. Such discourse might relate to ideas as nursing, professionalism education, ethics and so on.

This can become problematic because instead of listening with a detached curiosity to what is being said – and, through that process, really hearing the young person's story – his or her story can become 'entombed' with the professional narratives and belief systems. The client is then asked to enact a story told about them rather than his or her own story. To break out of our professional constructions and to reposition, it may be necessary to make an imaginative leap. We need to 'actively listen' in Egan's 1990 terms, repositioning ourselves so that we don't allow our professional knowledge and or personal prejudices to interfere with the flow of the young person's story.

Helping the story unfold

Wilkes & Belsher (1994) offer some key principles for working with adolescents. Although they were considering the work in terms of cognitive therapy, the principles can translate as general principles for working with young people.

Acknowledge the adolescent's narcissism

Narcissism refers to the tendency of adolescent patients to be somewhat egocentric in their interests and goals. This tendency should be seen as developmentally appropriate and can be used to develop the therapeutic relationship. Rather than using statements, questions can often be a good way of demonstrating we are listening. For example 'Would it be right to say you think …?' acknowledges the young person as the best judge of his or her own views and will reinforce the feeling that he or she is being listened to. Unless there is a specific need for them, avoid levelling comments such as 'I have heard that before' or 'You're not the only one that feels like that'. In short, the young person needs to feel at the centre of his or her world, so it makes sense to start the therapeutic process from where he or she actually is. Another way nurses can affirm the adolescent's self-importance is to offer choices every time it is possible to do so. This would be responding to what the evidence suggests adolescents want: more say and their views to be validated (RCPCH 2003).

Collaborative empiricism

This is a central tenet of the cognitive therapy approach but again it can be adapted to general communication with adolescents.

To collaborate is to join with, to cooperate with, and this is a particularly useful position to take up with the young person. The nature of the nurse's specialist knowledge, life experience and health may lead the young person to feel in a one-down, less powerful position. Such a position would leave the young person very sensitive to the feeling of being patronised and more likely to want to assert him- or herself by being conflictual and oppositional, or through passivity and withdrawal. Another way that demonstrates collaboration is to be a voice for the young person, this links with young people's view that an approachable adult will take things forward on their behalf (Lightfoot & Sloper 2000).

Empiricism means giving value to factual data and evidence. To excessively confront or challenge the evidence for the position the young person holds would be very unhelpful and lead to resistance and conflict; it would be an inappropriate form of Egan's tough listening. However a genuine desire to see things from the young person's perspective by checking out the evidence he or she has for taking up his or her present position will demonstrate respect and help the young person's story become more coherent.

Adopt an objective stance

This means having the capacity of being able to be somewhat removed from the intricacies of the young person's situation. This is different from being disinterested or defensively detached from the situation. Objectivity is an important factor in all helping relationships but it is – perhaps – sometimes harder to maintain with young people. Their high levels of emotionality and tendency to see things in black and white terms can draw nurses into a parental role or encourage them to overidentify with the young person and into collusion. One of the ways to maintain a helpful objective stance is not to be drawn into the role of problem solver but rather to act as a facilitator of the young person's problem-solving skills. Collaborative empiricism can help objectivity in that both parties are working together to find the evidence necessary to support whatever is being explored, therefore neither should need an emotional investment in a particular position or belief. These positions or beliefs stand or fall on the basis of the evidence there is to support them.

Include members of the social system

This links with Egan's 1990 reminder that active listening involves listening to the person within the context of his or her social system. Young people are rarely in a position to make important decisions without reference to their parents and other adults in positions of authority. Further, their parents and peer group have a powerful effect on how they see themselves and, as such, can be helpful or unhelpful in terms of the young person's self-esteem.

Chase the affect

To chase the affect is to pay particular attention to expressions and changes in emotional state. This means being sensitive to the verbal and non-verbal cues the young person gives and following them up: 'You seem to be thinking about something that has made you sad'. Such attention to the emotional expression is likely to convey empathy and a more accurate assessment of the overall situation leading to the most therapeutic response.

Socratic questioning

This style of questioning and exploration promotes the young person to think about what he or she is saying and feeling. Again, any challenge to the young person's beliefs and assumptions must be made in a sensitive manner of genuine enquiry. The nurse must be seeking to understand the young person's world and thus help the young person become clearer about things. An example might be: 'When the doctor was talking to your parents about your illness what were you thinking?' or 'What did you feel like doing at that moment?'

Model for the adolescent

This should be a subtle process in the relationship whereby the nurse models aspects of the behaviour that will be helpful. For example, a nurse who wants to help the young person be more tolerant of younger children in the environment will model tolerance towards the young person.

The therapeutic relationship

The therapeutic relationship is grounded in an interpersonal process that occurs between the nurse and the young person. It is a purposeful, goal-directed relationship aimed at advancing the best interests of the client. The way we help (our style) seems to be at least if not more important than how we help (the model or theoretical approach we use). George (1997), in a review of the therapeutic relationship in nursing, identified Peplau as the first nurse theorist who stressed the nurse–patient relationship as a vehicle for achieving health. In the same paper, George (1997) highlights the research from psychotherapy that suggests the therapeutic relationship to be the variable most highly correlated with outcome, and points out that other research has shown the qualities of the therapist style as influential. The qualities of the therapeutic relationship include active listening, trust, respect, genuineness, empathy and responding to client concerns. The requisite capacities for establishing a therapeutic relationship have been identified and defined as self-awareness, self-knowledge, empathy and awareness of boundaries and limits of the professional role (RNAO 2002b).

Requisite capacities for establishing therapeutic relationships

Self-awareness

Self-awareness is the ability to reflect on one's subjective thoughts, feelings and actions. Thus, to be aware of any attitude being conveyed that could impede the therapeutic process and would react to counteract any potential negative effect on the client.

Activity

You might want to consider an example from your own practice when you may have held an attitude or a view that impeded the therapeutic process.

Self-knowledge

With the development of self-knowledge, nurses are able to recognise that their own experience is shaped by nationality, race, culture, health, socioeconomic conditions, gender, education, early childhood experiences and development, as well as relationships, accomplishments, beliefs, issues and concerns. By gaining self-knowledge nurses are able to differentiate between their own experience and values and those of the client. In this way, they are able to appreciate the unique perspective of the client (his or her story), are able to avoid burdening the client with their own issues, and can prevent superimposing their own beliefs and preferred solutions on the client.

Empathy

Empathy is the ability of nurses to enter into the client's relational world, to see and feel the world as the client sees and feels it, and to explore the meaning it has for the client. Empathy involves nurses being able to attend to the subjective experience of the client and validate that their understanding is an accurate reflection of the client's experience.

Awareness of boundaries and limits of the professional role

Boundaries define the limits of the professional role. Nurses are obligated to place the client's needs before their own needs. Through self-awareness, nurses reflect on whether their actions are in the client's best interests. The supervision process should also be used to explore these issues. Sometimes, our own conscious or unconscious wishes make it hard to recognise boundary violations. Indications that boundaries may have been crossed include having special patients, spending extra time with patients, keeping secrets with clients and doing activities with clients that you do not share with colleagues.

WWW

For further exploration of these points visit the RNAO nursing guideline 'Establishing therapeutic relationships':

- http://www.rnao.org

The sequence of events in the relationship

For the sake of analysis, the therapeutic relationship can be seen in terms of a beginning, middle and end, although all three stages may occur in a single encounter. The beginning can be seen as the process of engagement, formulating the working alliance. The middle is the working phase during which how the work is structured is important. The end can be seen as the disengagement phase or letting go.

Models of helping

In her nursing model, Peplau (1952) describes three phases to the therapeutic relationship: orientation, working and resolution. In the beginning, both the nurse and the young person are strangers, each coming to the relationship with their own preconceptions of what to expect. These preconceptions will be based on their previous relationships, experiences, attitudes and beliefs. Peplau (1952) refers to the nurse and the client as being 'strangers' in this preorientation stage.

The orientation stage

In the orientation phase the parameters of the relationship are being established. The expectations of the young person and the nurse need to be explored and clarified. Consistency and listening are considered by clients to be critical at the beginning of a relationship. In this beginning stage, acceptance of the young person is important for the evolving relationship.

Activity

Are some young people and their families easier to accept than others? How can Stockwell's 1972 seminal work 'The unpopular patient' and subsequent research inform our practice on relationship building and patient acceptance?

The working phase

As the name suggests, this is the active phase where problems are identified and interventions decided on. How this is structured will depend on the helping model used, although the nurse should be involved in some key communication strategies. One of the common mistakes when working with distressed young people who are expressing negative or aggressive thoughts is to try to move them on to a more positive frame or want to offer alternative more constructive positions. Although this aim is laudable in itself the motivation is often to make the nurse feel more comfortable. Even if it is client focused, the timing is often wrong. One of the most important strategies, particularly with young people, is to validate the young person's thoughts, feelings and distress. This is not to collude with what in some cases might be a very distorted position (e.g. the anorexic stance) but to accept the young person's perspective and the distress caused by it. This working phase needs to be collaborative, led by the young person and facilitated by the nurse. The nurse needs to be the young person's advocate, ensuring that his or her views are considered in the overall care strategies.

The resolution phase

This final stage of the relationship is involved in completion of the relationship and endings. The process of ending is as important as the beginning but tends not to receive the same attention. It needs to be planned, talked about and should have been considered during the initial care planning: planning how and when the relationship should end. This is particularly important if the young person has a history of troubled or unreliable relationships. The nurse needs to be mindful of the experience of loss transition and change and the reactions of resistance, denial and ambivalence. While acknowledging the present, it may be helpful to be future orientated validating the young person's future plans.

Egan (1990), in 'The skilled helper', outlines one of the best known and most elaborated models of helping. It is important to remember that this model is designed for adults and that it would need to be sensitively adapted to the young person's developmental stage. It is also generally seen as a model of counselling. However, it could be argued that its structure allows it to adapt well to most helping situations. In its simplest form, the model has three stages:

- The present scenario (stage 1 the beginning stage): Helping the client identify, explore and clarify their problem situations and unused opportunities. Egan suggests that people can neither manage problem situations nor develop opportunities unless they identify and understand them.
- The preferred scenario (stage 2): Helping clients develop goals, objectives, or agendas based on an action-oriented understanding of the problem situation. Once clients understand either their problem situations or opportunities for development more clearly they may need help in determining what they would like to do differently. What things would look like if they were better than they are now?
- Getting there (stage 3): Help clients develop action strategies for accomplishing goals, that is, for getting from the present to the preferred scenario. Clients may know what they want to accomplish and where they want to go, but still need help in determining how to get there. This is the transition stage, dealing with ways of moving from the present to the preferred scenario.

Egan envisages the model as a very active process in which the client needs to act on his or her own behalf right from the beginning of the process. This can be a challenge if the young person feels disempowered and not in control of life's circumstances.

Activity

You might consider reading the chapter 'The overview of the model' in Egan (1990) 'The skilled helper' and judge how useful it could be for your nursing practice.

Development theory and therapeutic style

Aspects of developmental theory can be useful in an analysis of those qualities that help make a relationship therapeutic. Bowlby (1988) believed that the observation of normal development was relevant to psychotherapy and that, in getting a picture of what makes a good parent, we are likely to be in a better position to know what makes a good psychotherapist. This idea could be developed and extended to include the therapeutic style of all professionals in terms of their attachments and letting go of client/patient relationships. Adshead (1998) has outlined a number of ways in which professional carers act as attachment figures and utilise other aspects of developmental theory to achieve this.

Attachment theory

Attachment theory holds that humans are essentially social animals who need relationships for survival and whose first relationships with primary care givers have unique characteristics. Attachment behaviour is any form of behaviour that results in a person attaining or maintaining proximity to an attachment figure, usually a caregiver. Such behaviour is most obvious when people are frightened, fatigued or sick and is assuaged by comforting and care giving (Bowlby 1979a).

Previous attachment patterns will manifest themselves in any helping relationship and the helper is likely to be seen in terms of an attachment figure. The principle functions of any attachment figure are to provide a secure base and to modulate anxiety. In a helping situation both functions are achieved through an interactional process to which both the helper and the person helped contribute. Professional carers may be seen as providing the patient with a temporary attachment figure – the helper will provide a secure base. Bowlby argues for the importance of the secure base, stating that:

> Human beings of all ages are happiest and able to deploy their talents to best advantage when they are confident that, standing behind them, there are one or more trusted persons who will come to their aid should difficulties arise. The persons trusted, also known as attachment figure … can be considered as providing his (or her) companion with a secure base from which to operate
>
> (Bowlby 1979b p 103)

In childhood, the secure base is used as 'home' for what Bowlby calls 'a series of excursions', which continue throughout adulthood. As dependency decreases the excursions become longer, so that eventually the dependent individual can exist without anxiety away from the attachment figure. In the same way, within the helping relationship the professional carer provides a secure base from which the patient can make a series of excursions back to a level of optimal functioning.

It has been suggested that attachment figures simulate secure attachment by spending time in active reciprocal interaction (Rutter 1988). It seems that it is the quality of interaction more than the quantity that matters. In the first 3 months, mothers of secure infants respond more promptly when they cry, look, smile at and talk to their babies more, and offer them more affectionate holding. In the therapeutic relationship the degree of responsiveness of the helper is an important factor and mirrors the positive quality of earlier relationships as identified by Rutter.

Adshead (1998) suggested that the attachment figure can modulate anxiety in a number of ways: by acting as an effective container, by providing information and by providing consistent input. She suggests that the affective containment aspect of attachment can be seen as similar to the maternal containment function described by Bion (1962). The primary caregiver helps the baby to develop a capacity to think and tolerate anxiety by using his or her own mental processes to hold and digest the baby's internal projections. In this way, the baby's first cognitive and affective fragments are understood and contained, thus reducing anxiety. It is suggested that caregivers may be internalised cognitively and affectively by the person being helped in the relationship, and thus utilised to contain anxiety. At a conscious level, empathic listening may be experienced as soothing and comforting. Information giving and consistency, which help build trust, offer conscious containment of anxiety.

It is also possible to see the effective therapeutic environment in terms of Winnicott's (1987) phrase 'the holding environment' to denote not just the physical holding of the baby by the mother but the entire psychophysiological system of protection, support, caring and containing that envelops the child, and without which it would not survive physically or emotionally.

Again, with the unfolding of the young person's and family's narrative within the helping relationship there may be similarities with Stern's (1985) cross-modal attunement. In cross-modal attunement the mother follows the baby's babbling. Kicking, bouncing and so on with sounds or movements of her own that match and harmonise with those of the baby. In the use of accurate empathy and the ability to reflect back to the young person the sense that he or she has been seen and understood will create rhythms similar to those described in attunement.

What can the child health nurses do?

Applying theory to practice

PowerPoint

When you have completed this section, compare your responses to the information on the companion PowerPoint presentation.

Scenario

Katie is 15 years old and has cystic fibrosis. She has been readmitted following a chest infection and weight loss. During her stay she seems to be increasingly introspective and sad.

Activity 1

How would you respond and why to Katie's question 'Look at me, who is ever going to want me like this?'

Before referring to the PowerPoint presentation, you might want to at write down a response you might make and give a brief rationale for why you chose that response. It might be helpful to read the sections on core communication skills, listening to and helping the story unfold.

Activity 2

What might be the developmental issues for Katie?

You might want to speculate by interpreting her situation in terms of the developmental models outlined in the chapter.

Activity 3

What are the health risk factors in Katie's situation?

It might be helpful to look again at the section on adolescent health and apply this to Katie's situation.

Activity 4

How might Katie's sense of agency be influenced by ill health?

It might be helpful to link this to issues of self-esteem and the developmental tasks.

Activity 5

What is the likely interplay between Katie's illness and her transition through the adolescent developmental tasks?

When you have completed these activities, check your responses with a fuller account of the factors influencing Katie on the PowerPoint presentation.

Scenario

Shona is 13 years old and was admitted to the ward because of an overdose and continuing threats to self-harm. When the nurse first meets her she is taken aback by her physical appearance; Shona really looks as if she could be 18. This visual information comes on top of the narrative being told about her. She is sexually active, precocious and seductive in her manner. She declares in a dramatic way that she plans to take more tablets next time. Her relationship with her parents is different in that she acts as Mum's interpreter.

Activity 1

Reflect why at 13 you did not find yourself in Shona's situation. If you did have a troubled adolescence, identify those factors that allowed you to reach a point where you could successfully apply to train as a nurse.

Activity 2

Outline what this young person most needs from the nurse right now. Describe how it might be delivered and provide a rationale for the care given.

Activity 3

What factors in Shona's early development might have contributed to the situation she now finds herself in?

Activity 4

When listening to Shona's unfolding story, what elements of her story might indicate risk factors in terms of future self-harm?

Activity 5

Outline short- and long-term goals aimed at reducing Shona's health-risk behaviours linking the goals to the evidence base for practice.

Summary

The mental health of children and young people should be a central concern of the children's nurse. It may be helpful to refer to the key points below.

Key points

- There is strong and growing evidence for the fundamental inter-relationship between physical, mental and social health. Problems in adolescence in any of these areas indicate the likelihood of long-term adverse health and social consequences.
- It has been suggested that everyone in contact with young people should take the symptoms of emotional distress, behavioural difficulties and hyperactivity seriously, as they impair function and development and are unlikely to be transient.
- An understanding of the adolescent's developmental tasks will allow the nurse to focus care giving in the most effective manner.
- It is imperative to the promotion of child and adolescent health that nurses develop the skills that will enable them to successfully engage with the young person and ensure a nursing interaction that is rewarding both for the young person and the nurse.

References

Adshead, G., 1998. Psychiatric staff as attachment figures: understanding management problems in psychiatric services in the light of attachment theory. British Journal of Psychiatry 172, 64–69.

Ahmad, Y., Dalrymple, J., Daum, M., et al., 2003. Listening to children and young people. Faculty of Health and Social Care, University of the West of England, Bristol.

Bennett, D.L., Tonkin, R.S., 2003. International developments in adolescent health care: a story of advocacy and achievement. Journal of Adolescent Health 33 (4), 240–251.

Beresford, B, Sloper, P., 2003. Chronically ill adolescents experiences of communicating with doctors: A qualatitive study. Journal of Adolescent Health 33, 172-179.

Bion, W., 1962. Learning from experience. Heinemann, London.

Bowlby, J., 1979a. On knowing what you're not supposed to know and feeling what you're not supposed to feel. Canadian Journal of Psychiatry 24:403-408

Bowlby, J., 1979b. The making and breaking of affectional bonds. Routledge, London

Bowlby, J., 1988. A secure base: clinical applications of attachment theory. Routledge, London.

British Medical Association, 2003. Adolescent health. BMA Publishing, London.

Burt, MR., 2002. Reasons to invest in adolescents. Journal of Adolescent Health 31(6)(Suppl 1), 136–152. Online. Available at: http://www.sciencedirect.com

Buston, K., 2002. Adolescents with mental health problems: what do they say about health services? Journal of Adolescence 25, 231–242.

Carr, A., 1998. Michael White's narrative therapy. Contemporary Family Therapy 20 (4), 485–503.

Children's Society 2008 The Good Childhood Inquiry. Online: http://www.childrenssociety.org.uk

Coleman, J.C., 1989. The focal theory of adolescence: a psychological perspective. In: Hurrelmann, K., Engel, U. (Eds.), The social world of adolescence: international perspectives. De Gruyter, Berlin.

Collishaw, S., Maughan, B., Goodman, R., Pickles, A., 2004. Time trends in adolescent mental health. Journal of Child Psychology and Psychiatry 45, 1350–1362.

Cooper, M., Glasper, E., 2001. Deliberate self-harm in children: the nurse's therapeutic style. British Journal of Nursing 10 (1), 34–40.

Dehne, K.L., Riedner, G., 2001. Adolescence: a dynamic concept. Reproductive Health Matters 9 (17), 11–15.

Department for Health and Department for Education and Employment, 1995. A handbook on child and adolescent mental health. HMSO, Manchester.

Department of Health (DoH), 2003. National service framework for children, standards for hospital services. HMSO, London.

Department of Health (DoH), 2004. National service framework for children, young people, and maternity services. HMSO, London.

Department of Health (DoH), 2008. Child health promotion programme: pregnancy and the first five years of life. DoH, London.

Department of Health (DoH), 2008. Children and young people in mind: the final report of the CAMHS Review. http://www.dcsf.gov.uk/CAMHSreview/downloads/CAMHSReview-Bookmark.pdf

Department of Human Services Victorian Government, 2002. Evidence-based health promotion: resources for planning, no. 2: adolescent health. Online. Available at: http://www.dhs.vic.gov.au/phd/0003097

Egan, G., 1990. The skilled helper: a systematic approach to effective helping. Brookes/Cole, California.

Erikson, E.H., 1963. Childhood and society, 2nd edn. Norton, New York.

Ermisch, J., 2003. Does a 'teen-birth' have longer-term impacts on the mother? Suggestive evidence from the British Household Panel Survey. Institute for Social and Economic Research, Colchester.

George, L., 1997. The psychological characteristics of patients suffering from anorexia nervosa and the nurses role in creating a therapeutic relationship. Journal of Advanced Nursing 26, 899–908.

Goodman, R., Scott, S., 1997. Child psychiatry. Blackwell Science, Oxford.

Goossens, L., Marcoen, A., 1999. Relationships during adolescence: constructive vs. negative themes and relational dissatisfaction. Journal of Adolescence 22, 65–79.

Hay, I., Ashman, A.F., 2003. The development of adolescents' emotional stability and general self-concept: the interplay of parent, peers, and gender. International Journal of Disability, Development and Education 50 (1), 77–91.

Healthcare Commission 2004 Patient survey report. Online. Available at: http://www.healthcarecommission.org.uk/assetRoot/04/00/81/84/04008184.pdf

Heron, J., 1975. Six-category intervention analysis. Human Potential Research Project. University of Surrey/British Postgraduate Medical Federation, University of London, p 16-18.

Heron, J., 2001. Helping the client: a creative practical guide, 5th edn. Sage Publications, London.

Jacobs, M., 1998. The presenting past: the core of psychodynamic counselling and therapy. Open University Press, Buckingham.

Kroger, J., 1989. Identity in adolescence: the balance between self and other. Routledge, London.

La Voie, J.C., 1994. Identity in adolescence: issues of theory, structure and transition. Journal of Adolescence 17, 17–28.

Lightfoot, J., Sloper, A., 2002. Having a say in health: guidelines for involving young patients in health services development. SPRU, University of York, p 9. Online. Available at: http://www.york.ac.uk/inst/spru

Meltzer, H., Gatward, R., Corbin, T., et al., 2003. Persistence, onset, risk factors and outcomes of childhood mental health disorders. Report based on the analysis of a three-year follow-up survey of the 1999 national survey of the mental health of children and adolescents in Great Britain commissioned by the Department of Health, the Department for Education and Skills and the Scottish Executive Health Department. The Stationery Office, London.

Meltzer, H., Gatward, R., Goodman, R., Ford, T., 2000. Mental health of children and adolescents in Great Britain. A survey carried out in 1999 by the Social Survey Division of ONS. The Stationery Office, London.

Meltzer, H., Gatward, R., Corbin, T., et al., 2003. The mental health of young people looked after by local authorities in England. The Stationery Office, London.

Mental Health Foundation 1999 Bright futures: promoting children and young people's mental health. Mental Health Foundation Publications, London. Online. Available at: http://www.mentalhealth.org

Needham, J., 2000. The nurse specialist role in adolescent health. Paediatric Nursing 12 (8), 11–15.

NHS Health Advisory Service, 1995. Together we stand: the commissioning, role and management of child and adolescent mental health services. HMSO, London.

Norwich Union 2001 The views of adolescents and nurses on the provision of health care in hospitals. Online. Available at: http://www.norwichunion.co.uk/health/literature/gen662_06_02_teenage%20_health.pdf

Parry-Langdon, N. (Ed.), 2008. Three years on: survey of the development and emotional well-being of children and young people. ONS, Cardiff.

Peplau, H.E., 1952. Interpersonal relations in nursing. Putnam, New York.

Registered Nurses Association of Ontario 2002a Enhancing healthy adolescent development: nursing best practice guideline. RNAO, Toronto. Online. Available at: http://www.rnao.org

Registered Nurses Association of Ontario 2002b Establishing therapeutic relationships. RNAO, Toronto. Online. Available at: http://www.rnao.org

Royal College of Paediatrics and Child Health, 2003. Bridging the gaps: health care for adolescents. Council Report CR114. Online. Available at: http://www.rcpch.ac.uk

Rutter, M., 1988. Attachment and the development of social relationships. In: Rutter, M. (Ed.), Scientific foundations of developmental psychiatry. American Psychiatric Press, Washington, DC, pp. 267–279.

Rutter, M., Graham, P., 1968. The reliability and validity of the psychiatric assessment of the child. British Journal of Psychiatry 114, 563–579.

Rutter, M., Smith, D.J. (Eds.), 1995. Psychosocial disorders in young people: time trends and their causes. John Wiley for Academia Europaea, Chichester.

Shooter, M., 2005. Children and adolescents who have chronic physical illness. In: Williams, R., Kerfoot, M. (Eds.), Child and adolescent mental health services: strategy, planning, delivery, and evaluation. Oxford University Press, Oxford.

Stern, D., 1985. The interpersonal world of the infant: a view from psychoanalysis and developmental psychology. Basic Books, New York.

Stockwell, F., 1972. The unpopular patient. Royal College of Nursing, London.

Viner, R., Keane, M., 1998. Youth matters: best practice for the care or young people in hospital. Caring for Children in the Health Services, London.

Wilkes, T.C.R., Belsher, G., 1994. Ten key principles of adolescent cognitive therapy. In: Wilkes, T.C.R., Belsher, G., Rush, J., Frank, E. (Eds.), Cognitive therapy for depressed adolescents. Guilford Press, London.

Winnicott, D.W., 1987. Home is where we start from; essays by a psychoanalyst. Pelican Books, London.

World Health Organization, 1995. Adolescent health and development: the key to the future. WHO Global Commission on Women's Health, Geneva.

Section 4

Caring for children with special needs

Chronic illness and the family

44

Barbara Elliott Peter Callery Julie Mould

ABSTRACT

This chapter focuses on the issues arising from childhood chronic illness for children's families. Specific concerns for children suffering from particular diseases have been covered in previous chapters so will not be addressed here. Rather, the general areas of health-related quality of life for children and parents, issues of self-management and the role of nurses working with families with a child with a chronic illness will be considered.

LEARNING OUTCOMES

- Define chronic illness and related concepts.
- Appreciate the range of chronic illnesses affecting children, recognising common issues and concerns.
- Be aware of the concept of health-related quality of life and its application in childhood chronic illness.
- Discuss the concept of self-management and its application in childhood chronic illness.
- Consider children's involvement in self-management.
- Consider the involvement of parents and other lay carers in self-management.
- Comprehend the range of nursing interventions employed in supporting children with chronic illness and their families.

Definitions of chronic illness

There are a number of different definitions of chronic illness but all recognise the protracted nature of the disease and the consequences for the individual's life. For example, chronic illness has been defined as: a condition that is long term and incurable or involves limitations in daily living requiring special assistance or adaptation in function (Perrin 1985). Eiser (1990) defines chronic diseases as those that affect children for extended periods of time, often for life, and which can be managed in terms of symptom control but not cured.

Children may be born with a chronic condition, such as cystic fibrosis, or develop one during childhood, such as asthma or diabetes. Every chronic condition that affects children has the potential to restrict their lives, and therefore the lives of members of their family, and make children feel different from their peers.

Key features of chronic illness

- The symptoms interfere with many normal activities and routines.
- Medical treatment is restricted in its effectiveness.
- Treatment itself contributes to the disruption of daily living (Vessey 1999).

As with other areas of childhood illness, the sick child is no longer viewed in isolation but as an integral part of a family. Family-centred care is nowhere more important than in childhood chronic illness, when the family has to live with their child's illness and its repercussions for prolonged periods of time, if not the child's whole life. Enabling families to manage children's conditions on a day-to-day basis is an important goal of health care. In some chronic illnesses children may have a recognised disability which they and their families have to manage in order to live their lives to their full potential. 'Aiming High for Disabled Children' (DCSF, DoH 2008) is the government's transformation programme for disabled children's services in England and has the vision that all families with disabled children will have the support they need to live ordinary family lives as a matter of course.

Many studies of the effects of chronic illness on children and their families have focused on specific diseases such as cystic fibrosis, diabetes, epilepsy and asthma. However, classifying patients according to diagnostic labels is perhaps not appropriate when examining the wider issues of the effects of chronic illness on children and families. It may be argued

DOI: 10.1016/B978-0-7020-3183-0.10044-X

that the emotional demands of any chronic disease are more important predictors of adjustment than the specific demands of any particular disease, and there may be more variability in psychological, social and educational measures within diagnostic groupings than between them (Stein & Jessop 1989). This chapter will therefore consider the general issues associated with childhood chronic illness using particular diseases to illustrate points raised.

Activity

Make a list of the different chronic diseases in childhood that you have encountered in the last 12 months. Consider the particular needs and problems of the children and their families. Discuss in your study group those problems/needs common to all or many of the children and their families and those which were disease specific.

Now reflect on the merits of grouping patients with the same diagnosis as a useful way of predicting their needs compared with the non-categorical approach of considering general issues of chronic illness.

Chronic illness is by definition persistent: children and their families must live with the illness for an extended period of time, possibly for the child's life. We have chosen not to use the term 'chronic disease' because this implies a medical perspective where the principal concerns are with the signs and symptoms of the condition and how these might be cured or at least treated. Instead, we use the term 'chronic illness' to focus attention on the experience of living with the symptoms and problems of the condition. Some problems can arise from the treatment, for example parents' concerns about the potential long-term effects of steroid use in asthma management. The outcome of treatments and other interventions, such as education about management, may not be cure but increased independence or better control of the illness.

Incidence and prevalence

Information about the incidence, number of new cases of disease per unit of population in a defined period, and prevalence, number of new and continuing cases of disease, is limited. Statistics are more readily available for some chronic illnesses than others so overall rates are generally estimates. It can also be difficult to decide which chronic conditions to include in overall rates – for example should acne and otitis media be included? It is advisable to access information about the incidence and prevalence of specific chronic illnesses, for example it is suggested that there are currently 1.1 million children being treated for asthma in the UK (Asthma UK 2009) and 5–15% of children under 7 years suffer from atopic eczema (National Eczema Society 2009). There has been an increase in the incidence of certain diseases such as asthma and diabetes and an increase in the life expectancy of children with other chronic illnesses such as cystic fibrosis and cancer. Approximately one-fifth of children with chronic illness have more than one condition (Newachek & Stoddard 1994).

Completely new categories of chronic conditions are emerging as technology develops and childhood mortality rates improve. Preterm babies are surviving at earlier gestation and increasingly low birth weights. Organ transplants are enabling children to survive longer with previously fatal diseases and there are increasing numbers of ventilator-dependent children cared for both in hospitals and the community. Understanding of the hereditary influences on the incidence of chronic conditions is constantly developing and nurses need a sound knowledge of genetics in order to deliver excellent care and advice to families and to participate in the ethical debates about treatment (Valentine & Hazell 2007).

There is obviously a wide range in the severity of chronic illness both within disease categories and between them. Some diseases, such as atopic eczema, may be common but not always perceived as an illness. This can bring further problems to children and their families as their experiences and needs may not be understood and even trivialised. A study of the prevalence of atopic symptoms in the UK found that almost half of the 12–14-year-olds surveyed reported one or more of the symptoms, itchy flexural rash, rhinoconjunctivitis or wheeze – and 4% reported all three (Austin et al 1999).

Children with chronic illness may not only have the symptoms of the disease and consequences of treatment to contend with but they also have increased rates of mental health problems and psychological difficulties (Vessey 1999). It has been suggested that an appropriate assessment tool to detect such problems should be added to routine paediatric outpatient assessments to aid detection and appropriate referral to child mental health services (Glazebrook et al 2003). The importance of recognising and effectively managing psychological well-being is also supported by evidence that adults with persistent chronic illness from childhood which limit their daily life suffer more depression and lower self-esteem than those with non-limiting conditions or healthy controls (Huurre & Aro 2002).

Seminar discussion topic

Watch the PowerPoint presentation, including the short video clip, on living with atopic eczema. Consider the physical, psychological and social implications of this disease for children and their families.

There is now a considerable amount of information about specific chronic diseases available on the internet. Some of this information is aimed at health professionals and other information is more suitable for parents and children. Certain internet sources are not particularly relevant to families and health professionals in the UK but others are becoming an important resource. Useful evaluations of the use of the internet are provided by Pandolfini et al (2000) and Pandolfini & Bonati (2002). The following activities will help you to assess the usefulness of some specific websites.

www

Access the websites for specific childhood diseases such as:

- http://www.cftrust.org.uk
- http://www.eczema.org.uk
- http://www.diabetes.org.uk
- http://jdrf.org.uk
- http://www.asthma.org.uk
- http://www.arthritiscare.org.uk
- http://www.childrenfirst.nhs.uk/index.php

Compare the information found with that available on a generic site such as:

- http://www.kidshealth.org

Activity

Using a popular search engine such as Google, access internet sites related to five common childhood chronic diseases. Assess how useful they are for you as a nurse, parents and children. Do they have specific areas for children? How could they be improved?

Concept of health-related quality of life in childhood chronic illness

To assess the effectiveness of interventions by nurses and other healthcare workers, it is necessary to use outcomes that are consistent with the focus on the experience of childhood chronic illness. Quality of life (QoL) is therefore an important concept in chronic illness. Measures of quality of life can either be generic or specific to particular diseases. The advantages of generic measurement would be that comparison could be made with healthy children. However, this is not practical with the instruments currently available: generic measures cannot detect differences that arise from the effects of particular illnesses, for example the effect of eczema on appearance. Therefore QoL is usually measured in children with disease-specific instruments (Eiser 1997). For this reason we use the term 'health-related quality of life' (HRQoL) to recognise that the topics addressed relate to health-related aspects of quality of life.

A valid assessment of HRQoL could enable assessment of the impact of an illness and the effectiveness of treatments and other interventions, including education about management, often provided by nurses. Consideration of QoL recognises children's own ratings of their health and well-being and avoids over-reliance on physiological assessments, giving children a voice in their care and improving communication between children and practitioners (Eiser 2007).

Assessment of HRQoL is particularly challenging in children. The development of instruments must take account of the 'response burden', that is, the 'extent to which issues of scale length or type of response need to be adapted for children's language and cognitive skills' (Eiser & Morse 2001). Children must be able to read and understand questionnaires used to assess quality of life. It may be more appropriate to develop instruments that appeal to children's interests and do not demand high reading ages, for example computer games (Eiser et al 2000). It is also important to recognise that the meaning of QoL can be quite different for children and adults. Young children's QoL is about having very shiny hair, lots of friends or running like a sports star rather than achievement of basic functional tasks (Eiser 1997). When adults rate children's QoL their ratings are based on different frameworks to the children's ratings, and it might even be that very close parent–child agreement is indicative of poorer QoL because childhood is about gaining autonomy and independence from parental views (Eiser 1997). As children develop 'any measure needs to have an in-built sensitivity to accommodate the normative changes that would be expected to occur during childhood' (Eiser 1997). It may therefore be necessary to ask different questions of children at different times in their lives and these questions may differ from those asked of parents when assessing QoL. There are challenges for researchers to develop new approaches to QoL assessment if they are to be child-centred.

Evidence-based practice

There is clear evidence that children's self-assessments differ from those of their parents:

In children younger than 11, children's global rating of change in symptoms correlated strongly with changes in quality of life (QoL) but not with measures of airway calibre or asthma control, while parents' global ratings did not correlate with children's QoL but showed moderate correlations with airway calibre and asthma control (0.50). In children over the age of 11, correlations with all clinical variables were higher for their own than their parents' global ratings (Guyatt et al 1997).

Therefore children's own views about their symptoms and their QoL should be sought.

HRQoL measures can be used in routine practice to identify specific issues of concern to children and to parents (Mussafi et al 2007). Health professionals need the training and facilities to analyse and interpret responses (Eiser & Jenney 2007). Practitioners should be careful to consider the way in which a measure has been designed and tested when deciding how to assess QoL in children with chronic illness. Some questions that can help to decide on the appropriateness of a measure are:

- how have children's concerns been identified and integrated into the measure?
- is the measure designed to make appropriate demands on children, for example, reading age and cognitive ability?

Health-related quality of life for parents

Chronic illness in childhood occurs in a social context in which a supportive relationship between parent and child is essential for successful management. The impact of childhood chronic illness on the lives of parents, the adaptation processes required and their needs have been the focus of a considerable amount of research (e.g. Canam 1993, Elliott & Luker 1996, Fisher 2001, Gibson 1995, Hentinen & Kyngas 1998, Hodgkinson & Lester 2002, Lowes et al 2005, Young et al 2002a,b). There is an acceptance that parents are the main carers of children with chronic illness and considerable effort has been made in trying to understand the impact of this role on their lives and how healthcare professionals can support them in their role and facilitate successful coping. Better understanding of the experience of parenting a chronically sick child is thought to improve the relationship between health professionals and parents and ensure that care provided is appropriate and meaningful. Good relationships between health professionals and parents are considered to be beneficial both for children and parents. For example, a good relationship between doctors and mothers of children with atopic eczema was found to be the strongest predictor of adherence to skin-care treatment (Ohya et al 2001).

The emphasis on the inevitable negative impact of childhood chronic illness and disability has been criticised by some authors. It is not disputed that parenting a child with chronic illness is stressful at times but whether this causes distress in parents is being questioned. The focus of research and nursing literature on the tragedy of childhood illness and disability, parental stress, the burden of care and need for successful coping mechanisms is beginning to shift and the positive contributions to family life of children with disability is beginning to be recognised (Kearney & Griffin 2001).

Treatment of chronic illness may have a positive or negative impact on children's and parents' QoL. Successful management of a disease may be at odds with children's or parents' experience of the illness and it is important that treatment outcome measures include consideration of patient and parent reported outcomes. International instruments to measure parents' experience of childhood chronic illness, and which can be used to determine the acceptability and efficacy of pharmaceutical treatment, have been developed (Whalley et al 2002).

It is essential that any QoL instrument is developed from the perspective of those whose HRQoL it intends to measure. We have already suggested that a child's perspective of HRQoL may be very different from that of their parents. In the majority of cases, the HRQoL instrument is developed from the analysis of qualitative interviews with patients and parents (Henry et al 2003). Analysis of these interviews provides information about the impact of the child's disease on the family and their experience of living with childhood chronic illness. A distinction must be made between instruments that use parents to assess their child's HRQoL and those that focus on assessment of the parents' HRQoL.

Evidence-based practice

Instruments that purport to measure quality of life (QoL) are frequently used in research studies that assess the impact of a disease on a child and/or his or her family. They may also be used to evaluate treatment strategies. It is essential therefore that they are tested for validity and reliability. They must also measure aspects of QoL that are important to those on whom the instrument is being used. Many of the instruments used today have been developed from qualitative interviews and tested on large numbers of patients and carers. Several adult QoL instruments have been adapted for use with children or parents as proxy participants. Comparisons between parent and child ratings of QoL have been made, for example Vance et al (2001).

As well as influencing parents' HRQoL, the impact of chronic illness on families can be enormous. Efforts have been made to develop a scale to measure the impact of chronic illness on parents and families (Stein & Reissman 1980) and applied in specific diseases such as atopic eczema (Su et al 1997). Bonner et al (2006) developed and validated an instrument for measuring parents' experiences of child illness which focuses on four critical domains of parental adjustment: guilt and worry, unresolved sorrow and anger, long-term uncertainty and emotional resources.

Within disease categories, parents' estimate of the severity of disease has been found to be the single strongest predictor of family impact of the disease (Balkrishnan et al 2003). There may be differences in the perception of the impact of childhood illness between parents and paediatricians (Janse et al 2005) and it is important to recognise that it is the assessment of severity by the parents, and not by the professionals, that predicts the impact on the family. Chronic diseases considered as relatively minor by health professionals may in fact have a greater impact on the family than other more serious diseases. For example, Powers et al (2003) found that the QoL of children suffering from migraines as assessed by the children themselves and their parents was similar to that of children with arthritis and cancer. By contrast, assumptions of the negative impact on family life of children with severe disability are being challenged and the need for acceptance of the highly individual response of families must be recognised (Kearney & Griffin 2001). Some of the issues assessed by the measures are considered below.

Emotional responses

The emotional responses of parents to the diagnosis of chronic illness in a child are frequently linked to loss and grief. Parents may experience multiple losses, loss of their healthy child, loss of freedom and lifestyle, loss of confidence and support systems and potential loss of their child's life (Lowes & Lyne 2000). The grief reactions they may suffer have been studied in relation to many specific childhood diseases and are well documented in the nursing literature. For example, feelings of shock, anger, denial, sadness and frustration have been reported in parents of children newly diagnosed with diabetes (Hatton et al 1995) and it is suggested that these reactions are a result of an awareness of the discrepancy between expectation and reality for their child's world (Lowes et al 2005). Time-bound theories of grief have been applied to parents of children with chronic illness, suggesting that they progress through a series of stages culminating in acceptance of their child's condition and resolution of their grief. Such theories have been challenged and an alternative model of 'chronic sorrow' has been suggested as representative of parents' experience of childhood chronic illness. Teel (1991) describes chronic sorrow as a recurring sadness interwoven with periods of neutrality, satisfaction and happiness – suggesting that parents make a functional adaptation to childhood chronic illness but do not accept it. Lowes & Lyne (2000) provide a useful review of the literature on grief reactions to childhood chronic illness.

It must be remembered that diagnosis may also result in feelings of relief and hope, particularly if the parents have been concerned for sometime about their child's health. Parents may also be falsely accused of being in denial when they are trying to remain positive and optimistic about their child's condition. Kearny & Griffin (2001) quote a mother of a child with significant health problems:

> I knew her condition was serious and her prognosis poor but to me she was my firstborn, beautiful child.

When a child has a chronic illness, Larson (1998) describes how the mother has to embrace the paradox between loving the child as he or she is and wanting to erase the disability; between coping with the incurability of the child's illness and looking for solutions; between maintaining hope for the child's future and struggling with negative information and their own fears.

Scenario

David is a third-year child branch student who is caring for a 6-month-old baby girl with cystic fibrosis. She has a chest infection but is otherwise well and her mother is delighted with her weight gain and achievement of normal development. David overhears the mother telling a friend that she doesn't think there is anything wrong with her baby and is considering stopping giving her medication because she is so well.

Consider how David might deal with this situation. How might he ensure that the mother recognises her baby's need for treatment but maintain her positive approach and delight in her child's progress?

Parental health

Parental health and well-being may suffer as a consequence of caring for a child with chronic illness and, although not ill themselves, mothers in particular may suffer many of the consequences of chronic illness (Young et al 2002a). Mothers may experience stress in relation to caring for a chronically sick child and coping with the demands of the illness. Stress may be experienced in relation to decision making, the burden of care and accepting a change in identity (Hodgkinson & Lester 2002). Many research studies throughout the 1970s and 1980s explored the stress experienced by parents (in particular mothers) and the coping strategies they developed when dealing with chronic illness in a child (Faux 1998).

Financial consequences

Parents of children with chronic illness may find it difficult to sustain full-time employment. Time off work to care for their child and attend hospital appointments, as well as the extra cost of childcare for a child with additional needs, may make paid employment impossible. In addition, there are costs involved in bringing up and caring for a child with chronic illness that are extra to those for healthy children. A study of 273 parents who had responsibility for the day-to-day care of a severely disabled child found that it cost at least three times as much to bring up a child with severe disability from birth to 17 as to bring up a child without disability (Dobson & Middleton 1998). Additional costs result from clothing, bedding, laundry, food, equipment, furniture, transport, toys, toiletries and activities.

Scenario

Laura is a 6-year-old girl with atopic eczema. She requires frequent application of ointment to keep her skin hydrated. This makes her clothes greasy and sticky and she requires several changes of clothes each day. She can only wear pure cotton clothes next to her skin as man-made fibres irritate her. Her bedding needs to be changed every morning as it is soiled with skin cells, exudate and ointment.

Laura's condition deteriorates if she eats certain foods. Her mother has to prepare special food for her meals, much of which is wasted if Laura does not like it.

It is thought that house-dust mites contribute to Laura's skin condition so her parents have replaced the carpet in her bedroom with laminate flooring and her curtains with wooden blinds.

The benefits system in the UK recognises the additional costs involved in chronic illness and disability and parents can apply for a range of additional benefits. Some are extra amounts within existing benefits, such as the Disabled Child Premium in Income Support, and others are purely for disabled people such as Disability Living Allowance (DLA). However, for many families there is a considerable gap between their income and what they consider necessary to spend on their child (Dobson & Middleton 1998).

Children do not become eligible for certain benefits until they reach a specific age. For example, free nappies are available for children over 3 years old who are incontinent and children with mobility problems are eligible for the mobility component of DLA once they are 5 years old. Such age restrictions can seem unreasonable to parents and many may not be aware of their child's entitlements. Information about current financial support for families is available from the Department of Work and Pensions at http://www.dwp.gov.uk.

WWW

Access this website for current information about rights, support and benefits for disabled people:

- http://www.direct.gov.uk/en/DisabledPeople/index.htm

Activity

Consider a child with a chronic illness you have nursed recently. List the additional financial costs to the family involved in caring for their child. What help with these additional costs might the family receive?

Social consequences

The role of being a parent of a child with chronic illness may compromise the ability to function adequately in other roles such as friend, professional, spouse or partner and parent of other children. Childhood chronic illness may make parents reluctant to leave the child to pursue social and leisure activities. In addition, the disease may produce additional caring needs and treatment regimens for parents, such as regular injections or physiotherapy, which may reduce the time available to meet their own social needs.

There is evidence that the nature of normal childcare, such as bathing, feeding and entertaining, may be changed when a child has a chronic illness and normally enjoyable tasks may become difficult and onerous. Parents of children with atopic eczema have described the constant struggle to keep their child entertained to distract them from scratching and the difficulties of bathing and nappy changing when skin is excoriated, itchy and sore (Elliott & Luker 1996). There is evidence to suggest that parents can feel particularly stressed in relation to their parenting skills when a child has a chronic illness and may be less efficient in disciplining their affected child (Daud et al 1993).

Restricted social activities may lead parents to perceive that they have less social support (Daud et al 1993). This is a concern as ongoing social support is crucial for the successful adaptation of parents to their child's chronic illness (Whyte 1992). Perceived social support has been found to be a predictor of family coping and a factor that influences the resilience of high-risk groups of families with a child with chronic illness (Tak & McCubbin 2002).

Marital relationships

There is a belief that family dysfunction and marital problems frequently follow the diagnosis of chronic illness in a child. However, there is conflicting empirical evidence in this area and much anecdotal evidence to suggest that caring for a chronically sick child may bring parents closer together. Gender differences between mothers and fathers in how they cope with chronic illness in a child and from whom they receive their support have been reported (Katz 2002) and conflict may arise from these differences.

There are conflicting reports in the literature of the effects of caring for a chronically ill child on marital satisfaction and stability, with some studies showing a negative effect and others finding no differences. Most studies of parents of children with chronic health problems report decreased marital satisfaction compared with parents of healthy children. A recent study by Contact a Family found that, whereas one-quarter of the 2000 parents studied felt that having a disabled child had brought them closer together, nearly half felt that it had caused problems in their relationships and almost 10% believed that it had lead to separation from their spouse or partner (Contact a Family 2004). Childcare responsibilities and decision making are likely to cause conflict and are the most frequently cited stresses of parents of children with chronic illness (Quittner et al 1998). However, a study that compared 94 married parents caring for a child with chronic illness with over 3000 married parents of well children found no differences in perceived marital quality or satisfaction between the two groups (Eddy & Walker 1999). Similarly, Katz & Krulik (1999) found no difference in levels of marital satisfaction between fathers of healthy children and those of children with chronic illness, although the latter group did experience a greater number of stressful life events and lower self-esteem.

Decreased marital satisfaction does not necessarily result in decreased marital stability. It is suggested that marital stability is a product of net outcomes (rewards minus costs), barriers to leaving the relationship and alternative attractions (Eddy & Walker 1999). When parents have a child with chronic illness there may be more strain on the relationship, resulting in fewer rewards and greater costs but the barriers to leaving are increased and opportunities for alternative attractions reduced. All children, whether sick or healthy, constitute important marital capital in that they increase the barriers to leaving a relationship for the majority of parents.

Siblings

The family context in which children with chronic illness live inevitably means that their well siblings are affected by the disease and its management. Within families, the relationship between siblings may be just as important as the parent–child relationship, if not more so. Brothers and sisters spend a considerable amount of time together and children can be very distressed by chronic illness in a sibling. They may supply considerable emotional, social and physical support to the sick child, thus being a source of help to their parents. However, well siblings have their own unique needs and may themselves make additional demands at a time when their parents' attention is focused on the sick child.

There is no question that some chronic illnesses result in well siblings being separated from the sick child and one or both of their parents on a regular basis and sometimes for prolonged periods. Their daily routine is disrupted and they may have fewer opportunities for social activities and interactions with their parents. The sick child frequently becomes the centre of attention and siblings may feel neglected and deprived of attention as their parents try to deal with problems without involving them (Drotar & Crawford 1985). Parents often believe that it is the well siblings who suffer the most through not receiving their fair share of attention.

However, the research literature in this area is contradictory as to the consequences of chronic illness for well siblings (Blubond-Langner 1996, Eiser 1993). There is a great deal of research literature reporting the negative effects of chronic illness on well siblings. A whole range of problems have been reported including somatic and psychosomatic disorders, school problems, increased accidents, behaviour problems including hyperactivity and antisocial behaviour, emotional problems, aggressiveness, withdrawal and poor social adjustment. At the other end of the spectrum are studies that indicate that chronic illness does not have a negative effect on well siblings, indeed there may be positive consequences. Empathy, compassion, coping and communication skills have been reported in well siblings, as well as an increased maturity, appreciation of their own health and increased family cohesion.

Explanations of why having a sibling with chronic illness results in some children experiencing positive outcomes and others negative ones have been sought and it is apparent that factors other than the disease alone are influential. A number of factors have been considered by various researchers and summarised by Blubond-Langner (1996). Factors such as age, birth order, gender, socioeconomic status of the family, parents' marital situation, prior family problems, character of the disease and relationship with the sick child can all influence how a child copes with chronic illness in a sibling. It should be noted that much of the research to date has relied on parental, usually the mother's, reporting of the behaviour and health of their children, which may be influenced by many factors including the parents' own health and adaptation to their child's illness.

It is suggested that negative outcomes in well siblings should not be expected but that there should be an awareness of their unique relationship with the sick child and their individual needs. The adjustment of children to chronic illness in a sibling is best understood within the context of the family. Childhood chronic illness may be viewed as a stressor that, combined with other factors, may result in an increased risk of psychological problems for some siblings of sick children. The factors that mediate the effects of chronic illness on well siblings are poorly understood but it is believed that the quality of family functioning and relationships has both direct and indirect effects on siblings (Drotar & Crawford 1985).

Self-management in chronic illness

Self-management of chronic illness has the potential:

> ...to allow people with chronic diseases to have access to opportunities to develop the confidence, knowledge and skills to manage their conditions better, and thereby gain a greater measure of control and independence to enhance their quality of life
>
> (Department of Health (DoH) 2001)

The more we focus on chronic illness rather than chronic disease, the more essential it is to recognise the expertise of the people living with the condition. However, there are important issues to consider when applying these ideas in childhood chronic illness. The first of these is who is the 'self' involved in self-management? Children cannot be seen in isolation because parents have legal and moral responsibilities for their care and protection. However, parents are proxies: their experience of the illness is different to their children's. Important differences emerge when children and their parents report symptoms or QoL, and the impact of illness can differ between children and parents (Braun-Fahrlander et al 1998, Callery et al 2003, Renzoni et al 1999). To complicate matters further, the 'self' is not limited to one parent and one child. In addition to the adults in their family, children must deal with adult carers in other settings, for example at school. A variety of adults can contribute to the care of children in the absence of their parents, adding further elements to the 'self' involved in self-management.

The range of people involved in self-management will have differing objectives. Parents of children with asthma can judge asthma by its observable effects on their children's behaviour and its impact on parents' own lives, so that they may be most concerned about avoiding acute attacks (Callery et al 2003). They can accept a level of continuing symptoms and restriction of activity as 'tolerable' asthma. Children can be more concerned with the day-to-day effects of asthma and how these make them appear different to their peers (Callery et al 2003, Ireland 1997). Again, this can lead to acceptance of restriction of activity, for example to avoid appearing different by taking inhalers in public. These differences highlight the need to identify the objectives of children and of adult carers in planning self-management of chronic illness.

Guidelines on asthma management stress the importance of individualisation of self-management plans (British Thoracic Society (BTS) & Scottish Intercollegiate Guidelines Network (SIGN) 2008). However, it appears that little attention has been paid to identification of children's objectives, concerns and experiences in self-management plans used in practice. In a survey of 47 UK centres using 30 self-management plans for school-aged children with asthma, only two plans had apparent space for inclusion of individualised objectives and 21 did not identify objectives even implicitly in the title (Milnes & Callery 2003). Only three plans were clearly addressed to the child, the remainder were impersonal (six), addressed to an adult carer through the child (twelve), principally to an adult carer (four), ambiguous (four) or open ended (one). These findings suggest a lack of consensus about the role that children should take in self-management of asthma.

It is important to understand the meaning of chronic illness to both child and parent, or other adult carer, because it influences the ways in which they respond to advice from health carers. Peak flow recording by children aged 5–16 years has been shown to be unreliable with the 'percentage of correct peak flow entries decreased from 56% to <50% from the first to the last study week ($P < 0.04$), mainly as a result of an increase in self-invented peak flow entries' (Kamps et al 2001). One response to such findings is to describe the behaviours as 'non-compliant' and to obtain more control over the process, for example by using electronic peak flow meters that would not record self-invented entries. However, an alternative approach is to seek to understand the perspectives of children and their adult carers to explain their reasons for behaving in this way in order to adapt advice to their needs. The differences between professional and family perspectives are highlighted by the different meanings attached even to apparently straightforward terms such as 'wheeze' by parents and professionals (Cane et al 2000, Young et al 2002b).

Reflect on your practice

Think about a consultation between a child, parent and nurse or doctor that you have observed. How much of the time did each of those involved speak? What was the nature of the talk when each was speaking? Were the child's objectives for treatment discussed? Did the child have opportunities to influence decisions about treatment and/or care?

Self-management education is effective in adults (Gibson et al 1999). A review by Guevara et al (2003) concluded that:

> Educational programmes for the self-management of asthma in children and adolescents improve lung function and feelings of self-control, reduce absenteeism from school, number of days with restricted activity, number of visits to an emergency department, and possibly number of disturbed nights. Educational programmes should be considered a part of the routine care of young people with asthma

The effect of education was most marked in children with severe asthma, when interventions were directed at individuals rather than groups and when interventions were based on peak flow recording. However, none of the studies included in this review assessed QoL and other limitations in the study reports limited the conclusions that could be reached for various ages and other sub-groups of children. Further research is required to identify the best way to provide education for different groups of children. More child-centred approaches to self-management, which incorporate the objectives and perspectives of children as well as their adult carers, might be the most promising way to improve the effectiveness of self-management education.

The nurse's role

Most children with a chronic illness are cared for by their parents at home. The child and family with a chronic illness require an integrated approach between health, social care and education services, in addition to collaborative working with the voluntary and independent sectors, to ensure an holistic approach is taken to meet the child and family's physical, developmental, social and psychological needs (Valentine & Mcnee 2007).

On diagnosis few families realise the extent to which a chronic illness will change their lives (Eiser 1990) and adaptation to living with a chronic illness is a continual process. Valentine & Mcnee (2007) believe children's nurses need an in depth knowledge of the theories of grief, loss, adaptation and change to facilitate and support children and families with chronic illness to adapt and adjust their lives to incorporate the demands of disease management.

Nurses work with children with chronic illness and their families in a variety of roles. Hospital nurses may care for the child and family around the time of diagnosis and during periods of acute exacerbation of their illness. Community children's nurses may support the child and family at home, helping them to incorporate care and treatment into their daily routine and manage the child's illness on a day-to-day basis. Health promotion and assessment of child development may be undertaken by health visitors. Many areas now employ nurses for specific diseases, such as cystic fibrosis and diabetes specialist nurses. These nurses use their specialist knowledge and expertise to support children and their families, and may also act in an advisory role for other nurses and other professionals involved in their care.

PROFESSIONAL CONVERSATION

Julie is a clinical nurse specialist for children with cystic fibrosis

I base my role as the cystic fibrosis Clinical Nurse Specialist (CNS) on four inter-related components:

- clinical practice
- education
- research/audit
- change agent.

Fifty per cent of my time is practice based, when I am able to utilise my skills and knowledge with children and their families in the home, school, outpatient and inpatient settings. I work as an autonomous practitioner and am expected to exhibit high levels of judgement, discretion and decision making in clinical care within my area of specialist practice.

Education is a major part of the role. Various teaching methods, delivered in a timely way and pitched at an appropriate level, are chosen to suit each individual child and family to enable them to gain knowledge and understanding of the disease and to deliver treatment and care in the home. As an educator, I can increase the knowledge and understanding of different health professionals either formally in the classroom or informally by working alongside them.

Through the utilisation of research to develop teaching packages and guidelines, I endeavour to improve the standards of care delivered to the CF children and their families. By auditing against these guidelines I can determine which areas require improving and which areas can be seen as good practice.

As a change agent I see myself in an ideal position to affect change not only directly with CF children and their families and other health professionals but also indirectly with the NHS Trust. Using resources innovatively can benefit the organisation and CF children and their families.

It is important that the CNS is seen as a role model and leader and a visible part of nursing practice. The CNS requires depth and breath of knowledge of their speciality and expertise in nursing care. This is gained through experience, further training and postgraduate qualifications.

If the child's chronic illness results in considerable disability and a number of services are involved to provide complex health care, then it is advisable for a key worker to be identified as a single point of contact for the child and their family. The key worker needs be able to cross boundaries easily between different services in order to fully appreciate the care and treatment provided to the child and their family. Key worker standards for disabled children and their families can be found at http://www.ccnuk.org.uk.

A key worker will provide information and advice, identify and address needs, access and co-ordinate services, provide emotional support and act as an advocate for the child and family (Mukerjee et al 1999, Tait & Dejnega 2001). The DoH (2004 p 28) states that:

> studies of key workers consistently report positive effects on relationships with services, fewer unmet needs and greater family well being.

Key workers are an important aspect of care for children with chronic illness and disabilities requiring complex health care provision and in recent years have received considerable interest in policy and research (Beecham et al 2007, Children's Workforce Development Council 2007, DoH 2004, Greco et al 2004, 2006, National Collaborating Centre for Cancer 2005, Sloper et al 2005).

Whether nurses are acting as key workers or simply involved in the care of a child with chronic illness either in hospital or the community they will be part of a team of health professionals. Multidisciplinary and collaborative team working and sound communication skills are fundamental to good nursing care of children and families.

The following six factors may be helpful when caring for children with chronic illness and their families.

1. Finding out

Prior to caring for a child and family with a chronic illness, it is necessary to have some background knowledge and to be aware of previous medical, nursing, social and psychological issues and interventions. Information can be gained by reading case notes and contacting the health professionals and other support agencies involved in the care of the child and family. Although not definitive, the following list shows the range of information nurses may learn about a child and family prior to even meeting or working with them:

- any problems antenatal, during labour, postnatal
- bonding
- type of disease (e.g. genetic)
- stage of illness and course disease is likely to take
- reaction to diagnosis
- reaction to illness
- operations
- frequency of hospitalisation
- respite care
- acute exacerbations of illness
- remission
- growth and development:
  - height, weight, head circumference, body mass index, nutrition
  - vision, hearing, speech, communication
  - breathing
  - mobility
  - elimination
  - sleep patterns
  - skin
- independence/dependence
- sexuality
- schooling
- family set-up
- support agencies involved
- doctors and other health professionals involved
- key worker
- coping strategies
- treatment
- competencies
- medications
- concordance
- behaviour
- normalisation
- parenting style
- ethnicity and family culture/beliefs
- finance/benefits
- transport.

This information gathering is crucial to the first part of any assessment to give the nurse a framework and knowledge to work with the child and family. Some of the information gathered and shared may be based on another professional's subjective assessment so it is important that nurses remain non-judgemental at this stage.

Activity

During a clinical placement in the hospital or community, where you are involved in the care of children with chronic illness, select three children and look at their case notes. What picture and knowledge do you gain about these children and their families from the case notes alone?

2. Building up relationships

Continuity of care is the main component in building up a relationship with children with chronic illness and their families. It has been argued that parents with a child with disability need a professional approach from nurses, which acknowledges hope without labelling parents as unrealistic or in denial (Kearney & Griffin 2001).

Visiting children and their families at home is less formal than the hospital setting and the home environment makes it easier for them to discuss issues openly. When undertaking nursing interventions in the busy home environment there can be many distractions but these can provide useful information about the ongoing care and relationships. The children and family can communicate information and feelings that may have little to do with a current problem but have greater significance to their overall care.

It is important that nurses are mindful of the need to communicate effectively with children and their parents. The social position of children relative to adults means that communication between health professionals and children may be difficult and compromised by the influence of parents. Although parents have an important role in interpreting and facilitating communication between children and health professionals, they have been found to constrain communication and contribute to the marginalisation of children in encounters with health professionals (Young et al 2003). It is important, therefore, that nurses encourage children to communicate their needs effectively (Department for Education and Skills (DfES) 2005).

Nursing care of children with chronic illness does not always involve physical activities. Listening, seeing and feeling may be more appropriate actions. A positive attitude demonstrating an interest in the children and their families and not just the chronic disease is essential. Knowledge is gained by observation regarding habits of the family, such as smoking, safety in the home, cleanliness and hygiene, heating, availability of food, socioeconomic status and extended family and support. There may be many opportunities for health promotion and advice can be given when appropriate.

Through regular, direct and/or indirect contact with chronically ill children and their families, nurses can assist them in adapting to meet the challenges of the chronic illness and reduce their feelings of being different. Parents of chronically ill or disabled children face a number of common tasks in adapting to their child's condition (Canam 1993):

- Accept the child's condition
- Manage the child's condition on a day-to-day basis

- Meet the child's normal developmental needs
- Meet the developmental needs of other family members
- Cope with ongoing stress and periodic crises
- Assist family members to manage their feelings
- Educate others about the child's condition
- Establish a support system.

Parents who are not completing these tasks may not have the knowledge, skills or resources necessary. The nurse can be influential in providing appropriate support, services and resources and therefore promote effective coping strategies.

A variety of coping strategies used by parents of children with chronic illness can be elicited from the literature (Lowes & Lyne 1999) and these coping strategies will vary from one family to another. Nurses should support children and their families during any life transitions or crises. By having a shared understanding of the issues raised, nurses are in a position to listen to and value children and their families, increase self-esteem and reassure them of their strengths. In this way nurses can facilitate children and families in their development of strategies for overcoming the difficulties and problems they are facing. Nurses must also acknowledge their own limitations in knowledge and expertise and refer and work with other services when appropriate.

By building up relationships nurses are in a position to form the second part of an assessment that embraces the child and family in totality and over time an holistic therapeutic relationship can be developed. This relationship allows the child, family and nurse to discuss issues openly when fluctuations in the child's illness and family stability occur.

Activity

Compare and contrast the picture and knowledge you gained from the case notes of the three children in the previous activity with the picture and knowledge you gained from caring for them either in hospital or on home visits.

Consider how information gained from different sources can be used to form a holistic view of the child and family.

3. Education and nursing care

Chronic illness is dynamic. There may be acute exacerbations when hospitalisation is required, slow deterioration with new problems, and the need for palliative care in some cases. The dynamic nature of the illness means that children and their families need to be prepared in advance for possible changes in their child's condition and educated when changes occur in order to give the necessary care and treatment.

The term 'disease trajectory' is frequently used to describe the course of a disease and the work involved in its management. The disease trajectory is the developmental process involved in learning to live with a chronic disease and is characterised by stages through which an individual progresses to achieve responsibility for his or her disease management. For nurses to develop an understanding of chronic illness, it may be useful to view the illness in terms of stages with key triggers, which move individuals from one stage to the next. Such explanations provide neat frameworks for understanding illness behaviour and have been applied to a range of chronic illnesses, for example poliomyelitis (Davis 1963), diabetes (Thorne & Paterson 2001), juvenile rheumatoid arthritis (Pelaez-Ballestas et al 2006) and leukemia (Wills 1999).

There has been some questioning of the appropriateness of describing the development of childhood chronic illness in such a manner when there are so many individual differences and factors affecting the course and severity of individual illness experiences. However, understanding of disease trajectories for particular illnesses can help nurses prepare children and their families for changes in their condition and factors likely to affect its progression. Parents have a major responsibility for accurately diagnosing and managing changes in their child's condition and seeking assistance when appropriate. The vigilant monitoring of their child's condition, observing for complications and deterioration can be an onerous responsibility for parents (Ray 2002).

Families need education about the usual minor illnesses that occur in childhood as these may have a greater significance to children with chronic illness, for example they may be more vulnerable to infection. Information about the expected growth and development of their child is also important. Preparing families for changes in their child's condition aids them in developing strategies to adapt.

Although recognising that many children and families have detailed knowledge of their illness, nurses should never presume that they know everything about their illness. It is wise to explore their current knowledge and practical expertise regarding the illness before discussing new care and treatment. This helps clarify knowledge and identify any misconceptions held by children and families before new information is given. Information should be given clearly, concisely and honestly, based on the questions the family asks and on the context in which the conversation is held. Written information, videos, audiotapes, demonstrations, talking to other children and families can often reinforce any verbal information given.

Practical care can vary from basic nursing care, such as bed bathing, to highly technical care, for example, mechanical ventilation. Children and their families will inevitably be involved in such care but the level of their involvement should be negotiated on an individual basis. Nurses should negotiate care that has mutual aims and agree a plan of action with each child and family. Listening to their individual experiences helps nurses to plan interventions that are sensitive to the child and family's needs. Many treatment regimens are complex, time consuming and emotionally laden (Eiser 1990) and, consequently, it is important that nurses regularly review any practical care undertaken by the child and family to ensure that they are willing and confident to continue with such care.

A fundamental principle is that any care undertaken by children and their families at home must be negotiated, agreed and sometimes taught. Kirk (2001) found that parental obligations and the desire for discharge from hospital often made them naïvely accept responsibility for the care and treatment of their child at home, and that there was no effective negotiation. However, once they were at home, parents were in a more powerful position to negotiate their role and be assertive with professionals. Parents develop considerable expertise in caring for their child and in some cases have considerably more specialist knowledge than the community-based professionals who visit the child and family. However, parents highly regard professionals who admit the limitations of their knowledge as it provides the basis for trusting relationships (Kirk & Glendinning 2004). It is important that heath professionals acknowledge and recognise the expertise and knowledge a child and family possess to help develop holistic therapeutic relationships.

Activity

When on clinical placement, ask the senior nurse to identify an appropriate child with a chronic illness to whom you can talk (under supervision) about his or her knowledge of their disease and what care and treatment they undertake at home.

With the senior nurse's agreement and supervision, ask parents caring for a child with a chronic illness what they know about the disease and what care and treatment they undertake at home.

Discuss the information gained with your mentor or the senior nurse.

4. Advocacy

Advocacy means speaking out on behalf of a particular issue, idea or person (Waterson & Haroon 2008). Patients, and child patients in particular, are vulnerable and lack power when they enter the healthcare system, and nurses may frequently find themselves in the position of acting as the patient's advocate. However, it must be recognised that whereas nurses are almost compelled to act as patients' advocates because of the expectations of their practice, this role can put unrealistic demands upon them (Gates 1994). Nurses should act as advocates in certain situations but their decision to do so should be based on clear understanding of the possible consequences of such action, and on their limitations. Independent advocates who act on behalf of patients may be more appropriate than nurses in some circumstances, and nurses need to be aware of when it is appropriate to refer families to such services. Further discussion of advocacy in nursing is beyond the scope of this chapter and readers are recommended to refer to appropriate texts on the subject.

Nurses may have to act as advocates for those children with chronic illness and their families who lack the assertiveness, confidence and eloquence to represent themselves (Ellis 1995). In the early stages of a chronic illness a nurse may act as an advocate to interpret issues such as health service systems, medical terms, benefits and interaction with other professionals. As the child and family become more experienced in dealing with the chronic illness, and confident in asserting their needs, the advocacy role becomes less. Nurses can then empower children and their families by providing enough information and support to enable self-advocacy.

As the child moves into adolescence, the nature of family and peer relationships changes. Peer relationships become increasingly important during adolescence. Peers become more important in offering emotional support, companionship and social interaction which helps adolescents to form their own identity, social skills and self esteem (Tarrant 2002). Children with chronic illness may spend a considerable amount of time away from school/college or be in hospital which makes it difficult to maintain relationships with their peers – resulting in loneliness, low self-esteem, feelings of not being wanted and sometimes of being depressed (Farrant & Watson 2004). Many adolescents recognise the negative realities of their illness, including death, but tend not to talk about their illness unless forced to and usually put all these thoughts in the background in order to get on with life (Bluebond-Langer 2001). Adolescents with a chronic illness are adolescents first and ill second.

Conflict may arise within the family as the adolescent asserts his or her need for autonomy and independence and comes to terms with the restrictions imposed by the illness. Although such conflict is neither restricted to nor inevitable during adolescence, a number of studies have examined the issues facing adolescents with chronic illness. For example, adolescents with chronic illness still indulge in risky behaviours – Tyrell (2001) demonstrated that 21% of teenagers with cystic fibrosis smoked, compared to 56% of controls and Kyngas & Barlow (1995) found that adolescents with diabetes felt that adults could not perceive or understand their situation and that there was a worrying tendency of adolescents with poor metabolic control to lie about their level of management and self-care activities rather than be nagged by parents and health professionals. Non-adherence to treatment regimens may be problematic at this age and the result of feelings that their diagnosis is unjust (Hentinen & Kyngas 1992).

The shift of care from the family to the adolescent is a period of great adjustment. The family may be protective and not want to 'let go' of the care and treatment it has given the child, often for years. Family anxiety and protectiveness may impede healthy adolescent development (Blum et al 1993). The adolescent needs to gain independence from the family but has to accept the responsibilities of self-care, which they may not want to undertake (Edwards & Davis 1997). Adolescents need to be supported to assert autonomy in the management of their chronic condition but should not be expected to take on the whole responsibility for negotiating and navigating through the healthcare system (While et al 2004). A nurse must ensure that an adolescent is shown respect, listened to and their opinions valued in order to keep the channels of communication open between the adolescent, family and other professionals.

5. Support

Nurses need to work with children's existing support networks and help them to develop new ones to ensure that they and their families feel adequately supported. Family, friends, teachers, youth workers and others provide social support to all children. When a child has a chronic illness these support systems may be reduced and new support networks may need to be developed in order to provide for the needs of the child and family. Ellerton et al (1996) compared the social support networks of children with a range of chronic illnesses with those of healthy children. Healthy children reported more support overall than children in the illness groups and children with spina bifida reported the smallest support networks and the fewest number of peers in their networks.

Families provide much practical support in managing children's chronic illnesses and dimensions of family support have been studied in relation to specific diseases. For example, Siarkowski (1999) reviewed the literature on childhood adaptation to insulin-dependent diabetes mellitus and found that family guidance and control produced better glycaemic control but that other dimensions of family support, such as warmth and caring, had no influence on glycaemic control.

School is an important source of support for children with chronic illness. The school should be responsive to the emotional, social and educational needs of a child and should be a place of safety and normality for the child (Edwards & Davis 1997) and it is important that children who are chronically ill are facilitated to integrate the management of their condition into school life, participating in sports/activities and achieving their full academic potential (Valentine & Mcnee 2007). If appointed, the key worker should ensure that the school is aware of a child's illness and management. The school should take appropriate measures for children's individual needs and there should be one contact person at the school with whom the key worker can discuss each child and family's needs and concerns, and vice versa. As interventions in managing children with chronic illness are voluntary in many education settings, it is important that the school and staff feel supported, otherwise they may withdraw this voluntary care, which could restrict or deny such children an education in school (Watson et al 2002). Approaches that facilitate good communication between health professionals and school staff have been explored and joint meetings, shared documentation and local policies have been found to be beneficial (Mukherjee et al 2002). Problems in communication arise when the parent is used as the conduit for information, there are practical difficulties in arranging meetings and there is a lack of knowledge about professional roles (Mukherjee et al 2002).

Other professionals, whether employed by statutory or non-statutory agencies, have an important role to play in the support of children with a chronic illness and their families. The key worker or nurse together with the child and family identify issues that require referring to other agencies and coordinate services required. Services need to be planned in advance, not on a crisis basis, because of the lengthy processes involved in recruiting and training carers (Kirk 1999). It is frustrating to a family to find that services are not always designed and targeted to fit their child and family's needs. The key worker's knowledge of local, cultural, community-based services is essential.

Knowledge of national organisations for specific illnesses from which families can access information, raise funds for research and development and obtain help and support is important. Organisations for common chronic illnesses tend to have local branches. These provide support groups and can increase the availability of recreational and community-based activities. If the chronic illness is rare, a local branch may not be accessible and many families rely on postal mail, national support groups and the internet. These children and families are more vulnerable to isolation and lack of information, and often have to travel to tertiary centres for care and treatment. The latter can sometimes impose transport and financial constraints upon the family.

Contact a Family (http://www.cafamily.org.uk) produces an excellent list of support groups all over the UK, and some overseas, for families with children with chronic illnesses. They link families who can provide support for each other and provide information about support groups.

Seminar discussion topic

The Cystic Fibrosis Trust campaigns to improve the clinical and social care of those affected by cystic fibrosis, as well as raising public awareness of the condition. It funds medical and scientific research aimed towards understanding, treating and curing cystic fibrosis. It also aims to ensure that people with cystic fibrosis receive the best possible care and support in all aspects of their lives. The Trust has established branches and groups throughout the UK to raise funds. The support service provides advice and information for those affected by cystic fibrosis, their families and their carers. More information about national and local activities can be obtained from:

- http://www.cftrust.org.uk

In your seminar group, discuss the range of activities undertaken by charities such as the Cystic Fibrosis Trust and how these activities can complement the work of statutory organisations. Consider resources provided locally as well as nationally.

6. Outcome

By implementing factors 1–5, nurses should have a broad picture of each child and family, which incorporates understanding of their:

- management of the illness
- integration of the child with chronic illness into family life
- quality of life.

Children and families with a chronic illness should be confident in their abilities to recognise early signs and symptoms of changes in the illness so that they can initiate interventions themselves or be able to contact the appropriate professional to prevent or minimise exacerbations of the illness and to reduce hospital admissions.

Nurses are in a prime position to observe and monitor children with chronic illness at home, in school and at clinic appointments so that growth and development, physical and social activity are optimally maintained for each child. Any concerns noted by nurses should be reported to the multidisciplinary team. Decisions made by the multidisciplinary team based on the information provided can be fed back to the child and family to negotiate and plan any necessary interventions.

Children with chronic illness can deteriorate slowly and exacerbations or complications of the illness can have a major affect and quicken the deterioration. Medical or surgical treatment cannot always return the children to their original health status. At this stage children may need to be hospitalised and interventions from professionals can become more complex. Families have to reorganise and manage their lives as their child's lifestyle changes. Using factors 1–5, nurses must reassess each child and family and renegotiate care, treatment and support.

Activity

On your clinical placement, identify a child with chronic illness whose condition has worsened. Discuss with the nurse who is looking after this child and family:

- What care, treatment and support have been initiated for the child and family?
- Has the quality of life for the child and family changed? If so, to what extent?
- How do the child and family feel about these changes?

Summary

This chapter has considered the issues facing the families of children with chronic illness. Although it is important to recognise that each child with a chronic illness, and their family, is in a unique situation, common concerns and goals have been discussed, including health-related quality of life and self-management. Maintaining a reasonable quality of life for the whole family is important because this may help in strengthening their coping strategies. The range of nursing interventions employed with families and children has been explored, stressing the importance of a clear understanding of the illness and its effects on each individual child and their family. Building-up holistic therapeutic relationships to support children and families through the dynamic changes of chronic illness is an essential component of good nursing care.

References

Asthma, U.K., 2009. http://www.asthma.org.uk/all_about_asthma/asthma_basics/index.html [accessed 15 April 2009].

Austin, J.B., Kaur, B., Anderson, H.R., et al., 1999. Hay fever, eczema and wheeze: a nationwide UK study (ISAAC, international study of asthma and allergies in childhood). Archives of Diseases of Childhood 81, 225–230.

Balkrishnan, R., Housman, T.S., Carroll, C., et al., 2003. Disease severity and associated family impact in childhood atopic dermatitis. Archives of Diseases of Childhood 88, 423–427.

Beecham, J., Sloper, P., Greco, V., Webb, R., 2007. The costs of key worker support for disabled children and their families. Child: Care, Health and Development 33 (5), 611–618.

Blubond-Langer, M., 1996. In the shadow of illness: parents and siblings of the chronically sick child. Princeton University Press, Princeton, NJ.

Bluebond-Langer, M., Lask, B., Angst, D.B., 2001. Psychosocial aspects of cystic fibrosis. Arnold, London.

Blum, R.W., et al., 1993. Transition from child-centred to adult health-care systems for adolescents with chronic conditions. Journal of Adolescent Health Care 14, 570–576.

Bonner, M.J., Hardy, K.K., Guill, A.B., McLaughlin, C., Schweitzer, H., Carter, K., 2006. Development and validation of the parent experience of child illness. Journal of Pediatric Psychology 31 (3), 310–321.

Braun-Fahrlander, C., Gassner, M., Grize, L., et al., 1998. Comparison of responses to an asthma symptom questionnaire (ISAAC core questions) completed by adolescents and their parents. SCARPOL-Team. Swiss study on childhood allergy and respiratory symptoms with respect to air pollution. Pediatric Pulmonology 25, 159–166.

British Thoracic Society and Scottish Intercollegiate Guidelines Network, 2008. British guideline on the management of asthma. Thorax 63 (Suppl. 4), 1–121.

Callery, P., Milnes, L., Couriel, J., Verduyn, C., 2003. Qualitative study of children's and parents' beliefs about childhood asthma. British Journal of General Practice 53, 185–190.

Canam, C., 1993. Common adaptive tasks facing parents of children with chronic conditions. Journal of Advanced Nursing 18, 46–53.

Cane, R.S., Ranganathan, S.C., McKenzie, S.A., 2000. What do parents of wheezy children understand by 'wheeze'? Archives of Disease in Childhood 82, 327–332.

Children's Workforce Development Council (CWDC), 2007. The Lead Professional Managers' Guide. CWDC, Leeds.

Contact a Family, 2004. Relationships – no time for us. Online. Available at: http://www.cafamily.org.uk/relationships.html

Daud, L.R., Garralda, M.E., David, T.J., 1993. Psychosocial adjustment in preschool children with atopic eczema. Archives of Diseases of Childhood 69, 670–676.

Davis, F., 1963. Passage through crisis. Bobbs-Merril, Indianapolis, IN.

Department of Health (DoH), 2001. The expert patient a new approach to chronic disease management for the 21st century. DoH, London.

Department of Health (DoH), 2004. National Service Framework for Children, Young People & Maternity Services. DoH, London.

Department for Children, Schools and Families (DCSF) and Department of Health (DoH), 2008. Aiming high for disabled children. DCSF/DoH, London.

Department for Education and Skills (DfES), 2005. Common core of skills and knowledge for the children's workforce. Department for Education and Skills (DfES), Nottingham.

Dobson, B., Middleton, S., 1998. Paying to care: the cost of childhood disability. Joseph Rowntree Foundation, York.

Drotar, D., Crawford, P., 1985. Psychological adaptation of siblings of chronically ill children: research and practice implications. Journal of Developmental and Behavioural Paediatrics 6 (6), 355–362.

Eddy, L.L., Walker, A.J., 1999. The impact of children with chronic health problems on marriage. Journal of Family Nursing 5 (1), 10–31.

Edwards, M., Davis, H., 1997. Counselling children with chronic medical conditions. The British Psychological Society, Leicester.

Eiser, C., 1990. Chronic childhood disease. Cambridge University Press, Cambridge.

Eiser, C., 1993. Growing up with a chronic disease: the impact on children and their families. Jessica Kingsley, London.

Eiser, C., 1997. Children's quality of life measures. Archives of Disease in Childhood 77, 347–354.

Eiser, C., 2007. No pain, no gain? Integrating QoL assessment in paediatrics. Archives of Disease in Childhood 92, 379–380.

Eiser, C., Jenney, M., 2007. Measuring quality of life. Archives of Disease in Childhood 92, 348–350.

Eiser, C., Morse, R., 2001. Quality-of-life measures in chronic diseases of childhood. Health Technology Assessment 5 (4), 1–157.

Eiser, C., Vance, Y.H., Seamark, O., 2000. The development of a theoretically driven generic measure of quality of life for children aged 6–12 years: a preliminary report. Child Care Health and Development 26, 445–456.

Ellerton, M., Stewart, M.J., Ritchie, J.A., Hirth, A.M., 1996. Social support in children with a chronic condition. Canadian Journal of Nursing Research 28 (4), 15–36.

Elliott, B.E., Luker, K., 1996. The experiences of mothers caring for a child with severe atopic eczema. Journal of Clinical Nursing 6, 241–247.

Ellis, P.A., 1995. The role of the nurse as the patient's advocate. Professional Nurse 11 (3), 206–207.

Farrant, B., Watson, P.D., 2004. Health acre delivery: perspectives of young people with chronic illness and their parents. Journal of Paediatrics & Clinical Health 40, 175–179.

Faux, S.A., 1998. Historical overview of responses of children and their families to chronic illness. In: Broome, M.E., Knafl, K., Pridham, K., Feetham, S. (Eds.), Children and families in health and illness. Sage, San Diego, CA, pp. 179–195.

Fisher, H.R., 2001. The needs of parents with chronically sick children: a literature review. Journal of Advanced Nursing 36 (4), 600–607.

Gates, B., 1994. Advocacy: a nurses' guide. Scutari Press, London.

Gibson, C.H., 1995. The process of empowerment in mothers of chronically ill children. Journal of Advanced Nursing 21, 1201–1210.

Gibson, P., Coughlan, J., Wilson, A., et al., 1999. Self-management education and regular practitioner review for adults with asthma (Cochrane Review). The Cochrane Library. Update Software, Oxford.

Glazebrook, C., Hollis, C., Heussler, H., et al., 2003. Detecting emotional and behavioural problems in paediatric clinics. Child: Care, Health and Development 29 (2), 141–150.

Greco, V., Sloper, P., Barton, K., 2004. Care coordination and key worker services for disabled children in the UK. Social Policy Research Unit, University of York, York.

Greco, V., Sloper, P., Webb, R., Beecham, J., 2006. Key worker services for disabled children: the views of staff. Health & Social Care in the Community 14 (6), 445–452.

Guevara, J.P., Wolf, F.M., Grum, C.M., Clark, N.M., 2003. Effects of educational interventions for self management of asthma in children and adolescents: systematic review and meta-analysis. British Medical Journal 326, 1308–1309.

Guyatt, G.H., Juniper, E.F., Griffith, L.E., et al., 1997. Children and adult perceptions of childhood asthma. Pediatrics 99 (2), 165–168.

Hatton, D.L., Canam, C., Thorne, S., Hughes, A.M., 1995. Parents' perceptions of caring for an infant or toddler with diabetes. Journal of Advanced Nursing 22 (3), 569–577.

Henry, B., Aussage, P., Grosskopf, C., Goehrs, J.M., 2003. Development of the cystic fibrosis questionnaire (CFQ) for assessing quality of life in pediatric and adult patients. Quality of Life Research 12 (1), 63–76.

Hentinen, M., Kyngas, H., 1992. Compliance of young diabetics with health regimens. Journal of Advanced Nursing 17, 530–536.

Hentinen, M., Kyngas, H., 1998. Factors associated with the adaptation of parents with a chronically ill child. Journal of Clinical Nursing 7, 316–324.

Hodgkinson, R., Lester, H., 2002. Stresses and coping strategies of mothers living with a child with cystic fibrosis: implications for nursing professionals. Journal of Advanced Nursing 39 (4), 377–383.

Huurre, T.M., Aro, H.M., 2002. Long-term psychosocial effects of persistent chronic illness: a follow-up study of Finnish adolescents aged 16 to 32 years. European Child and Adolescent Psychiatry 12 (2), 85–91.

Ireland, L.M., 1997. Children's perceptions of asthma: establishing normality. British Journal of Nursing 6, 1059–1064.

Janse, A.J., Sinnema, G., Uiterwaal, C.S.P.M., Kimpen, J.L.L., Gemke, R.J.B.J., 2005. Quality of life in chronic illness: perceptions of parents and paediatricians. Archives of Disease in Childhood 90, 486–491.

Kamps, A.W., Roorda, R.J., Brand, P.L., 2001. Peak flow diaries in childhood asthma are unreliable. Thorax 56, 180–182.

Katz, S., 2002. Gender differences in adapting to a child's chronic illness: a causal model. Journal of Pediatric Nursing 17 (4), 257–269.

Katz, S., Krulik, T., 1999. Fathers of children with chronic illness: do they differ from fathers of healthy children? Journal of Family Nursing 5 (3), 292–315.

Kearney, P.M., Griffin, T., 2001. Between joy and sorrow: being a parent of a child with developmental disability. Journal of Advanced Nursing 34 (5), 582–592.

Kirk, S., 1999. Caring for children with specialised health care needs in the community: the challenges for primary care. Health and Social Care in the Community 7 (5) 350–335.

Kirk, S., 2001. Negotiating lay and professional roles in the care of children with complex health care needs. Journal of Advanced Nursing 34 (5), 593–602.

Kirk, S., Glendinning, B., 2004. Developing services to support parents caring for a technology-dependent child at home. Child: Care. Health & Development 30 (3), 209–218.

Kyngas, H., Barlow, J., 1995. Diabetes: an adolescent perspective. Journal of Advanced Nursing 22, 941–947.

Larson, E., 1998. Reframing the meaning of disability to families: the embrace of paradox. Social Science and Medicine 47 (7), 865–875.

Lowes, L., Lyne, P., 1999. A normal lifestyle: parental stress and coping in childhood diabetes British Journal of Nursing 8 (3), 133–139.

Lowes, L., Lyne, P., 2000. Chronic sorrow in parents of children with newly diagnosed diabetes: a review of the literature and discussion of the implications for nursing practice. Journal of Advanced Nursing 32 (1), 41–48.

Lowes, L., Gregory, J.W., Lyne, P., 2005. Newly diagnosed childhood diabetes: a psychosocial transition for parents? Journal of Advanced Nursing 50 (3), 253–261.

Milnes, L.J., Callery, P., 2003. The adaptation of written self-management plans for children with asthma. Journal of Advanced Nursing 41, 444–453.

Mukherjee, S., Beresford, B., Sloper, P., 1999. Unlocking key working. Joseph Rowntree Foundation & The Policy Press, Bristol.

Mukherjee, S., Lightfoot, J., Sloper, P., 2002. Communicating about pupils in mainstream school with special health needs: the NHS perspective. Child: Care, Health and Development 28 (1), 21–27.

Mussaffi, H., Omer, R., Prais, D., et al., 2007. Computerised paediatric asthma quality of life questionnaires in routine care. Archives of Disease in Childhood 92, 678–682.

National Collaborating Centre for Cancer, 2005. Improving outcomes in children & young people with cancer: the manual. National Institute for Health & Clinical Excellence, London.

National Eczema Society http://www.eczema.org/atopic.html [accessed 21 April 2009].

Newachek, P.W., Stoddard, J.J., 1994. Prevalence and impact of multiple childhood chronic illnesses. Journal of Paediatrics 124 (1), 40–48.

Ohya, Y., Williams, H., Steptoe, A., et al., 2001. Psychosocial factors and adherence to treatment advice in childhood atopic dermatitis. Journal of Investigative Dermatology 117, 852–857.

Pandolfini, C., Bonati, M., 2002. Follow up of quality of public orientated health information on the world wide web: systematic re-evaluation. British Medical Journal 324, 582–583.

Pandolfini, C., Impicciatore, P., Bonati, M., 2000. Parents on the web: risks for quality management of cough in children. Pediatrics 105 (1), e1.

Pelaez-Ballestas, I., Romero-Mendoxa, M., Ramos-Lira, L., Caballero, R., Hernandex-Garduno, A., Burgo-Vargas, R., 2006. Illness trajectories in Mexican children with juvenile idiopathic arthritis and their parents. Rheumatology 45, 1399–1403.

Perrin, J.M., 1985. Introduction. In: Hobbs, N., Perrin, J. (Eds.), Issues in the care of children with chronic illness, Josey-Bass, San Francisco, pp. 1–12.

Powers, S.W., Patton, S.R., Hommel, K.A., Hershey, A.D., 2003. Quality of Life in childhood migraines: clinical impact and comparison to other chronic illnesses. Pediatrics 112 (1), e1–e5.

Quittner, A., Opipari, L., Espelage, D., et al., 1998. Role strain in couples with and without a chronic illness: associations with marital satisfaction, intimacy and daily mood. Health Psychology 17, 112–124.

Ray, L.D., 2002. Parenting and childhood chronicity: making visible the invisible work. Journal of Pediatric Nursing 17 (6), 424–438.

Renzoni, E., Forastiere, F., Biggeri, A., et al., 1999. Differences in parental- and self-report of asthma, rhinitis and eczema among Italian adolescents. SIDRIA collaborative group. Studi Italiani sui Disordini Respiratori dell' Infanzia e l'Ambiente. European Respiratory Journal 14, 597–604.

Siarkowski, A.K., 1999. Children's adaptation to insulin dependent diabetes mellitus: a critical review of the literature. Pediatric Nursing 5 (6), 627–639.

Sloper, P., Greco, V., Beecham, J., Webb, R., 2005. Key worker services for disabled children: what characteristics of services lead to better outcomes for children and families? Child: Care, Health & Development 32 (2), 147–157.

Stein, R.E., Jessop, D.J., 1989. What diagnosis does not tell: the case for a non-categorical approach to chronic illness in childhood. Social Science and Medicine 29 (6), 769–778.

Stein, R.E.K., Reissman, C.K., 1980. The development of an impact-on-family scale: preliminary findings. Medical Care 18, 465–472.

Su, J.C., Kemp, A.S., Varigos, G.A., Nolan, T.M., 1997. Atopic eczema: its impact on the family and financial cost. Archives of Diseases of Childhood 76, 159–162.

Tait, T., Dejnega, S., 2001. Coordinating Children's Services. Mary Seacole Research Unit, De Montfort University, Leicester.

Tarrant, M., 2002. Adolescent peer groups and social identity. Social Development 11 (1), 110–123.

Tak, Y.R., McCubbin, M., 2002. Family stress, perceived social support and coping following the diagnosis of a child's congenital heart disease. Journal of Advanced Nursing 39 (2), 190–199.

Teel, C.S., 1991. Chronic sorrow: analysis of the concept. Journal of Advanced Nursing 16, 1311–1319.

Thorne, S.E., Paterson, B.L., 2001. Health care professional support for self-care management in chronic illness: insights from diabetes research. Patient Education and Counselling 42, 81–90.

Tyrell, J., 2001. Growing up with cystic fibrosis: the adolescent years. In: Bluebond-Langer, M., Lask, B., Angst, D.B. (Eds.), Psychosocial aspects of cystic fibrosis. Arnold, London.

Valentine, F., Hazell, S., 2007. The definition and aetiology of chronic illness. In: Valentine, F., Lowes, L. (Eds.), Nursing care of children & young people with chronic illness. Blackwell Publishing, Oxford, pp. 1–28.

Valentine, F., Mcnee, P., 2007. Context of care & service delivery. In: Valentine, F., Lowes, L. (Eds.), Nursing care of children & young people with chronic illness. Blackwell Publishing, Oxford, pp. 29–54.

Vance, Y.H., Morse, R.C., Jenney, M.E., Eiser, C., 2001. Issues in measuring quality of life in childhood cancer: measures, proxies, and parental mental health. Journal of Child Psychology and Psychiatry and Allied Disciplines 42 (5), 661–667.

Vessey, J., 1999. Psychological comorbidity in children with chronic conditions. Pediatric Nursing 25 (2), 211–214.

Waterston, T., Haroon, S., 2008. Advocacy and the paediatrician. Paediatric Child Health 18, 213–218.

Watson, D., et al., 2002. Exploring multi-agency working in services to disabled children with complex healthcare needs and their families. Journal of Clinical Nursing 11, 367–375.

Whalley, D., Huels, J., McKenna, S.P., Van Assche, D., 2002. The benefit of pimecrolinmus on parents' quality of life in the treatment of pediatric atopic dermatitis. Pediatrics 110 (6), 1133–1136.

While, A., Forbes, A., Ullman, R., Lewis, S., Mathes, L., Griffiths, P., 2004. Good practices that address continuity during transition from child to adult care: synthesis of the evidence. Child: Care Health and Development 30 (5), 439–452.

Whyte, D.A., 1992. A family nursing approach to the care of a child with a chronic illness. Journal of Advanced Nursing 17, 317–327.

Wills, B.S.H., 1999. The experiences of Hong Kong Chinese parents of children with acute lymphocytic leukaemia. Journal of Pediatric Nursing: Nursing Care of Children and Families 14 (4), 231–238.

Young, B., Dixon-Woods, M., Findlay, M., Heney, D., 2002a. Parenting in crisis: conceptualizing mothers of children with cancer. Social Science and Medicine 55 (10), 1835–1847.

Young, B., Dixon-Woods, M., Windridge, K.C., Heney, D., 2003. Managing communication with young people who have a potentially life threatening chronic illness: qualitative study of patients and parents. British Medical Journal 326 (7384), 305–309.

Young, B., Fitch, G.E., Dixon-Woods, M., et al., 2002b. Parents' accounts of wheeze and asthma related symptoms: a qualitative study. Archives of Disease in Childhood 87, 131–134.

Caring for children with critical illness

45

Marion Aylott

ABSTRACT

The primary aim of this chapter and the companion PowerPoint presentation is to explore fundamental issues and key concepts for children's intensive care nursing practice. Children's intensive care combines aspects of many specialities, for example anaesthesiology, paediatrics, microbiology, cardiothoracic surgery and cardiology, into one integrated and unique whole to provide care for the most severely ill children. Children whose very existence is immediately threatened have many multiple aspects of care they require in common, regardless of underlying illness. Thus children who have suffered trauma, heart disease, severe infectious disease, devastating medical illness or are recovering from complex surgery all benefit from the collaborative practice of critical care to provide respiratory support, haemodynamic control and holistic support of the child and family. Therefore, this chapter gives a detailed account of these three nursing practice issues and will include a clinical scenario, which will provide opportunities to apply critical care knowledge gained in this chapter to a clinical situation.

LEARNING OUTCOMES

- Demonstrate an understanding of the key concepts of children's intensive care nursing.
- Explain the principles of respiratory and cardiovascular support within the intensive care setting.
- Consider the role of the children's nurse as part of the multi-professional team in helping to maintain respiratory support and haemodynamic control.
- Discuss the physical and psychological care of the child with critical illness and their family.

Glossary

Afterload: The load against which the left ventricle ejects after opening the aortic valve.

Cardiac contractility: Contractile capability of the heart.

Cardiac output: The volume of blood that the heart pumps in 1 minute.

Central venous pressure: A measure of pressure in the right atrium.

Chronotropic: Agent that acts to increase heart rate.

Compensated shock: Blood flow is normal or increased and may be maldistributed; vital organ function is maintained.

Compliance: The ease with which the lungs and thorax expand during pressure changes.

Endotracheal intubation: Insertion of endotracheal tube into the trachea either through a patient's nose or mouth and directly through the larynx between the vocal cords into the trachea to open and maintain airway.

Fibrosis: Replacement of lung epithelium and elastic fibres with fibroplast scar tissue.

Frank-Starling's law: An increase in preload leads to an increase in stroke volume.

FRC: Functional residual capacity is the pool of air left in the lungs at the end of total expiration.

Heart rate: The number of cardiac contractions that occur in 1 minute.

Hypoxia: An inadequate supply of oxygen.

Inotrope: Agent that acts to improve myocardial contractility and enhance stroke volume.

Irreversible shock: Inadequate perfusion of vital organs; irreparable damage; death cannot be prevented.

Minute volume: Amount of gas inhaled and exhaled in 1 minute.

PEEP/CPAP: Positive end expiratory pressure, or continuous positive airway pressure, is the baseline pressure and controls functional residual capacity in the patient's lung.

PIP: Peak inspiratory pressure indicates the maximum pressure that has occurred during the last ventilatory cycle.

Preload: The load on the ventricle before ejection.

Shock: Circulatory system failure to supply oxygen and nutrients to meet cellular metabolic demands.

Stroke volume: The amount of blood ejected by both ventricles with each contraction.

Systemic vascular resistance: The resistance against which the left ventricle must eject to force out its content with each beat.

DOI: 10.1016/B978-0-7020-3183-0.10045-1

Tidal volume: The amount of gas or air breathed in or out in one breath.

Uncompensated shock: Microvascular perfusion is compromised; significant reductions in effective circulating volume.

Introduction

A paediatric intensive care unit (PICU) is a specifically designed and equipped multidisciplinary healthcare specialty for the treatment of critically ill children from early infancy to adolescence (British Paediatric Association (BPA) 1993), which has been shown to be important in achieving the best possible outcomes for children (Pearson et al 1997). Nurses are an important element of the team of staff that cares for the critically ill child, and this is reflected by the high nurse:patient ratio – ideally 1:1 – that is characteristic of intensive care. To understand what critical care is, we must focus on the social context in which it occurs. Thus critical care is where care is critical (Coombs 2001). The role encompasses an independent as well as interdependent element. Although critical care nurses work one to one so that they can truly focus on each patient, they will contribute as part of a team when the need dictates. Additionally, nursing and therapeutic intervention in critical care extends beyond the patient. It includes the interface with technology, for example the lines, the monitors, the organ support machinery and the drains.

What is critical illness?

There are around 12,000 admissions each year to PICU in England, which averages approximately 120 in each Health Authority area (NHS Executive (NHSE) 1997a). Critical illness is a derangement in physiology with the potential to result in significant morbidity and mortality without prompt and appropriate invasive and therapeutic intervention (Hazinski 1999). There are, however, many differences in healthcare facilities available in PICUs across the UK relating to the case mix of patients admitted and the intensive care resources available in particular units. The variety of disease seen in any children's intensive care unit depends on the population from which it receives patients (Duncan 1998). For example, a hospital with a cardiac surgery programme will increase the number of patients that unit admits with that condition. Although a wide variety of diseases may lead to critical illness, the fundamental interventions required are limited. The common pathway of deterioration in critical illness occurs as a result of progressive deterioration of respiratory and circulatory function with respiratory failure or shock as the pathophysiological expression with the final denominator being cardiopulmonary failure (Advanced Life Support Group (ALSG) 2001).

What constitutes an intensive care patient?

As we have seen, critical illness is characterised by acute loss of physiologic reserve but in many cases the course of illness is prolonged and often the underlying cause may be difficult to discern. Moreover, despite a child having a recognised critical illness there is great interpatient variability. In addition, until the very recent past children with critical illness were nursed in a range of settings including general adult intensive care units depending on geographical location. In Britain, paediatric intensive care developed in an ad hoc and fragmented way. Now, however, after 20 years of effort, Britain is moving towards a more integrated service.

Concerns about paediatric intensive care were first raised by the British Paediatric Association (BPA) in the 1980s, and again in 1993 when it published its report on paediatric intensive care. This report highlighted the fragmented configuration of paediatric intensive care provision, demonstrating that only 51% of children were cared for in paediatric intensive care units, 20% in adult intensive care units and 29% in children's wards (BPA 1993). Furthermore, only 36% of paediatric intensive care units provided a retrieval service. Concerns were also expressed regarding the lack of physical facilities, lack of education and training of both medical and nursing staff and poor staffing levels available to care for these critically ill children.

In 1996 an inquiry into the death of a child named Nicholas Geldard, who died in a paediatric intensive care unit in 1995 after inappropriate transport for management following a spontaneous cerebral haemorrhage, was published (Ashworth 1996). In response to this, the Department of Health (DoH) requested an inquiry into paediatric intensive care services with a view to developing a policy framework for paediatric intensive care (NHSE 1996). In 1997 'Paediatric intensive care: a framework for the future' was published (NHSE 1997a). This paper set out a strategy for developing and integrating the service for critically ill children within a geographical area and so centralise the skills and experience of medical and nursing staff. The central recommendations of this paper have been supported by others (Pearson et al 1997).

Today, children requiring intensive care are no longer cared for in general children's wards and centres that do not meet the standards as laid out by the NHSE framework document. Quality of paediatric intensive care is not only reliant on a centralised and standardised service but also – importantly – the effectiveness and appropriateness of treatment within a child- and family-orientated environment. To facilitate this, nurses working in paediatric intensive care units undertake a specifically designed, competency-based course to equip them with the knowledge, skills and understanding that underpins effective paediatric intensive care nursing practice.

WWW

Read the DoH papers Framework for the future and A bridge to the future online:

- http://www.doh.gov.uk/nsf/paediatr.htm

Children are admitted to PICU when one or more body systems cannot maintain physiological homeostatic equilibrium without intensive therapeutic support. However, there are varying degrees of organ failure and levels of intensive support (NHSE 1997a,b).

Activity

Analyse the categories of intensive care as defined by the DoH papers: A framework for the future and A bridge to the future. Discuss in your learning group how these levels of care and facilities, including staff skills and expertise, compare with a general paediatric ward.

Scenario

Introducing Daniel

The Badger ward paediatrician and nursing staff were concerned about the condition of 15-month-old Daniel, who weighed 13 kg and was developing increased respiratory distress since admission 4 hours earlier. Daniel had been admitted to Badger ward as a referral from his GP and was accompanied by his parents, Emma and Alan. Daniel had a 2-week history of an upper respiratory tract infection, which over the previous 2–3 days had worsened, with decreased appetite and fluid intake. Since admission to Badger ward, his respiratory distress had markedly increased. Initial treatment was directed towards alleviating his respiratory distress and included 30% oxygen via a head box and intravenous antibiotics. Despite this therapy there had been no evidence of improvement. The paediatrician contacted the PICU intensivist to review Daniel on Badger ward.

The paediatric intensivist and an experienced PICU nurse equipped with emergency bag and retrieval trolley responded immediately to this request. On assessment they found that Daniel was in obvious respiratory distress. He was irritable and reluctant to leave his mother's arms. His pulse rate was 180, respiratory rate 65 with grunting and sternal and intercostal chest recession. Inspiratory stridor and expiratory wheeze were readily audible and his tidal volume was decreased.

Daniel was transferred to PICU on the retrieval trolley on his mother's lap.

Activity

Consider Daniel's situation and the DoH categories for intensive care. What was the rationale for Daniel's admission to PICU?

Relating back to Chapter 27, consider why the critical care team who assessed Daniel decided to transfer him to PICU in his mother's lap, without further intervention on Badger ward.

Scenario

On admission to PICU, additional vital signs were obtained:

- Daniel was awake and irritable and appeared exhausted
- respiratory rate had increased from 60 to 70
- his recession appeared pronounced
- oxygen saturation: 95%
- pulse rate had increased from 174 to 200
- radial and dorsalis pulses were weak and thready
- his skin was cool, dry and pale
- capillary refill: 4 seconds
- blood pressure: 90/60 mmHg
- he was conscious and responding to his mother
- blood glucose: 1.7 mmol/L
- axilla temperature: 38.5°C
- no skin rash noted
- an arterial gas was obtained: pH 7.25, pCO_2 7.6, pO_2 22, base deficit −3.

Rapid cardiopulmonary assessment

Recognition of potential respiratory failure, based on clinical evaluation of the child is vital (ALSG 2001). Intubation and ventilation of a child with potential respiratory failure will be considered if a child fails to improve after initial oxygen therapy or if further deterioration is observed. An individual must be able to support three specific functions:

- Protect the airway
- Adequately ventilate
- Adequately oxygenate.

A failure to perform any one function will result in respiratory failure. Respiratory failure is defined as a major abnormality of gas exchange (Lissuer & Clayden 2001) and is an absolute indication for intubation and mechanical ventilation. However, not every patient who is intubated has a primary pulmonary pathology. Intubation and ventilation may serve to support the cardiovascular system. For example, for patients in cardiogenic shock the demands of the respiratory system may precipitate cardiovascular collapse. Supporting the patient with mechanical ventilation can reduce the demands on the heart, allowing it to recover. Intubation can also serve to protect the airway for those who cannot do it themselves, for example patients in coma as a result of a head injury. Moreover mechanical ventilation offers the option of hyperventilation for patients with intracranial hypertension.

Activity

Analyse the data collected during a rapid cardiopulmonary assessment of Daniel and arterial blood gas and list the factors that support the decision to intubate and ventilate.

Respiratory support

Intubation

Intubation and ventilation are always performed with caution, as anaesthetic agents as well as positive pressure ventilation will exacerbate hypovolaemia. Assessment of Daniel's perfusion indicates a degree of hypovolaemia therefore he was given 260 ml (20 mL/kg) of normal saline as an intravenous bolus with good effect observed by an improvement in his heart rate and perfusion. In addition, he was administered broad-spectrum intravenous antibiotics.

Intubation is a painful and unpleasant procedure and should never be performed on a conscious or semi-conscious patient. Unless the child has completely collapsed, the medical practitioner, usually an anaesthetist or intensivist, will perform

Action	Rationale
Suction apparatus with appropriate size suction catheter.	Relatively small amounts of mucus accumulation, oedema or airway obstruction can reduce airway patency or obscure view of the vocal cords for intubation.
Assemble appropriate sized and working bag valve mask device.	To ensure effective ventilation.
Positioning to achieve optimal airway patency is essential to bag valve mask. A shoulder roll may be used to help extend the neck and position the airway in a neutral position (nose perpendicular to the ceiling). An airway adjunct may also be used if head position is difficult to maintain	A child under the age of 2 years has a large, heavy head with prominent occiput, short chubby neck and a large tongue. Furthermore, sedation and CNS dysfunction will exacerbate these effects.
Assemble appropriate sized and working laryngoscope and blade. Check adequate illumination from bulb. 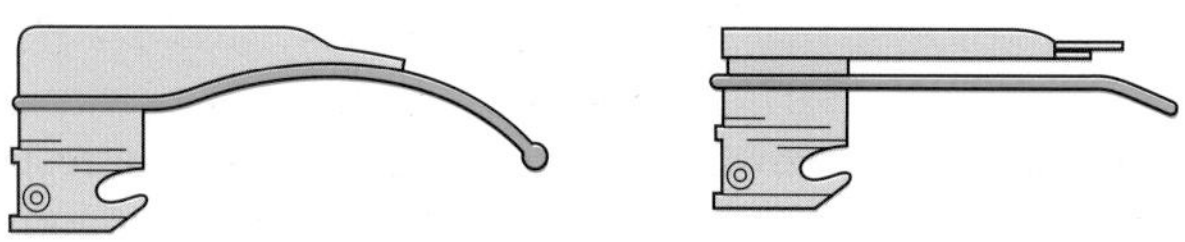	A straight laryngoscope blade is better in younger children as it is used to pick up the floppy epiglottis. A curved laryngoscope blade is better in older children who have a stiff epiglottis where the blade is placed in the vallecula.
Assemble the correct size endotracheal tube (ETT) plus one a size above and one size below. 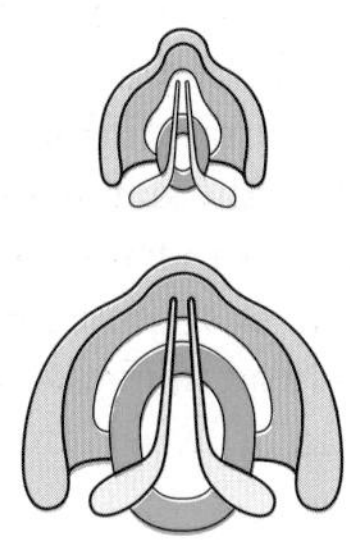	The narrowest part of the airway in a child under 8 years at the level of the cricoid cartilage which is cone-shaped. An ETT may pass through the volcal cords easily in the young child but be too large to pass through the cricoid cartilage. Select the correct size uncuffed tube carefully using a broselow tape, a recognised chart of the formulae; $\frac{\text{Age}}{4} + 4$ For the child under 2 years: Age — Kg — ETT Newborn — 3.5 — 3.5 3 months — 6.0 — 3.5 1 year — 10 — 4.0 2 years — 12 — 4.5
Assemble ETT with introducer if wanted. 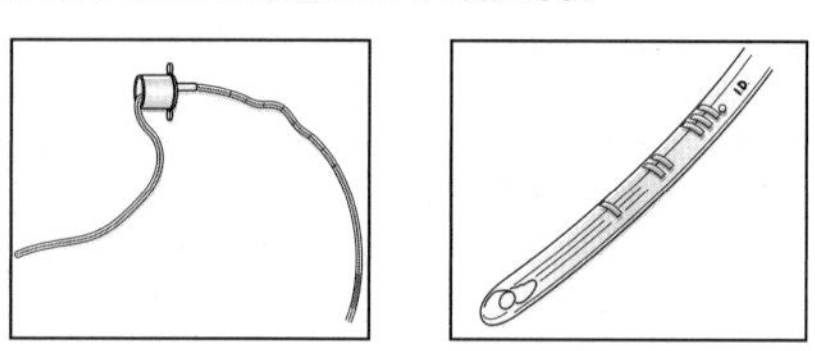	The practitioner intubating may request an introducer. This makes the tube more 'stiff' which makes intubating easier. When inserting the introducer take care to ensure that it does not protrude beyond the tip of the ETT itself as this may cause tissue trauma to the trachea. Many bend the top of the introducer over the connector after checking for profusion as a further safety mechanism.
Assemble tape ready cut to secure ETT in place.	This enables stability of the ETT in place. Various methods of securing an ETT exist. Find out how your PICU prefers to secure an ETT.
Stethoscope.	To confirm ETT placement prior to the formal confirmation of a chest X-ray.

Fig. 45.1 • The action and rationale for preparation prior to intubation.

what is called rapid sequence induction. This means inducing anaesthesia and giving muscle relaxants. Common drugs used in this age group are morphine, midazolam and atracurium. When the drugs are being prepared for rapid sequence induction, equipment should be prepared and checked to be in good working order to ensure a safe procedure, as displayed in Figure 45.1.

As the sedation and anaesthetic agent of choice is administered intravenously and the child starts to lose consciousness, the child will be preoxygenated with 100% oxygen using

Scenario

Daniel was intubated with a size 4.5 mm endotracheal. Initial ventilation parameters were:

- respiratory rate: 30
- inspiratory time: 0.8 seconds
- tidal volume: 180 mL
- PEEP: 5 cmH_2O.

Synchronised mandatory ventilation (SIMV) mode was selected; resultant peak inspiratory pressure (PIP) was 28 cm H_2O. Analgesia and sedation were maintained with continuous infusions of morphine and midazolam, respectively.

a bag-valve-mask device for at least 1–2 minutes. This ensures that the child is in optimum condition prior to the procedure of intubation. Once the child is assessed to be unconscious and bag valve mask ventilation is established the paralysing agent is administered intravenously. A nasogastric tube should be passed to empty gastric contents and left of free drainage thus preventing aspiration. It is also useful for decompression of gas accumulated in the stomach during bag-valve-mask ventilation. During the intubation procedure the medical practitioner may ask an assistant to apply cricoid pressure. This is external compression of the trachea to decrease the probability of aspiration and inflation of the stomach and also enhances visualisation of the glottis. Care must be taken to apply cricoid pressure symmetrically. Once the endotracheal tube is in place, observations are made to confirm that the tube is in the correct position. This is done by:

- observing for bilateral chest movement with ventilation
- auscultation using a stethoscope to ensure breath sounds heard clearly over the anterior and posterior chest and in both axillae
- confirming that there are no breath sounds over the stomach
- confirming that O_2 saturations are improving
- confirming that the heart rate is stable and within normal limits
- The endotracheal tube is then secured in place and a chest X-ray ordered for formal confirmation of tube placement.

Mechanical ventilation: physiological principles and effects

Mechanical ventilatory support is the major supportive treatment used in critical care. A mechanical ventilator is simply a machine used to replace or supplement the natural function of breathing. It is usually a temporary measure until the patient can breathe adequately without help. Ventilation is simply the movement of gas into and out of the lungs. To safely and effectively provide care for intubated infants and children receiving assisted ventilation it is necessary to have an understanding of the fundamental physiological principles of lung function and the physiological effects of assisted ventilation in terms of both gas exchange and pulmonary mechanics and an appreciation of the particular disease process leading to the need for assisted ventilation.

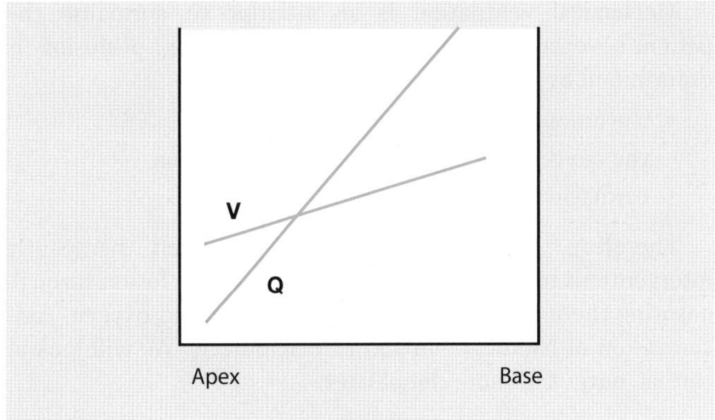

Fig. 45.2 • The ventilation (V) and perfusion (Q) relationship.

Ventilation and perfusion relationship

The primary function of the lungs is to enable gas exchange between inspired air that reaches the alveoli and the blood of the pulmonary capillaries. This process of gas exchange is crucial for homeostasis and is interdependent with the circulatory system's prime role of blood transport. To enable adequate gas exchange it is crucial that oxygen and carbon dioxide move between air and blood by simple diffusion across the alveolar surface. More specifically, there is a balance between ventilation (V) and perfusion (Q). However, it is more complicated than this. V and Q are not evenly distributed throughout the lung (Hazinski 1999). Figure 45.2 illustrates how V increases from apex to the base of the lung and Q increases from apex to base relatively more than perfusion. During normal quiet breathing in an upright position the bases of the lung receive about 50% more ventilation than the apices. This is due to:

- gravity
- variations in airways size (remember Poiseuille's law, Chapter 4)
- variations in alveolar elastic properties (surfactant – to be discussed later).

If oxygen is not delivered to alveolar capillaries, or the alveolar surface is damaged, oxygen and/or carbon dioxide elimination may be impaired, V and Q are not balanced and respiratory failure ensues. In a single lung unit V and Q must be matched to allow gas exchange (Fig. 45.3).

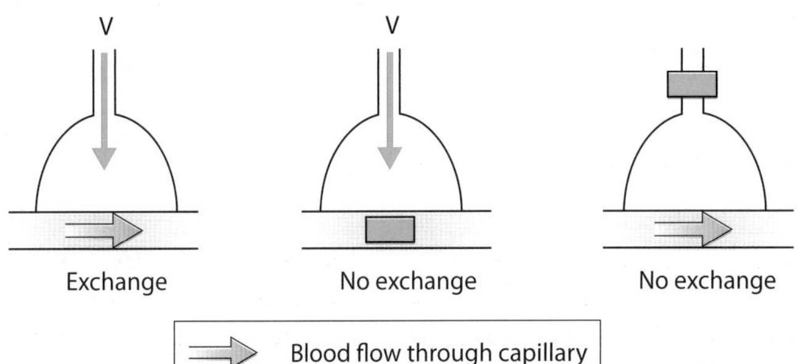

Fig. 45.3 • A simple illustration of V and Q mismatch.

Mechanical ventilation is an attempt to normalise the patient's ventilation-perfusion ratio. However, perfusion is determined by:

- the amount of oxygen in the blood
- the oxygen binding capacity of haemoglobin
- cardiac output.

Therefore, when a patient is being ventilated, therapeutic interventions must also be taken to optimise perfusion through ensuring there is a sufficient delivery of inspired oxygen, concentration of haemoglobin and cardiac output. We will look at cardiac output in more detail later.

The mechanics of breathing

Three factors affect the mechanics of breathing:

- Force (pressure)
- Displacement (volume)
- Rate of displacement (flow), which comprises compliance and resistance.

These factors are all interrelated:

$$\text{Pressure} = \text{Volume} \div (\text{Compliance} + \text{Resistance})$$

$$\text{i.e. Pressure} = \text{Volume} \div \text{Flow}$$

During normal inspiration the mechanical contraction of the inspiratory muscles causes the thoracic cage to enlarge in volume. This increased volume causes a pressure gradient between the lungs and the atmosphere. This pressure differential is enough to cause an in-rush of air into the lungs. The work that the inspiratory muscles perform represents the negative pressure applied. Figure 45.4a shows the changes in airway pressure in the mouth during spontaneous quiet breathing. Airway pressure during inspiration is negative, allowing air to enter the lungs, and is positive during expiration. Also, there is normally a brief pause, when airway pressure remains at atmospheric pressure. Figure 45.4b shows the upper airway pressures (measured at the mouth) during mechanical ventilation. In artificial ventilation, the ventilator must provide the inspiratory pressure provided by the inspiratory muscles in normal respiration. This is done by creating a positive intrapulmonary pressure whereby air is pushed out of the ventilator into the lungs of the patient, thus raising the pressure in the airways relative to atmospheric pressure. This resultant increase in intrapulmonary pressure forces the lungs to expand. It is important to remember that artificial ventilation fundamentally alters normal airway pressures. This fact accounts for most of its benefits and complications.

In the equation Pressure = Volume ÷ (Compliance + Resistance), compliance and resistance are assumed to remain constant and is illustrated by (a) in Figure 45.5. However, this is not the case in cardiopulmonary illness. With stiff lungs (reduced compliance) patients tend to take rapid, small breaths, to minimise elastic workload as in Figure 45.5b. With high airway resistance, for example in asthma, patients take large slow breaths (Figure 45.5c). As can be seen in Fig. 45.5, the inspiratory lung volume is low in both. Thus, their combined effect is a greater load presented to the ventilator.

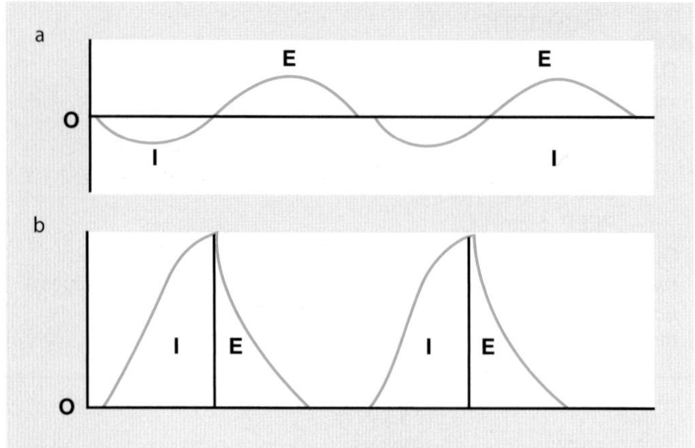

Fig. 45.4 • Changes in airway pressure during (a) normal spontaneous breathing versus (b) artificial mechanical ventilation.

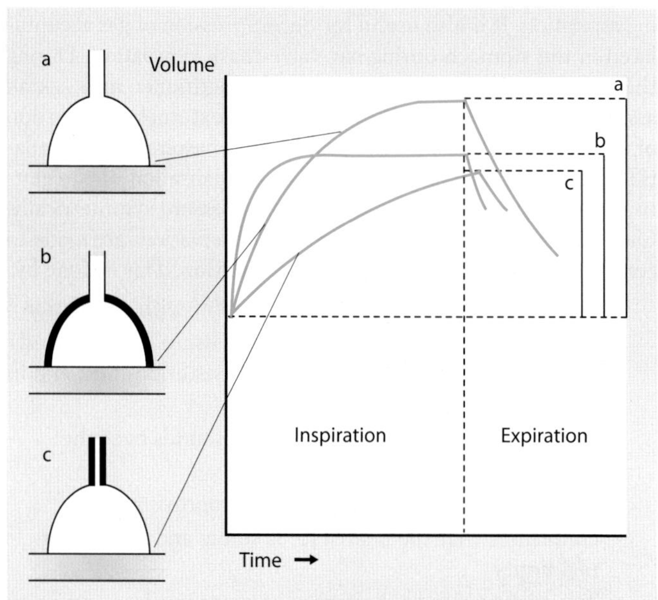

Fig. 45.5 • The effects of compliance and airway resistance on lung volume. (a) The effect of normal compliance; (b) the effect of reduced compliance; (c) the effect of increased airways resistance.

Pressure, volume and flow change over time in illness, therefore they are considered variable. From the equation of motion, the ventilator must control one of these variables. A mechanical ventilator will control airway pressure, inspired volume or inspired flow.

But there is more to compliance. To achieve compliance, alveolar lung units have an important lung property – they are elastic. They can be expanded by small forces and return to their resting state. Two components are responsible for their elastic behaviour:

- Elastic tissue consisting of elastic and collagen fibres embedded in alveoli walls and around bronchi

- The surface tension reducing effect of surfactant increases compliance.

Thus less pressure is required to inflate alveoli (Martini 1998). The lung contains a foamy phospholipid fluid commonly known as surfactant. Pulmonary surfactant is produced by type I and II alveolar pneumocytes, and is responsible for decreasing the surface tension of the lining fluid within the bronchial tree. Without surfactant, pulmonary airways become unstable and have decreased compliance. Surfactant decreases the surface tension of the alveoli in order to aid the diffusion of gases (Martini 1998). A reduction in production of surfactant will directly affect gas exchange. General causes of reduced surfactant production are:

- acidosis
- hypoxia
- hyperoxygenation
- pulmonary oedema
- atelectasis.

To help understand this concept, think about blowing up a balloon. At first it is difficult and then there is a 'give' and the balloon inflates easily. This occurs in the same way in the lungs. The greatest workload in the respiratory cycle is in early inspiration where the pressure–volume curve is relatively flat (Fig. 45.6).

Once the steep part of the pressure–volume curve (PVC) (the P_{flex}) is reached, the lung suddenly inflates easily; this is the inflection point. The PVC is flattest at low lung volumes and consequently the work of breathing is highest. If the lungs were left filled with air so that the resting state is at or above the inflection point, the work of breathing is reduced considerably. Going back to our analogy, this is like letting a balloon deflate incompletely and then re-inflating it. This is the basis for positive end expiratory pressure (PEEP), which is a continuous constant pressure of gas delivered to prevent alveolar collapse (PEEP will be discussed in more detail later).

Finally, the last physiological mechanism we must consider is closing volume. In health, the lungs dangle downwards in the pleural cavity supported by a vacuum of negative pressure. As you would expect, the magnitude of this negative pressure is greater in the apices than in the bases. The effect of this is to splint the airways open at the end of the tidal volume (normal expiration) – the expiratory reserve volume (ERV) (McCance & Huether 2002) (Fig. 45.7). Apical alveoli are more inflated at rest than basal. But during inspiration, because the latter are at a steep part of the pressure–volume curve, the gas turnover (see Fig. 45.6) is greater. However, in illness, further confounded by upper airway compromise, and especially when lying supine, there is a tendency for distal, particularly basal airways to collapse in expiration. This is known as the closing volume. If this is not addressed by delivering PEEP through the ventilator, eventually the closing volume will impinge on and begin to exceed functional residual capacity (FRC) and atelectasis (alveolar collapse) will occur at the end of quiet expiration.

As we have seen, artificial ventilation is unlike normal ventilation. Positive pressure ventilation can be injurious to the lungs, which were designed as a negative pressure circuit receiving oxygen at 21%. Moreover, artificial ventilation is most often required by patients with underlying lung or cardiovascular pathology which makes the lung tissue even more susceptible to ventilator-induced lung injury and cardiovascular complications.

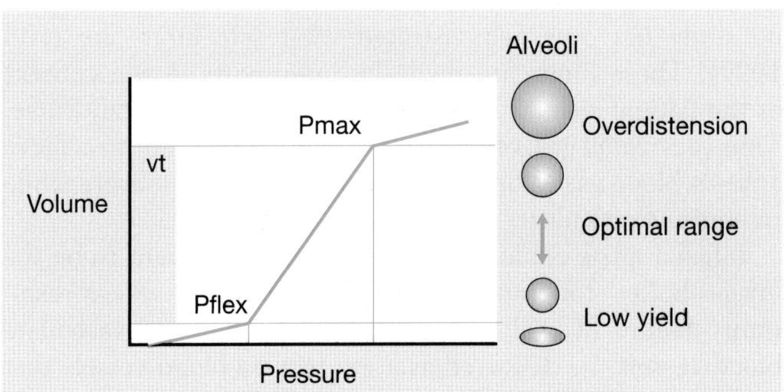

Fig. 45.6 • Alveolar compliance and the pressure–volume curve.

Evidence-based practice

Evidence has been mounting since the late 1980s that mechanical ventilation can cause and exacerbate lung tissue injury (Dreyfus et al 1985, Kolobow et al 1987). Although most of this evidence has originated from animal studies, clinical reports support this concern (Bohn 1998):

- Oxygen toxicity
- Barotrauma (pressure)
- Volutrauma (shearing forces)
- Insufficient humidification.

Ventilation: lessons learned

Accumulating evidence has revealed that high oxygen concentrations, high inflation pressures, large tidal volumes and low PEEP ventilation strategies are damaging to the lungs:

- Oxygen in supraphysiological concentrations is injurious to the lung, particularly in concentrations over an FiO_2 of 0.60 (Robb 1997a).
- Positive pressure ventilation is non-physiological and causes pulmonary injury. The higher the pressures used, the greater the injury. This is referred to as barotrauma and is typically associated with excessive airway pressures leading to extra-alveolar air and also includes pneumothorax, pneumomediastinum, pneumoperitoneum and subcutaneous emphysema. What exactly qualifies as a dangerous pressure is not known (Bohn 1998).
- Volutrauma is lung injury secondary to alveolar overdistension. It is manifested by disruption of the alveolar capillary membrane and alterations in gas exchange. The propensity for volutrauma is related to the volume of lung available and to regional differences

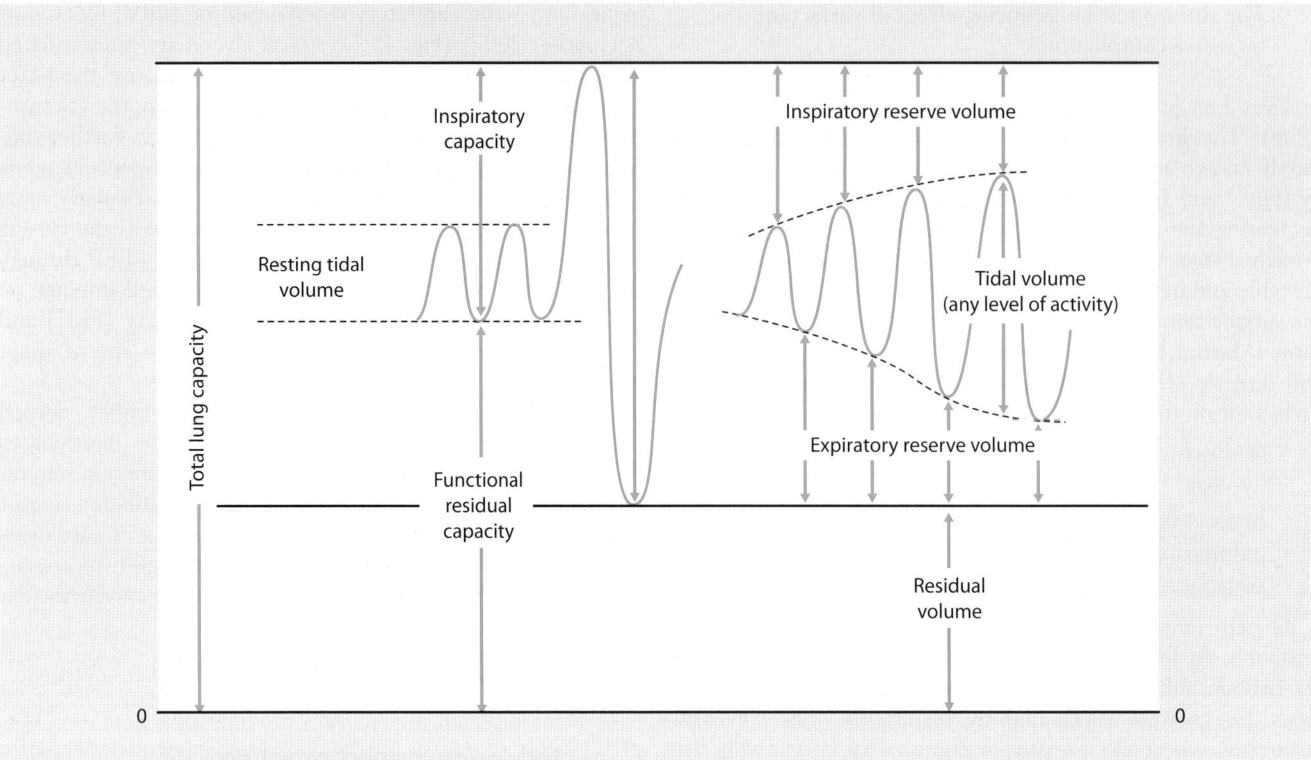

Fig. 45.7 • Lung volumes.

in compliance. In, for example, pneumonia where lung volume is significantly diminished and compliance is reduced, the risk of volutrauma is increased (Kerr 1997).

- Shearing forces caused by repeated expansion of collapsed alveoli is injurious to the lung by causing the release of inflammatory mediators independent of over-distension or oxygen concentration (Bohn 1998). The concept of 'shear' injury along with the increase in dead space to tidal volume ratio prevents the use of high rates to compensate for small tidal volumes/low pressures.

Strategies to reduce lung injury

In response to these findings, respiratory experts have espoused the use of lung protective ventilator strategies (Kerr 1997). One strategy is to use sufficient PEEP to raise FRC above closing capacity without compromising cardiac output and as a consequence oxygen delivery. This strategy keeps alveolar units on the steep part of the compliance curve (see Fig. 45.6). Higher levels of PEEP help to maintain:

- alveolar recruitment (the 'open lung' approach)
- reduce V/Q mismatch and progressive hypoxemia
- achieve lower tidal volumes (4–8 mL/kg).

Thus, higher levels of PEEP lead to reduced end inspiratory volumes preventing shear/stretch injury.

Another strategy advocated is the use of pressure-limited ventilation and increasing mean airway pressures by permissive hypercapnia and hypoxemia (Reynolds et al 1993). There is no research evidence to dictate what acceptable oxygen or carbon dioxide levels are. The general philosophy is that an acceptable level is determined by what intensivists are willing to do to get there considering the research findings available regarding the causation of lung injury. For example, if an oxygen saturation of 95% can only be achieved through using a PEEP of 12 cmH_2O and a FiO_2 of 1.0 (100%) this is not acceptable in the light of the best available evidence. Both high PEEP and high inspired-oxygen concentrations are injurious to the lung. However, if achieving a carbon dioxide level of 5.4 kPa results in a peak pressure of 30 cmH_2O, this might be acceptable as this carbon dioxide level is acceptable. In general (Parker et al 1993):

- peak pressures greater than 35 cmH_2O are not acceptable
- the upper limit for an acceptable FiO_2 is 0.60
- the upper PEEP limit is 15 cmH_2O.

It is recognised that these limits are arbitrary in nature and no study has ever demonstrated what safe limits are (Hill 1997). These limits are made by intensivists in the context of the patient's clinical situation and expected clinical course. Thus the overall goal of mechanical ventilation is not to achieve a target blood gas value but to maximise oxygen delivery while minimising pulmonary injury.

Inhaled nitric oxide (iNO) was originally thought to be the 'magic bullet' for improving V/Q mismatch in severe respiratory failure (Tibballs 1998). Given its ability to vasodilate blood vessels, be delivered as a gas (act on blood vessels that perfuse ventilated alveoli: selective pulmonary vasodilatation) and its short half-life (no systemic hypotension), it was studied with great interest. However, although iNO does improve oxygenation in acute respiratory distress syndrome, it does not improve outcome. It has more of a beneficial effect in patients with pulmonary hypertension, especially neonates with persistent pulmonary hypertension of the newborn or post-operative cardiac patients.

There are options, beyond adjusting the ventilator, which have implications for nursing. Body positioning affects ventilation/perfusion (V/Q) matching and therefore arterial oxygen levels. Accumulation of secretions and atelectasis can occur in the dependent regions of the lungs, therefore regular position changes will help to avoid problem areas developing. Position can also affect a child's FRC. A reduction in FRC will make a child more vulnerable to atelectasis and allow more rapid hypoxia. It is important to consider which positions may help to optimise oxygenation and this is a multi-professional decision made in consultation with a respiratory physiotherapist. It is well established that atelectasis develops in the dorsal areas of the lung when patients are in a supine position for any extended period of time (Ganong 2001). 'Prone positioning' a patient can help re-expand these collapsed areas, improve alveolar ventilation and hence gas exchange (Ball et al 2001). Additionally, the chest wall has a more favourable compliance curve in the prone position. Most patients will usually have improved oxygenation when prone and can tolerate being prone for 20 hours at a time, with regular pressure relief. It has not been established that prone positioning improves mortality but it can be useful in the patient that is difficult to oxygenate.

In normal circumstances the upper airway warms and humidifies air, so that it reaches core temperature and 100% saturation just below the carina. This process is known as gas conditioning (Williams et al 1996). During gas conditioning inspired air is also cleaned and filtered of foreign particles by the mucociliary transport system, which extends from the nasopharynx towards the bronchioles (Estes & Meduri 1995). Thus, gas conditioning optimises gas exchange and protects delicate lung tissue. The placement of an endotracheal tube bypasses this defence mechanism and the gas exchange function of the lung. The placement of the endotracheal tube physically shifts the conditioning, and heat and moisture recovery functions, further down the airway which would not normally be required to give up heat and moisture.

Hence in the intubated patient, the mucociliary transport system is the sole remaining mechanical defence system. The mucociliary transport system's function depends on the:

- thickness of the mucus
- depth of the aqueous layer
- cilia beat frequency.

If the temperature of inspired gas is less than core temperature the beat frequency of the cilia will reduce and the gas will be heated to a suboptimal temperature causing the relative humidity of the gas to be reduced. Less than optimal humidification results in a compromised mucociliary transport and pooling of mucus in the lower airways thus restricting gas exchange and being an ideal site for bacterial colonisation (Centers for Disease Control (CDC) 1994). Furthermore, the gel layer will lose moisture and become thicker. If suboptimal humidification is allowed to continue, cell damage might occur and the process of gas conditioning will move deeper into the lung. Increased thick mucus and reduced clearance of secretions from small airways results in reduced airway patency and lung compliance (Williams et al 1996). Thus the nurse must ensure that inspired gases are maintained at core temperature and humidity. Effective humidification will also maximise lung defence by reducing exposure to contaminants invading the airways by increasing clearance of contaminants through suctioning.

Cardiovascular complications: lessons learned

Mechanical ventilation through its delivery of positive intrathoracic pressure has an adverse effect on the heart. Consequently, patients require close assessment and monitoring of their cardiovascular function. Increasing intra-thoracic pressure decreases venous return to the right side of the heart and subsequently to the left side of the heart (Robb 1997b). Therefore patients may need additional fluid volume to maintain cardiac output. The nurse must be mindful to observe cardiovascular parameters in relation to ventilator airway pressure. Decreased cardiac output due to positive pressure ventilation is often ameliorated by fluid administration. The degree of cardiac compromise may often limit the amount of PEEP that a child can tolerate and hence what the intensivist is willing to use.

Modes of ventilation

The goals of assisted ventilation are to achieve adequate gas exchange while at the same time minimising damage to the lungs or interference to the circulation. The review of the risks and side effects of positive pressure ventilation possibly goes some way towards explaining why there are quite so many modes of ventilation available today.

This chapter will now turn to a brief synopsis of the common approaches to ventilation based on physiological principles. It is by no means exhaustive or complete, and is not intended to be. For a more exhaustive discussion of management issues surrounding mechanical ventilation of the sick child refer to one of the major intensive care texts, such as the 'Manual of pediatric critical care' (Hazinski 1999).

Ventilators (Fig. 45.8) deliver gas to the lungs using positive pressure at a certain rate. The amount of gas delivered can be limited by time, pressure or volume. The duration can be cycled by time, pressure or flow. The basic terms used with ventilators are the following:

- Peak inspiratory pressure (PIP): indicates the maximum pressure that has occurred during the last ventilatory cycle
- Positive end expiratory pressure (PEEP): is the baseline pressure and controls functional residual capacity (FRC)
- Pressure above PEEP (PAP)
- Mean airway pressure (MAP)
- Inspiratory time (Ti): shown in seconds
- Expiratory time (Te): shown in seconds

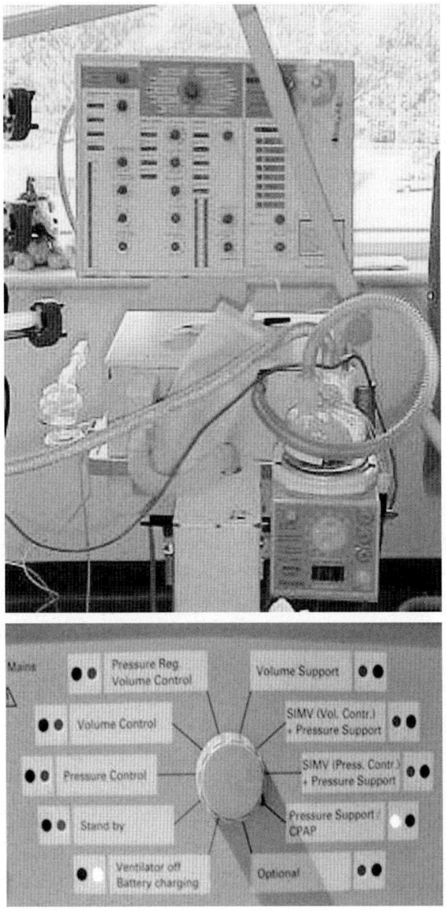

Fig. 45.8 • A ventilator (top) and a close-up of the control panel (below).

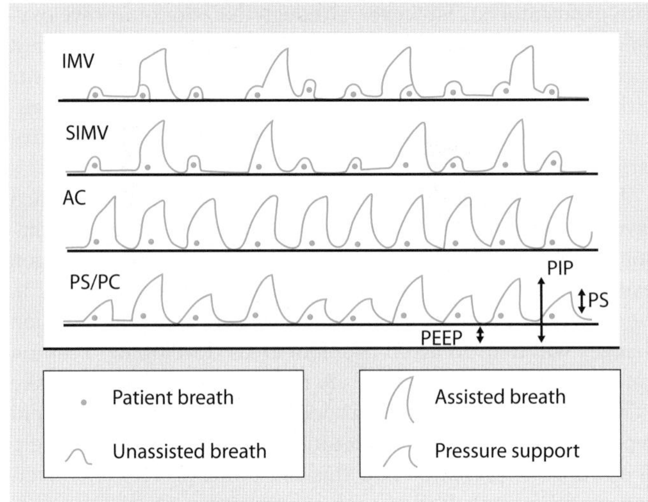

Fig. 45.9 • Ventilator modes.

- Tidal volume (Vt): amount of gas delivered with each breath
- Minute volume (MV): amount of gas breathed in or out over 1 minute = Vt ∞ Rate
- Continuous positive airway pressure (CPAP).

Note: CPAP is equivalent to PEEP, except the term is usually used when referring to patients who are not intubated but on what is called nasal CPAP (NCPAP).

The common ventilation modes illustrated in Figure 45.9 are the following:

- Assisted control mode (AC): the ventilator will guarantee that the patient receives a set tidal volume or peak airway pressure with every breath. The patient can breathe 'above' the set rate but will receive full support regardless of their effort.
- Intermittent mandatory ventilation (IMV): the ventilator supports breaths only at the set rate and interval. Breaths 'above' the set rate are not supported.
- Synchronised intermittent mandatory ventilation (SIMV): the ventilator synchronises an IMV 'breath' with the patient's effort. If, for example, the set rate is 10, then every 6 seconds the patient will receive a machine triggered breath. In between those 10 breaths, the patient is free to breathe but those breaths are not supported. These breaths can be supported if a 'pressure support mode' is added.
- Pressure support or pressure control mode (PS/PC): the ventilator supplies pressure support but no set rate. A patient needs to generate a certain amount of work to trigger it. Additionally, a patient has to breathe through an endotracheal tube that is almost always narrower than their own airway and ventilate the increased dead space imposed by the ventilator circuit. A patient may not be able to generate adequate tidal volumes for these reasons. To compensate for this increase in the work of breathing, pressure support is given.

Irrespective of mode, whenever a breath is supported by the ventilator, the limit of the support is determined by a preset pressure or volume. Thus, if volume is set, pressure varies and conversely, if pressure is set, volume varies according to the patient's lung compliance.

In CPAP, PEEP is elevated baseline airway pressure (Fig. 45.10). The two terms 'PEEP' and 'CPAP' are used interchangeably and can lead to confusion. They are in fact the same thing. The concept of PEEP is that a pressure is applied at the end of expiration to maintain alveolar recruitment and can, therefore, improve oxygenation and ventilation. Airway

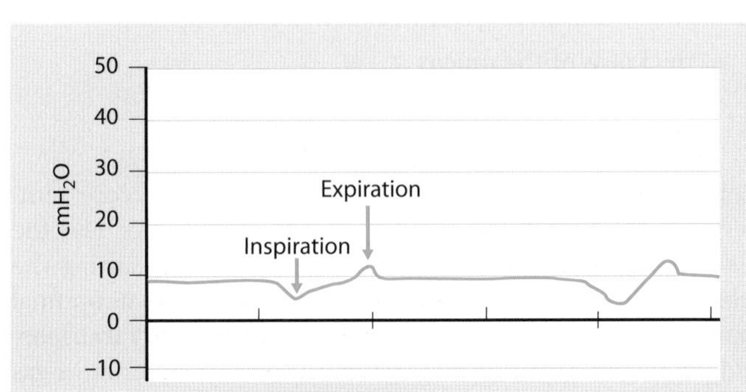

Fig. 45.10 • CPAP – pressure wave.

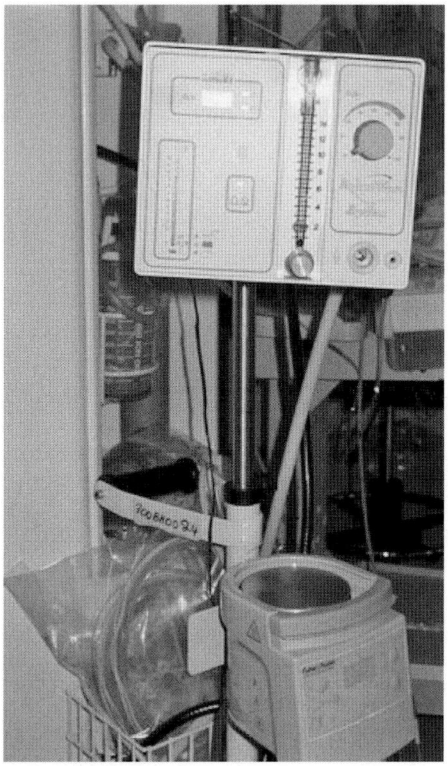

Fig. 45.11 • CPAP driver.

pressure is kept positive and not allowed to return to atmospheric. PEEP is usually set at between 4 and 10 cmH_2O, which is usually enough to ensure that the patient receives sufficient tidal volume (Pearson 2002). It can also stent open areas of trachea malacia (abnormal softening) and thereby improve ventilation and oxygenation even if these areas in of themselves do not participate in gas exchange. A great advantage is that CPAP can be delivered non-invasively either by nasal prong or mask (Fig. 45.11).

As ventilator technology has advanced, newer modes have been developed such as, pressure-regulated volume control (PRVC), volume support, inverse ratio (IRV), airway-pressure release ventilation (APRV) and high-frequency oscillatory ventilation (HFOV). Some are variations of volume or pressure modes and some are completely unrelated to conventional mechanical ventilation. It is important to recognise that none of these modes has yet been shown to be better than another or to reduce mortality for any disease.

Ventilator settings

The initial settings prescribed and set by the intensivist for both volume and pressure are similar. Except in volume control a tidal volume is set at usually 8–10 mL/kg and in pressure control the peak airway pressure is set. The starting peak airways pressure is set at what is needed to adequately inflate the patient's chest and generate breath sounds and is usually 15–20 cmH_2O above PEEP. The starting breath rate is usually one that would be physiologically appropriate for the age of the patient. Immediately after intubation patients are usually placed on a FiO_2 of 1.0 and are weaned down as long as the oxygen saturations remain acceptable. PEEP is usually set at 5 cmH_2O and then

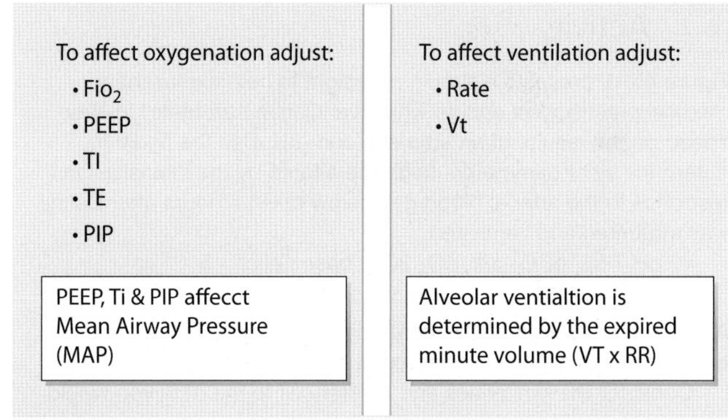

To affect oxygenation adjust:
• Fio2
• PEEP
• TI
• TE
• PIP
PEEP, Ti & PIP affecct Mean Airway Pressure (MAP)
To affect ventilation adjust:
• Rate
• Vt
Alveolar ventialtion is determined by the expired minute volume (VT x RR)

Fig. 45.12 • Simple paradigm to explain likely ventilation setting changes.

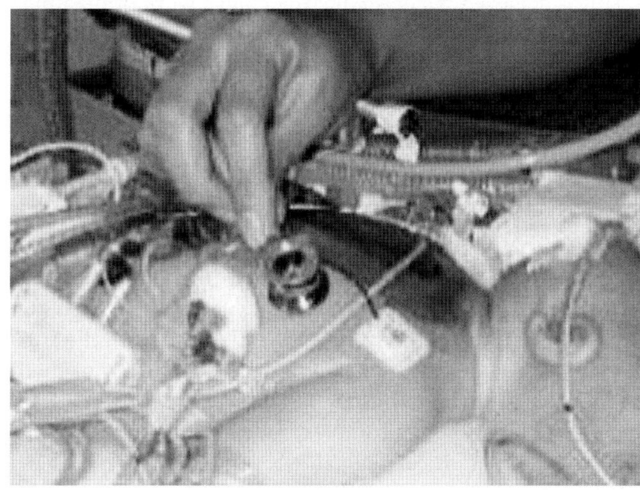

Fig. 45.13 • Nursing assessment.

increased as needed to achieve acceptable oxygen saturations with a FiO_2 less than 0.6 (Pearson 2002) (Fig. 45.12).

Respiratory assessment and monitoring of the ventilated child

Clinical observation of the ventilated child is mandatory. Generally it is the intensive care nurse who observes, assesses, communicates, monitors, analyses and interprets data in order to effectively care for the critically ill child 24 hours a day (Fig. 45.13). In addition to the usual respiratory and cardiovascular observations discussed in Chapter 4, the critical care team must observe adaptation of the ventilator to the child and the degree of harmony between these two partners.

Activity

To ensure patency of the airways, the nurse must ensure that active humidification is set to administer inspired gas at 37°C and 100% relative humidity in the lungs to assist lung clearance of secretions from the endotracheal tube by suctioning using an evidence-based technique. Trauma, infection and cardiopulmonary compromise are well-documented adverse events associated with a poor technique:

- Read the review by Pollard (2001).

Activity

Figure 45.12 presents a simple paradigm to help explain how medical practitioners decide which ventilation parameter to alter based on the results of an arterial blood gas. Use the figure to determine what parameters might be altered by the intensivist in response to the arterial blood gas below taken 4 hours after Daniel was intubated and ventilated:

- pH 7.56, pCO_2 3.2, pO_2 20.0, base deficit –5
- oxygen saturations were 100%.

Analyse your local intensive care observation chart and note the breadth of data that are collected at least hourly.

Consider the similarities and differences to the data you would collect on a child receiving oxygen therapy on a children's medical ward.

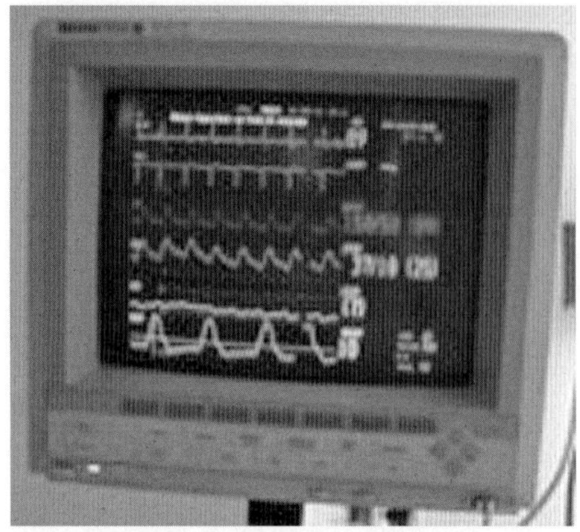

Fig. 45.14 • A monitor.

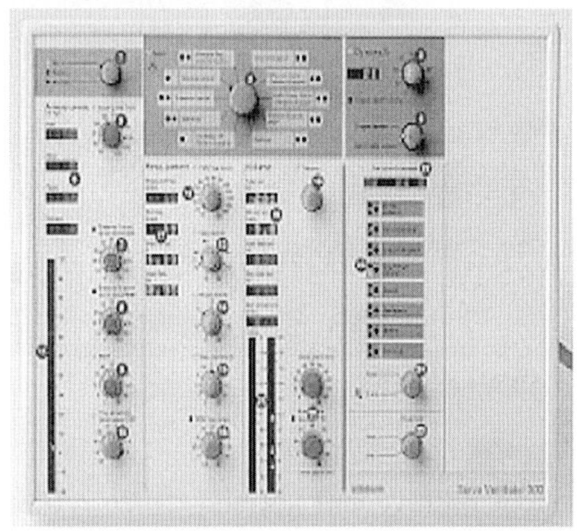

Fig. 45.15 • Ventilator board.

This is achieved by: observing the child's work of breathing and spontaneous chest movement against ventilator induced chest movement; regular 3–4-hourly blood gas analysis (as often as quarter-hourly if the child is unstable); constant cardiorespiratory observation; monitoring and hourly recordings together with ventilator observations. 'Monitoring' is a term usually reserved for automatic visual display of patient data such as temperature, pulse, respiration and blood pressure (Fig. 45.14). A continuous monitoring system, with safety alarm limits set, providing a minute-by-minute accurate picture of the child, means that effective decision making is carried out in 'real time' and at the 'right time' (Wheatley 2001). In the critical care environment the capabilities and complexity of modern technology are used to their best advantage. Deciding what needs to be monitored is complex but fundamentally essential in the care of the critically ill patient.

In addition to the respiratory monitoring techniques covered in Chapter 4, the nurse observing the ventilated child will monitor end tidal carbon dioxide ($ETCO_2$) and record ventilation parameters, which are analysed in the light of the child's vital signs, pulse oximetry and arterial blood gas results in collaboration with the medical team (Fig. 45.15).

Capnography is the measurement of carbon dioxide (CO_2) in each breath of the respiratory cycle. The capnograph displays a waveform of CO_2 (measured in kPa or mmHg) and it displays the value of the CO_2 at the end of exhalation, which is known as the end tidal CO_2 (Fig. 45.16). The capnograph sensor is placed between the endotracheal tube and the breathing circuit.

$ETCO_2$ provides a non-invasive method of evaluating ventilation and is helpful in assessing placement of the endotracheal tube. CO_2 is exhaled through the trachea and not usually from the oesophagus and so the measurement of CO_2 in the expired air distinguishes tracheal from oesophageal intubation. Provided the patient has a stable cardiac status and stable body temperature, an $ETCO_2$ with a normal capnograph trace approximates to the partial pressure of CO_2 in arterial blood ($PaCO_2$) (normal $PaCO_2$ is approximately 5.3 kPa) (Bhende 2001). The arterial PCO_2 is normally 0.3–0.7 kPa higher than the $ETCO_2$ reading and thus can be used to reduce the frequency of blood gas analysis required.

Figure 45.17 illustrates the different components of the capnograph trace. The first phase occurs during inspiration. The second phase is the onset of expiration, which results in a rapid increase in CO_2. The third phase, the expiratory plateau, occurs as the CO_2 is exhaled from all the alveoli. The highest point (4) of the plateau is known as the $ETCO_2$ and marks the end of expiration. Phase four is the onset of inspiration. If the waveform does not return to the baseline during inspiration this indicates that re-breathing of exhaled gas is occurring and is accompanied by a rise in $ETCO_2$ reading. Sudden loss of the capnograph, that is a decrease to zero, should alert the clinician to a catastrophic event such as oesophageal intubation, total obstruction, or ventilator malfunction. An exponential decrease of $ETCO_2$ can be seen due to loss of pulmonary blood

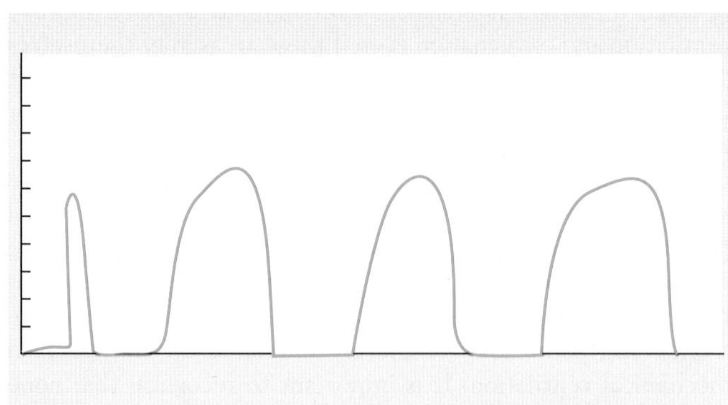

Fig. 45.16 • End tidal CO_2 showing on a caprogram display.

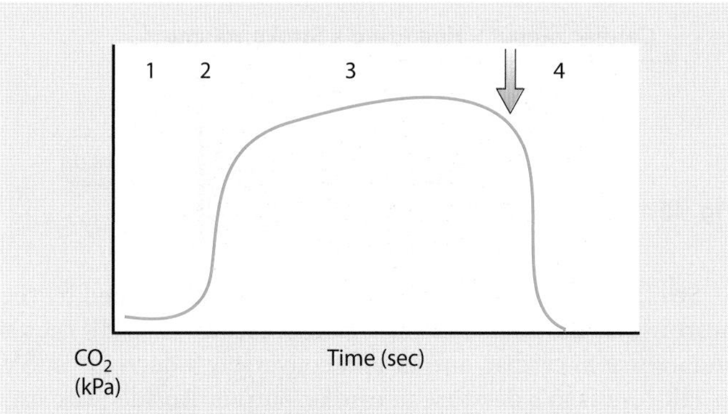

Fig. 45.17 • The capnograph trace.

flow as in cardiac arrest or sudden hypotension for example. A gradual decrease in $ETCO_2$ indicates decreased production such as in hypothermia. Rising $ETCO_2$ can be seen either due to increased CO_2 production, such as in sepsis, malignant hyperthermia, or due to decreased CO_2 elimination when there is decreased alveolar ventilation (Bhende 2001).

Scenario

One hour after intubation, the nurse noted that Daniel's heart rate was 145, blood pressure 130/92, respiratory rate 30 and oxygen saturation 100%. Ominously, the $ETCO_2$ that had been reading 5.6 kPa had increased to 9.7 kPa.

PROFESSIONAL CONVERSATION

Michael, a registered children's nurse new to PICU, summons his mentor for help and records this learning episode in his reflective diary.

Trouble-shooting

If after intubation or at any time during ventilation therapy a child's condition deteriorates the pneumonic 'DOPE' is a useful tool to help make a systematic patient assessment and perform appropriate interventions when waiting for the arrival of the intensivist who had been asked to attend Daniel. Is the deterioration as a result of:

- D = displaced tube?
- O = obstructed tube?
- P = pneumothorax?
- E = equipment?

Assess A: the airway first – is the tube still in? Is it in the right position? The endotracheal tube was still at 13 cm at the lips. Had the endotracheal tube not been in place it would have been removed and bag-valve-mask ventilation instituted.

Assess B: breathing next – is the chest rising? Had the chest not been seen to rise with ventilation Daniel would have been disconnected from the ventilator and bag valve inflations given to eliminate the ventilator circuit as the problem. 'Bagging' by hand can also allow the facilitator to gauge compliance.

Are breath sounds present and equal? Changes in breath sounds? Endotracheal tubes can become obstructed with secretions or be dislodged especially if the patient moves (or is moved)? Need for endotracheal tube suction? Mucus plugs can block lower airways as easily as they can obstruct the endotracheal tube. A suction catheter was placed through the endotracheal tube to be certain that it was patent and to rule out obstruction by mucous plug. It was patent and suction did not return any abnormal secretions. The chest rise appeared to be symmetrical bilaterally and breathe sounds were unchanged on auscultation. We noted the increasing blood pressure and administered sedation. Despite these actions the problem persisted.

The entire ventilatory circuit from the level of the endotracheal tube back to the ventilator was checked to find that the tubing was kinked thus restricting flow in the circuit. The tubing was repositioned to relieve the obstruction and Daniel's $ETCO_2$ started to decrease immediately back to its previous level. If this had not revealed a problem and the child's vital signs were stable we would have considered the potential of malfunction of the $ETCO_2$ device.

Extubation

As discussed earlier, children require respiratory support for many pulmonary and non-pulmonary problems. In the majority of cases, intubation and mechanical ventilation are necessary until the underlying cause of the respiratory failure is improved or resolved. The focus of management and care is thus facilitating the resumption of spontaneous ventilation that is 'weaning'. Weaning is essentially the transfer of demands from the ventilator to the child. It is important to assess the individual child's ability to handle the increased demands that extubation will place upon the child. In practice the critical care team is always weaning the child by progressively reducing ventilator support settings as the child's condition improves thus minimising the adverse effects of ventilation. Progressive reduction of rate, FiO_2 and PEEP demands that the child does more and is guided by arterial blood gas results. A child is usually ready to be extubated when he or she (Pearson 2002):

- is able to protect his or her own airway
- has a FiO_2 of less than 0.35
- is breathing at a comfortable physiological rate
- is receiving an pressure support that is just enough to compensate for the added work of breathing imposed by a ventilator circuit and ETT
- requires a PEEP less than 5 cmH_2O.

Haemodynamic control

Scenario

On admission to PICU, additional vital signs were obtained:

- Daniel was awake and irritable and wanting to remain in Emma's lap
- respiratory rate: 70
- marked sternal and intercostals recession
- oxygen saturation: 95%
- heart rate: 200
- radial and dorsalis pulses: weak and thready

- skin was cool, dry and pale
- capillary refill: 4 seconds
- blood pressure: 90/60 mmHg
- he was conscious and responding to his mother Emma
- he appeared exhausted
- blood glucose: 1.7 mmol/L
- axilla temperature: 37.5°C
- no skin rash noted
- an arterial gas was obtained: pH 7.25, pCO_2 7.6, pO_2 22, base deficit –3.

In this scenario, Daniel is admitted to PICU and a rapid cardiopulmonary assessment was undertaken by the admitting critical care nurse which was documented as above. You will note from the data collected that there are signs and symptoms of cardiovascular instability for example marked tachycardia, poor perfusion (capillary refill >2 seconds), hypoglycaemia and a reduced level of consciousness. In reality, Daniel's cardiovascular status would have been managed almost simultaneously with his respiratory failure by the critical care team following a systematic ABC approach. However, for the purposes of this chapter respiratory support and haemodynamic control has been artificially separated for ease of presentation and to facilitate learning in a step-by-step approach.

Haemodynamic principles

The management of critically ill patients is based on knowledge of fundamental physiological variables. Monitoring of the haemodynamic status of these patients has developed from the non-invasive monitoring of a single parameter to the more invasive technological monitoring of multiple parameters we see today. This allows a comprehensive analysis of haemodynamic status enabling healthcare practitioners to not only provide effective treatment but importantly to anticipate deleterious events and intervene proactively in advance.

Haemodynamics refers to the forces, such as preload and afterload that affect the circulation of blood throughout the body. Critical care nurses assess the stability of these factors when they take a blood pressure or palpate a pulse. Although the interaction of these forces is quite complicated, the concepts can be more easily understood by substituting the word, 'stretch' for preload and 'resistance' for afterload. Preload and afterload are closely related. Put simply, they reflect the heart's effectiveness in managing blood flow out of its chambers that is cardiac output. This chapter will now turn to a more detailed explanation and discussion of the determinants of cardiac output introduced above.

Cardiac output

Cardiac output (Fig. 45.18) is defined as the volume of blood pumped by the heart in 1 minute, and is represented by the equation:

$$\text{Cardiac output (CO)} = \text{Stroke volume (SV)} \times \text{Heart rate (HR)}$$

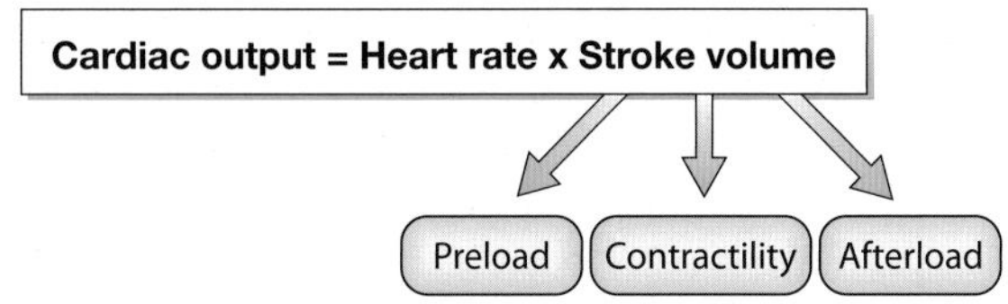

Fig. 45.18 • Determinants of cardiac output.

Stroke volume (SV) is the amount of blood pumped by the heart in one contraction. Thus, an increase in SV or HR causes an increase in cardiac output and conversely a decrease in SV or HR results in a decrease in cardiac output. An adequate cardiac output is essential to supply oxygen and nutrients to major organs and peripheral tissues. For example, a reduction in cardiac output may diminish blood flow to the brain and result in an altered level of consciousness. Alterations in heart rate, contractility, preload and afterload can affect cardiac output.

What is contractility?

Contractility is the force generated by the heart during each contraction. The contractility of the heart can be influenced by what is known as the preload. Preload is the force that stretches the contractile muscle fibres, the myofibrils, of the resting heart. This 'stretch' is determined by the amount of blood present within the left ventricle prior to contraction. The greater the volume of blood in the left ventricle, the greater the stretch on the myofibrils the greater the contractile force and thus, the greater the preload. An adequately filled and stretched left ventricle should briskly contract to eject blood. However, there is a point where the stretch (fill) is insufficient and cardiac output is diminished. Likewise there is a point where the stretch (fill) is too extreme that output is diminished. This relationship between preload (stretch) and contractile force is explained by the Frank-Starling mechanism (Fig. 45.19).

Starling's mechanism states that, up to a point, the more the myofibrils are stretched in diastole, the more forcefully the heart contracts in the next systole. A simple analogy is an elastic band. If we apply a moderate stretch to the elastic band it will 'ping' back with moderate force. Likewise, if we apply a strong stretch to the elastic band it will 'ping' back with greater force. However, if we repeatedly provide too great a force to

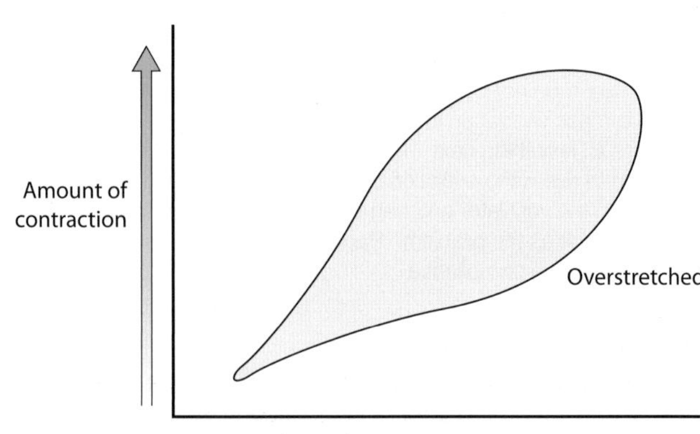

Fig. 45.19 • The Frank–Starling mechanism.

the elastic band it will very quickly lose its elasticity and fail to do its task. It is much the same with the myofibrils in the heart, if over-burdened, they will eventually fail; this is represented in Figure 45.19. It must be remembered, however, that children, particularly under the age of 8 years have insufficient myocardial contractile proteins to significantly increase contractility and are therefore largely dependent on an increase in heart rate to maintain cardiac output.

Stroke volume is affected by preload, contractile force and afterload. As discussed, preload is the amount of blood delivered to the heart during diastole but this is in turn dependent on venous return. Venous return can be affected by variable venous capacitance known as afterload, which can increase or decrease blood return to the heart (preload).

Understanding afterload

Afterload is the resistance against which the heart must pump. When the heart overcomes resistance, the blood can be ejected. Sources of resistance include blood pressure (BP), systemic vascular resistance (SVR), and the condition of the aortic valve.

$$\text{Blood pressure (BP)} = \text{Cardiac output (CO)} \times \text{Systemic vascular resistance (SVR)}$$

When there is arterial vasoconstriction, as in shock or aortic valve narrowing as in aortic stenosis, the ventricle has to create a greater amount of pressure, or afterload to overcome that resistance – a useful analogy is that it is akin to opening a door against a strong wind.

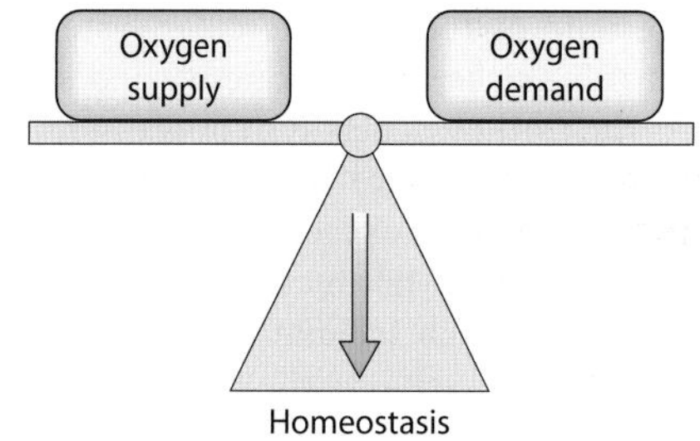

Fig. 45.20 • Homeostasis.

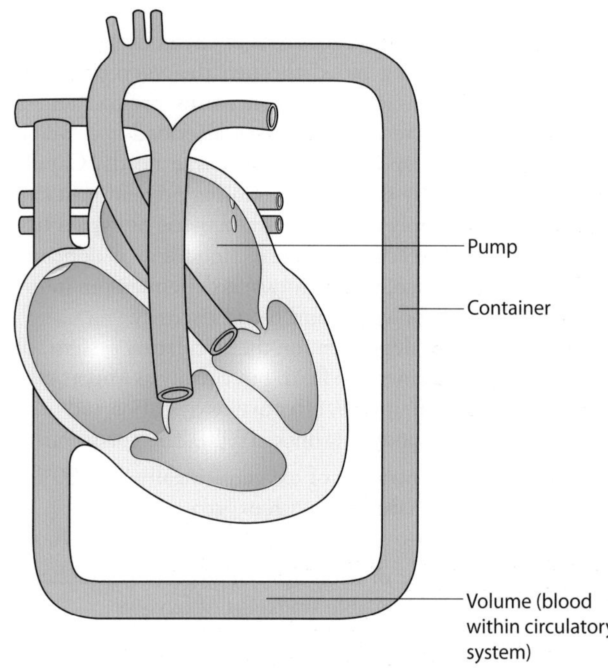

Fig. 45.21 • Pump, container and fluid analogy.

What is shock?

The body's cells require a constant supply of oxygen and nutrients and elimination of carbon dioxide and waste products. These needs are fulfilled by the circulatory system in conjunction with the respiratory system, central nervous system and gastrointestinal system. The ultimate goal of this integrated control of the circulation is to maintain blood flow to the tissues to the optimum extent. Normally the body can compensate for some reduction in tissue perfusion through a variety of compensatory mechanisms. However, when compensation fails, shock develops. Shock has been defined as '... a complex clinical syndrome that is the body's response to cellular metabolic deficiency' (ALSG 2001 p 111). It is characterised by inadequate delivery of oxygen and metabolic substrates to meet the metabolic demands of the tissues that is a state of imbalance, and a threat to homeostasis (Fig. 45.20).

Metabolism in normal conditions is aerobic. In contrast, metabolism in poor perfusion states is anaerobic and although glucose is broken down into pyruvic acid, there is not enough oxygen present to metabolise it and pyruvic acid accumulates along with other metabolic acids (Marieb 2002). Anaerobic metabolism uses glycogen and fat for energy leading to a build up of lactic acid and carbon dioxide. Shock occurs first at cellular level resulting in generalised cellular hypoxia (starvation) and widespread impairment of cellular metabolism. This process if unchecked leads to cell death, tissue death, organ failure, system failure and ultimately death (ALSG 2001). Using a well-known analogy (ALSG 2001) (Fig. 45.21), the characteristics of shock involve dysfunction of the body's:

- pump (heart)
- fluid volume (blood)
- container (blood vessels).

Inadequate tissue perfusion can result in derangement of any of these components. The heart is the pump of the circulatory system. Put simply, it receives blood from the venous system, pumps it to the lungs to be oxygenated and then pumps it to organs and peripheral tissues. When the heart 'fails' the output is reduced. The amount of blood pumped around the body by the heart is dependent on:

- heart rate
- ability to empty the heart, which depends on:
  - contractility
  - resistance to flow and blood pressure
- ability to fill the heart, which depends on:
  - amount of blood returning for re-circulation
  - filling pressures versus compliance.

Blood is the fluid of the cardiovascular system. Blood is a viscous fluid that is thicker, more adhesive and slower moving than water. As the cardiovascular system is essentially a closed system, an adequate volume of blood must be present to fill the system. Blood transports oxygen, carbon dioxide, nutrients, hormones, metabolic waste products and heat.

The blood vessels which include arteries, arterioles, capillaries, venules and veins, serve as the container for the cardiovascular system. This container provides a continuous, closed, pressurised pipeline that moves blood under the control of the autonomic nervous system, which delivers haemoglobin saturated with oxygen to diffuse into cells at end organs. The vessels regulate blood flow to different areas of the body by adjusting their size and re-routing blood through the microcirculation. Contraction of venous circulation increases preload and SV, but contraction of arterioles increases afterload and BP. The microcirculation is responsive to local tissue needs. Capillary beds can adjust size by opening and closing pre and post capillary sphincters to supply undernourished tissue or bypass tissue with no immediate needs. Therefore, blood flow is dependent on peripheral resistance, which in turn is dependent on internal diameter, length of the vessel and blood viscosity.

Tissue perfusion is dependent on the circulatory system, consisting of pump, container and fluid. But equally as important are conditions for optimal uptake, effective oxygenation and utilisation of oxygen in the body (Hazinski 1999). The conditions are:

- adequate concentration of oxygen – ideally 97–100% of haemoglobin is saturated with oxygen
- oxygen diffuses across the alveolar–capillary membrane
- adequate number of haemoglobin molecules attached to red blood cells to enable transport of oxygen
- adequate and efficient off-loading of oxygen at the tissue–cellular level.

These conditions are often referred to as the 'Fick principle'.

In summary, it can be seen that shock is a cellular state of imbalance resulting in inadequate tissue perfusion and can be caused by either one or a combination of the following components (Fig. 45.22):

- An inadequate pump:
  - inadequate preload
  - inadequate contractile strength
  - inadequate heart rate.

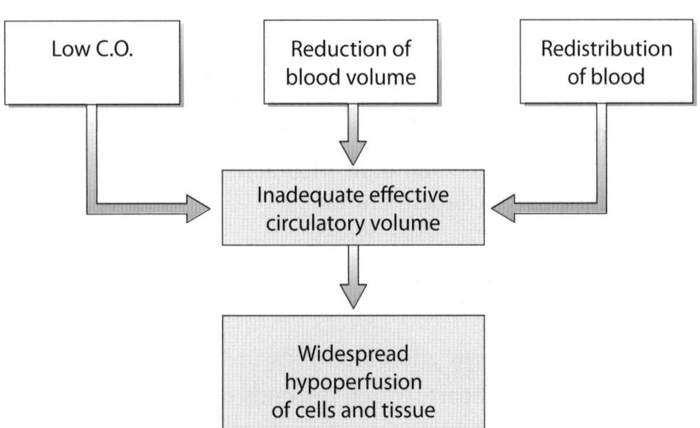

Fig. 45.22 • Common pathway.

- An inadequate fluid volume:
  - insufficient fluid volume.
- An inadequate container:
  - excessive dilation without increase in fluid volume
  - excessive SVR.

Stages of shock

The three recognised stages of shock (ALSG 2001) are commonly identified as:

- compensated shock
- decompensated shock
- irreversible shock.

Compensated shock

In the initial stage, cardiac output and perfusion are decreased and the body acts to defend itself and preserve major organs by way of a series of reflex mechanisms involving the central nervous system and neurohormonal systems. These reflex compensatory mechanisms occur in the macrocirculation, in the kidney and the microcirculation. For this reason, this stage is often referred to as 'compensated' shock. These subtle indicators make shock difficult to detect at this stage especially in children who, as a result of usually young healthy major organs, are efficient compensators.

Decompensated shock

If untreated, shock will progress to 'decompensated shock' where compensatory mechanisms fail and shunting of blood to vital areas becomes ineffective resulting in severe hypoperfusion. A loss of autoregulation of the microcirculation and increased capillary permeability causes reduced blood volume to the right side of the heart and reduced cardiac output. This in turn reduces blood pressure, which reduces coronary artery perfusion. Myocardial oxygen demand then exceeds myocardial oxygen supply. Imbalance of arterial blood supply to the myocardium causes arrhythmias, muscle ischaemia, and a self-perpetuating cycle of reduced cardiac output and cardiac failure occurs. Also in prolonged loss of cardiac output:

- cerebral blood flow is reduced
- renal tubules become ischaemic
- prolonged vasoconstriction causes ulceration of the stomach wall allowing bacteria and toxins to cross into the bloodstream
- bilirubin is not metabolised by the underperfused liver and waste products build up
- cell death causes release of enzymes from the pancreas, which depress the myocardium
- ischaemia of alveolar cells inhibits surfactant production in the lungs causing alveolar collapse, atelectasis, and reduced pulmonary compliance leads to acute respiratory distress syndrome (ARDS)
- increased pulmonary vascular permeability causes interstitial and intra-alveolar oedema.

Irreversible shock

The final stage of shock, sometimes also referred to as the 'refractory stage' is a profound condition where vital organs falter as a result of being starved of oxygen for too long:

- hypotension is unresponsive to drugs and fluids
- severe hypoxaemia is unresponsive to oxygen therapy
- anuria and build-up of toxic waste as the renal system fails
- liver causes hyperglycaemia and build-up of waste products and allows no metabolism of drugs
- pancreatic dysfunction further affects myocardial contractility, haematologically
- multiple emboli form, intravascular clotting and severe coagulopathy
- neurologically, there is reduced response to stimuli and sympathetic stress response due to failure of the medulla causing circulatory failure and death eventually occurs.

Early recognition of shock

Early recognition of shock is essential. The outcome of children once in decompensated shock is, in general, very poor (Pearson 2002). Early recognition of the child in compensated shock and prompt and appropriate intervention as a result has been shown to reduce mortality and secondary morbidity. As already stated, the early indicators of shock are subtle and difficult to detect largely because children who as a result of usually young healthy major organs are efficient compensators. To recognise the initial body response to a loss of cardiac output, the nurse must be fully cognisant of the compensatory mechanisms used by the cardiovascular system. In addition, a thorough knowledge and understanding of the pathophysiology of different types of shock together with a high index of suspicion facilitates recognition of these subtle signs and symptoms. It is to a physiological description of the compensatory mechanisms of shock that this chapter now turns.

Shock: compensatory mechanisms

Young children are able to maintain a normal cardiac output and thus remain normotensive until vascular and cardiac decompensation is imminent (Partrick et al 2002). To recognise the initial signs of shock a high index of suspicion can help to raise your awareness of the subtleties of compensation. Ask yourself if the child is at risk:

- Has the child got a history of diarrhoea, vomiting and decreased oral intake?
- Has he or she had surgery recently?
- Has he or she got allergic symptoms and recent exposure to a known allergen?
- Has he or she got a congenital heart defect?

The cardiovascular system is regulated by many feedback control loops and as a result, its responses are not simple. At the onset of shock, during the compensatory stage, the systemic and microcirculatory system work together and their activities tend to remain coordinated (Martini 1998). There is a combination of neural, hormonal, chemical and humoral mechanisms for defending cardiac output.

Mean arterial blood pressure (MAP) is sensed by baroreceptors located in the aortic and carotid bodies which monitor the circulation closely for changes in blood pressure. These receptors control arterial pressure mainly by adjusting heart rate and arteriolar vessel radius. Baroreceptors respond to small changes in vascular tone and pressure and message the sympathetic nervous system (SNS) to decrease vagal tone which increases heart rate and decreases coronary artery resistance thus improving myocardial oxygen supply (Fig. 45.23).

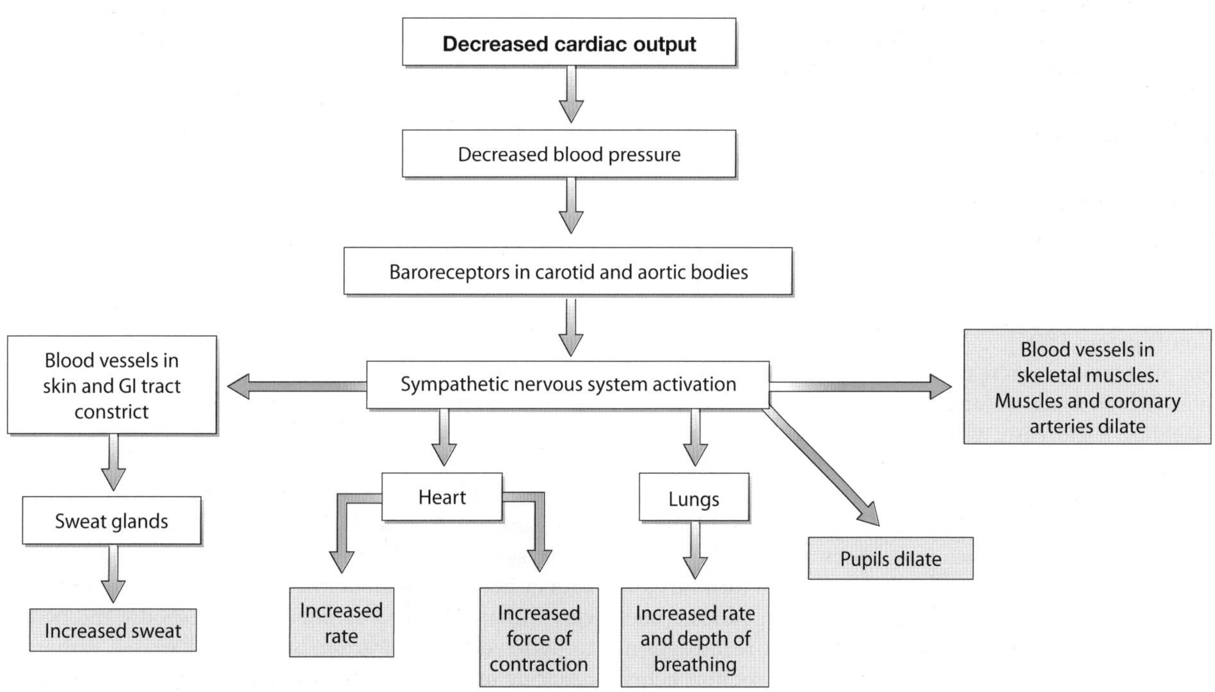

Fig. 45.23 • Neural compensatory mechanism.

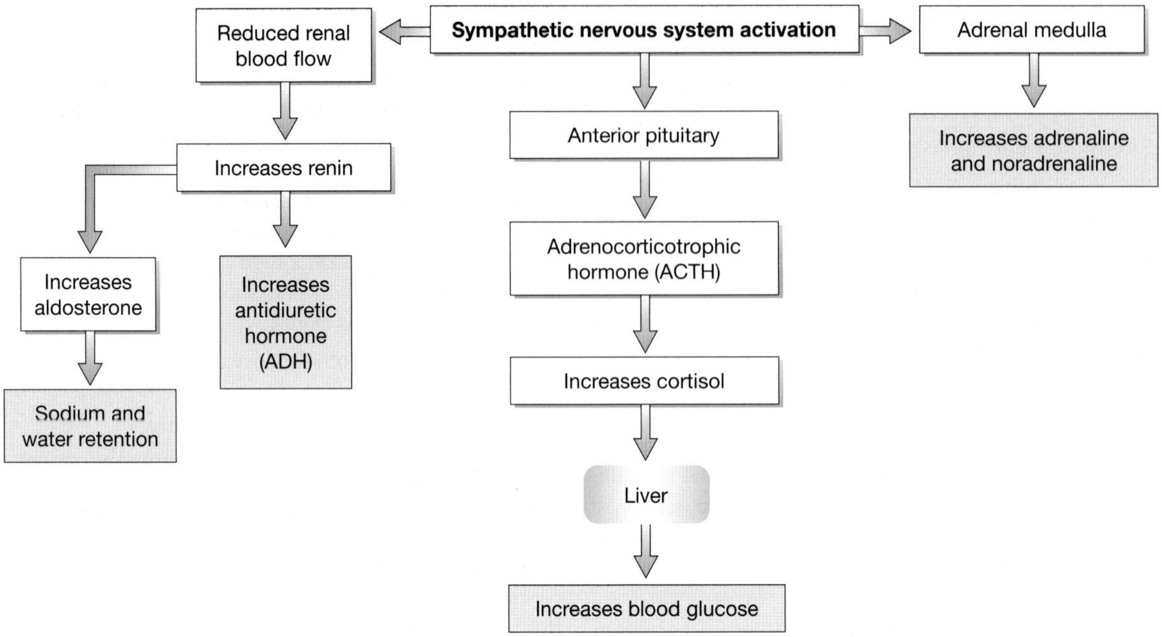

Fig. 45.24 • Hormonal compensatory mechanism.

MAP is also the basis for autoregulation by the heart, lungs and brain.

Autoregulation is the automatic adaptation of the radius of an arteriolar vessel in an organ to maintain constant blood flow over a wide range of mean pressures to protect functioning of that organ (Darovic 1995). Arterioles are the primary sites that contribute to systemic vascular resistance (SVR). In addition, in the microcirculation, adrenergic control of the arterioles is a major determinant of blood flow into the capillaries. The adrenal gland in response will increase catecholamine release. Catecholamines consist of adrenaline and noradrenaline which are endogenous vasoconstrictors which cause added vasoconstriction in an added attempt to improve cardiac output (McCance & Huether 1994). Catecholamines also enhance cardiac contractility and heart rate. Constriction of blood reservoirs such as the skin, skeletal muscle, liver and spleen disgorge blood to be shunted from the capillary beds to flow directly from arterioles into the venous system thus increasing circulating blood volume (Figs 45.24, 45.25). This arteriovenous shunting helps to redirect blood flow to vital organs. Arteriovenous shunting is one reason why blood pressure data alone are not a reliable indicator of peripheral tissue perfusion (Epstein 1997).

Renin production is increased as a result of decreased renal perfusion, which leads to angiotensinogen production eventually yielding angiotensin which is a potent vasoconstrictor. Antidiuretic hormone (ADH) is released from the posterior pituitary gland another potent vasoconstrictor which prevents the elimination of water. The continued failure of the kidneys to eliminate and excrete hydrogen ions causes a metabolic acidosis and consequent decrease in blood pH which in turn further impairs myocardial function and cardiac output. Aldosterone is released stimulated by ADH causing sodium reabsorption in the renal distal tubules and as water follows sodium helps to conserve both sodium and water. Retained sodium assists in the reabsorption of tissue fluids (Fig. 45.24). Decreased mean arterial pressure leads to arteriolar constriction, which together with decreased pressure in capillaries leads to decreased hydrostatic pressure that, due to reabsorbed sodium, is less than osmotic pressure assists increased reabsorption of fluid 15 mL/kg/hour from the tissues (Prior 1999).

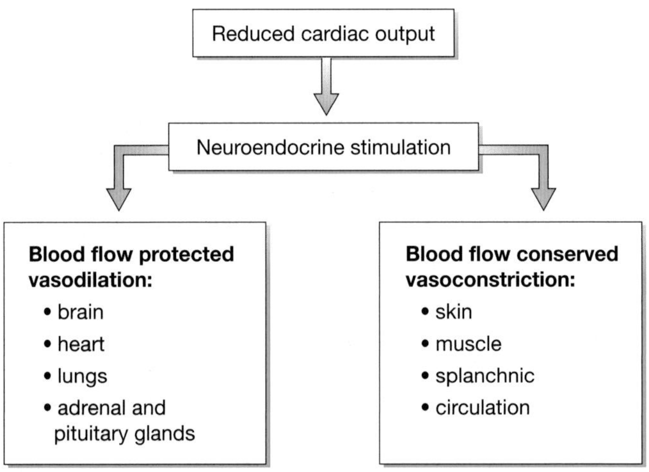

Fig. 45.25 • Chemical compensatory mechanism.

Chemoreceptors located locally in tissue beds sense the hypoxia due to the now inadequate blood flow to the tissues as a result of systemic circulation constriction and cause further vasoconstriction (Marieb 2002). The cells become starved of oxygen. Tissue begins to metabolise anaerobically and the patient becomes acidotic. Respiratory function during shock is very important in compensation. In response the body begins to hyperventilate in order to blow off excess carbon dioxide resulting in respiratory alkalosis (Fig. 45.25). This hyperventilation will also help to improve venous return (pump model).

In summary, the mechanisms for restoring cardiovascular homeostasis are:

- redistribution of blood flow: attempt to preserve perfusion to vital organs
- augmentation of cardiac output:
  - increased heart rate
  - increased peripheral resistance
- restoration of intravascular volume: arteriovenous shunting.

These protective mechanisms will eventually cease to function and circulatory failure will ensue if not recognised and intervention initiated aggressively (Edwards 1998). Again, blood pressure is not the key to deciding whether or not a child is in shock, although it does help to decide whether they are in compensated or decompensated shock. Much of the body's response revolves around the maintenance of normal aerobic metabolism and thus maintenance of viable cell function and measurement of the degree of tissue oxygenation in vital organs. The body's compensatory mechanisms are beneficial in the early stages but these homeostatic mechanisms soon become counterproductive. Nurses play a major role in recognising shock and play a direct role in influencing timely and appropriate intervention in conjunction with medical colleagues.

Types of shock

Any reduction of blood volume by whatever means (pump, container, fluid) can cause shock. Shock is classified according to the causes to three classes (Table 45.1):

- Hypovolaemic
- Cardiogenic
- Distributive.

It is important to be aware that more than one type of shock may be present at the same time.

Activity

Hypovolaemic shock is a volume problem:

- What signs and symptoms would you expect to see in a child in hypovolaemic shock?

Table 45.1 Classification and causes of shock

Classification	Clinical causes	Primary mechanism
Hypovolaemic	Circulating fluid volume loss	Exogenous blood, plasma, fluid or electrolyte loss
Cardiogenic	Pump failure	Myocardial ischaemia Cardiac arrhythmias Cardiac failure
Distributive	Increased venous capacitance and extra-cardiac obstruction of blood flow	Massive inflammatory response, e.g. septic and anaphylactic shock

Hypovolaemic shock

This is the most common form of shock in children (Maill et al 2003). It is caused by a loss of intravascular volume. The decrease in blood volume may be caused by:

- external blood loss, e.g. haemorrhage
- internal blood loss, e.g. ruptured spleen
- severe dehydration as a result of:
  - vomiting
  - diarrhoea
- excessive plasma loss, e.g. burn
- excessive diuresis, e.g. diabetic ketoacidosis
- third space loss, e.g. peritonitis.

A child's body can tolerate a loss of 20–25% circulating volume prior to a drop in blood pressure and cardiac output. In hypovolaemic shock the body attempts to maintain circulation despite the deficit.

Activity

Cardiogenic shock is a pump problem:

- What signs and symptoms would you expect to see in an affected child?

Cardiogenic shock

Cardiogenic shock is caused by an inability of the heart to pump sufficient blood. Inadequate function of the heart may be caused by heart failure that is weak cardiac contraction, from any cause. Cardiac output falls despite normal or elevated blood volume and cardiac pressures. Examples include:

- myocardial ischaemia
- arrhythmia
- congenital heart disease
- cardiomyopathy due to drug toxicity.

A major difference between cardiogenic and other types of shock is that pulmonary oedema secondary to heart failure is most usually present (McCance & Huether 2002).

Distributive shock

Distributive shock is a container problem and is caused by excess vasodilatation causing loss of afterload and SVR. Examples are:

- neurogenic shock (rare)
- anaphylactic shock, e.g. bee sting, peanuts
- septic shock.

Neurogenic shock occurs due to widespread and massive vasodilation due to imbalance of the parasympathetic (overstimulation) and sympathetic (understimulation) stimulation of vascular smooth muscle. Interruption of the sympathetic nervous system, which normally maintains muscle tone, results in persistent vasodilation. This overwhelming vasodilation results in pooling of the blood in the peripheries resulting in poor perfusion of the heart, brain and kidneys. The individual will have warm, dry skin and a slow heart rate. Neurogenic shock for example may be caused by trauma of the spinal cord and medulla above T6, which is extremely rare in children due to their immature anatomy and physiology (Maill et al 2003).

Anaphylactic shock is the widespread immune and inflammatory response (Hazinski 1999). The pathological response is similar to that of neurogenic shock that is vasodilation, increased vascular permeability causing peripheral oedema causing relative hypovolaemia and smooth muscle constriction leading to bronchoconstriction and dyspnoea. Individuals present with an almost immediate response to inciting antigen with any combination of the following: cutaneous manifestations such as urticaria, erythema, pruritis, angioedema; respiratory compromise with stridor, wheezing, bronchorrhea, respiratory distress; and varying degrees of circulatory collapse with tachycardia, vasodilation, hypotension.

Septic shock

Septic shock is classified as a distributive shock. However, it is a combination of problems with the pump, container and fluid and is characterised by a:

- loss of preload
- loss of afterload/SVR
- loss of contractility.

Septic shock is the most common cause of death in PICU (Pearson 2002). A well known cause of septic shock is meningococcal septicaemic which has a fatality rate of 50% if the patient is already in shock when they first receive medical help (BMA 2002). A purpuric rash known as purpura fulminans is usually seen in meningococcal disease and constitutes a medical emergency.

WWW

Link to this British Medical Association website and study the photographs of the non-blanching purpuric rash usually seen in meningococcal septicaemia:

- http://www.meningitis.orgdocs/GPleaflet

The terms sepsis, severe sepsis and septic shock are used to identify the continuum of the clinical response to infection (Bone et al 1997). An uncontrolled body system response to infection can rapidly escalate to severe sepsis and septic shock is causing acute organ dysfunction and ultimately death (Hazinski 1999). Although bacterial infection is the most common cause, fungal, viral and protozoa infections may also cause septic shock (Dolan 2003).

Whatever the initial cause of the infection, patients with septic shock have an overwhelming inflammation followed by a common pathway consisting of a systematic inflammatory cascade activated by inflammatory mediators (toxins) (Bone 1996). These mediators stimulate the release of cytokines, which act to amplify the inflammatory response and leads to systemic endothelial damage. Exposure of tissue and presence of cytokines stimulate the coagulation cascade. Coagulopathy leads to intravascular thrombus formation. In addition diffuse endothelial injury leads to vasodilation and increased capillary permeability resulting in extravasation of protein rich fluid and hence oedema (Gosling et al 1996). Therefore there is progressive vasodilation and maldistribution of blood flow, which ultimately causes organ hypoperfusion. A substance known as myocardial depressant factor (MDF) is secreted from white blood cells in response to endotoxin. MDF depresses the myocardial contractile function and results in ventricular dilatation thus further compromising cardiac output (Pathan et al 2004). To further complicate matters, in response to the pro-inflammatory mediators, excessive anti-inflammatory mediators are also released which then cause immunosuppression.

The clinical manifestations of septic shock depend on where the child is in the inflammatory response trajectory (Collins 2000). In the early phase of septic shock the child has a hyperdynamic circulatory state, often referred to as 'warm shock'. The initial mediators of inflammation lead to a marked reduction in SVR due to vasodilation and cardiac output increases. The child's heart rate increases, their pulses are 'bounding' and their skin is described as warm, dry and well perfused. In this situation a child is normotensive but may have a widened pulse pressure as vasodilation decreases diastolic blood pressure (DBP) and increased cardiac output raises systolic blood pressure (SBP). A progression from warm to cold shock occurs as hypovolaemia and ventricular dysfunction occur.

This progression can be rapid in small children because of their limited ability to maintain the increased cardiac output (Butt 1998). In response to a fall in cardiac output, catecholamines are released causing vasoconstriction. Increasing vasoconstriction compromises oxygen delivery and leads to anaerobic metabolism and lactic acid production. Acidosis in the capillary beds causes the arterioles to dilate and the venules to constrict causing pooling and stasis of blood. Hypotension develops as intravascular volume is further depleted from ongoing capillary leak and progressive myocardial depression occurs (Fig. 45.26). If the cycle of depleted intravascular volume, poor tissue perfusion, impaired oxygen utilisation, exhausted metabolic energy supplies and myocardial dysfunction is not broken, the child will progress to vascular collapse, irreversible multiple system organ failure and death (Butt 1998).

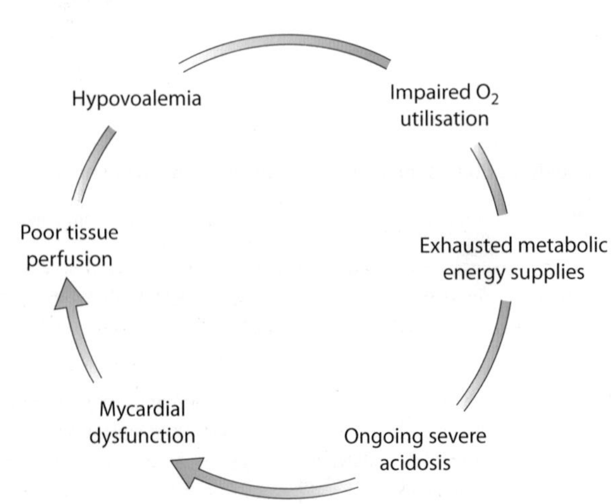

Fig. 45.26 • Pathophysiological cycle.

Haemodynamic monitoring

Haemodynamics is the state of the circulatory system as it relates to the perfusion of the body's tissues. Haemodynamic instability occurs when there is inadequate perfusion (global or regional) to support normal organ function. It has long been recognised that the physiological response of the patient to a stress or disease process will very largely determine the outcome (Webster 1999). It is important, therefore, to monitor the physiological responses of patients since this not only allows the assessment of physiological reserve but will also give a baseline against which the effectiveness of any applied treatment can be judged. Basic knowledge of the principles or monitoring and correct interpretation of data is important since a failure to do so can result in significant morbidity or, indeed, mortality of the patient. In the critically ill and haemodynamically unstable patient tissue oxygenation is determined by measuring components of cardiac output such as heart rate, arterial blood pressure, central venous pressure, arterial oxygenation and haemoglobin. In complex situations such as septic shock pulmonary artery pressure monitoring may also be used. We will now introduce the concepts of arterial blood pressure and central venous pressure monitoring.

Activity

Septic shock is a pump, container and fluid problem:

- What signs and symptoms would you expect to see in a child in 'cold' shock?

Arterial blood pressure (ABP) is measured by a catheter commonly placed in the radial, brachial or tibial artery and which is kept patent using a continuous infusion of intravenous heparin saline, 1 unit per mL at between 0.5 and 2 mL/hour depending on the size of the child. Arterial pressure is measured at its peak, which is the SBP, and at its trough, which is the DBP. The SBP is determined by the stroke volume, contractility, systemic arterial resistance and preload. The SBP is a clinical indicator of afterload. The DBP is affected by systemic arterial resistance and heart rate. Systemic mean arterial pressure (MAP) is defined as the mean perfusion pressure throughout the cycle:

$$\text{Mean arterial pressure (MAP)} = \text{Systemic vascular resistance (SVR)} \times \text{Cardiac output (CO)}$$

Pulse pressure is the difference between systolic and diastolic pressure and is normally about 40 mmHg. An increased pulse pressure may be the result of increased SV or contractility and is common during fever and anaemia. An acute decrease in pulse pressure may indicate an increase in SVR, decreased SV or decreased intravascular volume (McGhee & Bridges 2002). In summary, because of the multiplicity of factors that contribute to ABP, interpreting changes in arterial pressure and its components (SBP, DBP, MAP and pulse pressure) as indicative of any single factor may lead to an erroneous assessment of a patient's condition. Furthermore, however, numerically satisfactory ABP or MAP values are not necessarily related to adequate perfusion and organ system function. For optimal management of critically ill patients, ABP data must be integrated with information gained from clinical assessment of patient's status. This is particularly important in the management of the critically ill child. Children have significant physiological reserve and compensatory mechanisms and therefore may display an appropriate ABP for age even with significant circulating volume loss (Partrick et al 2002).

Central venous pressure (CVP) is measured by a catheter placed in the right atrium attached to a transducer which amplifies the energy signal and displays its wave form onto a monitor using a similar set-up to an arterial line as described above. Venous pressure is a term that represents the average blood pressure within the thoracic vena cava near to the right atrium. Thus, determination of the CVP provides a direct measurement of the changes in the pressure of blood returning to the heart. CVP is a useful tool for assessing the volume status of a patient. Since veins dilate and collapse passively depending on how much blood (volume) they contain, the pressure of blood in large veins depends directly on the patient's 'volume status'. The more fluid in the venous system the higher the central venous pressure is. A normal CVP is 2–8 mmHg in the self-ventilating patient (Darbyshire 1998). CVP is influenced by a number of factors including:

- cardiac output
- respiratory activity
- contraction of skeletal muscles (particularly legs and abdomen)
- sympathetic vasoconstrictor tone
- gravity.

A decrease in cardiac output either due to decreased heart rate or loss of heart contractility results in blood backing up into the venous circulation (increased venous volume) as less blood is pumped into the arterial circulation. The resultant increase in thoracic blood volume increases CVP. An increase in total blood volume as occurs in renal failure or with activation of the renin– angiotensin–aldosterone system will increase venous pressure. Venous constriction elicited by sympathetic activation of veins, or by circulating vasoconstrictor substances, for example, catecholamines, decrease venous compliance, thereby increasing venous pressure. It is important to remember that increased intra-thoracic pressure associated with positive pressure ventilation causes a reduction in CVP.

Treatment of shock: always starts with ABCs

Airway needs will vary depending on the aetiology of shock, from no intervention to aggressive intervention. In our scenario, Daniel was assessed to be in respiratory failure and was immediately intubated and ventilated. However, sometimes a patient can be in shock but be breathing adequately and oxygenating well. Given the knowledge that shock syndrome causes excessive oxygen demand, it is advised that these patients are always given 100% oxygen via a non-rebreathe bag regardless of good saturations (ALSG 2001). Often, these patients ultimately need intubation and respiratory support to help them compensate for profound metabolic acidosis.

Daniel had progressed rapidly to respiratory failure accompanied by signs and symptoms of shock. He exhibited marked tachycardia, cold extremities with delayed capillary refill and poorly palpable peripheral pulses; these are suggestive of hypovolaemia. However, Daniel's history of upper respiratory tract symptoms and fever suggested an infectious aetiology. The rapid deterioration to a shock state from what earlier in the day appeared to be a seemingly benign prodrome in an otherwise healthy child made the critical care team suspicious that this might be sepsis. Therefore, unless an alternative diagnosis is very clear, a third-generation cephalosporin antibiotic is given as soon as a blood culture is taken (ALSG 2001). As is often the case, the precise aetiology of Daniel's illness was not clear. Despite this, the clinical findings indicated the need for prompt intervention.

Scenario

On admission to PICU, Daniel's circulatory assessment found:

- heart rate: 200
- radial and dorsalis pulses: weak and thready
- skin was cool, dry and pale
- capillary refill: 4 seconds
- blood pressure: 90/60
- prior to intubation, 20 mL/kg normal saline was given rapidly

Activity

Refer to Chapter 22 in ALSG (2001) 'Advanced paediatric life support: a practical approach', where techniques for achieving vascular access are described.

Antibiotic therapy, although essential in addressing the underlying cause, does not treat septic shock as severe sepsis involves a disturbance in the immune system response to the original infection. Additionally, antibiotics do not directly improve tissue perfusion or the associated delivery of oxygen and nutrients. Furthermore, oxygen therapy is of limited benefit because the primary problem is not inadequate oxygenation but inadequate transport of oxygenated blood. Remember that in severe sepsis a patient has excess coagulation and inflammation and impaired fibrinolysis with disruption of the endothelial layer. The endothelial wall disruption includes markedly increased capillary permeability and venodilation. The venodilation that occurs causes a relative hypovolaemia. Therefore, treatment of septic shock must be aimed at recovering function at microcirculatory level in order that dysfunctioning organs can begin to function again.

Circulation

Irrespective of aetiology, initial shock therapy is directed at restoring circulating blood volume and perfusion. Fluid resuscitation is the mainstay of initial haemodynamic management. Optimal cardiac output is dependent upon volume, heart rate and contractile fibres in the myocardium achieving the appropriate amount of stretch. Therefore, replacing lost volume will support cardiac output by increasing preload, thus enhancing cardiac muscle stretch and subsequent contraction, the optimum effect of the Starling mechanism. Thus a simple fluid bolus helps to improve a patient's haemodynamic status.

If not already available, vascular access should be obtained as quickly as possible once a 'shock state' is recognised. The UK Resuscitation Council (2002) recommends that medical practitioners make three peripheral intravenous attempts over a maximum of 90 seconds and progress to immediate placement of an intraosseous needle if unsuccessful. Replacement must be made using a fluid bolus of 20 mL/kg of isotonic fluids given within a 10–20-minute period. Normal saline is the solution of first choice because it is ubiquitously available and carries minimal risks. However, repeated administration of iso-oncotic crystalloid solution boluses can lead to extravasation of fluid from the intravascular to the interstitial space especially in situations where there is increased capillary permeability, for example in septic shock. In these circumstances colloids may be administered as they have an important effect on the intravascular space. When infused, the osmotic colloid pressure on the intravascular space increases. As a result, fluid is drawn from the interstitial space into the intravascular space. Therefore, the blood is rehydrated by osmosis (Alderson et al 2001).

Activity

Read Docherty & McIntyre (2002), which includes a simplified interpretation of the arguments and discussion offered in the Cochrane Review (Alderson et al 2001).

Activity

Daniel is given 20 mL/kg normal saline over 10 minutes. His circulation should then be re-assessed:

- What will you assess, why and how?

Scenario

Despite a transient improvement after an initial bolus of 20 mL/kg normal saline with a heart rate of 130 and capillary refill of 3–4 seconds, Daniel requires further fluid therapy. After 60 mL/kg (3 × 20 mL/kg boluses). Daniel remains pale with a heart rate 160, SBP 70 mmHg, capillary refill of 5 seconds and pulse oximetry that is not picking up. A central line has been inserted and Daniel has a CVP reading of 4 mmHg. He is started on dopamine at 4.0 mcg/kg/min and dobutamine at 10 mcg/kg/min administered via the central venous line.

A 5 mL/kg bolus of 10% dextrose in addition to maintenance fluids commenced has improved his blood glucose from 1.7 to 4.2 mmol/L.

Activity

Refer to the 'UK Paediatric Formulary Medicines for children, 2nd edn' (RCPCH 2003) and review the actions, dosage and side effects and nursing implications for the administration of the following inotropic agents: adrenaline, noradrenaline, dopamine and dobutamine.

As severe sepsis worsens, the benefits of fluid therapy are reduced, mainly because fluid therapy alone cannot address the cellular problem of increased capillary permeability as seen in severe sepsis. The fluid bolus has little effect on CVP. The widespread endothelial damage, vasodilation and capillary permeability are so great that pressure cannot be developed in the system. Because myocardial depression and vasodilation may be features of the patient's septic shock, inotropic agents may be valuable in restoring adequate perfusion. An inotrope is an agent that improves myocardial contractility and enhances stroke volume.

In patients with no significant improvement after two or three fluid boluses, particularly if sepsis is expected, inotropic agents are used to maintain arterial pressure. The agents most commonly used are catecholamines. Dopamine and dobutamine are both catecholamines but have different profiles as they activate different specific receptors. Their main course of action is through adrenergic receptors:

- α: peripheral vasculature stimulation: vasoconstriction
- β_1: myocardium stimulation: inotropy and chronotropy
- β_2: lungs and peripheral vasculature stimulation: smooth muscle relaxation (vasodilation and bronchodilation).

Dopamine is the gold standard as the initial vasopressor support of septic shock because of its versatility and its activation of dopamine receptors, thus possibly protecting the kidneys and preventing acute renal failure due to tubular necrosis. Dopamine, a precursor of adrenaline (epinephrine), administered as a continuous infusion, affects preload by causing vascular constriction or dilation through its effect on the sympathetic nervous system. Dopamine acts on α, β and dopamine receptors. Low-dose dopamine, 2–4 mcg/kg/min, has peripheral vasodilating effects but causes little or no increase in force of myocardial contraction (positive inotropy). However, low-dose dopamine may help to maintain splanchnic circulation and promote renal perfusion via dopamine receptor action. Dopamine affects β receptors at 5–10 mcg/kg/min and α receptors at >10 mcg/kg/min. If unable to meet haemodynamic goals with dopamine, medical practitioners will have a low threshold for switching or adding other agents such as adrenaline, noradrenaline and dobutamine, which have been shown to be beneficial in the hemodynamic support of septic shock. Dobutamine, a synthetic catecholamine, is also administered as a continuous intravenous infusion and acts primarily on β_1 receptors. Dobutamine increases myocardial contractility (inotropic effect) and heart rate (chronotropic effect) and therefore increases stroke volume. It also causes peripheral vasodilation decreasing afterload. Overall dobutamine improves cardiac output.

Monitoring the child in shock

Seminar discussion topic

Shock is an altered state of tissue perfusion severe enough to induce derangements in normal cellular function. Neuroendocrine, hemodynamic and metabolic changes work together to restore perfusion. Treatment of shock is primarily focused on restoring tissue perfusion and oxygen delivery while eliminating the cause. The general goal is to maximise oxygen delivery and minimise oxygen demand and thereby enhance perfusion:

- Haemodynamic goals:
  - mean arterial pressure > 60 mmHg
  - heart rate within normal parameters
  - central venous pressure > 8 but < 15 mmHg
  - capillary refill < 2 seconds.
- Organ perfusion goals:
  - CNS: improved sensorium
  - skin: warm, well perfused
- renal: urine output > 1 mL/kg/hour
- Oxygen delivery adequacy:
  - arterial oxygen saturation > 95%
  - Hb concentration > 10 g/dL
  - lactate < 2 mmol.

Work with colleagues to determine the implications for nursing in working collaboratively to achieve these goals.

Family-centred critical care

The hospitalisation of a child with a life-threatening illness constitutes a major stress experience for both the child and parents endangering the child's and the parent's biological, social and psychological integrity. Infants and children admitted to intensive care (Fig. 45.27) require immediate stabilisation and life support that is frightening, invasive and likely to alter the appearance of the infant or child with an uncertainty about outcome. Nurses must be knowledgeable of the impact this phenomenon has on children and their families and the factors influencing their adjustment to this stressful experience to assist children and their families in developing positive, adaptive coping mechanisms. Contemporary health care, assessment of need at the level of the client group has become increasingly important (DoH 1999) and is hoped will enhance quality of care.

Much research has been carried out in an endeavour to understand parental experiences of intensive care. Therefore, the needs of family members of the critically ill child are well established, although maternally biased. A critique of this literature reveals that positivistic studies, which attempt

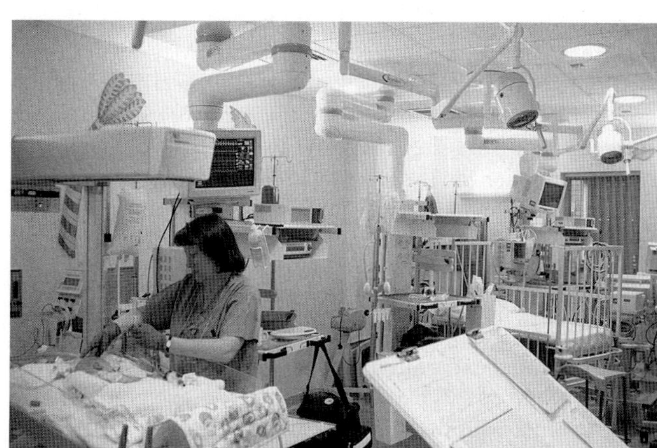

Fig 45.27 • PICU environment.

to quantify parental feelings and experiences, dominate the literature with the majority being American (Noyes 1998). The perceived needs of American parents can be expected to differ from those of British parents for a number of reasons, for example the differing healthcare delivery systems and philosophies, healthcare professional education and training, and the culture and expectations of parents (Temmink et al 2000), which are arguably not transferable to a British population. Therefore, we will focus on the results of British research.

Evidence-based practice

Studies of adult patient recollection of intensive care experience are plentiful and report disturbing accounts of hallucinations, inability to communicate, pain, anxiety and memory of vivid details relating to intensive care procedures and mechanical ventilation (Granberg et al 1996). Playfor et al (2000) provide the only research data of children's experiences. They investigated 44 children's recollections, aged between 4 and 16 years of their intensive care experience using semi-structured interviews. Only 15% of the recollections were negative. More specifically: no child treated with neuromuscular blocking agents remembered any period of paralysis; six children complained of a lack of sleep, of these, three complained about the noise and the other three complained of pain/discomfort; eight children remember feeling frightened; eight remember being thirsty; two had negative recollections of the nasogastric tube and one child had negative recollections of the endotracheal tube. Following discharge, two children experienced dreams but only one of these children described the dreams as frightening.

British positivistic researchers were concerned with the question: 'What are the most important needs and stressors of parents of children on intensive care?'. They consistently demonstrate the importance of certain features of the parents' stressor experience, such as, uncertainty about the child's condition, the environment and parental role alteration and establish the parental need for information, reassurance, and support to be near their child (Farrell & Frost 1992, Haines et al 1995, Heuer 1993). These researchers also defined variables that impacted on these stressors, for example, parental gender (Heuer 1993) and acuity of illness and need for intervention (Haines et al 1995). These studies clearly demonstrate that a child's need for intensive care is a major stressor and that parents have a hierarchy of concerns analogous with a hierarchy of needs (Maslow & Lowry 1998), that is, that the level of technological intervention has an impact on the nature of the stressors experienced. However, it is suggested that the use of scales in principle are inappropriate for the investigation of parental experience as they fail to establish any knowledge of parental situational meaning construction or a comprehensive understanding of parental needs (Aylott 2002). Understanding parental experience is a question of quality and nature rather than quantity. Subjectivist research using a qualitative methodology through its open-minded exploratory approach aims to understand the complex world of this lived experience from the point of view of the parents who lived it (Aylott 2000, Noyes 1999, Place 1997). These studies ask: 'What is it like to have a child in intensive care?'

Place (1997) in his ethnographic study of children's intensive care, offers a sensitive analysis of the relationship between the parent, their new parent role and their child's altered appearance. Place describes how the body is 'technomorphic', that is, revisable by connection to technological artifacts which in turn has an impact on social interaction, self and identity. He also makes a distinction between what he calls 'child data' that is what is happening within the body and 'data child' which is the physical manifestation of the body through its connection to surrounding technological artifacts such as monitors reading vital signs. The 'child data' and 'data child' explicate each other. In intensive care healthcare professionals and parents are all concerned to maintain the integrity of the 'technomorphic' body, which forms a key dimension in the interactions between health carer, child and parents.

Noyes (1999) conducted an exploratory study to elicit mother's lived experiences of their children's intensive care crisis and coping utilising a symbolic interactionism perspective (a philosophical perspective which views human experiences as an emergent process in which meaning arises from the interactions between subject and object). She reports on the impact of the initial shock and crisis, the child's appearance and the implications of being resident. Noyes (1999) demonstrated that mothers whose children are undergoing intensive care are in crisis and are vulnerable at this time and recommends that nurses proactively seek to address the psycho-emotional needs of parents prior to and immediately after admission and deliver family-centred care. Furthermore, this has long-term implications as mothers' stress-related symptoms and perception of their families as dysfunctional after discharge from hospital has been shown to persist as long as 6 months after a child's illness event (Board & Ryan-Wenger 2002).

Aylott (2000) conducted an exploratory study of parents' experience of their child's extracorporeal membrane oxygenation (ECMO) utilising a grounded theory approach. ECMO is an invasive technique that oxygenates blood outside the body, obviating the need for gas exchange in the lungs, and, if necessary, provides cardiovascular support. Children that require this treatment are extremely sick. Parents described: the horror of critical illness that was acute and sudden with a telescoped trajectory offering little chance to reflect and prepare for the experience; a sense of loss, an alienation of the mundane, which had altered significance from everyday life 'taken for granted-ness'; how the boundaries between their child's body and other technologies became blurred as the body was colonised and extended to include both the child and the technological elements; how understanding 'child data' as described by Place (1997) became important in communicating with staff and gaining 'control' and involvement in their child's care. This was also described as therapeutic in dealing with cognitive dissonance about the child's outward appearance once stabilised despite the internal disorder and disease.

These studies (Aylott 2000, Noyes 1999, Place 1997) are useful in showing that parents' accounts are more than 'stories about' they are importantly ways of 'seeing as'. Negotiation and partnership are important concepts as a means of cultivating parent trust in staff, maintenance of hope and their ability to cope. Although the clinical picture may vastly constrain physical involvement in their child's care, parents wish to challenge and collaborate in decision making and sometimes in procedures. This is in essence family-centred care.

Family-centred care moves beyond the rhetorical theoretical recognition of the centrality of the child and family in health care. A family-focused multiprofessional critical care team views the child and family as a unit to be cared for and organises care delivery around them as a unit as opposed to the more traditional patient-centred model (Henneman & Cardin 2002). However, providing family-centred care in a critical care setting is not a simple endeavour and is often misconceived as a list of interventions, for example open visiting. Family-centred care is a philosophical approach to care that recognises the needs of the family as well as the important role that they play during a child's critical illness therefore it should be more accurately referred to as family-centred critical care in this setting. Although providing family-centred critical care means that the critical care team recognise their responsibility to help the family, as well as the child, survive the crisis of an illness and have an obligation to endeavour to meet their fundamental needs, it is important to stress that meeting a child's needs should always be the priority for both the child's family and the critical care team (NMC 2002).

Research has indicated the fundamental needs of the family of the critically ill child as the need for honest and open information, the need for reassurance and support and the need to be in partnership with healthcare professionals regarding their child's care. These needs need to be ascertained from individual families and from individuals within a family and interpreted accurately. Thus it is important that nurses receive clarification about what these needs are and entail whilst at the same time recognising their dynamic nature. Empowering child and family participation in experiences that enhance control and independence and build on their strengths in the critical care environment demands advanced effective communication skills of the nurse and multi-professional team and the establishment of therapeutic relationships under stressful conditions.

Research indicates that it is important to a child's family that they are assured that their child is receiving the best possible care (Aylott 2000). Several investigators document the benefits of family presence during invasive procedures and resuscitation which includes: knowing that everything possible was being done for their child; reducing anxiety and fear; feeling of being comforting and helpful to their child and the staff; sharing critical information about their child and the child's condition; maintaining the child-family relationship; closure on a life shared together; and facilitating the grieving process in the critical care environment and later at home (Eckle & MacLean 2001, Jarvis 1998, Meyers et al 2000, Sacchetti et al 2000). Adult patient studies indicated that having family present provided comfort, helped with coping and pain control, maintained the family bond, and reminded health providers that the patient was a person with a family who deserved dignity and respect (Redley & Hood 1996, Robinson et al 1998) (Table 45.2). This has stimulated discussion about this controversial topic in both professional and consumer literature (Goldstein et al 1997, Powers & Rubenstein 1999, Rosenczweig 1998, Sacchetti et al 2000).

Activity

Analyse the evidence-based proposed advantages and disadvantages of family presence during resuscitation listed in Table 45.2. Consider the question:

- 'Do the advantages of allowing parents to be present during their child's resuscitation outweigh the potential disadvantages?'

Although many family members and healthcare providers support the option of family presence, family members frequently are not given the option to remain with their child during invasive procedures and resuscitation efforts. This separation during treatment occurs for a variety of reasons. Health professionals express concern that: the event may be too traumatic for the family; clinical care might be impeded; family members might become too emotional or out of control; staff may experience increased stress with family present; unit rooms are too crowded, staff are focused on the child and may not be available to assist family members; there is a shortage of nurses; and there is the risk of increased liability (Eckle & MacLean 2001, Jarvis 1998, Meyers et al 2000, Rosenczweig 1998). Yet, families reported that they would be present again if a similar event occurred (Meyers et al 2000). In addition, investigators reported that there were no adverse psychological effects among family members and the operations of the emergency care providers was not disrupted when the option of family presence was used (Meyers et al 2000, Robinson et al 1998, Sacchetti et al 2000).

Interestingly, parental presence at resuscitation has been fully supported by the UK Resuscitation Council since 1996,

Table 45.2 Advantages and disadvantages of family presence during invasive procedures and resuscitation

Advantages	Disadvantages
Holistic approach: acknowledges role of family	Family may disrupt procedure/resuscitation efforts
Child/family bond facilitated	Healthcare staff perceive that they may not be able to show emotion
Family can observe efforts of healthcare team	Fear of litigation due to lack of understanding
Family see that all that can be done is done	Observer effect may inhibit staff performance
Imagination is more fearsome than reality	May cause psychological damage to family
Reduce litigation because of openness	Long-term effects on family unit not known
Family can provide comfort	Increases stress of staff involved
Families perceive that they are participating in procedure/resuscitation	Child's privacy may be violated
Facilitates bereavement process	Resuscitation efforts may be unnecessarily prolonged
Facilitates relationship between family and staff	Interference of procedure/resuscitation
	Distraction of focus from child
	Family anger/violence towards staff

despite the controversy and in advance of much of this research. Every critically ill child is a member of a family system and is usually the major source of support for the child during times of stress, crisis and decision making. Research studies have shown that most families want the option to be present during invasive procedures, during their child's medical procedures and at the time of their child's death.

Summary

Topics for this chapter were chosen because of their importance to children's morbidity and mortality and their prevalence as problems in intensive care. This chapter has considered the respiratory support, haemodynamic control and family-centred critical care required by a child with life-threatening illness on a paediatric intensive care unit. It demonstrates the principles of intensive care, which require that nurses apply specialist evidence-based knowledge and skills in the direct provision of care to manage a dynamic and rapidly evolving illness process in collaboration with medical and allied profession colleagues. The challenge is to provide this technologically sophisticated care in a compassionate environment and facilitate in depth interaction between the critically sick child and their family.

References

Advanced Life Support Group (ALSG), 2001. Advanced paediatric life support: the practical approach, 3rd edn. British Medical Association, London.

Alderson, P., Schierhout, G., Roberts, I., Bunn, F., 2001. Colloids versus crystalloids for fluid resuscitation in the critically ill. The Cochrane Library, issue 4. Update Software, Oxford.

Ashworth, W., 1996. Inquiry into the care and treatment of Nicholas Geldard. North West Regional Health Authority, Manchester.

Aylott, M., 2000. Parents' experience of their child's extra-corporeal membrane oxygenation: a qualitative study. Nursing in Critical Care 5, 228–235.

Aylott, M., 2002. Interviewing as therapy: researching parents' experiences of their child's life threatening illness requiring ECMO. Nursing in Critical Care 7 (4), 163–170.

Ball, C., Dams, J., Boyce, S., Robinson, P., 2001. Clinical guidelines for the use of the prone position in acute respiratory distress syndrome. Intensive and Critical Care Nursing 17, 94–104.

Bhende, M.S., 2001. End-tidal carbon dioxide monitoring in pediatrics – clinical applications. Journal of Postgraduate Medicine 47, 215–218.

Board, R., Ryan-Wenger, N., 2002. Long-term effects of pediatric intensive care unit hospitalisation on families and young children. Heart and Lung: the Journal of Acute and Critical Care 31 (1), 53–66.

Bohn, D., 1998. New ventilation strategies. In: Duncan, A. (Ed.), Paediatric intensive care. BMJ Books, London, pp. 41–91.

Bone, R.C., Grodzin, C.J., Balk, R.A., 1997. Sepsis: a new hypothesis for pathogenesis of the disease process. Chest 112 (1), 235–243.

British Medical Association (BMA), 2002. Meningococcal meningitis and septicaemia: guidance notes. Meningitis Research Foundation, London.

British Paediatric Association (BPA), 1993. The care of critically ill children. Report of the Multidisciplinary Working Party on Paediatric Intensive Care. BPA, London.

Butt, W., 1998. Management of septic shock in children. In: Duncan, A. (Ed.), Paediatric intensive care, BMJ Books, London, pp. 236–266.

Centers for Disease Control (CDC), 1994. CDC guidelines. Respiratory Care 39 (12), 1191–1236.

Collins, T., 2000. Understanding shock. Nursing Standard 14 (49), 35–39.

Coombs, M., 2001. Critical care: where care is critical. Nursing in Critical Care 6 (3), 111–114.

Darbyshire, P., 1998. Making sense of central venous pressure monitoring. Nursing Times 84 (6), 36–38.

Darovic, G.O., 1995. Hemodynamic monitoring: invasive and non-invasive clinical application. WB Saunders, Philadelphia.

Department of Health (DoH), 1999. Making a difference: strengthening the nursing, midwifery and health visiting contribution to health and healthcare. HMSO, London.

Docherty, B., McIntyre, L., 2002. Nursing considerations for fluid management in hypovolaemia. Professional Nurse 17 (9), 545–549.

Dolan, S., 2003. Severe sepsis – a major challenge for critical care. Intensive & Critical Care Nursing 19, 63–67.

Dreyfus, D., Basset, G., Soler, P.S., Saumon, G., 1985. Intermittent positive-pressure hyperventilation with high inflation pressures produces pulmonary microvascular injury in rats. American Review of Respiratory Diseases 132 (4), 880–884.

Duncan, A., 1998. Paediatric intensive care. BMJ Publishing, London.

Eckle, N., MacLean, S., 2001. Assessment of family-centered care for pediatric patients in the emergency department. Journal of Emergency Nursing 27 (3), 238–245.

Edwards, S., 1998. Hypovolaemia: pathophysiology and management options. Nursing in Critical Care 3 (2), 73–82.

Epstein, O., 1997. Clinical examination. Mosby, London.

Estes, R., Meduri, G., 1995. The pathogenesis of ventilator associated pneumonia: 1 mechanisms of bacterial translocation and airway inoculation. Intensive Care Medicine 21, 365–383.

Farrell, M., Frost, C., 1992. The most important needs of parents of critically ill children: parent's perceptions. Intensive and Critical Care Nursing 8, 130–139.

Ganong, W.F., 2001. Review of medical physiology, 20th edn. Lange Medical Books, New York.

Goldstein, A., Berry, K., Callaghan, A., 1997. Resuscitation witnessed by relatives: has proved acceptable to doctors in paediatric cases [letter]. British Medical Journal 314, 144–145.

Gosling, P., Bascom, J.U., Zikria, B.A., 1996. Capillary leak, oedema and organ failure: breaking the triad. Care of the Critically Ill 12 (6), 191–197.

Granberg, A., Bergbom-Endberg, I., Lundberg, D., 1996. Intensive care syndrome: a literature review. Intensive and Critical Care Nursing 12, 173–182.

Haines, C., Perger, C., Nagy, S., 1995. A comparison of the stressors experienced by parents of intubated and non-intubated children. Journal of Advanced Nursing 21, 350–355.

Hazinski, M.F., 1999. Manual of pediatric critical care. Mosby, New York.

Henneman, E.A., Cardin, S., 2002. Family-centred critical care: a practical approach to making it happen. Critical Care Nurse 22 (6), 12–19.

Heuer, L., 1993. Parental stressors in a paediatric intensive care unit. Paediatric Nursing 19 (2), 128–131.

Hill, N., 1997. Complications of non-invasive positive pressure ventilation. Respiratory Care 42, 432–442.

Jarvis, A.S., 1998. Parental presence during resuscitation: attitudes of staff on a paediatric intensive care unit. Intensive and Critical Care Nursing 14, 3–7.

Kerr, M., 1997. Paediatric ventilatory care. In: Morton, M.S. (Ed.), Paediatric intensive care. Oxford University Press, Oxford, pp. 109–151.

Kolobow, T., Moretti, M.P., Fumagalli, R., et al., 1987. Severe impairment in lung function induced by high peak airway pressure during mechanical ventilation: an experimental study. American Review of Respiratory Diseases 135 (3), 312–315.

Lissuer, T., Clayden, G., 2001. Illustrated textbook of paediatrics. Mosby, London.

Maill, L., Rudolf, M., Levene, M., 2003. Paediatrics at a glance. Blackwell Science, Oxford.

Marieb, E., 2002. Essentials of human anatomy and physiology, 7th edn. Benjamin Cummings, San Francisco.

Martini, F.H., 1998. Fundamentals of anatomy and physiology. Prentice Hall, New Jersey.

Maslow, A.H., Lowry, R., 1998. Towards a psychology of being. John Wiley, London.

McCance, K., Huether, S., 2002. Pathophysiology: the biological basis for disease in adults and children. Mosby, London.

McCance, K.L., Huether, S.E., 1994. Pathophysiology: the biological basis for disease in adults and children, 2nd edn. Mosby Year Book, St Louis.

McGhee, B.H., Bridges, M.E.J., 2002. Monitoring arterial blood pressure: what you may not know. Critical Care Nurse 22 (2), 60–78.

Meyers, T.A., Eichhorn, D.J., Guzzetta, C.E., et al., 2000. Family presence during invasive procedures and resuscitation: the experience of family members, nurses, and physicians. American Journal of Nursing 100 (2), 32–42.

NHS Executive, 1996. Paediatric intensive care. NHSE, Leeds.

NHS Executive, 1997a. Paediatric intensive care: a framework for the future. Report of the National Co-ordinating Group on Intensive Care to the Chief Executive of the NHS Executive. NHSE, London.

NHS Executive, 1997b. Paediatric intensive care: a bridge to the future. Report of the Chief Nursing Officer's Taskforce to the Chief Executive. NHSE, London.

Noyes, J., 1998. A critique of studies exploring the experiences and needs of parents of children admitted to paediatric intensive care units. Journal of Advanced Nursing 28 (1), 131–141.

Noyes, J., 1999. The impact of knowing your child is critically ill: a qualitative study of mother's experiences. Journal of Advanced Nursing 29 (2), 427–435.

Nursing and Midwifery Council (NMC), 2002. Code of professional conduct. NMC, London.

Parker, J.C., Hernandez, L., Peevey, K., 1993. Mechanisms of ventilator induced lung injury. Critical Care Medicine 21, 131–135.

Partrick, D.A., Bensard, D.D., Janik, J.S., Karrer, M., 2002. Is hypotension a reliable indicator of blood loss from traumatic injury in children? The American Journal of Surgery 184 (6), 555–559.

Pathan, N., Hemingway, C.A., Alizadeh, A.A., et al., 2004. Role of interleukin 6 in myocardial dysfunction of meningococcal septic shock. The Lancet 363 (9404), 203–209.

Pearson, G., 2002. Handbook of paediatric intensive care. WB Saunders, London.

Pearson, G., Shann, F., Barry, P.W., et al., 1997. Should paediatric intensive care be centralised? Trent versus Victoria. The Lancet 349, 1213–1217.

Place, B., 1997. The constructing of bodies of critically ill children: an ethnography of intensive care. In: Prout, A. (Ed.), Childhood and the body. Macmillan, London, pp. 135–143.

Playfor, S., Thomas, D., Choonara, I., 2000. Recollection of children following intensive care. Archives of Disease in Childhood 83, 445–448.

Pollard, C., 2001. Endotracheal suction in the infant with an artificial airway. Nursing in Critical Care 6 (2), 76–82.

Powers, K.S., Rubenstein, J.S., 1999. Family presence during invasive procedures in the pediatric intensive care unit. Archives of Pediatric Adolescent Medicine 153, 955–958.

Prior, F.G.R., 1999. Plasma colloid osmotic pressure in the critically ill. Care of the Critically Ill 15 (5), 167–172.

Redley, B., Hood, K., 1996. Staff attitudes towards family presence during resuscitation. Accident and Emergency Nursing 4 (3), 145–151.

Resuscitation Council UK, 1996. Should relatives witness resuscitation? Resuscitation Council UK, London.

Reynolds, E.M., Ryan, D., Doody, D., 1993. Permissive hypercapnia and pressure controlled ventilation as a treatment of severe adult respiratory distress syndrome in a pediatric burn patient. Critical Care Medicine 21, 468–475.

Robb, J., 1997a. Physiological changes occurring with positive pressure ventilation: part one. Intensive and Critical Care Nursing 13:293–307

Robb, J., 1997b. Physiological changes occurring with positive pressure ventilation: part two. Intensive and Critical Care Nursing 13:357–364

Robinson, S., MacKenzie-Ross, S., Campbell-Hawson, G., et al., 1998. Psychological effect of witnessed resuscitation on bereaved relatives. Lancet 352, 614–617.

Rosenczweig, C., 1998. Should relatives witness resuscitation? Canadian Medical Association Journal 158 (5), 617–620.

Royal College of Paediatrics and Child Health (RCPCH), 2003. Medicines for children, 2nd edn. RCPCH, London.

Sacchetti, A., Carraccio, C., Leva, E., et al., 2000. Acceptance of family member presence during pediatric resuscitations in the emergency department: effects of personal experience. Pediatric Emergency Care 16, 85–87.

Temmink, D., Francke, A.L., Hutten, J.B.F., et al., 2000. Innovations in the nursing care of the chronically ill: a literature review from an international perspective. Journal of Advanced Nursing 31 (6), 1449–1458.

Tibballs, J., 1998. Clinical aspects of nitric oxide therapy. In: Duncan, A. (Ed.), Paediatric intensive care. BMJ Books, London, pp. 196–235.

Webster, N.R., 1999. Monitoring the critically ill patient. Journal of the Royal College of Surgeons 44, 386–393.

Wheatley, I., 2001. How can patient monitoring provide an effective tool to augment clinical judgement in the critical care environment? Nursing in Critical Care 6 (3), 145–147.

Williams, R., Rankin, N., Smith, T., et al., 1996. Relationship between the humidity and temperature of inspired gas and the function of the airway mucosa. Critical Care Medicine 24 (11), 1920–1929.

Care of the child requiring palliative care

Jayne Price Marisa McFarlane

ABSTRACT

The primary aim of this chapter is to examine the holistic needs of the child requiring palliative care in the context of the family. Palliative care for children has evolved as a distinct but specific field of practice over recent years and is an integrated approach to caring for children and their families within a variety of settings. As a continually developing field of practice palliative care for children it has experienced a number of developments in relation to policy and an ever-increasing research base since the first edition of this text. Throughout the course of this chapter and the companion PowerPoint presentation, the biopsychosocial and spiritual care needs of children with life-limiting illness, and their families, will be examined within a partnership approach to caring.

LEARNING OUTCOMES

- Examine the components that contribute to the philosophy of palliative care.
- Appreciate the importance of a family-centred and an interdisciplinary approach to care of a child with a life-limiting illness.
- Gain an insight and understanding into the biopsychosocial and spiritual needs of the life-limited child and family.
- Appreciate the needs of the family in bereavement.

Introduction

Palliative care for children is about quality of living ensuring the child and family live fully in the knowledge that early death is expected (Association for children with a life-threatening illness (ACT) 2004, Levetown and the Committee of Bioethics 2008). Over recent years, the care of children and young people with life-limiting illnesses has been the subject of growing interest (Hain & Wallace 2008) and as a result paediatric palliative care has evolved as a small but distinct area of practice across the UK and internationally (McNeilly et al 2004). Government strategy and policy within the UK have children with palliative care needs and their families central to their agenda (Department of Health (DoH) 2005, 2007, 2008). Knowing that a child is life-limited poses a particular challenge for parents and professionals (Armstrong-Dailey 1990).

The subsequent death of the child causes a devastating loss to families and communities, and in turn leads to one of the most profound and long-lasting of griefs. The death of the child defies the natural expected order of life events (Sourkes et al 2005).

Although it has been argued that the principles and ethics underpinning palliative care delivery are universal across age spans, the caring for children within this and other specialist areas of health care bring unique and different challenges, issues and dilemmas (Sourkes et al 2005). Whilst some of the principles of caring for the adult patient may be useful it is essential to recognise and acknowledge the very unique needs of the child requiring a palliative approach and their family (ACT 2003, Price et al 2005). One of the most distinctive differences within children's palliative care is the broad diagnostic diversity which results in the challenging uncertainty around prognosis experienced by children and families. Many of the disorders experienced by children are rare (Watterson & Hain 2003). Others may be familial and hence genetic counselling is crucial. In addition due to the degenerative nature of many of the life-limiting illnesses of childhood, palliative care services are traditionally involved with the child and family from an early stage, often over a long period of time (Hynson & Sawyer 2001).

The need for care can be unrelenting and can lead to social deprivation and extreme stress for the family (Corkin et al 2006). Burn-out in staff regularly caring for these children and families has also been noted (Costello & Trinder-Brook 2000).

Palliative care for children – a historical perspective

Palliative care for children is about quality of living for both the child whose life is limited and their family (ACT 2009, Liben et al 2008). The development of this specialty can be attributed

DOI: 10.1016/B978-0-7020-3183-0.10046-3

to the advent of … children's hospice movement and the further develo… of paediatric oncology outreach services. Born out of … re to improve care for dying people the hospice m… evolved as it had become accepted that the mod… …ical establishment was not fully addressing all the … dying people and their families. The need for expan… services was soon identified from simply providing care … adult cancer patients and in 1982 the first children's hos… …ce was opened in Oxford. Helen House developed from the special friendship between Sister Frances Dominica and a child called Helen, who had a life-limiting illness. Through this relationship, Sister Frances recognised the need of respite care and practical support for other families in similar situations. Her vision was for a haven where this practical support and respite care could be delivered. Helen House provided a 'home from home' where families could share the caring, providing them an environment where practical help, friendship and quality time were offered. This was to 'blaze a trail in the provision of hospice care for children and young people' (Worswick 2002 p 160). Helen House remains an exemplar for the development of children's hospice services world wide and the number of children hospices grew in conjunction with the development of 'hospice-at-home teams'. The growth generated an appraisal into the care delivered to children with life-limiting illnesses and their families. In 1992 the ACT (Association for Children with Life-Threatening or Terminal Conditions and their families), since renamed the Association for Children's Palliative Care, was set up to influence and promote excellence and equity in care provision and support for children and young people with life-threatening or life-limiting conditions and their families.

WWW

Visit the Association for Children's Palliative Care (ACT) website. Establish the work currently being carried out by ACT.

- http://www.act.org.uk

ACT work closely with other agencies, for example Children's Hospices UK (Formerly ACH), to promote excellence for all children requiring palliative care and their families (Price et al 2005). Although this philosophy of care has developed largely from within the hospice movement it has since permeated to a variety of additional settings – namely hospital and home. This being so, it is now referred to as paediatric palliative care or palliative care for children and the specialty has greatly developed in recent years through policy development and international networks (Hain & Wallace 2008). Despite the expansion and development of services in recent years, providing palliative care tailored to a child's individual needs has not been without its challenges. These challenges include difficulty recognising which children require palliative care, the variation in availability of services depending on geographical location, a lack of understanding by policy makers about what constitutes palliative care and the limited evidence base underpinning practice (Price et al 2005).

Palliative care for children – a distinct specialty

Although many of the terms used within the specialty are used interchangeably one of the most widely accepted definitions in the UK is from ACT (2009 p 9):

> Palliative care for children and young people with life limiting conditions is an active and total approach to care, embracing physical, emotional, social and spiritual elements. It focuses on enhancements of quality life for the child and support for the family and includes the management of distressing symptoms, provision of respite and care through death and bereavement.

Palliative care is not purely about dying but is about quality of living and is provided to children with life-threatening life-limiting condition. The above definition highlights the different attributes that contribute to the philosophy of palliative care for children. The ACT Charter outlines the needs of children and families and can be viewed on the companion PowerPoint presentation.

Palliative care for children requires an integrated approach and it has become widely accepted that a mixed model of care is essential. Within this model the principles of palliative care and cure-focused care are delivered concurrently, ensuring consistency throughout the child's illness (Michelson & Steinhom 2007).

WWW

Visit the Children's Hospices UK website. Establish the purpose of this organisation and the services it provides for children and their families:

- http://www.childhospice.org.uk.

At least 15,000 children require palliative care in the UK (ACT/RCPCH 2003) and a wide range of conditions renders their need for this type of care. Four broad groups of children have been identified as likely to require this unique type of care whose needs can change over time (ACT/RCPH 2003). Within the four groups of children many have complex chronic conditions and all the children have the possibility of an early death (Himelstein 2006). These groups are listed on the companion PowerPoint.

Reaction to a life-limiting illness

The diagnosis of a life-limiting/life-threatening illness rocks the most stable of families (Chad 2008). It is the start of a journey that can resemble a roller-coaster ride: the ups and downs along the uncertain road of the illness trajectory and can lead to a long-standing relationship with the healthcare team (Nuutila & Salantera 2006). The way the news is broken can stay with a family for many years and a variety of models have been established to assist healthcare professionals in this complex and challenging task (Price et al 2006). In addition other factors affect the psychological impact of facing a life-limiting illness.

These include the age and cognitive development of the child, the duration and type of treatment (if available), the prognosis, the degree of disruption to normal routine and education, the degree to which body image may be affected and the potential separation from siblings and main caregivers.

The overall reaction to the diagnosis of a child's life-limiting condition or the birth of a baby with a life-limiting condition is similar to that of bereavement as parents are grieving the loss of their 'well' child or the 'healthy baby' they wished for (Davies 2004). The child may also be grieving for the 'normal' life and the future which they may feel they have lost (Maunder 2004). Soricelli & Utech (1985) identify that grief symptoms are experienced from diagnosis and throughout the illness trajectory of a child with a life-limiting condition and highlighted four distinct phases of bereavement – firstly bereavement at the time of diagnosis, secondly bereavement during integration, thirdly renewed bereavement if curative options have been available and are exhausted and death is approaching, with the fourth phase being post-death mourning.

Kubler-Ross (1970) identified five reactions to dying; these can equally be applied to a diagnosis of a life-limiting or life-threatening illness. These are denial, anger, bargaining, depression and acceptance. The child and the family may experience a multitude of different feelings at different times and there is no set way for how the individual may feel at any particular time. Regardless of the type of feelings being experienced at any particular time, the child and family require cohesively planned care and support from an experienced team who are responsive to individual need. The family needs information and support at the time of diagnosis and afterwards (RCN 1999, Price et al 2006). Planning palliative care for children must therefore be tailored to the individual and changing needs of that child and their families (Beardsmore & Fitzmaurice 2002) and include a wide array of agencies and services within the NHS and outside to ensure a holistic quality care is provided (ACT 2003).

The team approach to paediatric palliative care

The need for an interdisciplinary team approach to paediatric palliative care is essential in the provision of a quality seamless service to children and their families (McNeilly & Price 2007). Providing palliative care for children requires thorough planning, effective communication as well as coordination and cohesiveness within the interdisciplinary team (Hynson et al 2003).

Clear, concise communication is a fundamental component of successful team working with each team member having a role to play. Members of the interdisciplinary team must share identical goals of care and respect the individual roles of team members and also family needs and values. A cohesive package is required with clarity of roles in order that conflicting information is avoided. Team variance can create an environment where confusion is present. The healthcare professional must function effectively and efficiently on an individual basis and as part of the team. The palliative care package for the child and family should have an identified key worker (ACT/RCPCH 2003). This worker will coordinate the care and ensures a seamless package is provided, that clarity of roles is established and good communication is maintained (ACT 2003). The key worker could be a CCN, palliative care nurse, hospice or paediatric oncology outreach nurse specialist (POONS). Vickers et al (2007) purport that the POONS is in an ideal position to act as the key worker for a child with advanced cancer. The team will be made up of different professionals, depending on the individual family and their circumstances. Examples of members of the interdisciplinary team are listed on the companion CD-Rom.

The importance of good team working cannot be understated this is supported by ACT (2003) who clearly stipulate that the assessment, planning, implementing and evaluation of plans of care including symptom control for children with a life-limiting illness needs to be interdisciplinary.

Symptom control for children

Symptom management has been identified as a major component of palliative care (Michelson & Steinhorn 2007). Parents have identified that children suffer multiple symptoms, particularly at the end-of-life (Wolfe et al 2000). It is essential to recognise that the symptoms experienced by children are rarely simply physical events. Symptoms should be regarded as more often a complex experience with physical, psychological, social and emotional elements (Brady 1996).

Reliable, valid and frequent assessment is central to successful symptom management (Brown 2007). Assessment regardless of the symptom is an ongoing process, which permits choice and flexibility when circumstances for the child and family change (Anghelescu et al 2006, DoH 2000). The child's stage of development must be central to assessment and management of symptoms. A variety of assessment tools can be used in the extracting and assimilating of information with children. Many assessment tools offer a combination approach using verbal and non-verbal indicators (see Chapter 17). Paediatric Pain Profile (Hunt 2003) is an example of an assessment tool for use with pre-verbal, unconscious and non-verbal children. Although a range of assessment tools exist, their under-use in practice with children with life-limiting conditions has been highlighted (McCluggage & Elborn 2006).

Adequate symptom control is viewed as the ultimate aim of palliative care regardless of the setting in which care is provided. Negotiation with and open lines of communication between the child, family and nurse are essential in achieving optimum symptom control. Symptoms experienced vary depending on the child and specific diagnosis and families have much to offer in the assessment and evaluation of symptom management. Symptom management plans should in addition be flexible, evidence based and include combinations of both pharmacological and non-pharmacological interventions (Anghelescu et al 2006). Education of parents and preparation regarding symptoms is crucial (Beardsmore & Fitzmaurice 2002) in order that they know what to expect. The nurse must consider that symptoms that may not be disturbing to the child can be very distressing to parents.

Scenario

Carol, an 8-year-old girl, was at the end-of-life stage – she was unconscious, settled and comfortable. Her parents were by her hospital bed and very involved with her care. A few days before her death, Carol developed noisy respirations. This caused her parents great distress and they found it extremely frightening. This symptom was managed by administering a hyoscine patch, which was placed behind Carol's ear. Explanations and reassurance was provided for the parents. The noise was reduced and parental anxiety was eased.

This scenario illustrates the importance of involving the parents, consideration of parental need and recognising that they suffer alongside their child. Many symptoms are managed pharmacologically which can be challenging given that many of the drugs used effectively for symptom management with adults are not licensed for use in children (McCulloch et al 2008). A number of routes of administration can be used and the chosen route depends on the age, condition of the child and any access devices that the child may have in place.

The oral route is usually first choice for administration of medication in child – many drugs are available in elixir form. The child and family should be involved in decisions about the preferred format. Intramuscular injections should be avoided in children where possible. Many children at this stage in illness may have a central line in position, which provides a useful alternative route for administration. Some children may have a nasogastric tube in place and this can be utilised successfully for administration of medication. Infusions can be given subcutaneously via syringe drivers (McNeilly et al 2004) or via an existing central venous catheter. In recent years the transdermal route has become another option for the delivery of some drugs. Rectal preparations are available for many drugs; they should be avoided in children with low platelet counts and repeated use can cause soreness in children.

The focus of complementary therapies in palliative care is on symptom control. Buckle (2003) discusses the value of aromatherapy and massage in children's palliative care. These techniques can aid in promoting communication with children, reducing anxiety, enhancing relationships and enhancing quality of life in terms of symptom management. Other types of complementary therapies include reflexology, guided imagery and hypnotherapy. These therapies can be used in conjunction with conventional medicine. As with all interventions the child's welfare must be paramount and underpin all care delivered.

Commonly occurring symptoms experienced by children and interventions are identified in Table 46.1. Further details of symptoms and their management are listed in Rainbow Children's Hospice Guidelines (see below). A study by Pritchard et al (2008) examining parents' perceptions of symptoms experienced by children with advanced cancer included changes in their child's behaviour and appearance. Healthcare professionals should prepare and support parents regarding these two distressing symptoms. ACT has a discussion forum which brings together those working within paediatric palliative care both nationally and internationally – this is a very good forum for sharing practice experiences about symptom control and other issues. Information on this is available at http://www.act.org.uk (click on 'networking' and then 'Paedpalcare').

WWW

Refer to Rainbow Children's Hospice guidelines – basic symptom control in paediatric palliative care at:

- http://www.act.org.uk/dmdocuments/Microsoft_Word_2008_Symptom_Control_Manual.pdf

for a detailed manual for symptom management for children.

Holistic care of the child and family

Palliative care to children and families is developed around an ethos of holistic care delivery – that is, care that addresses physical, psychological, social and spiritual needs of the child and family (Goldman et al 2006a). Seldom are the issues and symptoms experienced by children and families simply in one category, much more often they are complex and multi-faceted. The child with palliative care needs must be viewed within the context of a family system (McNeilly et al 2006). The philosophy of palliative care for children is thus premised on a holistic, individualised approach, which centres round the specific needs of each individual child and family during their limited life trajectory (Price et al 2005). The care should be assessed, planned, implemented and evaluated using a collaborative partnership approach and should address the biological, psychological, social and spiritual needs of the child and family (see Chapter 6 and 7).

The collaborative partnership approach should be based on a trusting, therapeutic relationship with families (Monterosso & Kristjanson 2008). Families should be welcomed as partners in all stages of the nursing process, parents should feel they have a choice and be in control of the situation (Vickers & Carlisle 2000).

The last days of a child's life particularly remain clear in the minds of parents (Postovsky & Ben Arush 2004). Memories – negative and positive – that parents have of their child's end-of-life care can have an effect on parental adjustment and theoretical perspectives on parental grief further support this (Davies 2004). Therefore the nurse has a professional responsibility to ensure that care is sensitively and carefully provided in response to the individual needs of both the child and family (Friedman et al 2005). The family includes parents, siblings and the wider family circle. Caring for a child with a life-limiting illness can have major emotional, psychological and social impact on the family unit.

Ensuring a robust family support network including social support systems is essential as a family face losing their child. Social isolation can be experienced when a child is ill; a study carried out by Steele (2005) gained insight of families experiences of living with a child who had a neurodegenerative life-threatening illness. Families expressed that they often disengaged themselves from previous relationships outside the immediate family as the ill child was the focus of parental time and energy. This in turn could lead to them feeling isolated and alone, particularly at times of crisis. Parents and other family members should be encouraged to continue involvement in their child's care even as the child's condition deteriorates. Continual assessment of the needs of the parent and their coping is required, as is the necessary support.

Table 46.1 Symptom management in children's palliative care

Symptom	Possible causes/exploration	Pharmacological management	Non-pharmacological management	Comments/special notes
Pain Pain is most feared by parents whose child is approaching death Freidman et al (2005) discuss that under-medication is a common issue relating to pain and other symptoms, particularly at the end of life	Pain is multifaceted, made up of physiological, emotional, spiritual and social aspects Each of these elements require consideration, as does the fact that the child continues to grow and develop	Analgesia should be selected for the type of pain being experienced Pain may be chronic and a combination of drug types may be used (Friedman et al 2005) Keep analgesia simple initially and gradually progress as necessitated by the specific need of the child (see WHO pain ladder on CD rom) A variety of routes can be used – oral, buccal, rectal, subcutaneous or IV infusion. Transdermal is a way of managing symptoms in children without needles and is increasingly being used (Hain & Wallace 2008)	Non-pharmalogical approaches to pain can include techniques such as guided imagery, relaxation, complementary therapies, distraction therapy, heat and cold (Anghelesca et al 2006) and positioning of the child Careful explanations to child and family and parental presence may have a positive affect in reducing fear and anxiety and thus may reduce the intensity of the pain experienced	Assessing and managing total pain is a priority when caring for the child and family Refer to Chapter 17 Anticipation is critical in managing pain in children (Himelstein 2006) Pain assessment must be developmentally and age appropriate (Himelstein 2006) Parental support will be required regarding the use of opioids and associated fear (Beardsmore & Fitzmaurice 2002)
Nausea and vomiting	This may be a result of constipation, raised intracranial pressure (ICP), intestinal obstruction, anorexia, cough, pain or as a side effect of opioid therapy	A wide range of antiemetics are available Antiemetics act on different sites so it is essential to recognise the potential cause of the nausea and vomiting in order that the correct antiemetic is selected If vomiting and nausea are not resolved combinations that work on different sites can be used in combination effectively Dexamethasone can be added to first line to enhance efficacy	Common sense measures include avoiding known stimuli to vomiting (McCluggage & Jassal 2009) These can include: Avoid strong odours Offer small amounts of food Good oral hygiene Distraction techniques including play	These drugs can be given orally often in elixir or tablet form Certain antiemetics come in melt form that can provide a useful alternative for children If the oral route is not suitable for a particular child, then rectal or subcutaneous routes can be used Many antiemetic drugs are compatible with opiates and can be added to syringe drivers and administered with analgesia (McCluggage & Jassal 2009) Nausea can contribute to weakness, inactivity and irritability. These non-specific signs can often be confused with pain (Himelstein 2006)
Respiratory symptoms: including cough, dyspnoea, congestion, respiratory distress, grunting	The cause of the respiratory symptom and the severity of the problem is dependent on the nature of the underlying disease In children with malignancies may be due to pleural effusion, SVC obstruction, anaemia or ascites Children with neurodegenerative disease and cystic fibrosis are most likely to experience problems related to the respiratory system in the terminal stage of illness	Diazepam to reduce the anxiety associated with breathlessness, simple linctus for an irritating cough and hyoscine can be used successfully for the management of excessive secretions Laboured respiration and grunting may occur in the latter stages of illness when death is imminent, the child is normally in a deep unconscious state, this may be treated with diamorphine, subcutaneous midazolam or rectal diazepam Parents require explanation and reassurance during this stage (Sourkes et al 2005) Oxygen therapy and nebulised bronchodilators may be useful	As anxiety can make breathlessness worse, calm reassurance for both child and family is important (McCluggage & Jassal 2009) Appropriate positioning of the child may also ease this symptom e.g. propping the child upright to permit optimal lung expansion Physiotherapy with or without suction may help to settle the child Use a fan to circulate air Use relaxation and deep breathing exercises Keep the room well ventilated	Breathlessness can be increased by anxiety Anxiety can exacerbate the physical symptoms. Anxiety of parents clearly affects the worries of the child

Continued

Table 46.1 Symptom management in children's palliative care—Cont'd

Symptom	Possible causes/exploration	Pharmacological management	Non-pharmacological management	Comments/special notes
Constipation	Constipation can result due to inactivity, dehydration, an obstruction (e.g. tumour involvement), nerve involvement or as a side effect of medication (e.g. opioids)	Where possible, the aim of treatment should be to avoid it in the first place (Himelstein 2006) If the child does develop constipation a variety of laxatives can be selected Oral laxatives should be used in the first instance and hopefully if they are successful the use of rectal treatments can be avoided	Enlist the help and support of the family who will be able to give information to the nurse about the child's normal bowel movements Encourage increased activity if appropriate given child's condition Attention to fluid intake and diet Provide privacy and maintain dignity during defecation	Prevention is key to management of constipation (Himelstein 2006) A laxative should be prescribed and administered at the commencement of opioid therapy (McCluggage & Jassal 2009)
Symptoms of central nervous system (seizures, agitation, twitching and restlessness)	Children with neurodegenerative conditions or brain tumour may suffer seizures Twitching and agitation may be caused by electrolyte imbalance, hypoxia and opioids Altered sleep pattern and depression can also lead to agitation	Rectal diazepam is particularly useful and effective for children having a fit Buccal midazolam is increasingly being used in older children or when the rectal route is difficult to access Midazolam can be added into the syringe driver to address the agitation, which can be experienced in the late terminal stages of life in children	Non-pharmacological interventions for agitation should include calm, reassuring, open communication to the child and the use of relaxation, guided imagery or massage	If the child who is prone to a seizure is being cared for at home the families should have a supply of diazepam and be given practical advice on seizure management (Beardsmore & Fitzmaurice 2002) The family should also be taught how to maintain their child's safety
Skin problems/pruritus	Children who are facing death are prone to this as a result of a decrease in oral intake and medication such as opioids (Himelstein 2006) Children who have biliary, renal or hepatic disease would also be prone to this skin irritation Children who have been on or are on steroids may be predisposed to skin problems, as their skin can be thinned and papery in appearance Skin breakdown can occur as a result of reduced mobility and also due to a decrease in the child's nutritional intake	Skin irritation can be managed by skin care products and antihistamines administered orally or intravenously. These may ease discomfort	Avoid harsh soaps, which may dry the skin Avoid the use of highly perfumed bath/shower products and moisturising products Keep fingernails short and discourage scratching to prevent excoriation (Sourkes et al 2005) Keep the child cool and dress child in cotton clothing Distraction and relaxation may help (Sourkes et al 2005)	Dry skin and pruritus are more common in children than breakdown of skin areas Regular assessment of a child's skin condition should be carried out to establish if any change has taken place Regular and accurate assessment of the child's skin integrity should be carried out and recorded. The parents or main caregivers should be educated as to how to carry this out Mobility should be encouraged as the child's condition dictates. If the child is confined to bed then their position should be changed 2-hourly. Air mattresses can be obtained by nursing staff (either hospital or community)

Fatigue Most common symptom reported by families whose child died with malignant disease (Hechler et al, 2008, Wolfe et al, 2000)	Causes in children with malignancies include anaemia, poor nutrition, metabolic disturbancies, medication and psychological factors (Frager & Collins 2006) Signs can include poor energy, weakness, altered sleep patterns or reduction in participation in usual activities (Himelstein 2006)	Specific drug therapy does not currently exist (Himelstein 2006)	Prioritise daily activities to conserve child's energy levels Plan and pace activities throughout the day	A thorough history should exclude other causes such as depression or anaemia (Himelstein 2006) Occupational therapists and physiotherapists may be able to assist with management programmes
Anxiety	Anxiety usually takes the form of separation anxiety, loneliness, procedure-related anxiety, fear of abandonment and 'death anxiety' (McCulloch & Hammel 2006). Organic causes such as pain, insomnia, breathlessness or weakness may heighten anxiety (Twycross & Wilcock 2001)	Midazolam and levomepromazine are the first two drugs of choice (although midazolam is known to cause paradoxical agitation). These can both be used via a syringe driver or midazolam can be given buccally or intranasally. Rectal diazepam or sublingual lorazepam are useful in acute cases of anxiety	Provide the environment and opportunity for the child to raise their concerns or fears Honesty, if offered gently is helpful. Ensure the question being asked is being answered – listen to what is being asked Consider complementary therapies, input from psychology or youth worker in the case of young person	The sedating effects of most of these drugs need to be discussed with parents – it may be a side-effect which parents will have difficulty with Parents need to be aware and comfortable with health professionals discussing anxieties with their child

This is only a selection of a few of the commonly experienced symptoms. Infections, bleeding, anorexia, muscle spasm are amongst other symptoms, that can be experienced by children. See Rainbows Children's Hospice Guidelines, 7th edn (2008) for a more exhaustive and detailed account of symptom management and Goldman et al (2006a) Oxford Textbook of Palliative Care for Children.

A social worker will be able to advise, direct and assist the family in identifying and securing suitable resources to promote overall family functioning (Sourkes et al 2005). Financial burdens can grip families who have to care for a child with life-limiting illnesses. The child's illness could necessitate one or both parents giving up work to care for the child. Families may be unaware of the help they are entitled to, which can include income support, care allowances and travel and other grants. Voluntary agencies may also provide help assistance with household chores. For example, CLIC Sargent Cancer Care for Children Northern Ireland provides a family support service whereby volunteers help with ironing, cleaning, etc., to allow the parents to spend more time with the sick child and siblings.

Other organisations may be able to offer holidays for the complete family unit in purpose-built facilities. The interdisciplinary team should work together in ensuring that the family is aware of the availability of services and their entitlement. The child's education is an important part of maintaining a quality life for the child with a life-limiting illness. Its importance is two-fold. First, education is an essential way of the child continuing to develop to his or her potential. Second, it allows continuing socialisation and integration with peers. As the child's condition changes, his or her educational needs will need to be re-assessed to see how best they can be addressed. Hospitals and hospices have teachers as part of the interdisciplinary team and home tutors can also be available if the child is unable to attend his or her own school (DoH & DFES 2004).

Psychological care

Learning that a child has a life-limiting illness launches a family into what Steele (2005) describes as 'unchartered territory'. Support is required as parents and the child can experience a range of emotions including fear, anxiety, anger, guilt, uncertainty, blame and shock.

Hope has been identified as one of the greatest coping mechanisms for families (De Graves & Aranda 2005) and can be defined as 'the subjective probability of a good outcome for ourselves or someone close to us' (Little & Sayers 2004, p 1329). Hope is something that has been cited as important to parents throughout their child's illness trajectory and even up to the moment of their child's death. Bereaved mothers who participated in a study by Laakso & Paunonen-Ilmonen (2002) identified that they expected nursing staff to maintain and provide hope as long as the child remained alive. However hope for a cure may be replaced by the hope for a good death when parents have an awareness that death is imminent (Little & Sayers 2004).

The emotional responses of the family impact on the care and support they give their child. Mothers appear to express their feelings more freely than fathers and it is often assumed by healthcare professionals that fathers can cope. It is essential that the different members of the interdisciplinary team ensure that the needs of the father are also addressed and that they are included in discussions and decision making.

Parents will have questions regarding their child and their child's care – examples of these questions as the child is nearing the end of life are listed on the companion PowerPoint. Beardsmore & Fitzmaurice (2002) caution the use of time scales if parents ask 'How long has my child got?'. Parents can hold on to time scales and if the child dies before or after the suggested time frame can feel cheated or frustrated.

Time should be permitted in order that parents can assimilate information before they can decide how to approach it. Family members need to be empowered with information to enable them to make decisions about care (Price 2003). Jones (2006) suggests that in addition to information families need control and advocacy for decisions they have to make. It is important to ensure that honest, accurate consistent responses and information are given. The family will have options but may require guidance when making decisions as parents are seen as the surrogate decision makers for their child (Hynson et al 2003).

The inclusion of siblings in each stage of the process of dying can greatly benefit the surviving sibling (Gibbons 1992, Mulhern et al 1983). Parents and healthcare professionals should ensure open, honest communication, inclusion and support for siblings as a child moves towards the end of life. Nurses can educate families on the importance of involving siblings as soon as possible when it is clear that the child is going to die, this has been identified in the literature as anticipatory guidance (Giovanola 2005).

Scenario

David is 8. His 11-year-old sister Clare was diagnosed with a brain tumour 2 years ago. This did not respond to treatment and she is now approaching death. Clare is being cared for at home and is unable to leave the house. Consider the changes David might be experiencing:

- in his family life
- in his relationship with his sibling and parents
- in his own feelings and emotions.

What strategies could these parents use to prepare David for Clare's imminent death?

An honest and truthful approach has been identified as one of the rights of the child and is viewed as an essential component of effective communication in quality palliative care. The understanding children have of death evolves gradually. Talking to children about illness and death is extremely difficult – the child's developmental stage must be given careful consideration (Hynson et al 2003) when communicating effectively with life-limited children.

Children with life-limiting illness are suspected as having an awareness of their impending death (Bluebond-Langner 1978). Bluebond-Langner's landmark study has shaped thinking on this issue and indicated that children as young as 3 were aware of their diagnosis and prognosis without having been told. It is understandable that parents want to protect their child from harm and distress. A situation of mutual pretence can arise where both the child and the parent pretend to be unaware of the situation to protect each other (Bluebond-Langer 1978, While 1989).

Evidence-based practice

Kreicbergs et al (2004) carried out a quantitative study in Sweden and used questionnaires to establish whether or not parents had spoken to their child about their impending death.

Results indicated that 429 parents out of 449 participants stated whether or not they had spoken to their child about death. None of the 147 parents who had talked about death regretted it, whereas 69 of 258 parents who did not talk about it regretted not having done so.

The nurse must accept that honesty can be extremely painful for families and that sensitivity must be central to this. In certain situations, some parents may still wish to withhold the truth in an attempt to protect the child. This can be a difficult situation for the healthcare professional, who must respect the family's right. Swaffield (1985) identified that many of the children whose parents had chosen not to tell them of their impending death were aware of it anyway. The nurse must work in collaboration with the other members of the interdisciplinary team creating a atmosphere that fosters truthfulness (Dunlop 2008) and should ensure the family are fully informed as to the knowledge that exists around child awareness of death. (Helpful tips for talking to children about death can be found on the companion PowerPoint slide.)

Scenario

John is an 11-year-old boy in the terminal stage of his illness. His parents want him to know the truth about his impending death. They think he probably knows but ask his named nurse to tell him. What would you do if you were that nurse?

Again, it is important to re-iterate that individuality is the key in palliative care. However, the named nurse in this particular situation endeavoured to facilitate and support the parents in their decision. She sat down with John and, holding his hand, asked him if there was anything he wanted to talk about or if there were any questions he wanted to ask. He simply asked 'Can you please make sure I am not in pain?' He did know and did not wish to discuss it any further. Levetown and the Committee on Bioethics (2008) concede that children who do not ask should be given the opportunity to receive information, however if they refuse it this should not be forced upon them.

Truth telling and talking to the dying child can cause the nurse to face an ethical dilemma, especially if it contravenes the family's wishes. Other ethical dilemmas in palliative care include withdrawing treatment, decisions around 'Do Not Resuscitate', and feeding and fluids in the child facing death. These can also cause distress for families and raise ethical issues for staff (see Chapters 20 and 21).

PowerPoint

Access the companion PowerPoint presentation and look at the case study.

A wide range of verbal and non-verbal communication strategies can be used when communicating with life-limited children. Touch, play, art and the therapeutic use of story-telling are important strategies in palliative care, aiding the child in expressing their concerns, fears and feelings (Done 2001). These strategies are also useful in aiding siblings to express their feelings and are useful media for preparing them for the impending death. Play is widely recognised as the language of the child and as such play is an important communication medium for the child (see Chapter 10). Play specialists in both the hospital and community have expert training to enable them to fully implement play packages in order to maximise benefit to the child and family (Price & Spence 2004).

Charitable organisations have a role to play in the psychological well-being of children with life-limiting illnesses and their families for example organisations such as Make-a-Wish, Dreams Come True and Dial A Dream. Wishes granted are wide ranging and can give the family happy memories, which can comfort them in bereavement.

www

Go online to the Make-a-Wish and Starlight Foundation websites and familiarise yourself with the mission statements of the charities and the ways in which they have in the past helped children and families. Read the personal stories of wishes that have been granted:

- http://www.make-a-wish.org.uk
- http://www.starlight.org.uk

Families and children can gain much psychological and social support from groups where they meet with other families whose children have the same condition. They also have experts and counsellors to assist the child and family in developing family and personal coping strategies. Examples of these groups are Contact-a-family, React and other local support groups.

The impact on the marital relationship, the interactions and communication between parents has also been examined. Evidence has indicated that a child's life-threatening illness can lead to strain on the relationship between parents as they focus on caring for the child and therefore can neglect their relationship (Steele 2005). This provides a useful insight into the possible changes in the dynamics of relationships and endorses the importance of ensuring that within the 'family systems approach' to care emotional support and communication is channelled to mothers, fathers, siblings and other family members.

Spiritual care

Many families have established sources for spiritual support and these will continue during their palliative journey and particularly at critical junctures – for example diagnosis, relapse or end-of-life.

The nurse must ensure that the spiritual needs of the child and family are addressed and take cognisance of the fact that spiritual needs can occur independently of religious needs (Davies et al 2002). Spiritual care should include the uniqueness of the child and family, and should address their needs, values and beliefs encompassing moral aspects and value systems possessed by a parent and a child – for example insight and wisdom, reliance on values and virtues such as hope, trust and love. Evidence suggests that parents find issues around spirituality as being a source of help as their child near the end of life. Prayer, faith, access to clergy and the transcendent quality of the child–parent relationship that endures beyond death were identified as important by parents whose child died in Intensive Care (Robinson et al 2006).

Evidence-based practice

Feudtner et al (2003) carried out a study of hospital chaplains working in 115 children's hospitals in America. A 67% response rate was received.

Spiritual distress experienced by children can include anxiety, fear and coping with symptoms.

For parents, spiritual distress can include questioning why this was happening and also feelings of guilt because they could not prevent their child experiencing suffering or dying.

Barriers in providing spiritual support were identified by the chaplains. The barriers noted were healthcare professionals who were inadequately trained to detect spiritual distress and in addition being asked to visit children and families too late to ensure all the care they needed was provided.

Some families who have previously had little or no religious faith or belief may wish to have contact with a minister/chaplain as they face the death of their child – they should be facilitated to this as early as possible (Feudtner et al 2003). The child too may wish to discuss ideas, views and fears from a spiritual stance. Some young people may wish to talk, discuss and plan the arrangements for their funeral with the minister before their death. If this is their wish, it is important that they are given the opportunity to do so. Anger 'against God' can be common in some parents whose child is dying – the minister/chaplain may be a channel by which they can vent their anger and a professional who may help and facilitate them working through their feelings and emotions. For some families, to have their child baptised may be important at this time and should be facilitated. Children and families should be given the opportunity, time and privacy to perform any religious acts that may provide them comfort, for example lighting a candle (obviously safety must be paramount).

We are now living in a very wide and diverse cultural society. It is essential that all members of the team caring for the child recognise the individuality of each child and family and recognise, respect and accept any specific spiritual wishes, beliefs or rituals surrounding death and beliefs of death.

Respite care

Respite care is an instrumental part of palliative care for children and young people (Corkin et al 2006). Caring for a child with a life-limiting illness is both physically and emotionally draining for the family (Maguire 2001). The care may involve 24-hour devotion of the parent to the sick child. It is essential that the family is offered some time away for the physical and emotional exhaustion that the tasks of caring can cause. Parents and families willingly undertake very complex care at home when their child has a life-limiting illness. Their ability to cope will decrease and their level of stress will increase unless they receive regular respite care. Judd (1994 p 218) defines respite care as:

> Complementary, flexible care in the home or home from home setting with appropriate medical and nursing support, offering parents or carers an interval of relief.

As with all other aspects of palliative care for children and families, the need and type of respite care required should to be tailored to the individual family. The range or respite provision offered is limited in certain parts of the UK (Thurgate 2005), however with an increase in the profile of the needs of children with life-limiting illness, and their families, new services continue to be developed in an attempt to meet the increasing demand.

End-of-life care

Identifying when a child enters the end-of-life phase is not easy (ACT 2004) and is dependant upon the child's condition, with clinical patterns being variable (Finlay et al 2008). For some families there is little time to acknowledge that death is imminent, for others there is a more clear move to this phase – for example where a decision may have been made to stop treatment or where treatment options are exhausted (ACT 2004). Families face many decisions throughout the whole palliative care journey but especially at the end-of-life stage. One of the primary choices is often the 'place of care' as the child approaches death. Improvements and developments within community services have led to many families choosing their own home as the place where they want their child to be nursed. Where appropriate, the child or young person should be included when the family considers the choice of where the child should be nursed. All their options should be outlined and again they may require time to discuss and make a decision (Brown 2002). Parents often prefer the palliative care of their children carried out at home (Hynson & Sawyer 2001, Vickers & Carlisle 2000, Vickers et al 2007).

Activity

Consider the advantages for the child and family if home is the place where the end-of-life care is delivered.

Children often prefer that they be cared for at home in their own familiar environment and home is also the place where the family may maintain greater control and a more normal family life can be managed (Friedman et al 2005). Despite support from the interdisciplinary team, caring for the child at home can place a heavy responsibility on the parents. Goldman et al (1990) assert that the hospital environment can provide security, although the environment may not be comfortable and parental control may be lacking. It is important that parents who are not able to choose the home care option should not be made to feel guilty (Friedman et al 2005). The hospice can provide a valuable alternative for families who cannot contemplate a home death (Watterson & Hain 2003). Hospices can offer a homely, less clinical environment for families with the security often desired by parents.

The components of care already discussed in this chapter are also crucial at the end of life. End-of-life care should be based upon an individualised holistic approach to care centred round the changing need of the child and family. Communication, good team working, a therapeutic relationship with child and family, good symptom management and a forum where family decisions are nurtured and facilitated are central aspects of quality end-of-life care. Stress and anxiety of families, often coupled with the reluctance to accept that death is imminent, can be particularly challenging. Changes in the child's behaviour and appearance were identified by parents as symptoms which caused them concern as they approached death (Pritchard et al 2008) – this finding has implications for healthcare professionals as addressing the likelihood of these with families in advance is important.

The ACT Care Pathway gives an excellent framework to guide and structure end-of-life plans and ensures that all the child and family needs are considered. The end of life component of this pathway can be viewed on the companion CD-rom.

Care of the child following death

The need for parental support and advice is never greater than at the time when the death occurs (see Chapter 10 for an introduction to communication in bereavement). Even if the death has been expected, the parents' reactions at the time of death are unpredictable. Parents who have just lost their child will usually require guidance from the healthcare professional. Parental choice and control is essential (ACT 2004). The professional must therefore be aware of the relevant issues and be knowledgeable and informed about the options facing the family at this sad time:

- Time and privacy should be given to parents when decisions have to be made.
- Death should be established by a medical officer/GP.
- Families should be able to stay with their child for as long as they wish and be encouraged to hold, cuddle, wash and dress their child if desired.
- Families should be prepared for how the child's appearance will change after death and the possible noises the body may make.
- Cultural and religious beliefs and practices should be respected (ACT 2004).
- Families should be given the opportunity to talk through procedures and not merely given the written information.
- Written booklets are useful to back up verbal information and guide parents to further support networks (Davey 1995).
- The family might want a handprint or lock of hair to keep (ACT 2004) consent should be obtained from the family.
- Families should be given time to spend with their child; this may include siblings. They should never feel rushed or hurried (Brown 2007).
- Parents should be informed of their choices regarding taking their child home following a planned death in hospice or hospital (Whittle & Cutts 2002).
- All those professionals who have contact with the family must be immediately informed about the child's death so that appointments, etc., are not sent for the child. This can cause considerable distress to the family (ACT 2004).
- Post mortems are not usual if the death is expected, however in some cases a post mortem may be useful if a diagnosis was not clear or to help gain insight into rare conditions. Parents will need support, reassurance and information to aid them to make decisions and choices (ACT 2004).

Activity

In the Clinical Companion to this book read McNeilly & Price (2008) Chapter 44 'Care of the child' in Kelsey and McEwing (eds) 2008 Clinical Skills in Child Health.

Bereavement care

The death of a child is a uniquely traumatic experience for a parent (Brewis 1995, Rando 1986). The grieving process following such a loss is complex and multifaceted. The definition of palliative care cited at the outset of this chapter includes bereavement support as one of the essential components of children's palliative care. This section therefore examines the needs of a family following the death of their child and the nurse's role in bereavement care. At this stage it seems appropriate to clarify the terms that are commonly used here. Hindmarch (2000) suggests that:

- bereavement is what happens
- grief is what one feels in reaction to the bereavement
- mourning is what one does to express grief.

Activity

Consider the factors that may affect an individual's grief.

The gendered differences in parental reaction to death of a child have been studied in a key work by Feeley & Gottlieb (1988). This study reported that mothers' grief reactions appeared angrier, despairing and much more isolating than that of fathers. Mothers were also more likely to talk about their feelings whereas fathers were more likely to keep busy. This finding is further supported in a discussion paper carried out by Duncombe & Marsden (1995) which referred to the 'tragedy of the inexpressive male' and in addition pointed out the more apparent willingness of mothers to 'recognise, label, express and disclose feelings'.

The devastation caused by a child's death is far reaching, affecting parents, siblings, grandparents, wider family circles, healthcare professionals and communities. Rando (1986) identifies that the loss of a child to a parent can seem like a physical loss (that is that they have lost a part of themselves), the loss of their role, loss of hopes, dreams and their identity as protector. Klass (1988) identifies two central features of parental grief following the death of their child. First, is that it represents to the parent a loss of self and, second, that is represents a loss of competence.

Worden (1991) describes the process of mourning as a series of tasks linked to stages. He identified four stages with inherent tasks, which the mourner must work through to resolve one's grief:

- to accept the reality of loss
- to work through the pain of grief
- to adjust to an environment in which the deceased is missing
- to emotionally relocate the deceased and move on with life (the task of resolution).

However, this staged approach can be seen as providing a very rigid approach to grief work, although it does permit individuality, moving in and out of different stages, and overall provides a very prescriptive framework. It is important to recognise that Worden's grief work does not necessarily state that the stages are experienced sequentially or that any time limit can be applied. Uniformity is not part of the grieving process. There are no rules in grief and both parents are likely to respond in different ways.

Goldman (1999) states that the progress through phases of grief is not straightforward or only in one direction and perspectives on parental grief would now indicate that in the case of bereaved parents negotiate the complexities of readjusted life with 'the dead child' and their continuing bonds with this child (Davies 2004).

Activity

Consider some roles that may negatively affect fathers when dealing with their grief. Check below.

William Schatz (1986) identified the following male roles as negatively affecting the way he dealt with his grief following the death of his son:

- The role of being strong, a macho man always in control of his emotions.
- The role of competing and winning in a crisis and being the best.
- The role of being protector of family and possessions.
- The role of being the family provider.
- The role of being problem solver, fixing things or finding someone who can.
- The role of controller.
- The role of self-sufficient standing on his own two feet.

The nurse who is coordinating the bereavement care of a family should be aware of these issues and patterns of grief.

Siblings require particular attention during the period leading up to the death of the child as mentioned earlier and following the death through bereavement. Following the death, even though it may have been expected, is a time of great turmoil, interruption and uncertainty for the siblings. The age and cognitive development will obviously affect their understanding. Children have very definite needs in bereavement. They require information, reassurance, time to express their feelings and the need to be involved (Brown 2002). Children need also to have some type of routine maintained – this, coupled with support from the adults around them, may be difficult as the parents are struggling to deal with their own loss and feelings. Parents may need help from the healthcare professional in coordinating the bereavement care to gain an insight into patterns of childhood grief and suggestions as to how the child may be helped through the process.

Fox (1988) has outlined four tasks for grieving children:

- To understand or begin to make sense out of what is happening.
- To grieve and express emotional responses to loss.
- To commemorate in some formal or informal way the life of the person who has died.
- To learn how to integrate the loss into one's life to continue with everyday activities of living and loving.

Children can be helped in bereavement by having a memento of the person who has died. This way the child is provided with a tangible reminder of the person who is gone, is reminded of their existence and reassured that life does go on. This could be a favourite toy, photograph, another item of value to the child who has died or even a selection of items in a designated memory box. A number of resources are available to help children experience a healthy grieving process (see the list of books available for children on the companion PowerPoint presentation).

Parents are often anxious about siblings attending the funeral. On one hand, they want to protect them and on the other the parent may feel unable to cope with their own feelings and the feelings of the child. Children should be involved in discussions about this, should be given information beforehand about what they should expect at the service, and their wishes and opinions should be listened to. If they do wish to attend, it may be appropriate for another adult to be assigned to look after them during the service (Black 1998). If they do not attend they should be told as soon afterwards what happened and be given the chance to visit the grave.

It can be very helpful if children are involved in bereavement support groups, which enable the child to work through their grief and to see that they are not alone. Many children's hospices run groups such as these. With support and guidance from family and professionals, the child will learn to adapt to their loss and live their own life.

It is also important to remember the extended family circle and community that may be affected by the death of the child. Grandparents not only lose their grandchild but also have the added burden of 'losing' their own child who is consumed with grief. Many grandparents may experience

WWW

Visit the Winston's Wish website and investigate ways in which this organisation helps support bereaved children.

- http://www.winstonswish.org.uk

'survivor guilt' and could ask 'Why am I still living when my grandchild is dead?'

The wider community is also affected by the death of a child and it is important that the healthcare professional coordinating the bereavement follow-up ensures that contact is made with the child's school. Teachers may feel uncertain how to support the other pupils and staff at this time and usually welcome advice at how to manage the grief and commemorate the child who has died.

The bereavement component of the palliative care may be coordinated and provided by a community children's nurse, Macmillan nurse, hospice nurse or other identified healthcare professional. The individual family should dictate the frequency of visits and type of support required. Contact may well decrease as the family develops coping strategies. The nurse may have to refer a parent to a psychologist or bereavement counsellor if they feel that the individual concerned needs further specialist bereavement support (Dunne 2004). Many hospitals and hospices hold annual remembrance services, which are important to families. Other ways organisations can assist with remembering the child are inclusion in the book of remembrance and sending cards and flowers on specials dates, for example the first anniversary of the child's death.

Activity

List some organisations that help bereaved families.
(Details of these can be found on the companion PowerPoint slide.)

The needs of the healthcare professional

Care of children who are life-limited can be a source of profound satisfaction for staff (Rushton 2005). However it can also be stressful for all those involved in the care package. The death of a child may lead to extreme guilt, anger, sadness and perhaps the feeling that the healthcare worker has failed the child and family (Michelson & Steinhorn 2007).

Evidence-based practice

Costello & Trinder-Brook (2000) carried out a study examining the experiences of 44 children's nurses who cared for dying children in hospital. Positive experiences highlighted by nurses included being able to give support to grieving parents, feeling they could give the child individual attention, controlling pain and other symptoms, as well as providing follow-up care after death. Negative experiences that came out of the study included poor staffing and skill mix, sudden death, emotional attachment to the child and involvement with the family. The study indicated that the death of the child in hospital has a major impact on the nurse and also highlights the importance of preparing nurses for the emotional impact that the death of a child will have.

Avoiding burn-out requires careful self-stress management strategies and awareness of the needs of oneself and others in the team (Baverstock & Finlay 2006). All members of the team must be remembered: porters, domestic assistants and student nurses also can develop a bond with the child and family and can sometimes be overlooked when a death occurs. It is important to consider that you may be a healthcare professional but that also you are a human being with real feelings and emotions. Armstrong (2007) reported that the need to grieve often went unrecognised and there was a lack of support to allow for the grieving process. Most nurses interviewed identified the need for formal mechanisms of support to be available such as debriefing or counselling. It is essential to recognise our feelings and pain at a loss and deal with this. An 'ostrich approach' is dangerous and ignoring one's own needs can have a detrimental effect in the long term. Organisations such as Child Bereavement Charity offer support and training for healthcare workers in this area.

Reflect on your practice

Reflect on ways that you have seen or consider may be useful strategies for staff coping with death of a child.

Check out suggestions for staff coping management strategies on the companion PowerPoint slide.

Summary

Palliative care is an integrated approach to care that addresses holistic care needs at different stages of the uncertain illness trajectory and focuses on quality of life for the child and family.

Quality palliative care for the child or young person requires a cohesive partnership approach, centred on the family with a collaborative interdisciplinary focus to care. Nurses play a key role within the team and are required to identify and address the needs, fears and anxieties of the child–family circle.

Although considerable development has occurred within children's palliative care over recent years and policy has recognised the distinct needs of children with life-limiting conditions, future developments are required. The implementation of the recommendations of these strategic documents (DoH 2007, 2008) will be a good place to start whilst ensuring services for all children regardless of where they live. In addition further substantive research is required and further educational opportunities nationally, and internationally, as we move forward in the continual provision of care based on the best evidence (Institute of Medicine (IOM) 2003, Price & McNeilly 2009).

Key points

- Palliative care for children can be delivered in a variety of care settings and has developed as a distinct specialty.
- The child and family should be central to decisions about the care delivered.

- The interdisciplinary team should address holistic needs of the child.
- Honest and simple responses are important in communicating to children about death.
- Parents and siblings need much support and information as death approaches.
- It is important to remember that for a parent who has lost a child bereavement is a long, complicated and very individual process.
- Nurses need to recognise that caring for children and families facing death is extremely stressful. They should be aware of the importance of developing their own personal management strategies.

References

Anghelescu, D., Oakes, L., Hinds, P., 2006. Palliative care and pediatrics. Anesthesiology Clinics of North America 24, 145–161.

Armstrong, D., 2007. Childhood cancer: the challenge of providing nursing care in the last days of life. Unpublished MSC dissertation. University of Ulster.

Armstrong-Dailey, A., 1990. Children's hospice care. Pediatric Nursing 164, 337–339.

Association for Children's Palliative Care (ACT), 2009. Guide to development of children's palliative care services, 3rd edn. ACT, London.

Association for children with a life-threatening illness (ACT), 2003. Assessment of children with life-limiting conditions and their families – a guide to effective care planning. ACT, London.

Association for children with a life-threatening illness (ACT) and Royal College of Paediatrics and Child Health (RCPCH), 2003. Guide to development of paediatric palliative care services, 2nd edn. ACT/RCPCH, London.

Association for children with life-threatening illness (ACT), 2004. Integrated multi-agency care pathways for children with life-limiting conditions. ACT, London.

Baverstock, A., Finlay, F., 2006. A study of staff support mechanisms within children's hospice. International Journal of Palliative Nursing 12 (11), 506–508.

Beardsmore, S., Fitzmaurice, N., 2002. Palliative care in paediatric oncology. European Journal of Cancer 38, 1900–1907.

Black, D., 1998. Bereavement in childhood. British Medical Journal 316, 931–933.

Brady, M., 1996. Symptom control in dying children. In: Hill, L. (Ed.), 1996. Caring for dying children and families, Chapman Hall, London.

Bluebond-Langer, M., 1978. Mutual pretence: causes and consequences. The private worlds of dying children. University Press, Princeton.

Brady, M., 1996. Symptom control in dying children. In: Hill, L., (Ed.), 1996 Caring for dying children and families. Chapman Hall, London.

Brewis, E., 1995. Issues in bereavement – there are no rules. Paediatric Nursing 79, 337–339.

Brown, E. (Ed.), 2002. The death of a child: care for the child, support for the family. Acorns Children's Hospice Trust, Birmingham.

Brown, E. (Ed.), 2007. Supporting the child and the family in paediatric palliative care, Jessica Kingsley Publishers, London.

Buckle, S., 2003. Aromatherapy and massage – the evidence. Paediatric Nursing 156, 24–27.

Chad, T., 2008. Losing a child to spinal muscular atrophy. Paediatric Nursing 203, 32–33.

Corkin, D., Price, J., Gillespie, E., 2006. Respite care for children, young people and families – are their needs addressed? International Journal of Palliative Nursing 129, 422–427.

Costello, J., Trinder-Booker, A., 2000. Children's nurses' experiences of caring for dying children in hospital. Paediatric Nursing 126, 28–32.

Davey, N., 1995. Paediatric bereavement care. Paediatric Nursing 79, 24.

Davies, B., Brenner, P., Orloff, S., Sumner, L., Worden, W., 2002. Addressing spiritual needs in pediatric hospice and spiritual care. Journal of Palliative Care 18 (1), 59–67.

Davies, R., 2004. New Understandings of parental grief: literature review. Journal of Advanced Nursing 46, 506–513.

De Graves, S., Aranda, S., 2005. When a child cannot be cured – reflections of health professionals. European Journal of Cancer Care 14, 132–140.

Department of Health (DoH), 2000. Framework for the assessment of children in need and their families. The Stationery Office, London.

Department of Health (DoH) and Department for Education and Skills (DfES), 2004. National Service Framework for children, young people and maternity services. Disabled children and those with complex health care needs. DoH, London.

Department of Health (DoH), 2005. National Service Framework for children, young people and maternity services – commissioning children's and young people's palliative care services. DoH, London.

Department of Health (DoH), 2007. Palliative care services for children and young people in England. An independent review for the Secretary of State for Health. DoH, London.

Department of Health (DoH), 2008. Better lives: better care. Improving outcomes and experiences for children, young people and their families living with life-limiting and life threatening conditions. DoH, London.

Done, A., 2001. The therapeutic use of story telling. Paediatric Nursing 133, 17–20.

Duncombe, J., Marsden, D., 1995. 'Workaholics' and 'whinging women': theorising intimacy and emotion work – the last frontier of gender inequality? Sociological Review 43, 150–170.

Dunlop, S., 2008. The dying child: should we tell the truth? Paediatric nursing 20, 828–831.

Dunne, K., 2004. Grief and its manifestations. Nursing Standard, 45–51 1845.

Feeley, N., Gottlieb, L.N., 1988. Parents coping and communication following their infant's death. Omega 191, 51–67.

Feudtner, C., Haney, J., Dimmers, M.A., 2003. Spiritual care needs of hospitalized children and their families: a national survey of pastoral care providers' perceptions. Pediatrics 111, 67–72.

Finlay, F., Lewis, M., Lenton, S., Poon, M., 2008. Planning for the end of children's lives – the lifetime framework. Child Health Care and Development 34, 342–344.

Fox, S.S., 1988. Good grief: helping groups of children when a friend dies. Cited. In: Langton, H. (Ed.), 2000. The child with cancer – family centred care. Baillière Tindall, London.

Friedman, D.L., Hilden, J.M., Powaski, K., 2005. Issues and challenges in palliative care for children with cancer. Current Pain and Headache Reports 9, 249–255.

Gibbons, M.B., 1992. A child dies, a child survives: the impact of sibling loss. Journal of Pediatric Health Care 6, 65–72.

Giovanola, J., 2005. Sibling involvement at the end of life. Journal of Pediatric Oncology Nursing 22, 222–226.

Goldman, A., Beardsmore, S., Hunt, J., 1990. Palliative care for children: home hospital or hospice. Archive of Disease in Childhood 65, 641–643.

Goldman, A., 1999. Care of the dying child. Oxford University Press, Oxford.

Goldman, A., Hain, R., Liben, S. (Eds.), 2006a. Oxford textbook of palliative care for children. Oxford University Press, Oxford.

Goldman, A., Hewitt, M., Collins, G., Childs, M., Hain, R., 2006b. Symptoms in children/young people with progressive malignant disease; UKCCSG/Paeditric Oncology Nurses Forum Survey. Pediatrics 117, 1179–1186.

Hain, R., Wallace, A., 2008. Progress in palliative care for children. Pediatrics and Child Health 18, 141–146.

Himelstein, B.P., 2006. Palliative care for infants, children, adolescents and their families. Journal of Palliative Medicine 9, 163–180.

Hindmarch, C., 2000. On the death of a child, 2nd edn. Radcliffe Medical Press, Oxford.

Hunt A 2003. Paediatric pain profile at www.ppprofile.org.uk

Hynson, J.L., Sawyer, S.M., 2001. Paediatric palliative care: distinctive needs and emerging issues. Journal of Paediatric Child Health 37, 323–325.

Hynson, J., Gillis, J., Collins, J., Irving, H., Trethewiw, J., 2003. The dying child: how is care different? Medical Journal of Australia 179, S20–22.

Institute of Medicine, 2003. When children die: improving palliative and end-of-life care for children and their families. National Academy Press, Washington DC.

Jones, B.L., 2006. companionship, control, and compassion: a social work perspective on the needs of children with cancer and their families at the end of life. Journal of Palliative Medicine 9, 774–788.

Judd, D., 1994. Give sorrow words – working with a dying child, 2nd edn. Whurr Publishers, London.

Klass, D., 1988. Parental grief, solace and resolution. Springer, New York.

Kreicbergs, U., Valdimarsdottir, U., Onelov, E., Henter, J., Steineck, G., 2004. Talking about death with children who have severe malignant disease. New England Journal of Medicine 351, 1175–1186.

Kubler-Ross, E., 1970. On death and dying. Tavistock Press, London.

Laakso, H., Paunonen-Illmonen, M., 2002. Mother's experience of social support following the death of a child. Journal of Clinical Nursing 11, 176–185.

Levetown M and the Committee on Bioethics, 2008. Communicating with children and families; from everyday interactions to skill in conveying distressing symptoms. Pediatrics 121, e1441–e1460.

Liben, S., Papadatou, D., Wolfe, J., 2008. Paediatric palliative care: challenges and emerging ideas. Lancet 371, 852–864.

Little, M., Sayers, E., 2004. While there's life, hope and the experience of cancer. Social Science and Medicine 59, 1329–1337.

Maguire, H., 2001. Developing a hospice service in Northern Ireland. Paediatric Nursing 138, 19–21.

Maunder, E.Z., 2004. The challenge of transitional care for young people with life-limiting illness. British Journal of Nursing 13, 594–596.

Michelson, K.N., Steinhorn, D.M., 2007. Pediatric end-of-life issues and palliative care. Clinical Pediatric Emergency Medicine 8, 212–219.

McCluggage, H.-L., Elborn, J.S., 2006. Symptoms suffered by life-limited children that cause anxiety to UK children's hospice staff. International Journal of Palliative Nursing 12, 254–258.

McCluggage, H.-L., Jassal, S.S., 2009. Symptom management. In: Price, J., McNeilly, P. (Eds.), Palliative care for children and families: an interdisciplinary approach. Palgrave MacMillan, Basingstoke.

McCulloch, R., Comac, M., Craig, F., 2008. Paediatric palliative care: coming of age in oncology? European Journal of Cancer in press.

McNeilly, P., Price, J., McCloskey, S., 2004. The use of syringe drivers: a paediatric perspective. International Journal of Palliative Nursing 108, 399–402.

McNeilly, P., Price, J., McCloskey, S., 2006. Reflection in children's palliative care: a model. European Journal of Palliative Care 131, 31–34.

McNeilly, P., Price, J., 2007. Interdisciplinary teamworking in paediatric palliative care. European Journal of Palliative Care 14, 64–67.

McNeilly, P., Price, J., 2008. Care of the child after death. In: Kelsey, J., McEwing, G. (Eds.), Clinical skills in child health practice. Elsevier, London.

Monterosso, L., Kristjanson, G., 2008. Supportive and palliative care needs of families of children who die from cancer: an Australian study. Palliative Medicine 22, 59–69.

Mulhern, R.K., Lauer, M.E., Haufmann, R.G., 1983. Death of a child at home or in the hospital: subsequent psychological adjustment of the family. Pediatrics 71, 743–747.

Nuutila, L., Salantera, S., 2006. Children with a long term illness; parents' experiences of care. Journal of Pediatric Nursing 21, 153–160.

Postovsky, G., Ben Arush, C., 2004. Care of a dying child of cancer – the role of the palliative care team in pediatric oncology. Pediatric Hematology and Oncology 21, 67–76.

Price, J., 2003. Information needs of the child with cancer and their family. Cancer Nursing Practice 2 (7), 35–38.

Price, J., Spence, N., 2004. Play in the community-quality care for the child with cancer. Cancer Nursing Practice 38, 31–34.

Price, J., McNeilly, P., McFarlane, M., 2005. Paediatric palliative care in the UK: past, present and future. International Journal of Palliative Nursing 113, 124–126.

Price, J., McNeilly, P., Surgenor, M., 2006. Breaking Bad News to parents – the children's nurses role. International Journal of Palliative Nursing 12 (3), 115–120.

Price, J., McNeilly, P. (Eds.), 2009. Palliative care for children and families: an interdisciplinary approach. Palgrave MacMillan, Basingstoke.

Pritchard, M., Burghen, E., Srivastava, D.K., et al., 2008. Cancer related symptoms most concerning to parents during the last week and last day of their child's life. Pediatrics 121, 1301–1309.

Rainbow Children's Hospice 2008 Guidelines – basic symptom control, 7th edn. Online. Available at: http://www.rainbows.eazytiger.net/symptom.htm

Rando, A.T. (Ed.), 1986. Parental loss of a child. Research Press, Illinois.

Robinson, M., Thiel, M., Backus, M., Meyer, E., 2006. Matters of spirituality at the end of life in the paediatric intensive care unit. Pediatrics 118, 719–729.

Royal College of Nursing, 1999. Supporting parents when they are told of their child's health disorder or disability: guidance for nurses, midwives and health visitors. RCN, London.

Rushton, C., 2005. A framework for integrated pediatric palliative care. Journal of Pediatric Nursing 20, 311–325.

Schatz, W.H., 1986. Grief of fathers. In: Rando, A.T. (Ed.), Parental loss of a child. Research Press, Illinois.

Soricelli, B.A., Utech, C.L., 1985. Mourning the death of a child; the family and group process. Social Work 30, 423–429.

Sourkes, B., Frankel, L., Brown, M., et al., 2005. Food, toys and love: pediatric palliative care. Current Problems Pediatric Adolescent Health Care 35, 350–386.

Steele, R., 2005. Strategies used by families to navigate uncharted territory when a child is dying. Journal of Palliative Care 21 (2), 103–110.

Swaffield, F., 1985. Protecting the parents? Nursing Times 31, 51–52.

Thurgate, C., 2005. Respite for children with complex health needs: issues from the literature. Paediatric Nursing 173, 14–18.

Twycross, R., Back, I., 1998. Nausea and vomiting in advanced cancer. European Journal of Palliative Care 52, 39–45.

Vickers, J., Carlisle, C., 2000. choices and control: parental experiences in pediatric terminal home care. Journal of Pediatric Oncology Nursing 171, 12–20.

Vickers, J., Thompson, A., Collins, G.S., Childs, M., Hain, R., 2007. Place and provision of palliative care for children with progressive cancer: a study by the Paediatric Oncology Nurses' Forum/United Kingdom Children's Cancer Study Group Palliative Care Working Group. Journal of Clinical Oncology 25, 4472–4476.

Watterson, G., Hain, R., 2003. Palliative care; moving forward. Current Paediatrics 13, 221–225.

While, A., 1989. The needs of dying children and their family. Health Visitor 62, 78–176.

Whittle, M., Cutts, S., 2002. Time to go home: assisting families to take their child home following a planned hospital or hospice death. Paediatric Nursing 1410, 24–28.

Wolfe, J., Grier, H.E., Klar, N., et al., 2000. Symptoms and suffering at the end of life in children with cancer. New England Journal of Medicine 342, 326–333.

Worden, J.W., 1991. Grief counselling and grief therapy. Tavistock Press, London.

Worswick, J., 2000. A house called Helen – the development of hospice care for children. Oxford University Press, Oxford.

Useful websites

http://www.act.org.uk – the Association for Children's Palliative Care
http://www.hospice-spc-council.org.uk
http://www.make-a-wish.org.uk – Make-a-wish organisation
http://www.childhospice.org.uk – Children's Hospice UK
http://www.chionline.org – Children's Hospice International
http://www.jessiesfund.org.uk – Jessie's Fund music therapy
http://www.cafamily.org.uk – Contact a family
http://www.dial-a-dream.co.uk – Dial a Dream
http://www.reactcharity.org
www.childbereavement.org.uk – Child Bereavement Charity
http://www.icpcn.org.uk/ – International Children's Palliative Care Network

47

Children with learning disabilities

Victoria Jones Ruth Northway

ABSTRACT

In nursing, more than one-third of all the people we come into contact with are disabled in some way (Disability Rights Commission and Department of Health 2004). People experience disability in many different ways, one of which is in the form of the intellectual impairment that is currently termed 'learning disability'. In virtually all areas of children's nursing there will be children and young people who have been labelled as having a learning disability. They may have additional health needs and require the support of a range of professionals and different agencies. Parents and other family members also require this support and it is important that it is provided in a coordinated manner.

LEARNING OUTCOMES

- Understand the importance of considering the child before their impairment.
- Define 'learning disability' and identify the factors that can give rise to learning disabilities.
- Understand the ways in which the presence of a learning disability can impact on the lives of children and their families.
- Appreciate the role of the nurse in supporting children with learning disabilities and their families in the context of an interprofessional and interagency approach to care.

Introduction

> It is essential that children with learning disabilities are regarded as children first and that their needs are met as well as those of the rest of the family. Their needs are the same as for any other child but in addition their special needs must also be addressed
>
> (Lindsay 1998 p 51)

This quote makes some very important points, which form the basis of this chapter. First, it stresses that children with learning disabilities are children first. Second, it recognises that they have additional needs and that their families may have additional needs. This chapter will, therefore, focus on identifying some of these additional needs and suggest some ways in which children's nurses can work together with the child, his or her family, and other professionals to ensure that these needs are both recognised and met.

It is also important to say that this chapter is written from the perspective of a social model of disability. In the past, society (which includes nurses and other members of the healthcare professions) tended to view disability and disabled people in terms of a medical or individual model of disability. This approach has meant that disabled people were viewed as not being able to do things because of their disability. In contrast, the social model of disability argues that whereas some people may have certain impairments (such as a visual, mobility or intellectual impairment) what actually prevents them from taking a full role in society is a range of physical, social, psychological and economic barriers. In other words, it is these barriers that disable them. This different view of disability has important implications for the way in which we respond to the needs of disabled people (Northway 1997). This chapter will therefore consider both the nature of the impairment that children and young people with learning disabilities are assessed as having as well as the barriers that they and their families may face. The emphasis when considering the nature of professional support should thus be on the identification and (where possible) removal of these barriers.

A final point, which it is important to stress, is that children and young people with learning disabilities, and their families/carers, are not a homogenous group. For example, their social circumstances, personal resources, cultural background and environmental circumstances will vary. In addition, the area in which they live may determine the support services available to meet their needs. This means that we must be wary of generalising and should seek to understand the particular circumstances of each child and his or her family.

DOI: 10.1016/B978-0-7020-3183-0.10047-5

The nature of 'learning disabilities'

Activity

- Write a list of all the words you have heard being used to refer to someone with a learning disability. Try to put them in two columns – positive and negative terms as we perceive them today.
- Which ones have been used in legislation?
- Make a list of terms you are not sure about. Try to investigate them.

Terminology and labelling

Some groups of people who have been given the label 'learning disabilities' have indicated that, if they must have a label at all, 'people with learning difficulties' is the most acceptable term for others to use for them. They emphasise that people with learning difficulties are people first and intellectually impaired second. Guidance from the government (Department of Health (DoH) 2001) reinforces this distinction but uses the term 'learning disability' to refer to the same group of people. The government goes on to reject the term 'learning difficulty' because it is used in legislation to refer to a group of people with a wider range of educational needs. The term 'learning disability' is thus the current term that is used to refer to individuals and groups of people who would previously have been referred to as having a 'mental handicap' or being 'mentally subnormal'. Such terms are no longer used because they are viewed as having negative connotations. Terminology is thus constantly changing and currently a further term, 'intellectual disability', is favoured and used by some. It may also be helpful to note that terminology varies across continents and when undertaking searches of literature you may want to include 'intellectual impairment' (Australasia) and 'mental retardation' (North America) as search terms.

The term 'learning disability' is a label applied to individuals and groups for many different reasons (e.g. to organise service provision, define a condition, or explain a delay in achieving developmental milestones). Throughout history, people who currently are labelled as having learning disabilities have had many labels applied to them. These tend to reflect the overarching social and economic climate of the day, dominant theoretical perspectives and the language incorporated into the law of the time. For example, the 1983 Mental Health Act replaced the term 'subnormal' with the terms 'mental impairment' and 'severe mental impairment'. Both the Act and these terms are still in use today in legal situations. To understand the nature of learning disability we therefore have to take account of the social and historical context. Different theoretical perspectives have been used to try to understand and explain the nature of learning disabilities. These include sociological, psychological, medical and anthropological perspectives (Gates 2007).

Activity

- Make a list of some of the ways that being labelled as 'learning disabled' could be helpful. Then make a list of some of the ways having such a label could be detrimental. It may be helpful to think about how we label other people and things.
- Consider how, in your role as a nurse, you can make best use of labels and terminology for all your clients whilst avoiding some of the negative impacts associated with being labelled.

Being labelled as having a learning disability can have negative consequences due to prevailing social attitudes. Others can view the person with a learning disability as being different and difference in this context is viewed negatively. They can have low expectations of people with learning disabilities and stereotype them as having a range of negative characteristics. This then has an impact on the life experiences of the person to whom the label is applied. For example, if they are viewed as not being able to learn they will not be provided with educational opportunities and, because they have not been given the chance to learn, their educational development will be delayed. The original view of others (that the person cannot learn) is thus reinforced. Social attitudes thus become one of the barriers that disable people who have impairments.

Having a label or a diagnosis can, however, also bring some benefits. For example, unless you are assessed as having a particular condition or need you may be unable to access certain services and support mechanisms. An example of this might be access to additional educational support in the classroom, which can only be accessed after assessment and diagnosis as having a learning disability.

Labels and diagnoses can also be seen to be of benefit to service planners and service providers. Epidemiological and demographic studies (which rely upon the identification, collation and quantification of certain characteristics) are used as a basis upon which to decide priorities for service development. Similarly, criteria are often applied by services to decide who should (and who should not) be able to access their service. They may thus serve as criteria for rationing of limited resources.

Formal criteria have been developed to 'identify' people who fit into the group of people labelled as having learning disabilities. These can be grouped under cognitive, social functioning and developmental approaches.

Cognitive functioning approach

Despite there being a lot of disagreement about exactly what intelligence is, and whether we can establish fair and equal ways to measure it, intelligence has been used as a factor to determine if someone has a learning disability since the early 1900s (see Gross (1991) for a critical discussion).

The intelligence quotient (IQ) is a standardised figure that makes it possible to compare how an individual performs against other people in the population when taking a test of their cognitive ability. IQ is worked out using the following formula:

$$[\text{Mental age (test result)}/\text{Chronological age (actual age)}] \times 100 = \text{IQ}$$

The World Health Organisation (WHO 1993) refers to IQ measurements to distinguish the degree of impairment experienced by people with learning disabilities. In this way a child's learning disability may be described as being:

- mild
- moderate
- severe
- profound.

Social functioning approach

This refers to the ability of an individual to adapt to the demands made by society and to hold roles in their community. For example, the ability of a child to meet his or her social needs in a classroom setting (communication, self-help, independence and relationships). However, measuring the degree of social functioning of an individual is difficult. If we refer back to the social model of disability it can be seen that the extent to which the child can function is going to be influenced by the degree to which appropriate supports are in place. For example, how many of us would find that our social functioning was impaired if we were unable to wear one form of support, namely our glasses or contact lenses? Similarly, a child may have some degree of intellectual impairment but his or her ability to be independent in a classroom setting may depend on the extent to which picture symbols are used to indicate where key facilities (such as the toilet) are. Additionally, many people who might have an element of impaired social functioning might not have a learning disability; some may also have physical or mental health needs that impair their social functioning. It is also important to take account of the age of the child and what would normally be expected in terms of their social development.

Reflect on your practice

Think about the situation of children with learning disabilities in the context of a children's ward in which you have worked. How could their social functioning have been improved in this context?

The developmental approach

The WHO (1993) refers to social functioning/ability in its current definition of learning disability, but also introduces a further element, namely the period during which the impairment occurred:

> Learning disability is a state of arrested or incomplete development of mind, which is especially characterised by impairment of skills manifested during the developmental period…
>
> (WHO 1993)

This distinguishes a learning disability from other forms of impairment of social and cognitive functioning that may arise later in life, such as those that result from brain injury or dementia.

Combining approaches

What tends to happen is that the cognitive, social and developmental approaches are combined when seeking to provide a definition of learning disabilities and when seeking to determine whether an individual has learning disabilities or not. This can be seen in the current definition used by the DoH (2001 p 14) in the White Paper 'Valuing people', which states:

> Learning disability includes the presence of:
>
> – a significantly reduced ability to understand new or complex information, to learn new skills (impaired intelligence), with;
>
> – a reduced ability to cope independently (impaired social functioning);
>
> – which started before adulthood, with a lasting effect on development.

Factors that can give rise to the presence of a learning disability

A learning disability can result from a single causative factor or from multiple interacting factors. Many children with learning disabilities do not receive a specific medical diagnosis (Department of Health and Department for Education and Skills (DoH/DfES) 2004). Indeed of all people who are labelled as having a learning disability it is often only possible to identify the specific causative factor for less than half. This figure, however, has increased in recent years due to advances in genetics.

Watson (2007) identifies four stages at which learning disabilities may occur. These are preconceptual, prenatal, perinatal (the first 28 days of life) and postnatal (28 days onwards). At each stage factors relating to heredity and the environment can exert an influence. Some causative factors are the following:

- Preconceptual: this might include the fact that genetic characteristics of the parents may give rise to an increased risk that the child will inherit a particular condition. In addition, the health of the mother may give rise to increased risks.
- Prenatal: this might include, for example chromosomal anomalies, genetic disorders, infection, irradiation, immunological and toxicological damage, maternal malnutrition.
- Perinatal: this might include, for example, difficult or abnormal labour, birth injury, prematurity and gestational disorders.
- Postnatal: this might include, for example, malnutrition of the child, sensory and social deprivation, blood chemistry imbalances, infection, ingestion of toxins and cerebral trauma.

Although it may be possible to identify key factors to explain the presence of a learning disability in some children it is often difficult to try and relate their level of cognitive or social functioning to one cause as it would be impossible to know the many other factors which may have had a chance to influence their performance.

In addition the link between the causative factor and the effects this has on the individual are often unclear. For example, in the case of children who have Down syndrome, the causative factor is known (i.e. trisomy 21) but exactly how this brings about the characteristic features of the syndrome is not so certain. It does, however, tell us that because the child has Down syndrome they are more likely to have certain health conditions such as cardiovascular problems, leukaemia, hypothyroidism and sensory impairments (NHS Health Scotland 2004). That is not to say that all children with Down syndrome will have these problems, but rather that they have an increased risk.

It is therefore unhelpful to apply a 'cause and effect' model that raises the risk of implying or offering a prognosis for a child that may be wholly inaccurate. Indeed, such an approach may even serve to deny children the opportunity to be the individuals that, both genetically and socially, we all are.

WWW

For information on specific conditions and syndromes, along with details concerning inheritance patterns visit the web site of the organisation Contact a Family at:

- http://www.cafamily.org.uk

The incidence of learning disability

The difficulties in determining precisely who might be considered to have a learning disability have been outlined above. Despite these difficulties, however, it is possible to try and identify how many people have a learning disability. For example, the DoH (2001) stated that in England alone about 1.2 million people have a mild learning disability. A further 210,000 people have a severe or profound disability and of these it is thought that approximately 65,000 are children or young people.

The prevalence of moderate and mild learning disability is generally higher among deprived and urban populations. The incidence of severe and profound learning disabilities, however, does not vary across regions or socioeconomic groups but the number of people with severe learning disabilities is expected to increase by about 1% per year until 2016 (DoH 2001). This is due to:

- greater life expectancy
- increasing numbers of children with complex and multiple disabilities surviving to adulthood
- a significant rise in the number of children with autistic spectrum disorders
- a greater incidence in the number of children with profound disabilities born to some families of South Asian heritage.

These last three factors have clear implications for children's nurses with regard to the skills and competencies needed to work effectively with learning disabled children and their families. There will also be implications for those managing and developing services, who will need to ensure they can meet the needs of this expanding population. The importance of ensuring that a skilled workforce is available to make services accessible for all disabled children has been recognised by the government (HM Treasury and Department for Education and Skills 2007).

The impact of learning disability on the child and the family

When considering the impact of learning disability on the child and his or her family, it is important to consider a number of different aspects from initial diagnosis and growing up through to transition to adult services. An understanding of each of these aspects is important if children's nurses are to provide an effective service to children with learning disabilities and their families. In addition it is important to consider the health needs of children with learning disabilities since children's nurses have a key role to play in identifying such needs and in ensuring that they are met. In thinking about the impact of a child with learning disabilities on the family it is important, however, to remember that this impact can be positive and that where difficulties do arise these can often be the result of a lack of support or inappropriate service provision (Maxwell & Barr 2003). As SCOPE notes:

> ...many of the difficulties that ensue when a child has a disability are largely a result of the way society responds to that fact rather than being an inherent part of the disability itself
>
> (SCOPE 1999 p 28)

This is clearly linked to an understanding of disability based on the social model. Barriers that can negatively affect the child with a learning disability and their family thus need to be identified and eliminated.

Activity

- Read the paper written by Maxwell & Barr (2003) for an excellent overview of the experience of one mother of a young person with Down syndrome over the early years of his life. Although this is only one mother's account, it clearly highlights a range of issues that are evident in the wider literature.
- When reading the article, try to identify some of the barriers which the child, the mother and the rest of the family have experienced.
- What helped the family and what caused them additional difficulties?

Initial diagnosis

Receiving the news that your child has a learning disability can be a difficult process. However, it can also be a point from which parents can begin to plan the future (Dobson et al 2001,

Maxwell & Barr 2003). Crucial to this process is the manner in which concerns regarding the child's development are shared with the family since problems occur when a carefully considered and planned approach is not taken (SCOPE 1999).

Unfortunately, there are many examples of parents receiving the news in an insensitive and inappropriate manner. In addition, it is not uncommon for parents to express concerns regarding their child only to have them dismissed or not taken seriously by professionals (SCOPE 1999). In its report 'Right from the start', SCOPE (1999) highlights the very difficult nature of the process and identifies that parents were sometimes told 'too little too late' or 'too much too soon'. As a result of its findings, SCOPE has undertaken a programme of work that seeks to improve this process. In its template for good practice, the key principles are identified as valuing the child and respecting the parents (SCOPE 2003). The key practice framework stresses the need for preparation, who should be present, tuning into the parents, the next steps (practical help and information), as well as the need for support for professionals. The importance of good practice at this stage cannot be overemphasised since it will influence the relationship which the family develops with service providers (Michael 2008).

Activity

Read online the work undertaken by the SCOPE 'Right from the start' project. How is information given to parents in your clinical area? Can you see ways in which it could be improved?

- http://www.rightfromthestart.org.uk

Having received the diagnosis, parents are then faced with the prospect of telling other people. Maxwell & Barr (2003) provide the example of when Virginia Maxwell and her husband were told by other people that their son was 'a gift from God' but that a family member also told them that 'he was from the devil' and that they were being punished for their sin. Such reactions from others give an indication of some of the difficulties that parents will face over and above having to adjust to the diagnosis themselves.

The importance of early intervention and support is highlighted since delays in such intervention can, for example, lead to a loss of function or ability without appropriate postural management (DOH/DfES 2004, HM Treasury/DfES 2007).

Growing up

In a study undertaken in 1998, Dobson et al gathered information by the use of questionnaires and diaries with 182 parents of severely disabled children (Dobson et al 2001). They found that the parents of disabled children spent almost twice as much as the parents of non-disabled children, resulting in many families having additional financial concerns. However, the project's original aim – to explore the financial implications of raising a severely disabled child – was expanded when it was recognised that the financial costs constituted only one element of the data that were analysed. The families reported a lack of emotional and practical support in raising their children and referred to a process of 'adjustment' in their family life.

For many families of disabled children, other factors also come into play. The experience of being stared at, being the topic of professional conversations and not feeling like a typical family were themes in Dobson et al's (2001) findings. Many parents felt that their family was viewed as both 'different' and as the victim of a personal tragedy. This denied them the 'emotional and social worth' attributed to most families. They concluded that it is vital that practitioners, services and policy makers make use of the expertise of parents to ensure the appropriate provision of services and efficient use of resources, which will benefit the whole community. Unfortunately, however, the knowledge and experience which parents have concerning their children with learning disabilities is not always valued by others (Maxwell & Barr 2003).

WWW

Read the Dobson et al (2001) report and other Joseph Rowntree Foundation research findings at:

- http://www.jrf.org.uk/publications/impact-childhood-disability family-life

Families have highlighted that relevant and accessible information is one of the aspects of services they most value (Sloper & Mitchell 2000). The policy context in health provision emphasises patient involvement in decision making but, despite this, it is an area many parents feel poorly served. 'Valuing people' (DoH 2001) thus states that, under the 'Quality protects' programme, children's social services will:

> ...provide more and better information for families and increase the availability of key workers and other measures designed to improve coordination
>
> (DoH 2001 section 3.5)

More recently the 'Aiming High for Disabled Children' Report (HM Treasury/DFES 2007) identified access to appropriate information for every disabled child and their families at every stage of the child's life as a key element of the 'core offer' which is to be made available. However, the fact that this needs to be made a priority some 6 years after 'Valuing people' perhaps suggests that this is still an area of service weakness.

Sloper & Mitchell (2000) worked with families to identify quality criteria for information. They interviewed 27 parents who cared for children with a range of disabilities. They also consulted a group of practitioners working in both health and social care settings. This relatively small number of participants could be a reason to limit the extent to which it is possible to generalise from the findings of the study. However, to try to combat this, the research was designed to recruit parents who made use of a range of services and were based in the north of England and practitioners who were selected from the south. They concluded that a three-tiered approach combining directories, in-depth booklets and local information key workers was the ideal way to meet the information needs of families. They also highlighted that quality presentation and clear information about the roles of different agencies were critical considerations in developing information for families of disabled children.

Parental access to information is essential when considering issues such as which school their child should attend. For example, it is current policy that children with learning disabilities should have their educational needs assessed, that educational placement should ensure that these needs are met, and that appropriate support mechanisms are in place. Wherever possible, the child should be educated alongside non-disabled peers in mainstream schools. However, some parents feel that their child would not receive appropriate support to meet their additional needs within mainstream schools. Likewise, there are others who, faced with the offer of an educational placement within a special school, argue their child's right to placement in mainstream education and stress the responsibility of the Local Education Authority to provide such a placement along with any additional support required.

Provision of information concerning the options available and the mechanisms in place to challenge decisions that they are not happy with is crucial to parents in such situations. For further information concerning educational provision for children with a learning disability and for information concerning the debates surrounding integrated and segregated education, see Willis (2007).

Seminar discussion topic

Examine the arguments for and against inclusive education. What are the philosophies that underpin these approaches?

It is important to remember that the presence of a child with learning disabilities within the family has an impact not only on the parents but also on other children within the family. Some work has thus been undertaken with siblings (see, for example, Burke & Montgomery 2001, Evans et al 2001).

Burke & Montgomery suggest that their pilot work indicates that having a disabled brother or sister can bring both benefits and disadvantages. Included in the latter is the fact that siblings may be asked to take on caring tasks. In addition, where the learning disability is due to an inherited genetic disorder then this may affect their future decisions concerning children of their own (Maxwell & Barr 2003). However, the provision of support groups can assist in promoting positive interaction with their learning disabled sibling as well as increasing self-esteem (Evans et al 2001). It is therefore important that, when working with families, all family members are considered.

The provision of respite care is one service which can reduce family stress and allow parents time with their non-disabled children (HM Treasury/DfES 2007). It can also provide a good developmental opportunity for children with learning disabilities. However, a recent report entitled 'Breaking Point' (Mencap 2006) details how families may have to reach breaking point before access to such support is forthcoming. Even then this support is not guaranteed. In the survey Mencap conducted for this report 6 out of 10 families were not getting any short break service provision or were receiving a service which was so minimal that it did not meet their needs. It would thus appear that this is a further area where greater service provision is required.

Transition to adult services

Reflect on your practice

Mrs Lewis is the mother of a 16-year-old girl with profound and multiple disabilities. She has been a frequent visitor to the children's ward over a number of years because her daughter has experienced a range of health problems. During this period of time you have got to know her well. During the most recent visit, however, she had appeared very concerned about the future. She said that at school they had been making plans for what would happen after her daughter left school but that she was very worried.

Given that planning is taking place for her daughter's future what do you feel might be causing Mrs Lewis's current anxiety? What might be the role of the children's nurse in addressing some of her concerns?

The transition from children's services to adult services can be a time of great stress for families. Although it is a process that should be carefully planned, research suggests that it can be a 'rather abrupt affair' (Ward et al 2003). Indeed respondents in a recent independent inquiry suggested that once a child reaches 18 support and coordination can vanish (Michael 2008). The research undertaken by Ward et al revealed that often parents and young people were told at one outpatient appointment that their next contact with services would be with adult services. Even when families did report that transition planning had taken place, more than half stated that transfer to adult health services had not been considered at all. On a more positive note the researchers indicate that 18% of respondents felt that transfer of responsibility for health had been addressed well. They suggest that this indicates that such planning can be undertaken effectively. To improve the situation they argue that health must be addressed as part of the wider process of transition planning and that health professionals who know the child must be involved in this process (Ward et al 2003). This has clear implications for children's nurses as well as for those working in adult services. Effective supports and services need to exist (NHS Health Scotland 2004).

The health needs of children with learning disabilities

NHS Health Scotland (2004) state that, compared with the rest of the population, people with learning disabilities have:

- a higher number of health needs and more complex health needs
- a higher level of unmet health needs

- a different pattern of health needs; the types of health needs they experience can differ and some are specific to people with learning disabilities.

Evidence-based practice

NHS Health Scotland (2004) has undertaken a major review of the evidence concerning the health needs of people with learning disabilities. This document both reviews the evidence regarding health needs across the lifespan and makes recommendations for the development of more responsive services. For further information visit:

- http://www.healthscotland.com

As has already been noted, people with Down syndrome, for example, are at increased risk of having certain health problems (NHS Health Scotland 2004). In addition, children with learning disabilities have an increased prevalence of epilepsy (with children with severe and profound learning disabilities having a greater prevalence), are at increased risk of visual and sensory impairments, and there is a reported high prevalence of mental ill health and problem behaviours (NHS Health Scotland 2004). However, although we know that the health needs of people with learning disabilities can be greater, and that some people have additional needs as a result of their specific impairment, these needs often go unnoticed and unmet. Over the past 20 years it has been increasingly recognised that people with learning disabilities have undetected and unmet health needs (Howells 1986, NHS Health Scotland 2004, Wilson & Haire 1990). As a result it is suggested that people with learning disabilities die as a result of preventable conditions (Barr et al 1999). Whilst these studies relate primarily to adults and whilst children may receive a better quality of health service when compared with adults (Michael 2008) many children with learning disabilities experience problems with accessing appropriate healthcare. This is particularly true for children with complex needs (Michael 2008). Before reading further, look at the case scenarios below.

Scenario

Jenny

Jenny is a 12-year-old girl who has severe learning disabilities. She lives at home with her parents and is a frequent visitor to her local children's ward as she has regular and severe epileptic seizures. She is currently in the ward for a review of her medication following a particularly severe seizure. When she had the seizure she was at home and had been found in the living room lying on the floor. When she recovered from the seizure she seemed very disorientated but did not appear to have otherwise injured herself as she got to her feet and started to walk around. While she was on the ward it was noticed that when she was assisted to bathe she would wince whenever her left hip was touched. She was X-rayed and she was found to have sustained a fracture during her seizure, which had not previously been detected.

Simon

Simon is a 15-year-old boy with mild learning disabilities. It has been suggested that he may suffer from autistic spectrum disorder. He is normally very active but he does not enjoy being in close contact with other people. However, he does appear to have good understanding of what other people say to him and, when his mood allows, he is able to converse with others. He is currently in hospital following appendectomy. When he was brought into the ward he was very withdrawn and obviously in pain but did not want anyone to go near him. His mother said that she had noticed him getting less active over the past couple of days and had tried to get him to tell her what was wrong. However, each time she did this he just got agitated and went to his room. Eventually, however, he had become so unwell that she took him to their GP. Their regular GP was away and so they saw a locum who appeared very hurried, did not take the time to examine Simon because he was uncooperative, and said that she thought that it was just to do with his condition (meaning his autism and learning disabilities). His mother then took him to the emergency department at the hospital where they (eventually) diagnosed him as having appendicitis. He has now been on the ward for a couple of days following his operation but the nurses are worried that he is not recovering as well as they would expect and they suspect that he is in pain. However, although he appears to understand what they say to him they cannot get him to tell them what is wrong. He is also beginning to display what they feel is strange behaviour. Although most of the nurses are trying very hard to meet Simon's needs, one nurse on the ward says that children like Simon shouldn't be on general wards – they should be looked after in specialist areas. In addition, another parent on the ward has complained to the ward staff about his behaviour, also believing that he shouldn't be on the ward.

- Consider each of the above scenarios – what barriers did these young people face in relation to having their health needs met? What could have been done to overcome these barriers?

WWW

For further information concerning autistic spectrum disorders please visit the website of the National Autistic Society:

- http://www.nas.org.uk

In reading through the above scenarios you will, hopefully have identified a number of key barriers that are commonly faced by people with learning disabilities in relation to their healthcare needs. These include the following:

- Communication: people with learning disabilities can find it difficult to communicate to others that they feel unwell. They may not be able to use verbal communication methods or they may have a limited vocabulary, which makes it difficult in a healthcare system which often relies upon the ability of the patient to describe their symptoms. Sometimes communication can take the form of what is perceived as 'difficult' behaviour and, unfortunately, this can be attributed to the fact that a person has a learning disability rather than that they may be unwell or in pain. It is not just people with learning disabilities, however, that have communication difficulties. Sometimes healthcare professionals also lack the skills required to communicate effectively with people with learning disabilities. They may use medical jargon, complex sentences, or be unable to understand augmentative forms of communication such as Makaton (a form of sign language).

- Time: determining whether someone with a learning disability has a health problem can be a long and complex process due to, for example, the communication difficulties outlined above and to other factors such as the fact that procedures may have to be introduced more slowly. However, within the healthcare system pressures of work can mean that time is not always made available for this process. This can result in health needs not being identified.
- Diagnostic overshadowing: what this means is that any change in behaviour or health need is viewed as part of the person's learning disability. This then means that professionals and services can fail to respond since they view it as not being amenable to change. This is clearly shown in the scenario where a locum GP said that Simon's difficulties were due to the fact that he has learning disabilities and autism.
- Negative attitudes: thankfully, these are relatively rare. Nonetheless, they are still prevalent among some members of society and also among nurses and other professionals. Negative attitudes and discrimination may not be as explicit as in the case study above. However, negative perceptions concerning the quality of life of children with learning disabilities may lead to a reluctance to offer certain forms of life-saving or life-enhancing treatments, such as adequate pain control.

A number of things can be done to overcome some of these barriers. For example, all health professionals need to be aware of the additional health needs that people with learning disabilities may experience, thus making them more alert to the possibility that they can occur and overcoming the potential for diagnostic overshadowing. Health professionals need to develop their skills in communicating with people with learning disabilities including the development of skills in augmentative forms of communication. The way in which services are structured also needs to be examined so that additional time is made available when children with learning disabilities require examination or treatment. Finally, negative attitudes, wherever they are found, need to be challenged. It is only by doing so that children with learning disabilities will be able to exercise their right to health care on an equitable basis with other children.

WWW

Look at some of the practical suggestions regarding combatting barriers to health inequalities for people with learning disabilities in the Department of Health (1999) publication 'Once a Day':

- http://www.dh.gov.uk/en/Publicationsandstatistics/Publications/PublicationsPolicyAndGuidance/DH_4006868

Working together

The Chief Nursing Officer's 'Review of the nursing, midwifery and health visiting contribution to vulnerable children and young people' (DoH 2004) notes that care is often fragmented 'between health, social care and education, between the hospital and between nurses, midwives and health visitors'. Because children and young people with learning disabilities clearly come within the group of children who are considered to be potentially vulnerable, this fragmentation is a source of concern. Collaborative working is required if appropriate support is to be provided for families of children with learning disabilities. An important step towards this is to understand the role of some of the professionals who might be involved.

The role of the learning disability nurse

The learning disability nurse is one of the professionals who might be involved with children with learning disabilities and their families (for further information see Northway & Jenkins 2007). Over many years there has been a great deal of debate as to the role of the specialist learning disability nurse. In 1995, the then Chief Nursing Officer for England commissioned a review of the role. In the report which resulted the following were identified as key roles for learning disability nurses (Kay et al 1995):

- Assessment of need
- Health surveillance and health promotion
- Developing personal competence
- The use of enhanced therapeutic skills
- Managing and leading teams of staff
- Enhancing the quality of support
- Enablement and empowerment
- Coordinating services.

Each of these roles may be seen as being relevant to working with children with a learning disability. For example, nurses may be able to undertake specialist assessments of behavioural needs and work with families to develop their confidence and competence in managing their child's behaviour. In other instances they may work with young people with learning disabilities in relation to sexual health promotion (Atkinson 2002). They might also be involved in the assessment of risk in relation to epilepsy and the development of appropriate management plans with families (O'Brien & Loughran 2004). As a coordinator of care, and due to their experience of working with people with learning disabilities across the lifespan, learning disability nurses may also have much to offer at the point of transition from children's to adult health services.

Activity

- For further information concerning the role of the learning disability nurse see Turnbull (2003)

Current policy advocates that people with learning disabilities, including children, should use generic health services wherever possible and receive specialist support (if required) to access such services. However, in some areas this has meant that the role of learning disability nurses in working with children has reduced over the past two decades. Not all children with a learning disability will require the support of a learning disability nurse and some may only require such support for a short period of time. However, others with more complex physical and/or behavioural needs may require support on a more continuous basis. In such instances it is important that the skills, knowledge and experience of the learning disability nurse are recognised and their involvement in working with children and families is actively sought. Indeed the Chief Nursing Officer's report (DoH 2004) argues that integrated children's teams should 'routinely' be seeking the involvement of learning disability nurses.

Collaborative working

Scenario

Louise

Louise is a 7-year-old who enjoys doing things with her family and who likes visiting her local fast-food shop for a milkshake. She also has very complex needs. She has severe learning disabilities and cerebral palsy. She has mobility problems and needs to use a wheelchair. She also has difficulties with swallowing.

Shaun

Shaun is a 14-year-old boy who likes doing all the things that other teenagers like to do. He spends each Saturday going to his local football club along with his dad and other mates and enjoys playing his music too loud in his bedroom. Shaun has moderate learning disabilities and also has epilepsy. Recently he has started to become very moody and argumentative. Only last week he lashed out at his younger sister. His family is getting very worried about his behaviour.

Reflect on your practice

Think about the two scenarios above:

- Which professionals might be involved with Louise, Shaun and their families at the moment?
- Is this likely to change over the next 5 years?
- What support might the learning disability nurse offer?
- What support might the children's nurse or school nurse offer?
- What difficulties could there currently be in relation to coordinating support to these two families?
- How might some of these be overcome?

The range of needs experienced by children with learning disabilities and their families means that no one profession is going to be able to provide all of the support required (Bollard 2003, Kay et al 1995). There has been much discussion and debate concerning the need for multi-professional and interprofessional working. For example the National Service Framework states:

> The quality of care that these children and young people receive, and the quality of their and their families' lives depends upon good multi-disciplinary care planning and treatment
>
> (Department of Health and Department for Education and Skills 2004; section 4.8)

However, such policy recognition does not always translate into effective service provision. Kerr (2001) identifies two key interfaces that need to be carefully managed in relation to children and young people with learning disabilities:

- The interface between services for children and those for adults.
- The interface between the range of agencies and professionals involved in the lives of people with learning disabilities.

Bollard (2003) distinguishes between multiprofessional and interprofessional working, arguing that the former does not require interaction between the professionals involved whereas the latter implies interaction. This is what is required if coordinated services are to be provided for children with learning disabilities and their families.

Interaction, collaboration and partnership do, however, need to extend beyond the need for professionals to work together with professionals. For services to really make a positive impact children and young people along with their families and carers all need to be viewed as important members of the team.

Summary

This chapter has explored the nature of learning disability, its effect on the child and their family, and the ways in which nurses can work together with the child, their family, and other professionals to ensure that needs are identified and met in an appropriate and timely manner. Finally, when attempting to think about children and the families of children who have 'learning disabilities' it may help to remember the following points:

- Children with a learning disability are children first. They have the same needs as other children but also have additional needs.
- A learning disability is a permanent condition. However, people with learning disabilities grow and develop as individuals just like everyone else but generally at a slower pace.
- People with learning disabilities have the same human rights as non-learning disabled people.
- Some people are born with a learning disability, and some acquire a learning disability as the result of an injury or illness.
- Some people with learning disabilities also have a physical or sensory impairment but many do not. Some are also at increased risk of certain health conditions.
- Children with a learning disability need to be seen in the context of their family and support provided to all

family members. Professionals need to be aware of the significance of key stages in the child's life such as initial diagnosis, commencing school and transition to adult services.
- People with learning disabilities have dreams and aspirations like all other people and many of them may be achievable if they are offered appropriate support by the multidisciplinary team and their communities.

Men and women with learning disabilities can be parents, employees, Olympic athletes, husbands and wives. Some have driving licences, GCSEs and teaching qualifications. A few have climbed to Everest's base camp. For others, their greatest triumph may be smiling or some act of self-determination. As it is for all children, it is impossible to know what kind of a person a child with a learning disability will be when he or she grows up. For this reason it is of paramount importance to remember that they are children and young people first, with a disability second, and will continue to grow and develop throughout their lives. It is simply that, due to impairment, these stages may take longer. The failure to recognise this in the past has contributed to making the experience of a learning disability more limiting than it might otherwise be. Nursing practitioners, as members of the multidisciplinary team, can play a key role in minimising the negative impacts a learning disability may have on an individual and their family and in promoting quality of life for all.

References

Atkinson, S., 2002. It's great to grow up. Learning Disability Practice 5 (10), 28–30.

Barr, O., Gilgunn, J., Kane, T., Moore, G., 1999. Health screening for people with learning disabilities by a community nursing service in Northern Ireland. Journal of Advanced Working 29 (6), 1482–1491.

Bollard, M., 2003. Inter-professional working: its relevance and importance to learning disability practice. In: Jukes, M., Bollard, M. (Eds.), Contemporary learning disability practice. Quay Books, Salisbury, pp. 20–30.

Burke, P., Montgomery, S., 2001. Brothers and sisters: supporting the siblings of children with disabilities. Practice 13, 27–38.

Department of Health (DOH), 2001. Valuing people. A new strategy for learning disability for the 21st century. DoH, London.

Department of Health (DOH), 2004. The chief nursing officer's review of the nursing, midwifery and health visiting contribution to vulnerable children and young people. The Stationery Office, London.

Department of Health (DOH) and Department for Education and Skills (DfES), 2004. National Service Framework for Children, Young People and Maternity Services: Disabled Children and Young People and those with Complex Health Needs. The Stationery Office, London.

Disability Rights Commission and Department of Health, 2004. You can make a difference – improving hospital services for disabled people. The Stationery Office, London.

Dobson, B., Middleton, S., Beardsworth, A., 2001. The impact of childhood disability on family life. York Publishing Services, York.

Evans, J., Jones, J., Mansell, I., 2001. Supporting sibling evaluation of support groups for brothers and sisters of children with learning disabilities and challenging behaviour. Journal of Intellectual Disabilities 5, 69–78.

Gates, B., 2007. The nature of learning disabilities. In: Gates, B. (Ed.), Learning disabilities: towards inclusion. Churchill Livingstone, Edinburgh, pp. 3–20.

Gross, R.D., 1991. Psychology: the science of mind and behaviour. Hodder and Stoughton, London.

HM Treasury and Department for Education and Skills, 2007. Aiming high for disabled children. The Stationery Office, London.

Howells, G., 1986. Are the medical needs of mentally handicapped adults being met? Journal of the Royal College of General Practitioners 36, 449–453.

Kay, B., Rose, S., Turnbull, J., 1995. Continuing the commitment. The report of the Learning Disability Nursing Project. Department of Health, London.

Kerr, G.R.D., 2001. Assessing the needs of learning disabled young people with additional disabilities: implications for planning adult services. Journal of Intellectual Disabilities 5, 157–174.

Lindsay, M., 1998. Signposts for success in commission and providing health services for people with learning disabilities. Department of Health, London.

Maxwell, V., Barr, O., 2003. With the benefit of hindsight. A mother's reflections on raising a child with Down syndrome. Journal of Learning Disabilities 7 (1), 51–64.

Mencap, 2006. Breaking point. A report on caring without a break for children and adults with severe or profound learning disabilities. Mencap, London.

Michael, J., 2008. Healthcare for all. The Stationery Office, London.

NHS Health Scotland, 2004. Health needs assessment report: people with learning disabilities in Scotland. NHS Scotland, Glasgow.

Northway, R., 1997. Disability and oppression: some implications for nurses and nursing. Journal of Advanced Nursing 26, 736–743.

Northway, R., Jenkins, R., 2007. Specialist learning disability services. In: Gates, B. (Ed.), Learning disabilities: towards inclusion. Churchill Livingstone, Edinburgh, pp. 105–123.

O'Brien, D., Loughran, S., 2004. Risk assessment and epilepsy. Learning Disability Practice 7 (3), 12–17.

SCOPE, 1999. Right from the start. Looking at diagnosis and disclosure – parents describe how they found out about their child's disability. SCOPE, London.

SCOPE, 2003. Right from the start template. Good practice in sharing the news. SCOPE, London.

Sloper, P., Mitchell, W., 2000. User friendly information for families with disabled children: a guide to good practice. York Publishing Services, York.

Turnbull, J. (Ed.), 2003. Learning disability nursing. Blackwell Science, Oxford.

Ward, L., Mallett, R., Heslop, P., Simons, K., 2003. Planning for health at transition. Learning Disability Practice 6 (3), 24–27.

Watson, D., 2007. Causes and manifestations of learning disabilities. In: Gates, B. (Ed.), Learning disabilities towards inclusion. Churchill Livingstone, Edinburgh, pp. 21–42.

Willis, A., 2007. Compulsory school education. In: Gates, B. (Ed.), Learning disabilities towards inclusion. Churchill Livingstone, Edinburgh, pp. 137–153.

Wilson, J., Haire, B., 1990. Health care screening for people with mental handicap living in the community. British Medical Journal 301, 1379–1381.

World Health Organization, 1993. Describing developmental disability. Guidelines for a multiaxial scheme for mental retardation (learning disability). WHO, Geneva.

Useful websites

http://www.viauk.org/
http://www.bild.org.uk
http://www.mencap.org.uk
http://www.library.nhs.uk/learningdisabilities/
http://www.learningdisabilities.org.uk/
http://www.intellectualdisability.info/home.htm

Index

D

M

N

O

P